Fundamentals of Basic EMERGENCY Care

THIRD EDITION

Richard Beebe • Deborah Funk, MD • Jules Scadden

Richard W. O. Beebe, MEd, RN, NREMT-P
Program Director
Bassett Healthcare
Center for Rural Emergency Medical Services Education
Cooperstown, New York

Clinical Assistant Professor
State University of New York
Cobleskill, New York

Deborah L. Funk, MD, FACEP
Assistant Professor/Attending Physician
Department of Emergency Medicine
Albany Medical Center Hospital
Albany, New York

Medical Director
Life Net of New York

Julie K. (Jules) Scadden, NREMT-P, Ps
CQI/IT/Data Coordinator
Sac County Ambulance
Sac City, Iowa

Adjunct EMS Instructor
Western Iowa Tech Community College
Sioux City, Iowa

Adjunct EMS Instructor
Iowa Central Community College
Fort Dodge, Iowa

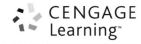

CENGAGE
Learning™

Australia • Brazil • Japan • Korea • Mexico • Singapore • Spain • United Kingdom • United States

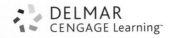

Fundamentals of Basic Emergency Care, Third Edition

Richard W. O. Beebe

Deborah L. Funk

Julie K. Scadden

Vice President, Career and Professional Editorial: Dave Garza

Director of Learning Solutions: Sandy Clark

Acquisitions Editor: Janet E. Maker

Managing Editor: Larry Main

Editorial Assistant: Amy Wetsel

Vice President, Career and Professional Marketing: Jennifer Baker

Marketing Director: Debbie Yarnell

Senior Marketing Manager: Erin Coffin

Marketing Coordinator: Shanna Gibbs

Production Director: Mark Bernard

Content Project Manager: David Plagenza

Art Director: Benjamin Gleeksman

For product information and technology assistance, contact us at **Cengage Learning Customer & Sales Support, 1-800-354-9706**

For permission to use material from this text or product, submit all requests online at **www.cengage.com/permissions**. Further permissions questions can be e-mailed to **permissionrequest@cengage.com**

Library of Congress Control Number: 2009923970

ISBN-13: 978-1-4354-4217-7
ISBN-10: 1-4354-4217-2

Delmar
5 Maxwell Drive
Clifton Park, NY 12065-2919
USA

Cengage Learning is a leading provider of customized learning solutions with office locations around the globe, including Singapore, the United Kingdom, Australia, Mexico, Brazil, and Japan. Locate your local office at: **international.cengage.com/region**

Cengage Learning products are represented in Canada by Nelson Education, Ltd.

To learn more about Delmar, visit **www.cengage.com/delmar**

Purchase any of our products at your local college store or at our preferred online store **www.ichapters.com**

NOTICE TO THE READER

Publisher does not warrant or guarantee any of the products described herein or perform any independent analysis in connection with any of the product information contained herein. Publisher does not assume, and expressly disclaims, any obligation to obtain and include information other than that provided to it by the manufacturer. The reader is expressly warned to consider and adopt all safety precautions that might be indicated by the activities described herein and to avoid all potential hazards. By following the instructions contained herein, the reader willingly assumes all risks in connection with such instructions. The publisher makes no representations or warranties of any kind, including but not limited to, the warranties of fitness for particular purpose or merchantability, nor are any such representations implied with respect to the material set forth herein, and the publisher takes no responsibility with respect to such material. The publisher shall not be liable for any special, consequential, or exemplary damages resulting, in whole or part, from the readers' use of, or reliance upon, this material.

Printed in the United States of America
4 5 6 7 8   15 14 13

Dedications

Without the love and support of our families, none of us could achieve our aspirations and dreams. I would like to thank my wife, Laura, for her boundless love and support, as well as my daughters, Heather and Amanda, for their inspiration.

I would like to dedicate this book to my students—past, present, and future—who challenge me every day to be the best educator I can be and to the Western Turnpike Rescue Squad, my home away from home for more than 25 years.

R.W.O.B.

I am deeply thankful that I have a career that puts me on the frontlines of society. I have the opportunity every day to meet new people who have different challenges. I consider it a good day if I can help someone with their challenges. I consider it a great day if I can learn something while doing that. I consider it an incredible day if I can help someone, learn something, and teach someone else about it. Always remember that there is something to learn in every situation, even if it is just that you have something new to learn!

D.F.

I have been blessed with many wonderful friends and mentors whose love, encouragement, and belief in me have provided constant inspiration. I would like to dedicate this book to those friends and mentors; to the EMS providers who work tirelessly in the streets providing excellent patient care; to my son Christopher, who not only gave up our time together but turned out to be a great researcher during the course of writing this book; and to the rest of my children and grandchildren, whose love, support, and sacrifice have enabled me to work and teach in a profession I love.

J.K.S.

Brief Contents

Table of Contents

CHAPTER 4:
GENERAL PRINCIPLES
OF PATIENT ASSESSMENT

366

About the Authors

Rich Beebe

Richard Beebe, MS, BSN, NREMT-P, is the program director for Bassett Health Care's Center for Rural Emergency Medical Services Education in Cooperstown, New York. He is also a Clinical Assistant Professor at the State University of New York at Cobleskill. Richard Beebe is a practicing field Paramedic with the Guilderland Police Department, since 1988. He has his Masters degree in education and is a Registered Nurse and a nationally registered Paramedic. Mr. Beebe has been an EMS educator for more than two decades and is a chapter member of the National Association of EMS Educators. He is a state and national speaker and author or editor of several textbooks who has been recently working in a leadership role on the committee for the National EMS Education Standards of the National Association of EMS Educators.

Deborah Funk

Deborah Funk M.D., FACEP, is an Assistant Professor of Emergency Medicine at Albany Medical College in Albany, New York, where she has been involved in EMS education and medical direction for more than a decade. Having completed an EMS Fellowship, Dr. Funk is a Medical Director for Life Net of New York and is involved in advancing EMS statewide.

Jules Scadden

Julie K. (Jules) Scadden, NREMT-P, PS, has been actively involved in EMS for 18 years as a volunteer and career EMS provider and educator. She is currently a Paramedic Specialist, CQI/IT/Data Coordinator for Sac County Ambulance Service in Northwest Iowa.

Ms. Scadden is an EMS instructor serving as adjunct faculty for Western Iowa Tech Community College in Sioux City and Iowa Central Community College in Fort Dodge. She has been a contributing author and reviewer for EMS textbooks and currently writes on issues effecting the rural provider and volunteer for her column "Rural Ramblings" for EMS1.com. She also is a frequent presenter at EMS conferences nationally, specializing in topics covering special patient populations and Children with Special Challenges.

An active advocate for EMS, Ms. Scadden had served on numerous advisory boards and committees, including the Iowa System Standards development committee and the Advocacy Committee for NAEMT. She is one of the founders and past Secretary of the National EMS Museum Foundation and the Iowa CPR Education Foundation, where she currently serves as its President.

Foreword to the Third Edition

I would like to welcome you into the profession of Emergency Medical Services! As you will find out, there are as many stories and reasons for entering into this noble profession as there are people who provide care to those who cannot care for themselves. The field of Emergency Medical Services (EMS) is a young one, with the modern age of EMS born of the 1966 National Academy of Sciences white paper *Accidental Death and Disability: The Neglected Disease of Modern Society*. There were many other influences on the development of the EMS systems we know today, from advances in resuscitation techniques and technology in the late 1950s and early 1960s to the first EMS Medical Directors working directly with the first EMTs. Federal funding in the 1970s and the development of trauma systems also left their mark on our profession.

The events of the post-September 11, 2001, world have highlighted the intersection of EMS between public health and public safety. Regardless of the model of delivery (fire, third service, police, volunteer, paid, hospital), this missions of public health and public safety converge. In reality, as an Emergency Medical Technician (EMT), you are often the first individual in the health care delivery system with whom the patient comes into contact. I would submit that the main function of the EMS professional at all levels and all types lies mainly in public health and health care delivery than in public safety. Our role is not only to rescue people, but care for them, often in a one-on-one setting where we can have a significant impact on the lives of patients. We are also on the front lines of public health surveillance, not only for threats of biological terror but for emerging infectious diseases, collectively providing early detection of a pandemic.

Our unique position within the community provides us access to patients in a way that can be used to help improve the public health, from follow-up visits to patients with chronic conditions in the community to child safety seat inspections, much in the same way firefighters have provided fire prevention services for decades. We also play an important role in the larger response to public health emergencies. These emergencies encompass incidents such as infectious disease outbreaks, pandemic preparation, mass immunization, and scene support for public health investigations.

How can we educate an EMT about his or her varied roles as a health care provider? How can we educate the new EMT to be an adaptable, well-educated individual with excellent critical thinking skills? One way to accomplish this goal is using the problem-based learning format that is the basis for this textbook and instructor materials. In this learning format, the students focus on solving a variety of real-life problems just as you will when you care for patients. Very few patients call for EMS to report, "I'm having a heart attack" or "I just ruptured my aneurysm." Patients provide us with a variety of clues, some pertinent and some not as pertinent. Our job is to sort these clues out and come up with the most likely cause for the patient's chief concern and treat appropriately. While a rigid cookbook approach to medicine may be of comfort to some people, EMTs face many situations where this approach will not work and may indeed be harmful to the patient. There is no doubt a lot of memorization of facts required for medical care. However, more important is the ability to critically think through a problem and develop an appropriate solution. This quality of critical thinking separates the good EMT from the excellent EMT. A problem-based approach will help the EMT student become the thinking EMT.

If I can leave you with 10 thoughts looking back on a 21-year career and then looking forward to another 21 years, I would ask you to remember these things:

◆ A career in Emergency Medical Services is a marathon, not a sprint. There is an overwhelming tendency to try to do it all. Don't! Make sure you leave time for yourself and your family.
◆ In order to provide the best possible care to your patients, you must first take care of yourself physically, emotionally, and spiritually. The job of

an EMT is both a physically and emotionally taxing job. Stay physically fit through exercise and avoid smoking. Stay emotionally and spiritually fit by developing rewarding relationships and engaging in activities outside your passion for EMS.

◆ Never accept anything as truth set in stone without evaluating the evidence yourself. Always press your teachers, preceptors, and colleagues to support what they say.

◆ Medical science is always changing. What you learn today may not hold true next year, five years from now, or ten years from now. All fields of medicine, including EMS, require lifelong learning and a continual update of knowledge.

◆ Treat your patients the way you want your family treated. Many of you have heard this directive in many forms. This is a nonnegotiable principle.

◆ Always carry yourself and act as if a respected family member is watching you. Maintain a professional manner at all times. You wouldn't want to embarrass your parent or grandparent, would you?

◆ Strive to perform your job to the best of your ability and go the extra mile for your patient. That extra compassion can make a huge impact in the lives of patients and their families.

◆ Always work toward improving your capabilities. Each situation we encounter is unique and provides us experience for the next situation. By learning from each call and finding one small thing you can do to improve what you do, you will grow and become an exceptional EMT.

◆ Be flexible and adaptable. The environment you work in is ever changing with new situations, patients, and challenges every day. Learn from the past and apply that knowledge to the future.

◆ Finally, admit when you are wrong, whether that is to your supervisor, medical director, colleague, or a patient. We are all human and make mistakes. Admitting a mistake not only builds credibility, but opens the door for improvement.

Again, I welcome you into the profession of Emergency Medical Services. My career has been enjoyable and rewarding. I hope you will find the same satisfaction as you embark on your career in Emergency Medical Services.

Jeff Myers, DO, EdM, NREMT-P, FAAEM
Clinical Assistant Professor Emergency Medicine
EMS Fellowship Director and Associate System EMS Medical Director
SUNY-Buffalo School of Medicine and Biomedical Sciences

Preface

DISCLAIMER

The EMT must be aware of the regional differences that will be encountered in practice. Not all areas of the country provide EMS in the same manner. This book cannot begin to encompass all of the regional differences throughout the United States. *Fundamentals of Basic Emergency Care*, Third Edition, provides learning of the national standard for care. The EMT student should actively seek out the standards set forth in his or her region through contact with instructors, medical directors, and state EMS agencies.

Throughout this text, the EMT student will be encouraged to problem-solve based on case studies. These are simulations and are not based on fact. There may be many solutions to a single case study. It is important for the student to realize that no one case is representative of a single method of assessment and treatment. This text provides concepts for patient care and treatment that are most commonly used. This is not the definitive source for all the answers to every patient encounter. This text provides a means for the EMT student to increase his or her problem-solving abilities to determine the proper course of action when in the field. However, the only definitive source for questions regarding specific patient care is the EMS instructor and the medical director.

The authors and publisher have made a conscientious effort to ensure that the drug information and recommended dosages in this text are accurate and in accord with accepted standards at the time of publication. However, pharmacology and therapeutics are rapidly changing sciences. Therefore, before administering any drug, students are advised to check the package insert provided by the manufacturer for the recommended dose, for any contraindications for administration, and for any added warnings and precautions.

TO THE STUDENT

Welcome to *Fundamentals of Basic Emergency Care*, Third Edition, a textbook for EMT students using problem-based learning. *Fundamentals of Basic Emergency Care*, Third Edition, is organized logically, beginning with EMS dispatch and ending with documentation, following the same steps of an EMS response. This format organizes the text with foundational material, followed by a step-by-step approach to emergency calls, and ends with typical emergency situations.

Chapter 1 is intended as a foundation for EMTs. There is an extensive discussion of the history of EMS, reflecting the authors' belief that EMTs need to know their roots. It also includes a thorough discussion of the EMT's general roles and responsibilities and legal responsibilities. In these times of increased personal responsibility and accountability, the new EMT must know what his or her vocation requires. The chapter ends with the important issue of maintaining the wellness of the EMT.

In Chapter 2, the authors purposely expanded the information on anatomy and physiology beyond what is typically found in other EMT textbooks. With the addition of the unit on pathophysiology, the EMT student can develop a more in-depth understanding of the human body, its functions and disease processes. This deeper look at pathophysiology gives the EMT who aspires to become a paramedic someday a foundation to better develop the more advanced knowledge and skills sets needed as an advanced life support (ALS) provider. The unit on lifespan development provides an added level of understanding for the EMT student on how the body changes throughout life. A solid foundation in anatomy, physiology, pathophysiology, and lifespan development is crucial to an EMT and future paramedic student.

Chapter 3 introduces the EMT to the ABCs of care. This chapter begins with the safety of the EMT through infection control, as the first step in preparation during an EMS response. It provides the material students need to learn the most essential components of patient care. A sound understanding of these principles is critical to the EMT's success.

Chapter 4 explores, in a methodical fashion, each of the components of an EMS call, starting with scene safety and ending with reporting and documentation. Over the years, EMS professionals have shifted to a more cautious, safety-oriented approach. The authors have identified this trend, expanding the chapter on safety to include both street and house calls. The basic assessments are then covered extensively to ensure that the EMT student walks away with a clear understanding of these important skills.

Chapters 5 through 9 develop the EMT's understanding of emergency care from trauma to medical emergencies. The number of deaths from trauma has dropped considerably, and medical emergencies have become more prominent in EMS in the past 25 years. To reflect these changes in emergency medicine, the authors have purposely chosen to emphasize the medical emergencies an average EMT is likely to encounter. There are also sections on maternity, newborn, pediatric, and geriatric medical emergencies, emphasizing the unique developmental differences at each stage of life. One unit is devoted to advance directives to reflect the changing demographics of the United States. As Americans get older, EMTs will have to become more competent in the care of the elderly patient, and Fundamentals of Basic Emergency Care, Third Edition, can help prepare them for the challenges ahead.

Finally, Chapter 10 discusses operational skills and the special circumstances an EMT may encounter, such as multiple-casualty incidents and scenes involving hazardous materials adhering the principles of the National Incident Management System (NIMS) and incident command. There is expanded information on the role of the EMT when working with advanced providers such as air medical personnel. Although most prehospital care is still provided by EMTs, they are often providing that care in cooperation with advanced providers, such as paramedics. The EMT who can provide assistance with ALS improves team efficiency and patient care, an important added value to an EMT.

SPECIAL FEATURES

◆ **Added Depth to the Curriculum:** This text follows the new National EMS Education Standards, designed to increase the flexibility and creativity in EMS education programs. Going beyond the curriculum, this text strives to truly cover all the fundamentals of emergency care, serving as a textbook for EMTs and a resource for EMS professionals.

◆ **Key Concepts/Key Concepts Revisited:** Key Concepts/Key Concepts Revisited open and close each unit with core information and concepts, giving a concise reference for key unit material.

◆ **Case Study/Case Study Revisited:** Case studies open and close each unit. They encourage critical thinking and problem solving, supporting the ability of EMT students to take what they learn to the streets.

◆ **Introduction to Medical Terminology:** EMTs must know certain medical terms and phrases in order to communicate with hospital staff; however, they must also be able to explain these terms to patients in plain English. *Fundamentals of Basic Emergency Care*, Third Edition, attempts to introduce the medical terms at appropriate times, in a manner that the EMT can understand and could explain to the patient.

◆ **Photographic Skill Sets:** Pictorial step-by-step skills allow you to see the proper methods used to perform the essential functions of your profession. Use these as a guide to practicing the skills in a lab along with the assessment checklist in your workbook.

◆ **Safety Tips:** Safety Tip boxes emphasize the importance of safety on the job and describe methods to maintain safe patient care, along with your safety and that of your team.

◆ **Street Smart:** Street Smart boxes allow students to benefit from the authors' years of field experience. This feature provides insight into handling various situations on scene as well as care of the patient.

◆ **Pediatric Considerations:** Pediatric Considerations highlight areas of special significance to young patients. It brings your attention to the variations in presentation, care, and management of the pediatric patient.

◆ **Geriatric Considerations:** Geriatric Considerations highlight areas of special significance to elderly patients. It brings your attention to the variations in presentation, care, and management of the elderly patient.

- **Cultural Considerations:** Cultural Considerations share manners, ways of providing care, communication, and relationships of various cultural and ethnic groups you may encounter in your area of practice.
- **Ask the Doc:** Ask the Doc boxes highlight information from the National Association of EMS Physicians. These boxes note position papers and research being conducted in the field on emergency services.

NEW TO THIS EDITION
Chapter 1
- A historical timeline has been added showing the beginning of EMS-like activities in the time of the Romans to the official beginning and growth of EMS up to today.
- Information on universal access has been updated to the most recent statistics and innovations being made in the public's ability to access the EMS system through 9-1-1 calls and services.
- The roles and responsibilities of the EMT are emphasized, and discussion has been added concerning the role of EMS in public health.
- Content related to certification and licensure has been expanded as well as the legal responsibilities of the EMT.
- Discussions of the Health Insurance Portability and Accountability Act and the Emergency Medical Treatment and Active Labor Act have been added.
- Discussion of the importance of the well-being of the EMT has been updated based on the latest research in this area.

Chapter 2
- This chapter continues to provide the most comprehensive coverage of anatomy and physiology found in any EMT–Basic textbook.
- A unit has been added addressing the pathophysiology of disease process using the Fick principle.

- Lifespan development has been added as a new unit, stressing the importance of understanding the changes that take place beginning with birth and throughout the aging process.

Chapter 3
- This chapter covers the essentials of emergency care beginning with current infection control criteria necessary to protect the EMT during patient contact.
- Basic airway control with high-quality photographic skills sets demonstrating the appropriate methods for opening and managing the airway are featured.
- Basic pharmacology for the EMT has been expanded.
- Lifting and moving of patients has been expanded to provide more in-depth information on back care for the EMT.

Chapter 4
- This chapter follows the steps of an EMS response from dispatch to documentation.
- Terminology changes based on National Education Standards for Primary and Secondary assessments are included.
- A comprehensive unit on therapeutic communications has been added.
- A full unit on EMS communications emphasizes the importance of this topic.
- A full unit on basic medical terminology has been added to help the EMT understand and accurately use the terminology spoken in the medical profession.

Chapter 5
- Information on altered mental status has been expanded to include information on headaches.
- Information on abnormal behavior has also been expanded.
- New units are included on bariatrics, rashes and fevers, and behavioral emergencies.

Chapter 6

◆ A new unit provides an overview on trauma, including expanded information on kinematics and mechanism of injury.
◆ The unit on traumatic brain injury, including face, skull, and dental injuries, has been expanded.
◆ Information on spinal injuries has also been updated and expanded.

Chapter 7

◆ The unit on prenatal care is expanded.
◆ Units covering emergency childbirth and flowing into care of the newborn have been combined.

Chapter 8

◆ The unit on pediatric medical emergencies is expanded.
◆ A new unit with expanded information on pediatric trauma is included.
◆ Other new units address child abuse and neglect and children with special health care needs.

Chapter 9

◆ Information on geriatric medical and traumatic injuries has been expanded.
◆ A new unit examines end of life issues.

Chapter 10

◆ The unit on emergency vehicle operations is expanded.
◆ New units on the National Incident Management System (NIMS) and air medical transport are presented.

New Features in This Edition

This text has been revised and follows the new National EMS Education Standards.

Revamped illustrations provide a fresher look with more depth than illustrations presented in previous editions.

The *Fundamentals of Basic Emergency Care*, Third Edition, is a comprehensive textbook that provides the EMT student with the raw materials needed to form a foundation in EMS. But as medicine and technology change, so does EMS. The EMT student is encouraged to use the information in *Fundamentals of Basic Emergency Care*, Third Edition, in combination with other sources, especially your medical director and your EMS educator.

This text follows the flow of an EMS response. The book begins with the roots of EMS, flowing into the preparatory information covering the medical and legal responsibilities of the EMT. Next the EMT learns the basic anatomy and physiology of the human body, pathophysiology of the disease process, and lifespan development. EMT students will gather the tools to understand their responsibilities and the workings of the human body, enabling them to perform the assessments necessary to determine appropriate field management for the ill or injured.

The book then logically takes the EMT into the flow of an EMS response. The EMT takes the tools he or she has learned and begins to apply it in a systematic approach, beginning with dispatch, scene size-up, the primary assessment, therapeutic communications and history taking, the secondary assessment, reassessment, communication with the hospital, and transfer of patient care, ending with documentation of the response.

New topics include: Air medical transport, bariatrics, children with special challenges, lifespan development, the National Incident Management System, pathophysiology, pharmacology, traumatic brain injury, a trauma overview, and therapeutic communications.

TO THE EDUCATOR

Have you ever stood on the sideline of an emergency call and watched your students? This can be an eye-opening experience. You may observe the following:
◆ Inability to think critically
◆ Inability to problem-solve
◆ Inability to respond quickly in a crisis situation

The authors, EMS providers with more than 45 years of street experience between them, noticed this trend among new EMTs and asked, "Why?"

The revision of the EMT curriculum to apply an assessment-based approach was certainly a step in the right direction. It narrowed the focus of an EMT's training, allowing educators more time to concentrate on fewer objectives instead of trying to touch on the entire universe of medicine. But something is still missing. The curriculum does not, and cannot, include two essential EMT skills—problem solving and critical thinking. Teaching EMT students these skills is not a function of the curriculum, but of instructional methodology.

Case Based Cooperative Learning

Problem-based learning (PBL) is an educational strategy. PBL involves giving a team of students a puzzling problem and asking the team to resolve it. The problem, structured within the context of a real-life scenario, forces students to refer to available resources for facts and to develop content knowledge in the process. Students must then develop a plan of action. This learning process leads to increased problem-solving abilities.

PBL is a student-centered educational strategy. Direct instruction by the educator is minimized. Instead, the student learns to become a self-directed learner, a role that will serve him or her for a lifetime. The educator assumes the roles of coach, resource guide, and subject matter expert, not lecturer.

PBL takes advantage of many sources of information other than traditional scholastic materials. Students can refer to senior EMTs for direction, but not instruction, as they try to resolve the problem. These senior EMTs become mentors as they share their similar experiences, or "war stories," with like problems. Students can also tap into the Internet for more "e-learning" about the problem.

PBL is about more than just accumulating facts to regurgitate at exam time; it is about learning how to learn. The student learns how to obtain information and apply it to an ill-structured problem with the aim of producing a meaningful result. One of the

wondrous discoveries often made by EMTs using PBL is that there is more than one approach to resolving a problem.

More information is available on PBL in the Electronic Classroom Manager that accompanies this text. There is also an abundance of information on PBL available on the Internet. Please take a moment to educate yourself about this novel approach to EMS education. Even a small effort at the end of EMT class to try "one problem" can produce remarkable results.

EXTENSIVE TEACHING AND LEARNING PACKAGE

The complete supplements package was developed to achieve two goals:

1. To assist students in learning the essential skills and information needed to secure a career in the area of EMS
2. To assist instructors in planning and implementing their programs for the most efficient use of time and other resources

Student Workbook

ISBN 978-1-4354-4218-4

An excellent resource to provide additional practice. The workbook includes the following:

◆ Fully updated to match the third edition.
◆ Review of key terms
◆ Exercises and activities to promote retention of unit material and further enhance critical-thinking skills
◆ Skills review checklists

Instructor Resources

ISBN 978-4354-4219-1

The Instructor Resources (IR) helps you, the educator, facilitate student learning. For the educator interested in implementing problem-based learning, case studies are provided and may be copied and distributed to the class or to assigned student teams, who are then encouraged to follow through the guiding questions.

Answers to the guiding questions accompanying the additional case studies are also provided. The educator is reminded that there may be more correct answers to a problem beyond those provided. And remember, how the students arrived at their answer is as important as the answer itself. The IR is intended to be a starting point, not an authoritative source. Educators are encouraged to develop their own personalized problems, using the case studies provided as an example. EMS educators are also encouraged to carefully analyze the student-team responses compared to good EMS practice.

The IR also includes the following:

◆ Instructor's Manual with lecture outlines, student outlines, answers to the text questions, additional case studies, skill checklists, a resource list, and student handouts;
◆ Modularized lesson plans;
◆ PowerPoint presentations correlated to the student outlines;
◆ An image library to enhance the PowerPoint presentations or to create custom presentations;
◆ Computerized test bank;
◆ Quick Reference Guides to correlate content to the National EMS Education Standards;
◆ Administration tools;
◆ Equipment checklists; and
◆ Progress log sheets.

ADDITIONAL RESOURCES
WebTutor Advantage

Designed to complement *Fundamentals of Basic Emergency Care*, Third Edition, Cengage Delmar Learning WebTutor Advantage on WebCT is a content-rich, Web-based teaching and learning aid that reinforces and clarifies complex concepts and provides an electronic test bank. The WebCT platform also provides communications tools to instructors and students, including a source calendar, chat, e-mail, and threaded discussions.

Join us on the Web at *www.cengage.community/ems*

ACKNOWLEDGMENTS

The authors would like to sincerely thank the following individuals and organizations for their contributions to *Fundamentals of Basic Emergency Care*, Third Edition. Without their kind assistance, *Fundamentals of Basic Emergency Care*, Third Edition, would not have become a reality. Each of them can be proud of their contribution to the overall success of the book that will surely follow.

Reviewers

The honest input of the reviewers served two purposes for the authors. First, it reminded the authors of the diverse practice of EMS across the United States. Clearly, at times EMS is as much an art as it is a science. In every instance, the authors tried to incorporate their ideas and experiences when they did not violate medical research.

Second, the reviewers' comments periodically forced the authors to review their facts. For this reason, the authors can say we feel strongly that the information in *Fundamentals of Basic Emergency Care,* Third Edition, is factually correct and scientifically supported, in every instance possible, at the time of publication.

We, the authors, sincerely want to thank these reviewers for their time and effort.

Third Edition Reviewers

Debbie Akers
    Regional Education Coordinator
    Western Virginia EMS Council
    Roanoke, Virginia
Scott Birdie, BS, EMT-CC, CIC
    EMS Instructor
    North Shore/Long Island Jewish Center for
        Emergency Training and Development
    Manhasset, New York
Tony Caliguire
    Instructor, Cardio Respiratory and Emergency
        Medicine
    Hudson Valley Community College
    Troy, New York
John Gosford
    EMS Coordinator
    Lake City Community College
    Lake City, Florida
Joe Grafft
    Immediate Past President

National Association of EMS Educators
Pittsburgh, Pennsylvania
Art Hsieh
Chief Executive Officer and Director of Education
San Francisco Paramedic Association
San Francisco, California
Shirley Jones, MSEd, MHA, BA, EMT-P
EMS Educator
Noblesville, Indiana
Mike Kennamer
Director of Workforce Development
Northeast Alabama Community College
Rainsville, Alabama
Mike McLaughlin
Director of Health Occupations
Kirkwood Community College
Cedar Rapids, Iowa
Beth McNeil
Adjunct Assistant Professor
Monroe Community College
Rochester, New York
Gregory S. Neiman, BA, NREMTP
BLS Training Specialist
Virginia Department of Health, Office of
    Emergency Medical Services
Richmond, Virginia
John Rinard
Program Supervisor
Texas Engineering Extension Service
College Station, Texas
Sandy Waggoner, BA, EMT-P, EMSI
Public Safety Coordinator
EHOVE Ghrist Career Center
Milan, Ohio

Accuracy Checkers
for the Third Edition

Beth Ann McNeill, BFA, MS (c), EMT-B, NYS
Regional Faculty
    Monroe Community College
    Rochester, New York
Les Hawthorne BA, NREMTP
    Instructional Designer
    Maryland Fire and Rescue Institute Headquarters
    College Park, Maryland

Medical Advisor Third Edition

Deborah Funk M.D., FACEP
    Assistant Professor of Emergency Medicine
    Albany Medical College
    Albany, New York

Photo Acknowledgments

The authors would like to thank the following
organizations and individuals for their support and
assistance in the production of *Fundamentals of
Basic Emergency Care*, Third Edition.

Organization Acknowledgements
for the Third Edition

Charleston County EMS
    Don Lundy, Director
    Charleston, South Carolina
Clive Fire Department
    Rick Roe, Chief
    Clive, Iowa
Henry County Health Center-EMS
    Jerry Johnston, Director
    Mt. Pleasant, Iowa
Hobart Fire Department
    Robert Lamprecht, Director
    Hobart, Indiana
Montgomery County Hospital District
    Jason West, Paramedic-in-charge
    Houston, Texas
National Association of EMTs
    Patrick Moore, President
    Clinton, Mississippi
New England Ambulance Service
    Neal J. Costigan, RN, NREMT-P
    Vice President of Corporate Compliance
    Cranston, Rhode Island
Norwalk Fire Department
    Douglas Richardson, Captain
    Norwalk, Iowa
Portland Fire Department
    Terry Walsh, Deputy Chief
    Portland, Maine

Raleigh Fire Department
John McGrath, Chief
Raleigh, North Carolina
Sac County Ambulance Service
Scot McDonough, EMT-P, Director
Sac City, Iowa
Six Forks EMS-Cover
Daniel Cline, Chief
Raleigh, North Carolina
Story County Medical Center-EMS
John Halbrook
Johnston, Iowa
Wake County EMS
Skip Kirkwood, Chief
Raleigh, North Carolina
Wake Forest University Baptist Medical Center
Ricky Harold, Program Manager
Winston-Salem, North Carolina

Additional Organization Acknowledgements

Albany Medical Center Hospital
Department of Emergency Medicine
Albany, New York
Dr. Mara McErlean, Chair
Albany MedFLIGHT
Albany, New York
Dean Dow, RN, Program Director
Bassett Healthcare
Center for Rural EMS Education
Cooperstown, New York
Scott Bonderoff, Administrative Director
Shalom Nursery School
Karen Ekstein, Director
Guilderland Police Department
Guilderland, New York
James Murley, Chief of Police
Guilderland Emergency Medical Services
Guilderland, New York
Thomas Deleon, EMT Director
Watervliet Fire Department
Watervliet, New York
Brian Carroll, Fire Chief
Western Turnpike Rescue Squad
Albany, New York
Scott Bowman, EMT-P, Chief

Individual Acknowledgements for the Third Edition

Dr. Lou Romig, FAAP, FACEP
Team Life Support, Inc
Miami, Florida
Linda Adams, EMT-P
Des Moines, Iowa
Heather Carleton, EMT-P
Portland, Maine
Gordon Cochran, EMT-I
Lake View, Iowa
Michael Forschler, EMT-P
Colfax, IA
Terry Gilpatrick, EMT-P
Portland, Maine
Steven "Kelly" Grayson,
NREMT-P, CCP
KatyBeth Grayson
Kinder, Louisiana
Brian Hellund, NREMT-P
West Des Moines, Iowa
John Holbrook, NREMT-P
Johnston, Iowa
Jerry Johnston, BA, NREMT-P
Mt. Pleasant, Iowa
Lt. Eric Kalleum, EMT-P
Dallas Center, Iowa
Joshua Ledoux, EMT-P
Des Moines, Iowa
Mike Legeros
Wake County EMS Photo Units
Raleigh, North Carolina
Scot McDonough, EMT-P, PS
Sac City, Iowa
Paul Nyane Family
Iowa City, Iowa
Rick Roe, EMT-P
Clive, Iowa
Nicholas Scadden Family
Illinois City, Illinois
Joshua Schut, EMT-P
Clive, IA
Tony Sposeto, EMT-P
Waukee, Iowa
Scott Struchen, EMT-B
Sac City, IA

Larry Torrey, RN, EMT-P
    Westbrook, Maine
Brooke Wilson
    Ohlinger Publishing
    Delaware, Ohio

Additional Individual Acknowledgements

Dr. Michael Dailey, FACEP
    Albany Medical Center
Michael Galletelli
    Metroland Photo, Inc.
    Albany, New York
Geraldine Oakley
Dr. Kevin Reilly, FACEP
    Albany Medical Center
David J. Reimer Sr.
    Emergency Services Photography
    Kutztown, Pennsylvania
Dr. Ronald Stram, FACEP
    Albany Medical Center
Dr. Wayne Triner, FACEP
    Albany Medical Center

Technical Advisors

The authors would like to thank the technical advisors for their perseverance and determination to "get the job done." Their valuable contributions to the quality and accuracy of the photographs are clearly evident throughout the book.

Jonathan Behrens AAS, EMT-P
Lab Coordinator
Bassett Paramedic Program
Town of Colonie EMS
    Colonie, New York

Brian Booth, NREMT-P
Western Turnpike Rescue Squad
    Albany, New York

Geoff Ekstein, BA, CC-NREMT-P
Guilderland Emergency Medical Services
    Guilderland, New York

Chapter Opener Photos

Chapter 1: Courtesy of Sac County Ambulance, Sac City, Iowa

Chapter 2: Courtesy of Henry County Health Center EMS, Mt. Pleasant, Iowa

Chapter 3: Courtesy of Montgomery County Hospital District, Conroe, Texas

Chapter 4: Courtesy of Montgomery County Hospital District, Conroe, Texas

Chapter 5: Courtesy of Norwalk Fire Department, Norwalk, Iowa

Chapter 6: Courtesy of Wake County EMS, Raleigh, North Carolina

Chapter 7: Courtesy of John Halbrook & Story County Medical Center, Story City, Iowa

Chapter 8: Courtesy of Hobart Fire Department, Hobart, Indiana

Chapter 9: Courtesy of Wake County EMS, Raleigh, North Carolina

Chapter 10: Courtesy of Charleston EMS, Charleston, SC

Cover: Courtesy of Six Forks EMS, Raleigh Fire Department & Mike Legeros (Photographer) Raleigh, NC

Delmar-Cengage Learning

The authors would also like to extend our sincere appreciation to the entire staff at Delmar/Cengage Learning. While the list of individuals at Delmar/Cengage Learning who helped this book become a reality is long and distinguished, there are a few individuals that we would like to single out for special recognition.

We would first thank Dawn Gerrain, who initially saw our vision and agreed to help us achieve our dream, an EMT textbook that was written for the street EMT by EMS providers. We would also like to thank Janet Maker, our acquisitions editor, who provided valuable guidance, and Benj Gleeksman, art director, for their expertise and guidance. We would also like to thank Monica Ohlinger, Ohlinger Publishing, for her direction and insight from the beginning of this project.

Finally, we would like to extend a very special thank you to Brooke Wilson, our developmental editor. Brooke's tireless patience and drive for the highest quality matched that of the authors. She was the driving force and served as a constant inspiration to keep this project moving forward to its completion.

How to Use This Book

National Education Standards
The Emergency Medical Technician (EMT) will have the fundamental depth and foundational breadth of understanding consent/refusal of care, confidentiality, advance directives, tort and criminal actions, evidence preservation, statutory responsibilities, mandatory reporting, and ethical principles/moral obligations of prehospital care.

NATIONAL EDUCATION STANDARD
The new National EMS Education Standards are designed to increase the flexibility and creativity in EMS education programs and to facilitate and improve alternative delivery methods, such as problem-based learning.

Key Concepts

- The legal responsibilities of the EMT.
- The EMT's duty to patient's right to confidentiality.
- The patient capacity to refuse care.
- Important components of the EMT's responsibility when a patient refuses care against medical advice.
- Three types of advance directives.
- The differing types of consent.
- The legal importance of documentation.
- The circumstances under which resuscitation may be withheld.
- The EMT's role in reporting suspected abuse.
- The most common allegations that may be raised against an EMT in a court of law.
- The laws in place to help protect EMTs from litigation.

KEY CONCEPTS/ KEY CONCEPTS REVISITED
Key Concepts/Key Concepts Revisited open and close each unit with core information and concepts, giving you a concise reference for key unit material. Key Concepts at the beginning of each unit provide an advance organizer, highlighting the key material to be learned in that unit. Use the Key Concepts Revisited to refresh and measure your understanding of the unit material.

CASE STUDY/ CASE STUDY CONTINUED
Real-life case scenarios frame each unit, allowing you to problem-solve a patient encounter that you may be faced with in the field. A case study opens each unit, giving you enough information to

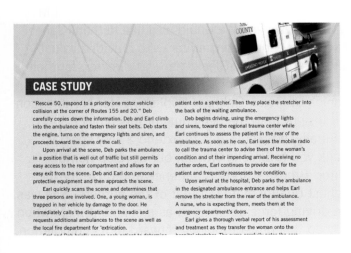

CASE STUDY

"Rescue 50, respond to a priority one motor vehicle collision at the corner of Routes 155 and 20." Deb carefully copies down the information. Deb and Earl climb into the ambulance and fasten their seat belts. Deb starts the engine, turns on the emergency lights and siren, and proceeds toward the scene of the call.

Upon arrival at the scene, Deb parks the ambulance in a position that is well out of traffic but still permits easy access to the rear compartment and allows for an easy exit from the scene. Deb and Earl don personal protective equipment and then approach the scene.

Earl quickly scans the scene and determines that three persons are involved. One, a young woman, is trapped in her vehicle by damage to the door. He immediately calls the dispatcher on the radio and requests additional ambulances to the scene as well as the local fire department for "extrication."

Earl and Deb briefly assess each patient to determine

patient onto a stretcher. Then they place the stretcher into the back of the waiting ambulance.

Deb begins driving, using the emergency lights and sirens, toward the regional trauma center while Earl continues to assess the patient in the rear of the ambulance. As soon as he can, Earl uses the mobile radio to call the trauma center to advise them of the woman's condition and of their impending arrival. Receiving no further orders, Earl continues to provide care for the patient and frequently reassesses her condition.

Upon arrival at the hospital, Deb parks the ambulance in the designated ambulance entrance and helps Earl remove the stretcher from the rear of the ambulance. A nurse, who is expecting them, meets them at the emergency department's doors.

Earl gives a thorough verbal report of his assessment and treatment as they transfer the woman onto the hospital stretcher. The nurse carefully notes the care

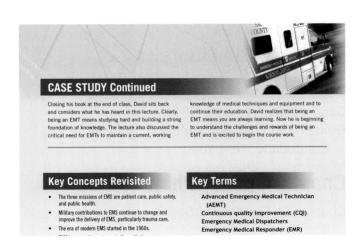

CASE STUDY Continued

Closing his book at the end of class, David sits back and considers what he has heard in this lecture. Clearly, being an EMT means studying hard and building a strong foundation of knowledge. The lecture also discussed the critical need for EMTs to maintain a current, working

knowledge of medical techniques and equipment and to continue their education. David realizes that being an EMT means you are always learning. Now he is beginning to understand the challenges and rewards of being an EMT and is excited to begin the course work.

Key Concepts Revisited

- The three missions of EMS are patient care, public safety, and public health.
- Military contributions to EMS continue to change and improve the delivery of EMS, particularly trauma care.
- The era of modern EMS started in the 1960s.

Key Terms

Advanced Emergency Medical Technician (AEMT)
Continuous quality improvement (CQI)
Emergency Medical Dispatchers
Emergency Medical Responder (EMR)

begin the process of critical thinking needed to manage the encounter. The case study resumes at the end of the unit, bringing together the real-life scenario and unit information. These case studies are designed to bridge the gap from student to practitioner.

SKILLS

Pictorial step-by-step skills sets allow you to see the proper methods used to perform the essential functions of your profession. Use these skills sets as a guide to practice the skills in a lab setting along with the assessment checklist in your workbook.

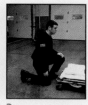

Skill 14-1 Proper Lifting Techniques

PURPOSE: To allow the EMT to lift objects without causing back injury.
STANDARD PRECAUTIONS:

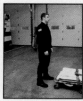

☑ Appropriate personal protective equipment
☑ Appropriate back support
☑ Proper footwear
☑ Adequate numbers of trained assistants

1 The EMT positions his feet about shoulder length apart, facing forward.

2 The EMT lowers his body by bending at the knees, one knee down, keeping the back straight.

BOXED FEATURES

Highlighted boxed features throughout the text call your attention to special circumstances, heightening awareness of special populations, cultural differences, and tips from the professionals.

Street Smart

Street Smart boxes allow you to benefit from the authors' years of field experience. This feature provides insight into handling patient care and various situations on scene.

Safety Tips

Restless patients can easily fall from stretchers if preventive action is not taken. A fall can be prevented if the side rails are in the upright position whenever someone is not at the bedside. The EMT should never leave a patient's bedside without first putting up the side rails. A patient's falling out of bed translates to broken hips or other injuries, angry family members, and maybe even a claim of negligence. Prevent a patient from sustaining a preventable injury by always double-checking before leaving the room to be sure that the side rails are up. Then document that the side rails were up on the prehospital care report.

Safety Tips

Safety Tips emphasize the importance of safety on the job and describe methods to maintain safe care of patients—and the safety of the EMT.

Pediatric Considerations

Pediatric Considerations highlight areas of special significance to young patients. These boxes call attention to the variations in presentation, care, and management of the pediatric patient.

Geriatric Considerations

Geriatric Considerations highlight areas of special significance to elderly patients. These boxes call attention to the variations in presentation, care, and management of the elderly patient.

Cultural Considerations

Cultural Considerations share manners, ways of providing care, communication, and relationships of various cultural and ethnic groups you may encounter in your area of practice.

Ask The Doc

Ask the Doc boxes highlight information from the National Association of EMS Physicians. These boxes note position papers and research being conducted in the field on emergency services.

Key Terms

Power TakeOff (PTO)	Silos
Rollover protective structure (ROPS)	Toxic organic dust syndrome (TODS)sss
Silage	

KEY TERMS

Key Terms familiarize you with medical language as well as demonstrate for you how to translate the medical terms into language that your patients will be able to understand.

Review Questions

1. What are some common mechanisms of injury on a farm?
2. When do most farm injuries occur?
3. What are the general principles of farm rescue?
4. What hazards do livestock represent?
5. What are the hazards of farm machinery?
6. What are the injuries that can be seen from
7. What are the dangers of silo rescue?
8. How might rescuers be injured in grain bin rescues?
9. What gases may be found in a manure storage facility?
10. What dangerous chemicals can be found on a farm?

REVIEW QUESTIONS

Review Questions at the end of each unit help test your knowledge and emphasize key unit material. You can use the review questions to test yourself on the key concepts learned at the completion of each unit.

Further Study

Desafey Liller, Karen. *Injury Prevention for Children and Adolescents: Research, Practice, and Advocacy*. Washington, DC: American Public Health Association, 2006.

Glasgow, Nina, Nan Johnson, and Lois Wright Morton. *Critical Issues in Rural Health*. Hoboken, NJ: Wiley-Blackwell, 2004.

Jones, R. *Textbook of Primary Medical Care*. New York: Oxford University Press.

FURTHER STUDY

Further Study selections are available at the end of each unit. Use these resources to take your learning one step further and explore topic-related reference material.

Fundamentals of Basic EMERGENCY Care

THIRD EDITION

Richard Beebe • Deborah Funk, MD • Jules Scadden

CHAPTER 1

Foundations of Emergency Medical Services

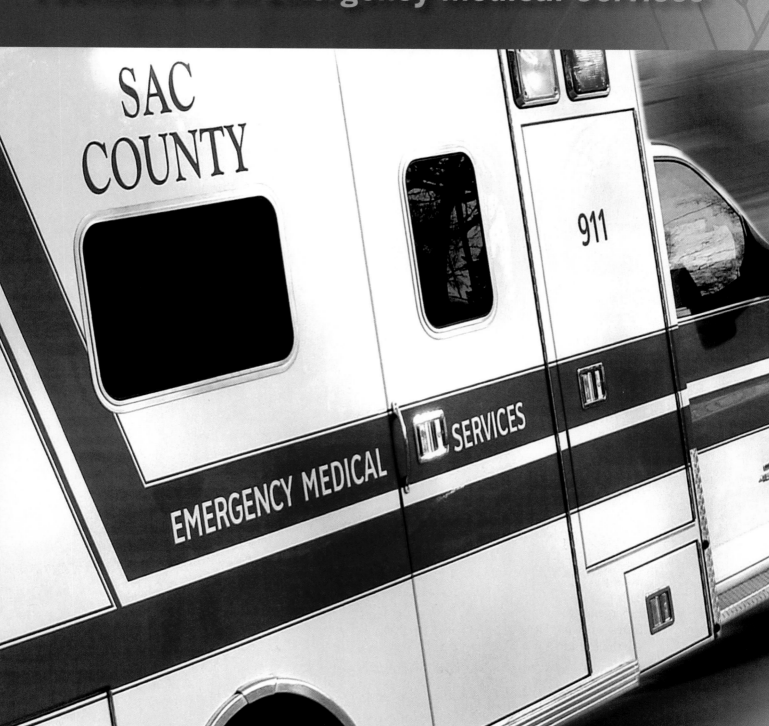

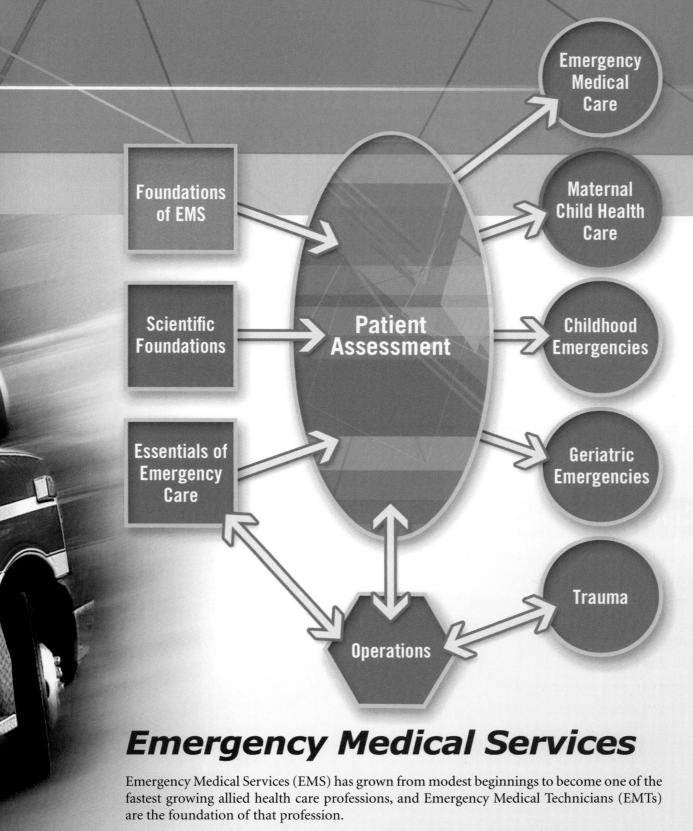

Emergency Medical Services

Emergency Medical Services (EMS) has grown from modest beginnings to become one of the fastest growing allied health care professions, and Emergency Medical Technicians (EMTs) are the foundation of that profession.

In many cases, EMTs are the public's first contact with the health care system. As a part of the health care team, the EMT is expected to deliver high-quality medical care from the scene, through transport, and until the patient is delivered to the hospital emergency department.

This chapter introduces emergency medicine as a specialty of medicine and emergency medical service as a profession. It also explores the roles and responsibilities of an EMT.

UNIT 1 Introduction to Emergency Medical Services

Emergency Medical Services (EMS) has grown from modest beginnings when funeral homes used hearses as ambulances to become one of the fastest growing allied health care professions in the United States. Emergency Medical Technicians (EMTs) are at the forefront of that profession and serve as its foundation. In many cases, EMTs are the first contact that the public has with the health care system. As a part of the health care team, the EMT is expected to deliver high-quality medical care from the scene until the patient is delivered to the emergency department of the hospital and to represent the health care profession. This unit introduces emergency medicine and emergency medical services.

National Education Standard
The Emergency Medical Technician (EMT) student shall have a simple depth and a foundational breadth of knowledge of EMS systems and the history of EMS.

Key Concepts

- The impact of historical events on the evolution of EMS.

- The evolution of emergency medical care.

- The place of modern EMS in the health care system.

- Key scientific and position papers that directly influenced EMS systems development.

- Elements of an EMS system.

- Evolution of emergency medicine and EMS.

- Professional challenges that face the EMT in the future.

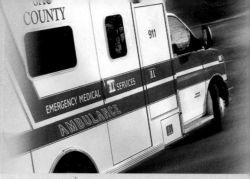

CASE STUDY

David's mother is an Emergency Medical Technician (EMT) for a local ambulance company, and she really seems to enjoy the job. It offers flexible hours and, perhaps more importantly, a chance to provide patient care. David admires his mother's dedication to her work and is thinking about taking the EMT class. He tells himself that even if he doesn't like it, he'll still earn at least six college credits.

Today is the first day of class. The instructor, Deb, an older woman with red hair and full of energy, is talking to several older students. She seems animated, and they all seem energized as they talk about a recent call.

David recognizes some of the students, fellow high school classmates who he remembers as aspiring paramedics. As students introduce themselves one by one, David is impressed with the diversity of the class. One retired gentleman, Paul, is taking the course so he can help his local volunteer rescue squad during the day. Two students about David's age, Bill and Nick, are hoping to take the municipal fire department entrance examination for several surrounding cities. They must earn their EMT certification before they can apply. Another student, Monica, explains that she is studying geology and thinks being an EMT might be handy in some of the remote mountainous areas she expects to travel. Several other students work for the local ambulance company, like David's mother, and want the formal training to improve their job skills and patient care.

After the student introductions, the lead instructor Deb introduces the rest of the faculty. The faculty, like the class they will teach, come from a variety of backgrounds, some from the fire service, some from municipal EMS, and some from volunteer First Aid Squads. One works in mall security and teaches EMS as a side job. Clearly there are a good number of faculty to mentor the students through the class.

With introductions out of the way Deb calls for a break. David meets several fellow students in the hallway near the drinking fountain, and they talk about their expectations and concerns about taking an EMT class. One student, Mary, says, "Being responsible for someone's life is an awesome responsibility." David thinks about his mother, who brought four lives into this world and is now trying to make it a safer place for everyone else.

Critical Thinking Questions

1. What are some of the various delivery systems for EMS locally?
2. What is the primary mission of EMS?
3. What is the history of EMS?
4. How does an EMS system work?
5. What challenges can be expected to EMS?

INTRODUCTION

Welcome to **Emergency Medical Services (EMS),** a coordinated network of professionals whose function is to provide a variety of medical services to people in need of emergency care. Many people from across the country and from all walks of life have chosen to become a part of this health care team.

EMS is rooted historically in the lifesaving mission of fire services. However, changes in modern health care have transformed EMS providers from being lifesavers to being the health care system's frontline ranks.

The mission of EMS is three-fold. Perhaps its most well-known mission is to provide out-of-hospital patient care in anticipation of transport to more definitive care at the hospital. This prehospital emphasis is becoming increasingly more important as medicine has begun to use EMS as an "early alert system" for heart attacks, strokes, and trauma.

The second mission of EMS involves public safety. Public safety includes a variety of subjects from injury and illness prevention to disaster preparedness. The goal of all public safety personnel is to create a situation in which citizens are free from risk and harm. EMS programs such as the PIER program (Public Information, Education and Relations) demonstrate EMS involvement in public safety.

The third and most recent addition to the EMS mission is public health. Public health is more than caring for individual citizens—it is caring for the entire community. In its capacity on the frontline of health care, EMS is in an ideal position to identify public health concerns and to work with the public health system to resolve these issues.

HISTORY OF EMERGENCY MEDICAL SERVICES

Perhaps the start of emergency medical service can be attributed to the Good Samaritan, a name given to that ancient wanderer who stopped to help an injured traveler on the roadside. The concept of first aid continued when the Roman military selected soldiers to be medical orderlies (*miles medicus*) to tend to the wounded on the battlefield. Later, religious groups (*apostolic orders*) had members who served the people's needs, particularly in healing the sick. An example of these religious orders still exists today in the Sisters of Mercy.

In most cases emergency medical care grew out of necessity. If drowning was a problem, as it was in many seaports, then lifesaving techniques such as barrel-rolling and other resuscitation techniques were developed to try to respond to the problem. Special groups, such as the United States Life Saving Service (USLSS), practiced these resuscitation skills and became legendary for their heroism.

In some cases, groups such as the Royal Society for the Resuscitation of the Apparently Dead were formed to advance the science of resuscitation and to teach others approved lifesaving techniques. This tradition continues today by such volunteer organizations as the American Red Cross and the American Heart Association.

MILITARY CONTRIBUTION TO EMS

There is no greater need for methods to care for the ill and injured than during a war. Before the advent of antibiotics and immunizations, many wars saw more death from disease, such as Yellow Fever, than from mortal wounds from firearms. Military physicians, surgeons, medics, and corpsmen have all made a significant contribution to EMS. The timeline in Figure 1.1 illustrates their contributions.

1500 B.C. Roman Wars
- Evidence of first treatment protocols
- Romans and Greeks use chariots to remove wounded from the battlefield

1797 The Napoleonic Wars
- Napoleon's Chief Surgeon Baron Dominique-Jean Larrey constructs a horse-drawn carriage called the *ambulance volante*, or "flying ambulances."

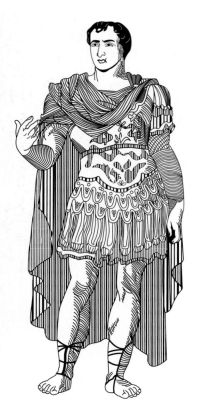

Figure 1.1 Timeline of military history

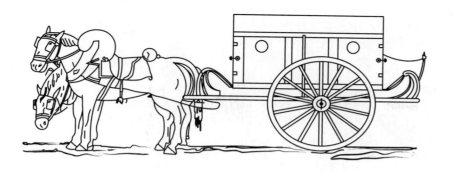

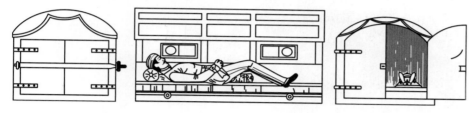

1860s The U.S. Civil War

- The First Ambulance Service in the United States is developed by U.S. Army Surgeon Jonathan Letterman. Letterman reorganized the Army Medical Corp. to include ambulances, similar to Larrey's flying ambulances.
- Clara Barton volunteers on the Civil War battlefields and sees the mayhem firsthand. Returning from the Franco–Prussian war, where she witnessed the good work of the Red Cross on the battlefield, Barton founds the American Red Cross.

1910–1940 The World Wars

- 1917 sees the first air medical transport utilizing an unmodified French Fighter Aircraft to transport wounded in the retreat of the Serbian army from Albania.
- The advent of the "combat medic" to care for the wounded in the field brings to the frontlines advanced procedures, including intravenous solutions, crude antibiotics, and intraosseous (bone) needles.
- Improved systems for trauma care are established, including field hospitals and forward first aid stations.
- Mechanized ambulances with the characteristic Red Cross emblem on the side are used, signaling the arrival of the era of the "ambulance driver."

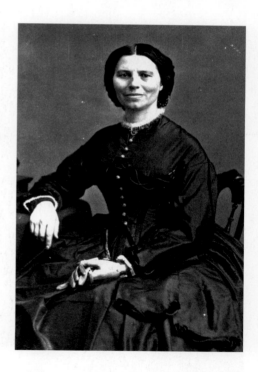

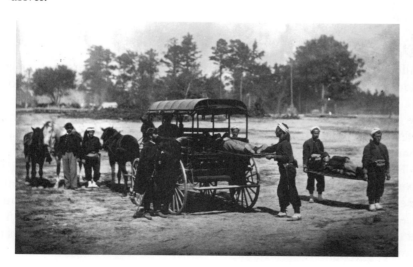

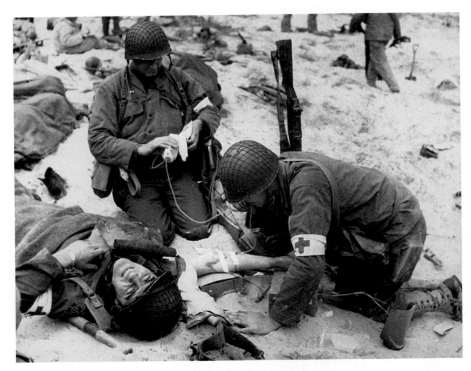

1950–1970 Korean and Vietnam War

- Mobile Army Surgical Hospitals (MASH) are developed during the Korean and Vietnam conflicts in an attempt to save the most seriously injured patients through a transportation-dependent method of triaging.
- Transportation of wounded soldiers by helicopter to medical units is used first during the Korean War, the genesis of modern aeromedical transportation.
- The HU-1, Huey, helicopter is deployed during the Vietnam War; its large patient compartment allows emergency care to begin while in flight.

1970s–Present (Iraq War)

- The 68W, health care specialist, that is, Army medic, is introduced; with an advanced skill set, the 68W is prepared to treat combat casualties as well as civilian combatants.
- Advances include development and deployment of special blood-stopping dressings, one-handed tourniquets, and special surgical procedures for extremity injuries and burns.

CIVILIAN CONTRIBUTION TO EMS

While the methods of out-of-hospital care and transport were making great strides in the military, the civilian sector was moving at a much slower pace. Ambulances used for solely transporting the sick and injured were rare (Figure 1.2). By 1966, more than half of the ambulances in the United States were still owned and operated by funeral homes, which used hearses for ambulances.

During the 1960s rescue squads began emerging out of existing fire departments or as independent third-party services. Despite the advent of these volunteer Life Saving and First Aid Squads, Rescue Squads, and Ambulance Corps, patient care consisted of basic and advanced first aid such as that taught by the American Red Cross. The timeline in Figure 1.3 shows the history and progress of EMS.

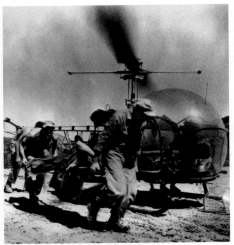

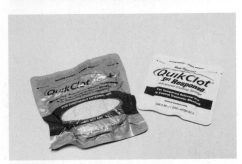

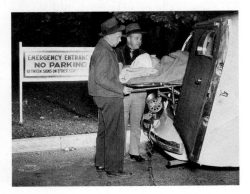

Figure 1.2 Modern civilian EMS

1865–1950 U.S. Ambulance Services

- 1865 Cincinnati establishes the first civilian ambulance service
- 1869 New York City establishes an ambulance service with hospital interns riding in horse-drawn carriages designed specifically for the sick and injured.
- 1910 One of the first ambulances, called the "Invalid's Car," runs out of Iowa Methodist Hospital, Des Moines, staffed with a nurse and resident from the hospital.
- The Roanoke Life Saving and First Aid Squad is formed in 1928 as the first volunteer rescue squad in the United States.

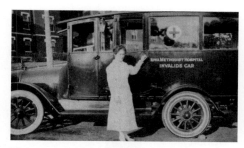

Figure 1.3 Timeline of civilian EMS

1950s Out-of-Hospital Medical Advances

- American Red Cross takes the lead in providing basic medical training, making classes such as Standard and Advanced First Aid the standard of care for rescue squad members.

    In 1958 mouth-to-mouth ventilation is demonstrated by Dr. Safer using volunteers from the Baltimore Fire Department, who agreed to be paralyzed.

- Cardiopulmonary resuscitation (CPR) is taught to civilians for the first time in the late 1950s and early 1960s.
- In 1958 Dr. Joseph K. "Deke" Farrington, known as the Father of EMS, and Dr. Sam Banks start a trauma training course for the Chicago Fire Department in what will become the prototype of the EMT-Ambulance course.

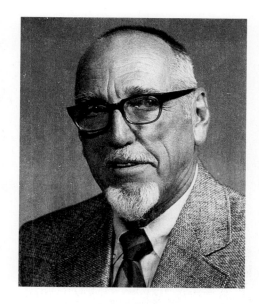

1960s Development of an EMS System

- In 1966 the National Academy of Sciences produces a white paper on "Accidental Death and Disability: The Neglected Disease of Modern Society" for President Kennedy. It states that, to that date, more Americans have died on American highways than in all U.S. wars to date.
- The National Highway Safety Act of 1966 encourages states to begin organized EMS programs.
- In 1968 St. Vincent's Hospital in New York City establishes the first coronary care unit in the United States, and Columbus, Ohio, establishes mobile coronary units, staffed with cardiology fellows from Ohio State University. Both soon replace physicians with advanced trained EMTs.
- In 1969 the first nationally recognized EMT course is held in Wausau, Wisconsin, with Dr. Farrington serving as the course medical director.
- First paramedic services are established in Miami, Florida, using the first telemetry units designed by Dr. Eugene Nagel in 1967–68.
- Dr. Leonard Cobb, Harborview Medical Center, and Seattle Fire Department establish the Medic One paramedic program in 1969.

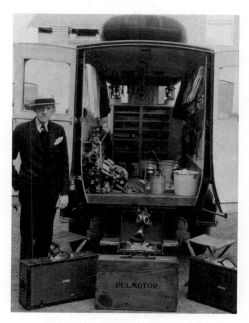

1970s The Star of Life & Voices of EMS

- In 1970 the National Registry of EMTs (NREMT), a national EMS certification organization that maintains a registry of certifications, is established.

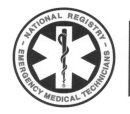

National Registry of Emergency Medical Technicians®
THE NATION'S EMS CERTIFICATION™

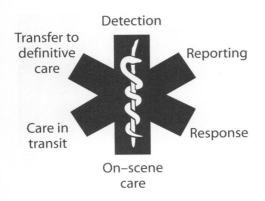

Detection
Transfer to definitive care
Reporting
Care in transit
Response
On–scene care

- In 1971 "Emergency!" debuts on television, putting a public face on EMTs and paramedics as providing expert medical care on the scene of an accident, increasing public awareness of EMS and possibly influencing government funding of EMS.
- In 1973 Star of Life is adopted as the national EMS symbol, representing the six points of the complete EMS system: detection, reporting, response, on-scene care, care in transit, and transfer to definitive care. The central staff with a serpent wrapped around it represents medicine and healing.
- In 1973 U.S. Congress passes the Emergency Medical Services System (EMSS)Act (PL93-144), identifying 15 essential components of an EMS system and allocating federal funding for individual EMS regions to address these components.
- In 1975 the National Association of EMTs (NAEMT) is formed to represent the needs of all EMTs to the public and government.
- In 1979 the American Ambulance Association (AAA), a representative organization for the ambulance service industry and legislation affecting EMS, is founded

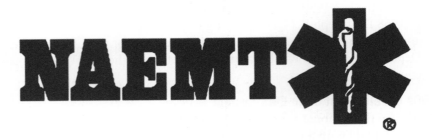

1980–2006 Agenda for the Future—Education and Federal Funding

- The Omnibus Budget Reconciliation Act of 1981 consolidates EMS funding into state preventive health and health services block grants. Funding under the EMSS Act is eliminated.
- Medical Priority Dispatching begins in Salt Lake City, Utah, in 1984.
- In 1984 the EMS for Children (EMS-C) program, under the Public Health Act, is established, providing funds for enhancing the EMS system to better serve pediatric patients.
- In 1985 the National Research Council publishes "Injury in America: A Continuing Public Health Problem," describing deficiencies in the progress in addressing the problems of accidental death and disability.
- The Comprehensive Omnibus Budget Reconciliation Act (COBRA) prevents patient "dumping," transferring patients incapable of paying for services.
- In 1988 the National Highway Traffic Safety Administration initiates the Statewide EMS Technical Assessment program based on 10 key components of EMS systems.
- The Trauma Care Systems and Development Act of 1990 provides funding to states for trauma system planning, implementation, and evaluation, encouraging development of inclusive trauma systems.
- In 1993 the Institute of Medicine publishes "Emergency Medical Services for Children," pointing out deficiencies in the health care system's ability to address the emergency medical needs of pediatric patients.
- In 1996 "The EMS Agenda for the Future" is released, outlining 14 essential attributes for future EMS development.

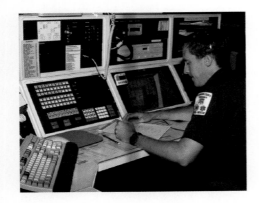

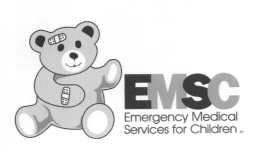

EMSC
Emergency Medical Services for Children℠

- In 2006 the controversial report, "The Future of Emergency Care: Emergency Medical Services at the Crossroads" is released by the Institutes of Medicine.

MODERN EMS

The modern EMS system is a complex organization of public first responders, communications networks, and emergency medical responders. These different aspects of the Emergency Medical Services system are represented by the Star of Life®, which symbolizes detection, reporting, response, on-scene care, care in transit, and transfer to definitive care.

Each of these spokes in the Star of Life® is important to patient care and a positive outcome from an emergency. The first step in EMS is detection and reporting.

UNIVERSAL ACCESS

In the past, it was standard across the country to use a seven-digit number to access emergency medical care, police, or fire assistance. Each community had different emergency access numbers, so it was difficult for travelers to obtain help quickly. Even members of the community who had to find the appropriate number in the phone book suffered delays because of this system.

The idea of a three-digit universal access number for emergency services was initiated in 1968 by AT&T. Since then, communities across the United States have adopted 9-1-1. It was hoped that an easily remembered three-digit number (9-1-1) would remedy the problem of accessing emergency medical services quickly. Today, many 9-1-1 dispatch centers have enhanced capabilities to help determine the exact location of the caller through the use of a computerized system that identifies the location of the telephone used to place the phone call. In addition, this computer-aided dispatch (CAD) system identifies the police, fire, and medical units closest to the location. This enhanced 9-1-1 system makes it possible to dispatch emergency response units rapidly and accurately.

The National Emergency Number Association (NENA) reports that, on average, 200 million calls are made each year to a **public safety access point (PSAP)** by citizens using 9-1-1. A PSAP is a communication center where calls are routed to emergency response units. Answering those calls are call takers in approximately 6,121 primary and secondary regional PSAPs throughout the United States. These regional PSAPs provide 9-1-1 coverage to more than 99% of the American population and 96% of the United States landmass. Presently, 9-1-1 service is being expanded to include cellular telephones, using global positioning satellite (GPS) technology, to exactly pinpoint the caller's location of the call.

EMERGENCY MEDICAL DISPATCH

Answering the 9-1-1 call at the PSAP is the emergency medical dispatcher, in some places called the communication specialist (COMSPEC) or the medical communicator (MEDCOM). An **emergency dispatcher** is a trained call taker who can take down the caller information while alerting emergency services such as fire, police, and emergency medical services. Many PSAPs try to have their dispatchers answer the 9-1-1 call within 30 seconds more than 95% of the time. They also aim to dispatch appropriate first responding emergency units within 90 seconds from the time the call is received, in accordance with the National Fire Protection Association (NFPA) standards.

In the past, well-meaning dispatchers would give simple instructions to the injured or ill or to family members waiting for the wail of a distant siren. They would advise the family to turn on the porch light or to roll the unconscious patient onto his or her side. Having a dispatcher give more extensive instructions to a caller had not yet become routine until one night in 1976. On that night a paramedic was in the alarm room in Phoenix, Arizona, when a call came in for an infant who was not breathing. The dispatcher, aided by the paramedic, gave the family instructions over the telephone to care for the child until the emergency medical personnel arrived. The baby survived, and EMS saw the birth of **emergency medical dispatch (EMD).**

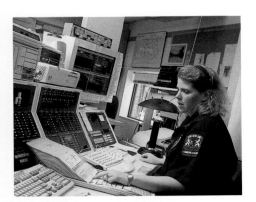

Figure 1.4 Emergency Medical Dispatcher

Specially trained call takers provide specific pre-arrival medical care instructions to callers while emergency crews respond. These instructions can range from how to control bleeding from a wound to how to deliver a baby to how to perform CPR. Thanks to the pioneering work of Dr. Jeff Clawson of Utah, medical expertise was added to the abilities of dispatchers. Using these techniques, trained communications specialists will question the caller and give lifesaving instructions while sending the closest and most appropriate aid units to the scene (Figure 1.4). Emergency medical dispatchers are truly the "first-first responders."

The practice of evaluating the nature of the illness or injury and assigning it a priority based on strict protocols is an important part of modern dispatch procedures. This practice allows the most appropriate use of sometimes-limited resources within an EMS system. In addition, the type of response by the units assigned to the scene can be prioritized. For example, flashing warning lights and sirens are used for only the most serious emergencies. EMD is rapidly becoming the standard of care in EMS, with the majority of PSAP (9-1-1) centers using such a program.

EMERGENCY MEDICAL RESPONDERS

In almost every medical emergency there is someone standing nearby who could provide assistance. With proper training, these people might have a significant impact on the outcome of an injury or illness. The American Red Cross (ARC) and American Heart Association (AHA) sought to take advantage of this reality when they launched their programs for training citizens in CPR and first aid.

The first person who arrives at the scene of an injury or illness can be referred to as a **first responder (FR).** Often, first responders are police officers, security guards, or members of the fire department—citizens who have a duty to help. The classes offered by the ARC and AHA were useful in providing basic training to these individuals, but a more expanded course in immediate lifesaving techniques was needed. The need for advanced training for first responders led to the development of a nationally recognized level of training called **Emergency Medical Responder (EMR).** The EMR learns basic assessment, simple airway management, oxygen administration, bleeding control, rescuer CPR, and defibrillation. An average EMR course would be about 50 hours. Law enforcement officers, such as the one shown in Figure 1.5, are frequently trained to be EMRs.

EMERGENCY MEDICAL TECHNICIAN

A person who has completed the basic entry level of training for the pre-hospital care is referred to as an **Emergency Medical Technician (EMT).** Traditionally, an EMT is found aboard an ambulance. In fact, in most jurisdictions there must be at least one EMT in attendance of the patient at all times. However, EMTs work in many different environments other than an

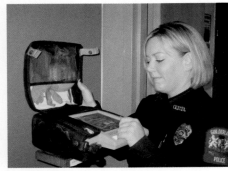

Figure 1.5 Emergency Medical Responder

ambulance— as part of a SWAT team, in wilderness medicine, or in public events venues, for example.

All EMTs bring the same skills to a patient's side, whether they work on board an ambulance, as part of a security detachment at a mall, or in the field as soldiers. The skills an EMT learns include airway maintenance, oxygen administration, bleeding control, CPR, defibrillation, patient assessment, and limited medication administration. The EMT's knowledge covers the basics of many illnesses as well as the proper management of a patient during transport to a hospital, as shown in Figures 1.6 and 1.7.

Since the first EMT curriculum was introduced in 1969, then called the EMT-Ambulance, the public has come to recognize EMT as the minimum standard of care for EMS. As the profession has changed, and technology with it, the National Standard Curriculum (NSC) for the EMT has also undergone substantial changes. The most recent changes are outlined in the **National EMS Education Standards.** These standards are broad educational statements that state the objective of EMS education at each level and that recognize EMS as a rapidly changing profession requiring flexibility within limits.

ADVANCED EMERGENCY MEDICAL TECHNICIAN

The next immediate level of EMS provider above the EMT is the **Advanced Emergency Medical Technician (AEMT).** The AEMT level represents an effort at standardization of so-called "intermediate" levels that exist across the nation. These intermediate levels, some 44 different levels across the country, represent local and regional efforts to expand the scope of practice of an EMT to include specialized or advanced procedures.

The first effort at standardization occurred in 1999 when the NSC for the EMT-I was developed; it included higher-level patient assessment skills; advanced airway management techniques, including endotracheal intubation; cardiac arrest management skills, such as electrocardiogram (ECG) interpretation and drug administration; intravenous therapy, including intraosseous infusions; and advanced trauma care.

After the experiences of Hurricane Katrina, the EMS community determined that cross-jurisdictional standardization of medical care was needed for all EMS responders, a concept called **interoperability.** The federal government, through its EMS office in the National Highway Traffic Safety

> ## Consider This....
>
> In the past, the title was EMT–A, and the A stood for ambulance. Over time, professionals in EMS came to realize that EMTs work in more than just the ambulance setting, and thus the designation was changed to EMT–B (for basic). Now everyone recognizes that an EMT is the entry level into EMS, and the accepted terminology is EMT.

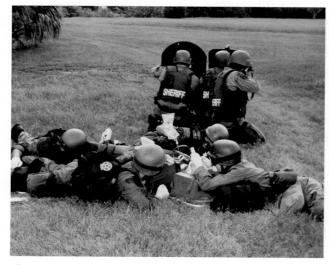

Figure 1.6 An EMT can be part of a Police Special Weapons and Tactics Team

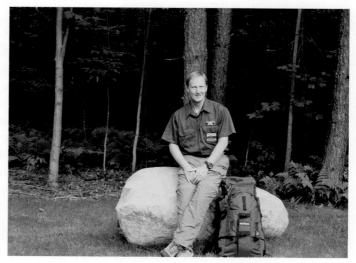

Figure 1.7 Some EMTs work in wilderness surroundings (Photo courtesy of Clark Hayward)

Administration (NHTSA), emergency medical physicians, and state EMS administrators sought to create a new level of responder universally known as the AEMT.

The AEMT is first an EMT who can provide basic emergency care. An AEMT can also provide some advanced medical care. This expanded **scope of practice** permits the AEMT to perform procedures that an EMT is not permitted to perform. A scope of practice is a legal description of the limits of care that an EMS provider can offer to a patient. The scope of practice of an AEMT includes non-intubating airways, deep suctioning of the lungs, intravenous (IV) access, intraosseous access in children, administration of intravenous fluids, and a limited number of intravenous drugs.

The extra skills that an AEMT can provide are medically proven to be of benefit to the patient. In other words, the skills of an AEMT are of high benefit and low risk to the patient. The idea of an AEMT is to provide some EMS systems, such as rural, frontier, or volunteer services that cannot afford paramedic level service but want an advanced level of EMS, a viable option. The AEMT level was specifically intended to be an add-on module to the EMT. That is, it could be completed as additional training immediately following an EMT class.

An accurate description of the role of an AEMT is an EMT who can expertly manage the first 10 minutes of a life-threatening emergency in the prehospital setting, using advanced skills and specialized equipment often seen in an emergency department.

PARAMEDIC

The highest level of prehospital EMS education is the **Paramedic.** Most paramedic education programs are offered at local community colleges or teaching hospitals. The paramedic training program is usually between 1,000 and 1,500 hours in length and includes expanded training and education in the management of the ill or injured patient. The National Registry of EMTs has announced that soon only graduates of accredited paramedic programs will be eligible for national certification.

Paramedic skills include comprehensive patient assessment, advanced airway management, intravenous access techniques, expanded medication administration, and cardiac arrest management.

As does the EMT and AEMT, a paramedic works closely with a physician and follows the physician's instructions regarding patient care. These instructions are often in the form of written protocols.

ORIGINS AND PRACTICE OF EMERGENCY MEDICINE

In the past, a friend or family member might have brought a patient to the back door of the hospital during the off hours when the doctor's office was closed. A nurse would be called down from the hospital floors to the "emergency room" to attend to the patient while a doctor was summoned. In smaller hospitals, the medical residents, or doctors in training, would also respond to the emergency call. In larger city hospitals, a young and inexperienced doctor who had just started a private practice might work nights "moonlighting" to make extra money. These inexperienced doctors often had no special training in acute medical care.

EMERGENCY MEDICINE

Inadequately trained physicians and even more poorly equipped emergency rooms became more problematic when the highly mobile U.S. public started to rely less on the family doctor and more on hospitals. The need for a specialized physician was recognized, and physicians who were specially trained in rapid assessment and diagnosis of acutely ill or traumatically injured patients, called **Emergency Physicians,** began to staff specially equipped emergency departments. An emergency physician is shown in Figure 1.8.

In 1968 emergency physicians banded together to form the American College of Emergency Physicians (ACEP). The organization's mission was to advance the cause of emergency medicine as a medical specialty. The belief was that specialized training was necessary for a physician to effectively care for acutely ill and injured patients. In 1979 emergency medicine was recognized as the 23rd specialty in medicine.

Emergency rooms quickly became more appropriately referred to as emergency departments, entities that interacted with both hospital services, such as radiology and cardiology, and prehospital services, such as EMS. The emergency department came to be defined as the emergency medical center for a hospital. An emergency department is a place to which people with medical emergencies can go, unscheduled, and receive immediate care. By its very definition, the emergency department had to be open 24 hours a day, seven days a week.

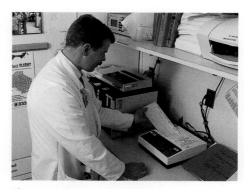

Figure 1.8 The Emergency Physician is the leader of the EMS team

SPECIALTY CARE CENTERS

With the integration of the emergency department into the hospital's operations, other physicians started to look at the emergency department, traditionally at the rear of the hospital, as the front door of the hospital.

Working closely with their emergency physician colleagues, cardiologists, neurologists, and surgeons began to see the potential of rapid intervention in medical emergencies and rapid triage of patients to special facilities. Today there are interventional cardiac centers and stroke centers that depend on the rapid assessment and triage of patients by the EMT and transport to the appropriate facility to improve survival of these special patient populations. The first specialty center may have been the trauma center.

TRAUMA CENTERS

It was soon recognized that even these newly restructured emergency departments were not capable of caring for the most severely injured patients. Physicians such as R. Adams Cowley of Baltimore Shock Trauma and the University of Maryland, researched the factors contributing to trauma death and concluded that trauma patients needed expert surgical care within the first hour of their injury. Proper surgical care within this so-called "golden hour" is associated with the best chance of survival for a seriously injured patient. As a result, special trauma emergency departments were created.

In 1980 the U.S. Department of Health and Human Services released a position paper on trauma centers. It called for the categorization of hospitals and systems of trauma care. Hospitals that were known to have the capability to properly manage severely traumatized patients (persons with severe injuries) were designated as **trauma centers.** Modern patient care protocols call for EMTs to transport certain seriously injured patients to such a designated trauma center.

AEROMEDICAL TRANSPORTATION

As hospitals have continued to specialize, partially as a result of an increasingly competitive health care industry, another need was created. Health care systems needed to be able to transfer patients from community hospitals or

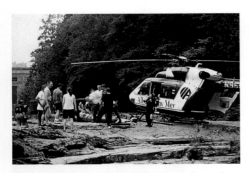

Figure 1.9 Aeromedical services is another aspect of EMS

critical access health facilities to the medical centers where specialized services would be available. To provide this rapid transport, rotary wing (helicopters) and fixed wing aircraft were used.

Today, more than 250 aeromedical services exist in the United States. The missions of these services are a mix of prehospital emergency response and interfacility transport. Because of this mix, many flight teams are made up of a registered nurse and an Emergency Medical Technician-Paramedic (EMT-P) with specialized aeromedical training. Figure 1.9 shows a standard flight configuration of a flight nurse, a flight paramedic, and a pilot.

THE FUTURE OF EMS

Although EMS has come a long way in the last 50 years, changes are needed to accommodate the changing needs of the populations being served and to adjust to new financial and medical developments. Increasing elderly and homeless populations, decreasing health care resources, tightening finances, increasing demands for quality, and a need for organized research all contribute to the challenges that EMS faces today and will face in the future.

AGING AMERICANS

After World War II, there was a huge increase in the number of births in the United States, which came to be called the *baby boom*. Today, these children of the baby boom, known as *baby boomers*, are becoming middle-aged and elderly. As people age, they are likely to develop significant health problems. These increasing health problems often lead to an increased use of medical services. Accordingly, the number of EMS calls to the elderly is increasing. Older adults have special needs that must be recognized, and treatment of the elderly may differ from treatment of younger patients. The special needs of the elderly are addressed later in Chapter 9.

HOMELESSNESS

With the increasing use of medications to treat psychiatric illnesses and a shift away from institutionalization for all but people who cannot care for themselves or who may pose a threat to others, many people with psychiatric conditions live independently. These persons sometimes are unable to properly care for or house themselves. In addition, the nation's changing economy has made it impossible for some Americans to provide food or shelter for themselves or their families. Shelters designed to house such homeless people are usually overcrowded. The social services system often cannot satisfy the needs of all the people in need of help. Because of their lack of regular health care and adequate housing, the homeless have come to rely on the EMS system and emergency departments for their medical care.

INFECTIOUS DISEASES

Infectious diseases such as Methicillin-resistant *Staphylococcus aureus* (MRSA) and Avian Flu have made headlines and raised special concerns for the EMS profession. Both new strains of infectious agents and some long-standing diseases that are increasingly resistant to antibiotics are challenging the way that EMTs perform their functions, increasing the importance of infection control practices and preventive immunizations.

OPERATIONAL CHALLENGES

Contributing to the challenges in EMS are operational issues. Operational issues are those concerns and problems that exist within the EMS system and do not include patient-driven priorities, such as staffing, financial, and accountability issues.

HUMAN RESOURCES

In many suburban and rural parts of the United States, EMS is provided by volunteers. These volunteers provide an invaluable service to their communities that, nationwide, would cost in the billions of dollars to replace with paid providers. However, modern demands, such as the need for two incomes to maintain an average lifestyle, have made it difficult for the average citizen to find time to volunteer for EMS. Declining membership is a problem that has been identified by many national EMS groups and continues to pose a significant challenge for EMS.

FINANCIAL RESTRICTIONS

The requirements for equipment, training, insurance, and other costs in today's out-of-hospital health care system can be overwhelming. Small volunteer organizations may find it difficult to fulfill these requirements with the minimal funding they have at their disposal. The budgets in many municipalities have not increased proportionately to the rising cost of managing an EMS system.

Organizations that represent EMS at a national level are constantly trying to resolve the issues that have forced the closing of volunteer EMS agencies across the country. The EMS community must continue to fight for better financial support to continue the mission of emergency care in the field.

ACCOUNTABILITY

Accountability for expenses is being demanded of every governmental or quasi-governmental organization, including EMS. Citizens want to know that their tax dollars are being spent wisely and cost-effectively. EMS has recognized this demand and has responded appropriately with programs of total quality management.

Most EMS agencies are involved in either quality assurance or **continuous quality improvement (CQI)** programs, which are designed to find and address areas in need of improvement within the agency. These types of programs help ensure that the EMS system is able to provide high-quality patient care at a reasonable cost. Both state and federal laws are starting to require that all EMS agencies that accept public monies have these types of programs in place.

ADVENT OF EMS RESEARCH

For years, the practice of EMS has been largely based on in-hospital experience and the opinion of physicians. This anecdotal experience has led to some errors and misadventures. To improve the quality of care and decrease the number of errors, emergency physicians have turned to evidence-based medicine (EBM). Physicians using EBM apply evidence from research that uses the scientific method to ascertain what the best practice of medicine is. Practices of questionable efficacy or safety have been discarded, and new procedures that have been proven beneficial by research are being implemented. Some of the techniques and practices that EMTs will learn in this text will be different from what may have been previously taught due to information gained from EBM.

For example, research studies have determined that rapid defibrillation is the key to survival in cardiac arrest. This research has led to the addition of defibrillation to the scope of practice of the EMT. Training in the use of the AED is now available not only to EMTs but also to the general public through CPR training.

Unfortunately, carefully designed scientific studies have been rare in the field of EMS. However, such research has been gradually increasing since the 1990s. Although issues such as lack of funding and difficulties in obtaining consent in emergency situations have made conducting quality EMS research difficult, it is by no means impossible. Emergency physicians and EMTs have to make evidence-based practice a priority. Well-designed studies are being completed every day that help the EMS community shape its practices on the basis of scientific fact rather than anecdotal experience or popular opinion.

CONCLUSION

The rich past of EMS is filled with examples of individual heroism and leadership. We share our heritage with emergency physicians, emergency nurses, and other allied health professions. This association does not diminish EMS; it only amplifies the importance of teamwork.

The future of EMS depends on vigilant attention to trends in emergency medicine and the challenges they may present. To face these challenges, the EMT should insist on research-based practice and refine daily practices accordingly to provide the best quality of patient care.

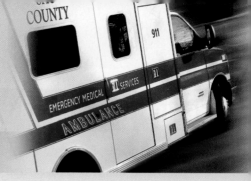

CASE STUDY Continued

Closing his book at the end of class, David sits back and considers what he has heard in this lecture. Clearly, being an EMT means studying hard and building a strong foundation of knowledge. The lecture also discussed the critical need for EMTs to maintain a current, working knowledge of medical techniques and equipment and to continue their education. David realizes that being an EMT means you are always learning. Now he is beginning to understand the challenges and rewards of being an EMT and is excited to begin the course work.

Key Concepts Revisited

- The three missions of EMS are patient care, public safety, and public health.
- Military contributions to EMS continue to change and improve the delivery of EMS, particularly trauma care.
- The era of modern EMS started in the 1960s.
- EMS is a complex system, starting with the emergency medical dispatcher and ending with delivery to definitive care. This complexity is illustrated in the eight points of the Star of Life.
- The professional EMT is part of a larger health care delivery system
- There are many challenges to the future of EMS.

Key Terms

Advanced Emergency Medical Technician (AEMT)

Continuous quality improvement (CQI)

Emergency Dispatchers

Emergency Medical Dispatch (EMD)

Emergency Medical Responder (EMR)

Emergency Medical Services (EMS)

Emergency Medical Technician (EMT)

Emergency Physician

First responders (FR)

Interoperability

National EMS Education Standards

Paramedic

Public safety access point (PSAP)

Scope of practice

Trauma centers

Review Questions

1. What are the three missions of EMS?
2. What are three historical documents that significantly impacted EMS?
3. What are three key legislative acts that help start EMS?
4. Who are three EMS medical leaders?
5. What are the six elements of an EMS response as represented in the Star of Life?
6. Who are the EMS providers in an EMS system?
7. What are three current specialty care centers?
8. What are the three social challenges to EMS?
9. What are the three operational challenges to EMS?

Further Study

Committee on the Future of Emergency Care in the United States Health. *Emergency Care for Children: Growing Pains.* Washington, DC: National Academy Press, 2007.

Committee on Trauma and Committee on Shock, Division of Medical Sciences, National Academy of Sciences, National Research Council. *Accidental Death and Disability: A neglected disease of society.* Washington, DC: National Academy Press, 1966.

Page, James O. *Making a Difference: The History of Modern EMS.* 2d ed. New York: Elsevier, 2004.

Post, Carl. *Omaha Orange: A Popular History of EMS in America.* Sudbury, MA: Jones and Bartlett, 2002.

UNIT (2) Roles and Responsibilities of the EMT

The Emergency Medical Technician (EMT) is an important part of the prehospital health care team. Professionalism, training, continuing education, and appropriate medical direction are essential components of an EMT's career. This unit discusses these issues in detail.

National Education Standard

The Emergency Medical Technician (EMT) will have a simple depth and foundational breadth of knowledge of the roles and responsibilities an EMT, EMS professionalism, quality improvement, and patient safety.

Key Concepts

- The roles and responsibilities of the EMT.
- The importance of personal, public, and patient safety.
- The professional attributes of an EMT.
- Professional EMS organizations.
- The EMT Code of Ethics.
- The process of continuous quality improvement (CQI).
- The importance of medical direction.

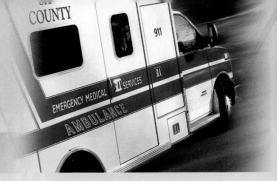

CASE STUDY

"Rescue 50, respond to a priority one motor vehicle collision at the corner of Routes 155 and 20." Deb carefully copies down the information. Deb and Earl climb into the ambulance and fasten their seat belts. Deb starts the engine, turns on the emergency lights and siren, and proceeds toward the scene of the call.

Upon arrival at the scene, Deb parks the ambulance in a position that is well out of traffic but still permits easy access to the rear compartment and allows for an easy exit from the scene. Deb and Earl don personal protective equipment and then approach the scene.

Earl quickly scans the scene and determines that three persons are involved. One, a young woman, is trapped in her vehicle by damage to the door. He immediately calls the dispatcher on the radio and requests additional ambulances to the scene as well as the local fire department for "extrication.

Earl and Deb briefly assess each patient to determine who needs attention first. The woman who is trapped is still secured by her seat belt. Earl assesses her airway and breathing and gives her oxygen. Continuing in his assessment, he finds that she has the physical signs of shock. Earl immediately calls for assistance in rapidly removing her from the vehicle.

The woman is removed from the vehicle and placed onto a backboard, with the help of several firefighters. Deb maintains restricted cervical movement while Earl, with continued assistance from the firefighters, places the patient onto a stretcher. Then they place the stretcher into the back of the waiting ambulance.

Deb begins driving, using the emergency lights and sirens, toward the regional trauma center while Earl continues to assess the patient in the rear of the ambulance. As soon as he can, Earl uses the mobile radio to call the trauma center to advise them of the woman's condition and of their impending arrival. Receiving no further orders, Earl continues to provide care for the patient and frequently reassesses her condition.

Upon arrival at the hospital, Deb parks the ambulance in the designated ambulance entrance and helps Earl remove the stretcher from the rear of the ambulance. A nurse, who is expecting them, meets them at the emergency department's doors.

Earl gives a thorough verbal report of his assessment and treatment as they transfer the woman onto the hospital stretcher. The nurse carefully notes the care provided. After quickly cleaning up and placing new sheets on the stretcher, Deb and Earl document the call and clean and restock the ambulance, in preparation for another call.

Critical Thinking Questions

1. What roles do the EMTs in this case play?
2. What are the EMTs' responsibilities in this case?
3. What should be included in an EMT's job description?

INTRODUCTION

The public turns to Emergency Medical Services (EMS) for help in times of crisis. This need has led to the creation and development of the modern EMS system. The EMT within this system must aspire to the highest levels of professionalism, including continuous self-improvement and ethical behavior.

ROLES OF THE EMT

The EMT has many roles and responsibilities, but the first and most important role is that of **caregiver.** A caregiver is a person who assists in the identification and treatment of an illness and helps to alleviate suffering, both mental and physical.

Although all the skills that an EMT brings to the patient's side are helpful, perhaps the most important skill or attribute is compassion. **Compassion** is the ability to be aware of another person's suffering and to want to help relieve it. In some cases an EMT is limited in what she can physically do for a patient, but in every case the EMT can show that she understands the patient's situation or feelings—that is, show empathy for the patient—and take the opportunity to demonstrate compassion through therapeutic communications.

Another role of the EMT is that of **steward.** A steward is someone who cares for the affairs of another. EMS, as a practice, is shared with physicians, and EMTs, as allied health providers, represent not only themselves but their medical director and their service.

One way that EMTs can show that they accept responsibility as a steward, as a representative of their service, is in their appearance. Clean and neatly dressed EMTs show respect to both their service and their service medical director but also instill confidence in the patient and the patient's family. A team of well-dressed EMTs are shown in Figure 2.1.

EMTs, in their role as one of the three public safety services, are also in a position to provide **leadership.** Leadership is that quality of causing others to follow in one direction to accomplish a goal. Often chaos occurs during a medical crisis, and the patient turns to EMS for help. It is the EMT's responsibility to bring calm to the situation and provide considerate care to the patient. That care usually requires that the EMT set priorities for care. In some instances the EMT may elect to care for the patient on scene. In other cases the EMT may decide to have the team "package" the patient—that is, place the patient on a stretcher and into the ambulance for immediate departure. In both cases the EMT's decision is a demonstration of that EMT's leadership, as shown in Figure 2.2.

RESPONSIBILITIES OF THE EMT

The EMT is an integral part of the **prehospital health care team.** This team is made up of many different members, including medical personnel, firefighters, and law enforcement officers, all of whom must be thoroughly familiar with their own roles and responsibilities (Figure 2.3). When all members of the team work together, the common goal will be realized. In this case, the goal is to deliver professional care in a timely manner.

The EMT is given the responsibility of bringing quality medical care to patients wherever they may be. This care may range from lifesaving procedures to simply comforting the patient. Regardless of the scenario, the EMT is expected to provide a high quality of basic medical care to the patient in a professional manner while maintaining her own safety and the safety of coworkers.

The EMT's responsibility goes beyond simply caring for the patient. Accurate and thorough patient assessment is necessary to guide appropriate treatment. The EMT must also understand the principles of safe lifting and movement of patients. Decision making is also a key skill. The EMT must be able to quickly and accurately set priorities for patient care and determine the mode of transport and the appropriate destination hospital.

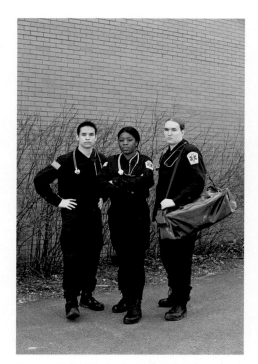
Figure 2.1 Well-dressed EMT prepared for duty

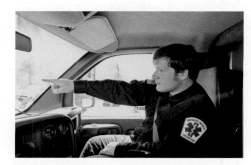
Figure 2.2 EMT leading a team

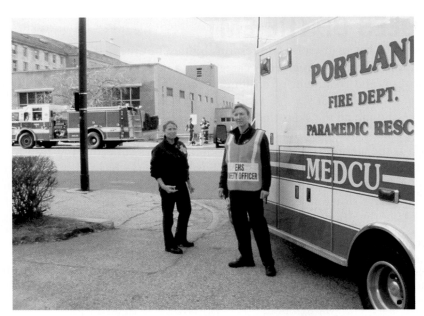

Figure 2.3 Public safety team member (Courtesy of Larry Torrey and MEDCU, Portland, Maine)

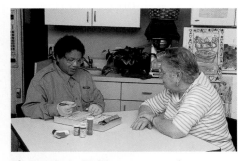

Figure 2.4 EMT documenting patient care

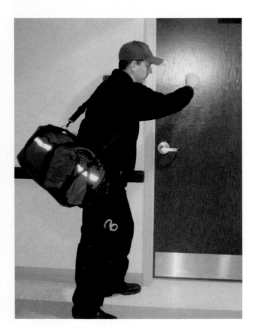

Figure 2.5 Tactical approach to a potentially dangerous scene

As in any other health care profession, thorough documentation of all assessment findings and interventions is necessary upon completion of patient care. Both written and verbal reports must be provided to the receiving hospital staff at the time of patient transfer. Written reports must include all necessary data to allow for later review of the details of care and transport. Figure 2.4 shows an EMT completing a patient care record, the final duty of an EMT during patient care.

Above all, EMTs must remember that their job is to do what is best for patients. A certain amount of flexibility is required to provide individualized care to each patient.

TEAM SAFETY

Safety is crucial in many jobs, including that of an EMT. During the course of normal duties, an EMT may be placed in many difficult-to-control environments. The EMT must learn to control those aspects of the situation that can be controlled and anticipate any problems that may arise. Considerable time will be spent during EMT training to ensure that the skills and procedures students learn will be performed in a safe manner.

PERSONAL SAFETY

The first priority of any prehospital team member must be personal safety. The patient's needs are of high priority. However, these needs should not be allowed to place the EMT or other team members in unreasonable danger.

It is senseless for trained medical professionals to allow harm to come to themselves. If an EMT is injured, she becomes another patient, compounding the problem. The EMT must always be aware of potential hazards and take necessary steps to avoid them.

Safety precautions may be simple, such as wearing gloves for protection against potentially infectious bodily fluids, or they may be more complicated, such as delaying entry into a possible crime scene until appropriate law enforcement agencies have arrived and determined the safety of the scene. Figure 2.5 shows an EMT using a tactical approach to a potentially dangerous scene. The subject of delaying entry to a crime scene will be dealt with in more detail in Unit 3.

CREW, PATIENT, AND BYSTANDER SAFETY

In addition to taking steps to protect themselves, EMTs must be aware of potential danger to the patient, the crew, and bystanders on the scene. If a member of the team is no longer able to perform duties because of an injury, the team is no longer efficient. It is the responsibility of every team member to ensure her own safety and the safety of the other team members.

Some situations may call for the EMT to protect the patient from further harm. If a patient is in a potentially dangerous situation, the EMT must make it a priority to remove the patient from the danger as soon as safety permits.

The EMT must also take the appropriate steps to protect the patient from self-inflicted harm while maintaining personal safety. To protect the patient while maintaining personal safety, the EMT may have to involve other team members.

Emergencies often draw significant attention from laypeople. An EMT must always be aware of potential hazards to private citizens such as bystanders and members of the media. Crowd control may be assigned to another team member, such as a law enforcement officer, but the EMT may need to initiate the call for this assistance (Figure 2.6).

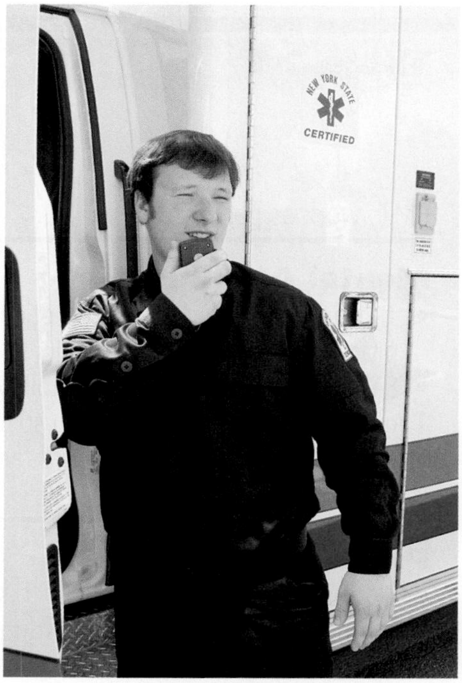

In short, the EMT is responsible for providing medical care to the patient while maintaining personal safety as well as the safety of the crew and bystanders. It is always better to anticipate safety issues and prevent problems than to deal with the results of an unanticipated incident.

Figure 2.6 EMT asking for police assistance

JOB DESCRIPTION

The EMT is expected to perform a wide variety of duties in many different circumstances. The work of the EMT requires particular skills and attributes to perform the functions of the job. The description of those physical skills and mental attributes are listed in a functional job description. A functional job description is developed after completion of a functional job analysis.

The National Highway Traffic Safety Administration (NHTSA) has completed a functional job analysis and described the characteristics for the EMT, shown in Table 2-1. Many states have adopted a similar functional job analysis to develop a functional job description for the EMT.

OPERATIONAL DUTIES

It is important that the EMT work in a manner that reassures both patient and bystanders. From maintaining a clean, well-stocked ambulance to attending appropriate training and continuing education, a prehospital health care provider has a variety of procedural duties that contribute to effective performance on the job. See Table 2-2.

PATIENT CARE PROCEDURES

EMTs may find themselves in many situations that have not been accurately described to them. For this reason EMTs and other EMS team members must be well trained and prepared for a wide variety of situations.

On the basis of assessment findings, an EMT will provide emergency medical care to ill or injured adults, infants, and children. Specific patient care duties are shown in Table 2-3. This text provides detailed discussions of these duties to assist you in your initial training.

Table 2-1 NHSTA Functional Job Analysis

EMT Characteristics

EMTs work as part of a team.

Mental Attributes
- Thorough knowledge of theoretical procedures and ability to integrate knowledge and performance into practical situations are critical.
- Self-confidence, emotional stability, good judgment, tolerance for high stress, and a pleasant personality are essential characteristics of the successful EMTs at any level.
- EMTs must be able to deal with adverse social situations, which include responding to calls in districts known to have high crime rates.

Physical Demands
- Aptitudes required for work of this nature are good physical stamina, endurance, and body condition that would not be adversely affected by lifting, carrying, and balancing at times, patients in excess of 125 pounds (250, with assistance).
- EMTs must be able to work long hours.
- Motor coordination is necessary for the well-being of the patient, the EMT, and the coworker over uneven terrain.

Communications
- Driving the ambulance in a safe manner, accurately discerning street names through map reading, and the ability to correctly distinguish house numbers or business locations are essential to task completion in the most expedient manner possible.
- Use of the telephone and radio for transmitting and responding to physician's advice is essential.
- The ability to concisely and accurately describe orally to physicians and other concerned staff one's impression of the patient's condition is critical because EMTs work in emergency conditions in which there may be no time for deliberation.
- EMTs must be able to accurately summarize all data in the form of a written report. Verbal and reasoning skills are used more extensively than math. Math does play a part, however, in determining medication ratios per patient's body weight.

(Adapted from Appendix A, National Standard Curriculum for EMT)

Table 2-2 Operational Duties of an EMT

- Maintains a clean, fully stocked vehicle.
- Is able to quickly locate and use any piece of equipment on the vehicle.
- Receives dispatch information accurately.
- Drives to the scene quickly but safely, observing all traffic laws.
- Safely parks the vehicle.
- Performs a scene assessment.
- Determines the need for further assistance.

(continued)

Table 2-2 Operational Duties of an EMT (*continued*)

- Determines the mechanism of injury or the nature of the illness.
- Assesses the patient and provides appropriate care.
- Calls for additional help if necessary.
- Moves the patient to the ambulance.
- Continues patient care during transport to the hospital.
- Chooses the appropriate hospital for the patient's condition.
- Involves medical control when needed.
- Provides the destination facility with sufficient advance notification.
- Continually reassesses the patient.
- Continually reassures the patient.
- Safely transports the patient to the hospital and transfers care.
- Provides the hospital staff with concise verbal and written reports.
- Restocks the ambulance and returns to service.

Table 2-3 Patient Care Duties

Airway and Breathing
- Insertion of airway adjuncts intended to go into the oropharynx or **nasopharynx**
- Use of positive pressure ventilation devices such as the bag-valve-mask or manually triggered ventilators and **automatic transport ventilators**
- Suction of the upper airway
- Supplemenal oxagen therapy

Pharmacological Interventions
- Use of unit dose auto-injectors for the administration of lifesaving medications intended for self or peer rescue in hazardous materials situations (e.g., atropine auto-injectors)
- **Assist patients in taking their own prescribed medications**
- **Administration of the following over-the-counter medications with appropriate medical oversight:**
  - **Oral glucose for suspected hypoglycemia**
  - **Aspirin for chest pain of suspected ischemic origin**

Medical/Cardiac Care
- Use of an automated external defibrillator

Trauma Care
- Manual stabilization and splinting of suspected cervical spine injuries
- Manual stabilization and splinting of extremity fractures
- Bleeding control
- **Application and inflation of the pneumatic anti-shock garment (PASG/MAST) for fracture stabilization**

Emergency Moves

(NOTE: Items in bold type are those skills within the scope of practice for an EMT but outside the scope of practice of an Emergency Medical Responder)

PROFESSIONAL ATTRIBUTES OF AN EMT

As members of the prehospital health care team, EMTs are held to the same standard of professionalism as any other member of the team, regardless of level of training, area of practice, or pay scale. Patients who access EMS deserve to receive the same quality of care in their homes as they would receive in a hospital or in their doctor's office.

An EMT must strive to maintain professional conduct by demonstrating a caring, confident, and courteous demeanor on the job. The same level of professionalism that is expected of an emergency department physician or nurse is expected of an EMT.

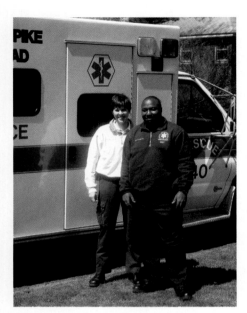

Figure 2.7 EMT with the soft look uniform

PROFESSIONAL APPEARANCE

It has been said that "a picture speaks a thousand words," and in the case of an EMT's appearance, nothing is more true. A clean, neat uniform projects a professional attitude. An easily identifiable uniform and a name tag help citizens identify the members of the prehospital medical team. Some systems use military-style uniforms that command authority; others use a "softer" look, wearing polo shirts, for example. An EMT who takes care in her appearance, like the EMT in Figure 2.7, conveys the message that she will exercise the same care in managing a patient.

PHYSICAL PREPAREDNESS

Many of the EMT's duties require some physical exertion. The EMT who maintains good physical condition will be best suited to complete these tasks safely. Unit 4 discusses further benefits physical fitness can have on the EMT's well-being.

PERSONALITY TRAITS

Although anyone can train to become an EMT, certain personality traits are better suited to this role. The EMT should be kind and compassionate as well as willing to help others, regardless of personal prejudices.

EMTs often find themselves in highly sensitive situations. Persons who call for emergency assistance from an EMS team deserve to receive compassionate and confidential care regardless of their condition or background. Remaining nonjudgmental is crucial, although it may sometimes be difficult.

ETHICAL BEHAVIOR

The National Association of Emergency Medical Technicians (NAEMT) is an organization that represents EMS professionals across the United States. Its primary mission is to promote the advancement of EMS as an allied health profession.

An important part of maintaining the necessary professionalism within a group or organization is the ethical principles by which it operates. The EMT Code of Ethics is reproduced in Table 2-4. The values and principles set forth within the EMT Code of Ethics are crucial in the makeup of the prehospital health care professional.

EMS EDUCATION

The first step toward becoming a professional EMS provider is proper educational preparation. Since the inception the National Standard Curriculum (NSC) and, more recently, the National EMS Education Standards (NEMSES), EMT courses across the country have adhered to this prescriptive set of objectives that help standardize the knowledge of an EMT.

Table 2-4 EMT Code of Ethics

- The Emergency Medical Technician respects and holds in confidence all information of a confidential nature obtained in the course of professional work unless required by law to divulge such information.
- The Emergency Medical Technician, as a citizen, understands and upholds the law and performs the duties of citizenship; as a professional, the Emergency Medical Technician has the never-ending responsibility to work with concerned citizens and other health care professionals in promoting a high standard of emergency medical care to all people.
- The Emergency Medical Technician shall maintain professional competence and demonstrate concern for the competence of other members of the Emergency Medical Services health care team.
- An Emergency Medical Technician assumes responsibility in defining and upholding standards of professional practice and education.
- The Emergency Medical Technician assumes responsibility for individual professional actions and judgment, both in dependent and independent emergency functions, and knows and upholds the laws that affect the practice of the Emergency Medical Technician.
- An Emergency Medical Technician has the responsibility to be aware of and participate in matters of legislation affecting the Emergency Medical Service System.
- The Emergency Medical Technician, or groups of Emergency Medical Technicians, who advertise professional service, do so in conformity with the dignity of the profession.
- The Emergency Medical Technician has an obligation to protect the public by not delegating to a person less qualified any service that requires the professional competence of an Emergency Medical Technician.
- The Emergency Medical Technician will work harmoniously with and sustain confidence in Emergency Medical Technician associates, the nurses, the physicians, and other members of the Emergency Medical Services health care team.
- The Emergency Medical Technician refuses to participate in unethical procedures and assumes the responsibility to expose incompetence or unethical conduct of others to the appropriate authority in a proper and professional manner.

Written by Charles Gillespie, M.D., Adopted by The National Association of Emergency Medical Technicians, 1978.

EMT TRAINING

To provide quality patient care, the EMT must first participate in a basic training course to learn the principles of emergency care. State and federal agencies regulate the initial training courses for the EMT. The educational standards are outlined by the U.S. Department of Transportation EMS Education Standards.

Many national organizations contributed to the preparation of these documents, which are revised regularly to mirror changes in practice and research. Each state adds to or enriches the curriculum in a way that is felt to be most appropriate for the state's needs. This curriculum serves as a basis upon which training courses are designed.

Because the duties of EMTs will place them in many different situations, their initial training will include different types of learning opportunities. Classroom, or didactic, teaching will be standard to prepare students with the required cognitive (knowledge-based) objectives. Practical hands-on instruction will enable students to learn assessment and treatment in a controlled environment. These psychomotor skills are the backbone of an EMT's practice. Figure 2.8 shows several EMT practicing skills in a lab scenario.

Clinical requirements may include observation time in the hospital and in the prehospital environment to enable the EMT to learn how to put this new knowledge into practice.

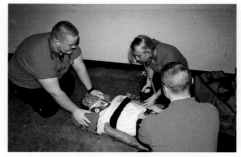

Figure 2.8 EMT practicing in lab

CERTIFICATION AND LICENSURE

To reassure the public that the person responding to the emergency is a minimally competent EMT, each state provides for a process of examination that can lead to licensure as an EMT in that state. All EMTs must successfully complete this standardized examination of both skills and knowledge to attain this licensure to practice as an EMT.

Once the EMT is licensed, she can practice as an EMT within the scope of practice as defined by state law. Each state has statutes that define the scope of practice of all health care professionals, including the EMT, and they are usually found in the public health law or the medical practice act.

In some cases the state itself provides the certification examination that leads to licensure as an EMT. In those states EMTs are permitted to practice once they are certified by the state.

In other circumstances the state depends on a national examination for certification. A nationally recognized **certification** demonstrates that the EMT has attained a certain level of competency as recognized by her peers. For EMS, the National Registry of Emergency Medical Technicians (NREMT) certifies EMS providers.

The NREMT has certified more than 1 million EMTs in the United States, and the National Registry examination is used as the certifying examination, at one level of EMS provider or another, in 46 states (Figure 2.9). The NREMT examination's test plan, called a test blueprint, is developed based on the result of the EMT Practice Analysis conducted periodically and generally is considered to be a reliable test instrument.

States Accepting National Registry Certification for EMT

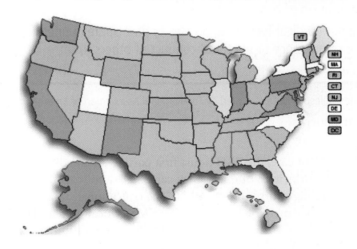

- ◯ All Levels Available
- ◯ Basic
- ◯ Paramedic
- ◯ Non Registry
- ◯ Basic & Paramedic
- ◯ In Discussion with the Registry

Figure 2.9 States accepting National Registry Certification for EMT

The NREMT's mission statement is to certify and register EMS professionals throughout their careers by a valid and uniform process that assesses their knowledge and skills for competent practice. Many EMS providers take serial examinations as they attain each new level of EMS: EMT, AEMT, and Paramedic.

EMS providers are sometimes confused about the distinction between the terms *certification* and *licensure*. In a legal opinion delivered to the NREMT, and available online, the distinction was made clear. Certification is a voluntary process that is completed with a private organization, such as the NREMT. States may elect to use this certification as the basis for their permission for an individual to practice. States may also elect to test the EMT themselves. In those cases the examination, despite the use of the term certification, is a licensing examination. The distinction is: whenever the state gives an EMT the right to practice as an EMT, it has licensed that EMT.

LIFELONG LEARNING

Once initial certification has been achieved, the requirements for education have not ended. All health care professionals must make a commitment to lifelong learning through continuing medical education. It is important not only for the EMT to be aware of new information but also to participate in its development and dissemination, when possible. As do other areas of medicine, prehospital care continues to change as researchers find new and more efficient ways to provide emergency medical care.

In a rapidly changing world, where new technologies are introduced every day, the professional EMT is always learning. This lifelong learning can be divided into two categories: competency assurance and professional development. Competency assurance ensures the EMT maintains those skills and knowledge necessary to perform the duties of the profession. Typically an EMT attends refresher training and obtains recertification on a periodic basis as a demonstration of competency assurance.

CONTINUING EDUCATION FOR COMPETENCY ASSURANCE

As with any education, after a period of time, some material may be forgotten and may need reviewing. Most states have prescribed time lines with requirements for refresher training. These requirements vary greatly in form but all serve the same purpose—to ensure that the provider has reviewed the core components of the curriculum since initial training.

One requirement may be a refresher course that reviews the core components of the curriculum every 2 or 3 years. Another way of ensuring review is to require participation in a regular continuing education program that covers the core components. Some states require that a test be taken every 2 or 3 years for recertification. Regardless of the form of the review, EMTs must prove regularly that they continue to remain skilled in the procedures and in the assessment and treatment techniques for which they were originally trained.

SKILL MAINTENANCE

The initial training introduces EMTs to many skills that will be perfected after much practice. As do other skills, these will degenerate if not practiced frequently. It is the responsibility of the EMT to maintain a certain level of proficiency with regard to important skills.

CONTINUING EDUCATION FOR PROFESSIONAL DEVELOPMENT

Professional development goes beyond the core content in an EMT course and involves additional learning. Leadership training or learning about emergency management are examples of professional development. Professional development also includes learning about new medical technologies or treatment procedures. EMTs should read trade journals such as those shown in Figure 2.10 to stay abreast of new medical technologies.

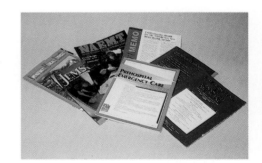

Figure 2.10 EMTs should read trade journals for new medical information

QUALITY IMPROVEMENT

The prehospital health care field of EMS is constantly undergoing change. Many of these changes will affect the everyday practice of the EMT. It is the responsibility of all health care providers to be aware of and to contribute to, as they are able, the changes that their profession undergoes. Professional organizations such as the NAEMT provide the structure for creating change that is beneficial to the EMT and to the ability to provide quality patient care.

The EMT should also be aware of the professional magazines and journals that support the advancement of quality patient care by prehospital providers. These journals provide a way to keep up to date on national EMS events and current literature relevant to the practice of medicine by the EMT.

CONTINUOUS QUALITY IMPROVEMENT

The EMS system is an integral part of the emergency management of a sick or an injured patient. The process by which such care is provided needs to be closely examined on a regular basis to ensure timely, cost-effective care. This examination can be done through careful quality review and by completing quality research that focuses on prehospital care. It is the responsibility of the EMT to participate in research projects that are designed to examine current practices and that ultimately serve to improve patient care.

The ultimate goal of every EMS team member is to provide quality medical care in a timely manner while maintaining team safety. The recognition of that goal is the first step in quality management within the EMS team. Quality management can be thought of as a continual process that involves the planning, execution, assessment, review, and improvement of the overall plan.

PLANNING

Ensuring that the desired goal is commonly realized by all members of the team requires that a clear system be in place. All members of the team must be familiar with this system to ensure its effectiveness.

Within EMS, the system is usually organized by protocols and standard operating procedures. These documents provide a plan that, if followed, will lead to the common goal of quality delivery of care. The EMT is responsible for knowing these elements.

Over time, the overall plan may need to be adjusted. It is the responsibility of the EMT to help alter the plan as needed and to adapt to any changes that may be made.

PERFORMANCE

The system must be set up in a manner that allows execution of the plan without difficulty. If components of the plan are unreasonable or difficult to accomplish, it is unlikely that the plan will be followed regularly. For example, if the plan includes a response time to emergencies of fewer than 8 minutes but the ambulance station is located more than 8 minutes from a majority of the calls, this response time will not likely be accomplished.

ASSESSMENT

To advance, the team must have a method of assessing the quality of the care provided. This assessment is often accomplished by a specific committee of providers that may include administrative personnel, field providers, and the medical director of the organization. This assessment may occur prospectively (before or during a call) or, more commonly, retrospectively (after the call).

Prospective quality assessment is usually accomplished by a member of the assessment team accompanying a crew on an emergency call and observing the care provided. This is useful because it provides a clear picture of the quality of the care given. Such assessment is time and labor intensive and is not always possible, but it should be a part of every quality management program.

Retrospective quality assessment is often accomplished by review of the documentation by the team, with identification of strengths and weaknesses. This review of run reports may be comprehensive, or it may be focused on one particular area during specific audits.

This method of assessment is more easily accomplished than is prospective quality assessment, but it obviously provides a limited view of the actual care provided to the patient. This review can be made more effective by ensuring that the providers use a standard method of documentation and that the method incorporates all of the factors that would be important in determining quality of care.

Many states or regions have produced a standard patient care report (PCR) for use as a documentation tool. This report must be fully completed to be useful in quality assessment.

Another method of retrospective review is to gather feedback. The patients and their families can be surveyed to identify problems or strengths they may perceive. Other users of the system, such as hospital receiving staff or staff at other frequently visited sites (e.g., local nursing homes, special centers) should also be asked for feedback. The EMT in Figure 2.11 is helping with a patient care record audit.

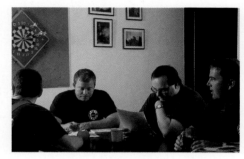

Figure 2.11 EMT helping with patient care record audit

Feedback from patients and facility staff can serve to identify potential problem areas that may need improvement, but it also can identify areas in which the system is highly effective. Being aware of both weaknesses and strengths is important to ensure that the needs of the patient and the public are being correctly identified and fulfilled to their satisfaction.

PERFORMANCE IMPROVEMENT

Once the assessment has been completed, areas in which the plan was met are identified and reinforced. For example, if part of the plan is to deliver compassionate patient care and a patient writes a letter praising an EMT for her kind and compassionate treatment during a recent event, the EMT should be praised and the positive feedback should be shared with all members of the team. Factors that allowed the EMT to deliver this quality of care should be identified and used to improve the entire system.

On the other hand, areas of the plan that clearly were not met should be identified and explored further. The reason for the failure to meet the goal should be determined or that particular goal should be reexamined. For example, if response times are consistently above the recommended time limit, perhaps the time limit is unrealistic for the current situation. Either the limit should be changed or the cause for the extended response time should be determined and corrected.

The findings on quality assessment should be used to improve the ultimate delivery of care. Training can be geared toward areas needing more emphasis. Retraining can be instituted if appropriate. This process is called *quality improvement.*

Once a system is in place that identifies a clear goal and includes a plan for its execution, assessment, and improvement, it should not remain static. As everything in medicine changes with the identification of new means of providing care and current research within the field, this process of quality management must be continuous. The EMT should take responsibility for the level of care practiced and should continually strive for improvement of her own abilities and the improvement of the entire EMS team.

MEDICAL DIRECTION

An essential component of all EMT training is appropriate medical direction provided by a higher medical authority. Physicians should be involved in all aspects of EMS training and practice. A medical director can serve as a medical expert, consultant, and educator. Physicians can receive specialty training in the field of emergency medical service and can serve as an invaluable resource for all prehospital care providers.

EMS physicians are required to provide medical direction in several areas of prehospital practice. A physician's input is essential in establishing treatment protocols and in the preparation of training programs and continuing education events. The ultimate goals of the EMS medical director are to help ensure the safety and well-being of the EMTs; to maintain the delivery of quality patient care; and to assist in the proper education, training, and certification of EMTs.

In the prehospital setting it is rare for a physician to be present on the scene when an EMT is caring for a patient, nor is the physician's presence necessary. A physician who has been involved in the training process, the establishment of treatment protocols, and the quality review of calls can be sure that the EMT will provide quality patient care. Truly the EMT is the eyes and hands of the physician in the field.

This process of preparing protocols and standards of care is referred to as **off-line medical control.** The term indicates that the physician does not have to be physically present while the EMT is caring for a patient but, through protocols and procedures, has control over each patient's care.

If an EMT has a question about the care needed by a patient, or if the issue is not clearly addressed in the protocols, then **on-line medical control** is utilized. This involves communication between the EMT and the physician while care is being rendered in the field. On-line medical control can be established with the system's medical director or, more commonly, with a physician in the local emergency department.

The medical director is ultimately responsible for the medical actions of the EMTs on the team. The EMTs are essentially acting as the physician's designated agents while caring for patients under the physician's direction. It is therefore necessary for the physician to be involved in training, retraining, continuing education, and quality management procedures within the system.

CONCLUSION

The EMT is a specially trained health care provider. As a prehospital health care provider, the EMT must be prepared to provide quality care in a multitude of environments and to initiate treatment on the basis of minimal information.

The unique abilities of the EMT to provide calm, compassionate, quality health care in an otherwise chaotic situation is what makes the EMS system successful. The EMT brings to the patient the same quality medical care that would be available from a physician in an office or from staff in a hospital.

Prehospital health care providers must continue to maintain the same level of professionalism that is expected of any other health care provider. This professionalism involves education, ethical care, and quality management, all done with the involvement of a knowledgeable physician.

Ask the Doc

The National Association of EMS Physicians in its position paper on "Physician Medical Direction in EMS" outlines the essential, desirable, and acceptable qualifications for a medical director as well as the medical director's responsibilities for out-of-hospital care, including communications, field clinical practice, and administration of EMS systems.

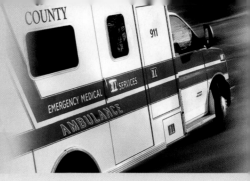

CASE STUDY Continued

"What a busy call," Deb tells Earl as they head back to the office. "That woman was seriously injured. She was going into shock. She could have lost her life if it were not for the quick actions of the team. And the trauma team acted so quickly. It seemed like a hundred people were doing a thousand things in perfect synchrony."

What impressed Deb most was that, amid all the chaos, the attending surgeon was carefully listening to her description of the mechanism of injury and the physical findings they had on scene. Deb has a flashback to class when her instructor told her that she would be the eyes and hands of the physician in the field. She realized how true that statement is.

Key Concepts Revisited

- The roles of an EMT include compassionate caregiver, steward, and leader.
- The responsibilities of an EMT include personal safety, team safety, and public safety.
- The duties of an EMT are found in the functional job description, agency standard operating guidelines, and the scope of practice documents of the state.
- The professional attributes of an EMT include professional appearance, physical conditioning, positive personality traits, and ethical behavior.
- The preparation of an EMT includes original education that leads to certification and licensure.
- The continued preparedness of an EMT includes a commitment to lifelong learning, competency assurance, skills maintenance, and professional development.
- Excellence in EMS demands performance improvement that includes a process of continuous quality improvement.
- Continuous quality improvement is a cyclical process of planning, execution, and evaluation.
- The EMT, as an allied health care provider, is under the control and direction of physicians.
- An EMT holds a special place in the health care system as a prehospital care provider.

Key Terms

Caregiver
Certification
Compassion
Leadership
Off-line medical control
On-line medical control
Prehospital health care team
Steward

Review Questions

1. What are some of the roles and responsibilities of an EMT?
2. Whose safety is the responsibility of the EMT?
3. Whose safety comes first, and why?
4. From the start of a call for EMS to return to service, what are the operational duties of the EMT? (Hint: There are 20.)
5. What patient care procedures are within the scope of practice of an EMT?
6. What are three professional attributes of an EMT?
7. Name three elements of the EMT Code of Ethics. (Hint: There are 10.)
8. What is the difference between certification and licensure?
9. What are the components of EMS quality improvement?
10. What is medical direction?

Further Study

Angle, James S. Occupational Safety and Health in Emergency Service. 2d ed. Clifton Park, NY: Thomson Delmar Learning, 2006.

National Highway Traffic Safety Administration. *A Leadership Guide to Quality Improvement.* Washington, DC: Author, July, 1997.

Walz, Bruce. *Introduction to EMS Systems.* Clifton Park, NY: Thomson Delmar Learning, 2002.

UNIT ③ Legal Responsibilities of the EMT

The EMT has many legal responsibilities. Under certain circumstances the EMT has a legal duty to provide care in a specific manner. The EMT should be familiar with the laws regarding job responsibilities relevant to prehospital patient care. This unit discusses the responsibilities of a prehospital health care provider, including issues surrounding a duty to act, patient rights, consent, documentation, resuscitation decisions, collaboration with law enforcement, physical restraint of patients, and the reporting of suspected abuse. In addition, the most common allegations brought against EMTs and the means by which EMTs can protect themselves against lawsuits are examined.

National Education Standards

The Emergency Medical Technician (EMT) will have the fundamental depth and foundational breadth of understanding consent/refusal of care, confidentiality, advance directives, tort and criminal actions, evidence preservation, statutory responsibilities, mandatory reporting, and ethical principles/moral obligations of prehospital care.

Key Concepts

- The legal responsibilities of the EMT.
- The EMT's duty to patient's right to confidentiality.
- The patient capacity to refuse care.
- Important components of the EMT's responsibility when a patient refuses care against medical advice.
- Three types of advance directives.
- The differing types of consent.

- The legal importance of documentation.
- The circumstances under which resuscitation may be withheld.
- The EMT's role in reporting suspected abuse.
- The most common allegations that may be raised against an EMT in a court of law.
- The laws in place to help protect EMTs from litigation.

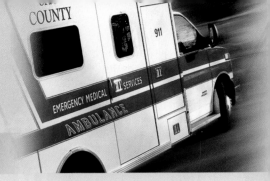

CASE STUDY

Bryce is dispatched to the local pharmacy for a female who passed out. When he arrives, he is taken to the back of the store near the pharmacy counter, where he sees a young woman lying on the floor being attended by a young man. As Bryce approaches, he notices a pair of crutches lying on the floor next to her. The patient has what appears to be abrasions and contusions on her face and arms and a brace on her left knee.

The patient is awake and able to answer questions. Bryce asks her what happened, and she tells him that she was in a car accident earlier today. She came to the pharmacy from the hospital for pain medication. She says she has a mild concussion and left knee sprain in addition to the visible injuries.

She states that while waiting for her prescription, she suddenly became dizzy and felt like she was going to pass out. Her friend helped her to sit down on the floor. She denies losing consciousness but states she still feels weak and dizzy.

Bryce asks her how old she is and explains that he will need to assess her for further injuries. She tells him she is 16 years old. She states she is starting to feel better and doesn't need to go to the hospital, where she had already spent several hours today. Her boyfriend states he will take her home and stay with her until her parents get home from work.

Critical Thinking Questions

1. Can an underage patient give consent to care? Are there any exceptions?
2. Who can consent for a minor?
3. What if the person who is legally able to give consent for a minor is not available at the scene?
4. When can a minor legally refuse care?
5. What duty does the EMT have in this situation?

INTRODUCTION

The EMT has many legal responsibilities. Under certain circumstances the EMT has a legal duty to provide care in a manner that is the same or similar to the care that another EMT would provide. The EMT needs to be familiar with the laws regarding job responsibilities relevant to prehospital patient care.

This unit discusses the responsibilities of a prehospital health care provider, including issues surrounding a duty to act, collaboration with law enforcement, physical restraint of patients, and the reporting of suspected abuse. In addition, the common allegations brought against EMTs and the means by which EMTs can protect themselves against lawsuits are examined.

THE LEGAL RESPONSIBILITIES OF AN EMT

An EMT is a health care professional who provides high-quality medical care to patients. An EMT's practice is limited to what is permitted by the physician medical director overseeing the EMS service. The physician provides direct authority for the individual procedures that an EMT can perform; in addition, the potential group of those skills and procedures is further restricted by law.

The laws that define the scope of practice for an EMT are found in medical practice acts or health regulations, depending on the state. In some cases, state laws refer to those skills and procedures that are contained within the National Education Standards for the EMT as the limits of an EMT practice. Therefore, a physician could not order an EMT to perform a cesarean section because it is outside the scope of practice for an EMT.

It is impossible for physicians to attend every patient in the field. Therefore, EMTs tend to patients at the scene of an accident or illness, acting as a physician extender. On the scene, the EMT's practice is limited to lifesaving and immediately needed procedures. Physicians define the limits of an EMT's practice through off-line medical control using written instructions. The most common example of off-line medical control is **medical protocols,** a set of written regulations that specify the proper procedure for caring for the patient. These medical protocols direct EMTs to which actions they can perform on the scene. If a patient's needs exceed what is outlined in the EMT's written protocols, the EMT may need advice on how to proceed with a particular situation and should consult a physician. This direct contact with a physician during actual patient contact is called *on-line medical control*, as discussed in Unit 2.

Physicians who are engaged in a medical relationship with a patient have a duty to care for that patient until the patient no longer wants care or the care has been properly turned over to another health care provider of equal or greater training. This responsibility to patients also pertains to an EMT.

KNOWLEDGE OF STANDARD OF CARE

The emergency nature of many EMS calls requires that the EMT be proficient at certain skills. In addition to performing at a moment's notice, the EMT must always know his role in patient care. The law requires that an EMT act within the guidelines that are recognized as appropriate for others with the same level of training. These guidelines are known as the **standard of care.**

The standard of care is established through a combination of sources such as state statutes, local ordinances, treatment protocols, National EMS Educational Standards, and textbooks such as this one. It is the responsibility of the EMT to be familiar with the sources outlining how he is expected to perform in a medical emergency. Clearly, the standard of care is not a single textbook, protocol, or governing law but that expectation held by the public regarding how an EMT should behave when caring for a patient. In a court of law, when it might be alleged that an EMT did not provide adequate treatment, the EMT would be held to the standard of what another equally trained EMT would do in the same or similar situation. In every instance, if the EMT keeps the patient's best interests as the highest priority, the EMT will be, in large part, performing to the standard of care.

LEGAL DUTY TO ACT

An EMT who has agreed to respond to calls, whether as a paid provider or volunteer, has a legal obligation to provide service when requested. This **legal duty to act** requires that the EMT treat any patient encountered within the recognized standard of care. In most states, an EMT does not have a legal duty to act when off duty; however, there can be exception in local or state regulations. Every EMT should be aware of the state laws regarding off-duty health care providers rendering assistance at the scene of a medical emergency. EMTs may feel a moral or ethical obligation to render assistance to persons in need regardless of the existence of a legal duty to act.

Once an EMT has initiated patient care, he must continue to care for that patient until care can be relinquished to an equally or higher trained provider. Failure to continue care or to properly turn the patient over to an appropriate provider may constitute patient **abandonment,** a form of EMT misconduct.

RESPECT FOR PATIENTS' RIGHTS

Every person in the United States has a right to emergency health care. This health care must be provided within the standard of care and in a confidential manner. Every competent adult has the ability to accept or refuse medical care as part of his or her patient's rights. Although at present there is no formal document for the prehospital circumstance, every hospital has a **patient's bill of rights** that outlines the rights and privileges of patients. The EMT must be familiar with issues of patient confidentiality, consent, refusal of care, and other patient rights as noted on the patient's bill of rights.

RIGHT TO CONFIDENTIALITY

Historically, patients have enjoyed a sacred trust, enforceable in a court of law, with their physician that allows medical information to be kept private. This trust cannot be broken without compelling reasons. The EMT, as an agent of the physician, is usually required to maintain the same confidentiality. The personal details of the patient's health history that an EMT is privy to during the course of an emergency call should be held in the strictest confidence at all times. Information regarding the nature of the care provided should not be shared with anyone who is not involved in the immediate care of the patient. When an EMT turns a patient over to another EMT or other health care provider, it is expected that all pertinent information will be shared. Insurance groups may also have a limited right to patient information for billing purposes.

Patient information must not be disclosed to non-privileged persons such as family, friends, or the public without the patient's permission. Even law enforcement personnel may not be privy to details of patient care unless written authorization from the patient or a court order is provided. Accordingly, EMTs should be cautioned against discussing details of EMS calls in public places, where they may be overheard by non-privileged parties.

In some states, EMTs are required to report certain situations to legal authorities, such as suspected child abuse or other violent crimes (this topic is discussed in more detail later). Even if not legally obligated to do so, the EMT may feel morally compelled to report suspicions of such incidents. It is acceptable, and encouraged, for EMTs to report suspicions of abuse or of violent injury to receiving hospital personnel who are directly involved in patient care; therefore, they are authorized to be given such information. In some states licensed health care workers may be mandated by state law to report incidences of suspected abuse or violent injury to the receiving hospital. The sharing of such suspicions will assist the hospital providers in protecting the patient.

It is common practice to use details of an incident to illustrate a learning point for other prehospital providers. In those cases care must be taken to withhold any identifying information to protect the confidentiality of the patient involved.

A failure to maintain the confidential nature of detailed patient information is referred to as a **breach of confidentiality** and can have legal implication. These actions are taken very seriously in the legal system. Lives can be seriously affected, and public opinion of EMTs is diminished by such acts. When in doubt, avoid discussing patient information.

HEALTH INSURANCE PORTABILITY AND ACCOUNTABILITY ACT

The **Health Insurance Portability and Accountability Act** of 1996 (HIPAA) was signed into law by President Clinton on August 21, 1996. This law addresses three main issues related to health care. The first seeks to allow insurance portability and continuity. The second requires the standardization of administrative and financial data exchange. Third, and perhaps most relevant to the

EMT on a daily basis, relates to the protection of privacy, confidentiality, and security of health care information. While the health insurance reform section of this law has been in effect for some time, the administrative simplification and required privacy protection became enforceable only recently.

On April 14, 2003, the HIPAA privacy rules were enacted, requiring strict confidentiality of all patient information. Additionally, these new standards provide patients with access to their medical records and more control over how their personal information is used and disclosed. HIPAA applies to health care agencies/providers who conduct certain financial and administrative transactions electronically; many EMS agencies fall into this category.

These regulations call for any data that identify a patient and the patient's health status to be kept in strictest confidence. Patient permission is required to share this "protected health information (PHI)" in many circumstances. PHI may be used as necessary for treatment, payment, and health care operations without a patient's specific consent. However, the information that is shared in these circumstances must be limited to what is necessary for the purpose. For example, although quality assurance (QA) records contain information about a patient's health and the care provided, the name and other identifiable demographic information are not needed for effective QA. Therefore, the EMS service must take reasonable care to remove such information from QA documents. These regulations are not meant in any way to hinder or limit a provider from freely communicating with other health care staff providing care to the patient—that is, advanced life support (ALS) (i.e., paramedics) providers intercepting with basic life support personnel (i.e., EMT), or hospital staff taking over care of the patient. However, the EMT must take reasonable precautions to maintain the privacy of a patient's PHI.

Further, HIPAA requires that patients be given a notice of privacy practices in use by the agency. Signed acknowledgment of receipt of this notice is also required when it is reasonably obtained. In an emergency situation, the law allows for the EMT to delay the notification and acknowledgment until a more appropriate time.

HIPAA regulations are meant to protect patients' privacy while maintaining the health care providers' ability to appropriately manage emergencies. The EMT is encouraged to discuss agency-specific policies regarding HIPAA with the agency's designated privacy officer or corporate compliance officer.

OBTAINING PATIENT CONSENT

When approaching a patient, an EMT should routinely ask for permission or consent to care for the patient. **Consent** refers to voluntary agreement by a person to allow something to take place. Consent can be obtained in a number of ways. Most EMTs do not ask the patient directly, "Do you consent to my examination?" When EMTs approach the patient, they should identify themselves as an EMT and ask the patient what the problem is. When the patient engages the EMT in a conversation about the illness or injury, the patient has in essence consented to the assessment. While initiating a physical assessment, the EMT should explain to the patient what is being done and the purpose of each action. This explanation will help the patient understand the need for further assessment and agree with the treatment plan.

TYPES OF CONSENT

Once the initial assessment has been completed, the EMT should explain to the patient the benefits and possible risks or consequences of treatment, using language that the patient will understand. Consent given following explanation of the risks and benefits of treatment is called **informed consent**.

A patient who verbally agrees to treatment has given express consent. **Express consent** must be obtained from every patient who is of legal age, 18 or 21 years of age in most states, and has the mental capacity to make a rational decision after being informed of the risks and benefits of the treatment plan. Most patient care is provided after the patient has given express consent.

Implied consent is assumed when treating unresponsive or incompetent patients who have potentially life-threatening injuries and are unable to make rational decisions (e.g., head injury). In most cases, the law assumes these patients would consent to treatment if they were able. Implied consent also applies for patients who have initially refused care, but then become unresponsive or incompetent to make a rational decision due to illness or injury.

CHILDREN AND CONSENT

Children are not legally permitted to give consent for medical treatment. In most situations, the EMT can obtain consent from a parent or a guardian who has been appointed by a court to make decisions for the child. When a parent or guardian is not immediately available, an adult sibling or close relative can give permission under the doctrine of **in loco parentis,** which translates as "local parent." Sometimes parents sign permission papers that authorize another individual to consent on their behalf. Coaches of team sports may often be given such permission by parents for use during special activities.

When no parent or legal guardian is immediately available and the child has a life- or limb-threatening injury or illness, an exception to consent must be made. In those emergent cases, the law assumes that the parents would want their seriously ill or injured child to be treated. Such treatment would be possible under implied consent.

As with most rules of law, laws pertaining to children and consent have exceptions. Certain minors are legally entitled to make decisions regarding medical care. Although definitions may differ in each state, common situations in which a minor may be considered to be an **emancipated minor** are a minor who is married, pregnant, in the military or financially independent, and no longer living with a parent or guardian. They are legally responsible for their own decisions and any consequences that result from those decisions.

Legal documentation of emancipation may be provided to the individual by the court. The EMT should request verification from the patient if any doubt exists. Laws can vary by state; therefore the EMT should be familiar with local statutes.

In some states, a minor can consent to medical treatment in certain situations. For example, a minor can seek treatment for a sexually transmitted disease without parental permission. In these cases, the courts have decided that the parents' rights are outweighed by the public need to control outbreaks of communicable disease.

PRISONERS, MENTALLY DISTURBED PERSONS, AND CONSENT

Although an individual who is imprisoned does not lose the right to make decisions regarding medical treatment, many states have enacted laws regarding medical treatment of incarcerated individuals. Some states require that prison officials provide consent for medical issues concerning prisoners. EMTs who frequently service prisons should clarify these laws in their state.

The **emergency doctrine** is a legal principle that allows for emergency treatment of prisoners or children if they are incapable of giving consent as a result of injuries or another condition. If treatment will potentially be life-saving, then the EMT may initiate treatment and transport despite the lack of express consent. If, however, the prisoner refuses treatment, further care may not be provided unless another individual is authorized to consent on the prisoner's behalf.

There are times when a court will authorize specific treatment despite the patient's refusal if the court finds that the patient is not competent to make a reasonable decision and that the treatment is in the patient's best interest. This authorization may be given in the case of a prisoner or in the case of a mentally disturbed person who is in need of medical care. The EMT who is faced with providing care for a patient who is refusing should determine whether such authorization has been given and should request the appropriate legal documentation. The assistance of law enforcement personnel should be obtained if it is necessary for the safety of the medical crew. Medical control should also be consulted if a question arises as to a patient's ability to refuse care.

Often, individual situations require specific responses that can be determined only by collaboration between law enforcement and medical personnel. Experience carries a great deal of weight in resolving such situations positively. Nevertheless, the opinion of the medical director, with counsel from an attorney, about how to handle predictable situations should be sought before such a situation occurs. This kind of preplanning can prevent legal problems later.

RIGHT TO REFUSE CARE

Any competent adult may refuse medical assistance. Whenever emergency medical care is refused, the EMT must act carefully, balancing the patient's rights against the possible harm that might befall the patient if left untreated.

A patient's refusal of care can be clear and direct, such as "I do not want your help," or something as simple as pulling an arm away as the EMT is trying to take a blood pressure reading. Whatever the patient's action, the EMT cannot use force, or even a threat of force, to gain the patient's agreement.

There are criteria that must be met in order for the EMT to recognize a patient's right to refuse care. First, the patient must be an adult. In legal terms that means the patient must be of the **age of majority,** the age at which a person may act without parental consent and be treated as an adult. In most states, the age of majority is 18 or 21 years old.

The patient must also be considered to be competent, or able to act in a responsible manner and comprehend the decision at hand. A person who has been determined to be unable to sufficiently comprehend the situation cannot consent to medical care. This lack of competence may be due to a permanent medical condition such as mental retardation or dementia. In these circumstances, a **guardian,** an individual given the legal authority to act on behalf of the patient, is usually appointed by the courts to make decisions for the patient.

Other conditions that may render a person temporarily unable to make rational medical decisions include head injury, alcohol or drug intoxication, and mental illness. The EMT must decide whether the patient is capable of making responsible decisions and of understanding the situation. When in doubt as to the patient's competence, the EMT should contact a medical control physician for advice.

AMA vs. RMA

With some experience and knowledge of local protocols, the EMT may differentiate between a refusal of medical assistance (RMA) and a refusal against medical advice (AMA). A refusal of medical assistance may occur when EMS is dispatched to a low priority, or nonemergency situation. The EMT may find a competent adult who was not aware EMS had been called and does not need help. However, there are situations when nonemergency transport may be appropriate. In these circumstances, the EMT should follow local protocols.

In the case of refusal against medical advice, the patient has a potentially life-threatening illness or injury, and the refusal of care would likely have an immediate harmful consequence. Patients who are refusing against medical advice should be approached carefully. The EMT should try to understand why the patient is refusing. Sometimes emotions such as fear of additional pain can be a greater motivator than the thought of the complications that could arise from the untreated illness or injury. Calm and rational explanations of the care being offered must precede any action, and the patient should understand that the EMT is advocating for the patient. When dealing with the patient, the EMT should start by offering minimally invasive therapies such as measuring vital signs. If the patient allows vital signs to be taken, the EMT should then explain the need for further treatment. Eventually the patient may trust the EMT enough to allow transportation to the hospital.

If a patient is thought to have the capacity to refuse care, the EMT must then inform the patient of the reasonable and foreseeable consequences of the refusal. For example, it is possible for a patient to die from a minor wound, but it may be considered unlikely. What is more likely is that the wound could become infected and cause the patient pain and even loss of function. The patient must be advised of the potential consequences of lack of evaluation and treatment for the concern.

The EMT must offer medical care to the limit that the patient will accept. For example, if the patient refuses to go to the hospital in an ambulance for treatment of an injury but will accept a bandage, the EMT must make the bandage available.

The EMT must encourage the patient to seek further medical attention if the problem persists or worsens. Patients should also be reminded that if they desire further treatment or transport later on, they can call EMS back to the scene.

Despite the EMT's best efforts, there may be times when the patient still refuses care and the EMT is forced to leave the patient in a potentially dangerous situation. Whenever possible, the EMT should leave the patient in the care of another competent adult. This person may convince the patient of the need for further medical treatment and can monitor the patient for complications.

In all cases of refusal, the liability for the decision to leave the patient rests with the EMT, the EMT's service, and the service's physician director. In the case of a refusal against medical advice, an EMT should contact medical control, explain the situation calmly and objectively, and let the physician try to convince the patient of the need for further treatment. If the patient chooses to refuse after this process, the EMT must thoroughly document the events. Unit 23 details the necessary documentation needed in this case.

ADVANCE DIRECTIVES

Despite advances in medicine, some patients have a terminal disease. Others, having lived a long and full life, may decide they do not wish to prolong their life, particularly if living would mean being a burden on their families or would result in prolonged suffering. These patients have a right to self-determination.

Normally, it is safe to assume that an unconscious patient would allow all medical treatment if conscious. However, consistent with their right to refuse treatment, patients can decide in advance of a medical emergency not to accept life support. Several mechanisms have been developed to facilitate the wishes of such patients. The directions a person leaves for family and caregivers in advance of a life-threatening situation are called **advance directives.** An advance directive may be of several forms. A more detailed discussion of advance directives can be found in Unit 47.

One such means patients have of conveying their wishes to caregivers is through the use of a **living will.** A document drawn up in private or in consultation with an attorney, a living will simply expresses the patient's wishes regarding specific treatment options in the event of a serious illness or injury. Some states allow prehospital personnel to recognize this document as binding; others do not. The EMT must know the state laws regarding recognition of a living will.

Another form of advance directive is the **do not resuscitate order (DNR).** This order is signed by a physician, after consultation with the person or with the family, if the person is unable to discuss treatment options. The order directs that resuscitative efforts not be initiated in the case of cardiac or respiratory arrest if it has been determined that resuscitation would be futile or would prolong suffering. In some states, only a specific prehospital DNR can be honored by EMTs. In other states, EMTs can honor any type of DNR. Some patients wear a bracelet, necklace, or other indicator that they have a DNR order.

It is important for the EMT to realize that a DNR order applies to the patient who is in cardiac or respiratory arrest. By no means does this order imply that treatment should be withheld to an ill or injured patient. Many times, routine prehospital treatment such as oxygen administration can provide comfort to a terminally ill patient while not contradicting a DNR order. An EMT who is faced with an unclear situation is best advised to begin resuscitation and call medical control for guidance.

A third type of advance directive is the **health care proxy.** The documentation of a health care proxy permits a person previously designated by the patient to make decisions in the event the patient becomes incapacitated. This person, having been chosen by the patient, usually is aware of the patient's beliefs and wishes.

DOCUMENTATION

The EMT is responsible for keeping careful written records of every patient interaction. It is recommended that the record be completed as soon as possible after patient interaction to avoid any loss of information over time.

The documentation done by an EMT will become a part of the patient's medical record and will be referred to by other health care providers who care for that patient. Accuracy and completeness are essential. Unit 23 discusses the details of proper prehospital documentation.

INITIATING RESUSCITATION

In general, an absence of pulse and breathing requires that an EMT start CPR unless the patient has a DNR order or if unambiguous signs of death or signs of injury inconsistent with life are present. Most states have clear regulations regarding when it is inappropriate to begin resuscitation. For example, an EMT will not attempt resuscitation if the patient meets any of the conditions listed in Table 3-1. All EMTs must be familiar with the policies regarding initiation of resuscitation in their particular state.

After death, a body begins to cool, and blood pools at the lower, or dependent, parts of the body. The patchy purple mottling seen on the skin is called *lividity*. After a period of time, the body will become stiff. This condition is called *rigor mortis*. Rigor mortis starts with the short muscles, like the jaw, and progresses to the larger muscles. Therefore, if it is difficult to open the airway on a patient who has no pulse, the EMT should suspect rigor mortis. Rigor mortis is usually present within 1 or 2 hours of death under normal temperatures. Lividity and rigor mortis are considered to be signs of death. No amount of resuscitation offered at this point would be effective.

Street Smart

There are situations in which a dying patient needs the comfort and convenience of an ambulance yet does not need emergency medical care. EMS and other hospital systems, such as hospice, should meet and discuss how to best serve such patients before the need arises. This kind of collaborative preplanning can prevent uncertainty in the field.

Table 3-1 Unambiguous Signs of Death
Decapitation (separation of the head from the body)
Severe lividity (pooling of blood in the dependent areas of the body)
Rigor mortis (stiffening of the muscles in the body after death)
Decomposition (actual disintegration of skin and muscle)

Bodies exhibiting decapitation or decomposition are also considered to be dead and should be left for the police to handle. Other wounds, such as head injuries with large amounts of brain matter exposed, may constitute mortal wounds. The EMT should contact medical control for instructions on cases that are questionable. When in doubt, the EMT should initiate resuscitation, and the medical control physician can decide on the next course of action.

If the decision is not to pursue resuscitation, then it is important to leave the scene as if it were a crime scene. In the event of a death outside of a hospital, law enforcement personnel may want to make a report for future reference.

COLLABORATING WITH LAW ENFORCEMENT

Crime scenes represent a special challenge to EMTs. On the one hand, there is the patient who is hurt and needs help. On the other hand, a crime has been committed, and the person or persons who committed the crime must be caught. A scene that requires law enforcement to be present is a potential crime scene.

A challenge may exist for an EMT if the patient is also suspected to have participated in the crime. The EMT must remember that it is up to the courts to decide the guilt or innocence of an individual. Every EMT must be nonjudgmental and render care without prejudice.

Another challenge faced by EMTs at a crime scene is to provide appropriate care to the patient while trying not to disturb any evidence that the police may find valuable in investigating the crime. Of course, if evidence must be altered to care for a patient, the EMT should not hesitate to provide the necessary care. In this case, the EMT should take note of the position of any item moved and relay this information to the investigating officer as soon as possible. It is also important to try to limit the number of EMS responders to a crime scene.

Table 3-2 lists some actions that an EMT should not take at any potential crime scene. The key problem for an EMT is to know when a scene is a crime scene. Sometimes, police are already on scene; in other cases, the EMT may have a feeling that something is just not right. In fact, many innocent-appearing scenes turn into crime scenes; therefore, the EMT should incorporate these considerations into daily practice.

An EMT who discovers the criminal nature of a scene after the fact may assist law enforcement by writing down any observations. For example, were there newspapers at the door and was the mail picked up? Upon entering the room, did the EMT notice any unusual smell such as natural gas or cigarette smoke? Were the lights on when the EMT entered the room? Was the television playing, or was a radio on? Were doors open, closed, or locked?

Both EMS and law enforcement have very important jobs. A good working relationship between the agencies can be important in many circumstances.

Table 3-2 What Not to Do When Dealing with a Crime Scene

Do not allow unneeded personnel on scene.
Do not move a deceased patient.
Do not cover the body with anything.
Do not unnecessarily move objects.
Do not touch any weapons (guns, knives, etc.).
Do not touch the following objects: Telephones Answering machines Sinks Toilets Light switches Televisions
Do not leave waste at the scene (gloves, etc.).

For the EMT, patient care takes priority over evidence collection, but such care can often be given without destroying evidence. Attention to a few details can save hundreds of hours of police work, improve the chance of police success in apprehending the criminal, and support a good working relationship between EMS and law enforcement.

MOTOR VEHICLE COLLISIONS

Many communities are viewing motor vehicle collisions that involve serious injury or a drunk driver as criminal acts. Therefore, EMTs are increasingly being asked to testify about the conditions on the scene. EMTs are well advised to consider these scenes as potential crime scenes and to carefully document their observations as soon as possible after patient care responsibilities are over. Table 3-3 lists some of the observations that an EMT might want to make. In every case, the EMT should be **evidence conscious** (aware of the importance of preserving items and conditions that pertain to a crime scene).

THREAT OF VIOLENCE ON THE SCENE

EMTs must be aware of the potential for violence against emergency service providers on the scene. One source of such violence is gang violence. Personal safety is always the first priority for the EMT when responding to any scene. The EMT should never enter a scene that is potentially unsafe without police assistance. Remember that only law enforcement officers are legally permitted to use force. EMTs should never consider physical force as a viable option.

Safety Tips

In some cases, injury of a gang member can result in retaliation and further violence. When this situation is suspected, the patient should be removed as quickly as possible from the scene. This escape from an unsafe situation is similar to the act of quickly rescuing a victim from a burning building.

Table 3-3 Evidence Worth Noting from a Motor Vehicle Collision

Scene evidence

Skid marks

Direction of travel

Piles of grass or rust debris

Puddles of fluids

Downed trees and poles

Tracks in snow or mud

Vehicle evidence

"Spidered" or "starred" windshield

Steering wheel position

Gear position

Seat belt position

Airbag deployment

Open alcohol bottles

Drugs in plain view

Position of patients

Any scene involving an injury due to an act of violence continues to be a potentially dangerous crime scene. Examples include the scene of a suicide or suicide attempt, homicide, drug overdose, domestic dispute, rape, abuse, riot, or injury from gunshots or other potentially dangerous weapons. Local law enforcement agencies will often provide EMS providers with education on the specifics of dealing with these potentially dangerous situations.

In addition to identifying bodily injuries during a head-to-toe survey, the EMT should note the presence of any weapons or dangerous instruments, such as ice picks, needles, or razor blades that may be hidden in clothing. Patients should never have a weapon in the back of an ambulance. Law enforcement personnel should be asked to remove the weapon from the patient before transport.

PHYSICAL RESTRAINT OF COMBATIVE PATIENTS

The first rule of medicine regarding treatment of a combative patient is to assume that the cause of the combativeness is medical until proved otherwise. Many medical conditions can cause a patient to be uncooperative, agitated, and even combative. These conditions are discussed in detail in later units.

The EMT must remember that only police officers are allowed to use physical force and only under certain conditions. The EMT may use **physical restraint** (a means of restricting freedom of movement) to prevent a patient from hurting himself or others. The police can be helpful in assisting EMTs

Ask the Doc

An excellent discussion about under what conditions restraints may be necessary is contained in the NAEMSP position paper entitled "Patient Restraint in EMS Systems." The paper describes the three types of restraint, techniques, verbal de-escalation, physical restraint and chemical restraint, the need for a uniform, and a protocol-driven approach to these emergencies.

with restraining patients because they are usually well trained in techniques of safe physical restraint.

REPORTING OF ABUSE

EMTs are in a unique position in that they are invited into people's homes. They have the advantage of being able to observe patients in their personal surroundings. Interactions with family members in the home environment can also be witnessed. Because hospital staff do not have access to a patient's home, they do not have the opportunity to witness the home situation and evaluate its safety. The EMT must observe the situation carefully and report any situations that appear to involve abuse or that are potentially unsafe for the patient to hospital or law enforcement personnel for further investigation.

CHILD ABUSE

Child abuse is any act of physical, sexual, or psychological maltreatment of a child or the failure of a parent or legal guardian to minimally provide necessities such as food, clothing, shelter, and medical care.

An EMT has a special role in detecting and reporting child abuse. Emergency department personnel cannot see the scene; they cannot match the **mechanism of injury,** or the instrument or event that results in harm, to the **pattern of injury,** or injuries characteristic to a particular mechanism. Emergency department personnel depend on the accurate observations of EMTs to help detect child abuse. Child abuse is discussed further in Unit 44.

Many states require that an EMT report any suspicion of child abuse to local authorities, such as child protective services. This requirement makes the EMT a **mandated reporter.** Not only is the EMT obligated, by law, to report suspicious circumstances, but the EMT may even be held criminally responsible for failing to report such suspicions. It is important that every EMT know how local reporting laws affect them.

No matter how obvious the likelihood of abuse may seem, the EMT must not accuse the parents of wrongdoing or make statements that are inflammatory. These types of statements may put the EMT, the EMS crew, and the child in further danger. Care and treatment of the child should be the primary focus.

DOMESTIC VIOLENCE

The public is becoming increasingly aware of the prevalence of **domestic violence** (acts of violence against a spouse, partner, or family member) in the United States. Victims of domestic violence may need psychological support and immediate medical attention for potentially life-threatening injuries, in addition to a safe haven from their attackers.

Typically, a victim of abuse is afraid of the abuser. Such fear may prevent the victim from seeking assistance or attempting to leave the situation. Many women are battered or abused during pregnancy, and many do not seek help until the situation is desperate. On average, the battered woman will return home seven times before permanently leaving the situation.

The EMT must remain nonjudgmental and demonstrate empathy toward the patient. It is the job of the police to investigate and arrest the abuser. Compassionate care and nonjudgmental treatment will encourage the abused woman to trust the EMT. This trust will perhaps make her more likely to call again if she needs help. A patient who is treated in a negative manner may lose confidence in EMS as a means of getting help when she is injured. Health care providers must be encouraging and supportive of a woman who has demonstrated the courage to call for help.

Pediatric Considerations

The EMT should observe the interactions between the child and the parent or caregiver. Does the child appear to be afraid? Is the parent attempting to comfort the child? Does the child act as though he doesn't expect the parent to comfort him? Is the child ignoring pain that is usually associated with an injury?

These subtle clues are usually only seen during unguarded moments when the parent and child are out of the public view, such as in the back of the ambulance. Report exactly what is observed to hospital personnel after the child's care has been turned over.

ELDER ABUSE AND NEGLECT

The most likely people to be battered and abused are the vulnerable and the infirm. The elderly fall into this category.

The patterns of injuries that are seen in **elder abuse** (an act of violence toward or neglect of an elderly person) are similar to the patterns of injuries seen in child abuse. Inconsistent stories, injury patterns that do not match the mechanism of injury, and attempts to hide an injury are typical. This issue is discussed in more detail in later units.

Whenever elder abuse is suspected, the first priority is patient care. However, after the call is over, help for the patient and the family is needed. Many EMS agencies have a social services referral system in place that puts the right people in touch with the patient and family.

COMMON ALLEGATIONS AGAINST EMS

Many members of the EMS community fear litigation. Although the possibility of a lawsuit against you or your service is certainly disconcerting, the reality is that most EMS calls do not result in litigation.

Although mistakes are possible, the EMT will find that the best way to stay out of legal trouble is to provide good patient care in a conscientious manner. This type of work ethic will minimize the chances of an EMT's contributing to a situation that may result in legal action.

AMBULANCE COLLISIONS AND LIABILITY

When driving an emergency vehicle, the EMT has a responsibility to the crew, patients, other motorists, and pedestrians to operate in a safe manner. Most state laws require that an emergency vehicle operator show due regard for others. The operator can be held responsible for any damages or injuries incurred as a result of lack of due regard. This legal responsibility is known as **liability.**

The most common source of lawsuits against EMTs is emergency vehicle accidents. Unfortunately, advances in driver training have not matched advances in attendant training. Driver safety programs such as the Ambulance Accident Prevention Seminar (AAPS) and Emergency Vehicle Operations Course (EVOC) are available but not universally required of emergency vehicle drivers.

Emergency vehicle drivers should be familiar with these statistics and should use care when operating in emergency mode. Many EMS systems have begun to limit the number of responses completed with lights and sirens in an effort to decrease this risk. Unit 48, Emergency Vehicle Operations, provides more information.

NEGLIGENCE

Malpractice is a term most often associated with physicians who have been found to have caused damage to a patient in their care. Malpractice also pertains to other health care providers, including nurses and EMS providers.

EMTs could face legal liability from both civil and criminal claims. A criminal liability case occurs when the government accuses an EMT of violating a criminal law. Conviction on criminal charges may result in incarceration, probation, and/or fines. A civil liability case occurs when a private individual files a lawsuit against an EMT, EMS service, or others, such as a medical director. Civil suits are based on tort law. **Tort law** is the area of law involving civil wrongs against another, and a finding of liability in a civil case typically results in the award of monetary damages. According to recent literature, claims of negligence in medical care result in the second largest monetary payout for EMS providers, after motor vehicle collisions. Negligence is a tort in which there was no intent to harm but there was a breach in the duty to act.

Claim of Negligence

Driving in the early morning, Mr. Miller falls asleep at the wheel and loses control of his truck. The truck runs off the road and crashes into an old oak tree.

Dazed for just a moment, Mr. Miller uses his cell phone to call 9-1-1. After some time Mr. Miller grows tired of waiting for EMS and exits the vehicle. He is intent on walking to the nearest farmhouse for help.

As he stands up, he gets light-headed, his legs buckle under him, and he collapses to the ground. When Mr. Miller regains consciousness, he is no longer able to feel anything below the waist.

On-duty EMTs from the local volunteer rescue squad respond, from their homes, to the EMS call. Upon arrival, they immediately survey the scene, decide that the situation is a trauma, and promptly proceed to manually stabilize Mr. Miller's head and neck.

After completing an initial assessment and a rapid trauma assessment, the EMTs correctly conclude that he may have suffered a neck injury. The EMTs carefully apply a cervical collar to protect his cervical spine, and they logroll him onto a backboard. Afterward, they assess his extremities for feeling and motion. The assessment is unchanged from the initial assessment.

After turning Mr. Miller over to the emergency department staff, the rescue squad returns to service. Several months later Mr. Miller's attorney serves the rescue squad with an "intent to sue" notice. The notice alleges that the EMTs were negligent in their treatment and that this negligent treatment caused or aggravated Mr. Miller's condition, resulting in the permanent paralysis of his legs.

1. What are the elements of a civil action necessary to prove a case? Are all of those elements here in the case that is presented?
2. What is the weakness in the patient's case against the EMTs?
3. What should be included in the EMTs' documentation of this call?

Negligence refers to the delivery of care in a manner that is considered to be below the established standard of care, or care that a reasonably prudent EMT would provide under the same or similar circumstances. There are four elements of negligence: duty to act, breach of duty to act, causation of injury, and damages. All four elements must be met to prove that negligence occurred.

DUTY TO ACT

Duty to act is an EMT's legal obligation to conform to a certain standard of care. Duty is the first thing that must be established for negligence to be considered. Responsible vehicle operation, equipment maintenance, and patient care are among an EMT's duties.

As described earlier in the unit, an EMT's legal duty is somewhat different depending upon whether the EMT is on duty or off duty. It is important for the EMT to know the state's laws regarding duty to act. When a duty does exist, the EMT may be held liable for failure to act reasonably. If a duty to act does not exist, the EMT cannot be faulted for failing to perform a task.

BREACH OF DUTY TO ACT

Breach of duty to act means a failure to perform in accordance with the standard that is expected. Once an actual duty has been established, if it is not carried out appropriately, a breach of duty exists. Negligence has occurred whenever **nonfeasance,** a failure of an EMT to fulfill a duty, or **misfeasance,** errors in the care an EMT provides after establishing contact with the patient, takes place. **Malfeasance,** or gross negligence, occurs when an EMT willfully, wantonly, or recklessly performs below the standard of care.

EMTs who provide care that is dangerous to the patient can be charged with gross negligence if the intent to cause harm is proven. Criminal charges can be brought against an EMT who is found to have been grossly negligent. Other examples of a breach of duty may include irresponsible vehicle operation and failure to maintain equipment.

CAUSATION OF INJURY

The third required element of a negligence claim involves proximate cause or causation of injury. Because the laws regarding negligence are meant to compensate those who are injured, actual injury is required to claim negligence. Further, it must be shown that the breach of duty directly caused the injury. If injury exists but was not a result of the EMT's breach of duty, then the EMT is not responsible for compensation. Regardless of duty and breach of duty, if no injury resulted, then there is no negligence.

DAMAGES

Finally, in a claim of negligence, it must be proved that an actual loss or damage has occurred. Such things as lost wages, medical expenses, and property damage are easily proven. Pain and suffering, emotional distress, and loss of companionship are more difficult to prove but are considered to be worthy of compensation. This type of damage allowance is known as compensatory damages.

Another, less common, type of damages that a person found guilty of negligence may be required to pay is known as punitive damages. Such remuneration is meant to punish the defendant and to set an example for others.

PATIENT ABANDONMENT

An EMT who has established an EMT-patient relationship by beginning emergency medical care for a person has a duty to continue that care until relieved by someone of equal or higher training. This relief usually comes when the patient is delivered to the hospital and the EMT's report is given to the accepting staff.

There are times when a patient is not transported by the first arriving EMT but by another provider. In such a case, the first EMT will give a report to the EMT who is taking over care of the patient.

There are some circumstances in which the patient does not require further care after initial treatment by the EMT. EMTs should have knowledge of local protocols because state regulations may vary regarding this situation. The EMT's documentation of the situation should clearly reflect that both the EMT and the patient find that there is no need for further medical care.

As discussed previously, sometimes a patient will refuse further medical care. If the patient is competent to refuse, then it is the patient who terminated the EMT-patient relationship. The EMT must document the situation carefully to avoid later accusations of abandonment.

An EMT who inappropriately leaves a patient without having been relieved of patient care responsibility by a provider of equal or higher training may be guilty of patient abandonment. This unilateral severance of the EMT-patient relationship is a form of EMT misconduct. If it is found that the EMT intentionally and unjustifiably terminated the EMT-patient relationship, then the EMT can be held responsible for any injuries that resulted.

ASSAULT AND BATTERY

The EMT must remember that every patient who is capable of making decisions has the right to refuse treatment or transport. An EMT who treats or transports a patient without consent or against the patient's will could be held liable.

Charges that may surface regarding the treatment or transport of a patient without consent include assault, battery, and false imprisonment. **Assault** refers to the case in which a patient is afraid that he or she may be touched without having given consent. **Battery** refers to actually unlawfully touching the patient against his or her wishes. The intentional confinement of a patient without the patient's consent and without an appropriate reason is called **false imprisonment.**

Each of those charges can be brought against an EMT, who may then face liability. The EMT should therefore be sure to obtain the appropriate consent before attempting to provide treatment to any person.

BREACH OF CONFIDENTIALITY

As mentioned previously, an EMT who holds knowledge of private information regarding a patient is expected to keep it in the strictest confidence.

EMTs who release information publicly about a patient, through spoken or written form, could be charged with **defamation** if that information is found to be damaging to the patient's character or reputation. The two forms of defamation an EMT could be accused of are the spoken form, **slander,** or the written form, **libel.** Disclosing patient care information to anyone who does not have a right to know can be called a breach of confidentiality. All EMTs must be mindful of who is nearby when patient information is being discussed. Patient records should always be kept in a confidential manner as specified under HIPAA regulations.

THE EMERGENCY MEDICAL TREATMENT AND ACTIVE LABOR ACT

In 1985 Congress enacted the original Emergency Medical Treatment and Active Labor Act (EMTALA) as a part of a larger law called the Consolidated Omnibus Budget Reconciliation Act (COBRA). This law has also become known as the "antidumping" law and is intended to protect patients whom hospitals might refuse to care for based on financial reasons. Having undergone several revisions, this law requires that any patient who comes to a hospital emergency department requesting care be provided with appropriate emergency treatment within the capabilities of the facility. If a hospital does not have the capability to definitively manage a particular patient, arrangements must be made for an appropriate transfer. Several conditions that must be met for transfers to occur in emergency situations, and the EMT who will be participating in the interfacilty transfer of patients should become knowledgeable regarding the specifics of EMTALA as it relates to the situation.

PROTECTION AGAINST LAWSUITS

Although most EMTs will never actually be involved in a legal claim, it is certainly helpful for all prehospital health care providers to be familiar with the relevant laws and means of protection. Although there are many means of defending against lawsuits, each state differs significantly in its legislation.

GOOD SAMARITAN LAWS

With the prevalence of medical lawsuits, health care professionals may be reluctant to help people who suddenly become ill or are injured while in public. In an effort to encourage health care providers to assist such people, the legislatures of many states have enacted laws called **Good Samaritan laws.**

The care provided must be offered freely and given without expectation of compensation. The care rendered must be to the level that another reasonable and prudent caregiver would have provided. Although Good Samaritan laws exist in all 50 states and the District of Columbia, each state has specific conditions that a provider must meet to be protected under these laws. EMTs should know the laws in their state if they expect to offer care when not on duty.

IMMUNITY STATUTES

All states have Good Samaritan laws; some states also have **immunity statutes.** An immunity statute protects a group of people, such as prehospital health care providers, from having to pay damages for acts performed as part of the job. Essentially, an immunity statute protects the EMT who will be compensated for assisting an injured person. The Good Samaritan laws, which apply specifically to uncompensated performance, generally do not provide this coverage. There are several elements of an immunity statute that must be met for the EMT to qualify for protection, such as maintaining the standard of care. The EMT should be familiar with the state's specific statutes.

BEST PRACTICES

The best strategy to avoid being involved in litigation is to use common sense in everyday practice. The EMT who knows and follows protocols, performing his duty in a compassionate manner, will be unlikely to be involved in a legal claim.

An EMT who is uncertain as to what treatment to provide should always provide care that is in the best interest of the patient. If ever in doubt, the EMT should involve the EMS supervisor or a medical control physician in assessment and management of the patient.

CONCLUSION

This unit is an overview of the relevant concepts that may be helpful in understanding the legal roles and responsibilities of the EMT. It is not intended to direct the EMT on how to act in every situation.

Specific legal responsibilities vary from state to state, and the EMT should inquire as to the state's laws regarding specific duties and liabilities. The advice of an attorney regarding these matters can be invaluable.

Most EMTs are never required to go to court; however, EMTs must do all that they can to protect themselves from the threat of legal action. The best protection against lawsuits is good patient care provided by a conscientious EMT.

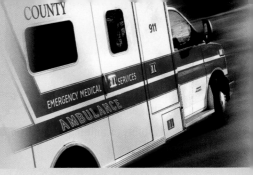

CASE STUDY Continued

Bryce explains to the patient that since she is under the age of majority and cannot give legal consent, he will need to transport her to the hospital for further evaluation. As he begins assisting her to the cot, a woman arrives stating she is the patient's mother. The store had called her at work concerning her daughter. After talking with her daughter, the mother tells Bryce that she does not want her taken back to the hospital by ambulance. Bryce discusses the possible consequences of her refusal of care and has her mother sign the appropriate refusal documents. He leaves the patient in the care of her mother, encouraging them to return to the hospital for further evaluation. Bryce returns to the station and begins documentation of the run, being sure to include a copy of the refusal documentation signed by the patient's mother.

Key Concepts Revisited

- EMTs should be familiar with the laws regarding job responsibilities relevant to prehospital patient care, including
  - ○ Knowledge of the standard of care
  - ○ Legal duty to act
  - ○ Patient's rights
    - Patient's have a right to have their medical information kept private.
    - HIPAA addresses the main issues related to health care information
      - ○ Allows insurance portability and continuity
      - ○ Standardization of administrative and financial data exchange
      - ○ Protection of privacy, confidentiality, and security of health care information
    - Patient's right to refuse care
      - ○ Against medical advice
      - ○ Refusal of medical assistance
    - Advance Directives
      - ○ Living Will
      - ○ Do Not Resuscitate
      - ○ Health Care Proxy
  - ○ Patient consent
    - Informed consent
    - Express consent
    - Implied consent
    - Children and consent
      - ○ In loco parentis
      - ○ Emancipated minors
    - Prisoners, mentally disturbed persons, and consent
      - ○ Emergency doctrine
  - ○ Initiating resuscitation
    - Unambiguous signs of death
  - ○ Collaborating with law enforcement
    - Dealing with a crime scene
    - Motor vehicle collisions
    - Threat of violence on the scene
    - Physical restraint
  - ○ Reporting abuse
    - Child abuse
    - Domestic abuse
    - Elder abuse and neglect

- Although most EMS calls do not result in litigation, the most common allegations against EMS are
  - Liability of ambulance collisions
  - Negligence
    - Duty to act
      - Malfeasance
      - Nonfeasance
      - Misfeasance
    - Breach of duty to act
    - Causation of injury
    - Damages
  - Patient abandonment
    - Assault and battery
  - Breach of confidentiality
    - Defamation
      - Slander
      - Libel
  - The Emergency Medical Treatment and Active Labor Act
  - Protection against lawsuits
    - Good Samaritan Laws
    - Immunity statutes
    - Best practices

Review Questions

1. What are the legal responsibilities of the EMT?
2. What is the EMT's duty to act?
3. What are some of the elements in the patient's bill of rights?
4. What is the patient's right to confidentiality?
5. What is meant by the capacity to refuse care?
6. What are the important components of the EMT's responsibility when a patient refuses care against medical advice?
7. Define three types of advance directives.
8. From whom is consent obtained for
   a. a conscious adult?
   b. an unconscious adult?
   c. a child?
   d. a prisoner?
9. What is the legal importance of documentation?
10. Under what circumstances may resuscitation be withheld?
11. What are several situations in which EMTs collaborate closely with law enforcement personnel?
12. What is the EMT's role in reporting suspected abuse?
13. What are the most common allegations that may be raised against an EMT in a court of law?
14. What are some laws that help protect EMTs from litigation?

Key Terms

Abandonment

Advance directive

Age of majority

Assault

Battery

Breach of confidentiality

Child abuse

Consent

Defamation

Domestic violence

Do not resuscitate order (DNR)

Duty to act

Elder abuse

Emancipated minor

Emergency doctrine

Evidence conscious

Express consent

False imprisonment

Good Samaritan laws

Guardian

Health care proxy

Health Insurance Portability
  and Accountability Act (HIPAA)

Immunity statute

Implied consent

Informed consent

In loco parentis

Legal duty to act

Liability

Libel

Living will

Malfeasance

Malpractice

Mandated reporter

Mechanism of injury

Medical protocols

Misfeasance

Negligence

Nonfeasance

Patient's bill of rights

Pattern of injury

Physical restraint

Slander

Standard of care

Tort law

Further Study

To learn more about the latest HIPAA regulations, visit http://www.hipaa.org or http://www.hipaadvisory.com.

For additional information and resources related to advance directives, visit http://www.partnershipforcaring.org.

Cid, D., & Maniscalco, P. Integrating Criminal Investigation into Major EMS Scenes. *Journal of Emergency Medical Services,* 1999. *24,* 68–69.

Colwell, C. B., Pons, P., Blanchet, J. H., & Mangino, C. Claims Against a Paramedic Ambulance Service: A Ten-Year Experience. *Journal of Emergency Medicine,* 1999. *17,* 999–1002.

UNIT **4** Stress and Wellness in EMS

The EMT will regularly witness tragedy and human suffering the like of which the average person rarely encounters. This opportunity to be involved and make a difference in people's lives is rewarding, but it also has consequences. This unit will review those consequences and provide recommendations on how the EMT can deal with them.

National Education Standard
The Emergency Medical Technician (EMT) shall have a fundamental depth and foundational breadth of knowledge of stress and wellness principles.

Key Concepts

- The definition of stress.
- Common stressors.
- The stress response, both physical and emotional.
- The body's reaction to stress.
- Specific EMS stressors.
- Work-related stressors.
- Recognizing stress.
- Managing stress.

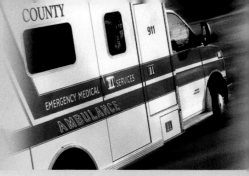

Just as Dan and Kris sit down to eat, the alert tones sound. As they hastily depart the restaurant, Dan wonders if he will have a chance to eat at all that day. Dan gingerly slides into the front seat, remembering that his back is still sore from this morning's rescue. He fastens his seat belt and acknowledges the call on the mobile radio. The dispatcher advises, "Car fire, possible persons trapped, fire-rescue dispatched, corner of Palma Boulevard and Gipp Road, time out 13:40."

This is the type of call that Dan dreads. His brother died from burns due to a fire, and Dan remembers how much pain his brother was in before he died. This memory causes his stomach to become instantly queasy. Attempting to put the painful memory out of his mind, Dan tries to concentrate on the task at hand. "Focus on the basics," he tells himself. "Remember, critical trauma patients are extricated in less than 10 minutes; stick to the ABCs." He can almost picture his EMT instructor over his shoulder. His heart is pounding, and his back is getting stiff from the combination of stress and the morning's exertions.

Arriving on scene Dan and Kris find that the car has crashed into the side of a tractor-trailer. The gas tank

on the truck has ruptured and caught fire. The fire was quickly extinguished by fire-rescue, but through the smoke the hands of the driver can be seen thrashing around. Fire-rescue is already busy cutting the car apart as Dan dons his protective gear.

"Will I remember what to do?" Dan thinks as he enters the car. The palms of his hands are already slick with sweat. He reminds himself, "Airway. Airway is always first." In the meantime, Kris has climbed into the backseat. She yells out over the loud din of power tools, "Hey, do you want me to take head stabilization first?" Frustrated, Dan thinks to himself, "I know that I am supposed to take manual stabilization first. How could I forget?" Wondering if Kris can see how red his face is, Dan quickly checks the driver for breathing and a pulse.

Critical Thinking Questions

1. What stressors is Dan experiencing?
2. What are Dan's physical and emotional responses to those stressors?
3. What triggered Dan's response?

INTRODUCTION

The EMT will be faced with many situations that may be emotionally charged. Patients and family members are often unable to cope with the emergency situation or the chaotic environment. It may be overwhelming, and the patient may respond very emotionally to the situation. The EMT is susceptible to the same emotional upheaval that the patient and family are experiencing.

These effects should not be denied or ignored, but they can be anticipated. If prepared, the EMT may find a way to continue to provide the medical care she is trained to provide, despite occasional overwhelming emotional stress. This unit prepares the student to understand and recognize common stressors an EMT may encounter in the field and offer recommendations on how to handle these issues effectively.

STRESS DEFINED

Stress is the physical, emotional, and behavioral response of the body to changing external conditions. This response is the body's way of adapting to these changes. Stress is a necessary part of our lives and can provide challenges that can keep life interesting.

The events that trigger stress are known as **stressors**. A stressor can occur suddenly, such as a sudden change in the environment, or it may be more prolonged, either in the form of multiple smaller events or one slowly building event.

The effects of everyday stress constantly challenge the body to respond. In a sense, stress can be compared to going to the gym. Working out at the gym is part of a regular fitness program that helps to tone and condition the body. Regular, moderate amounts of exercise help keep the body in shape and ready to respond to the daily duties of work and home life—and occasional greater demands that require extraordinary physical exertion, like digging out after a blizzard or stacking sandbags when a flood threatens. People who work out regularly are more prepared to withstand both the daily toll of physical activities and unexpected challenges than those who lead a sedentary lifestyle. People who are physically fit also know the limits of their endurance, and they know how to pace themselves, so they come through extraordinary challenges in better shape than people who are unprepared. The same principles of physical preparation and fitness apply to emotional health. The key to good mental health is to learn how to deal effectively with minor and moderate stressors while avoiding larger stressors.

Stress can be the result of many types of stressors. Table 4-1 identifies common factors that can cause stress. The way an individual thinks and feels about an event is what causes a stress response. Each person thinks about an event in a different way; therefore, an event that is perceived as stressful to one person may not be stressful to another individual.

STRESS RESPONSE

Although each individual may react differently to a particular stressful situation, everyone experiences similar strong emotions and characteristic physical responses to a stressful situation.

EMOTIONAL RESPONSE

The feelings we experience during a stress response may be powerful, sometimes even overwhelming. It is important to realize that stressors are not always undesirable. An example of a positive stressor is an EMT waiting to meet a good friend she hasn't seen in many years. She might be feeling strong emotions such as happiness, excitement, or anticipation, which are positive. Those emotions are certainly different from the emotions of fear, anxiety, and dread that the EMT may have felt while en route to a multiple victim motor vehicle collision.

As one can imagine, many different emotions may be experienced during a stress reaction. Table 4-2 lists some of the many emotions an EMT may experience as a response to stress.

PHYSICAL RESPONSE

Despite the individual factors involved in the perception of stress, a person's physical response to stress tends to be quite similar from person to person. When a person is faced with a stressor, the body's physical reaction is to prepare to defend itself either by fighting the perceived aggressor or running away from the stressor. This is sometimes called the *fight-or-flight response*.

This fight-or-flight response originates in the sympathetic nervous system. The effects on the body include increased heart rate, increased blood pressure, increased respiratory rate, increased use of oxygen and glucose, tensing of muscles, sweating, dilation of pupils, and the shunting away of blood from the skin, toward the muscles and core organs. The results of these effects are the feeling of

Table 4-1 Common EMT Stressors

Type of Stressor	Examples
Physical	Trauma Illness Poor nutrition Sleep disturbances Hunger Discomfort Pain
Psychological	Worry Fear Anger Happiness
Mental	Thoughts Perceptions Interpretation of events Personal significance of events
Environmental	Temperature (weather) Air pollution Noise pollution Crowding Time pressures
Sociocultural	Job loss or promotion Work situations Changes in interpersonal relationships Interpersonal conflict

Adapted from DeLaune, S., & Ladner, P. *Fundamentals of Nursing: Standards & Practice.* 2d ed. Clifton Park, NY: Thomson Delmar Learning, 2002.

a rapid heartbeat, sweatiness, tenseness, cool and clammy skin, and sometimes anxiety. Table 4-3 highlights common physical responses to stress.

Some of the hormones released during this response can last in the body for hours, days, or even weeks. Consequently, the physical effects may continue to be felt for several weeks after the stressful incident (Figure 4.1). EMTs must learn to expect these feelings and cope with them as much as possible to allow continued performance of necessary duties.

SPECIFIC EMS STRESSORS

Several specific circumstances are known to cause stress for EMTs while on the job. These tend to be situations that are emotionally charged. Being prepared for your body's reaction to situations you may encounter will be the first step you take in effectively managing the effects of stress in your life.

Table 4-2 Stress-Related Emotions

Anger	Pressure
Anxiety	Distress
Fear	Boredom
Competitiveness	Affection
Embarrassment	Intimacy
Defeat	Love
Confusion	Hopefulness
Jealousy	Superiority
Disappointment	Trust
Regret	Satisfaction
Guilt	Joy
Depression	Happiness
Despair	Exhilaration
Suspicion	Delight
Defensiveness	Silliness
Frustration	Pensiveness
Hurt	Shyness
Inferiority	Thoughtfulness
Rejection	Moodiness
Repulsion	

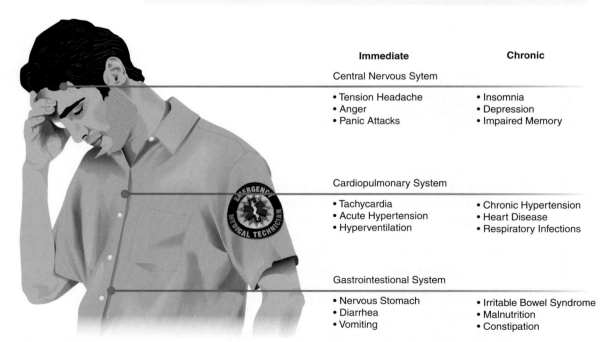

	Immediate	Chronic
Central Nervous Sytem		
	• Tension Headache • Anger • Panic Attacks	• Insomnia • Depression • Impaired Memory
Cardiopulmonary System		
	• Tachycardia • Acute Hypertension • Hyperventilation	• Chronic Hypertension • Heart Disease • Respiratory Infections
Gastrointestional System		
	• Nervous Stomach • Diarrhea • Vomiting	• Irritable Bowel Syndrome • Malnutrition • Constipation

Figure 4.1 Stress has numerous physical effects. Some reactions are immediate, whereas others are delayed

Table 4-3 Common Physical and Psychological Responses to Stress

Physiological

Cardiopulmonary
- Increased pulse
- Increased blood pressure
- Rapid, shallow breathing

Gastrointestinal
- Nausea
- Altered appetite
- Diarrhea or constipation

Neurological
- Dizziness
- Headache
- Dilated pupils

Genitourinary
- Frequent urination

Musculoskeletal
- Tension
- Twitching

Endocrine
- Increased blood glucose

Cognitive
- Impaired memory
- Confusion
- Impaired judgment
- Poor decision making
- Delayed response time
- Altered perceptions
- Inability to concentrate

Behavioral
- Pacing
- Sweaty palms
- Rapid speech
- Insomnia
- Withdrawal
- Exaggerated startle reflex

Psychological
- Irritability
- Increased sensitivity
- Sadness, depression
- Feeling "on edge"

Spiritual
- Alienation
- Social isolation
- Feeling of emptiness

Adapted from DeLaune, S., & Ladner, P. *Fundamentals of Nursing: Standards & Practice.* 2d ed. Clifton Park, NY: Thomson Delmar Learning, 2002.

DEATH

Encountering death while on the job is considered to be one of the most stressful events an EMT will experience. Feelings of sadness or grief are expected and are considered healthy for an EMT when faced with the death of a patient. Feelings of helplessness, despair, or even of failure are also common when an EMT tends to a dying patient.

In the course of patient care, an EMT may be faced with a situation in which a life cannot be saved. It is certainly a powerful situation and would be considered by most to be stressful, whatever the provider's level of experience.

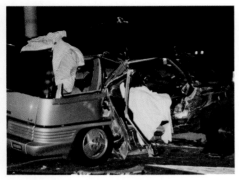

Figure 4.2 Terrible suffering can invoke powerful feelings in an EMT (Courtesy of Craig Smith)

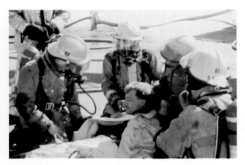

Figure 4.3 The death or serious injury of a coworker is a stressful event for an EMT

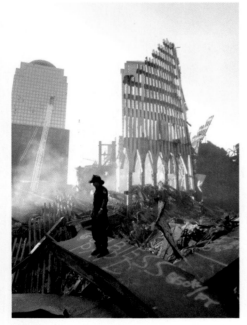

Figure 4.4 Terrorist acts, like the September 11, 2001, attacks in the United States, are examples of extreme disasters (Photo by Andrea Booher/FEMA News Photo)

If a positive aspect of the event is identified, the stress response may be lessened. For example, an EMT may feel sad about the death of a terminally ill patient but at the same time recognize that she has been able to comfort the family. The realization that there are positive aspects of most stressors will help EMTs manage the stress in their lives more effectively.

DEVASTATING TRAUMA

Situations involving traumatic injuries may be stressful to EMS providers. Trauma often affects young and older people alike and has the potential to devastate many lives (Figure 4.2). The EMT may experience feelings of fear or anxiety when faced with such a situation. If prepared, the EMT may be able to quickly dispel those feelings and return to the task of caring for the injured patient.

The emotions an EMT may experience at such a scene may be overwhelming. It is sometimes necessary for the EMT to step back from the situation for a moment to clear her thoughts before she can effectively care for the patient. Some specific situations that may evoke particularly powerful emotions include motor vehicle collisions, amputations, shootings, decapitations, and injuries to children.

ILLNESS OR INJURY OF COWORKERS

EMTs will sometimes be required to care for ill or injured coworkers (Figure 4.3). It is very difficult to have to care for someone with whom you have emotional ties. The EMT may experience overwhelming feelings of fear, anxiety, and frustration when faced with such a situation and may be reminded of her own vulnerability. It is crucial, however, that she be able to continue to work effectively. An EMT who feels that she cannot work effectively should immediately make arrangements for another EMT to take over.

VIOLENCE IN THE COMMUNITY

Another stressful situation EMTs may encounter is that of caring for a potentially abused individual. Whether that patient is an infant, child, adult, or elder, the feelings of suspicion, anger, and sadness cannot be avoided. It is important for the EMT to withhold blame and treat all involved nonjudgmentally. It is beyond the scope of an EMT's duty to determine the guilt or innocence of a suspected abuser.

The responsibility of the EMT is to remove the patient from a potentially harmful environment and care for any injuries. The specifics of how to recognize and report abuse will be discussed in more detail in later units. Understanding that a strong emotional reaction is likely will help the EMT to continue to function in such a situation.

DISASTERS

An incident involving multiple injured patients, or a multiple casualty incident (MCI), is a high-stress situation. These situations are often the result of a natural disaster, cataclysmic event, or an act of terrorism (Figure 4.4). The first arriving teams are often overwhelmed and unable to adequately care for everyone injured.

Special training is also needed to learn to handle such an incident. Handling MCIs is covered in detail in a later unit. It is important for the EMT to realize that she will not be alone in managing such a scenario.

Before the terrorist attacks of September 11, 2001, most EMS providers assumed that terrorism only occurred in other countries; the likelihood of large-scale terrorism occurring in their community seemed remote. That expectation has changed for many Americans. EMS providers must be ever-vigilant of the potential for events related to weapons of mass destruction, such as biological, nuclear, incendiary, and chemical weapons as well as explosives—a range of threats sometimes referred to by the acronym B-NICE.

Although special training for an emergency response to terrorism can help to mitigate the fear caused by weapons of mass destruction, the addition of another stressor, and the constant attentiveness that this threat demands, can lead to fatigue and eventual exhaustion.

STRESS RELATED TO WORK CONDITIONS

Several aspects of a job in emergency services are inherently stress producing. The need for constant training, long hours, and relatively low pay add to the stress of recurrent exposure to high-stress events interspersed by sometimes long inactive periods.

The often less-than-ideal working conditions of the EMT certainly do not foster a stress-free work environment. It is important for the EMT to recognize the source of job stressors; identifying stressors is the first step toward developing a response and coping mechanism.

LIFELONG LEARNING

The training of all health care providers is continuous. Initial training and then continuing education with frequent updates are essential to continue to provide quality medical care. This schedule of training may be stressful for persons who are not comfortable in a classroom environment. Altering the method of classroom instruction may reduce stress brought on by recurrent classroom activities.

WORK HOURS

In many regions of the United States, EMS providers work 12-hour or 24-hour shifts. This means that they spend long periods of time with coworkers, away from family and friends. In a busy system, such long shifts can be physically and emotionally exhausting.

SALARY AND WAGES

In light of the important role emergency medical services plays in society, EMTs are compensated rather poorly in many areas of the country. There certainly are exceptions, but for the most part, EMT salaries are on the low end of the pay scale. Because of their low pay, some EMTs have to hold down several jobs or work overtime to earn enough to support themselves and their families.

POOR SLEEP AND POOR EATING HABITS

During a tour of duty, an EMT must find time to eat and sleep (on longer shifts). This time is often interrupted by emergency calls or other job requirements. Lack of adequate time for sleeping and rushed eating habits can cause an EMT to be more susceptible to other stressors (Figure 4.5).

LACK OF FORMAL REWARDS

Despite the intense dedication of many EMTs to their work, formal rewards are received infrequently in emergency medical service. The EMT will learn that the most satisfying reward is to be told "thank you" or to see a patient smile. Regular reward programs can also make a sometimes relatively thankless job more fulfilling.

STRESS OFF WORK

Many EMTs have significant responsibilities at home as well as at work. Maintaining personal relationships, parenting, caring for elderly parents, and running a household are only some of the key issues many adults face at home.

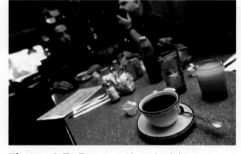

Figure 4.5 Poor eating habits can contribute to the body's inability to adequately cope with stressors

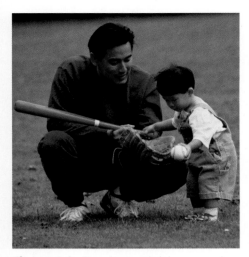

Figure 4.6 Family activities may be a useful break from the stress of the job

The family of an EMT may not be able to fully comprehend the daily stressors of a job in emergency services. This lack of understanding may lead the EMT to be reluctant to share with her family the events of her day. This reluctance may cause her family to feel ignored or frustrated. Attempting to relate some of her experiences to her family may provide the EMT with a needed release and will fulfill her family's need to share in her life.

TIME ISSUES

The EMT will often work long hours. A shift is not always over at its scheduled time because of the unexpected nature of emergency calls. Overtime is sometimes required. This type of shift work may pose hardships for the EMT's family.

Some EMTs remain "on call" while at home, responding when needed. Being on call makes planning family or personal events difficult for family members. Minimizing changes in work schedules will allow the EMT and her family to become accustomed to a particular schedule and may reduce some of this stress.

It is important for the EMT to keep a significant period of time completely free for family activities (Figure 4.6). This commitment gives the EMT some necessary time to relax and spend uninterrupted time with family.

SOCIAL LIFE

In addition to spending time with family members, it is important for the EMT to find time to spend with friends. These social contacts provide a necessary break from work and personal responsibilities. Taking time to unwind can be a means to reduce the effects of daily stress on the EMT. This time should include participation in hobbies or favorite sports or other forms of exercise (Figure 4.7). The importance of relaxation and physical exercise is discussed later in this unit.

MANAGING PERSONAL STRESS

An EMT will be repeatedly exposed to multiple stressors daily, both at work and at home. It is crucial for the EMT to learn to expect stress and prepare for it as much as possible. A variety of techniques and strategies are available for stress management.

PERSONAL WELL-BEING

Stress can exert an emotional and physical toll on the body. Mental and physical preparations are both key elements in reducing those effects. It is important for the EMT to maintain the best emotional and physical condition she can.

Allowing enough time for nonstressful activities such as hobbies or exercise is crucial. The EMT profession tends to attract people who prefer to be

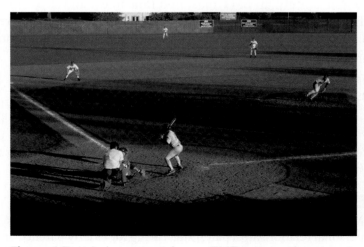

Figure 4.7 It is important for an EMT to take time to relax

busy and on the run. This constant, hectic pace allows stress to build up without an avenue for release and can lead to significant health issues.

Persistent stress can actually decrease the body's immune capabilities, leaving the individual susceptible to infectious disease. Other physical conditions associated with prolonged stress include high blood pressure, heart disease, migraine headaches, and stomach ulcers. Table 4-4 highlights some

Table 4-4 Stress-Related Disorders

Respiratory disorders
   Emphysema
   Chronic bronchitis
   Asthma

Cardiovascular disorders
   Hypertension
   Cardiac arrhythmias
   Migraine headaches

Endocrine disorders
   Thyroid problems
   Diabetes
   Excessive weight gain or loss

Musculoskeletal disorders
   Chronic back pain
   Arthritis

Genitourinary disorders
   Loss of bladder control
   Urinary frequency

Sexual and reproductive disorders
   Low libido
   Impotence
   Menstrual irregularities

Gastrointestinal disorders
   Colitis
   Chronic constipation
   Ulcers
   Gastritis

Integumentary disorders
   Eczema
   Hives
   Psoriasis

Adapted from DeLaune, S., & Ladner, P. *Fundamentals of Nursing: Standards & Practice.* 2d ed. Clifton Park, NY: Thomson Delmar Learning, 2002.

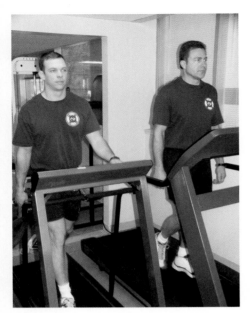

Figure 4.8 Exercise is a great way to relieve stress and maintain a healthy body

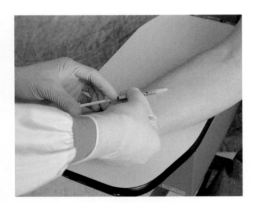

Figure 4.9 Health checkups and immunizations are part of an EMT's healthy lifestyle

common disorders related to stress. The EMT must be aware of these possibilities and take control of her life to prevent such complications.

HEALTHY LIFESTYLE

The first step in physical and mental preparation for frequent exposure to stress is to maintain a healthy lifestyle. This includes exercise, a balanced diet, and elimination of unhealthy habits such as smoking. If you start with a healthy body, stress will have less of an effect on your physical and mental well-being.

Some form of regular exercise can be helpful in keeping your body in shape and reducing the actual physical effects of a stressor (Figure 4.8). A balanced diet with limited amounts of sugar, caffeine, and alcohol can also prepare your body to respond well to stress.

Tobacco has been shown to negatively affect the body in many ways, one of which is to increase the physical response to stress. It is best not to smoke. Maintaining a balance between work, recreation, family, and health is important in preparing yourself to handle a stressful situation most effectively.

IMMUNIZATIONS

Part of advance preparation for a job in health care is to protect your body as much as possible from infectious diseases by staying up to date on recommended immunizations. An EMT may be exposed to several disease processes for which vaccines are available to help prevent disease transmission. Hepatitis B, tetanus, measles, mumps, rubella, influenza, and pneumonia are the most common diseases for which an EMT can receive vaccinations. Regular testing for tuberculosis is also recommended for people in the health care field (Figure 4.9). Other means of effective infection control are addressed in Unit 8.

INFECTION PROTECTION

Even with adequate vaccination, it is crucial for EMTs to take measures to protect themselves from infectious diseases such as tuberculosis and hepatitis A, C, and D and from exposure to HIV. Washing hands frequently and wearing gloves, masks, and gowns when appropriate protect EMTs from potentially infectious body substances. Specifics of such body substance isolation are discussed in Unit 8.

SCENE SAFETY

Every emergency scene involves many potential hazards. Potentially infectious body fluids are certainly not to be ignored, but before even coming into contact with the patient, the EMT must address other issues for safety reasons.

The EMT must take every precaution necessary to prevent harm from coming to herself, her crew, the patient, and bystanders. The scene survey, discussed in an upcoming unit, is the initial evaluation of a situation for potential dangers. It is only by constant vigilance to possible hazards that an EMT will protect herself and remain healthy and able to continue performing her job efficiently.

RECOGNIZING STRESS

An EMT's ability to recognize situations that cause a stress response will help her prepare for such an event. Once the cause of stress is identified, the EMT can find ways to minimize its harmful effects.

ACUTE STRESS

An acute stress is a single event that creates a stress response. Once having identified known stressful events, the EMT may attempt to reduce her exposure to them as much as possible. If the offending stressor consists of being awakened by loud radio tones, the EMT may choose not to work nights or may plan to sleep before and after her shift so that she can stay awake for the duration of the shift. Some stressful events cannot be avoided, but others can be anticipated and eliminated or at least alleviated.

CHRONIC STRESS

Over time, repeated stressors result in chronic stress, which can have a significant effect on the EMT's physical and emotional well-being. If not properly managed, these effects can lead to impairment of the EMT's ability to function on the job and even at home.

When an EMT no longer feels able to perform her duties because of the effects of such chronic stress, we describe this condition as **burnout.** If recognized early, burnout can be addressed and managed. If not recognized by the EMT or coworkers, burnout may lead to significant physical and emotional consequences. In some circumstances, formal psychological counseling is required to prevent further deterioration.

It is crucial that all emergency service providers be aware of the telltale signs and symptoms of chronic stress and burnout. Table 4-5 lists some of the classic warning signs of chronic stress and possible burnout.

Table 4-5 Signs of Chronic Stress and Burnout
Physical
Increased heart rate
Gastrointestinal discomfort
Anxiety
Headaches
Insomnia
Fatigue
Muscle tension
Emotional
Feeling on edge
Depression
Irritability
Anger
Behavioral
Avoidance
Withdrawal
Aggression
Procrastination
Increased alcohol and/or tobacco use
Drug abuse
Overeating

If an EMT recognizes these signs and symptoms in herself or a coworker, the situation must be addressed immediately. Most employers have means by which to address such issues. It is important to take action quickly. The ideal situation is to avoid the cumulative effects of chronic stress by managing issues as they arise. But, if physical and emotional burnouts do occur, they should be immediately addressed so the EMT can return to her previous level of functioning—equipped with more effective stress management skills.

STRESS RELIEF TECHNIQUES

Several techniques can be used to help to diffuse or reduce the emotional and physical responses to a highly stressful situation. Relaxation exercises can be employed at any time during or after a stressful event.

One such technique involves taking several deep, deliberate breaths while thinking a simple repetitive thought such as "Relax and let go; I am in control." This deep breathing procedure can be initiated when a stress response is first noted and can help the EMT regain focus and decrease or abort the stress response.

Diversionary techniques are also useful for dissipating the effects of an acutely stressful event. Physical exercise such as jogging, swimming, walking, washing the car, or cleaning a room can be useful to release some of the energy and hormones the stressor has created or released. Other diversionary techniques that can be employed after an event are participation in hobbies, social activities, or traveling.

No matter the method used, an EMT should have some form of stress release available at any time. Allowing the effects of stress to build up will only result in a more intensified response to the next stressor.

STRESS MANAGEMENT PROGRAMS

It is especially important for organizations in high-stress professions, such as EMS, to have a recognized plan to identify and lessen the effects of stress in the workplace. The first step in such a stress management program is to realize that prevention is the best option. If stressors can be identified and avoided or minimized, the need for relieving the effects of stress will be lessened.

Many aspects of a job in emergency services will continue to stimulate a stress response. Even though high-stress events are not totally avoidable, an EMT may be able to decrease the number of times she may encounter them. Even distribution of the stress load among team members should be a goal in every EMS system. In a busy system, the heavier assignments should be rotated. If possible, employees should be cross-trained to allow them to work in several different environments as a way of decreasing exposure to high-stress assignments. For example, an EMT might work in the field for one month then work on a community outreach program the next month.

Another way to manage unavoidable stress is to change the way the stimulus is perceived. This can be thought of as changing the quality of the stressor. The EMT should try to think about bothersome situations in a different manner. If a positive aspect of the event can be found, the EMT should focus on that aspect. This positive focus will help to reduce the stress response. For example, if an EMT finds that calls to a local nursing home remind her of her grandmother's death and become quite stressful for her, she should try to focus on a positive aspect of visits to this facility. Perhaps there are interesting paintings on the walls or the nursing staff is particularly helpful. Some aspect of the situation can often be found that will offset the previously unpleasant experience.

Talking about bothersome issues can also help the EMT to lessen the stress response. Coworkers should expect to share such feelings with one another as part of a stress management plan (Figure 4.10).

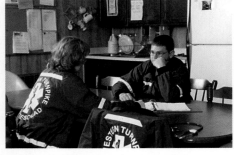

Figure 4.10 It is often useful to discuss difficult situations with coworkers as part of stress management

One form of relaxation exercise is called *guided imagery*. The following instructions are a guide to this technique.

- Assume a comfortable position in a quiet environment.
- Close your eyes and keep them closed until the exercise is completed.
- Breathe in deeply to a count of 4.
- Hold breath for a count of 4.
- Breathe out to a count of 4.
- Continue to breathe slowly and deeply.
- Think of your favorite place and prepare to take an imaginary journey there. Select a place in which you are relaxed and at peace.
- Picture in your mind's eye your favorite place. Look around you and see all the colors, the light and shadows, and all the pleasant sights.
- Listen to all the sounds. Pay attention to what you hear.
- Feel all the physical sensations—the temperature, the textures, the movement of the air.
- As you take in a deep breath, smell the aromas of your favorite place. Savor each aroma fully.
- Focus all your attention totally on your favorite place.
- Breathe in deeply to a count of 4.
- Hold breath for a count of 4.
- Resume your usual breathing pattern.
- Slowly open your eyes and stretch, if desired.

This procedure works best when all five senses are used. Like all other relaxation exercises, guided imagery becomes more effective with repetition. (Adapted from DeLaune, S., & Ladner, P. *Fundamentals of Nursing: Standards & Practice*. 2d ed. Clifton Park, NY: Thomson Delmar Learning, 2002.)

Comprehensive health and safety programs that are provided or encouraged by an employer can also significantly decrease the effect of the accumulation of stress on employees. Regular physical exercise should be encouraged to help decrease the levels of hormones that are released in a stressful situation. This decrease in stress reactivity can positively affect the EMT. Such an exercise program also will serve to strengthen the body and improve resistance to disease.

Supervisors should be trained to recognize the signs of stress overload and should have feasible options for managing such a situation. Finally, the EMT should not be afraid to speak up and share her thoughts and concerns about the impact of stress on her life. Once a stressor has been identified, it can be addressed and effectively managed.

Table 4-6 Incidents That Produce Strong Feelings in Responders

- Multiple casualty incident
- Death of an infant or a child
- Injury or death of an emergency service provider
- Severe traumatic injuries
- Prolonged response to any situation (e.g., a hostage situation)

CRITICAL INCIDENT STRESS DEBRIEFING

After an incident that seems to have had a particularly strong emotional impact on any member of the team, such as those incidents listed in Table 4-6, some form of psychological debriefing may be in order. In the past, formal debriefing programs such as **Critical Incident Stress Debriefing (CISD)** or Critical Incident Stress Management (CISM) sessions have been conducted in the immediate post-event period. Programs such as these are structured sessions facilitated by trained personnel meant to review the incident in detail and encourage the involved group of providers to discuss their experience during and after the incident. After these discussions, the group is provided with education regarding stress reactions and stress management techniques. This type of group debriefing session has been thought to decrease the chance of long-lasting psychological impact of a traumatic event.

The EMS experience with psychological debriefing has increased significantly since the terrorist attacks on September 11, 2001. Although most people who have been through a CISD session report that it seemed helpful, long-term studies do not show a clear benefit of CISD in terms of reduction of psychological consequences. Some experts believe that such a process might actually impede the natural recovery that most people experience. Several recent publications report a review of the existing literature that finds conflicting results from CISD. As a result of these newer findings, many professionals are no longer recommending formal CISD sessions. Research on this subject is ongoing.

What does seem clear is that in the days following a traumatic event, psychological support, education, and screening to detect those in need of more complex intervention is appropriate. The presence of severe psychological symptoms one to two weeks after the event may predict the need for individual help. EMS supervisors should be attentive to their staff in this time period and be able to direct individuals toward further treatment when appropriate.

SUICIDE IN EMS

EMTs do not always share their feelings or problems. Some emergency service providers become so overwhelmed by chronic job, home, and social stressors that they take their own lives. Suicide is not uncommon in high-stress professions. It is therefore crucial for each EMT to be aware not only of her own response to stressors but also of the responses of coworkers.

The EMT must learn to address these issues before friends or coworkers become so overwhelmed that they consider suicide. The EMT should know that a job in emergency services is high in stress. Every opportunity must be taken to reduce the effects of this stress and to maintain a constant vigilance to recognize signs of decompensation in others.

MANAGING STRESS IN PATIENTS

Understanding the causes of her own stress response is the first step the EMT can take toward understanding and dealing with the emotions experienced by a patient. It is expected that when faced with a painful and frightening experience, the average person will feel stressed. Most people have feelings of fear, anxiety, loss of control, and sometimes anger when faced with a personal emergency.

EMTs must remember that despite the seemingly routine nature of a call for them, the incident is stressful and unsual for the patient and his or her family. Treating patients with dignity and respect will often gain their confidence. It is crucial that the EMT provide honest explanations and answers to questions.

The EMT must also make every attempt to maintain a patient's privacy and dignity throughout the encounter. Sensitive questions should be asked in a private area, and exposure during examination should be minimized when possible.

Allowing patients to have control over some aspect of their care may help to make them feel more in control. Something as simple as asking whether the patient prefers to sit up or lie down during the transport may return a sense of control and therefore decrease any perceived stress.

Remember that part of the EMT's job is to comfort patients. Comfort may be provided in simple ways—by providing blankets in cold weather, ensuring that the patient's home is secured before leaving, or just holding the patient's hand. These are meaningful actions to many patients (Figure 4.11).

A patient's family members also experience significant stress when their loved one is ill or injured. It falls within the duties of the EMT to reassure family members. The family may be experiencing fear, anger, frustration, denial, or depression. Truthful information can be comforting to the family but must be given with regard to a patient's privacy. Listening to a family member's thoughts and fears may provide information useful in the care of the patient and will also reassure the family that the EMT cares about their loved one (Figure 4.12). Providing information and listening to family members will likely help reduce their stress.

CONCLUSION

Stress is the body's emotional, physical, and behavioral response to our changing environment. The EMT should be aware of her own response to stressful situations and should learn to prepare herself in such a way that the consequences of the stressful exposure are minimized.

Because each individual's response to stress is different, the EMT must also be sensitive to the reactions of her coworkers. An effective stress management program will include prevention techniques, relaxation and diversionary techniques, and a comprehensive health and safety program. Understanding that in the emergency services stress is not entirely avoidable, mechanisms for critical incident stress debriefing must be in place in every EMS system.

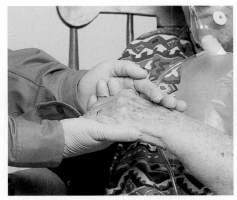

Figure 4.11 Simple comforting measures can help to decrease a patient's stress

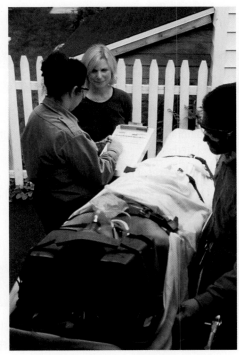

Figure 4.12 Taking a moment to reassure a patient's family can help decrease their anxiety

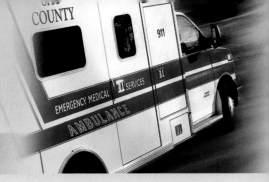

CASE STUDY Continued

After delivering the patient to the trauma center, Dan and Kris sit outside the ambulance bays quietly. Another crew exits, ready to go in service. Dan asks for a cigarette, but Kris reminds him quietly that he has been trying to quit. With that Dan is reminded that it is almost quitting time. He tells Kris he thinks he wants to go to the local "watering hole" for a drink. Kris acknowledges that it might seem like a good idea, but she is going to the gym to work out. She explains that the workout seem to help calm her down after a stressful work shift and also helps her sleep better. She invites Dan to join her at the gym.

Key Concepts Revisited

- Stress is a function of everyday living.
- Common physical and emotional stressors in EMS are job related.
- The body responds to these stressors.
- The body's reaction to stress can be pathological.

- EMS is prone to special stressors wrought by human suffering.
- The EMT must learn to recognize and respond to these intense stressors.

Key Terms

Burnout
Critical Incident Stress Debriefing (CISD)

Stress
Stressors

Review Questions

1. What is the definition of stress?
2. List some common physical, psychological, mental, and environmental effects of stress.
3. List some the common responses to stress.
4. What are some common EMS specific stressors?
5. What are some common work-related stressors?

6. What are some common off-work stressors?

7. What are some of the elements of healthy living for an EMT?

8. When is a critical stress debriefing important?

9. What EMS calls might cause strong reactions and necessitate critical stress debriefing?

10. Why is it important for EMTs to watch for signs of stress in their coworkers?

Further Study

DeLaune, S., & Ladner, P. *Fundamentals of Nursing: Standards & Practice.* 2d ed. Clifton Park, NY: Thomson Delmar Learning, 2002.

Everly Jr., George, & Mitchell, Jeffrey. *Critical Incident Stress Management.* Ellicott City, MD: Chevron, 1999.

Mitchell, Jeffrey. *Critical Incident Stress Debriefing.* 3d ed. Ellicott City, MD: Chevron, 1999.

Seaward, Brian Luke. *Managing Stress.* Sudbury, MA: Jones & Bartlett, 2000.

CHAPTER 2

The Human Body

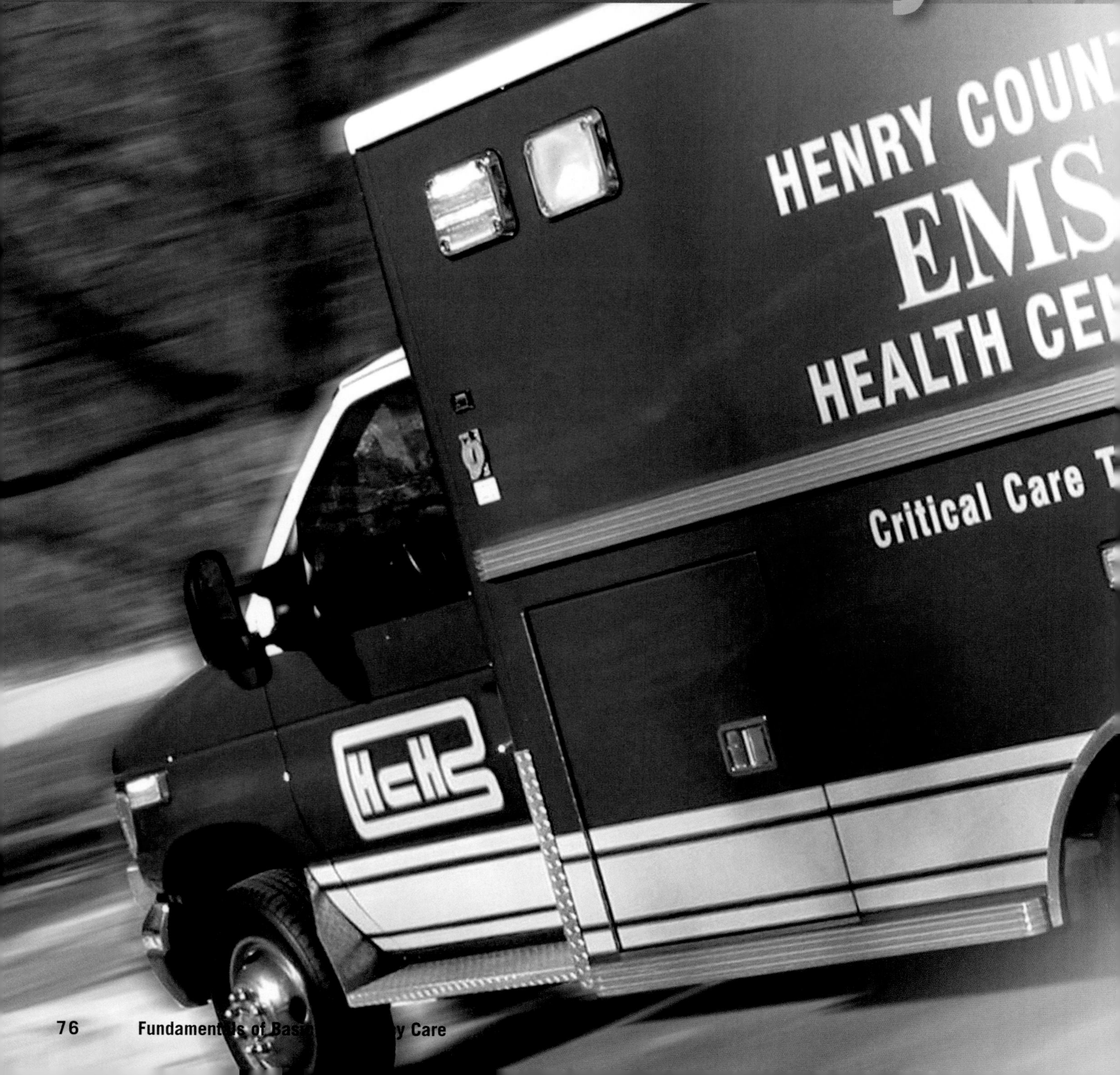

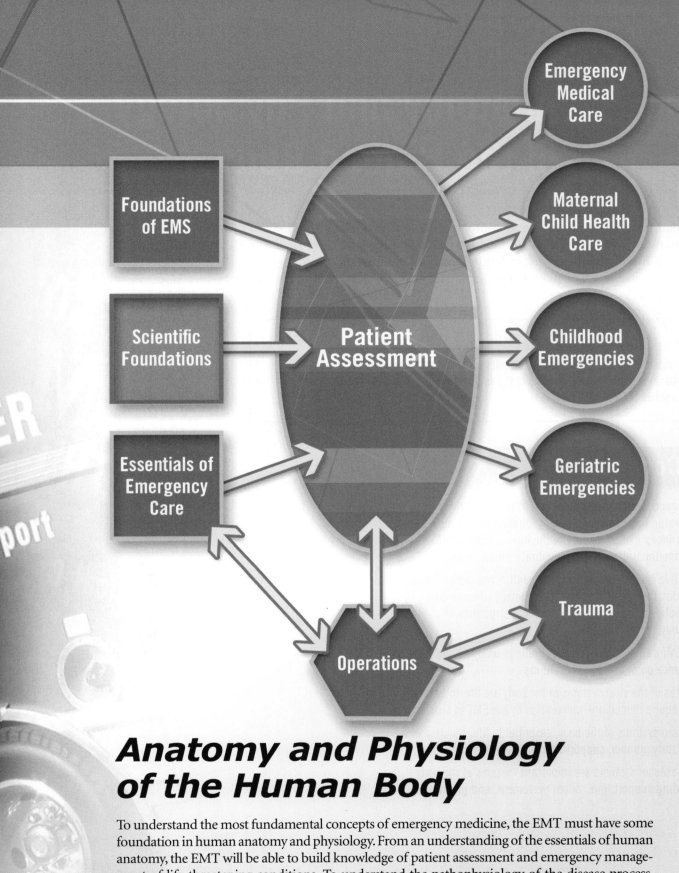

Anatomy and Physiology of the Human Body

To understand the most fundamental concepts of emergency medicine, the EMT must have some foundation in human anatomy and physiology. From an understanding of the essentials of human anatomy, the EMT will be able to build knowledge of patient assessment and emergency management of life-threatening conditions. To understand the pathophysiology of the disease process, the EMT must also have a basic understanding of how the systems of the body function together to support life. This chapter is an overview of the basics of human anatomy and physiology of the human body and the pathophysiology of disease processes that can occur to endanger life.

The human body is a wondrous and complex organism made up of billions of small structures working together for the life of a single large structure. The EMT must have a foundational understanding of human anatomy and physiology to provide the patient assessment and emergency care essential to prevent the loss of life and disability.

National Education Standards

The Emergency Medical Technician (EMT) shall be able to apply a fundamental depth and foundational breadth of understanding of the anatomy and function of all human systems to the practice of EMS.

Key Concepts

- Emergency Medical Technicians (EMTs) need an understanding of basic anatomy, anatomical terminology, and concepts of physiology of the human body to effectively manage the nature of an individual's illness or injury.

- Effective communication among health care professionals includes the use of standard terminology when referring to the motions and different anatomical structures of the body.

- The EMT can describe physical findings using an accepted reference point and direction terms.

- Failures of the vital systems of the body are life-threatening and require immediate intervention by the EMT to sustain life.

- The core systems of the body, essential to life, function in a regulatory manner, supporting the vital systems.

- The assessor systems are important systems of the body providing support, protection, movement, and procreation.

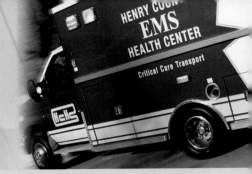

CASE STUDY

Joshua, Jeremy's partner, is throwing terms around again—terms like *unilateral* and *proximal* and names of organs, like *pancreas.* Joshua even volunteers that the job of the pancreas is to create insulin. Joshua has just finished an anatomy course at the local college while preparing to enter the paramedic program. Joshua seems to have learned so much useful information that Jeremy starts to think he might be a better EMT if he takes an anatomy class. Jeremy recalls feeling a little embarrassed recently when giving the patient care report to the nurse at the bedside. She used some terms he was not familiar with and he felt that he should have known those terms, but he was too embarrassed to ask. His EMT teacher

taught him a little anatomy, just enough to get by, but he kept saying there wasn't enough time in the EMT course to go into the details of anatomy and physiology.

Critical Thinking Questions

1. How does an understanding of anatomy and physiology help the EMT care for a patient?
2. How much anatomy should an EMT know?
3. About what vital systems should an EMT be knowledgeable?
4. Trace a drop of blood from the heart to the body and back to the heart.

INTRODUCTION

To begin understanding the nature of a patient's illness, the Emergency Medical Technician (EMT) must have a basic knowledge of human anatomy and physiology. This unit explores the basic anatomy, anatomical terminology, and concepts of physiology of the human body.

ANATOMY AND PHYSIOLOGY

Anatomy refers to the study of the structure of an organism. **Physiology** refers to the study of the function of the organism. Recognition of signs of disease and the ability to appropriately intervene are dependent upon a basic understanding of normal anatomy and physiology. After learning what is normal, the EMT can begin to recognize abnormalities and learn how to manage them.

This material may seem difficult to understand, and the terminology may seem foreign to an EMT student. Nevertheless, it is important that EMT students learn basic anatomy and physiology in order to effectively communicate with other health care professionals. In short, EMTs should be able to "speak the language" of other health care professionals, using correct medical terminology.

TOPOGRAPHIC ANATOMY

All health care providers use standard terminology when referring to different parts of the body. Some of these anatomical terms are based upon the landmarks that exist on every person's body. Other terms use a conceptual framework that is widely accepted among health care professionals. The study of the relationship of one body part to another is called **topographic anatomy.**

Whenever an EMT describes a patient, he is comparing the patient with a person in the **standard anatomical position.** As depicted in Figure 5.1, the person is facing forward, legs slightly apart, with feet pointing forward,

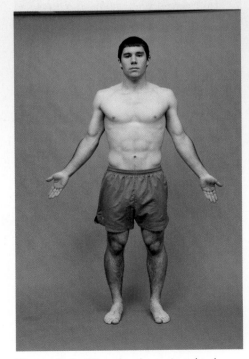

Figure 5.1 Standard anatomical position

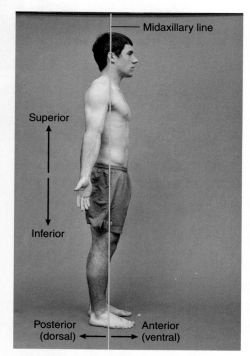

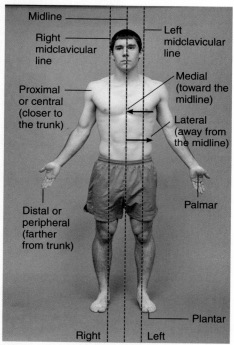

Figure 5.2 The standard planes of reference and directional terms

arms straight and extended a few inches away from the side, and palms facing forward.

LINES OF REFERENCE

Imagine the body with several invisible lines across it. These lines of reference can be used when describing an injury. The first line to imagine is the **midline.** The midline runs down the center of the body, equally dividing it into a right half and a left half. To either side of the midline are the right and left **midclavicular lines.** These lines start at the midpoint of each collarbone, or **clavicle,** and run parallel to the midline.

Another useful imaginary line is the **midaxillary line.** The midaxillary line runs from the middle of the armpit, or **axilla,** parallel to the midline. These are a few of the more common examples of the lines used in topographic anatomy (see Figure 5.2).

DIRECTIONAL TERMS

With an accepted reference point, the EMT can describe physical findings, such as injuries, in a precise manner. The following describes directional terms, which refer to a landmark or to a line of reference. These terms are illustrated in Figure 5.2. Notice that each term has an opposite.

Any point that is above the reference landmark is considered **superior.** For example, the mouth is superior to the chin. Therefore, any point below the chin must be **inferior** to it. *Superior* and *inferior* can be used to describe any injury or other physical finding provided the reference point is noted, which in this case is the chin.

Similarly, any point that is toward the front of the body is referred to as **anterior,** and any point that is toward the back of the body is called **posterior.**

The patient's flanks (sides) are *lateral* to the umbilicus (belly button). Conversely, the umbilicus is *medial* to the flanks. As can be seen in Figure 5.2, **medial** describes a point closer to the middle of the body, and **lateral** refers to a point farther from the midline.

Many parts of the body are in pairs. For example, ears, eyes, and arms all come in right and left. When describing injury to one but not both, use the term **unilateral,** meaning one side only. Conversely, if both right and left wrists are injured, then say that the patient has **bilateral** injuries.

EMTs often use the terms *proximal* and *distal* to describe a location where an injury exists between two points on an extremity. For example, "The cut on the forearm was proximal to the wrist but distal to the elbow." **Proximal** describes something that is closer to the trunk; **distal** describes something that is farther from the trunk. Sometimes the term **central** is also used to describe something that is toward the center of the body, and the term **peripheral** is used for something farther away from the center of the body.

The term **ventral** refers to the front of the body, and **dorsal** refers to the back or to the top surface of any body structure, such as the hand. Other terms that are used to describe position are **plantar,** meaning the sole of the foot, and **palmar,** meaning the palm of the hand.

Directional terms are also used to describe the location and relationship of organs in the body. The heart and lungs, for example, have a triangular shape and can be described as having an **apex** and a **base.** The apex is the "point" of the triangle, and the base is the flat bottom. The apex of the lungs is at the top, and the apex of the heart is toward the bottom. See Figure 5.3 for an illustration of this concept.

Directional terms are also used to describe the severity of injuries, such as injuries to the skin. The terms **superficial** and **deep** may be used to describe

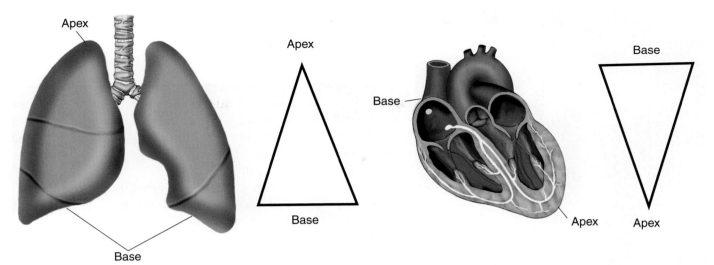

Figure 5.3 Apex and base

the degree of injury. Superficial describes an injury close to the surface; a superficial injury is less severe than a deep one. See Figure 5.4 for an example of this contrast.

ANATOMIC POSITIONS

The position that a patient is found in or is placed into can also be described using standard terminology. A patient found face down is said to be **prone** (Figure 5.5A). The patient who is placed flat on a backboard facing up with his backbone or spine on the backboard is **supine** (Figure 5.5B).

Some patients may prefer to sit upright. The EMT may place the patient on the stretcher in **Fowler's position** (Figure 5.5C). This is a semi-sitting position with the head and chest elevated to between 45 and 60 degrees. A patient who is sitting upright at 90 degrees is in **high-Fowler's position** (Figure 5.5D).

Patients suffering from shock may be placed in the **modified Trendelenburg,** or **shock position** (Figure 5.5E). In this position, the patient is supine with the legs elevated 12 to 16 inches. This position is thought to improve blood flow to the brain and other vital organs. Shock and its treatment are discussed in a later unit. True Trendelenburg position inclines the entire body so that the feet, legs, and abdomen are above the head, but it is often difficult to accomplish in an ambulance.

If a patient is found unconscious but does not appear to have any spinal injury, the EMT may turn the patient toward one side. This position encourages natural drainage of the secretions from the mouth and is referred to loosely as the **recovery position.** In Figure 5.5F, the patient is lying on the left side or is said to be in the **left lateral recumbent position.**

RANGE OF MOTION

The movement of the arms and legs permits walking as well as lifting, carrying, and holding. The arms and legs have a range of motion that enables us to perform these actions. Sometimes injuries limit that range of motion. During a patient assessment, an EMT should note any limitation to the range of motion caused by an injury. Therefore, it is important for an EMT to know the common terminology used to describe motion.

Putting your arm out to shake another person's hand is called **extension.** During extension, the movement widens the angle at the joint between two bones. When a hand is pulled back, with elbow bent, then the arm is in

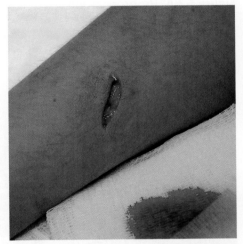
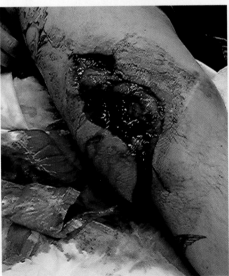

Figure 5.4 Superficial and deep injuries (Courtesy of Deborah Funk, MD, Albany Medical Center, Albany, NY)

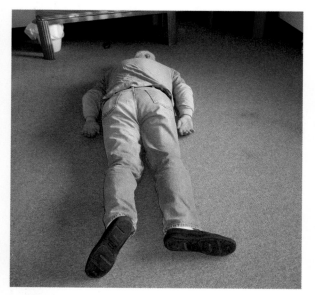

Figure 5.5A Prone position

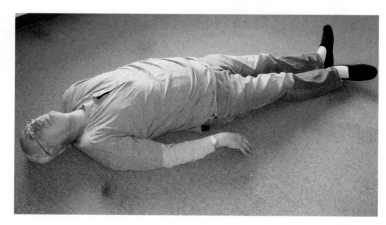

Figure 5.5B Supine position

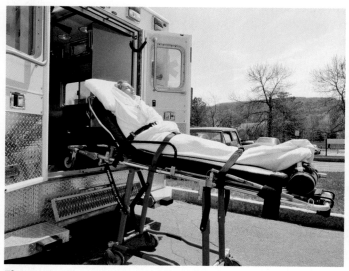

Figure 5.5C Fowler's position

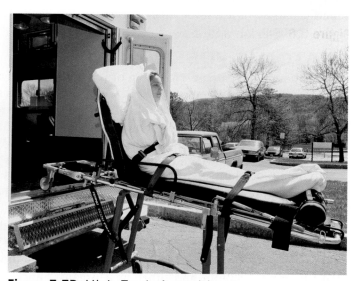

Figure 5.5D High-Fowler's position

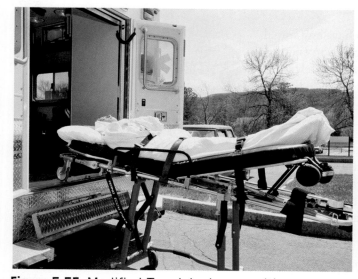

Figure 5.5E Modified Trendelenburg position

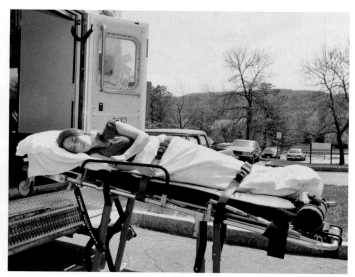

Figure 5.5F Left lateral recumbent position

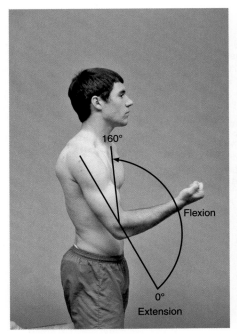

Figure 5.6 Flexion and extension

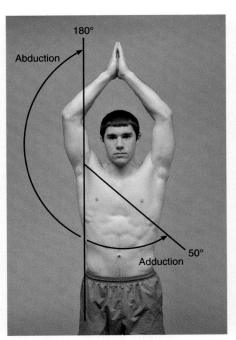

Figure 5.7 Adduction and abduction

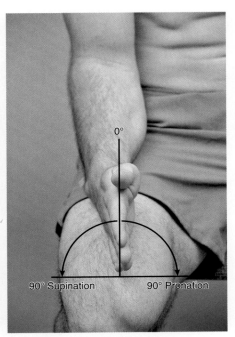

Figure 5.8 Supination and pronation

flexion. During flexion, the movement narrows the angle at the joint between two bones. Extension and flexion are illustrated in Figure 5.6.

An arm raised straight away from the midline is in **abduction;** when the arm is returned to the side, it is in **adduction.** An example can be seen in Figure 5.7.

To hold a bowl of soup in the palm of your hand, you must turn your palm upward in **supination.** Turning the palm of the hand downward is called **pronation.** See Figure 5.8 for an example.

Athletes often injure their ankles, and the EMT may be called onto the playing field. If the athlete's foot is turned outward, this is called an **eversion** injury. It is more likely that an athlete will twist his ankle inward and sustain an **inversion** injury. Figure 5.9 illustrates these two mechanisms for ankle injury.

The new EMT should practice using these terms in documentation and then have the report reviewed by an experienced EMT. The accurate use of these terms is important. When in doubt as to how to describe an injury, an EMT should use plain English. Other health care professionals will be more impressed with a simple but accurate description than with a "flowery" but vague or even inaccurate description of an injury.

THE VITAL SYSTEMS

The systems of the body can be categorized by how the body is affected if that organ or system is damaged through injury or illness. Organs essential for life are vital organs. An understanding of the structures, location, and function of these systems serves as a foundation to understanding how disease affects the body and how drugs help decrease the damage done by disease.

THE NERVOUS SYSTEM

The **nervous system** controls and coordinates all bodily functions. This complex task involves interactions between three main subdivisions of the nervous system. These subdivisions are the central, peripheral, and autonomic nervous systems. Figure 5.10 illustrates this interaction.

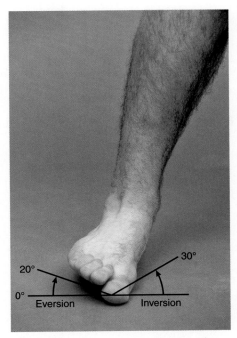

Figure 5.9 Eversion and inversion

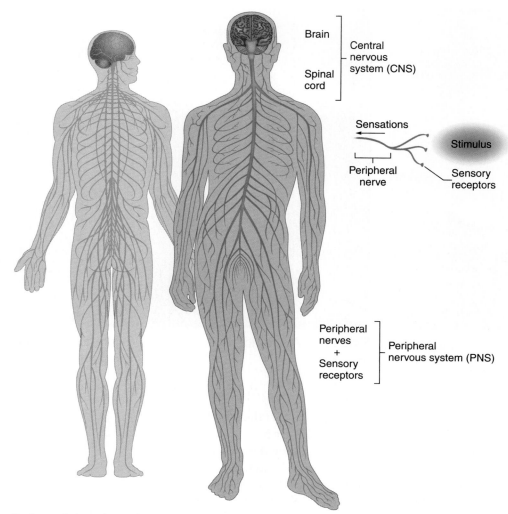

Figure 5.10 Central, peripheral, and autonomic nervous systems

EQUILIBRIUM

The body strives to maintain a steady optimal state for growth and development and resists any influence, internal or external, that would upset this balance. This constant state of internal equilibrium is called **homeostasis.**

Two organ systems are specifically involved in maintaining homeostasis: the nervous system and the endocrine system. The endocrine system is responsible for the more general adjustments in the body's internal organs, whereas the nervous system is responsible for the moment-to-moment fine adjustments.

THE CENTRAL NERVOUS SYSTEM

The **central nervous system** is made up of the brain and the spinal cord and is involved in the initiation and transmission of all control-oriented messages throughout the body.

THE BRAIN

The seat of all higher intellect, the human brain is thought to make us different from other creatures. However, in many ways our brains are very similar to those of other mammals. The human brain consists of a brainstem, cerebellum, and cerebrum. These areas of the brain have further subdivisions, each of which has its own unique functions. Figure 5.11 shows these subdivisions.

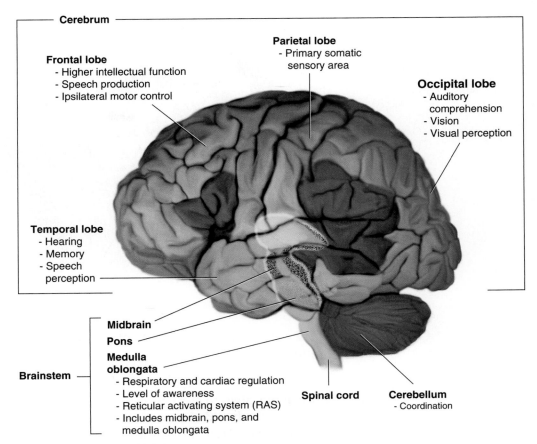

Figure 5.11 The brain and its subdivisions

THE BRAINSTEM

The most basic part of the human brain is the brainstem. The **brainstem** acts like a junction box for the complex wiring system of the central nervous system. The upper regions of the brain send all signals to the brainstem to be passed to the spinal cord for distribution to the body. The brainstem consists of the midbrain, pons, and medulla oblongata. All mammals have a brainstem that is involved in the control of life-sustaining functions such as breathing and heartbeat.

THE CEREBELLUM

The word **cerebellum** means "little brain." Actually, it can be thought of more as the "athletic brain." The cerebellum controls muscular coordination and complex actions, such as shooting a basketball or driving a car. When a police officer stops a car and tests the driver's sense of balance, as part of a drunken driver assessment, the police officer is testing the person's cerebellar functions.

THE CEREBRUM

The seat of all higher thinking is the **cerebrum.** The cerebrum is the largest area of the brain and occupies the majority of the cranial vault. The cerebrum is divided into a right and a left hemisphere. The cerebrum can be further divided into different lobes with each having its own specific duties and functions.

THE MENINGES

We can use the analogy of an egg to describe the organization of the brain. The brain is protected by a hard bony shell. Inside the shell are membranes, called **meninges,** that surround the brain and continue along the spinal cord. These meninges pad the brain from impact. The innermost layer is called

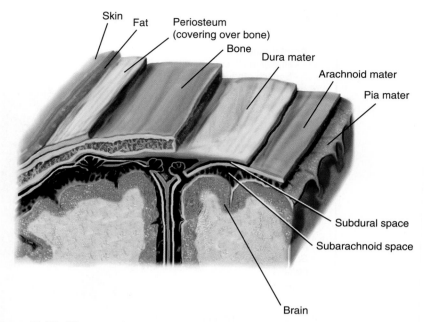

Figure 5.12 The meninges are made of pia mater, the arachnoid, and the dura mater

the pia mater and clings to every surface of the brain. The next layer of the meninges is the **arachnoid.** The arachnoid spreads weblike over the entire brain. The outermost layer is called the **dura mater,** which literally means "tough mother." Together, the pia mater, arachnoid, and dura mater act to "pad" the brain from injury.

As in an egg, there is a great deal of fluid, called **cerebrospinal fluid (CSF),** within the skull that further absorbs impact. The CSF also carries nutrients to and removes some wastes from the brain cells.

The combination of the bony skull, the protective meninges, and the shock-absorbing CSF protects the brain itself from impact and injury. These protective layers are seen in Figure 5.12.

THE SPINAL CORD

The spinal cord originates at the base of the skull and runs down the spinal column. All messages between the body and the brain pass along the spinal cord. The spinal cord can be compared to the trunkline of a telephone company. Cut the trunk line and all outgoing and incoming calls stop.

The cross section of the spinal cord is about the diameter of a dime in some areas. The space between the spinal cord and the surrounding bony spinal canal can be as little as the thickness of a pencil's lead. This sometimes precarious positioning can lead to injury to the spinal cord in accidents involving spinal trauma.

THE PERIPHERAL NERVOUS SYSTEM

The **peripheral nervous system** is made up of nerves that originate in the spinal cord and take messages to the body. Some nerves originate in the body's organs and tissues and transmit information back to the spinal cord, where it is then relayed to the brain. These peripheral nerves are very important and necessary for movement and sensation. Figure 5.13 illustrates the actions of the peripheral nervous system. The part of an EMT's exam that tests for movement and sensory function will be testing the interactions between the peripheral and central nervous systems.

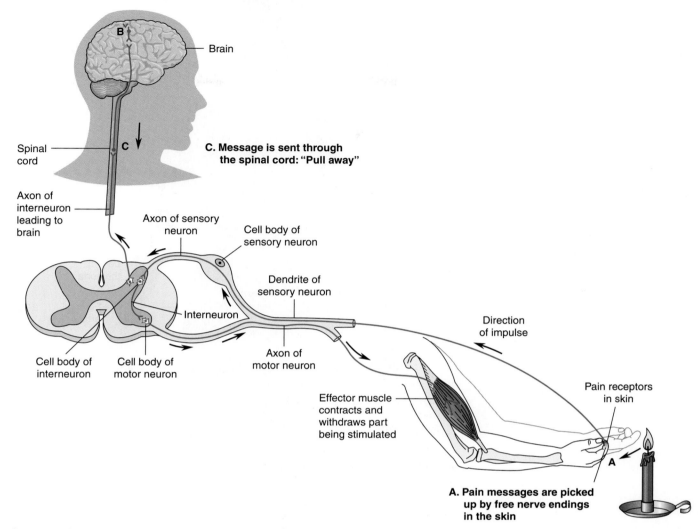

B. Message arrives in the brain: "Ouch! Hot"

Brain

Spinal cord

C. Message is sent through the spinal cord: "Pull away"

Axon of interneuron leading to brain

Axon of sensory neuron

Cell body of sensory neuron

Dendrite of sensory neuron

Interneuron

Direction of impulse

Cell body of interneuron

Cell body of motor neuron

Axon of motor neuron

Effector muscle contracts and withdraws part being stimulated

Pain receptors in skin

A. Pain messages are picked up by free nerve endings in the skin

Figure 5.13 The peripheral nerves provide the brain with information about the environment in which we live

THE AUTONOMIC NERVOUS SYSTEM

The heart muscle, smooth muscles of the body, and certain other structures controlling automatic body functions are under the control of the **autonomic nervous system.** This is a collection of nerves that originate in the brainstem and transmit vital impulses to these organs of the body. Many medicines that doctors prescribe affect the functioning of the autonomic nervous system.

THE CIRCULATORY SYSTEM

Every day the heart pumps gallons of blood around the body one beat at a time. The distribution of blood vessels around the body and back to the heart is called a circuit, and the action of blood flowing in that circuit is called **circulation.**

The purpose of this regular flow of blood is to transport oxygen and other nutrients to all of the organs of the body and to simultaneously remove their metabolic wastes. The **heart** acts as the pump for this amazing system to ensure adequate flow throughout the body. The **blood vessels** are the pipes. Their size and the distribution of blood flowing in them can be altered depending on the area most in need of blood flow. The **blood** is the medium for transport of oxygen and vital nutrients and removal of waste products. It also carries disease-fighting white blood cells, stabilizes body temperature,

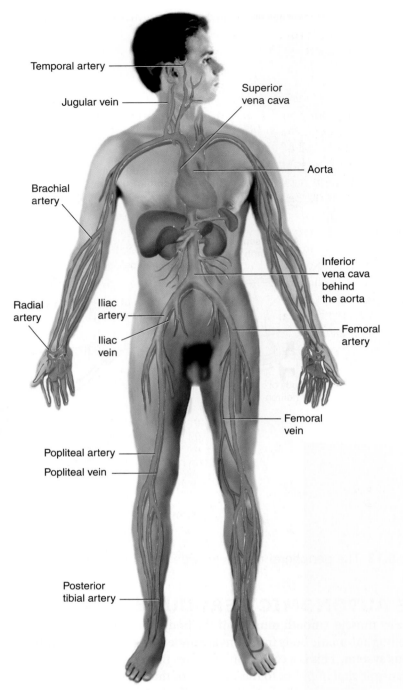

Temporal artery

Jugular vein

Superior vena cava

Brachial artery

Aorta

Radial artery

Iliac artery

Iliac vein

Inferior vena cava behind the aorta

Femoral artery

Femoral vein

Popliteal artery

Popliteal vein

Posterior tibial artery

Figure 5.14 Circulatory system (the heart is the center of the circulatory system)

restricts fluid loss through clotting, and regulates acid levels. The circulatory system is illustrated in Figure 5.14.

The life-sustaining activity of the circulatory system is often taken for granted. However, the circulatory system is so essential to life that any interruption of the function of the heart or damage to the integrity of the blood vessels can have serious and even life-threatening consequences. It is important that EMTs understand the circulatory system and be able to recognize when it is not functioning properly.

THE HEART

The heart is a unique muscular organ located slightly left of center in the chest, between the sternum and the spine.

The heart is surrounded by a tough fibrous covering called the pericardium (*peri-* means "around"; *cardium* refers to the heart) that separates it from the lungs on either side of it within the chest cavity.

CARDIAC FUNCTION

The heart is a remarkable feat of engineering. In fact, two muscular pumps operate independently yet in tandem. The first pump, the right pump, circulates blood through the **pulmonary circuit** so that it may pick up oxygen in the lungs and be rid of carbon dioxide and other wastes. The pulmonary circuit consists of the lungs and the blood vessels within them. This is a very short route and requires very low pressures.

The left side of the heart pumps blood to the entire **systemic circuit** so that oxygen and other nutrients may be brought to the tissues of the body and metabolic wastes may be removed. The systemic circuit involves all the body organs and tissues except the lungs. Therefore, the left side of the heart must pump effectively from the tip of the nose to the tip of the toes. This is a very long pathway and requires the left heart to pump at great pressures to provide adequate flow to all these areas. The pulmonary and systemic circuits are pictured in Figure 5.15.

The pumps of the heart are two-staged pumps. Each pump has a receiving chamber, called the **atrium,** which serves to prime the pump. The primary chamber for each pump, called the **ventricle,** actually performs the

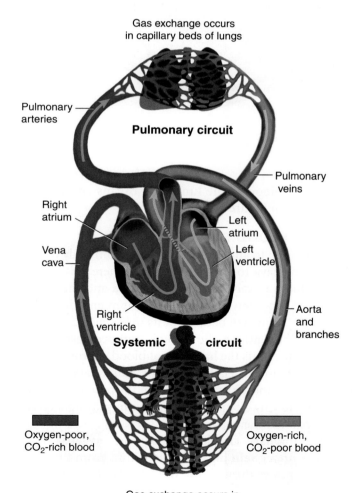

Gas exchange occurs
in capillary beds of lungs

Pulmonary arteries

Pulmonary circuit

Pulmonary veins

Right atrium

Left atrium

Vena cava

Left ventricle

Right ventricle

Aorta and branches

Systemic   **circuit**

Oxygen-poor, CO_2-rich blood

Oxygen-rich, CO_2-poor blood

Gas exchange occurs in
capillary beds of all body tissues

Figure 5.15 Pulmonary and systemic circulation

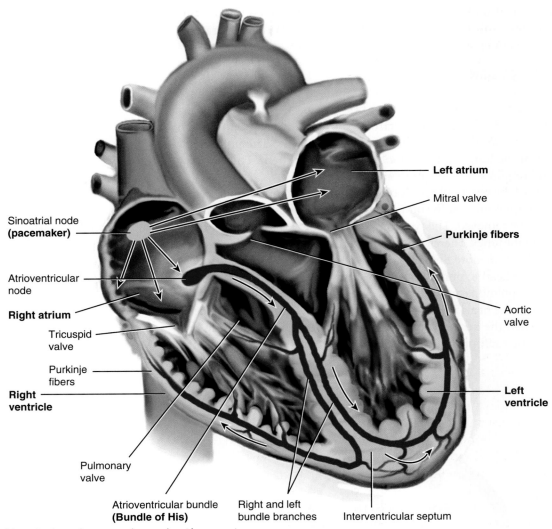

Left atrium

Mitral valve

Purkinje fibers

Sinoatrial node
(pacemaker)

Aortic
valve

Atrioventricular
node

Right atrium

Tricuspid
valve

Purkinje
fibers

**Right
ventricle**

**Left
ventricle**

Pulmonary
valve

Atrioventricular bundle
(Bundle of His)

Right and left
bundle branches

Interventricular septum

Figure 5.16 Heart chambers and conduction system

work of circulating blood to the lungs and organs and tissues. This relationship is depicted in Figure 5.16.

DIRECTION OF BLOOD FLOW

After delivering oxygen to and removing wastes from body tissues, the blood returns via the vena cava to the right atrium, where it is pumped into the right ventricle. One-way valves between the atria and the ventricles ensure continued forward flow. Between the right atrium and the right ventricle is the **tricuspid valve**, so named because of its three-cusp construction.

Once in the right ventricle, the blood is pumped past another valve, the **pulmonary valve** (prevents the backflow of blood), through the **pulmonary artery** (the artery that transfers blood to the pulmonary circuit for oxygenation) and into the pulmonary circulation. In the pulmonary circulation, the blood passes close to tiny air spaces, where it can pick up oxygen and be rid of carbon dioxide and other wastes.

From the pulmonary circulation, the now-oxygenated blood passes through the **pulmonary vein** into the left atrium. From the left atrium, this oxygenated blood passes through the **mitral valve** (also prevents backflow) and into the left ventricle.

The left ventricle contracts strongly about 70 times each minute, pumping blood rich in oxygen through the **aortic valve** into a large artery called the aorta and out to the body organs and tissues, where the oxygen and nutrients may be utilized. Once the nutrients have been delivered, the blood returns to the right atrium via a large vein called the vena cava. Now deoxygenated, or without oxygen, the blood is ready to begin another cycle. This continuous cycle is depicted in Figure 5.15.

ELECTROPHYSIOLOGY

The heart is unique as muscles go, because it is able to generate its own electrical impulses. This feature is referred to as *automaticity* and is unique to the heart muscle.

Specialized cells within the heart muscle, known as the *conduction system*, are designed to provide the most efficient means of electrical stimulation of the heart muscle. These unique conduction cells possess several other properties that allow them to do their job efficiently. They not only have the ability to generate their own electrical impulses but also can accept impulses from the cells around them and in turn transmit the message to surrounding cells.

The conduction system within the heart has several distinct cell types (refer to Figure 5.16). The **sinoatrial node,** or **SA node,** is the primary pacemaker of the heart. It generally initiates the electrical impulse that will result in an electrical response from the rest of the heart muscle and lead to a heartbeat.

From the SA node, the electrical impulse will travel down the most efficient pathway through internodal atrial pathways to the **atrioventricular node,** or **AV node.** The AV node slows the electrical impulse momentarily to allow for the mechanical contraction of the heart to catch up to its electrical activity.

From the AV node, the impulse travels into the ventricles by way of the **bundle of His** and then into the right and left **bundle branches.** The impulse will then be distributed through the ventricles via an extensive conductive pathway called the **Purkinje fibers,** which are located throughout the ventricles.

This conduction pathway allows for the efficient and orderly contractions of the atria and the ventricles, leading to an effective heartbeat. It is important for the EMT to understand the concept of the electrical activity within the heart so that he may intervene when an abnormality exists, as in cardiac arrest.

THE BLOOD VESSELS

The heart is connected to pipelines, called *blood vessels*, that transport blood to the organs and the tissues of the body.

A blood vessel is a hollow pipe that carries blood. Blood vessels that carry blood away from the heart are called **arteries.** The blood vessels that carry blood back to the heart are called **veins.**

With one exception, arteries carry oxygenated blood and veins carry deoxygenated blood. The pulmonary artery carries deoxygenated blood away from the right heart and into the lungs, and the pulmonary vein returns to the left heart with oxygenated blood from the lungs.

Capillaries are tiny blood vessels that receive blood from arteries and pass it into adjacent veins. They are so small that **red blood cells,** the oxygen-carrying cells, must pass through them in single file. This may seem like a very ineffective method of circulating blood, but it provides tissues in those capillary beds the opportunity to extract oxygen and excrete carbon dioxide. The relationship of the arteries, veins, and capillaries is exhibited in Figure 5.17.

THE ARTERIES

The largest artery of the body is the **aorta.** The aorta carries all of the blood from the left side of the heart to the body. As the aorta travels downward through the chest, it is referred to as the thoracic aorta. From the point where this large artery passes into the abdomen, it is then called the *abdominal aorta*.

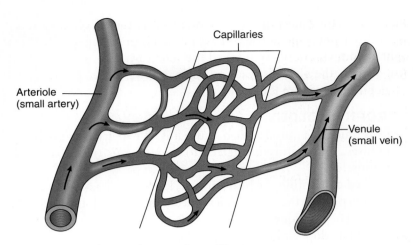

Figure 5.17 Arteries, veins, and capillaries

Many smaller arteries branch off the aorta. Figure 5.14 illustrates many of the major arteries of the body.

Each of the terminal arteries is named after a bone that lies close to the artery. Because of the proximity of arteries to bones, a pulse can be felt at each of these points. Perhaps even more important, if a pulse can be felt, then, with gentle direct pressure, circulation can be stopped. Therefore, rapid arterial bleeding beyond these **pressure points** could be halted. It is important that all EMTs know the exact location of the major pressure points in the body, shown in Figure 5.18. It should be noted that new research indicates that severe arterial bleeding should be controlled with an arterial tourniquet rather than pressure points. The EMT should follow local protocol regarding bleeding control.

THE VEINS

Blood is returned to the heart via blood vessels called *veins.* Some veins are visible, like those on the back of the hand, and are called superficial veins. Those veins that originate from internal organs are said to be deep veins. Bleeding from a deep vein can become life threatening in a very short time. One of the few deep veins that come to the surface is the **jugular vein** in the neck. An injury to the jugular vein is a serious wound.

Veins and arteries run together next to bones. As are the partner arteries, most veins are named after the bone they parallel. This system makes identifying veins and arteries easier for the EMT.

The largest vein in the body is called the **vena cava.** It has a superior and an inferior portion. The superior vena cava drains the deoxygenated blood from the brain, the neck, and the arms; the inferior vena cava drains the majority of the rest of the body.

Veins from the legs (iliac veins), the kidneys (renal veins), the liver (hepatic vein), and the intestines (mesenteric veins) all drain into the inferior vena cava. Figure 5.14 shows the main venous structures of the body.

THE BLOOD

The purpose of this elaborate human plumbing system is to transport blood. Blood has many functions, all of which serve to continue the life of the body.

The human body is a machine. To run such a machine requires fuels such as glucose, or sugar, and oxygen. The use of such fuels by the body is referred to as **metabolism.** There has to be a means to get these fuels to the individual cells in the tissues and organs of the body. Blood is that means of transportation.

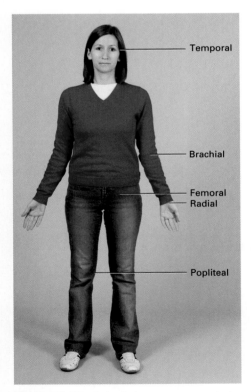

Figure 5.18 Arterial pressure points of the body

Blood that circulates to all the tissues of the body is perfusing the body. **Perfusion** is a Latin term meaning "to pour through," and that is exactly what blood does in the body.

Beyond the transportation of oxygen-carrying red blood cells, the blood also circulates disease-fighting white blood cells.

Finally, the blood has a self-repair mechanism. Whenever there is bleeding, as seen with many injuries, a coagulation cascade is activated, allowing a clot to form and bleeding to stop. Coagulation prevents the loss of blood and helps maintain its steady supply. This entire process of blood clotting is called **hemostasis,** which literally means to stop bleeding.

THE RESPIRATORY SYSTEM

An important mission of the circulatory system is to distribute oxygenated blood. Naturally, the next question should be, how does the blood get the oxygen? The answer is through the respiratory system.

The term **ventilation** refers to the actual movement of air into and out of the lungs. The mechanism that produces this air movement is discussed later in this chapter. The term **respiration** refers to the exchange of gases, such as oxygen and carbon dioxide, at the capillary level. The EMT will be able to improve a patient's ventilation but will often have no direct impact on the actual respiration at the cellular level.

The respiratory system can be easily divided into the upper airway and the lower airway. Essentially, the lower airway is the start of the "sterile airway." That means that one of the main burdens of the upper airway is to clean the outside air of any contamination before it enters the lungs.

THE UPPER AIRWAY

The largest opening, or orifice, of the body is the mouth. The mouth permits large volumes of air to enter into the airway and eventually into the lungs.

The inside of the mouth is referred to as the **oropharynx.** It is the portion of the airway that is visible to the EMT when the mouth is opened wide, such as when suctioning the airway.

The nose also permits the movement of air into the lungs. The nostrils of the nose have fine hairs, called cilia, that clean the air as it passes over them. The nasal passage, also called the **nasopharynx,** is also coated with a thick sticky liquid material, mucus, that traps and holds dirt, dust, and any other particulate contamination. The nasal passages also are rich in blood vessels that serve to heat the air that passes over them to a warm 98.6 degrees Fahrenheit (37°C), or body temperature. Figure 5.19 shows the structures of the upper airway.

The windpipe, or trachea, is a long funnel that channels air into the lungs. It starts at a structure called the **larynx.** The larynx is a cartilaginous boxlike structure that contains the vocal cords; hence, it is sometimes called the *voice box.* The vocal cords vibrate when air passes over them and create sound. In males, the voice box is larger than in females and externally can be identified as the Adam's apple.

Above the larynx is the **epiglottis.** The epiglottis is a cartilaginous structure that protects the trachea from foreign bodies. When the epiglottis fails and a foreign body enters the trachea, it may block the passage of air. The maneuvers to remove a foreign body airway obstruction (FBAO) must be performed so that air may pass again. These techniques are vital for the EMT to know.

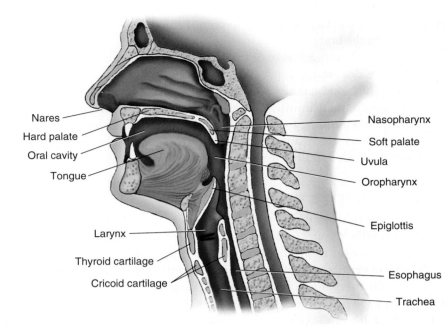

Figure 5.19 The structures of the upper airway

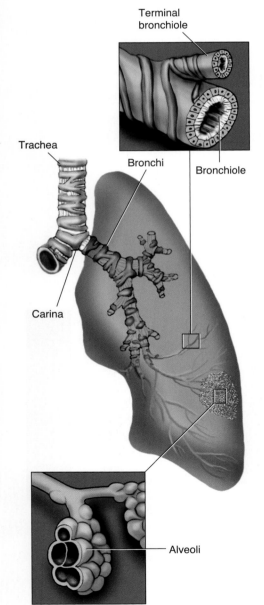

Figure 5.20 The lower airway structures

The warmed, filtered air continues to pass into the lungs via the trachea. The trachea is a semirigid tube that can be felt anteriorly in the midline of the neck. The trachea and its related structures are illustrated in Figure 5.19.

THE LOWER AIRWAY

The trachea ends at a division, or bifurcation. This point is called the **carina.** The right and left mainstem **bronchi** start here and continue deep into the lungs. The bronchi are cartilaginous tubes that divide into smaller passages called **bronchioles** and keep dividing into smaller passages until they become very narrow **terminal bronchioles.** Lining the inside of the bronchioles are **goblet cells** and **cilia.** The goblet cells produce a mucous blanket that is designed to entrap particles and microorganisms, such as bacteria, and prevent them from entering the alveoli. This thick mucous blanket is constantly moving upward, propelled by small hairlike projections called *cilia*, into the back of the throat to be coughed up. Toxins in cigarette smoke, for example, can paralyze the cilia and allow the bacteria-laden mucous blanket to stagnate, causing an infection called *bronchitis*. Attached to the terminal bronchioles are the clustered **alveoli.** These structures are shown in Figure 5.20.

RESPIRATION

It is inside the alveoli that the critical exchange of carbon dioxide and oxygen occurs. The small saclike alveoli are clumped together like clusters of grapes at the end of a vine. Tiny pulmonary capillaries surround these air spaces, allowing deoxygenated blood to pass closely by the oxygen-filled spaces. As the blood passes by these alveoli, carbon dioxide is released into the air space and oxygen is taken up into the blood. This process of gas exchange is referred to as *pulmonary respiration*. It is in this manner that certain wastes are removed from the blood and oxygen is taken on. This process is illustrated in Figure 5.21.

THE PLEURAE

Surrounding the lungs are two membranes called *pleurae*. One membrane, the **visceral pleura,** is found on the surface of the lungs themselves. The other membrane, the **parietal pleura,** lines the inside of the rib cage. These two pleural linings move against each other as the lungs expand and deflate with ventilation. A very small amount of fluid reduces friction by lubricating the space between them. Figure 5.22 shows the pleurae and their relationship to the lungs and chest wall.

THE DIAPHRAGM

The **diaphragm** is a large muscle that lies within the lower part of the chest and is unique in that it is similar to other skeletal muscles in structure but is not completely under voluntary control. It is controlled by the brainstem via nerves from the cervical spinal cord. A complex interaction of signals between the body and the brain signals how often the diaphragm needs to contract. Figure 5.23 illustrates the nervous control of the diaphragm.

VENTILATION

When the diaphragm contracts, it is pulled down into the abdomen, creating a negative pressure, or vacuum, within the thoracic cavity. This negative pressure then forces the intake of air through the mouth and nose into the lungs to equalize the pressure. When the diaphragm then relaxes, it is pushed back up into the chest and a positive pressure is created that forces the air out of the lungs. This is how we inhale and exhale. Figure 5.24 illustrates this physiology.

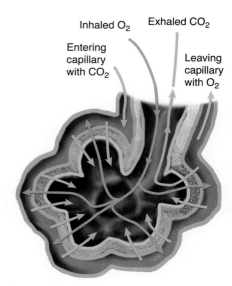

Figure 5.21 Exchange of oxygen and carbon dioxide takes place in the alveoli

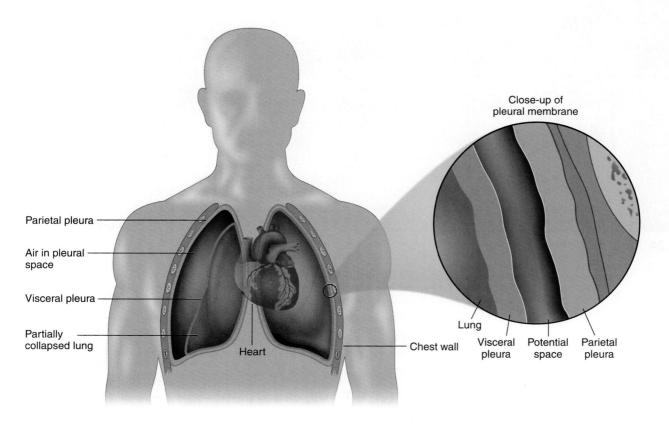

Figure 5.22 The pleural membranes allow the lungs to move smoothly within the chest

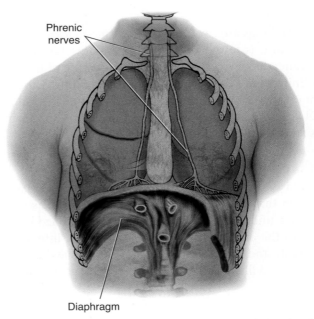

Phrenic
nerves

Diaphragm

Figure 5.23 The diaphragm is controlled by the phrenic nerves

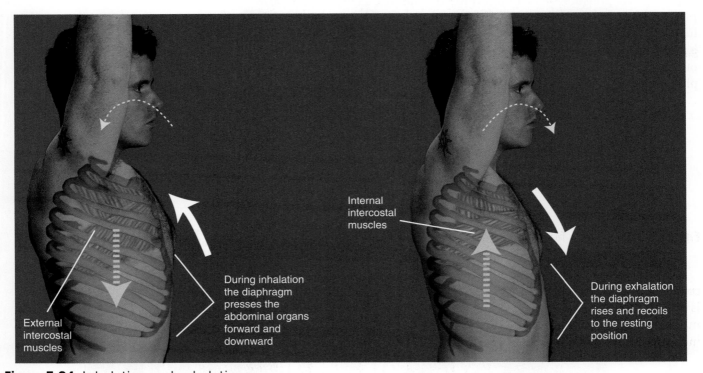

Internal
intercostal
muscles

During inhalation
the diaphragm
presses the
abdominal organs
forward and
downward

During exhalation
the diaphragm
rises and recoils
to the resting
position

External
intercostal
muscles

Figure 5.24 Inhalation and exhalation

THE CORE SYSTEMS

The core systems of the body are also essential to life but function in a more regulatory manner, supporting the functions of the vital systems. The EMT can have direct intervention when a vital organ fails. When an organ of the core systems is affected, the EMT's intervention is more to support and treat the symptoms enroute to more definitive care.

THE DIGESTIVE SYSTEM

Ventilation and respiration account for part of the intake of fuels and removal of wastes, but the remainder of this metabolic process is maintained by

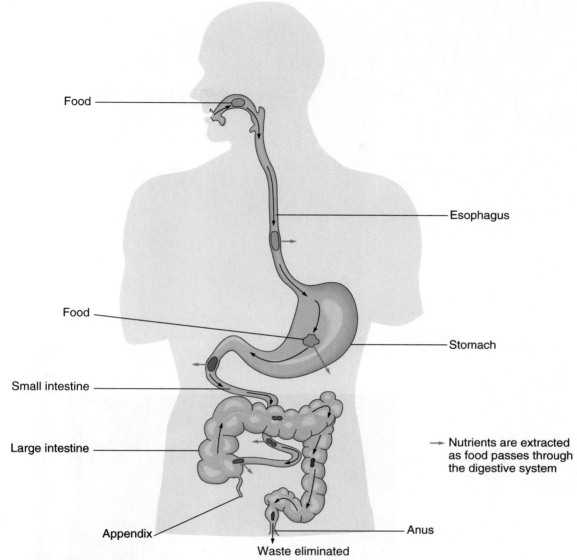

Food

Esophagus

Food

Stomach

Small intestine

Large intestine

Nutrients are extracted as food passes through the digestive system

Appendix

Anus

Waste eliminated

Figure 5.25 Nutrient flow in the gastrointestinal tract

organs involved in digestion and elimination. By digesting foods, the body is able to extract the sugars and other nutrients that it needs to survive. The nutritional flow starts at ingestion and ends with elimination of wastes and indigestible substances. This process is illustrated in Figure 5.25.

THE ABDOMINAL CAVITY

The organs of digestion are contained, for the most part, within the **abdominal cavity.** The abdominal cavity is bordered inferiorly by the pelvic floor, superiorly by the diaphragm, and anteriorly and laterally by abdominal wall musculature, as shown in Figure 5.26.

The abdominal cavity can be thought of as a large shallow bowl. Unfortunately, the only reliable distinguishing landmark on the anterior abdominal wall is the umbilicus. This point is used as a point of reference for describing areas of injury or pain. With the umbilicus as the center point, the abdomen has been divided into four quadrants. Each quadrant is named either left or right and upper or lower. This description is the most commonly used in emergency medicine and is pictured in Figure 5.27.

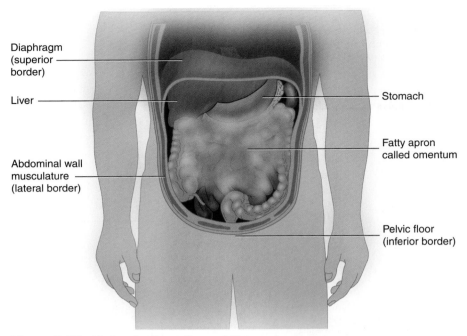

Figure 5.26 Abdominal cavity and its contents

Diaphragm (superior border)

Liver

Abdominal wall musculature (lateral border)

Stomach

Fatty apron called omentum

Pelvic floor (inferior border)

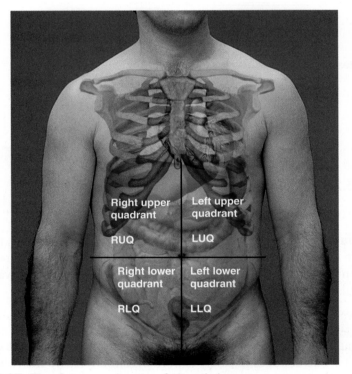

Figure 5.27 The four quadrants of the abdomen

Right upper quadrant

RUQ

Left upper quadrant

LUQ

Right lower quadrant

RLQ

Left lower quadrant

LLQ

THE DIGESTIVE ORGANS

The first portion of the digestive process occurs in the mouth. It is in the mouth that food is chewed, or masticated, mixed with digestive enzymes found in saliva, and swallowed as a mass, or a bolus. This bolus is then passed down the oropharynx, past the closed epiglottis, and swallowed into the

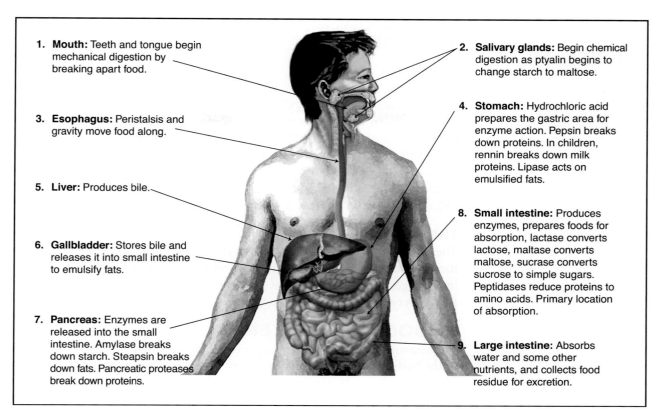

1. **Mouth:** Teeth and tongue begin mechanical digestion by breaking apart food.

2. **Salivary glands:** Begin chemical digestion as ptyalin begins to change starch to maltose.

3. **Esophagus:** Peristalsis and gravity move food along.

4. **Stomach:** Hydrochloric acid prepares the gastric area for enzyme action. Pepsin breaks down proteins. In children, rennin breaks down milk proteins. Lipase acts on emulsified fats.

5. **Liver:** Produces bile.

6. **Gallbladder:** Stores bile and releases it into small intestine to emulsify fats.

7. **Pancreas:** Enzymes are released into the small intestine. Amylase breaks down starch. Steapsin breaks down fats. Pancreatic proteases break down proteins.

8. **Small intestine:** Produces enzymes, prepares foods for absorption, lactase converts lactose, maltase converts maltose, sucrase converts sucrose to simple sugars. Peptidases reduce proteins to amino acids. Primary location of absorption.

9. **Large intestine:** Absorbs water and some other nutrients, and collects food residue for excretion.

Figure 5.28 The gastrointestinal system

esophagus. The esophagus, approximately 10 inches long, is a collapsible muscular tube that directs food into the stomach.

Once past the thoracic cavity and safely in the stomach, the bolus of food is further broken down by stomach acids and digestive enzymes. The stomach then empties its contents into the **small intestine.** About 90% of digestion (the breakdown and absorption of sugars and nutrients) occurs in the small intestine.

The small intestine is the largest digestive organ, taking up the majority of the abdominal cavity. The small intestine can be found in all four quadrants.

Other digestive enzymes excreted from the **gallbladder,** such as bile, aid in the process of digestion. The gallbladder is found in the upper right quadrant under the liver and is an important aid to digestion of fatty foods.

The large intestine encircles the abdominal cavity. At the end of the small intestine, the **large intestine** ascends within the right side of the abdomen and then crosses the superior abdomen and descends in the left side. The large intestine terminates at the midline **rectum.** The rectum forms and stores the feces that is eventually expelled out of the **anus.** This material consists of indigestible or unusable food products as well as other metabolic waste products. The pathway of digestion and gastrointestinal elimination can be seen in Figure 5.28.

THE APPENDIX

The **appendix** is a tubular organ attached to the large intestine that has no known function. Generally, most people go through life unaware that they have an appendix until this small pouch becomes inflamed by material trapped within it, a condition called *appendicitis.*

Externally, the appendix can be found in the lower right quadrant of the abdominal cavity. More specifically, if a mental (imaginary) triangle starting at the umbilicus (belly button) extending to the crest of the hip then to the pubis bone and then back to the umbilicus is formed, the appendix can be found in the middle of that triangle at a position called McBurney's point. Pain and tenderness at McBurney's point is highly suspicious for appendicitis.

THE LIVER

The **liver** is a solid organ in the right upper quadrant that serves to create the digestive bile stored in the gallbladder and has a number of other functions. All blood from the intestines must first pass through the liver before it can be circulated to the rest of the body. The liver neutralizes, or detoxifies, any poisons (toxins) in the bloodstream.

The liver also contributes to the production of factors that allow blood clotting (coagulation). Finally, the liver stores an emergency sugar supply called *glycogen* that is released whenever a person's blood sugar gets too low.

THE PANCREAS

The **pancreas,** a large gland located in the center of the abdomen and under the liver, creates some of the most powerful digestive fluids, or enzymes, in the digestive tract. In fact, the pancreas can create up to 2 quarts of these fluids every day as well as the hormone insulin.

ENDOCRINE SYSTEM

The nervous system provides the immediate moment-to-moment control of the body. Helping the nervous system maintain a more constant control of the body is the **endocrine system.**

The endocrine system is probably best known for the hormones that it produces. **Hormones** are chemicals that are produced by certain organs called **glands** and excreted into the bloodstream.

Once in the bloodstream, these hormones affect certain **target organs** or cells and change the way that organ or cell is functioning. This sort of chemical message transmission can be affected by prescription medicines. Figure 5.29 depicts many of the glands and target organs of the endocrine system.

An example of an endocrine gland and its hormone that will be relevant to the EMT is the pancreas. The *pancreas* is responsible for production of the hormone insulin, which is needed to control blood sugar levels in the body.

Insulin helps the body to use glucose. The pancreas produces more insulin when glucose levels are high, as is typical after a meal. Diabetics cannot produce insulin as needed and are therefore unable to use their glucose, resulting in high blood glucose levels. Diabetics are treated with insulin injections to replace the insulin that their pancreas cannot produce.

THE RETROPERITONEAL CAVITY

Clearly, the majority of the vital organs are contained within the cranial cavity, the thoracic cavity, and the abdominal cavity. There is another, often-overlooked, cavity—the retroperitoneal cavity.

The retroperitoneal cavity is located in the posterior of the abdomen. It is separated from the abdominal cavity by a thin lining called the peritoneum. Some of the intra-abdominal structures lie partially in the retroperitoneal cavity. Several structures lie completely within the retroperitoneal cavity— namely, the kidneys, the abdominal aorta, and the inferior vena cava.

THE KIDNEYS

The **kidney** is an organ that is densely packed with blood vessels. The purpose of the paired kidneys is to filter blood and from that filtrate eliminate unnecessary volumes of fluid, salts, and other wastes as urine. These organs are located on either side of the spine in the retroperitoneal cavity, well protected by the overlying lower rib cage.

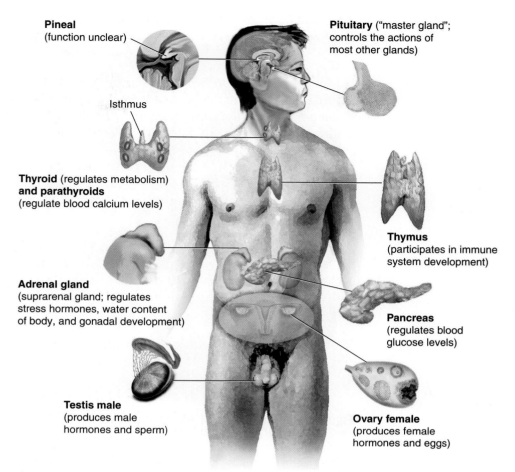

Figure 5.29 The endocrine system

Each kidney collects this urine in a collecting chamber within its center, called the *renal pelvis*. From the renal pelvis, the urine flows into pipelike structures called the **ureters.** The ureters are pencil-lead thick and may easily become blocked by solid collections of salts known as kidney stones.

The ureters are safely buried within a bed of muscle and fat within the retroperitoneal cavity. They empty into the **bladder,** which is an expandable container in the pelvis that can hold up to a quart of fluid. The kidneys and their associated structures are pictured in Figure 5.30.

THE LYMPHATIC SYSTEM

Paralleling the circulatory system is another circulatory system of sorts called the **lymphatic system,** which is often referred to as the *immune system.* The lymphatic system is filled with an almost colorless fluid that is very similar to blood plasma. This fluid, called **lymph,** carries away infectious microorganisms such as bacteria to the lymph nodes, solid glandlike bodies such as the tonsils, where white blood cells destroy them. **Lymph nodes** can be found in the neck, armpits, chest, spleen, abdomen, and pelvis.

The lymphatic system also assists the circulatory system to drain the body's tissues of excess fluids, returns that fluid to the central circulation, and discharges it into the vena cava via the lymphatic duct.

SPLEEN

The **spleen** is a solid, highly vascular organ made up of lymphatic tissue. It is located in the left upper quadrant of the abdomen, below the diaphragm and behind the stomach. The spleen serves to store blood, destroy old red blood

Pediatric Considerations

The spleen produces red blood cells in a fetus. When the long bones are fully developed, they take over the production of red blood cells, making the spleen's production of red blood cells insignificant in adulthood.

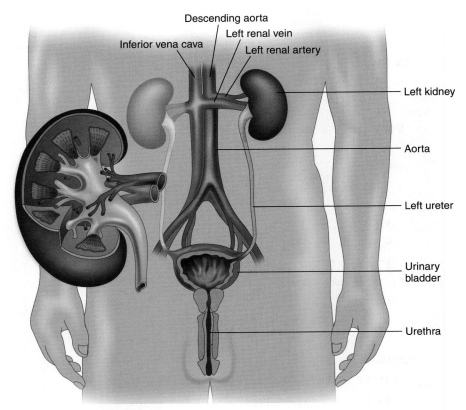

Figure 5.30 Structure of the urinary system

cells, filter foreign substances from the blood, and produce lymphocytes. Since the spleen is a highly vascular organ, trauma can produce severe bleeding. The spleen also plays a significant role in the immune system; therefore, individuals who have had their spleen removed due to trauma or disease may be at a higher risk for infections.

ACCESSORY SYSTEMS

The accessory systems are important systems, though not essential to life, that provide protection, support, and movement of the body, as well as the continuation of the species. The EMT may often be called to provide care for individuals who have an illness or injury to one of these systems.

THE INTEGUMENTARY SYSTEM

The skin is made up of many different tissues working together as a system. The skin is called the **integumentary system,** which means "covering."

The skin's outermost layer, the **epidermis,** is actually made up of layers of dead cells. These dead cells are constantly being rubbed, or abraded, off the body. At points where wear is intense, the skin actually develops calluses, or areas of thickened epidermis, to protect the underlying tissues.

Beneath the top skin layer is the **dermis.** Within the dermis are tiny blood vessels called capillaries and nerve endings that can sense heat, cold, pain, and pressure. The ability to feel these sensations is an important safety mechanism. Feeling heat or pain allows an individual to sense a potentially dangerous situation. Without the nerve endings found in the dermal layer of the skin, these useful warnings would be missed, putting individuals at greater risk for serious injury.

Sweat glands and hair follicles are also found within the dermis. These structures are important in temperature regulation. Sweat glands produce a

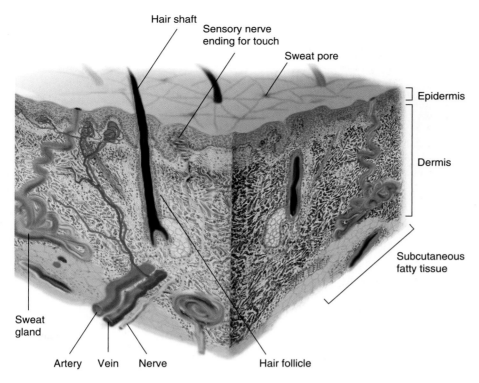

Figure 5.31 Structures of the skin

liquid that can bathe the skin and then evaporate to rid the body of excess heat. In cooler environments, hair serves as an insulator to maintain warmth.

Beneath the dermis is the **subcutaneous tissue** (*sub-* means "beneath," *cutaneous* means "skin"). The subcutaneous tissue connects the skin to the underlying muscular layer. Fat is also stored within this layer, serving not only as an energy reservoir but also as insulation to protect against extremes of temperature. Figure 5.31 shows the layers of the skin and important structures.

The skin has many functions. Perhaps one of its most important functions is that it protects the underlying structures from the external environment. One of the greatest environmental hazards the skin protects us from is disease-causing organisms. Bacteria and viruses do not usually penetrate intact skin. This is a protective mechanism against some types of infection.

Whenever an EMT approaches a patient, one of the first things he may notice about that patient is the appearance of the skin. Careful examination of the skin can provide the EMT with a wealth of information about the patient's condition, such as the quantity of blood circulating. The color of the patient's skin can reveal a lack of oxygen, liver failure, or severe carbon monoxide poisoning. The use of skin color as a diagnostic tool is discussed more in Unit 12.

THE MUSCULAR SYSTEM

Our ability to walk upright is a function of the unique musculoskeletal makeup of the human body. The ability of muscles to shorten, and in doing so to move the associated bone ends, is what permits movement. There are 206 bones in the human body and more than 650 muscles. An EMT should know a few of the larger muscles and bony structures. Most muscles can be remembered by either what they do or where they are. For example, the temporal muscle is attached at the temple of the forehead and moves the jaw. This muscle helps to chew food.

The **sternocleidomastoid muscle** is named for its points of origin and insertion. This muscle, also called the strap muscle, connects the sternum with the clavicle and the mastoid process and helps to lift the chest

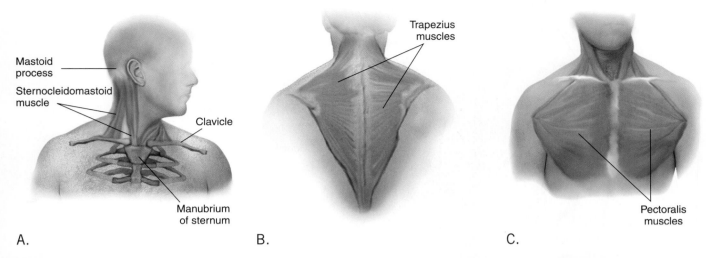

Figure 5.32 Muscles of the thorax A. Sternocleidomastoid muscle. B. Trapezius muscles. C. Pectoralis muscles

A.

B.

C.

Mastoid process

Sternocleidomastoid muscle

Clavicle

Manubrium of sternum

Trapezius muscles

Pectoralis muscles

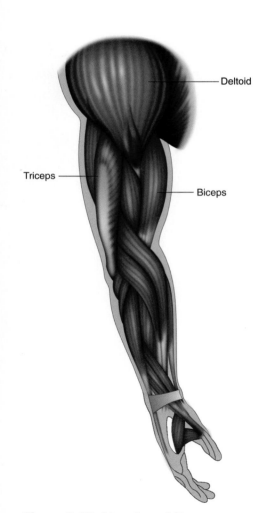

Deltoid

Triceps

Biceps

Figure 5.33 Muscles of the upper arm

wall. Because of this action, it is often referred to as an accessory muscle of breathing as it aids in expansion of the chest wall in times of respiratory distress.

The upper chest wall is blanketed, front and back, by large muscles. The triangular **trapezius muscles** cover the upper back and help to lift the shoulders. The **pectoralis major muscles** cover the anterior chest wall and help to lift the sternum and upper ribs. These important muscles of the thorax are shown in Figure 5.32.

Each shoulder and upper arm is covered and protected by a **deltoid muscle.** The deltoid muscle forms a triangle over the shoulder, with the base covering the shoulder and the apex pointing toward the elbow about two-thirds down the length of the upper arm. This is a site commonly used for intramuscular injections.

The **biceps muscle** is probably the best-known muscle. The request to "flex your muscles" usually means to display the biceps muscle of the upper arm as the elbow is bent and the muscle is contracted. The antagonist (a muscle that works in opposition to another muscle) to the biceps muscle is the **triceps muscle,** which straightens out the arm at the elbow. A depiction of the muscles of the upper extremity is found in Figure 5.33.

The anterior abdomen is protected by several strong layers of muscles. The diaphragm is another important muscle; it anatomically divides the abdominal cavity from the space enclosed within the rib cage, also known as the *chest cavity,* or the **thoracic cavity.** This muscle is vital in allowing normal breathing and is discussed in more detail later in this unit. These structures are shown in Figure 5.34.

The legs have a number of muscles that permit a person to stand, walk, and run. The larger muscles of the buttock, called the **gluteus muscles,** are important in allowing proper leg movement. Because of their easy identification, they are also another common site for intramuscular injections.

The **quadriceps muscle** runs down the anterior portion of the upper leg and permits us to extend our leg, such as when kicking a ball. The **gastrocnemius muscle,** or calf muscle, has been called the toe dancer's muscle because it enables a person to stand on his toes. Figure 5.35 shows the muscles of the lower extremity.

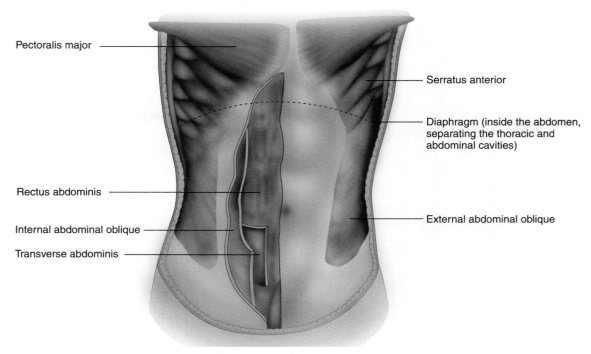

Figure 5.34 Muscles of the anterior abdominal wall

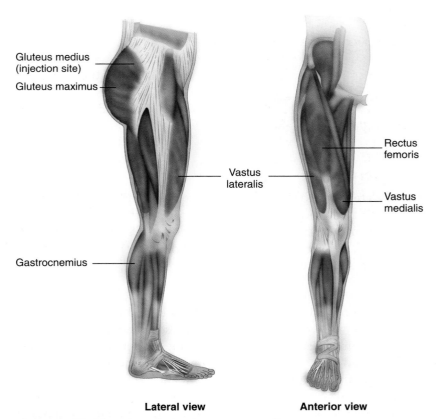

Lateral view   **Anterior view**

Figure 5.35 Muscles of the lower extremity

THE SKELETAL SYSTEM

The skeletal system constitutes the bony framework of the body. This framework serves two distinct purposes. The skeleton protects vital organs of the body and provides support for erect posture.

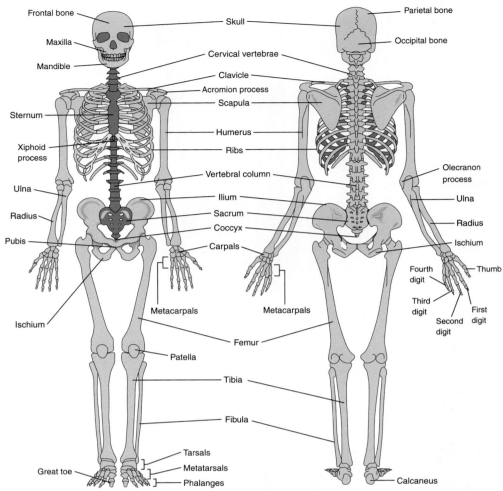

Figure 5.36 Axial (highlighted in blue) and the appendicular skeleton

THE AXIAL SKELETON

The **axial skeleton** includes the skull, the spinal column, and the bony ribs that are attached. These form the axis, or core, of the support structure of the body. The primary function of these bones is to protect the underlying brain, spinal cord, and thoracic and abdominal organs. The axial skeleton is illustrated in blue in Figure 5.36.

THE SKULL

The skull actually consists of multiple facial bones and several bones that make up the cranium itself. Figure 5.37 shows these in detail.

The face contains several large bones that provide support and a form to the jaw, cheeks, and nose. They are also involved in the act of chewing. The lower jawbone, or the **mandible,** is semicircular and contains teeth.

The **maxillae** are actually two bones that fuse at the midline to form the upper jaw. Attached to these bones is the anterior portion of the **hard palate** (the bone that forms the roof of the mouth).

The cheekbones are two bones that give shape and definition to the face. The cheekbones, or **zygomatic bones,** are attached at the temples and arch of the nose. The zygoma forms part of the eye's bony housing, or **orbit.** Parts of the orbital bones are thin and easily broken.

The **cranium** itself is an oblong egg-shaped collection of bones that is designed to protect the important anatomic structure underlying it, the brain.

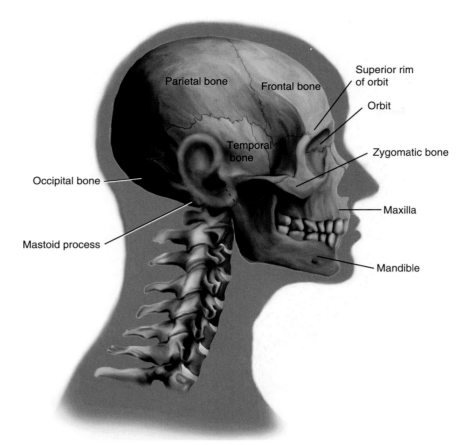

Figure 5.37 Bones of the skull and face

The anterior bone that makes up the forehead is called the **frontal bone,** and it is very strong. The **temporal bone,** which makes up the sides of the skull, along the temples, is weaker and more easily fractured with a direct blow. Located in the temporal bone, behind the ears, is the **mastoid sinus,** sometimes called the mastoid process. The term *sinus* means a cavity within a bone.

The posterior bone in the cranium is the **occipital bone.** The spinal cord passes through the occipital bone through a large opening called the **foramen magnum,** which translated means "big hole."

The largest of the bones of the skull is the **parietal bone,** which, by nature of its size and lateral position, protects a large part of the brain.

All the cranial bones are joined at immovable joints called **sutures.** The infant skull is not yet completely fused, and the sutures actually allow the skull to expand as the child's brain grows. Soft, flexible fibrous regions exist where several suture lines meet. These regions, called **fontanels** (Figure 5.38), are easily felt at the front and back of the head as "soft spots." Fontanels normally close and are no longer easily felt by about 18 months of age.

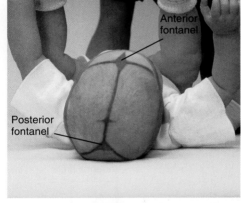

Figure 5.38 Fontanels of an infant's skull

THE SPINAL COLUMN

The **spinal column** is made up of a series of bones stacked one on top of another in a strong, yet flexible column. This unique design permits the spinal column to act as a series of joints, permitting bending, and to bear the weight of the entire body. The spinal column serves to support the head and provides for attachment of the ribs. Another important function is to protect the spinal cord, which lies within it.

The individual bones are called **vertebrae.** Each vertebra, except for the first two, has a drum-shaped center, called the *vertebral body,* that bears weight. A fibrous pad called an **intervertebral disk** cushions each vertebra. Posterior to the vertebral bodies are rings of bone that create the **vertebral foramen,** which houses the **spinal cord** (a collection of nerves that runs from the brain through the spinal column and branches to body organs and tissues). Figure 5.39 illustrates the anatomy of the spinal column.

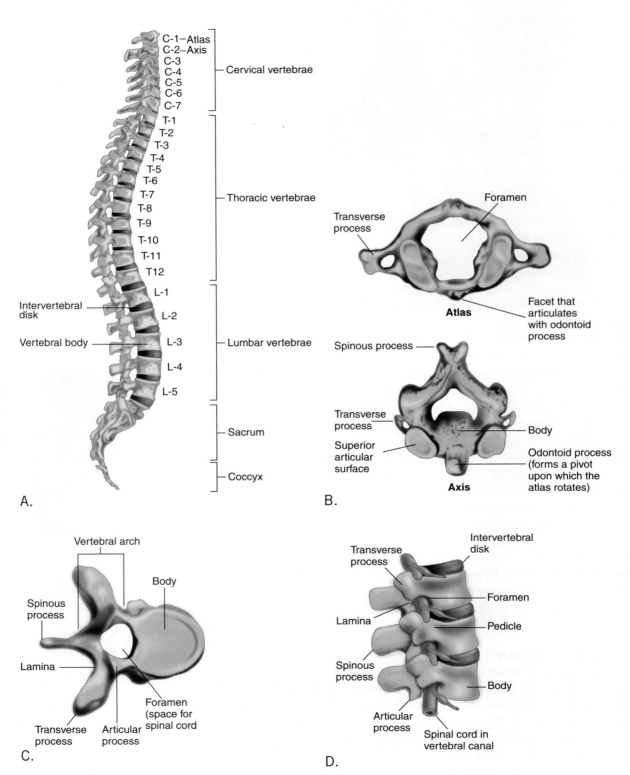

Figure 5.39A-D Anatomy of the spinal column

The spinal column has five distinct sections. The first is the cervical spine (or curvature), then the thoracic spine, followed by the lumbar spine, and finally the sacrum and coccyx.

The **cervical spine** (the uppermost section of the spinal column) is of particular importance to EMTs because it is particularly susceptible to injury during any traumatic event. In total, there are seven cervical vertebrae.

The posterior portion of the vertebra is called the **spinous process.** The spinous process of the seventh cervical vertebra can be easily felt, or palpated, at the base of the neck.

The first cervical vertebra, called the **atlas,** holds up the entire weight of the skull, like the mythical giant who is depicted as holding up the weight of the world. The second cervical vertebra is called the **axis.** This vertebra allows the head to turn from side to side, as the axle in a car allows the wheels of the car to go around.

An injury to any area of the cervical spine is potentially lethal if it damages the cervical spinal cord. The cervical portion of the spinal column is supported by muscles and ligaments but is not as well supported as the remainder of the spinal column, thus leaving it open to injury. To visualize the relative fragility of this portion of the spinal column, imagine a 22-pound bowling ball on the end of a broom handle. This would be analogous to the skull and the cervical spine (refer to Figures 5.36 and 5.37).

With a sudden force, such as might occur in a motor vehicle collision, either the muscles of the neck are strained or torn or the bones break. The broken bones may then protrude into the spinal canal and injure the fragile spinal cord, or the injury may produce such instability in the vertebral column that injury to the spinal cord may result.

The next 12 vertebrae are called the **thoracic vertebrae.** There is one spinal vertebra for each rib. These ribs originate at the spine and come together at the front of the chest, forming the **rib cage,** the bony structure that surrounds and protects the organs of the chest.

The next portion of the spinal column is the workhorse of the spine. The five **lumbar vertebrae** support the weight of the entire upper body. When an EMT bends and lifts a patient, he can put several hundred pounds of pressure on just a few of the five lumbar vertebrae. This pressure can cause quite a strain and, if done improperly, can result in serious injury.

The **sacral vertebrae** are actually a portion of the pelvic girdle. The five sacral vertebrae are usually joined or fused together to form a more solid point of contact for pelvic bones.

The last portion of the spinal column is called the tailbone, or the **coccyx.** If this bone were broken, for example after a fall, sitting would likely be very painful. The relationship between the cervical, thoracic, lumbar, sacral, and coccygeal vertebrae can be seen in Figure 5.39.

THE THORACIC CAGE

The heart and lungs, both vital organs, are protected and surrounded by a bony cage. This cage is called the rib cage and is made up of bony ribs, cartilage, and the sternum. Figure 5.40 shows the thoracic cage.

In the middle of the chest is the breastbone, also called the **sternum.** During CPR classes, all students are taught to identify the sternum and its landmarks. To review, the sternum has a **sternal body** or midportion. This is the section of the sternum upon which external cardiac compressions are performed. Logically, then, the heart must be under the body of the sternum.

The top section of the sternum is called the **manubrium.** The manubrium meets the body of the sternum at a bony ridge called the **sternal angle;**

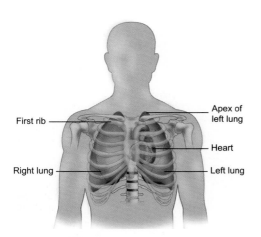

Figure 5.40 The thoracic cage. Note how it protects the heart and lungs

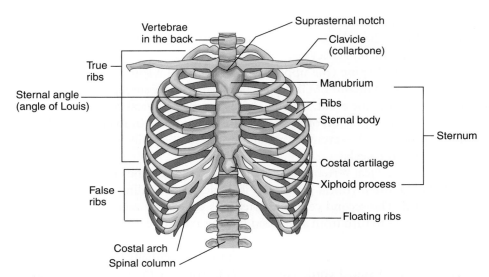

Figure 5.41 Anatomy of the rib cage and sternum (the sternum and rib cage are connected by cartilage)

it is also called the **angle of Louis** and is an important anatomic landmark on the chest wall.

Located at the uppermost border of the manubrium is the **suprasternal notch** (*supra-* is a prefix meaning "above"). Underneath the suprasternal notch lies the windpipe, or **trachea,** a cartilaginous tube that serves as the passageway for air to get to the lungs.

Returning to the main body of the sternum and running the fingers to the inferior portion, the EMT will palpate the **xiphoid process.** This bony protrusion is occasionally broken during external cardiac compressions if the hands are placed too low on the sternum. Underneath the xiphoid process lies the edge of the liver. Pieces of broken bone can injure the liver if external cardiac compressions are improperly performed. Figure 5.41 shows the anatomy of the rib cage and sternum.

The bulk of the rib cage is made up of ribs. These ribs attach posteriorly to the thoracic vertebrae. The top seven pairs of ribs are attached anteriorly to the sternum by cartilage. These seven pairs of ribs are called the **true ribs.** The next three pairs of ribs are attached anteriorly by cartilage to the seventh rib, not directly to the sternum. These are naturally called the **false ribs.** The false ribs form an umbrella-appearing curvature anteriorly called the **costal arch.** The remaining two ribs are unattached anteriorly and are therefore called the **floating ribs.**

The true ribs actually protect the vital organs in the thoracic cavity. The false ribs protect other important organs, such as the liver and the spleen, that are parts of the abdominal cavity, or the space between the chest and the pelvis, but do extend up into the chest. The diaphragm divides these two cavities. See Figure 5.42 for an illustration of this division.

Posteriorly, where the 10th rib and spine meet is the **costovertebral angle.** Underneath the costovertebral angle lies the kidney, somewhat protected from injury by the overlying ribs. The kidneys lie within the posterior part of the abdomen called the **retroperitoneal cavity.**

THE APPENDICULAR SKELETON

The remainders of the bones are a part of the appendages, or limbs, and are used primarily for support and movement. This **appendicular skeleton** is composed of the shoulder girdle, arms, pelvic girdle, and legs (refer to Figure 5.36).

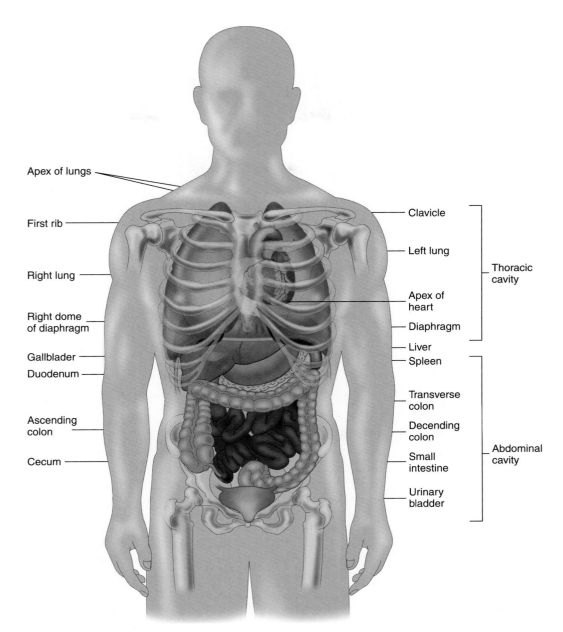

Figure 5.42 Abdominal and thoracic cavities are separated by the muscular diaphragm

THE SHOULDER GIRDLE

The shoulder girdle consists of two sets of bones, the clavicles and the scapulas. These bones create an insertion point for the arm to attach to the trunk.

The first bony prominences at the superior, anterior part of the chest that the EMT should identify are the collarbones, or clavicles. The clavicles protect the thoracic organs from blows from above.

Another pair of bones that lie over the top of the rib cage are located posteriorly and superiorly. These are the shoulder blades, or **scapulas.** The scapulas—a term related to the word for *blades*—are large flat bones that protect the posterior rib cage. Together, the scapula and the clavicles create the point of insertion for the arms, forming the shoulders. Figure 5.43 shows the scapula and the clavicles and illustrates the interrelation between the two sets of bones.

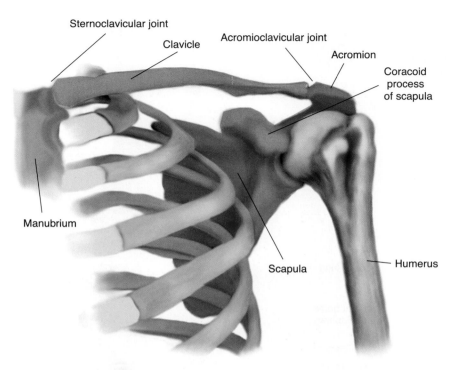

Figure 5.43 The shoulder girdle

THE ARMS

The arms, or **upper extremities,** and particularly the hands, provide us with the ability to perform uniquely human functions such as grasping and carrying. The arms can be divided into three sections: the upper arm, the forearm, and the hand.

The Upper Arm   The upper arm has only one bone, called the **humerus.** This long bone attaches to the body at the shoulder joint. The forearm attaches to the upper arm at the elbow. Along the shaft of the humerus run veins, an artery called the brachial artery, and nerves. The humerus protects these important structures. Almost all the long bones of the body have veins, arteries, and nerves running next to them. This association is shown in Figure 5.44.

When a patient strikes an elbow against a hard surface, the nerve along the humerus is pinched between the surface and the bone. Laypeople call this "hitting your funny bone," but the pain created by the impact of the humerus upon the nerve is anything but funny to those who have experienced it.

The Forearm   The forearm has two bones that are attached at the elbow and to the wrist. The bones of the forearm are the **ulna** and the **radius.** These bones are sometimes fractured during falls on an outstretched hand.

The ulna lies on the medial side, closest to the little finger of the hand. This bone provides firm support for the forearm.

The radius attaches to the wrist proximal to the thumb. The radius turns around the ulna whenever the palm of the hand is turned over. When the palmar surface of the hand is facing downward, in pronation, the ulna and radius are crossed. When the hand is turned upward, in supination, the radius bone completes a radius, in a circular motion, and the bones are parallel. The bones of the lower arm are labeled in Figure 5.45.

The brachial artery that parallels the humerus divides, or bifurcates, at the elbow, and one artery runs down each of the bones of the forearm. EMTs often take a count of the heartbeat, called a **pulse,** at the point where the

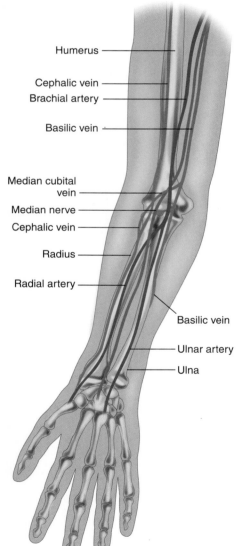

Figure 5.44 The arm

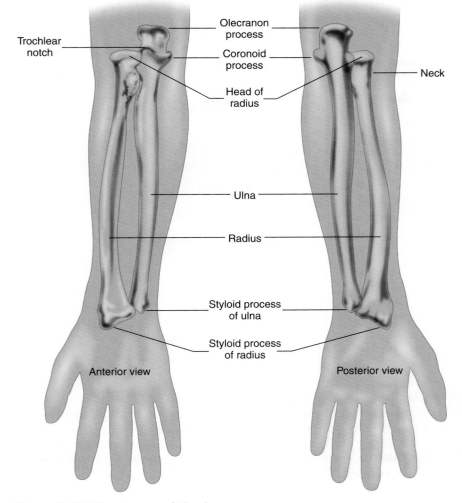

Trochlear notch

Olecranon process

Coronoid process

Head of radius

Neck

Ulna

Radius

Styloid process of ulna

Styloid process of radius

Anterior view

Posterior view

Figure 5.45 The bones of the lower arm

radial artery crosses over the radius bone in the wrist. A heartbeat felt at this site is called a radial pulse.

The Hand   Each hand is made up of 27 bones. These bones have been divided into carpals, metacarpals, and phalanges. Together, these small bones enable an individual to perform complex and intricate tasks.

Starting at the wrist, the **carpal bones** form two rows consisting of four bones each. The **metacarpals** form the framework for the palm of the hand. The fingers are formed by bones called **phalanges.** These bones are identified by their position relative to the wrist. The most distal bones are called distal phalanges; the most proximal to the metacarpals are the proximal phalanges. All the fingers except for the thumb have a third phalanx in the middle, called the middle phalynx. The bones of the hand are identified in Figure 5.46.

THE PELVIC GIRDLE
The bony pelvis supports the organs of digestion, elimination, and reproduction. This bony bowl-like structure is made up of the ilium, ischium, and pubis. The spine inserts into the pelvis at the rear; consequently, all the weight of the body is supported by the pelvis.

The Ilium   The most easily recognized part of the pelvis is the "hip bones," or the **iliac bones.** The superior portions are referred to as the iliac wings because of their shape. The iliac crests, at the top of the wings, can be felt on

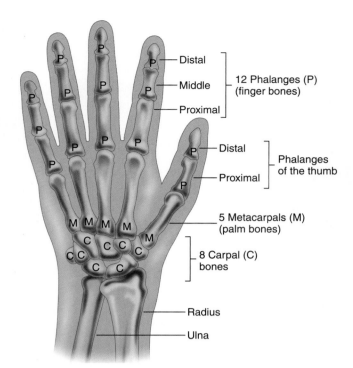

Figure 5.46 Bones of the hand

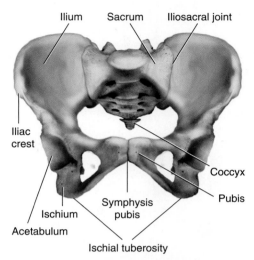

Figure 5.47 The pelvic girdle

most patients at the point where it is common to put the hands on the hips. The iliac bones create the main shape of the pelvis. The female pelvis is wider than the male pelvis and is well adapted for childbirth.

The Ischium   The portion of the pelvis that supports our weight as we sit is called the **ischium.** A bony prominence of the ischium is used as a point of fixation for splints of the lower legs.

The Pubis   At the very front of the pelvis is the **pubis,** consisting of two bones that complete the pelvic ring anteriorly. The joint formed by the union of the two pubis bones is called the **symphysis pubis.** Directly underneath the symphysis pubis lies the urinary bladder. EMTs may sometimes apply a gentle downward pressure to the symphysis pubis, while assessing for injury, to see if the pelvic ring has been disturbed. The bony pelvis is shown in Figure 5.47.

THE LEGS

The legs, or **lower extremities,** permit us to stand erect, walk, and run. Performance of all these activities requires a large number of well-coordinated muscles as well as the support of some major bones. Like the arm, the leg can be divided into upper and lower portions.

The Upper Leg   The upper leg has only one bone, like the upper arm, and it is called the **femur.** Found deep within the thigh, the femur is the longest and strongest bone in the body. The femur turns inward at the hip and inserts into its socket in the pelvis, called the **acetabulum.** The area where the femur meets the acetabulum is referred to as the hip. These structures can be seen in Figure 5.48.

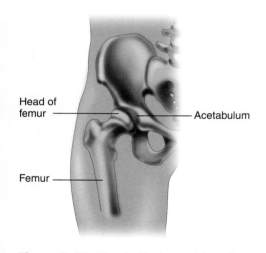

Figure 5.48 The ball-shaped head of the femur fits smoothly into the socket-shaped acetabulum to form the hip joint

The Patella   The **knee** is the joint between the femur and the lower leg. The **patella,** or kneecap, is a bony disk that lies over the anterior aspect of the knee, helping to protect the inner joint. Many people accidentally displace or dislocate their kneecap. However, it takes a great deal of force to dislocate the knee itself. A dislocated knee is a surgical emergency, whereas a dislocated kneecap is not. The patella is labeled in Figure 5.49.

The Lower Leg   Many people have "skinned the shin bone" in a fall. The shinbone, or the **tibia,** is the bone along the front of the lower leg, and it is covered anteriorly with only a thin layer of skin and fat. The other bone in the lower leg is the **fibula,** which is found at the lateral aspect of the lower leg.

On both sides of the ankle are bony prominences of the distal tibia or fibula called the medial and lateral **malleolus.** There is a pulse point posterior to the medial malleolus called the **posterior tibial pulse.** Figure 5.50 illustrates these structures of the lower leg.

The Foot   The saying goes "man is like a monkey; his feet are like his hands." This is true of the bones of the foot with one exception. Instead of being called carpals, the bones are called **tarsals.** The largest bone in the foot is the **calcaneus,** or heel bone. Figure 5.51 shows the bones of the foot in detail.

THE JOINTS

Joints are the points where bones meet bones. Joints permit a degree of movement called the *range of motion.* Each joint has its own normal range of motion. An injury to a joint may result in a decrease in this range of motion.

THE REPRODUCTIVE SYSTEM

There are obvious differences between male and female reproductive anatomy. Both sexes have organs of reproduction called glands or **gonads.** In the

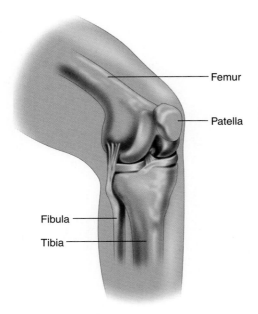

Figure 5.49 The knee and patella

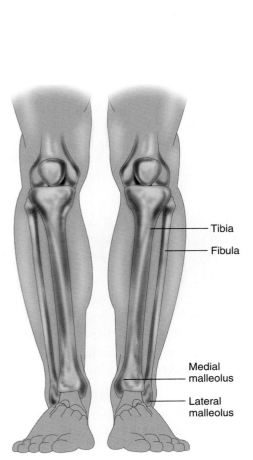

Figure 5.50 The lower leg

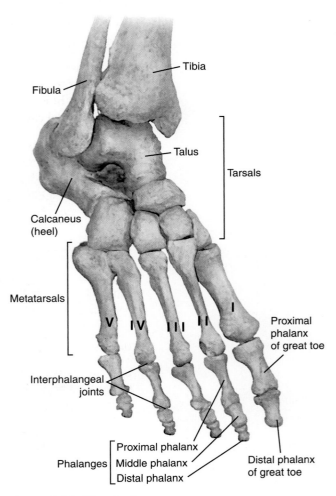

Figure 5.51 The foot

male, these are the testes, and in the female, the ovaries. All other features of these two systems are distinctly different between male and female.

MALE REPRODUCTIVE ORGANS

The male reproductive organs are situated outside of the abdominal cavity and consist of the testes and penis.

THE TESTES

The **testes** are the main sex hormone–producing glands in the male and are suspended outside of the body in a pouch called the **scrotum.** This pair of gonads produces the hormone called testosterone. Testosterone is responsible for the secondary sex characteristics of the male. These include facial hair, deep voice, broad shoulders, and profuse body hair. The testes are also responsible for producing the sperm that will fertilize a female's egg during conception.

THE PENIS

The **penis** is a conduit for the passage of both urine and semen. Semen is the fluid that contains not only the sperm (male reproductive material) from the testes but also fluid from the seminal vesicles and the **prostate gland** that assists in transport of the sperm.

The prostate gland also serves to block urine flow while it assists with the expulsion of semen, called *ejaculation.* If this gland becomes enlarged, as sometimes occurs in old age, then normal urine flow may become interrupted.

Because of the relatively unprotected location of the male genitalia, the penis and testes are prone to injury from trauma. Figure 5.52 shows the structures of the male genital system.

FEMALE REPRODUCTIVE ORGANS

The female reproductive organs are located in the pelvic cavity. This positioning protects these organs somewhat during nonpregnant states. During pregnancy, however, the enlarged uterus extends out of the pelvis and into the abdominal cavity.

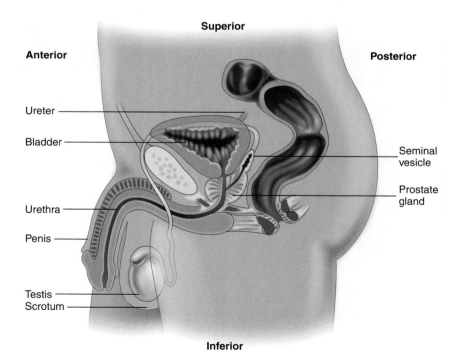

Figure 5.52 The male reproductive system

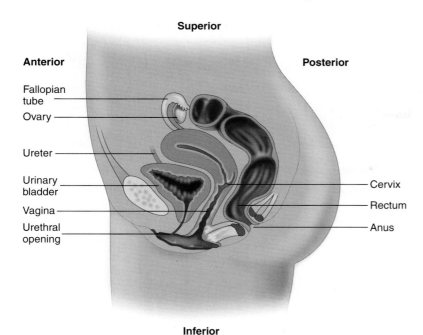

Superior

Anterior

Posterior

Fallopian tube

Ovary

Ureter

Urinary bladder

Vagina

Urethral opening

Cervix

Rectum

Anus

Inferior

Figure 5.53 The female reproductive system

THE OVARIES

The primary female gonad is the **ovary.** The ovary produces characteristic female sex hormones, such as estrogen and progesterone. These hormones are responsible for the development of female secondary sex characteristics such as breasts, wide hips, and typical distribution of fat.

The ovaries contain a woman's entire life supply of eggs. On average, every 28 days a mature woman's ovary releases an egg for fertilization. The egg passes through a structure called the **fallopian tube.** It is usually inside the fallopian tube that an egg may unite with a sperm and become fertilized, resulting in pregnancy.

THE UTERUS

The **uterus** is a muscular pouch that is known to the layperson as the womb. It is inside the uterus that the fertilized egg becomes implanted and where it grows and becomes a fetus. Stages of pregnancy are discussed further in Unit 40.

If the egg is not fertilized or the implantation is incomplete, then the egg and the uterine lining are swept out of the uterus in a menstrual flow. This flow occurs monthly and is referred as **menstruation.**

THE VAGINA

The **vagina** serves several functions. First, it is the path by which the menstrual flow exits the body. Second, it is the conduit for the acceptance of the male penis during coitus, the act of sexual intercourse.

Finally, the vagina serves as the birth canal. When an infant is ready to be delivered, the head passes down the vaginal canal and out of the vaginal opening. Figure 5.53 shows the structures of the female genitalia.

CONCLUSION

Although this review has been brief, it is important for the EMT to be familiar with basic anatomy and to know the normal functioning of the human body. Only with this knowledge can the EMT begin to recognize when a physical problem exists and how to go about remedying that problem.

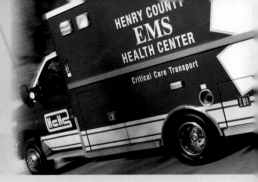

CASE STUDY Continued

Jeremy stops, thinks, and remembers that an anatomy course is a prerequisite for the paramedic program. He wants to become a paramedic eventually. "Perfect," he thinks to himself, "I can take an anatomy course while I'm working as an EMT. That way I can get more experience with patient care while preparing for paramedic school without wasting time." Jeremy resolves to call the college and find out when the next anatomy class is to begin.

Key Concepts Revisited

- Emergency Medical Technicians (EMTs) need an understanding of basic anatomy and concepts of physiology of the human body to effectively manage the nature of an individual's illness or injury.

- The use of standard terminology when referring to the motions and different anatomical structures of the body include:
  - Topographical anatomy
  - Standard anatomical position
  - Anatomical positions

- The EMT can describe physical findings using an accepted reference point and direction terms.
  - Lines of reference
  - Directional terms
  - Range of motion

- The organs and function of the vital systems are required for life:
  - The nervous system controls and coordinates bodily functions. The subdivisions of the nervous system include:
    - The central nervous system, which is responsible for the initiation and transmission of all control-oriented messages throughout the body. The structures include:
      - The brain
      - The spinal cord
  - The peripheral nervous system, which is responsible for the relay of messages between the spinal cord and the organs and tissues of the body.

  - The autonomic nervous system, which is responsible for the transmission of vital impulses from the brainstem to the organs of the body, including the heart.

  - The circulatory system, which transports oxygen and other nutrients to the body's organs and removes the metabolic wastes of cellular metabolism. The circulatory system includes:
    - The heart
    - The blood vessels
    - The blood

  - The respiratory system, which is responsible for breathing and the exchange of oxygen for carbon dioxide. The structures of respiration include:
    - The upper and lower airways
    - The structures of the chest
    - The process of ventilation
    - The process of respiration

- The structures and function of the core systems of the body are essential to life, serving to regulate and support the vital systems. The core systems include:
  - The digestive system, which serves to deliver a nutritional flow, providing the body with extract sugars and other nutrients it needs to survive.
    - The abdominal cavity holds the organs of digestion
  - The endocrine system, which helps the nervous system maintain constant control of the body.

○ The retroperitoneal cavity, which provides the space and protection for the vital organs of circulation (abdominal aorta and inferior vena cava) and the kidneys (the organs that maintain a balance of fluids, salts, and other wastes)

○ The lymphatic system (immune system), which protects the body from disease through development of immunities, transporting infectious microorganisms to structures within the system to be destroyed by white blood cells and draining excess fluids from tissue spaces.

• The assessor systems are not essential but are important systems of the body providing support, protection, movement, and procreation. The assessor systems include:

○ The integumentary system, the skin, which serves to protect the body from the environment and disease-causing organisms and regulate body temperature.

○ The muscular system, which is responsible for movement of the skeleton, food through the digestive tract, blood through the circulatory systems, and specialized cardiac muscle causing the heart to contract.

○ The skeletal system, which protects the vital organs of the body and provides support for erect posture.

○ The reproductive system, which is necessary for the continuation of the human species.

Key Terms

Abdominal cavity
Abduction
Acetabulum
Adduction
Alveoli
Anatomy
Angle of Louis
Anterior
Anus
Aorta
Aortic valve
Apex
Appendicular skeleton
Appendix
Arachnoid
Arteries
Atlas
Atrioventricular (AV) node
Atrium
Autonomic nervous system
Axial skeleton
Axilla
Axis
Base
Biceps muscle
Bilateral
Bladder

Blood
Blood vessels
Brainstem
Bronchi
Bronchioles
Bundle branches
Bundle of His
Calcaneus
Capillaries
Carina
Carpal bones
Central
Central nervous system
Cerebellum
Cerebrospinal fluid (CSF)
Cerebrum
Cervical spine
Cilia
Circulation
Clavicle
Coccyx
Costal arch
Costovertebral angle
Cranium
Deep
Deltoid muscle
Dermis

Diaphragm

Distal

Dorsal

Dura mater

Endocrine system

Epidermis

Epiglottis

Esophagus

Eversion

Extension

Fallopian tube

False ribs

Femur

Fibula

Flexion

Floating ribs

Fontanels

Foramen magnum

Fowler's position

Frontal bone

Gallbladder

Gastronomius muscle

Glands

Gluteus muscles

Goblet cell

Gonads

Hard palate

Heart

Hemostasis

High-Fowler's position

Homeostasis

Hormones

Humerus

Iliac bones

Inferior

Insulin

Integumentary system

Intervertebral disk

Inversion

Ischium

Jugular vein

Kidney

Knee

Large intestine

Larynx

Lateral

Left lateral recumbent position

Liver

Lower extremities

Lumbar vertebrae

Lymph

Lymph node

Lymphatic system

Malleolus

Mandible

Manubrium

Mastoid sinus

Maxillae

Medial

Meninges

Menstruation

Metabolism

Metacarpals

Midaxillary line

Midclavicular lines

Midline

Mitral valve

Modified Trendelenburg

Nasopharynx

Nervous system

Occipital bone

Orbit

Oropharynx

Ovary

Palmar

Pancreas

Parietal bone

Parietal pleura

Patella

Pectoralis major muscles

Penis

Perfusion

Peripheral

Peripheral nervous system

Phalanges
Physiology
Pia mater
Plantar
Posterior
Posterior tibial pulse
Pressure points
Pronation
Prone
Prostate gland
Proximal
Pubis
Pulmonary artery
Pulmonary circuit
Pulmonary valve
Pulmonary vein
Pulse
Purkinje fibers
Quadriceps muscle
Radius
Recovery position
Rectum
Red blood cells
Respiration
Retroperitoneal cavity
Rib cage
Sacral vertebrae
Scapulas
Scrotum
Shock position
Sinoatrial (SA) node
Small intestine
Spinal column
Spinal cord
Spinous process
Spleen
Standard anatomical position
Sternal angle
Sternal body
Sternocleidomastoid muscle

Sternum
Subcutaneous tissue
Superficial
Superior
Supination
Supine
Suprasternal notch
Sutures
Symphysis pubis
Systemic circuit
Target organs
Tarsals
Temporal bone
Terminal bronchioles
Testes
Thoracic cavity
Thoracic vertebrae
Tibia
Topographic anatomy
Trachea
Trapezius muscles
Triceps muscle
Tricuspid valve
True ribs
Ulna
Unilateral
Upper extremities
Ureter
Uterus
Vagina
Veins
Vena cava
Ventilation
Ventral
Ventricle
Vertebrae
Vertebral foramen
Visceral pleura
Xiphoid process
Zygomatic bone

Review Questions

1. Define the standard anatomical position.
2. What is the most important function of the skin?
3. What is the name of the hormone responsible for the metabolism of sugar? What organ produces this hormone?
4. What is the function of the nervous system?
5. What are the vital systems of the body?
6. What are the assessory systems?
7. What is the function of the kidneys?
8. Define respiration.
9. Name the structures of the upper and lower airway.
10. Describe the direction of blood flow.

Further Study

Scott, A. S., & Fong, E. *Body structures and functions.* 10th ed. Clifton Park, NY: Thomson Delmar Learning, 2004.

UNIT ⑥ Pathophysiology

Many diseases, disorders, and syndromes can affect physical health and the body's susceptibility to illness or injuries. The EMT should have a basic understanding of some common causes of illness and the body's response to illness and injury. Understanding the processes of disease will aid the EMT in applying appropriate assessment and management techniques. Specific illnesses and injuries are discussed more thoroughly throughout this book.

National Education Standards
The Emergency Medical Technician (EMT) will be able to apply a fundamental understanding of the pathophysiology of respiration and perfusion to patient assessment and management.

Key Concepts

- An understanding of pathophysiology, or the functional changes associated with or resulting from disease or injury, is necessary for effective management of that illness or injury.

- Predisposing risk factors can make an individual more susceptible to disease.

- Hypoxia, insufficient oxygen available for the body's tissues, is the number one chemical cause of cellular injury.

- The brain, which is the life center of the body, requires sufficient glucose-rich, oxygenated blood to function.

- Every known disease interferes with the process known as the Fick Principle.

- Adequate oxygen concentration of air is necessary for life.

- An intact and functioning respiratory system is necessary for oxygenation to take place.

- Diseases that impair or arrest ventilation and respiration upset homeostasis, leading to hypoxia without intervention.

- Diseases that affect any of the components that make up the circulatory system can result in decreasing the available gases for diffusion.

- Cellular metabolism is a vital chemical reaction required in the production of energy required by cells to survive.

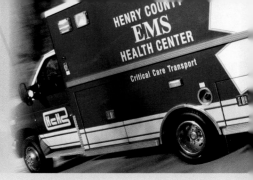

CASE STUDY

As Beth rolls the stretcher down the hall of the nursing home, she quickly scans the patient's medical record for details that might help explain the patient's sudden shortness of breath. The patient has a history of emphysema, probably from years of smoking. She looks down and thinks to herself, "He was probably a World War II veteran." She remembers her grandfather telling her that during the war the U.S. Army actually gave soldiers cigarettes in small packs and told them to "smoke'm if you got'em" when they paused for break. This small reward was often a welcome relief from the drudgery of marching. As a result, many soldiers became lifelong smokers, unable to "break the habit."

Beth also notes that the patient has heart damage from a heart attack several years ago that left him with heart failure. Knowing that the heart and lungs work together, Beth wonders if this might be the cause of the patient's shortness of breath.

Then she sees the diagnosis of lung cancer. Lung cancer can be devastating. Beth watched her grandmother die from it and remembered how she struggled for a breath toward the end and eventually died drowning in her own blood. The memory makes Beth tremble, but she smiles reassuringly at the old man on the stretcher.

Critical Thinking Questions

1. Why would smoking cause lung damage?
2. How does a heart attack lead to heart failure?
3. How does heart failure cause shortness of breath?
4. Why would a patient drown in his or her own blood from lung cancer?

INTRODUCTION

Pathophysiology (PATH-oh-FIZ-ee-ol-oh-jee) is the study of the functional changes associated with, or resulting from, disease or injury. It is the junction of normal human physiology and pathology, as they apply to the study of the nature and causes of disease or injury. Thus, an understanding of the changes caused by a disease or injury enables the EMT to determine the appropriate management of that illness or injury.

Pathology (pah-THOL-oh-jee) is defined as the study of disease. **Pathogens** (PATH-oh-jens) are the agents (microorganisms) of disease such as bacteria, viruses, and fungi that cause the pathogenic reaction. For example, bone disease such as osteoporosis can cause weakened bones to fracture. These types of fractures are considered pathologic fractures because they are a result of the disease process. To effectively treat the symptoms and remove the cause of disease requires an understanding of the **pathogenesis,** which refers to how the disease begins and progresses and what occurs at the molecular and cellular level.

DISEASE

Disease is a term often used to describe a condition in which abnormal symptoms occur. The term may also be used to describe an abnormal change in the structure or function of cells, tissues, or organs of the body. The body strives to maintain a state of sameness or normalcy, a concept called *homeostasis* (HOME-ee-oh-STAY-sis). When changes in the structure and function of cells interfere with homeostasis, the body becomes diseased.

The term **disorder** is used to explain a pathologic condition of the body and mind. The term is used when describing a condition involving a deficiency, such as nutrition as seen in an eating disorder. *Disorder* can also be used to refer to problems with the structure of the skeletal system (bone disorders) or other condition in which the term *disease* does not apply, such as an autistic disorder. *Disease* and *disorder* are closely related and often used synonymously.

Syndrome refers to a group of similar features, including certain signs, symptoms, and characteristics that occur together. These similar characteristics are caused by a specific disease or related problems, such as seen in persons with Down syndrome.

ETIOLOGY OF DISEASE

The cause or origin of a disease is called the **etiology** (EE-tee-OL-oh-jee) of that disease. As an example, disease-causing bacteria is the etiology of an infection is a microorganism or microbe, such as bacteria. The etiology of a disease may be from a fungus, virus, or bacterium. Other compounding factors, such as malnutrition, poor living conditions, or lack of immunizations, may influence the type and severity of disease.

There are times when the cause of a disease is of "unknown etiology" or **idiopathic** (ID-ee-oh-PATH-ik). The cause of an emerging disease is unknown until several cases have occurred, providing a sufficient number to be studied to identify the source of the disease and develop a treatment.

RISK FACTORS

Risk factors are predisposing factors that can make a person more susceptible to disease. These factors can include age, gender, environment, lifestyle, and heredity. Lifestyle behaviors are risk factors that people can modify or change, while others, such as age and gender, cannot be changed. Every person has some risk factors, making that person more or less susceptible to a disease when compared to another person.

Lifestyle behaviors are examples of risk factors over which people have some control. We can reduce our risk for disease and improve overall health by avoiding such risk factors as smoking, alcohol consumption, lack of exercise, and excessive stress. Additionally, practicing healthy behaviors to prevent contamination and transmission of disease by using standard precautions and thorough hand washing are also important.

Heredity and gender are both examples of risk factors that cannot be changed. Some diseases occur more often in one gender or the other. Breast cancer is far more common in women, although it does occur in men. Additionally, a woman with a family member who has had breast cancer has a higher chance of developing breast cancer herself. Knowledge of these risk factors provides individuals the opportunity to decrease overall risks by modifying their lifestyle behaviors.

PROGNOSIS

Prognosis (prawg-KNOW-sis) is the expected or predicted outcome of a disease. The prognosis for the common cold is that the patient should feel better in 3 to 5 days without specific therapy.

A disease is usually classified as being *acute* in nature if it has a rapid onset and short duration. A chronic disease, on the other hand, persists for a long time and may have begun slowly, initially without symptoms.

The occurrences of chronic diseases, such as hypertension (high blood pressure), increase with age. Chronic and acute disease can be mild or life threatening.

> ### Street Smart
>
> The use of tobacco was originally thought to be safe. Many people were engaged in tobacco use, unaware of the adverse effects of such behavior. Smoking and other tobacco use is a risk factor now known to cause disease, such as lung cancer.

A prognosis is subject to change throughout the progression of a disease. If a person develops a complication, such as the onset of a second disease or disorder, the prognosis will change to include the effects of these complications. An example would be a person with a common cold who is expected to feel better in 3 to 5 days but then develops bacterial pneumonia. The prognosis may change considerably with the additional infection.

PREDICTABLE OUTCOMES OF DISEASE

There are three predictable outcomes when a person is affected by disease: recovery, survival with remission, or death.

Recovery generally means the person has returned to health, with no remnant of the disease. The patient's recovery may include some physical or chemical changes called **residuals,** such as weakness or paralysis on one side of the body following a stroke. Some infectious diseases, such as tuberculosis, can become **dormant** or in a state of biological rest, until favorable environment exist for them to become active again.

Some patients live with a disease that has gone into a nonactive state called **remission.** Remission does not mean the patient is cured of the disease, but rather that the disease as been stopped.

Diseases that commonly lead to the death are said to have a high mortality rate. Death occurs when the body's defense mechanisms become overwhelmed and the body can no longer fight the progression of the disease.

CELLULAR INJURY

The causes of cellular injury in disease can be broken down into **extrinsic** (external) causes and **intrinsic** (internal causes). External causes such as infections, inflammation, or chemical and physical agents of disease are contracted from an organism or force originating outside the body. The internal causes originate from within the body, such as genetic derangement.

Hypoxia is the number one chemical cause of cellular injury and will be discussed later in this unit. Trauma is an example of a physical cause of cellular injury and includes any mechanism involving heat, cold, radiation, electrical injury, or **barotrauma,** which results from rapid or extreme changes in air pressure. An exaggerated inflammatory response as well as an inappropriate autoimmune response, such as arthritis, can also cause disease.

Necrosis (nee-CROW-sis) is cellular death and may involve a group of cells or tissues. The most common causes of cellular death are **anoxia** (an-NOCK-see-ah), no oxygen, and hypoxia, insufficient oxygen. Cells that are not getting enough oxygen cannot produce needed energy and eventually die.

HYPOXIA

Hypoxia (HIGH-**POCK**-see-ah) is a condition in which insufficient oxygen is available for the body tissues. Insufficient oxygen affects the disease process in two ways. Hypoxia can occur when the delivery of oxygen is disrupted by the disease process, whereas **hypoxemia** (high-**POX**-SEE-me-ah) refers to cell damage that results when there is insufficient oxygen in circulating blood to perfuse the cells. The effect of hypoxia on the disease process makes resolution of this condition a priority in the treatment of disease.

THE FICK PRINCIPLE

The brain, as the control center of the body, needs a sufficient circulation of glucose-rich, oxygenated blood to function. Therefore, the brain is the first to be affected by any disorder causing a deficiency of three essential elements: oxygen, **glucose** (sugar), and adequate circulation (blood flow). It takes an entire organism—that is, the whole body—to effectively deliver these essential elements to the brain.

Hypoxia (low oxygen concentration), **hypoglycemia** (low sugar), and **hypoperfusion** (inadequate blood flow) or shock must be aggressively managed to halt the progression of disease and ultimately avoid severe injury or death.

The mission of the body is to get the oxygen that is outside of the body in the ambient air into the body and down to the cell. The **Fick Principle** describes this process. First, there must be sufficient oxygen in the ambient air (oxygenation). Then it must enter the body (ventilation). Then it must pass across the alveoli, the blood membrane in the lungs (respiration), and enter the blood. Once the oxygen is in the blood, it must be carried to the cells (circulation) and deposited next to the body's cells, especially brain cells, for diffusion into the cells (cellular respiration) to occur.

When any components of the Fick Principle are interrupted—ventilation, respiration, oxygenation, circulation, or cellular respiration—cellular function is compromised. A number of causes, including disease, can compromise this process, any of which can result in a state of cellular injury called shock. Cellular injury, tissue death, organ failure, and death will occur if shock is not corrected. Many diseases that an EMT will encounter can interfere with the process described by the Fick Principle. Figure 6.1 illustrates the essential components of the Fick Principle.

OXYGENATION

The first element of the Fick Principle is oxygenation. **Oxygenation** refers to the amount of oxygen available in the atmosphere (air) that is inspired into the lungs. Earth's atmosphere, or ambient air, contains 21% oxygen. Oxygen is a small portion of the gases that make up air. The remaining portion of air consists of 78% nitrogen and 1% other trace gases. Oxygen-poor environments, as seen in smoke-filled buildings (higher level of carbon dioxide than oxygen), areas of high altitude (lower atmospheric pressures of oxygen), or confined spaces (lower oxygen concentrations), affect the amount of oxygen inspired and can lead to hypoxia (Figure 6.2).

CAUSES OF OXYGEN DEFICIENCY

The concentration of oxygen in ambient air may be affected by several processes, including the displacement of oxygen by other gases, consumption of available oxygen within a confined space, and the lowered atmospheric pressures at higher altitudes.

When air containing other gases such as pure nitrogen, carbon dioxide, or helium is inhaled, oxygen is replaced in the lungs by that gas. Blood flowing through the lungs receives insufficient oxygen and, in an effort to equalize the oxygen content in the lungs, gives up what oxygen it has to the lungs. This oxygen-deficient blood then travels to the brain. The tissues of the brain rapidly become oxygen-deficient, and the human body begins to experience certain physiological effects, including mental confusion, loss of coordination, weakness, nausea, and, without intervention, death.

The EMT may treat individuals suffering from the effects of an oxygen-poor environment. The need to understand the possible causes of oxygen deficiency is important not only to the management of the patient affected, but to ensure the safety of the responders who may be at risk for becoming affected by oxygen deficiency themselves.

CONFINED SPACE

Confined spaces, such as tanks, storage bins, manholes, and silos, exist in many occupations. Because there is a fixed amount of oxygen in a confined

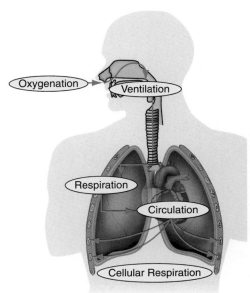

Figure 6.1 The essential components of the Fick Principle include oxygenation, ventilation, respiration, circulation, and cellular respiration

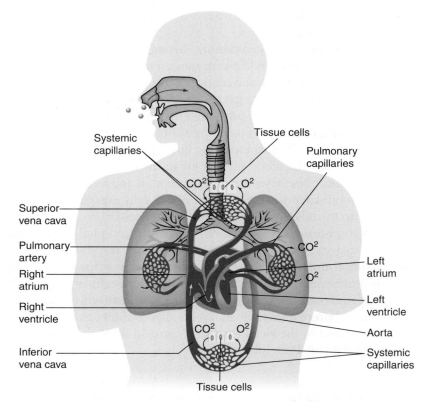

Figure 6.2 The path of an oxygen molecule to the cells

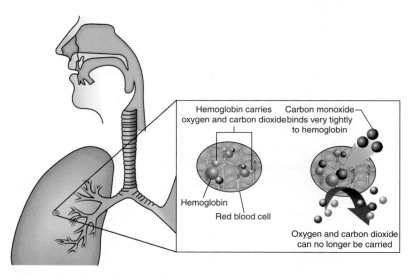

Figure 6.3 When oxygen is displaced in the cells by other gases, such as carbon monoxide, hypoxia can occur

space, the consumption of oxygen and subsequent displacement of oxygen with increased carbon dioxide leads to oxygen deficiency. Individuals working within these confined spaces are at risk for hypoxia (Figure 6.3).

RESPIRATORY SYSTEM

Oxygen enters the body by way of the structures of the upper airway and is transported to the alveoli in the lungs, where it moves into the capillaries and attaches to the hemoglobin in red blood cells. The red blood cells then transport the oxygen to the cells of the body through the arteries and capillaries of the circulatory system. When the cells and capillaries interface, oxygen moves from the blood in the capillary into the cell, displacing carbon dioxide, the waste product of cellular metabolism. Carbon dioxide moves from the cell into the capillaries for transport to the lungs via the venous system, where it is removed from the body through exhalation.

If the available oxygen is decreased due to an obstructed airway, inadequate ventilation, or poor gas exchange in the lungs, or if circulation to the cells is compromised, the cells become hypoxic and eventually die.

THE AIRWAY

An unobstructed and secure airway is vital for oxygenation and ventilation, the second element of the Fick Principle. The EMT must be knowledgeable about the structures of the upper and lower airway to effectively assess for and manage compromised ventilation.

ANATOMIC CONSIDERATIONS

As described in the previous unit, the structures of the airway are divided into the upper and lower airways. Air typically enters the body by way of the nose or mouth, moving through the *nasopharynx* (nasal portion) or *oropharynx* (oral portion) of the *pharynx* (throat). At the lower end of the pharynx, the passageway is divided into the *trachea* (windpipe) and the *esophagus*, the passageway for food.

The *epiglottis*, a small valve that closes over the larynx while swallowing food and liquid and opening to permit breathing, protects the trachea. Air then moves through the *larynx* (voice box), into the trachea, where it continues into the lower airway, consisting of the right and left bronchi, and bronchioles ending in the tiny *alveoli* (air sacs) of the lungs, where gas exchange takes place.

The *thoracic cavity* (chest cavity) holds the organs of the lower respiratory system and the circulatory system. The thorax is bordered inferiorly by the *diaphragm*, which separates it from the abdominal cavity. The **mediastinum,** an area between the right and left lungs, houses the trachea, the *venae cavae* (the two great veins that collect blood from the upper and lower body and return it to the heart), the *aorta* (great artery carrying blood from the heart to the body), the esophagus, and the heart.

The thorax is lined with a thick, elastic tissue called the *parietal pleura*. The outer surface of the lungs is covered with a thin layer of connective tissue, called the *visceral pleura*. The two pleural layers are separated by a lubricating serous fluid that reduces friction between the lungs and the chest wall, and a tiny space called the **pleural cavity,** or **potential space.** During inhalation, the pull of the parietal pleura on the visceral pleura creates a negative pressure that acts as a vacuum, allowing the lungs to stay inflated.

Muscles essential to breathing are the diaphragm and the **intercostal muscles,** the muscles between the ribs that contract and relax, changing the size of the thoracic cavity during ventilation. When ventilations are impaired through physical obstruction or a disease process, accessory muscles become more pronounced in an attempt to assist and maintain adequate ventilation. Accessory muscles of ventilation are located in the neck and head and include the *sternocleidomastoid (stûr'nō-klī'dǝ-mǎs'toid) muscle*, responsible for flexing and rotating the head; the **scalene** (skā'lēn') **muscles,** which elevate the sternocleidomastoid muscle; the wing of the nose, responsible for nasal flaring; and other small muscles in the neck and head. Accessory muscles anchor the sternum and upper ribs and do not contract during normal breathing. When the airway is obstructed or during exercise, accessory muscles can contract vigorously, actively pulling up on the rib cage and effectively expanding the thoracic cavity.

AIRWAY OBSTRUCTION

Partially or completely obstructed air passages can occur at any anatomic levels of the airway. Airway obstructions can be the result of a foreign body (food, fluid, or mucous) becoming lodged, swelling as seen in an allergic reaction, or the relaxation of muscles that control the structures of the airway (tongue). Obstruction of the airway results in the lack of adequate ventilation and oxygenation, leading to hypoxia.

FOREIGN BODY AIRWAY OBSTRUCTION

The upper airway can become obstructed by any foreign body that becomes lodged in any structure of the airway, preventing air from traveling to the alveoli for gas exchange. A partial foreign body airway obstruction (FBAO) allows for some air movement around the obstruction, which may or may not be adequate. A complete FBAO means all air exchange has stopped because the airway is completely occluded by the object. A particle of food is an example of a foreign body that can become lodged in the throat, creating a blockage in the upper airway.

The muscles controlling structures within the airway, such as the tongue, relax in patients who are experiencing an altered level of consciousness or are unresponsive. The tongue falls back, occluding the upper airway and preventing air from moving beyond the oropharynx. The muscles controlling the epiglottis also relax in the unconscious patient, allowing the epiglottis to fall over the opening of the glottic opening, occluding air movement into the trachea.

The *larynx* (voice box) is a common site of airway obstruction. When the epiglottis fails to close, food, liquids, or any foreign object in the airway can enter the larynx and become lodged or cause the larynx to spasm, preventing air from entering the trachea.

VENTILATION

Ventilation (breathing) is the mechanical process of moving air into and out of the lungs. Breathing is both an active and passive process requiring intact airway passages and the contraction and relaxation of the skeletal muscles, the external intercostal muscles, and the diaphragm.

Ventilation is a complex process, involving both inhalation and exhalation. Ventilation is controlled by sensors in the carotid and aortic arteries that supply the brain, the aorta, and the medulla located in the brainstem with the stimulus for ventilation to occur.

The **chemoreceptors,** sensors that measure the chemical changes in the body, detect the rise and fall in carbon dioxide, oxygen, and hydrogen levels in arterial blood and spinal fluid. The **central chemoreceptors** in the medulla are most sensitive to changes in carbon dioxide levels and the pH of blood, whereas **peripheral chemoreceptors** in the carotid arteries and aortic arch are more sensitive to changes in arterial oxygen levels.

As carbon dioxide levels rise, chemoreceptors send a message to the brainstem, triggering the **phrenic nerve,** located in the third, fourth, and fifth cervical segments of the spinal cord, to contract the diaphragm and the intercostal muscles. The diaphragm moves downward, increasing the volume of the thoracic (chest) cavity, and the intercostal muscles pull the ribs up, expanding the rib cage and further increasing the volume of the chest. This increase of volume lowers the air pressure in the alveoli to below atmospheric pressure. Because air always flows from an area of higher pressure to an area of lower pressure, air moves in through the respiratory tract and into the alveoli. The change of pressure inside the lungs compared to the pressure of the outer atmosphere is called **negative pressure ventilation.**

Expiration is mostly a passive function with increase in lung volume and relaxation of the diaphragm and intercostal muscles. The thoracic cavity returns to its original volume, increasing the pressure within the lungs, and forcing the air out.

The respiratory system responds primarily to changes in carbon dioxide levels, increasing the rate and depth of respiration to eliminate the higher levels of carbon dioxide. Oxygen is less of a stimulus for breathing in healthy people who breathe on a **hypercarbic** (high carbon dioxide) drive. Individuals with diseases of the respiratory system who experience high carbon dioxide levels chronically, such as emphysema, may actually breathe on a hypoxic (low oxygen) drive where the chemoreceptors rely on oxygen levels in the blood to regulate breathing. Put another way, individuals with a **hypoxic drive** breathe to increase their oxygen levels, not to reduce their carbon dioxide levels.

MINUTE AND TIDAL VOLUME

Adequate ventilation is achieved when there is an adequate respiratory rate and volume of air taken into the body. It is important to understand the relationship involving the rate a person is breathing and the amount of air being taken in with each breath, to determine whether adequate ventilation is taking place.

Respiratory rate is the number of breaths a person takes in 1 minute. The volume or amount of air inhaled and exhaled in one breath is called **tidal volume** (V_T). The amount of air breathed in and out in 1 minute is the **minute volume.** Minute volume deals with both the depth and rate of breathing and is a measure of the adequacy of an individual's breathing. Minute volume is calculated by multiplying the tidal volume by the respiratory rate.

$$\text{Minute Volume} = \text{Tidal volume} \times \text{Respiratory rate}$$

A decrease in either the tidal volume or the respiratory rate may decrease minute volume to the point at which adequate air per minute is no longer being moved in and out of the lungs. Inadequate minute volume leads to a decrease in gas exchange at the alveoli level, causing the cells to become hypoxic.

An increased respiratory rate only increases minute volume when the depth of each breath remains normal or increased. As the respiratory rate increases, if the depth of each breath lessens, tidal volume decreases, resulting in a lower volume of air reaching the alveoli for gas exchange.

ALVEOLAR VENTILATION

Alveolar ventilation is the amount of air breathed in that reaches the alveoli in the lungs. The trachea and bronchi in the lower airway do not participate in gas exchange; therefore, only the air that reaches the alveoli can be used.

The volume of air that stays in the respiratory tract, never reaching the alveoli, is known as **dead air space** (V_D). Whereas minute volume is only the amount of air breathed in and out in 1 minutes, alveolar ventilation is the amount of air breathed in and out in 1 minute that reaches the alveoli to be used in gas exchange. The average adult has a dead air space equaling approximately 150 ml out of the 500 ml (tidal volume) that is inhaled. Therefore, the amount of air that actually reaches the alveoli for gas exchange is 350 ml.

Dead air space is constant; if the volume of air inhaled decreases, dead air space will continue to use up the same volume of air, but the volume of air reaching the alveoli will be decreased. An individual with a normal respiratory rate of 12 breaths a minute but a lower volume of air taken than normal will

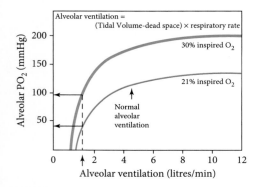

Figure 6.4 Alveolar ventilation is the volume of gas made available for use

not have an adequate amount of air reaching the alveoli. Thus, a patient with a respiratory rate of 12 but a tidal volume of only 300 ml has only 150 ml of air reaching the alveoli for gas exchange. This patient will require assisted ventilations to increase the volume of air being taken in, even though the respiratory rate is within the normal range of 10 to 20 breaths per minute.

High respiratory rates affect the volume of air taken in and decrease alveolar ventilation. If an individual is breathing very fast, the lungs do not have time to fill fully, inhalation time is decreased, breaths become shallow, and tidal volume is reduced. As an example, an adult breathing at 40 breaths per minute with only 250 ml of air taken in with each breath will require assistance because 150 of the 250 ml of air is entering the dead air space. This leaves only 100 ml available for gas exchange when it reaches the alveoli.

In cases involving both normal and rapid respiratory rate and shallow ventilations, lower tidal volumes equal decreased volume of air reaching the alveoli. Blood becomes oxygen poor, carbon dioxide increases, cells become hypoxic, and acid builds up. Individuals with inadequate respiratory rate or poor tidal volume with a normal respiratory rate require assisted ventilation to ensure that adequate air is reaching the alveoli for gas exchange. Figure 6.4 shows the equation for alveolar ventilation.

OBSTRUCTIVE DISEASE OF VENTILATION

Obstructive sleep **apnea** (OSA), from the Greek word meaning "without breath," is a disorder in which a structure of the upper airway causes an individual to stop breathing during sleep. The apneic phase can last for a minute or longer and may occur numerous times during the night. Of the three types of sleep apnea—obstructive, central, and mixed—obstructive is the most common. Obstructive apnea can be either a complete obstruction of the airway or a partial obstruction causing **hypopnea,** slow shallow breathing, both of which can wake the individual up.

One risk factor for OSA is excessive weight gain. Excessive fat accumulating on the sides of the upper airway can cause narrowing and closure of the airway when muscles relax during sleep. Additional risk factors include age, due to the loss of muscle mass common with aging; male hormones causing structural changes in the upper airway, leaving men at a higher risk than women for OSA; neuromuscular disorders; hypothyroidism; and syndromes such as Marfan's and Down syndrome. Inflammation, swelling, and narrowing of the upper airway are often seen in individuals who smoke. The use of alcohol and sedative drugs can relax the muscles surrounding the neck and are risk factors that can be modified to reduce the onset of OSA.

Positive pressure therapy is an effective treatment for obstructive sleep apnea. There are three forms of positive pressure therapy: autotitration, bi-level positive airway pressure (BiPAP), and continuous positive airway pressure (CPAP), the most common of the three therapy options. **Continuous positive airway pressure (CPAP)** applies positive pressure to the upper airway using a machine that sends pressurized air through a nasal or facial mask worn at night. The upper airway is essentially "splinted" open and prevented from collapsing.

Diseases of the lower airway most often involve the structures of the lungs. Chronic Obstructive Pulmonary Disease (COPD), characterized by abnormalities that make it difficult to exhale normally, involves two diseases, emphysema and chronic bronchitis. Both of these diseases cause an excessive inflammatory process that lead to abnormalities in the structures of the lungs, obstructing airflow.

Tobacco use is the number one risk factor for COPD, with cigarette smoking a greater risk than other forms of tobacco use. Additional risk factors for COPD are occupational exposures, pollutants, recurring respiratory infections, and genetic predisposition.

In chronic bronchitis, the major problem is the swelling and thickening of the lining of the bronchi and bronchioles and an increase of mucus production. The lower airways become narrowed, increasing resistance to air flow. The narrowed lower airway and thick mucus production prevents adequate airflow to the alveoli. The alveoli do not fully expand, causing respiratory distress and hypoxia.

Emphysema, like chronic bronchitis, restricts air flow in the lower airways, but emphysema directly affects the elasticity of lung tissue. The loss of elasticity causes air to become trapped and the alveoli to become distended, destroying the walls of the alveoli. Gas exchange is significantly disrupted when the alveoli surface area in contact with pulmonary capillaries, the site of gas exchange, is lost. The primary problem in emphysema is hypoxia and the retention of carbon dioxide. Breathing becomes increasingly difficult due to increased airway resistance; however, with emphysema, exhaling becomes an active process rather than passive, as the individual works to rid the excess of carbon dioxide (Figure 6.5). The assessment and treatment of COPD will be discussed further in Unit 26.

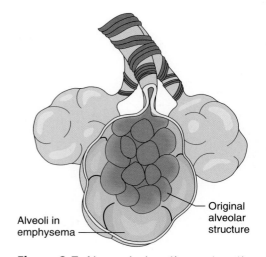

Figure 6.5 Normal alveoli vs. alveoli in emphysema

RESPIRATION

Respiration, the third element of the Fick Principle, refers to the exchange of gases between an organism and its environment. The exchange of oxygen (O_2) and carbon dioxide (CO_2) takes place in the alveoli of the lungs. The alveoli are surrounded by capillaries that deliver blood to the alveoli. The blood being carried by the capillaries is deoxygenated, low in oxygen concentration and high in carbon dioxide. Because both carbon dioxide and oxygen will move from areas of high concentration to areas of low concentration, oxygen moves from the alveoli into the capillaries and carbon dioxide moves from the capillaries into the alveoli. This process is called **diffusion.**

The blood in the capillaries is now oxygenated, meaning it contains a high concentration of oxygen and low carbon dioxide. **Hemoglobin,** found on the surface of red blood cells, is responsible for transporting oxygen via the arterial system for delivery to the cells. The carbon dioxide left behind in the alveoli is exhaled out of the lungs.

The capillaries surrounding the cells contain high levels of carbon dioxide and low levels of oxygen from normal cell metabolism. Again, diffusion takes place as the higher level of oxygen in the oxygenated blood entering the capillaries surrounding the cell move to those of lower concentration into the cell and the carbon dioxide move out of the cells into the capillaries. The oxygen-poor blood moves out of the capillaries into the venous system where it returns to the lungs for gas exchange.

In order for diffusion to take place, there must be a higher concentration (or pressure) of oxygen in the alveoli than the concentration of oxygen in the blood. When these conditions exist, diffusion occurs and the levels of gases in the alveoli and the blood equalize (Figure 6.6).

RESPIRATORY DEFICIENCY

Respiration can also be interrupted, impaired, or arrested by any one or more pathologies that upset homeostasis. The muscles of respiration—the external intercostals and diaphragm—can become injured or paralyzed. The loss of

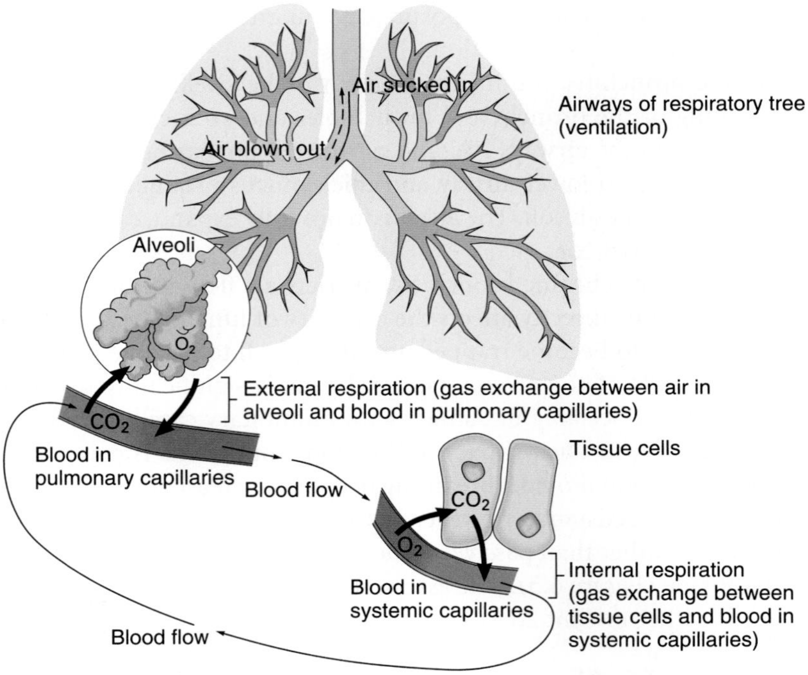

Figure 6.6 The process of gas exchange through respiratory diffusion

function of these muscles prevents the thorax from adequately expanding and relaxing, decreasing tidal volume and interfering with gas exchange.

NEUROMUSCULAR DISEASE

Amyotrophic Lateral Sclerosis (ALS), sometimes called Lou Gehrig's disease, is a neuromuscular disease caused by the degeneration of **motor neurons,** the nerve cells in the central nervous system that control voluntary muscle movement. Although voluntary muscle movement is primarily affected, as the disease progresses, all muscles within the body weaken and atrophy.

The rate of progression varies, but eventually all persons with ALS develop difficulty swallowing and chewing food, putting them at higher risk for airway obstruction. As the diaphragm and intercostal muscles weaken, forced vital capacity and inspiratory pressure diminish.

Bi-level positive pressure ventilation (BiPAP) is commonly used to support breathing for a period, with prognosis of long-term mechanical ventilation as the muscles of respiration continue to weaken and atrophy. Individuals with ALS die of respiratory failure or pneumonia because of the disease.

TRAUMA

Trauma refers to a physical injury or wound caused by external force or violence, such as blunt, penetrating, and blast forces, including burns. Trauma injuries can affect external structures such as the skin and internal structures ranging from bone to the organs of the body.

A **flail chest** occurs when a segment consisting of at least two ribs are broken in at least two places, causing the chest wall to move independently from the rest of the chest. The flail segment moves in the opposite direction as the rest of the chest wall in what is referred to as **paradoxical motion.** Flail chest is commonly seen in cases of significant blunt trauma and is a serious, potentially life-threatening injury, commonly accompanied by pulmonary contusion (Figure 6.7).

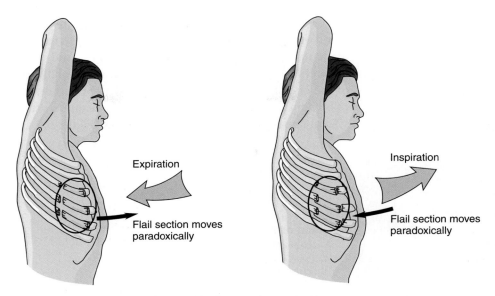

Figure 6.7 Paradoxical motion can impair ventilation and respiration

As discussed previously, during normal inspiration, the diaphragm contracts and the intercostal muscles push the rib cage out, causing the pressure inside the thorax to decrease and air to be brought in. The paradoxical motion occurs because the flail segment cannot resist the decreased pressure and will appear to push in as the rest of the rib cage expands. During expiration, the flail segment will be pushed out as the rib cage contracts.

The motion of the ribs in the flail segment is extremely painful, causing the injured person to increase the respiratory rate but take shallower breaths, thus decreasing the volume of air entering the lungs. Additionally, a **pneumothorax,** air in the pleural space outside the lung, can occur when the sharp edges of the fractured ribs puncture the pleural sac and lung, causing the lung to collapse (Figure 6.8).

Treatment of a flail chest includes support of ventilation to improve tidal volume and increase blood oxygenation, using positive pressure ventilation. In the hospital, tubes may be inserted into the pleural space to evacuate a pneumothorax and allow more effective lung expansion.

CIRCULATORY SYSTEM

The circulatory system is a closed system, made up of the heart, blood vessels, and blood, responsible for the transport of blood to all parts of the body. *Circulation* is the action of blood flowing in the body's blood vessels and heart. The blood is responsible for delivering oxygen, nutrients, and other essential chemicals to the tissues and removing carbon dioxide and other waste products of cell metabolism.

Systemic circulation, as the name indicates, supplies blood to the organs of the body's systems. The systemic circulation has two significant subdivisions: the coronary circulation, which supplies the myocardium of the heart, and the hepatic portal circulation, through which blood travels back and forth from the intestines to the liver.

Pulmonary circulation, vital to respiration, is the route of blood from the right ventricle to the pulmonary arteries and into the lungs where gas exchange takes place.

Cerebral circulation supplies the brain with oxygen and nutrients, removing waste. **Fetal circulation** refers to the temporary circulation between the mother and developing fetus during pregnancy.

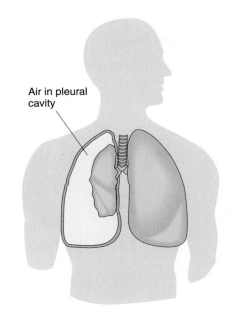

Air in pleural cavity

Figure 6.8 Pneumothorax

Circulation can be described simply in terms of a series of pipes (the blood vessels), connected to a pump (heart) forcing vital fluid (the blood) made up of cells that carry the fuels (oxygen) and wastes (carbon dioxide) throughout the body for distribution and removal. Damage to the structures of the circulatory system prevents the oxygen/carbon dioxide exchange and cells begin to die. Therefore, an intact and adequately functioning circulatory system is vital to maintaining homeostasis (Figure 6.9).

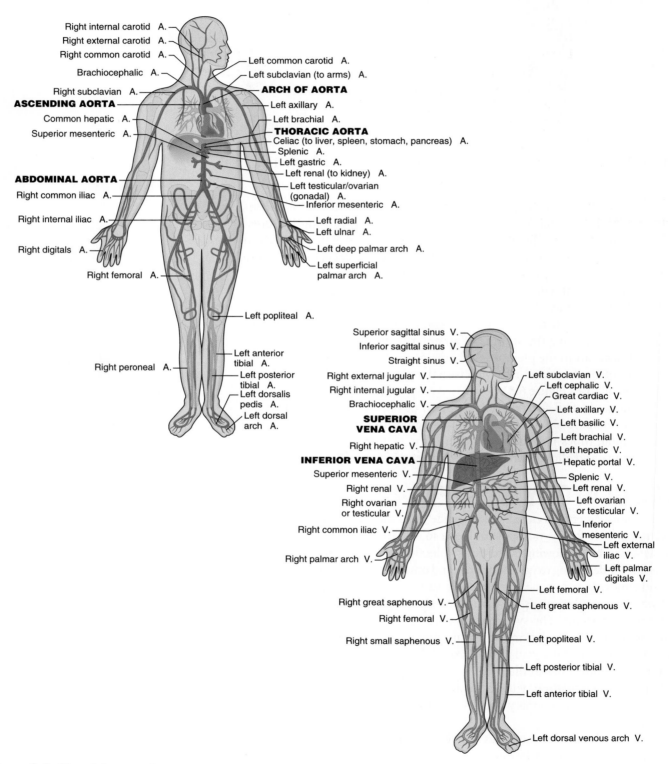

Figure 6.9 Circulatory system

THE PIPES

The *blood vessels* are the pipes that carry blood throughout the body. In general, arteries carry oxygenated blood away from the heart, and veins carry deoxygenated blood back to the heart. There are, however, two notable exceptions: The *pulmonary artery* carries oxygen-poor blood to the lungs for oxygenation, and the *pulmonary vein* takes oxygenated blood from the lungs and delivers it to the heart to be pumped out to the body through the aorta.

Capillaries are the tiny blood vessels that connect the veins and arteries. Oxygen and nutrients are exchanged for carbon dioxide and waste at the cellular level in this area.

The arteries and veins have walls composed of three layers:
- The inner layer called the **tunica intima** (TYOO-nih-kah IN-tih-mah), a single layer of **endothelial cells** that line the circulatory system;
- The middle layer, **tunica media,** made up of smooth muscle; and
- The outer layer, **tunica adventitia** (ad-vin-TISH-ee-ah), made up of white fibrous connective tissue (Figure 6.10).

THE ARTERIES

Artery walls are made up of the three coats or **tunics** surrounding a hollow core called a **lumen** (LOO-men) that allows blood flow. The walls of arteries are thicker and stronger than veins; they are elastic and able to contract, expanding to accommodate the large amount of blood injected into the aorta

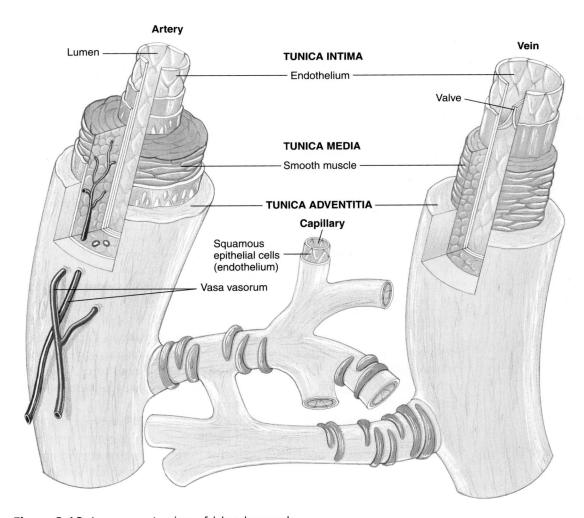

Figure 6.10 Layers or tunics of blood vessels

from the ventricles of the heart. As the ventricles of the heart relax, the elastic walls of the arteries recoil, pushing the blood forward through the numerous branches of arteries throughout the body.

The arteries serve to carry oxygenated blood away from the heart, with the exception of the pulmonary arteries, which return oxygen-poor blood to the lungs for oxygenation.

The major arteries of the body include the *aorta*, which supplies all other arteries with blood; the *coronary arteries*, supplying the heart; and *carotid arteries*, which supply the head and brain. The lower body and extremities are supplied by the *femoral artery* (thigh, groin, and legs), *dorsalis pedis* arteries (foot), and *posterior tibial* arteries (calf). Blood supply to the upper extremities is through the *brachial artery* (upper arm) and *radial artery* (distal arm).

The **arterioles** (ar-TEE-ree-olz) are the smaller arteries that supply blood to the capillaries.

THE VEINS

The veins are made up of the same three *tunics* (coats) as the arteries. However, because the blood flow is not as strong as in the arteries, veins contain less smooth muscle and elastic tissue but more white fibrous connective tissue. Veins are also capable of expanding to accommodate the varying blood pressure and volume. Unlike arteries, veins contain valves that ensure blood flows in a direction toward the heart.

The veins serve to carry deoxygenated blood back to the heart, with the exception of the pulmonary veins, which carry oxygenated blood from the lungs to the left atrium. The pulmonary veins are the only veins that carry oxygenated blood.

The major veins in the body follow the courses of the major arteries and share the same names. For example, the femoral artery and femoral vein lie close to each other within the thigh. The vena cava is the largest vein in the body and is referred to by the location of the body it drains. The superior vena cava carried oxygen-depleted blood from the head and upper body, entering the top of the right atrium of the heart. The inferior vena cava carries the deoxygenated blood from the lower body, entering the heart through the bottom of the right atrium. The deoxygenated blood is then pumped into the right ventricle and carried into the lungs for oxygenation via the pulmonary artery.

The **venules** connect the capillaries and veins, draining the collected blood from the capillaries into the veins.

SYSTEMIC VASCULAR RESISTANCE

The arterioles are sometimes referred to as the resistance vessels in the body. As the heart contracts, blood is pumped into the arteries faster than it can leave and the arteries stretch from the pressure. When the heart relaxes, the vessels return to their normal state, but the heart will contract again before all the blood has flowed into the arterioles. The pressure in the arteries is prevented from being fully relieved by the arterioles, creating **systemic vascular resistance (SVR),** also known as **total peripheral resistance.** The sympathetic and parasympathetic divisions of the autonomic nervous system directly affect systemic vascular resistance.

In times of stress, the sympathetic division increases the heart rate, breathing rate, and blood pressure. The fight-or-flight response of the sympathetic division is a compensatory mechanism preparing the body for an increased energy expenditure. The constriction of blood vessels is necessary to "shunt" the oxygen-rich blood to the vital organs of the body—that is, the heart, lungs, and brain.

Following a fight-or-flight response, the parasympathetic division, sometimes referred to as the *rest and repose system*, works to restore the body to its normal, nonstressful conditions. The parasympathetic division slows heart rate and breathing. The smooth muscles of the vessels relax and blood pressure is lowered as the vessels dilate to their normal size. Some drugs, such as nicotine found in tobacco, constrict blood vessels and ultimately increase vascular resistance.

BLOOD PRESSURE

The amount of pressure placed on the walls of blood vessels by the circulatory system is referred to as **blood pressure**. The **systolic blood pressure** is the pressure exerted against the walls of the vessels when the heart contracts. The **diastolic blood pressure** is the pressure within the vessels when the heart is at rest. Blood pressure is dependent on cardiac output and systemic vascular resistance. When either cardiac output or systemic vascular resistance increases, blood pressure will increase. When either cardiac output or systemic vascular resistance decreases, blood pressure will decrease. To provide adequate oxygen-rich blood to the brain, maintaining normal brain function, the body works to maintain an adequate blood pressure.

BARORECEPTORS

Baroreceptors, located in the arch of the aorta and internal carotid arteries, detect the pressure of blood flow and send messages to the central nervous system to increase or decrease systemic vascular resistance and cardiac output. They are stretch-sensitive receptors that respond to changes or distortions of normal pressure running through them. Baroreceptors can be divided into high-pressure, arterial baroreceptors and low-pressure, cardiopulmonary receptors. Baroreceptors help to maintain mean arterial blood pressure, allowing tissues to receive the right amount of blood.

Arterial baroreceptors lie in the arch of the aorta and internal carotid arteries. They detect changes in blood pressure, sending signals to increase or decrease heart rate. Baroreceptors detect the amount of stretch applied to the arteries where they are located. The more the walls are stretched, the more frequently they fire signals. If blood pressure falls, baroreceptors decrease the rate at which they fire signals (Figure 6.11).

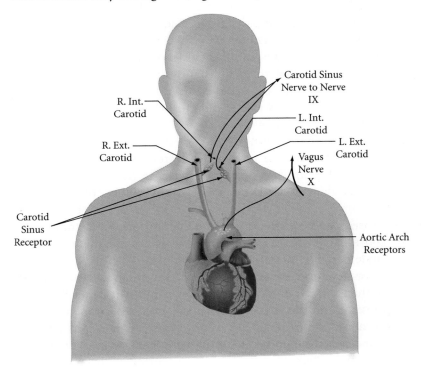

Figure 6.11 Baroreceptors

Baroreceptors located in veins and the walls of the atria of the heart are low-pressure receptors and are involved in regulation of blood volume. Blood volume determines mean pressure throughout the system, especially in the venous part of the system where most of the blood is held. Low-pressure baroreceptors affect both circulatory and renal function, producing changes in hormone secretion, which affect the retention and intake of salt and water.

Baroreceptors respond quickly to stabilize blood pressure. However, over the long term, they will reset; therefore, in people with hypertension, the baroreceptors eventually adapt as if the higher pressure is normal and will work to maintain this new pressure.

DISEASES AND DISORDERS OF BLOOD VESSELS

When the vessels of circulation (pipes) are disrupted or blocked, circulation slows or comes to a standstill. A disease process such as **atherosclerosis** (plaque in the pipes) can reduce or block blood flow. Distributive events such as anaphylactic shock, septic shock, **psychogenic shock (vasovagal shock)** or neurogenic shock cause the pipes to expand or leak fluids, reducing effective blood pressure in the pipes.

ARTERIOSCLEROSIS AND ATHEROSCLEROSIS

Arteriosclerosis is a group of diseases characterized by a loss of elasticity and thickening of the artery wall. Atherosclerosis and arteriosclerosis are often used to describe the same condition, as is the term "hardening of the arteries," a lay term for the same condition.

The loss of elasticity of the artery wall in arteriosclerosis results in the narrowing of the vessels *lumen* (hollow center), slowing or completely blocking the flow of blood to the organs they supply.

Atherosclerosis also causes the artery to lose elasticity or harden due to fatty, cholesterol-containing deposits (plaque) pushing into the inner endothelium, damaging the Teflon-like lining and allowing the plaque to stick. The wall of the artery thickens due to the plaque, resulting in a partially or completely occluded lumen. Plaque may also form in one area of a vessel and then break loose forming an **embolus** (EM-boh-lus), material floating in the blood. The embolus may travel a distance through the vessel, reaching an area of the vessel that has been narrowed. At that point it sticks to the vessel wall, occluding blood flow and leading to ischemia (tissue injury) of the organ it supplies.

The result of the narrowed lumen of an artery is increased blood pressure, increased workload on the heart, and decreased blood flow to the organs. The increased blood pressure then stretches the hardened arteries, causing further damage and increasing the workload on the heart even more.

Atherosclerosis may be caused by a combination of risk factors, some of which are controllable whereas others are not. Risk factors that cannot be controlled include heredity, a family trend for high cholesterol; age, with an increasing risk for development over the age of 30; gender, with men being at a higher risk than women until menopause, when the incidence becomes equal; and diabetes. Controllable risk factors may be altered through lifestyle changes, such as a healthy, low-fat, low-carbohydrate diet, increased exercise, reduced stress, and reduced blood pressure. Perhaps the most important controllable risk factor is not smoking.

DISTRIBUTIVE DISEASES AFFECTING BLOOD VESSELS

Blood vessel size is controlled by the autonomic nervous system in an effort to keep blood pressure within a certain range for each individual. Blood pressure ranges change automatically in response to the body's activity, stress, and oxygen demand. The brain and spinal cord are the parts of the autonomic nervous system responsible for control of the size of blood vessels and heart rate. The autonomic nervous system acts to decrease the diameter of blood vessels to control blood pressure; therefore, damage to the spinal cord or the brain can cause inappropriate changes in the size of blood vessels.

Neurogenic shock can occur when injury to the spinal cord damages the nerve cells of the autonomic nervous system. The blood vessels of the body that are controlled by those damaged nerves no longer receive the message to maintain their tone, causing them to relax and dilate. If damage occurs over a significant portion of the spinal cord, the size of the circulatory system increases, causing blood pressure to drop as the container (circulatory system) becomes too large for the available blood volume. Additionally, blood pools below the injury site, decreasing the volume returning to the heart. The decreased volume of blood returning to the heart causes a decrease in cardiac output and blood pressure.

Psychogenic shock is a sudden reaction of the nervous system from a sudden fright or severe pain rather than a direct injury. This reaction causes temporary, generalized dilation of the blood vessels; as a result, blood pools in the dilated vessels, reducing cardiac output, lowering blood pressure, and decreasing blood flow to the brain. The reduced perfusion to the brain can result in a sudden loss of consciousness or fainting (syncopal) event. Psychogenic or vasovagal shock is a non-life-threatening situation that is temporary. If unconsciousness persists longer than a few minutes, the EMT should suspect another diagnosis.

An extreme allergic reaction characterized by a severe inflammatory response is call **anaphylactic shock.** An inflammatory response immediately protects the body from a foreign invader, such as microorganisms, through isolation, destruction, and elimination, resulting in promotion of healing.

When the body comes in contact with an **allergen,** a substance to which it is allergic, the mast cells (found in all tissues of the body) release histamine, a substance that causes the arterioles, venules, and capillaries at the site of the injury to dilate. That response increases blood flow, called **hyperemia,** to the area. Hyperemia brings additional white blood cells (leukocytes) to line the walls of the vessels in anticipation of moving into the tissue to fight the intruder.

In anaphylaxis, when a person comes in contact with an allergen, antibodies react by binding to the surface of mast cells, causing the cells to release histamine into the tissues. As the histamine causes the capillaries to dilate, they become leaky, drawing fluid from the vascular space. The fluid shift causes edema and hyperemia, seen as hives, on the skin. Anaphylaxis can be life threatening because the blood vessels in the entire body can dilate, causing a significant fluid shift that results in shock. Edema of the airway and spasms of the smaller airways cause obstruction of breathing. Immediate and rapid intervention is required to stop the progression and reverse the inflammatory response. Individuals who know they are allergic to such things as bee stings, as an example, carry epinephrine pens to treat a life-threatening anaphylaxic reaction.

THE PUMP

The heart is a four-chambered pump made up of specialized muscle and an electrical conduction system that moves nutrient-rich blood throughout the body. The heart pumps blood through two separate pathways: the systemic

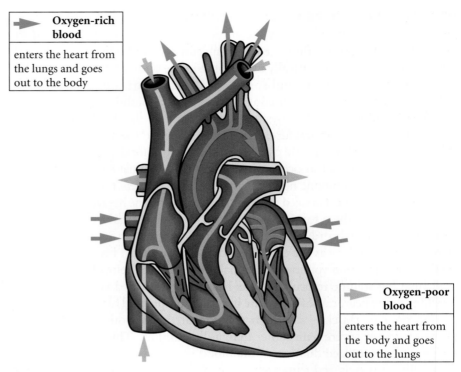

Figure 6.12 Circulation of blood through the heart

pipeline of blood vessels providing blood to the many systems of the body and the pulmonary pipeline of blood vessels that pass through the lungs, facilitating oxygenation and the removal of carbon dioxide (Figure 6.12).

HEART RATE

The cardiac cycle begins with the electrical stimulation of cardiac muscle by the sinoatrial (SA) node and passes to the atrioventricular (AV) node to the bundle of His and Purkinje fibers. The heart generates its own impulses, unlike the respiratory system, which relies on the brain for stimulus to breathe. The cardiac cycle repeats approximately 60 to 100 times each minute.

The *pulse* is the surge of blood through the arteries each time the left ventricle contracts. It can be felt by a hand over the chest or fingertips over an artery. The pulse rate, or the number of times the heartbeat is felt over 1 minute, can be a measure of how effective the left ventricle is functioning as a pump.

CARDIAC OUTPUT

Cardiac output is the amount of blood ejected from the left ventricle every minute. Adequate tissue perfusion is dependant on cardiac output. Cardiac output can be calculated by multiplying the stroke volume (milliliters of blood pumped by the left ventricle each beat) by the heart rate. Cardiac output adequate for good tissue perfusion requires ample **preload,** blood volume to be delivered to the heart and a heart that is contracting sufficiently.

Preload is increased when the volume of blood returning to the heart is increased, as seen in fluid overload. The **Frank-Starling law,** or more simply, *Starling law*, describes how the contractibility of the cardiac muscle is relative to the amount of stretch placed on the muscle by additional blood volume (Figure 6.13). Think of a rubber band stretched as far as possible before breaking. The force of tension placed on the rubber band has a direct effect on the

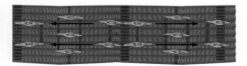

Greater Stretch = Greater Contraction

Figure 6.13 Frank-Starling law illustrates that the contractibility of the heart is relative to the amount of stretch placed on the muscle by increased blood volume

strength of recoil or snap when the tension is released. The heart muscle will stretch to accommodate the additional blood volume. The heart muscle then contracts with greater force in order to pump the additional blood out of the chamber. The Starling process is the compensatory mechanism for additional blood volume entering the right side of the heart. The greater the preload, the stronger the force of ventricular contraction; however, too much volume can result in dilating the ventricle and weakening the ability to contract.

Afterload is the amount of force the ventricle must overcome to provide blood flow to the circulatory system. In a fluid overload situation, the heart has to pump harder to overcome the increased fluid volume. Afterload is increased when peripheral vascular resistance is increased due to vasoconstriction, as seen in the fight-or-flight reaction of the sympathetic nervous system. A decreased blood volume, as seen in hemorrhage and vasodilation, decreases peripheral vascular resistance and ultimately decreases afterload.

Cardiac muscle requires sufficient oxygen and glucose to produce the energy needed to maintain cardiac output. According to the Starling law, the greater the preload (blood volume) delivered to the heart by the venous system, the greater stretch of the muscle. The muscle exerts a greater force on the contraction to pump the additional blood out of the heart. The heart must be healthy and well nourished for this mechanism, which is vital to sustaining perfusion during times of exertion, to occur.

Unhealthy cardiac muscle can more easily become ischemic. The damaged tissue affects cardiac output, indirectly affects blood pressure, and may result in cardiac failure. With no intervention to restore perfusion to injured cardiac tissue quickly, the cells begin to die.

PUMP FAILURE

Failure of the heart (pump) causes a domino effect leading to *hypoperfusion* (shock) and cellular death. There are many different causes for pump failure, which also affects respiratory function.

Pump failure can result from tissue damage to the heart muscle itself through **acute myocardial infarction (AMI),** or heart attack. An AMI is a dysfunction of the internal structures such as the valves of the heart. It can also be caused by disease processes such as an infection of the heart muscle or by systemic compromise such as high blood pressure (hypertension) and diabetes. Additionally, the pump can be compromised by damage to the nerves affecting impulses to the heart (vagus nerve) or conduction of the electrical system that can cause **dysrhythmias,** or abnormal electrical rhythms of the heart.

ACUTE MYOCARDIAL INFARCTION

Diseases of the heart are often caused by narrowing of the coronary arteries due to atherosclerosis. As the coronary arteries narrow through the disease process, perfusion to the heart muscle decreases, resulting in **angina,** or chest pain. The narrowed artery fails to deliver sufficient oxygen to the area of cardiac muscle it supplies, and *ischemia* (cellular hypoxia) begins to occur. If the artery becomes completely occluded, blood supply and oxygenation stop, causing **infarction** (death) to the cells of the heart unless circulation and oxygenation are restored quickly. Decreasing the risk factors of atherosclerosis, as described earlier, through lifestyle changes decreases the risks for heart disease.

Acute myocardial infarction (AMI) or heart attack, occurs when the oxygen supply to the heart is compromised due to a decreased blood supply, increased oxygen demand, or a combination of both. The decreased blood supply caused by plaque buildup in atherosclerosis is the most common cause of coronary artery disease, leading to an AMI.

As ischemia continues, myocardial cells become damaged, changing how they conduct electricity through the heart. These damaged cells do not contract efficiently, causing a change in cardiac output and, indirectly, blood pressure. The damage to the cells can be minimized if blood flow and perfusion are restored rapidly.

Cardiac tissue that does not receive oxygenated blood within that period will begin to die (infarct), and the resulting damage is no longer reversible. The infarcted area heals with a type of scar tissue that does not contract like muscle and will not function as normal cardiac tissue does. The failure of the scarred area of tissue to function adequately increases the workload on the rest of the heart muscle. The size of the infarcted area can lead to **congestive heart failure,** a condition in which the heart does not pump adequately, creating a buildup of fluids in the lungs and eventually the rest of the body.

HEART VALVE DISEASE

The valves of the heart and circulatory system function to prevent a backflow of blood, which causes an additional workload on the heart because it then has to repump the blood. Valvular heart disease is commonly due to malfunctions of the heart caused by congenital abnormalities or diseases such as rheumatic fever or **endocarditis** (inflammation of the inside of the heart). Valves may malfunction due to **stenosis,** a narrowed valvular opening, or valvular insufficiency, when the opening is too large to close sufficiently (Figure 6.14).

Valvular defects can lead to the formation of clots, or thrombus. If the thrombus breaks loose, becoming an embolus, it can occlude the arteries leading to the major organs, such as the lungs, causing a pulmonary embolism, or the brain, causing a cerebral vascular accident (stroke). Defects such as valvular insufficiency can also cause congestive heart failure, due to the increased workload on the heart.

CARDIAC DYSRHYTHMIAS

The term *dysrhythmia* describes a change in the normal electrical rhythm the heart produces. A normal sinus rhythm is the heart, functioning normally, producing an electrical impulse in the sinus node (SA) that travels through the heart's electrical system. When the impulse originates in the sinus node, the heart rate is normally between 60 and 100 beats per minute. If the SA node generates no impulse, the rhythm is sinus arrest and reduced cardiac output results due to the atria of the heart no longer contracting. In most cases, when the SA node fails to fire, the atrioventricular (AV) node or ventricular pathways will take over, producing a slower rate than normal. When the AV or ventricular pathways fail to take over, asystole, the absence of electrical activity occurs and the heart stops all function (Figure 6.15).

Dysrhythmias can originate in any of the pathways of the electrical system of the heart beyond the SA node and normal pathway. Atrial dysrhythmias include premature atrial contractions, atrial tachycardia, multifocal atrial tachycardia, atrial flutter, and atrial fibrillation. **Atrial fibrillation** occurs when the atria fire in chaotic or unorganized impulses, causing blood to stagnate in the atria. A clot or thrombus can break loose from this stagnant blood, moving downstream and occluding a smaller vessel. If this happens to be in the cerebral circulation, it will cause a stroke (Figure 6.16).

Ventricular tachycardia (VT), or rapid heart rate, is an example of a dysrhythmia originating in the ventricles of the heart. Ventricular tachycardia occurs when irritation in the ventricles causes them to fire faster than normal. The ventricles of the heart do not fill sufficiently due to the abnormally rapid contractions of the ventricles. Individuals with heart disease or prior infarction

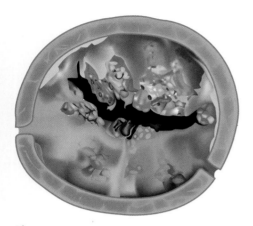

Figure 6.14 A heart valve with too large an opening may not close sufficiently, allowing blood to flow back into the atria, reducing the amount of blood pumped into the systemic circulation

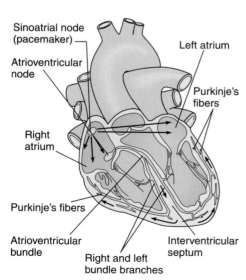

Sinoatrial node (pacemaker)

Atrioventricular node

Left atrium

Purkinje's fibers

Right atrium

Purkinje's fibers

Atrioventricular bundle

Right and left bundle branches

Interventricular septum

Figure 6.15 Normal electrical pathway through the heart

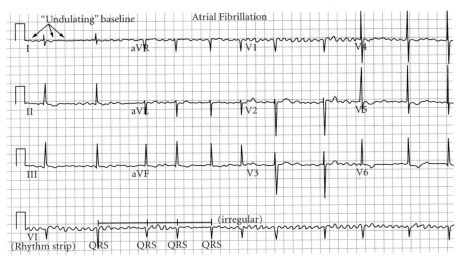

Figure 6.16 Atrial fibrillation

cannot tolerate this dysrhythmia for long. Most individuals with VT will deteriorate into ventricular fibrillation or pulseless VT, which will lead to death without immediate intervention. Ventricular tachycardia with a pulse present is treated with **cardioversion,** a process used to restore the heart's normal rhythm for unstable patients showing signs of shock, while stable patients are typically treated with medication, depending on prior heart functions. Once ventricular tachycardia becomes pulseless or deteriorates into ventricular fibrillation, both lethal dysrhythmias, the most effective treatment is **defibrillation,** an electrical shock applied to the heart to interrupt an abnormal rhythm (Figure 6.17).

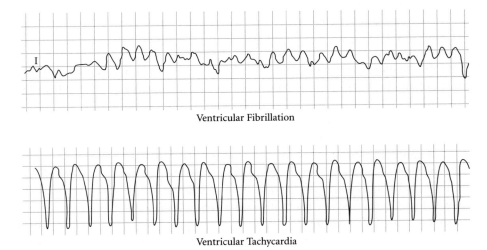

Ventricular Fibrillation

Ventricular Tachycardia

Figure 6.17 Ventricular fibrillation and ventricular tachycardia

THE FLUID

Blood is a multi-cell fluid made up of formed elements such as the red blood cells, containing hemoglobin, white blood cells, and platelets. Blood, pumped by the heart, travels through the pipes, carrying the fuels necessary for sustaining life, namely glucose (sugar) and oxygen. Glucose and oxygen fuel the individual cells that make up the tissues and organs of the body. **Metabolism** is the use, or "burning," of these fuels by the body.

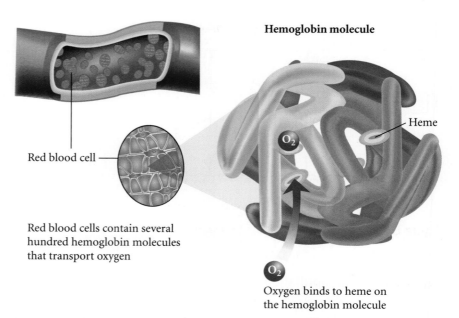

Hemoglobin molecule

Red blood cell

Heme

O₂

Red blood cells contain several hundred hemoglobin molecules that transport oxygen

O₂

Oxygen binds to heme on the hemoglobin molecule

Figure 6.18 Red blood cells contain hemoglobin necessary for carrying oxygen to the cells

Red blood cells carry hemoglobin, necessary for oxygen transportation to the tissues of the body (Figure 6.18). A decrease of hemoglobin in red blood cells results in poor, or inadequate, tissue perfusion (hypoperfusion) or *shock*.

Almost all oxygen (98%) in the blood is bound to and transported by hemoglobin; the balance (1.5%) is dissolved in plasma. For this reason, the partial pressure of oxygen combined with hemoglobin saturation (the percent of hemoglobin molecules carrying oxygen) is important.

Hemoglobin saturation, or *oxy-hemoglobin dissociation curve,* is simply the amount of hemoglobin in the blood and the amount of O_2 in the blood, in combination.

At a higher partial pressure of O_2 (above 40 mmHg), hemoglobin saturation normally remains high. This plane, or plateau of the curve, is significant because it tells us that under resting conditions only about 20% to 25% of hemoglobin molecules release their oxygen in the cells. This also indicates there is a substantial reserve of oxygen.

When the body becomes more active and the cells require more oxygen, the hemoglobin molecules in the blood provide the levels necessary for normal cellular respiration. As the body becomes more active, the oxygen levels in active cells can drop below 40 mmHg. As the oxy-hemoglobin dissociation curve in Figure 6.19 shows, as oxygen levels drop, hemoglobin releases oxygen to active cells, requiring it to sustain the energy; as a result, the hemoglobin saturation declines sharply.

DISEASES AND DISORDERS OF CIRCULATION

A break in the pipes of the circulatory system causes bleeding and the loss of the vital fluid needed to maintain perfusion. Whether the bleeding occurs externally or internally, the loss of hemoglobin-carrying red blood cells can cause hypoperfusion, or shock. Capillary injury is normally not serious; however, compromise of larger blood vessels can cause severe bleeding, or hemorrhage. If not reversed or halted, this will contribute to a life-threatening condition, known as hypovolemia. **Hypovolemia** is a systemic compromise that can result through both bleeding and loss of body fluids through dehydration.

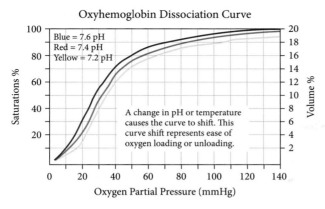

Figure 6.19 Oxy-hemoglobin dissociation curve

EXTERNAL BLEEDING

External bleeding usually occurs because of traumatic injury such as lacerations seen in stabbings, gunshot wounds, and amputations. The severity of blood loss depends on several factors, including the amount of blood lost, other injuries or preexisting conditions, existing medical problems, and the patient's age. The size of individuals can also affect the severity of the blood loss. Larger adults losing 500 ml of blood are not usually as adversely affected as a smaller adult or child losing the same amount.

When an artery, rich in oxygenated blood, is damaged or severed, arterial bleeding may occur. This type of bleeding is usually characterized by "spurting" with each beat or contraction of the heart. **Arterial bleeding** is under pressure and difficult to control. When the individual's blood pressure decreases, a late sign of shock, the spurting will also decrease; however, bleeding will continue as a steady flow of blood.

Bleeding that does not spurt with each heartbeat but is a steady flow from a wound usually indicates a severed or damaged vein. **Venous bleeding** is under less pressure and is easier to control than arterial bleeding, but it still may be severe and life threatening.

Capillary bleeding is typically slow, oozing, and easily controlled. This type of bleeding usually clots, and bleeding stops on its own. Capillary bleeding is not usually life threatening, but if a large surface area of the body is involved, bleeding can be severe.

INTERNAL BLEEDING

Internal bleeding can occur in both blunt force trauma and disease processes. Impact or crush injuries to the torso can cause bleeding of the heart, lungs, and internal organs. Disease processes such as aneurysms, abnormal clotting, or diverticulitis can also cause significant internal blood loss.

Diverticulosis is a condition of the colon in which little pouches called **diverticula** form. These pouches may become packed with fecal matter, becoming inflamed and causing pain and fever. **Diverticulitis** is an inflammatory disease that may lead to an obstruction of the colon, perforation, and hemorrhage.

Hemophilia (heem-o-FILL-ee-ah) is a rare, inherited bleeding disorder in which blood does not clot normally. Hemophiliacs have a deficiency or absence of either of two clotting elements in the blood. Hemophiliacs may bleed longer than others following an injury, and internal bleeding within the joints, especially the knees, ankles, and elbows, may also occur. Internal bleeding seen with hemophilia can damage organs or tissues due to inadequate perfusion and can sometimes lead to fatal hemorrhage.

Internal bleeding is more difficult to recognize because it is not visible, and severe blood loss can occur that rapidly progresses into hypoperfusion and death, sometimes within a matter of minutes. Like external bleeding, the severity of internal bleeding depends on the individual's overall health, age, other medical conditions, and cause of bleeding. Internal bleeding should always be suspected when unexplained signs of shock exist.

DEHYDRATION

Dehydration can result from lack of fluid intake and conditions that cause sustained or excessive vomiting and diarrhea. It can also be caused by environmental exposures such as heat exhaustion and medical treatments such as chemotherapy. **Dehydration** is the loss of too much body fluid, causing an imbalance of electrolytes, the salts and minerals affecting the amount of water in the body, and muscle activity. The fluid volume needed to carry the molecules of water, foods, gases, wastes, and ions (electrically charged particles) to maintain fluid balance must be replaced to maintain homeostasis.

Diarrhea, or loose, watery stools, is one of the most common causes of dehydration due to loss of body water. Diarrhea is usually acute and caused by bacteria, as seen in contaminated food or water. Diarrhea can also be caused by viral and parasitic infections, as well as a reaction to medications. Chronic diarrhea is usually due to diseases that affect the intestines, such as inflammatory bowel disease, Crohn's disease, and celiac disease. Diarrhea can be a symptom of irritable bowel syndrome.

Diarrhea is not usually harmful, but if it persists for more than 3 days without replenishment of both the fluid volume and electrolytes, dehydration can become severe and hypovolemic shock ultimately occurs.

CELLULAR RESPIRATION

Cells require energy to survive. Their continued functioning depends on chemical reactions within the cells. Biologically useable energy is required for these chemical reactions to take place. ATP (adenosine triphosphate) is the energy source available to cells for these chemical reactions to maintain cellular structure and function. **Cellular metabolism,** also called **cellular respiration,** is the process that describes the chemical changes that take place within a cell.

There are two categories of *metabolism* (chemical and physical changes taking place within the cells): **anabolism** (an-AB-oh-lizm), a process requiring energy that builds larger molecules by combining smaller molecules, and **catabolism** (ka-TAB-oh-lism), a process in which energy is released to break down large molecules into smaller ones. **ATP (adenosine triphosphate),** energy required by cells, is made within the cells through *catabolism* (decomposition) of the organic molecules of carbohydrates, fats, and proteins. The formation of ATP during the breakdown of organic molecules requires molecular oxygen, or cellular respiration (Figure 6.20).

As we have noted previously, respiration requires an exchange of gases between the cell and its surroundings to allow oxygen into the cell and carbon dioxide to move out of the cell. Cellular respiration is the **aerobic** (requiring oxygen) **metabolism** process of ATP production. *Glucose,* a simple sugar molecule, is the most common substance broken down in the cells to produce ATP, or energy at the cellular level.

Glucose metabolizes when there are adequate amounts of oxygen present, producing large amounts of energy for the cells to use. The product of glucose metabolism is water and carbon dioxide, which is transported to the lungs for elimination. This type of metabolism is called *aerobic metabolism.*

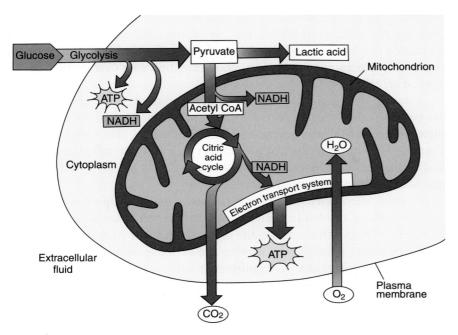

Figure 6.20 Cellular respiration (metabolism)

When oxygen is not available while the cell is metabolizing glucose, very little energy is produced for the cell. The process of metabolizing glucose with little energy production is called **anaerobic** (without oxygen) **metabolism.** When very little oxygen is being delivered to the cells, very little energy is being produced. The by-product of anaerobic metabolism, acid, causes muscle fatigue, which in turn requires more energy to produce ATP. Aerobic respiration is required to produce the needed energy; however, if oxygen cannot be supplied to the muscle from the bloodstream quickly enough, lactic acid begins to accumulate from anaerobic metabolism. The response of the body is to accelerate heart and breathing rates to get more oxygen into the body. Once the oxygen reaches the muscle, the lactic acid is broken down, relieving muscle fatigue.

Cellular respiration can be adversely affected by the inhalation of toxic gases, such as cyanide or carbon monoxide, and certain biological agents, such as anthrax and tuberculosis. **Toxins** are poisons capable of causing cellular injury and death. Toxins compromise cells through one of two mechanisms—direct reaction with the cell or metabolites. **Metabolites** are usually small molecules left over from chemicals after the cells have reacted with them. In other words, they are a by-product of metabolism.

DISEASES AND DISORDERS OF CELLULAR RESPIRATION

A toxin can affect cellular respiration by internal or external means. External toxins, such as cyanide, carbon monoxide, and bacteria, enter the body through food, water, air, or physical contact with skin or mucous membranes. Internal toxins, such as free radicals, are produced by the body through the metabolic process.

EXTERNAL TOXINS

Carbon monoxide is a colorless, odorless gas that is the by-product of incomplete combustion. The most common sources of carbon monoxide are exhaust from motor vehicles, smoke from fires, and nonelectric heaters, such as furnaces and hot water heaters. When carbon monoxide is inhaled, it directly binds to the hemoglobin approximately 200 times better than oxygen does, thereby displacing oxygen and decreasing tissue oxygenation. Carbon monoxide may also be directly toxic to the myocardium, with some patients complaining of angina (chest pain) and presenting with dysrhythmias indicative of an AMI.

Cyanide poisoning can be a by-product of smoke inhalation involving the burning of substances such as rubber, plastic, and silk. Products used in photography, metal processing, and other industries also contain cyanide. Certain plants, such as apricot pits and a type of potato called cassava, naturally contain cyanide. Only chronic or massive ingestion of any of these plants can lead to serious cyanide poisoning.

Cyanide affects virtually all body tissues by inactivating an enzyme, cytochrome oxidase, needed in cellular respiration, even when adequate oxygen is present. Without this enzyme, the cells cannot make ATP. In simple terms, cyanide suffocates the cells by making the available oxygen useless. The tissues with the highest oxygen requirement—the brain, heart, and liver—are most profoundly affected.

Bacteria, such as streptococcus, can secrete a protein, called **exotoxins,** into the interstitial fluid, where they are absorbed into the surrounding cells. Exotoxins can affect specific cells. As an example, the toxins produced by the streptococcus bacteria affect vascular tissue. Group A streptococcus infections have been associated with shock and organ failure. Complications of group A streptococcal infections can be severe and include **bacteremia** (bacteria in the blood) associated with aggressive soft tissue infections such as **necrotizing fasciitis,** also known as the "flesh-eating disease."

INTERNAL TOXINS

Internal toxins are produced through cellular breakdown following the death of bacteria. **Endotoxins,** the fragments of bacterial cell wall membrane released following the death of the bacteria, are attracted to other cell wall membranes. For example, bacteria such as *Clostridium tetanus* can produce *phospholipase*, an enzyme that breaks down cell walls.

Free Radicals   **Free radicals** such as hydrogen peroxide and other reactive oxygen chemicals are the by-product of incomplete metabolism, which causes cellular injury. The oxygen we breathe is used by mitochondria within our cells to convert sugars, fats, and inorganic phosphate (ADP) into ATP. During the chemical processes of metabolism, a small amount of leftover oxygen loses electrons, creating free radicals.

Most stable chemical compounds in the body possess a pair of electrons. Free radicals are produced when one electron is stripped from the pair. The free, unstable electron seeks out and combines with another element to form a new stable compound. This process breaks up a stable compound, releasing another free radical and continuing the cycle.

Reactive oxygen chemicals can connect with amino acids within the DNA, causing cellular destruction, or they can pair with **lipids** (fats that are not soluble in water), causing a chain reaction called *lipid perioxidation*, which also results in cellular destruction. The result of cellular injury caused by free radicals is the inability of damaged cells to produce proteins and reproduce themselves. The weakened cell walls permit an increase of intracellular sodium, leading to **autolysis,** or the biological self-destruction of cells.

The result of free radicals over time is weakened tissues and organs. The body is less able to fight off diseases, such as cancer, stenosis of arteries, and other disorders. To protect the body, the mutation of cells by free radicals needs to be prevented or repaired by **antioxidants,** photochemicals found in plants. Antioxidants essentially deactivate potentially dangerous free radicals, breaking the chain reaction before cellular injury occurs or progresses.

CONCLUSION

Understanding diseases and disorders affecting homeostasis—the balance of oxygenation, ventilation, respiration, circulation, and cellular respiration—is vital to the EMT's understanding of patient assessment and management in the field.

Recognizing compromise of these processes will help EMTs treat patients appropriately in the out-of-hospital setting and assist prehospital health care providers in determining the need for advanced life support (ALS) interventions.

Street Smart

Each cell produces its own antioxidant, but the ability to produce antioxidants decreases with age. A diet rich in fruits and vegetables supplemented with vitamins and minerals can supplement the production of antioxidants. Vitamins A, C, and E, known as the ACE trio, are antioxidants, with vitamin C considered the most powerful of the three.

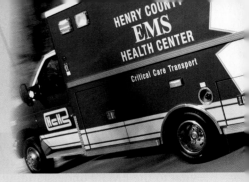

CASE STUDY Continued

Beth understands the pathophysiology of lung cancer and heart disease and knows the elderly man will die eventually from those conditions. This knowledge does not make it any easier to care for him. But rather than dwell on the negative, Beth elects to look for positive ways to interact with her patient. He is a veteran, proud to have served his country with honor, and he has lived a full life, so Beth engages him in conversation about his military service, his family, and his country. She hopes this might, for a moment, take his mind off his suffering and make life a little more bearable.

Key Concepts Revisited

- An understanding of pathophysiology, the functional changes associated with or resulting from disease or injury, is important to effective management of that illness or injury.

- Changes in the structures and functions of cells interfere with homeostasis, causing the body to become diseased.

- Predisposing risk factors can make an individual more susceptible to disease, or they can be modified to lessen susceptibility to disease.
  - o Risk factors that cannot be modified include age, gender, and heredity.
  - o Risk factors that can be modified include lifestyle choices, smoking, obesity, lack of exercise, excessive alcohol consumption, environment, and excessive stress.

- Three predictable outcomes of disease are:
  - o Recovery, or a complete return to health with no remnants of disease;
  - o Residuals, or recovery with physical or chemical changes remaining; and
  - o Remission, nonactive, or dormant disease state.

- Hypoxia, the number one chemical cause of cellular injury, results from:
  - o Extrinsic causes, including trauma and environment, or
  - o Intrinsic causes, including disease.

- The brain, as the life center of the body, requires sufficient glucose-rich, oxygenated blood to function.

- Every known disease interferes with the five components of the process known as the Fick Principle:
  - o Oxygenation—oxygen content in ambient air
  - o Ventilation—the process of bringing oxygen into the body
  - o Respiration—gas exchange to oxygenate blood and eliminate waste
  - o Circulation—process of bringing oxygenated blood to body cells for gas exchange
  - o Cellular respiration—process of metabolizing oxygen and glucose into energy

- Adequate oxygen concentration in the air can be compromised by
  - o Displacement by other gases such as nitrogen, carbon dioxide, and helium,
  - o Lower atmospheric pressures, and/or
  - o Consumption within confined spaces.

- An intact and functioning respiratory system is necessary for oxygenation to take place.

- Ventilation, a complex process of bringing oxygen into the lungs and eliminating carbon dioxide, is dependent on:
  - o Chemoreceptors measuring the chemical changes of respiration: carbon dioxide, oxygen, and hydrogen levels;
  - o Minute volume, the amount of air breathed in and out in 1 minute;

- Tidal volume, the amount of air inhaled and exhaled in one breath; and
- Alveolar ventilation, the amount of air breathed reaching the alveoli in the lungs for gas exchange.

- Disease and physical injury affect ventilation, leading to respiratory compromise, through
  - Obstructions of the structures of the upper airway by foreign body obstruction or swelling, or
  - Obstruction of lower airways by a disease process such as COPD.
- Gases diffuse across the capillary/alveoli membrane in the process called respiration.
- Diseases or injuries that impair or arrest ventilation and respiration upset homeostasis, leading to hypoxia without intervention. These conditions include
  - Neuromuscular disease such as ALS and
  - Traumatic injury to any of the structures of respiration.
- Oxygenated blood must circulate to the cells using the pump, pipes, and fluid of the circulatory system.
  - The pipes are the blood vessels responsible for transporting oxygen to and carbon dioxide away from the tissues and organs of the body.
  - The pump or heart is responsible for getting the nutrient-rich fluid, vital for all functions of life, into the pipeline and throughout the body.
  - The blood, or fluid of the body, contains the essential elements needed for cellular function and fuels (glucose and oxygen) necessary for sustaining life.
- Diseases of the any of the components that make up the circulatory system can result in decreasing or preventing available gases for diffusion:
  - Blood vessels (pipes) can be disrupted or blocked by
    - Diseases such as arteriosclerosis that narrow the vessel and decrease blood flow
    - Autonomic nervous system disruption
      - Neurogenic shock
      - Psychogenic shock
    - Inflammatory response
      - Anaphylactic shock
  - The heart (pump) can fail, preventing blood to be pumped out to the cells
    - Cardiac output disruption
      - Decrease in preload
      - Decrease in afterload

- Acute myocardial infarction (AMI)
  - Occlusion of blood vessels causes damage to the muscle
  - Cardiac muscle infarcts and cannot contract
  - Heart cannot pump enough blood out to the system
  - Fluid backs up into the lungs and pools in the system
- Heart valve defects lead to clot formation, possible emboli, occluding arteries, and decreasing blood flow to organs
  - Increases workload on the heart through fluid backup
- Cardiac dysrhythmias
  - Disruption of the electrical current stimulating the heart to contract
- A break in the pipes causes bleeding and a loss of the multi-celled fluid carrying the fuels of life (oxygen and sugar)
  - Hypovolemia is the systemic compromise that results in loss of blood and body fluids
  - Dehydration is the result of lack of fluid intake or excessive fluid loss
    - Fluid volume is required to carry the molecules of water, food, gases, wastes, and electrons to maintain homeostasis
  - Diseases such as diverticulosis and hemophilia can cause excessive internal bleeding leading to hypovolemic shock
- Cellular metabolism is a vital chemical reaction required in the production of energy cells need to survive.
  - Aerobic metabolism requires oxygen to break down glucose and produce high levels of energy.
  - Anaerobic metabolism occurs when oxygen is not available, producing little energy and producing acid.
- Internal and external toxins, resulting in cellular destruction, may adversely affect cellular respiration.
  - External toxins such as carbon monoxide and cyanide displace oxygen in the blood cells and decrease oxygen for cellular metabolism
    - Bacteria produce exotoxins affecting specific cells and vascular tissue

- Internal toxins are produced during cellular breakdown following the death of bacteria
  - Endotoxins are fragments of bacterial cell wall membranes that are attracted to other cell wall membranes

- Free radicals are the by-products of incomplete metabolism
- Recognition of compromises of any of the processes within the Fick Principle will help the EMT manage patients appropriately in the prehospital setting.

Key Terms

Acute myocardial infarction (AMI)

Adenosine triphosphate (ATP)

Aerobic metabolism

Afterload

Allergen

Alveolar ventilation

Amyotrophic lateral sclerosis (ALS)

Anabolism

Anaerobic metabolism

Anaphylactic shock

Angina

Anoxia

Antioxidants

Apnea

Arterial bleeding

Arterioles

Arteriosclerosis

Atherosclerosis

Atrial fibrillation

Autolysis

Bacteremia

Baroreceptors

Barotraumas

Blood pressure

Capillary bleeding

Cardiac output

Cardioversion

Catabolism

Cellular respiration (cellular metabolism)

Central chemoreceptors

Cerebral circulation

Chemoreceptors

Congestive heart failure

Continuous Positive Airway Pressure (CPAP)

Dead air space

Defibrillation

Dehydration

Diastolic blood pressure

Diffusion

Disease

Disorder

Diverticula

Diverticulitis

Dormant

Dysrhythmia

Embolus

Endocarditis

Endothelial cells

Endotoxin

Etiology

Exotoxin

Extrinsic

Fetal circulation

Fick Principle

Flail chest

Frank-Starling law (Starling law)

Free radicals

Glucose

Hemoglobin

Hemoglobin saturation

Hemophilia

Hypercarbic

Hyperemia

Hypoglycemia

Hypoperfusion

Hypopnea

Hypovolemia

Hypoxemia

Hypoxia

Hypoxic drive

Idiopathic

Infarction

Intercostal muscles

Intrinsic

Lipids

Lumen

Mediastinum

Metabolism

Metabolites

Minute volume

Motor neurons

Necrosis

Necrotizing fasciitis

Negative pressure ventilation

Neurogenic shock

Oxygenation

Paradoxical motion

Pathogenesis

Pathogens

Pathology

Pathophysiology

Peripheral chemoreceptors

Phrenic nerve

Pleural cavity/potential space

Pneumothorax

Preload

Prognosis

Psychogenic shock (vasovagal shock)

Pulmonary circulation

Recovery

Remission

Residuals

Respiratory rate

Risk factors

Scalene muscles

Stenosis

Syndrome

Systemic circulation

Systemic vascular resistance (SVR)

Systolic blood pressure

Tidal volume

Total peripheral resistance

Toxin

Trauma

Tunics

Tunica adventitia

Tunica intima

Tunica media

Venous bleeding

Ventricular tachycardia

Venules

Review Questions

1. Define pathophysiology and explain why an understanding of the disease process is important to the EMT.
2. How does hypoxia affect the cells of the body?
3. What are the five elements of the Fick Principle?
4. Name two possible causes of obstruction of ventilation.
5. What is the difference between ventilation and respiration?
6. Name a disease process that affects the muscles of ventilation and respiration.
7. Name three causes of circulatory failure.
8. Define cellular respiration.
9. How do both internal and external toxins adversely affect cellular respiration?
10. What elements of cellular metabolism are required for high-energy production?
11. What adverse affects do free radicals have on the body?
12. Explain how failure of the first four elements of the Fick Principle affects cellular respiration.

Further Study

Brown. K. *Emergency Dysrhythmias and ECG Injury Patterns.* Clifton Park, NY: Thomson Delmar Learning, 2003.

Dalton, A., Limmer, D., Mistovich. J., & Weiman. H. *Advanced Medical Life Support.* 3d ed. Upper Saddle River, NJ. Pearson/ Prentice Hall, 2007.

Myer, J., Neighbors, M., & Tannehille-Jones. R. *Principles in Pathophysiology and Emergency Medical Care.* Clifton Park, NY: Thomson Delmar Learning, 2002.

Rizzo. D. *Fundamentals of Anatomy and Physiology.* 2d ed. Clifton Park, NY: Thomson Delmar Learning, 2006.

UNIT ⑦ Life Span Development

The developmental age of a patient, physically, mentally, and emotionally, will affect almost every aspect of an EMT's care of that patient. Basic vital signs vary by age. The patient's developmental age must be taken into account when the EMT interacts with the patient during an encounter. Having a fundamental understanding of human development over a life span is essential to good patient assessment and management.

> ## National Education Standard
> The Emergency Medical Technician (EMT) shall apply a fundamental understanding of life span development to patient assessment and management.

Key Concepts

- Human development over a life span involves physical, mental, and psychosocial changes.

- Changes in human development affect how an EMT interacts with a patient.

- Knowledge of human development can help the EMT understand how injury and illness may affect the patient.

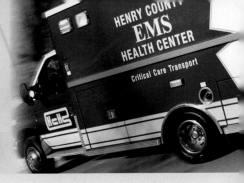

CASE STUDY

While en route to the nursing home, Jeff and his partner start to discuss what it is like to be elderly and how they would want to live when they are elderly. Looking out the window, as the siren blares, Jeff is thinking about his daughter and how quickly she has changed from infant to preschooler to teenager. Especially when your children grow up right before your eyes, he realizes, life seems to fly right past a person.

Jeff is also thinking that he is starting to feel his age. He wonders how long he can keep doing EMS. At age 50, he feels the aches and pains after a day of lifting stretchers.

His thoughts turn to his mother, who moved in with his family last year after breaking her hip. She was just standing in her kitchen when she fell. She is increasingly frail, and though her mind is still sharp and full of wit, her short-term memory fails her more and more often. Jeff and his wife have talked about the potential health and safety problems that might result when his mother is home alone. They have discussed whether to talk with her about moving to a nursing home for her own safety.

Jeff's attention is diverted as he turns into the approach to the nursing home. Clean and modern looking, the nursing home looks more like a hospital than a home. The dispatcher advises the crew that the patient has expired and their services are no longer needed. They are back in service. The silence after the siren is turned off seems especially quiet.

Critical Thinking Questions

1. What physical changes occur in childhood, adulthood, and the elder years?

2. What mental changes take place in childhood, adulthood, and the elder years?

3. What psychosocial changes can be expected in childhood, adulthood, and the elder years?

INTRODUCTION

Injury and illness affect patients differently. This difference is, in part, due to age and associated changes of aging. For example, an upper respiratory infection that is an annoyance to an adolescent could be deadly for an elderly patient. By understanding the physical, mental, and psychosocial changes that take place over a lifetime, an Emergency Medical Technician can better assess the impact of illness and trauma upon the patient.

HUMAN DEVELOPMENT

The three areas of human development are mental (cognitive), physical (psychomotor), and psychosocial (psychological). Mental development involves growth and changes in intelligence, which allows us to learn and adapt to our environment to survive. The second area, physical development, encompasses growth and changes of the body and the ability to perform tasks at home, school, work, and play. The final area, psychosocial development, involves emotional growth and control.

Positive growth and change within any of these three areas, or domains, is called **maturation.** As people mature, they grow and learn, through practice, new knowledge, skills, and emotions. Disease can affect normal maturation negatively.

CONCEPTION

Remarkable growth occurs in a human beginning from the moment of conception through the moment of birth. During this time the foundations for all the body's organ systems are laid down. What starts as two cells develops into a human being.

Disease can occur during pregnancy and can have an impact on the brain, impairing cognitive growth, and on nerves, bones, and muscles, or psychomotor growth. For example, measles (rubella) can cause congenital anomalies and even result in premature labor and miscarriage.

Certain chemicals, called **teratogens** (tear–rat–O–jens), can also affect fetal development in the womb. Examples of teratogens include certain medications, illicit drugs, tobacco smoke, and alcohol. Alcohol use during pregnancy can lead to a condition called fetal alcohol syndrome (Figure 7.1). Maternal alcohol use may result in stunted growth and permanent brain damage. Adverse effects on the developing fetus may occur as the result of maternal drinking in any of the three trimesters of pregnancy. Stillbirths and deaths of infants at birth have also been linked to alcohol use.

INFANCY

When an infant is born has a great impact on survival and future growth. An infant born before 28 weeks from conception, or who weighs less than 1,500 grams (approximately 3 pounds), may not be mature enough to survive. One problem in particular for premature infants is the development of their lungs. At that early stage of development, the infant's lungs may have not matured enough for the infant to survive. Inadequate lung function may result in a period of prolonged hypoxia that leads to brain damage.

The changes that occur during the **neonatal** (nee–oh– nay–Tall) period, from birth to 30 days, are remarkable. For example, after birth the heart rate of a newborn is almost too fast to count, or greater than 150 beats per minute. Within minutes the heart rate drops to around 120 beats per minute. It is important that the infant's heart rate remain fast during these early moments. If a newborn's heart rate is less than 100 beats per minute, then blood flow is too slow, hypoxia ensues, and resuscitation is necessary.

Neonates, or infants less than 30 days old, may have trouble adjusting to life outside the womb, called *problems of transition*. These problems are the result of the neonate's unique physiology. For example, infants accustomed to a constant 98.6°F (37°C) temperature within the womb need to produce their own heat to survive. They do this by burning special energy stores, called brown fat, that keeps their temperature between 98° and 100°F. Premature infants have little or no brown fat and thus cannot produce heat well and are prone to hypothermia (low body temperature).

Another weak point in infants' physiology is their pulmonary system. Starting at the top and working down, neonates have shorter and narrower airways that can be easily obstructed. Furthermore, neonates are nose breathers, breathing through their nose unless they are in pain or experience air hunger from a lack of oxygen, or hypoxia. In addition, infants have weak intercostal muscles, the muscles between the ribs that act as accessory muscles of breathing, and depend almost entirely on the diaphragm to breathe. Finally the infants' lungs have fewer alveoli, the functional units that exchange oxygen and carbon dioxide in the lungs. Any problem with these three areas of the pulmonary system can lead to pulmonary failure. If an infant's nose were to become obstructed, for example from mucus produced during an

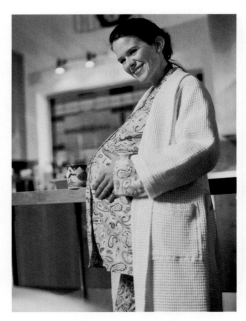

Figure 7.1 Alcohol consumption during pregnancy can lead to complications such as fetal alcohol syndrome

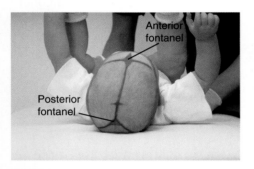

Figure 7.2 The infant's fontanels, or soft spots, allows the brain to expand within the skull

upper respiratory infection, the neonate would have to breathe through his mouth. This would result in faster heat loss, resulting in hypothermia; faster moisture loss, resulting in weight loss; and increased work at breathing, leading to energy loss.

As a result of the normal work of breathing, maintenance of body temperature, and other factors, it is normal for a neonate to lose 5% to 10% of body weight in the first week of life. Most neonates quickly regain that lost weight within weeks.

FIRST YEAR PHYSICAL DEVELOPMENT

An infant grows rapidly from head to toe. The brain develops rapidly, achieving 50% of adult capacity within the first 2 years. To accommodate this growth the skull has open fissures, called *sutures*, that allow the skull to be flexible, and two fontanels, the anterior and posterior fontanel. These fontanels, shown in Figure 7.2, also called the soft spots, areas of the brain covered only by soft tissue. This soft tissue allows the brain to expand without fracturing the skull. As the child matures, these fontanels close, as the skulls bones come together. The posterior fontanel closes at about 3 months but the anterior fontanel, at the crown of the skull, remains open for 9 to 18 months.

Because the infant's head is so large, about 25% of the body's size, the infant is top heavy and prone to falls. Infants learn to walk usually within the first year of life, and they take plenty of tumbles in learning to do so. Fortunately any swelling of the brain, as a result of a blow to the head, can be partially compensated by the elastic fontanel.

Without the capacity to think, infants rely heavily on primitive reflexes for survival. Examples of these reflexes include the rooting reflex. Touch the infant on the cheek and the infant will reflexively turn toward the stimulus. The infant also has a suckling reflex. Place a nipple in the infant's mouth and a series of coordinated muscular contractions designed to draw milk into the mouth occur. The infant also has a gag reflex to help protect the airway. This reflex, unlike some others, remains with the infant for life. The gag reflex develops around the 34th week of gestation in the womb. Therefore premature infants do not have a gag reflex and are more prone to aspiration.

As the infant's spinal cord develops, these primitive reflexes are replaced by voluntary actions. This maturation of spinal cord by myelination also occurs in a head to tail, or **cephalocaudal** (seff–ah–Lo–KAWD–al) pattern. This is evidenced by the psychomotor tasks the child accomplishes. First, at about 1 to 2 months, the infant pulls up the head, then the chest; at 6 to 8 months, the child can sit erect without support. Within several months the child crawls, cruises, and then awkwardly begins to walk. This unique walk, or gait, is referred to as a toddle and is the source of the name *toddler*. Most infants toddle by their first birthday.

Notice the use of the modifier *most*. Not all infants achieve common indicators of physical development, called *developmental milestones*, within that time span. An infant's failure to meet a developmental milestone is a red flag for health care providers and parents alike and bears further investigation into the cause of the developmental delay.

MENTAL DEVELOPMENT

As the infant's body develops, so does the brain. Initially the infant's only means of communication is to cry. Infants cry if they are hungry, in pain, or simply in need of reassurance that a caregiver is present and the infant is safe. As the brain develops, the infant starts to utter his or her first sounds, which are precursors to simple words. Most infants respond to words they hear frequently from their parents and siblings before they actually say them, and they say their first words between 10 and 15 months, a developmental milestone. By two years of age, most toddlers have a rich vocabulary that allows them to express their needs.

PSYCHOSOCIAL DEVELOPMENT

Like cognitive development, the psychosocial development of the infant corresponds to the physical growth of the brain. Initially, the infant only has primitive reflexes, such as withdrawal from pain, for example.

An infant's vision is fairly limited at birth. As time progresses and the brain develops, the infant starts to recognize patterns, including the mother's face. Eventually the infant responds to their mother's smile by mimicking the smile, called reflexive smiling. Reflexive smiling is the start of a pattern of social referencing and shows that the infant has a positive regard for the mother.

Social referencing—smiling to please others, for example—is the start of the human emotional experience. This positive experience is reinforcing to the infant and cannot be better illustrated than by the phenomena of failure to thrive.

Failure to thrive is a condition in which the infant fails to grow because of parental neglect or abandonment. A description of a condition, and not a disease, failure to thrive may suggest child abuse or neglect, although it may be secondary to an occult disease state, a state not readily recognized through obvious signs and symptoms. Any child who fails to meet normal milestones should be evaluated by a pediatrician.

SUDDEN INFANT DEATH

The sudden and unexplained death of an apparently healthy infant may be because of **Sudden Infant Death Syndrome (SIDS),** also known as *crib death*. The cause of SIDS remains unknown, but it tends to occur in infants from 1 month to 1 year of age. A recent "back to bed" campaign encouraging parents to place infants on their backs in their cribs has helped to reduce the number of SIDS deaths.

TODDLER

From 1 year to 3 years of a child's life may be some of the most wondrous and trying years for parents. The child, able to walk, starts to explore the world and its dangers. Frustrating behaviors have earned this period of child's life the title "the terrible twos." For some of the same reasons the child may be at greater risk for child abuse.

PHYSICAL DEVELOPMENT

As the child's brain continues to develop, it will attain 90% of its adult size. The child starts to improve gross motor skills, such as walking, and begins to acquire fine motor skills through activities such as play. Correspondingly the child's bones and muscle mass increase to accommodate the new demands.

Also during this time, the spinal cord completes its myelination and the child learns to control his or her bladder and bowels. While the child may be physiologically capable of toilet training at 1 year, most children do not complete toilet training until age 2 or later.

Toddlers actively explore the environment. As a result major health concerns during this period of child development include drowning, choking, burns, and poisoning. The child's developmental age should be considered

Street Smart

Healthy infants are attentive to their parents. An infant who lies lifeless in his or her parent's arms, like a limp Raggedy Ann doll, is seriously ill. This condition is sometimes referred to as appearing *toxic*.

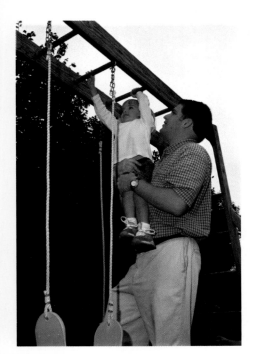

Figure 7.3 A child's developmental age should be considered when assessing a traumatic injury. Does the mechanism of injury match the developmental age? If not, the EMT may suspect child abuse

when assessing a traumatic injury. For example, would the child in Figure 7.3 be capable of running into an end table and sustaining a facial bruise?

MENTAL DEVELOPMENT

During the toddler years children learn mastery of their primary language. Through interaction with others and their environment, toddlers learn cause and effect and begin to appreciate that their actions have consequences.

PSYCHOSOCIAL DEVELOPMENT

The temperament of a toddler also manifests itself during this time. Temperament is a basic dimension of personality. Although temperament can change as a person matures, the toddlers' temperaments have a major impact on their social interactions with others, including an EMT. Elements of temperament include mood, attention span, task persistence, adaptability, and level of comfort with people, which determine whether a child will approach or withdraw from others.

The latter issue, approach or avoidance, is displayed in a child's behaviors. Some children offer signaling behaviors, such as extending a toy, while others cling to their mothers. When separated from their mothers, children may become upset and cry or throw a tantrum. These are normal behaviors that are a part of separation anxiety. Most children grow out of separation anxiety by age 3.

PRESCHOOLER

The term *preschooler* refers to children ages 3 to 5. This is the developmental stage when most children leave the protection of home and enter the world. This is a time of great psychosocial growth, but it also a time when children are exposed to new dangers not typically found at home, such as head lice and other communicable diseases passed from child to child in the preschool or day care setting.

PHYSICAL DEVELOPMENT

The physical growth of the child starts to slow in the preschool years and will not markedly increase until adolescence. The lungs of the preschooler are almost fully developed, but the terminal airways continue to branch and the alveoli continue to develop. The musculoskeletal system, in combination with the heart and lungs, permits the preschooler to actively participate in athletic activities. Table 7-1 lists the normal parameters of vital signs for a child from birth through 10 years of age.

Table 7-1 Vital Signs of Children (Normal Parameters)							
Average Pulse and Blood Pressure							
Age	Birth	6mo	1yr	2yr	6yr	8yr	10yr
Pulse	140	130	115	110	103	100	95
Systolic BP	70	90	90	92	95	100	105

It is also at this time the child's immune system becomes challenged by new disease-causing pathogens. Passive immunity, passed from mother to child, is gone, and children start to develop their own active immunities from exposure to disease. Many preschoolers develop pulmonary and gastrointestinal infections, with accompanying symptoms of cough, vomiting, and diarrhea. Childhood immunizations, which begin in infancy, continue to be important measures in preventing disease (see Figure 7.4).

MENTAL DEVELOPMENT

Preschoolers continue to learn about their environment as it enlarges beyond the home. Called the *pre-operational stage* by psychologists such as Piaget, the preschool years are the time when children start to understand that symbols have meaning and that they can draw on past experience to understand their present situation. For example, the child understands that a needle for a blood glucose sample will hurt—simple cause and effect based on previous experience.

PSYCHOSOCIAL DEVELOPMENT

Play is very important for the psychosocial development of preschoolers. The ability to play simple games and, more importantly, follow the rules helps to establish the importance of social interaction and accepted behavior. Play is central to the school-aged child, as shown in Figure 7.5. It is also at this age that children begin to display competitiveness.

SCHOOL AGE

Middle childhood, ages 6 to 12, are called the school years. School is a time of profound intellectual and psychosocial development. The impact of adult supervision and guidance, in the form of adult role models, starts to mold school-aged children into young adults.

PHYSICAL DEVELOPMENT

Many factors affect the physical development of school-aged children, including heredity, nutrition, and even emotional well-being. By age 6 all of the body functions and structures are intact, and children's builds are predictive of their adult bodies. Their athletic ability improves and muscle mass correspondingly increases. It is at this age that gender differences appear. Girls are physically more advanced than their male counterparts.

MENTAL DEVELOPMENT

The brain continues to develop, specifically with areas of the brain associated with focused attention. School-aged children are now able to "pay attention" to an adult speaking in a crowd. This ability to single out the speaker requires higher-level mental functioning. Children with attention deficit disorders are unable to focus on the speaker and tend to be easily distracted.

Typically school-aged children can also concentrate and follow instructions. For example, a school-aged child will participate in care if given instructions by an EMT. This ability to work with others while caring for oneself can be useful in the field.

PSYCHOSOCIAL DEVELOPMENT

School-aged children have learned how to read the emotional responses of others, called *social cues*, and respond accordingly. This phenomenon, called *social referencing*, may be observed by the EMT. The school-aged patient, generally hoping to please the adult, is compliant with requests and cooperative

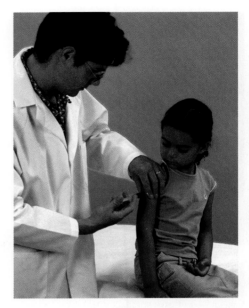

Figure 7.4 Children should receive a full program of immunizations

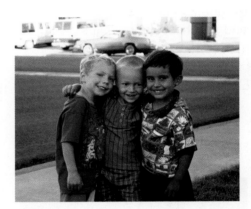

Figure 7.5 Play and friends become more central in a preschooler's life, but home remains the most important influence

Street Smart

The importance of play to preschoolers has implications for the EMT. It may be helpful if the EMT offers the child a stuffed toy and demonstrates the physical examination using the stuffed toy, such as listening to the chest of the toy before listening to the chest of the child.

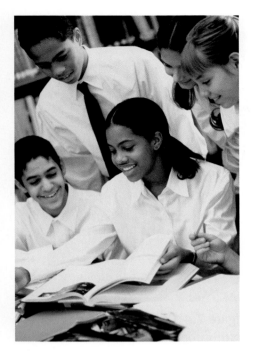

Figure 7.6 School-aged children experience many physical, mental, and psychosocial changes

with care. For the same reason these children are very aware of their peers and the response of their peers. In some cases, it may be important to separate the child from peers to get a sincere response to questions. The changes in a school-aged child, as illustrated in Figure 7.6, are remarkable.

ADOLESCENCE

A person's self-identity tends to emerge during adolescence. Dramatic changes of puberty and personal challenges tend to change children into what they will become as adults. Words that symbolize adolescence include rebellion and independence.

PHYSICAL DEVELOPMENT

Adolescents aged 13 to 19 years experience tremendous growth and development during this time, the most since infancy. These growth spurts start distally, at the hands and feet and progress to the trunk. The changes of adolescence—from breast buds to axillary hair—signal the start of sexual maturation. These sexual changes bring with them a number of associated health concerns, including sexually transmitted diseases and teenage pregnancy.

A part of sexual maturation is redistribution of fat. Girls tend to redistribute their body fat to the hips, thighs, and breasts, whereas boys tend to decrease their body fat and redistribute it to the abdomen. A current health concern is the development of obesity during adolescence. A more sedentary lifestyle and changes in diet have combined to increase the percentage of body fat in teenagers by 10% or more.

Dramatic physical development in this age-group tends to make adolescents more concerned about their body image. This concern is translated into modesty when the EMT asks to examine the patient. The EMT must respect the patient's modesty and make efforts to preserve the patient's privacy.

Injury and disability are foremost on adolescents' minds when they are sick or injured. An incapacity, no matter how seemingly minor, may be viewed as devastating. Adolescents may repeatedly ask the EMT if they are going to be all right or whether they will be disabled.

Adolescents also tend to be attracted to risky behaviors thought to be "grown up," such as alcohol abuse and illicit drug use (Figure 7.7). These behaviors have a number of associated health risks, some which are potentially life threatening.

MENTAL DEVELOPMENT

The mental development of an adolescent is almost adult-like. Adolescents can interact effectively with the EMT at three levels. First, they can articulate their concerns, speaking clearly to the EMT when describing their situation. Next, they can ask questions for clarification. These questions are

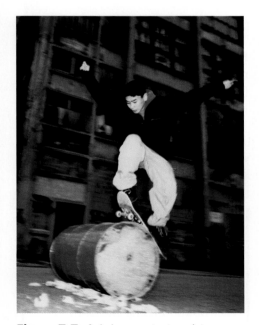

Figure 7.7 Adolescents tend to engage in risk-taking behaviors with potentially lifelong consequences

often insightful and intelligent. Finally, adolescents can assert themselves. Through strong and directed words, they can accept or refuse care that is being offered.

Because adolescents can articulate their concerns, ask insightful questions, and assert their rights as a person and patient, the EMT must enter into a careful negotiation with these young patients to obtain consent for care.

PSYCHOSOCIAL DEVELOPMENT

During adolescence a child learns how to collaborate with and to conform to others. The collaboration can be positive, such as participation in sports teams or science projects, or negative, such as membership in a gang. It is during these collaborations that adolescents' identity develops.

Some adolescents see themselves as productive citizens, able to volunteer in community services, such as EMS. Other adolescents, unfortunately, become antisocial and are labeled juvenile delinquents.

One significant question for adolescents to resolve is the question of sexuality. Personal appearance and social networking demonstrate adolescents' interest in sexuality (Figure 7.8). It is during adolescence that sexual exploration can occur, including, for some teenagers, questions about gender identity and sexual orientation.

EARLY ADULTHOOD

The key events that separate adolescence from early adulthood is the completion of high school and entry either into the workforce or postsecondary education and, perhaps more importantly, moving away from home. The single most important indicator of adulthood may be financial independence.

PHYSICAL DEVELOPMENT

A person is in peak physical condition during his or her early adult years and often has few health concerns. The neuromuscular and skeletal system is at its full adult growth.

But while young adults can bounce back more easily from illness and injury, this patient population still has considerable health concerns. Perhaps the number one health risk today is obesity. Exercise can help young adults deal with stress and maintain a healthy weight (Figure 7.9). Another health risk is drug use; the use of illicit drugs, such as methamphetamines and cocaine, the abuse of alcohol, and smoking cigarettes all have long-term implications for young adults.

One particular health risk of concern for young adults is trauma. As a result of risk-taking behaviors, such as high speed or drunken driving and gun violence, young adults suffer a disproportionate number of traumatic brain injuries and incidents of spinal cord trauma. The majority of these patients are male.

MENTAL DEVELOPMENT

Although it would seem that young adults would be at the peak of their intellectual capacity, in fact they shift their thinking away from concrete thinking about facts and figures to more abstract thinking about theories and truth. The latter, truth, speaks to the young person's ability to consider alternatives and options and to decide not the right answer but the best answer among many good answers. This type of thinking, thinking within context, is more pragmatic and tends to concentrate on critical thinking and problem solving.

PSYCHOSOCIAL DEVELOPMENT

Trust is the key term in the psychosocial development of the young adult. While risking rejection, the young adult must learn how and when to trust others. This is a constant in intimate relationships as well as work relationships.

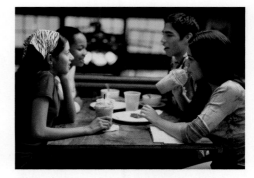

Figure 7.8 Social networking and personal appearance are important to adolescents

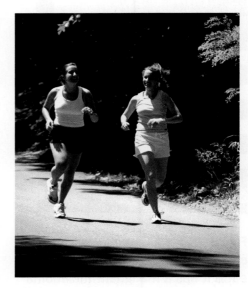

Figure 7.9 Exercise helps the young adult resist stress and avoid obesity

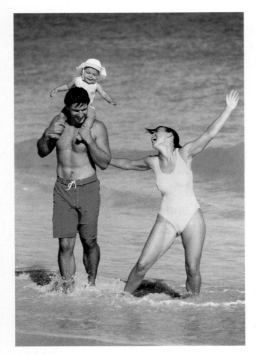

Figure 7.10 Early adulthood is a time to start families

As a result, young adults tend to be more decisive and persistent. They feel less like victims of life and more in control of their lives. It is important for the EMT to understand these developments and offer full disclosure of exam findings to young adult patients so that they can make an informed decision/consent.

Young adults are often new parents (Figure 7.10). Parenthood brings with it a number of new opportunities—and a variety of new stressors. These stresses can hamper an individual's health and response to disease.

VIOLENCE IN THE COMMUNITY

Intimate partner violence, also known as domestic violence, and child abuse are often first observed during young adulthood. These examples of violence in the community are the result of a cycle of violence. The first stage in the cycle of violence is tension building. For a number of reasons, such as stressors like unemployment and alcohol abuse, tension builds up and the batterer becomes increasingly irritable. The victim tries to keep the peace, until the batterer explodes and violence occurs. Immediately following the violence, the batterer feels guilty, is profusely apologetic, and makes hollow promises. Eventually the tension builds again and the cycle of violence is repeated.

Many batterers learned the behavior from their parents and may have been abused themselves. While the batterer understands that the behavior is unacceptable, the cycle of violence tends to persist.

Street Smart

Even as they enter adulthood, many young people are inexperienced with medical emergencies and unsure of their options. It is important for the EMT to be forthright in explaining care and to allow the patient to ask questions so that he or she can make an informed decision.

MIDDLE ADULTHOOD

The middle years, from age 40 to 65, are often the most productive years of one's life but also the years that see great changes in physical health. As the body ages, it tends to accumulate "errors" in cell division that can subsequently be the start for cancers of the breast, colon, and prostate. Cancer, such as the melanoma (Figure 7.11), tends to manifest in middle adulthood.

PHYSICAL DEVELOPMENT

One of the first signs of aging, besides graying of the hair, which can occur in a person's 20s, is loss of nearsightedness. The medical term for this condition is *presbyopia*, which is the result of decreased lens elasticity. Presbyopia is treated with reading glasses.

Accompanying presbyopia is *presbycusis*, a loss of hearing for high-pitched sounds. This hearing loss can be accelerated by loud sounds, such as sirens. The use of earplugs can help to prevent the early onset of presbycusis.

A classic sign of middle age for women is the onset of menopause. Menopause signals the end of a woman's reproductive life and is accompanied by a number of physical changes, including osteopenia.

Osteoporosis is a loss of bone density that occurs in old age, causing brittle bones and fractures to even minor trauma. Before osteoporosis occurs, the

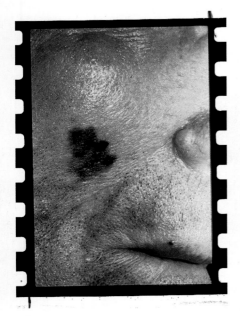

Figure 7.11 Cancer is a serious concern in middle adulthood. This patient has a malignant melanoma as a result of overexposure to the sun

patient may experience osteopenia in middle age. **Osteopenia** (Oss–tee–oh–pee–knee–A) is a loss of bone mineral density. There are several treatments for osteopenia, such as calcium supplements, that can help prevent or slow the arrival of osteoporosis. One of the treatments, hormone replacement, is controversial because it may increase the risk of breast cancer.

MENTAL DEVELOPMENT

As adults age, the way they think changes as well. In their youth adults demonstrate fluid intelligence, an ability to take new information and, in the absence of experience, apply it to a situation. Older adults have more crystallized knowledge, meaning they have the ability to use experience, apply it to the facts, and temper their decisions accordingly. This type of thinking may be thought of as wisdom. It has been suggested that middle-aged adults do not suffer a decline in intelligence but rather a rebalancing of intelligence, depending more on crystallized knowledge than fluid knowledge.

PSYCHOSOCIAL DEVELOPMENT

The term *midlife crisis* has been applied to middle-aged adults who are no longer parenting, also known as *empty nesters*, or who are parenting both their children and their elderly parents. With a heightened awareness of their aging, these middle-aged adults are attempting to prepare for their own retirement while trying to ensure the success of their children and the happiness of their parents.

LATE ADULTHOOD

Late adulthood could be considered to start at retirement. Retirement is a relatively recent social construct. In past centuries, people worked until they could no longer do so physically. However, work began to involve less and less arduous physical labor. At the same time, employers began to introduce pension programs as a way to retain workers, and the federal government introduced Social Security to provide retirement income. Today, most Americans retire between the ages of 62 and 65, but, depending on the state of the economy and their personal circumstances, some people continue to work well into their 70s.

While chronological age must be considered, a more accurate measure of late adulthood might be a person's physiologic age. A person's physiologic age is a function of the patient's ability to adapt to the environment. While some people may have the chronological age of 70, for example, their physical vitality may equal that of a 50-year-old. This vitality may be a function of a healthy diet and an exercise regimen that includes stretching exercises and the like (Figure 7.12).

As a result of the baby boom following World War II, the first half of the 21st century will be influenced in many ways by an aging American population. By 2050, there will be a projected 18.2 million people over age 85, compared to 3.6 million in that age range today. With advances in health care leading to longer lives, there may be as many as 800,000 Americans over the age of 100 by 2050.

PHYSICAL DEVELOPMENT

Numerous physical changes are associated with aging (see Table 7-2). The cardiovascular system starts to decline. A combination of thickening blood vessels, arteriosclerosis, and narrowed blood vessels from arthrosclerosis increases the work of the heart, gradually leading to heart failure. This is often shown by a decreased tolerance for exercise and an increase in coronary artery disease.

Like the heart, the lungs also change. For example, the cilia, those microscopic hairs that move bacteria-laden phlegm to the back of the throat for expectoration, decrease and, combined with a weakened cough, leave the patient predisposed to bronchial infections and pneumonia.

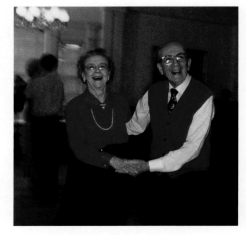

Figure 7.12 Activities, such as dancing, are important to the psychosocial health of the elderly as well as their physical health

Table 7-2 Changes and Effects of Aging in the Elderly

Cardiovascular
- Decreased heart muscle
- Loss of 25% to 30% of cardiac output
- Heart failure
- Increased hypertension
- Stroke
- Loss of up to 50% of lung capacity
- Shortness of breath

Musculoskeletal
- Loss of bone density
- Osteoporosis
- Pathologic fractures
- Decreased cartilage flexibility
- Degenerative joint disease
- Arthritis

Neuromuscular
- Loss of muscle mass
- Loss of 25% to 40%
- Loss of strength
- Decreased nerve conduction
- Slowed reactions

Metabolic
- Decrease in basal metabolic rate
- Decreased energy

Renal
- 30% to 50% loss of renal function
- Diminished excretion
- Risk of medication toxicity

The elderly, particularly women, are prone to osteoporosis, weakened spinal ligaments, and a characteristic curvature of the spine called **kyphosis** (kīfō'sis). With its forward head position, this condition can make it difficult for the EMT to place the patient on a backboard, and the pressure of a hard backboard on the spine may cause the patient considerable pain.

MENTAL DEVELOPMENT

Popular opinion aside, there is no evidence of loss of cognitive function—that is, mental decline—as a result of aging. Any loss of the ability to think or to maintain attention span may be linked to stroke or diseases such as Alzheimer's.

There is, however, an age-associated loss of memory, or senescence. This memory loss typically is not problematic unless it interferes with the patient's activities of daily living (ADL). However, severe memory loss may indicate the onset of dementia or other organic brain syndromes.

PSYCHOSOCIAL DEVELOPMENT

A common misperception is that most elderly people live in adult assisted living communities or nursing homes. In reality, only 5% live in these special circumstances. Most older adults live in the community with family or alone.

The elderly who live alone, especially if they are isolated and/or limited by physical impairments that diminish activity, can become depressed. An estimated one third of the elderly experience depression.

Untreated depression can lead to suicide. The suicide rate among the elderly is second only to that of adolescents. The majority of suicides involving elderly people, 84%, are by men, and the most common means of suicide is use of a firearm.

ACTIVITIES OF DAILY LIVING

The physical and mental health of an elderly patient can be assessed by observing the patient's **activities of daily living (ADL),** those tasks of self-care. Activities of daily living are those actions and behaviors people must perform to survive, such as eating, drinking, and elimination, along with routine tasks such as food preparation and personal grooming. Impairment of one's ADLs can lead to illness and death.

The fundamental ADL can be summarized by the mnemonic DEATH, which stands for dress, eat, ambulate, toilet, and hygiene. An impairment of any one these tasks requires immediate intervention by social services. If another person is responsible for the patient, and the patient has an impairment of these fundamental ADLs, then the EMT should suspect elder abuse and report the findings to the appropriate authorities.

DEATH AND DYING

A person's life span is a function of the era in which she or he was born. Current life expectancies for people born near the beginning of the 21st century could extend as long as 120 years. But eventually everyone dies. One of the grimmer realities of being elderly is the death of friends and loved ones.

CONCLUSION

Understanding the developmental age of their patients and customizing their care to patients' individual circumstances help EMTs provide higher-quality emergency care. Life span development encompasses changes in physical, mental, and psychosocial functioning and affects how patients respond to illness and injury. It also has an impact on how patients interact and communicate with the EMT. The application of the basic understanding of life span development should occur on every EMS call that an EMT attends.

Street Smart

Death is a reality of life for the elderly. While every EMT should receive training in grief counseling, what is most important is that the EMT demonstrate empathy and compassion for the patient who has lost a loved one.

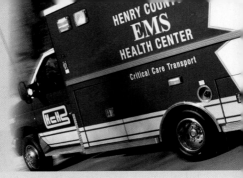

CASE STUDY Continued

After work, Jeff returns home to his wife and kids, says hello to his mother, and starts to work on "safe proofing" the house by adding grab rails in the bathroom and removing dangerous throw rugs on the smooth hardwood floors that present a trip hazard for his mother. His wife, smiling, tells him that her mother is coming next week to visit the grandkids, and he will need to have these projects done before then.

Key Concepts Revisited

- The EMT should be knowledgeable about the many physical, mental, and psychosocial changes that occur in a patient's lifetime.

- An EMT should know how these changes in human development will affect the patient care that the EMT renders

and how to adjust the care according to the patient's stage of development.

- The EMT should have a basic knowledge of human development to understand how trauma or illness can uniquely affect a person at each stage of life.

Review Questions

1. What are the three areas of human development?
2. What are chemicals that affect fetal development called? Give one example.
3. What are two major problems of transition that a neonate experiences?
4. What are the "soft spots" on an infant's head called, and when do they close?
5. When do most infants toddle (begin to walk)?
6. When is a child at greatest risk of child abuse?
7. What age is most common for attention-seeking behaviors?
8. Describe the cycle of violence seen in intimate partner violence.
9. Define physiologic age.
10. What is the name of the characteristic arching of the back seen in the elderly, often referred to as Dowagers hump?

Key Terms

Activities of daily living (ADL)
Cephalocaudal
Kyphosis
Maturation

Neonatal
Osteopenia
Sudden infant death syndrome (SIDS)
Teratogens

Further Study

For more information about development through the lifespan, visit http://www.learner.org/discoveringpsychology/development/

Cronin, A., & Mandich, M. B. *Human Development and Performance throughout the Lifespan*. Clifton Park, NY: Thomson Delmar Learning, (2005).

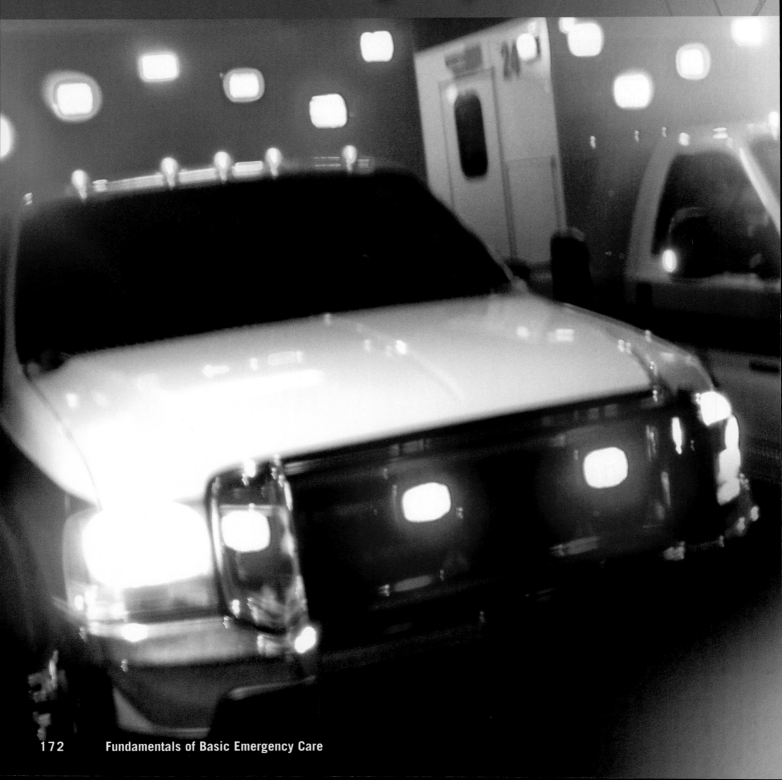

CHAPTER 3

Essentials of Emergency Medical Care

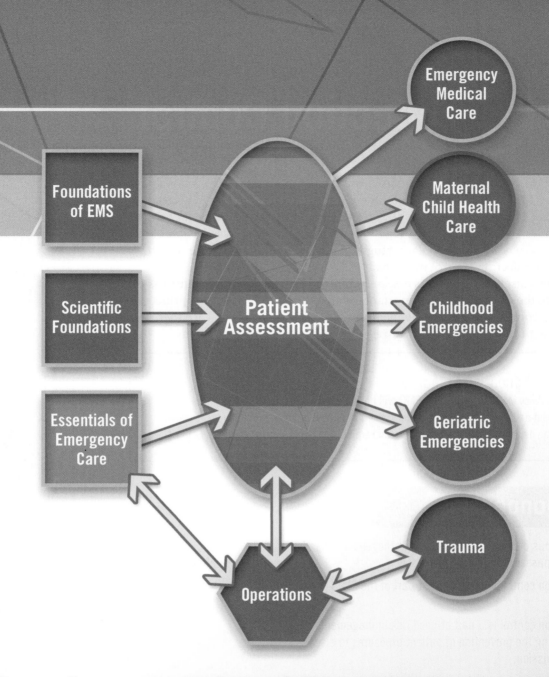

Foundations of EMS

Scientific Foundations

Essentials of Emergency Care

Patient Assessment

Operations

Emergency Medical Care

Maternal Child Health Care

Childhood Emergencies

Geriatric Emergencies

Trauma

Fundamentals of Emergency Medical Care

The foundation of an EMT's practice is laid upon several fundamental skills, such as airway management and bleeding control. Often these basic skills are all that is needed to save a patient's life. In every case, these basic skills must be performed before the EMT can use more advanced skills to care for the patient.

All EMTs, from the EMT–Basic to the EMT–Paramedic, must practice these fundamental skills until they become second nature. Only then can an EMT expect to be able to provide competent emergency medical care.

Infection control, airway management, ventilation, and bleeding control are reviewed in this chapter, along with the processes of taking vital signs and lifting and moving patients. All of these topics include skills that are a part of the emergency medical care an EMT provides to every patient.

UNIT (8) Infection Control

When an EMT approaches a sick or an injured patient, there is always a possibility of exposure to disease. Some patients carry infections that may be inadvertently transmitted to health care workers if preventive measures are not taken. Over the past 2 decades, health care workers have become increasingly knowledgeable about this issue. Today, EMTs are regularly taught about prevention of disease transmission through infection control measures.

This unit discusses infectious disease and how EMTs can prevent transmission of disease in the workplace. It is important for an EMT to understand the principles of infection control and prevention measures. The EMT who fails to learn these lessons may be putting her life and the lives of those she cares for in jeopardy.

> ## National Education Standards
> The Emergency Medical Technician (EMT) will have a simple depth and breadth of the assessment and management of a patient who may have contracted an infectious disease and how to decontaminate the ambulance and equipment after treating a patient.

Key Concepts

- Infectious diseases are caused by pathogens and can be easily passed from person to person.

- Infection control is an important part of the EMTs personal safety.

- Infection control is a part of good risk management, including the prevention of patient exposures to disease transmission.

- Identifying transmission pathways of infectious disease is important to effective infectious disease management.

- EMTs may routinely encounter a variety of common infectious diseases while on duty.

- Standard precautions, including body substance isolation through the use of personal protective equipment, reduce or eliminate the chance of infectious disease transmission.

- Hand washing and immunization are important elements of infection control.

- The type of personal protective equipment used by EMTs can be determined on scene based on the patient's chief concern and the treatment methods to be used.

- EMS is an important link in disease surveillance and notification.

- Medical follow-up for an infectious disease exposure includes evaluation of effective treatment, ongoing disease effects, and post-exposure prophylaxis treatment as required.

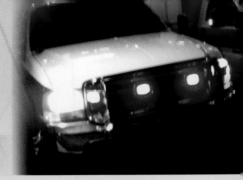

CASE STUDY

"We were called to a motor vehicle crash, involving two vehicles," Tim explains to his boss. Tim had experienced a "blood exposure" during a call and is in the process of filling out the necessary documentation for reporting a possible infectious exposure.

"I was working in the yard today, not officially on call, when the tones went off. I heard there were two vehicles involved and several patients. I knew the volunteer crew on duty would need extra hands while waiting for the next closest ambulance 20 miles away, so I responded to the scene from home. I was thinking about all the possibilities, number of people, injuries, if we'd have to extricate, as I left the house. I wanted to get to the scene to help as soon as I could, and didn't stop to change out from the shorts I was wearing."

After arriving on scene, Tim went down into a ditch through the tall grass and weeds to check on the patient still in the vehicle. The first victim had been walking around on the road when he arrived on scene. That patient was being attended by one of the two EMTs on the fire department.

Tim helped the volunteer firefighter get the patient out of the car. The patient was covered in blood, but Tim could not tell where the blood was coming from or if it was from this patient or the one on the road. The patient was moaning but not responsive enough to tell them what happened or where he was hurting.

After Tim turned the patient over to the ALS unit that had arrived while they were getting the patient out of the car, he noticed his legs were covered in blood. Shrugging it off as just something that happens on calls like this, he didn't think much about it until he got back to the station and took a quick shower. At the time, Tim felt stinging on his legs as he began washing the blood off and noticed numerous small cuts from the tall grass he'd had to walk through to get to the patient. It was then Tim realized he had exposed himself to a possible infectious disease through the open scratches on his legs and the blood from the patient or patients from the car.

Critical Thinking Questions

1. Why should this EMT be concerned?
2. What could he have done to prevent this from happening?
3. Was this a significant exposure? Why or why not?

INTRODUCTION

The duty of EMTs is first and foremost to protect themselves, their partners, and the patient when called to the scene of an illness or injury. Understanding what an infectious disease is and how disease is transmitted is vital in order to follow proper procedures in prevention, protection, and management of potential infectious diseases outbreaks and exposures.

INFECTIOUS DISEASE

An infection is a disease that is caused by some type of **microorganism,** a microscopic life form that flourishes in the body, sometimes causing illness. Infections can be acquired in many different ways, all requiring the microorganism to contact the person and enter the body. Each microorganism has a particular mode of **transmission,** or moving, from one place to another.

The EMT should be familiar with two basic types of disease. Infectious or *extrinsic* diseases are **contagious** or **communicable,** passed from one person to another. Diseases that are **intrinsic** are not contagious to others. It is important to understand there is a difference between infectious diseases and infection. An individual can get an infection, such as salmonella, a form of food poisoning, that will not necessarily be passed to another individual through personal contact. Communicable or infectious diseases range from colds and flu to sexually transmitted diseases and human immunodeficiency virus (HIV), the virus that can lead to AIDS. All of these diseases are spread through shared contact of the pathogen between individuals.

The benefits of simple infection control measures were described by Dr. Semmelweis, an Austrian obstetrician, in 1847. He reported a significant drop in infection rates when health care providers washed their hands before caring for each patient. Before hand washing was common, 18% of young mothers died in the hospital from postchildbirth infections (Figure 8.1). After Dr. Semmelweis insisted that all providers wash their hands between patients, the maternal death rate dropped to less than 1%. This simple infection control measure had dramatic results in preventing the spread of disease in these patients.

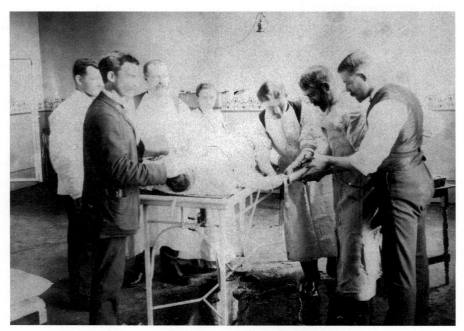

Figure 8.1 Doctors were slow to accept infection control principles

When an EMT understands the most common means of transmission of infectious disease, measures can be taken to prevent infection. Attempts to prevent the spread of infectious disease can be referred to as **infection control** measures.

PERSONAL SAFETY

The EMT's personal safety is one of the reasons why infection control is necessary. EMS is a profession with many potential risks. It is important that measures be taken to prevent the EMT from acquiring an infectious disease on the job and potentially spreading that disease to others.

The smart EMT looks for potential dangers in the work environment and takes preventive action. This kind of behavior is called **risk management.** Infection control plays a major role in risk management for all health care professionals.

When an EMT is evaluating the risk of infectious disease in the work environment, the potential for infection in the community served should be considered. Is there a large homeless population that may not have easy access to medical care? Is there a large immigrant population that may not have received immunizations considered routine in the United States or that is a population known to have a high incidence of a certain infectious disease?

When an EMT considers the potential for disease process within the community, she is creating a **risk profile**. An EMT who operates in a community known to have a high incidence of a particular infectious disease or injury risk would regularly take specific precautions to prevent transmission of that disease or to prevent that type of injury. The more that is known about the health of the community, the more specific the EMT can be about infection control of locally prevalent diseases. The local or county health departments can be helpful in determining a community's risk profile (Figure 8.2).

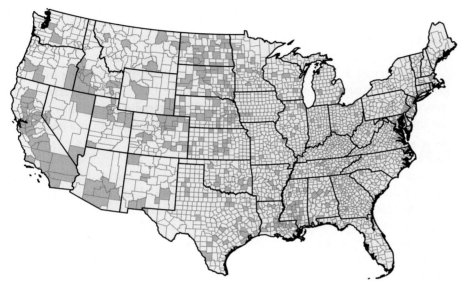

Figure 8.2 County health departments are a rich source of information about disease and local outbreaks of disease. This map shows reports of West Nile virus as collected by the U.S. Geographical Survey and the Centers for Disease Control and Prevention (Courtesy of the Centers for Disease Control and Prevention, West Nile Virus Map 2008)

The major diseases of concern to EMTs are seen on a broad basis, and the EMS profession has adopted general approaches to managing these risks. Agencies that specialize in the study and management of infectious disease, such as the *Centers for Disease Control and Prevention* (CDC) and workplace safety such as *Occupational Safety and Health Administration* (OSHA), have provided invaluable information and guidelines to EMS providers to lessen the chances of infectious disease exposures.

PATIENT SAFETY

An essential principle of medicine is to "do no harm." The assistance an EMT renders should not cause the patient more health problems. This issue is exemplified in the observations of Dr. Semmelweis. All medical professionals, including doctors, nurses, and EMTs, should avoid transmitting an infectious disease to the patient.

Infection control is a two-way street. Just as the EMT does not want to get exposed to an infectious disease through interaction with the patient, the patient does not want to be exposed to an infectious disease through interaction with the EMT. Most of the patients an EMT will care for are in a stressful situation. This stress can make the patient's body more susceptible to infection.

Even without the added stress of an emergency, some medications and disease processes can leave a patient with a weakened immune system and little or no resistance to disease. A person with a weakened immune state is said to be **immunocompromised.** Infections that would not make an average healthy person sick can cause serious illness in the immunocompromised patient.

FAMILY SAFETY

An EMT who is exposed to an infectious disease at work may inadvertently bring it home. The EMT may not become ill after exposure to the organism, but a significant concern is the potential of transmitting an infectious disease to family members. Children, who have immature immune systems; elderly parents, who have declining immune systems; and any ill persons in the household are all at a greater risk of becoming ill when exposed to an infectious disease. To protect these loved ones, the EMT needs to take infection control precautions to avoid becoming a disease **carrier.**

A carrier of an infectious disease harbors within the body the microorganism that causes an illness but may not become ill as a result. Carriers of an infectious disease may not even be aware of their carrier state, yet they can pass the microorganism along to other people who may become ill as a result.

CAUSES OF DISEASE

The agents of infectious diseases, microorganisms, exist just about everywhere. Microorganisms that can cause infection and disease, known as *pathogens,* include parasites, such as Helminthes (worms and protozoa), viruses, bacteria, and fungi. These agents can spread in a number of ways.

Although the study of microbiology is vast, an EMT needs to know about a few of the more common disease-causing agents. Chickenpox, measles, strep throat, and influenza are diseases that are commonly known to the public (Figure 8.3). Except under special circumstances, these illnesses are eliminated by the body over a relatively short period of time and pose no long-lasting threat to the EMT.

Patients with other infections, such as HIV and Hepatitis B (HBV), may pose a threat to the EMT in certain circumstances. EMTs are often in direct contact with a patient's blood or other bodily substances through which these diseases are transmitted. Table 8-1 lists common diseases an EMT may encounter during the course of routine patient care.

DISEASE TRANSMISSION

Infectious diseases can be easily transmitted from person to person. The pathogens that cause disease can be transmitted in a number of ways, including through **direct contact** with blood or other bodily fluids, through **indirect contact** through the air, food, or water, or by being injected by an infected vector (parasite).

CONTACT TRANSMISSION

Contact transmission occurs where there is direct contact with a substance harboring an infectious agent, such as blood or another body substance, including blood-to-blood contact and contact with open wounds, exposed tissue, and the mucous membranes of the eyes and mouth. HBV and HIV infection are examples of diseases transmitted through direct contact.

Transmission can also take place both directly and indirectly through a contaminated object, such as a needle, scissors, or any "sharps" that may have come in contact with bodily fluids.

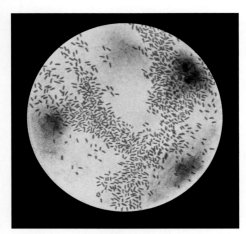

Figure 8.3 Most disease-causing agents are too small to be seen with the naked eye, such as Haemophilus influenza, as seen in this microscopic image (Courtesy of the Centers for Disease Control and Prevention Public Health Image Library)

Table 8-1 Common Disease-Causing Organisms and Infectious Illnesses

Organism/Illness	Signs and Symptoms	Mode of Transmission
Adenovirus (common cold)	Runny nose, cough, sore throat, congestion	Contact with droplets
Varicella virus (chickenpox and shingles)	Rash (itchy or painful)	Contact with open lesions, airborne
Mycobacterium tuberculosis (tuberculosis)	Cough, sweats, weight loss	Airborne
Hepatitis Type A virus	Fever, nausea, vomiting, yellow skin color	Contaminated food or water
Hepatitis Types B, C, D viruses	Fever, nausea, vomiting, yellow skin color, abdominal pain	Direct contact with blood or other body fluid
Herpes simplex 1 virus (oral herpes)	Painful lesions, usually around the mouth	Contact with saliva or wound
Herpes simplex 2 virus (genital herpes)	Painful lesions, usually in genital area	Contact with lesions
Human immunodeficiency virus (cause of AIDS)	Multiple infections such as pneumonia, thrush, herpes	Contact with blood or body fluids
Influenza virus (causes the flu)	Cough, fever, headache, vomiting, diarrhea, general malaise	Airborne
Methicillin-resistant Staphylococcus aureus (MRSA)	None (a bacterium that can inhabit a wound or healthy skin) or infection of wound	Contact with contaminated area
Neisseria meningitidis (a bacterium, one cause of meningitis)	Fever, rash, headache, stiff neck	Airborne respiratory secretions
Plasmodium malariae (blood parasite causing malaria)	History of exposure; fever, chills, headache, weakness, vomiting, and diarrhea	Bite from a malaria-infected female mosquito
Enterobius vermicularis (*round/pin worms*)	Mostly asymptomatic; perianal itching, especially at night, causing skin tears, which can lead to bacterial infections	Ingestion of eggs, can be airborne, environmental contact, hand to mouth, contaminated clothing, bedding

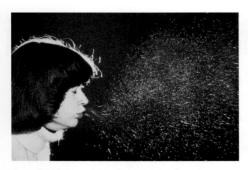

Figure 8.4 Airborne particles can travel far and contaminate many inanimate surfaces (Courtesy of Lester V. Bergman/Corbis)

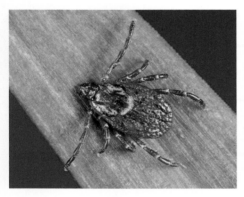

Figure 8.5 Disease is spread rapidly with the help of vectors such as the tick (Courtesy of the Centers for Disease Control and Prevention Public Health Image Library)

AIRBORNE TRANSMISSION

Coughing and sneezing produces a common means of disease transmission via droplets in the air. These particles are carried in the air until they settle onto a surface or are inhaled by an individual standing near the infected person when the droplets are expelled. Airborne and direct contact with respiratory secretions are the transmission mode for serious diseases such as Tuberculosis (TB). Sneezing and coughing are also the means by which less serious airborne diseases such as the common cold and influenza are transmitted (Figure 8.4).

VEHICLE TRANSMISSION

An indirect method of disease transmission is one in which food or water is a vehicle or carrier of the disease-causing organism. Food poisoning is actually the result of ingestion of food contaminated with a bacterium such as Salmonella.

Cholera, a water-borne disease caused by a bacterium found in dirty wells and rivers, was seen in the United States and England prior to the implementation of sanitation systems. Cholera can still be found in areas that have underdeveloped sanitation systems, and it can be transported into developed countries by travelers who bring in food products from areas where the disease is still prevalent.

VECTOR-BORNE TRANSMISSION

Around the world, a common source of disease is animals or insects. Ticks and mosquitoes transmit diseases such as Rocky Mountain Spotted fever, Lyme disease, West Nile virus, and malaria. A living creature that is involved in the transmission of disease is called a **vector.** Deer ticks carry the organism that causes Lyme disease and transmit it to humans when they bite. The deer tick is the vector for Lyme disease (Figure 8.5).

PORTAL OF ENTRY

To cause illness in a person, an infectious organism must first enter the body. The means of entry for the organism is called the **portal of entry.** There are many possible portals into the body. A common portal of entry is through the relatively unprotected mucous membranes in the mouth, nose, and eyes. An infectious agent that comes into contact with the well-vascularized mucous membranes can settle onto the surface and multiply or work its way into the superficial blood vessels and move throughout the body.

Another common, but often preventable, portal of entry for disease is through broken skin. The skin normally serves as a fairly impenetrable defense system, but broken skin can allow bacteria and other infectious organisms to enter the body.

SUSCEPTIBILITY TO DISEASE

The body does not necessarily become infected every time it is exposed to a disease. Actual illness caused by exposure to an infectious agent is dependent upon two factors: the strength of the organism, or its virulence, and the strength of the person's immune resistance. To create an illness, the organism must be virulent enough to overcome the resistance of the host.

Often, a virus or bacterium is weakened as a result of contact with air, drying in the environment, or other physical degradation. This weakened infectious particle may not have the strength to cause an infection. Hand cleaners and other cleaning solutions chemically weaken bacteria and viruses and may even kill them. These cleaning agents are often labeled *antibacterial.*

Whenever a pathogen, such as a virus or bacterium, enters the body, the body's defenses are set in motion. Disease-fighting white blood cells engulf the bacterium and subsequently remove it from the system. This immune defense is very effective against small numbers of microorganisms. However, if the number, or dose, is large, then these defenses may become overwhelmed and illness may result. For example, one cubic centimeter of blood can have as many as 100 million HBV particles. The larger the number of particles present, the harder the immune system must work to overcome the invasion.

An EMT can transmit a disease to others once she has been exposed to a pathogen of sufficient dose and virulence to overcome her immune system. This process can take days, weeks, or, in rare cases, years. The time when the EMT is contagious and can transmit the disease is the time when the EMT is a potential danger to family, friends, coworkers, and patients. Certain diseases such as influenza (flu) are highly contagious, and EMTs should take measures to protect themselves and others from contamination.

One method of protection is isolation. An EMT should not work when suffering from a contagious illness. A doctor's advice is helpful when deciding when to return to work after any illness.

DEFENSE AGAINST DISEASE

The skin is a remarkable organ. It not only helps regulate our internal body temperature but also protects the body from the outside environment. The uppermost layer of skin is composed of dead cells. These cells shed regularly, carrying any surface contamination away. The skin represents the first barrier to disease. Unless there is a break in the skin, this barrier is relatively impenetrable to most infectious microorganisms.

The surfaces of the respiratory and gastrointestinal tracts that come into contact with the outside environment are lined with **mucous membranes.** A mucous membrane creates liquid, called mucus, that can wash bacteria off the surface. However, these mucous membranes are quite porous and well lined with blood vessels. These features allow for an easy portal of entry for an infectious agent.

A healthy body is the best defense against disease. Annual physicals and ongoing health assessments are rapidly becoming standards in the health care industry. Employers, and the health care organizations to which they pay insurance premiums, have learned that it is less expensive to prevent disease than to treat it.

EMTs can also try to augment their immune system with regular immunizations. The body develops certain defense cells within the blood, called **antibodies,** that attack specific types of microorganisms. These antibodies need prior exposure to the microorganism to mount the most effective attack.

People are routinely provided exposure to common disease-causing agents (*pathogens*) in an attenuated, or weakened, form in order to allow the body to develop these specific antibodies. This process of exposing or inoculating the body to weakened pathogens is called **immunization.**

Every EMT should receive a broad spectrum of immunizations. Some immunizations are given only once in a lifetime. Others, such as the tetanus vaccine, must be given regularly to maintain immunity. **Immunity** refers to protection from a disease as a result of exposure or immunization.

OSHA requires that every EMT have the opportunity to receive the hepatitis B vaccine. If used as recommended, this vaccine is helpful in preventing hepatitis B infection after an exposure to the virus. Any time a vaccination is made available in this way, the EMT should seriously consider the risks for being exposed to the disease and the benefits and protection for the immunization.

Not all diseases have immunizations available. For example, there is no vaccine to protect against (TB) or HIV. The EMT is advised to get regular testing for these infections if she is at risk for exposure to them. Early diagnosis can lead to early treatment. Early treatment can have a dramatic impact on the quality of life that an EMT enjoys or can cure certain diseases entirely.

STANDARD PRECAUTIONS

Although the body has natural mechanisms to protect against pathogens and fight against infections once exposed, an EMT can and should take a number of precautions to protect themselves from contracting and transmitting infectious disease.

OSHA guidelines require emergency medical care personnel to protect against the transmission of disease through exposures to blood, bodily fluids, and other potentially infectious substances. Personal protective equipment (PPE) is used to provide for body substance isolation (BSI) and will be discussed in more detail later in this unit.

HAND HYGIENE

Proper hand hygiene is an important but often overlooked aspect of an EMT's practice. Throughout the day, germs accumulate on the hands from numerous sources and can be spread to others through hand-to-hand contact or by touching a common surface. Inadequate hand washing contributes to foodborne illnesses through such pathogens as *E. coli* and salmonella. Hand washing can remove most contaminants, largely preventing the spread of diseases such as the common cold, flu, and gastrointestinal illnesses.

Many soaps claim to be "antiseptic" or "antibacterial," but the type of soap used is not nearly as important as the hand-washing technique. The single most important action in hand washing is the scrub. The vigorous scrubbing for 20 seconds under running water washes away the top layer of dead skin, along with any bacteria.

Soap dispensers and faucets should be the kind that can be operated hands free. Paddle faucets can be turned off with an elbow to avoid using freshly washed hands to touch the "dirty" faucet. However, if neither of these types of plumbing is available, the faucet should be turned off with a clean paper towel. It is important to never use the freshly washed, bare hand to turn off the faucet to avoid recontamination. Skill 8-1 at the end of this unit demonstrates the proper procedure for hand washing.

Hand washing is part of the routine care of every patient. After every patient contact, after removing the gloves worn during patient contact and before the next patient contact, the EMT must wash her hands. In addition, open wounds must be covered because they are a portal of entry for an infection. An EMT should not work if an open wound exists on the hands that cannot be effectively covered or that is draining and soaking through an applied bandage.

The convenience of soap and running water is not always available to the EMT. In those cases, alternatives, such as waterless cleansers, should be available and used. Alcohol-based hand rubs are fast acting and significantly reduce the number of harmful pathogens such as viruses, bacteria, and fungi on skin.

Alcohol-based hand washes should be used after removing gloves, such as occurs between procedures, and after each patient contact. A common example is during a multiple casualty incident, when soap and fresh running water may not be readily available. The EMT should completely coat the hands with the alcohol-based hand wash and perform a vigorous 1-minute rub to reduce the majority of pathogens. If the EMT's hands are visibly soiled, then the use of soap and water is necessary. Furthermore, the EMT should wash

Street Smart

Rigorous hand washing several times per day can cause hands to become dry, sore, and cracked. The crack or break in the skin caused by the dryness is a portal of entry for disease. The use of unscented, moisturizing hand lotions by the EMT can help to reverse the drying effect and help the skin maintain its protection against disease-causing pathogens.

her hands with soap and water after every call regardless of whether waterless cleansers were used at the scene.

PERSONAL PROTECTIVE EQUIPMENT

The question most often asked by EMTs is, "When do I protect myself?" An obvious answer would be, "Whenever there is a risk for exposure!" However, the most appropriate answer is "Always!"

EMS has a "dress-up" philosophy when it comes to **personal protective equipment (PPE):** When you need it, you put it on. EMTs have equipment such as gloves, facemask, goggles, and a gown to be used as protection against pathogens when needed (Figure 8.6). EMTs should use dispatch information and the time before arriving on scene to don the PPE needed upon arrival.

The first rule of infection control in EMS is to treat all bodily fluids as if they are potentially infectious. Table 8-2 lists potentially infectious body fluids with which an EMT should avoid direct contact. Remember that "an ounce of prevention is worth a pound of cure." Whenever an EMT asks herself whether she needs personal protective equipment, she probably does. This level of protection was formerly called **body substance isolation,** referring to protection against any body substance that could be considered potentially infectious. That term has been replaced with **standard precautions.** This terminology describes the need to assume that all patients have the potential to have some form of infectious disease; therefore, protective measures should be considered standard for every patient encounter. It is important that the EMT minimally don gloves upon arrival on scene. Further PPE may be donned as the situation dictates.

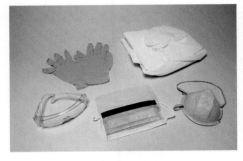

Figure 8.6 A variety of personal protective equipment is available for the EMT to use in infection control

Table 8-2 Potentially Infectious Body Fluids
Blood
Amniotic fluid
Vaginal discharge
Semen
Cerebrospinal fluid
Pleural fluid
Synovial fluid
Peritoneal fluid
Pericardial fluid
Fluids with little potential to transmit blood-borne diseases*:   • Tears   • Nasal discharge   • Vomitus   • Sputum   • Saliva   • Feces   • Urine

*Any bodily fluid that is blood-tinged should be treated as if it were blood.

BARRIER DEVICES

Barrier devices are any articles that create a physical partition between the EMT and the environment. These devices act like a second layer of skin, affording the EMT another layer of protection.

GLOVES

Because so much of what an EMT does involves the hands, the barrier devices used most often are gloves. A glove, when it is used properly, is an excellent barrier to transmission of disease by direct contact. Gloves are a routine measure used in the everyday practice of health care, protecting not only health care providers but also the patients they encounter.

Surgical gloves fit very snugly and are preferred by doctors and nurses for certain procedures. These special gloves are sterilized. Sterile gloves have gone through the process of sterilization, in which they are treated to remove any microorganisms. In general, sterile gloves are expensive and not necessary for daily use by EMTs, except under specific situations.

Gloves can be made from several different materials and come in different sizes. EMTs should ensure the appropriate type and size of gloves are available at the start of their duty shift. Gloves made of latex were once commonly used by health care providers; however, there has been an increase in the number of people, including EMTs, who have sensitivity to latex. Vinyl, latex-free, or other synthetic gloves are recommended to avoid a potentially serious allergic reaction.

Nonsterile gloves, the type EMTs commonly use, should never be washed off or reused. They are designed for one-time, one-patient-only use. A new pair of gloves must be worn with each new patient contact to avoid cross-contamination between patients.

Gloves that become torn when caring for the patient must be replaced with new gloves immediately following a thorough hand washing and before the EMT returns to patient care. In some cases it may be prudent to wear two pair of gloves, or "double glove," if there is a strong chance that the gloves will be torn.

If soap and water are not readily available, then waterless hand cleaners or antiseptic towelettes should be used. The EMT responsible for driving the emergency vehicle should deglove and wash the hands before beginning transport. Once at the emergency facility, the EMT should then reglove before handling and transferring the patient.

Hand washing after wearing gloves in all instances is essential. Although gloves provide a substantial amount of protection, they do not provide perfect protection, and microscopic tears sometimes occur. These microscopic tears may allow small amounts of blood or other material through, where they may come into contact with the EMT's skin. Any tiny breaks in the skin can then serve as a portal of entry.

GOGGLES

The eyes represent one of the largest exposed mucous membranes of an EMT. The eyes have many special self-protective capabilities that other mucous membranes do not have. Despite this fact, the eyes remain vulnerable to splashes with body fluids if the EMT is unprotected. Goggles should be worn whenever there is a possibility that blood or other bodily fluids could splash into the EMT's face, such as during suctioning.

Keeping the concept of barrier devices in mind, the EMT can protect the eyes by using goggles or protective safety glasses. Eye protection is a large concern in many industries in addition to EMS. Responding to this demand, manufacturers have created dozens of styles and types of protective eyewear.

An EMT should shop around for the eyewear that fits the best and then practice wearing it regularly.

Some EMTs wear eyeglasses for reading and other everyday activities. These glasses are satisfactory, provided they also fulfill their primary purpose in EMS, splash protection (Figure 8.7). Without side-splash protection, the EMT with eyeglasses is at risk for an accidental exposure.

MASKS

Masks provide protection from blood and other fluids splashing into the open mouth of the EMT. This problem is most common when an EMT is performing a procedure that requires the EMT to be close to the patient.

Masks provide another protection as well. A mask will protect the EMT from inhaling airborne infectious particles. These particles are often carried on microscopic water droplets in the air around the patient when the patient coughs or sneezes.

One specific airborne disease, a drug-resistant strain of TB, has become a problem to all health care workers in recent years. This systemic illness is discussed in greater detail later in this unit.

The increased incidence of resistant TB makes it necessary that any EMT caring for a patient with a cough must wear a protective mask. A protective mask, such as the N95 mask, should be carried with the EMT so that it is readily available (Figure 8.8). The mask is another barrier device that prevents exposure of the EMT to disease.

Some masks come as a mask/eye protection combination device (Figure 8.9). These "face shields" are convenient for the EMT. They provide mouth, nose, and eye protection and speed the process for application of PPE. EMTs should refer to their agency infection control manual to determine the appropriate type of mask to use for a given situation.

POCKET MASK

An EMT who comes upon a nonbreathing patient must always consider her own protection by using a pocket mask to ventilate the patient (Figure 8.10).

If a pocket mask is not readily available, the EMT should have a transparent shield device at hand. Both the pocket mask and the shield are barrier devices that allow effective ventilation while preventing direct contact of the rescuer's mouth with the patient's oral secretions.

GOWNS

Most EMTs depend on their duty uniform to provide the first layer of protection against accidental blood or body fluid splatter. Gowns provide added protection and should be worn anytime there is the potential of blood or bodily fluid splatters, such as in childbirth or major trauma.

Most gowns tie in the back and are impermeable to fluids. Some of these gowns are made of specially coated paper material. The more durable gowns are made of cloth and can be recycled. For the limited use that EMTs make of gowns, most EMS services provide the paper style of gown.

In the few cases in which more head-to-toe protection is needed, an EMT should consider wearing a disposable one-piece jumpsuit. These garments are used frequently in hazardous materials spills and are relatively inexpensive.

In the majority of high-risk cases, the EMT should wear a long paper gown. This will usually provide more-than-adequate protection while still being functional. Table 8-3 illustrates the use of different personal protective gear as a part of standard precautions.

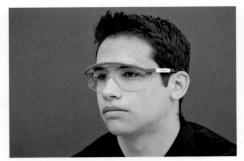

Figure 8.7 Without side guards, regular eyeglasses provide incomplete protection against splashes

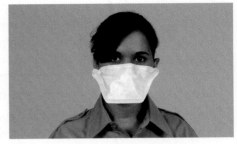

Figure 8.8 A mask provides the EMT with protection from airborne diseases

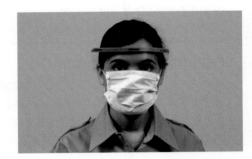

Figure 8.9 A mask and eye shield combination is both practical and effective

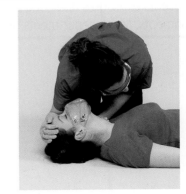

Figure 8.10 Barrier devices provide the EMT another margin of safety when performing cardiopulmonary resuscitation (CPR)

Table 8-3 Standard Precautions for Infection Control

Wash Hands (Plain soap)

Wash after touching blood, body fluids, secretions, excretions, and contaminated items.

Wash immediately after gloves are removed and between patient contacts.

Avoid transfer of microorganisms to other patients or environments.

Wear Gloves

Wear when touching blood, body fluids, secretions, excretions, and contaminated items.

Put on clean gloves just before touching mucous membranes and nonintact skin.

Change gloves between tasks and procedures on the same patient after contact with material that may contain high concentrations of microorganisms. Remove gloves promptly after use, before touching noncontaminated items and environmental surfaces, and before going to another patient. Wash hands immediately to avoid transfer of microorganisms to other patients or environments.

Wear Mask and Eye Protection or Face Shield

Protect mucous membranes of the eyes, nose, and mouth during procedures and patient-care activities that are likely to generate splashes or sprays of blood, body fluids, secretions, or excretions.

Wear Gown

Protect skin and prevent soiling of clothing during procedures that are likely to generate splashes or sprays of blood, body fluids, secretions, or excretions. Remove a soiled gown as promptly as possible and wash hands to avoid transfer of microorganisms to other patients or environments.

Patient-Care Equipment

Handle used patient-care equipment soiled with blood, body fluids, secretions, or excretions in a manner that prevents skin and mucous membrane exposures, contamination of clothing, and transfer of microorganisms to other patients or environments. Ensure that reusable equipment is not used for the care of another patient until it has been appropriately cleaned and reprocessed. Single-use items must be properly discarded.

Linen

Handle, transport, and process used linen soiled with blood, body fluids, secretions, or excretions in a manner that prevents exposures and contamination of clothing and avoids transfer of microorganisms to other patients or environments. Many departments use a red bag system; the red bag indicates a potential biohazard.

DONNING AND DOFFING PROTECTIVE APPAREL

EMTs are told what personal protective apparel to wear, but seldom are they told how to apply these articles or how to take them off. Improper application or careless removal of soiled protective apparel can result in accidental exposures. Before putting on other personal protective apparel, the EMT should first put on a mask and eye protection. The ties should be tight, and the mask secure so that it will not fall down accidentally. The EMT should then put on a gown, if necessary. Assistance tying the back of the gown is often needed. Finally, gloves should be applied over the sleeves of the gown.

To take off the personal protective apparel, the EMT should go in reverse order. First, the EMT would remove her gloves, then the gown, mask, and eye protection. In the case of gross contamination from blood or other fluid, the risk of accidental exposure is too great for an EMT to disrobe alone. The assistance of another EMT should be requested to ensure better safety and to decrease the risk of self-contamination. Specific instructions on application and removal of personal protective equipment are provided in Skills 8-2 and 8-3 at the end of this unit.

INFECTION CONTROL PREPARATION

Before an emergency call occurs, it is important that the EMT be prepared. EMS training, education, and equipment readiness are all part of being prepared for an emergency call. An infection control plan is also a part of that preparation.

Emergency service agencies will have written plans relating to infection control practices, usually found in the infection control manual or the EMS service's standard operating guidelines (SOG) manual. An infection control manual should list typical situations that may be encountered and how the EMT would protect herself from potential disease exposure in each case.

At the start of every shift, the EMT should be sure that there is an adequate supply of gloves, gowns, and masks and prepare the ambulance or emergency response vehicle (Figure 8.11). Floors should routinely be mopped with a cleaning solution that includes a disinfectant such as bleach. The entire interior of the vehicle must be cleaned regularly, according to departmental standards contained within the infection control manual.

Many EMTs reside at a station during their shifts. The rules listed in Table 8-4 represent good health practices, resulting in a work environment safe from unnecessary contamination.

RESPONDING TO A CALL

Prearrival instructions from the communications center can offer the EMT an opportunity to prepare PPE. On the basis of the information given, the EMT can decide what PPE to use.

For example, a patient with a cough, fever, and chills would represent several potential hazards to the EMT, including blood-borne and airborne

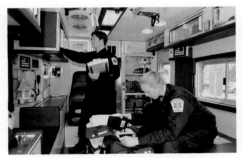

Figure 8.11 All emergency response vehicles must have an adequate stock of personal protective equipment for all personnel on board

Table 8-4 House Rules

1. EMTs may not eat food, apply makeup, or smoke until after hands have been washed thoroughly.
2. No hand washing is allowed in the same sink in which food is prepared.
3. Hands must be washed after:
   - every EMS call
   - whenever a toilet is flushed
   - whenever hands are soiled
4. All contaminated clothing must be removed before entering the dayroom.
5. Any potential infectious disease exposures must be reported immediately.

Table 8-5 Common Chief Concerns and Personal Protective Equipment

Chief Concern	Gloves	Mask	Eyewear	Gown
Fever	X	X		
Rash	X	X		
Seizures	X	X		
Coughing	X	X	X	
Bleeding wounds	X	X (if spurting)	X (if spurting)	X (if spurting)
Neck stiffness	X	X		
Vomiting	X	X	X	

infections. The EMT would minimally need a pair of nonsterile gloves and a mask that also offers eye protection.

ON THE SCENE

Infectious disease precautions taken upon arrival to the scene are usually based on the patient's chief concern (CC) or on the emergency medical procedures that are required. Concern-driven PPE assumes that the EMT spoke to the patient and has considered the patient's CC and the PPE that should be used. Table 8-5 lists common patient concerns and the PPE the EMT should use.

While assessing a patient, an EMT may discover certain signs of disease. For example, a person with a rash and fever may have an infectious disease and should be assumed to be contagious. The EMT must have PPE readily available at all times. Eye protection left in the ambulance cannot protect the EMT in the house.

Procedure-driven PPE implies that the first step of every emergency medical procedure performed by an EMT is to don PPE. For example, whenever suction is used, the EMT should minimally have on gloves, eye protection, and a mask. Table 8-6 lists common emergency medical procedures performed by EMTs and the PPE that must be used.

DISPOSAL OF WASTE

Bloody bandages and other contaminated waste must be disposed of properly before leaving the scene. These potentially infectious materials are considered a biohazard. A **biohazard** is any material that is potentially contaminated with biological waste. There are strict rules regarding the collection and management of biohazardous waste.

Biohazardous waste must be placed in a red plastic bag that is clearly marked with the biohazard sign. The red-bagged waste must be treated as infectious waste and placed in a proper disposal unit.

Not all waste on a scene is a biohazard. Oxygen masks, clear plastic wrappers, and the like should be put into regular garbage containers. Table 8-7 illustrates potentially infectious items typically used on the scene and how they should be disposed. Of course any item that is covered with blood or

Safety Tips

After the team leaves with the patient, someone must always follow up to be sure that anything that is potentially dangerous is removed and the scene is safe for the public.

Table 8-6 Common EMS Tasks and Personal Protective Equipment

Task	Gloves	Mask	Eyewear	Gown
Taking pulse rate	X			
Measuring blood pressure	X			
Controlling bleeding	X			
(Minimal visible blood)	X			
Giving an injection	X			
Inserting oropharyngeal/ nasopharyngeal airway	X	X	X	
Suctioning	X	X	X	
Intubation	X	X	X	
Arterial bleeding control	X	X	X	X
Assisting childbirth	X	X	X	X
Disinfecting equipment	X	X	X	X

other body fluids should be considered biohazardous waste and disposed of properly. It is wise to treat all medical waste as potentially biohazardous if unsure into which class of waste it falls.

NEEDLE DISPOSAL

EMTs will often work side by side with paramedics who are using IV needles and other sharp instruments. Some EMTs will assist a paramedic with the administration of certain drugs that require a needle to inject them into the skin.

The single largest risk for occupational exposure to blood-borne diseases is by accidental needle stick. It is important for EMTs to know how to handle any needle, syringe, or sharp blade. These groups of potentially hazardous instruments are commonly referred to as **sharps.**

Needles must always be handled carefully and discarded safely in an appropriate **sharps container,** as shown in Figure 8.12. These containers, usually bright red with a biohazard label on the side, are essentially puncture proof. Carrying a sharp any distance for disposal is risky; therefore, a sharps container must be readily accessible. Small sharps containers are frequently carried to the scene by paramedics for immediate and safe disposal of needles.

Needles or other sharp instruments must never be recapped by the EMT. Injury or contamination from blood on the needle can occur while replacing the cap and is an unnecessary risk to everyone.

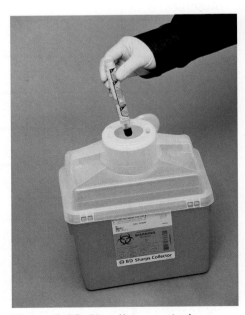

Figure 8.12 Needles must always be discarded safely in appropriate sharps containers

Table 8-7 Disposal of Potentially Infectious Materials

Item	Regular Waste (white bag)	Biohazardous Waste (red bag)	Sharps Container (hard plastic box)
Airway equipment	X		
Tissues		X	
Nasal cannula	X		
Oxygen mask	X		
Bag-valve-mask	X		
Plastic wraps	X		
Gloves	X (unless bloody then (X))		
Paper gowns	X		
Filled emesis basin		X	
Bloody dressing		X	
Vaginal pads		X	
Absorbent pads		X	
Soiled adult undergarments		X	
IV needles			X
Injection needles			X
Blood-filled glass tubes			X

It is the responsibility of all EMTs, both basic and advanced, to be accountable for all sharps. The scene must be clear of all sharps before it is considered safe. In some EMS systems, the person responsible for the sharps calls out "all sharps clear" to indicate to other team members that the scene is safe.

TRANSPORT AND INFECTION CONTROL

EMTs are often called to treat and transport patients with a known infectious disease such as TB or MRSA. Using standard precautions—that is, gloves, goggles, and masks—will protect against most known infectious diseases.

However, diseases such as tuberculosis require some additional protection a regular mask doesn't provide.

OSHA has adopted protective procedure standard recommendations for diseases, such as tuberculosis, that call for the use of a HEPA or N-95 respirator (Figure 8.13). These special masks are made to prevent any contact with infected droplets from a cough or sputum from the infected patient. If a HEPA mask or N-95 respirator is not available, or a disease such as TB is suspected but unconfirmed, a surgical or regular mask should be used.

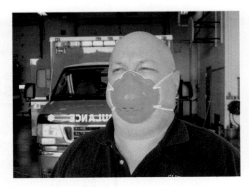

Figure 8.13 HEPA masks and N-95 respirators (Courtesy of Clive Fire Department, Clive, Iowa)

RESISTANT INFECTIOUS DISEASE

Multidrug-resistant organisms are pathogens that have adapted to and developed the ability to resist the antibiotics normally prescribed. Patients who are especially at risk for infection from these pathogens typically live in long-term care facilities or have spent an extended time in intensive care units or other medical care facilities.

Methicillin/oxacillin-resistant Staphylococcus Aureus (MRSA) and Vancomycin-resistant Enterococci (VRE) are two of the most common types of these pathogens. Patients may develop serious infections, including pneumonia and peritonitis (infection of the lining of the abdomen), which are resistant to standard antibiotic therapy.

Transmission is usually through direct person-to-person contact, and many medical facilities that treat these patients have instructions on personal protection that should be used during transport. EMTs should always use standard infection control procedures (body substance isolation) at a minimum with all patients with known infections.

PANDEMIC PRECAUTIONS

With the advent of diseases such as Avian Flu, planning for a potential flu pandemic has taken on a renewed urgency. A **pandemic** is a global disease outbreak, as seen in the 1918–1919 influenza pandemic. In 1918, a fifth of the world's population was infected with a virulent strain of influenza that is believed to have killed somewhere between 20 million and 40 million people over 2 years.

A flu pandemic occurs when a new influenza virus emerges. People have little or no immunity and there is no vaccine, allowing the disease to spread easily from person to person. The lessons learned from prior pandemics, especially the influenza pandemic of 1918–1919, are invaluable to planning and implementing infectious disease plans today.

It is important to remember that during an influenza pandemic, patients will require transport to health care facilities. OSHA's recommended guidelines were developed to protect EMTs and other health care workers, during prehospital care and transport. The recommendations should be used routinely, regardless of symptoms, when pandemic flu has been identified in the community or when patients have symptoms consistent with influenza-like illnesses. Table 8-8 lists OSHA guidelines for prehospital care and transport of influenza patients.

These guidelines should be followed for all patients suspected of an infectious disease, such as influenza or other potentially infectious illness transmitted through the air, even when a pandemic is not suspected.

AFTER THE CALL

After the patient has been turned over to another health care professional, the EMT must turn her attention to getting back in service.

The EMT should remove any contaminated clothing and put on a clean change of clothes. Being careful to avoid further contamination, the EMT should place her soiled clothing into the proper bin for soiled laundry.

Table 8-8 OSHA Guidelines for Prehospital Care and Transport of Influenza Patients

	Influenza-Like Illness with Patient Screening	Suspected Influenza without Patient Screening
Engineering Controls (Vehicle)	• Optimize the vehicle's ventilation to increase volume of air exchange during transport. The vehicle's ventilation system should be used in nonrecirculating mode and should bring in as much outdoor air as possible. • When possible, use vehicles that have separate driver and patient compartments that can provide separate ventilation to each area. In this situation, drivers do not require particulate respirators.	• Optimize the vehicle's ventilation to increase volume of air exchange during transport. The vehicle's ventilation system should be used in nonrecirculating mode and should bring in as much outdoor air as possible. • When possible, use vehicles that have separate driver and patient compartments that can provide separate ventilation to each area. In this situation, drivers do not require particulate respirators.
Administrative Controls	• Educate health care workers engaged in medical transport about the risks of aerosol-generating procedures. • Notify the receiving facility as soon as possible, prior to arrival, that a patient with suspected pandemic influenza infection is being transported to the facility and of the precautions that are indicated. • Minimize the opportunity for contamination of supplies and equipment inside the vehicle (e.g., ensure that all cabinetry remains closed during transport). • Continue to follow standard infection control procedures, such as standard precautions, recommended procedures for waste disposal, and standard practices for disinfection of the emergency vehicle and patient care equipment.	• Educate health care workers engaged in medical transport about the risks of aerosol-generating procedures. • Notify the receiving facility as soon as possible, prior to arrival, that a patient with suspected pandemic influenza infection is being transported to the facility and of the precautions that are indicated. • Minimize the opportunity for contamination of supplies and equipment inside the vehicle (e.g., ensure that all cabinetry remains closed during transport). • Continue to follow standard infection control procedures, such as standard precautions, recommended procedures for waste disposal, and standard practices for disinfection of the emergency vehicle and patient care equipment.
PPE	• If tolerated by the patients, place a surgical mask on all patients with respiratory illness to contain droplets expelled during coughing. If this is not possible (i.e., would further compromise respiratory status, or is difficult for the patient to wear), have the patient cover the mouth and nose with a tissue when coughing, or use the most practical alternative to contain respiratory secretions.	• Consider routine use of surgical or procedure masks for all patients during transport when pandemic influenza is in the community.

	Influenza-Like Illness with Patient Screening	Suspected Influenza without Patient Screening
PPE	• Health care workers transporting patients with influenza-like illnesses should use a respirator (N-95 or better). If respirators are not available, health care workers should wear a surgical mask.	• Health care workers transporting patients should use a respirator (N-95 or better). If respirators are not available, health care workers should wear a surgical mask.

Source: Appendix Q-OSHA Guidance—*Pandemic Influenza Preparedness and Response Guidance for Healthcare Workers and Healthcare Employers.*

The EMT should then wash her hands thoroughly, in the same manner as described previously. It is imperative to wash hands before doing anything else. An EMT should not apply any makeup, smoke, or eat any food until she has washed her hands.

If a sink with running water is not immediately available, the EMT should use either a waterless, alcohol-based cleansing gel or an antiseptic cloth made for that purpose.

DOCUMENTATION

Documentation is a critical part of an EMT's responsibilities. Documentation of infectious disease can be divided into patient reporting and exposure reporting.

When an EMT is reporting a patient's condition on the patient care report, all signs and symptoms considered significant must be listed, even if they do not appear to be related to the chief concern (Figure 8.14).

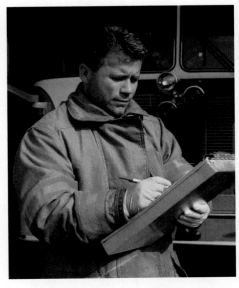

Figure 8.14 Documentation of the symptoms that the patient gave provides other health care providers a basis for continued treatment

CLEANUP

When the paperwork has been completed or while it is being done, the emergency equipment must be returned to service. This process includes cleaning equipment, noting defective or damaged equipment, and reporting it or replacing it.

One of the essential tasks before a piece of equipment can be returned to service is removal of obvious contamination, or **decontamination.** Decontamination is the use of either chemical or physical means to remove or neutralize any disease-causing organisms. After completing the decontamination process, the equipment must not be capable of transmitting disease to another person. There are several levels of decontamination.

The lowest level of decontamination amounts to old-fashioned housekeeping. If there is no visible blood or body fluids, then the object is simply wiped down with an EPA-approved, hospital grade disinfectant or germicide.

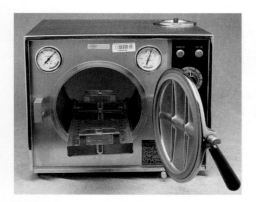

Figure 8.15 Sterilization, using an autoclave, is the highest level of disinfection

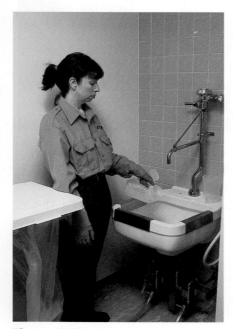

Figure 8.16 Liquid waste should be disposed of in a toilet or similar device, such as the hopper shown here, and flushed into the sanitary system

High-level disinfection requires sterilization. **Sterilization,** as the name implies, kills all microorganisms on the surface. Sterilization is required for any piece of equipment that might enter into another person's body, such as an IV catheter. Obtaining this level of decontamination often involves special procedures such as hot steam and pressure processing, autoclaving, or gas sterilization, with expensive equipment (Figure 8.15).

Occasionally, EMTs who either work with paramedics or who perform special procedures, such as intubation, need to sterilize individual pieces of equipment. In those cases, special chemicals are used. This process can take up to 12 or 24 hours, depending on the chemical sterilant.

It is often more cost effective to use disposable equipment. Disposable equipment is discarded into appropriate waste receptacles once it has been used. Regardless of the method of decontamination used, strict adherence to cleaning guidelines is required.

EMERGENCY EQUIPMENT CLEANUP

A majority of the cleanup concerns EMTs have are related to handling equipment contaminated with blood or other body fluids. First, the EMT should don a pair of gloves (heavy-duty kitchen-type gloves are preferred). An impermeable apron or gown may be required if splashing can reasonably be anticipated.

The removal of gross contamination with plain soap and water begins the process of equipment decontamination. The equipment should be cleaned down to the surface, and no visible blood should remain.

The next step depends on the intended use of the piece of equipment. If the equipment would touch only a patient's skin, then only intermediate-level disinfection is necessary. If the equipment would touch a patient's mucous membranes, then high-level disinfection is required.

With intermediate disinfection, the surface is wiped down with an Environmental Protection Agency (EPA) registered germicide. A cleaner that can kill pathogens, as written on the product label, is considered to be a germicide.

Alternatively, many EMTs use a bleach-and-water solution, containing one quarter cup of bleach to one gallon of water (per OSHA standards). This is a cost-effective and practical method of achieving intermediate-level disinfection. Table 8-9 lists the types of equipment an EMT might use and the level of decontamination that is necessary.

CLEANING AREAS

In all emergency departments and EMS stations, there is an area that is usually referred to as the "dirty utility room." This area is marked with a biohazard sign that warns people that inside are dangerous chemicals as well as potentially infectious materials. This specialized room is where all decontamination of portable equipment should take place.

This room or area is usually well lighted and ventilated, with a large, nonporous work surface, as well as hoses and sprayers for washing contaminated equipment from bedpans to backboards. All drains from large sinks or hoppers, toilets, and floor drains empty into a separate sewer system for proper disposal (Figure 8.16). Equipment may also be dried in the dirty utility room, but once the decontamination process is complete, the equipment will be moved to appropriate storage for use.

CLEANING THE AMBULANCE

After all contaminated equipment and waste have been removed, it is important to clean the vehicle. The rules for cleaning an ambulance are the same as for cleaning the equipment.

Table 8-9 Decontamination of EMS Equipment

Item	Low	Intermediate	High
Stretcher		X	
Linen	X	X	
Surfaces	X		
Benches	X		
Stethoscope		X	
Blood pressure cuff		X	
Splints		X	
Cervical collars		X	
Backboards		X	
Intubation equipment			X

If no visible blood or other body fluids are present, the exposed surfaces should be wiped down with a hospital disinfectant and allowed to air dry.

If blood or other biohazard is visible, soak up any blood or other body fluids with an absorbent towel, taking care to dispose of it properly. Then scrub the surface with soap and water to further remove grossly visible contamination (Figure 8.17). This initial cleaning should be followed by disinfecting the surface with either a bleach solution or a germicidal solution.

Next, air out the vehicle until all exposed surfaces are dried. This step usually takes only 10 or 15 minutes.

It is important that the ambulance be cleaned thoroughly on a regular basis, from the driver's compartment to the patient compartment and all of the equipment therein. Many EMS agencies have instituted a mandatory cleaning schedule that includes such tasks as wiping down the underside of the ambulance stretcher and cleaning the walls and ceiling of the ambulance. Small blood splashes, invisible to the naked eye, can harbor infectious diseases such as hepatitis B for weeks.

The final step of every EMS call is restocking the vehicle. Do not forget to replace the PPE that was used. Glove boxes need to be full. All portable kits need to be complete with eye protection, gloves, masks, and gowns.

LEGAL OBLIGATIONS

The Centers for Disease Control and Prevention (CDC) is an organization within the federal government that monitors outbreaks of infections and advises affected groups on how to handle the situation and control the spread

> **Street Smart**
>
> Avoid wiping down clear plastic surfaces with bleach solution because it can fog the surface.

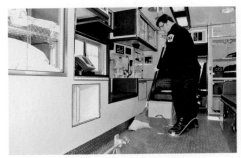

Figure 8.17 Cleaning the ambulance is part of the regular routine of every EMT

Table 8-10 OSHA Standard 1910.1030, Occupational Exposure to Bloodborne Pathogens

Intent: To eliminate or minimize occupational exposures to bloodborne pathogens.

Applicable to: All employees with potential for occupational exposure to blood or other potentially infectious material.

Requirements:
- Exposure control plan
- Exposure determination
- Methods of compliance
- Universal precautions
- Engineering controls
- Work practice controls
- Personal protective equipment
- Housekeeping/waste disposal
- Hepatitis B vaccination
- Signs and labels on hazardous materials
- Training
- Postexposure follow-up

Source: 29 Code of Federal Regulations 1910.1030.

of disease. The CDC has issued many advisories regarding common disease outbreaks such as hepatitis B caused by HBV and TB.

To encourage compliance with these advisories, another federal agency, the Occupational Safety and Health Administration (OSHA), produces standards for infection control practice in EMS. One of the first standards and practice rules published was the Bloodborne Pathogens Rule (29 CFR 1910.1030). This set of rules had clear provisions for employers regarding infection control practices. Table 8-10 outlines the rules and regulations of this standard.

The fire service also has an interest in the health and welfare of its members, because the majority of EMS has been and still is provided by EMTs working in the fire service. Senior fire service leaders and other fire service experts periodically meet to discuss and agree upon the standards of practice that the fire service should use. The National Fire Protection Association (NFPA) Standard 1581 specifically addresses the issue of infection control (Table 8-11).

SAFETY OFFICER

There are such a large number of state and federal rules, standards, and laws that the average EMT could easily become overwhelmed. Most progressive EMS agencies have created a position called the **infection control officer** or **safety officer.** The infection control officer is responsible for reviewing publications from agencies such as the CDC, OSHA, and the NFPA for new rules and standards that could affect EMS operations.

The position of infection control or safety officer is so common in fire departments and EMS agencies that there is a National Association of Safety

Table 8-11 NFPA Standard 1581, Fire Department

Infection Control

Intent: To reduce the exposures to infectious diseases by responders in both emergency and nonemergency situations.

Applicable to: Any organization providing rescue, fire suppression, and other emergency service functions.

Requirements: Describes minimum standards for infection control programs:
- Policy
- Training and education
- Infection control liaison person
- Immunization and testing
- Exposures
- Cleaning and disinfecting areas
- Storage rooms
- Infection control garments and equipment
- Personnel handling of sharp objects
- Skin washing
- Disinfectants
- Emergency medical equipment
- Protective clothing
- Disposal of material

Officers. These officers discuss methods of obtaining and distributing important information about infection control to their members.

The infection control or safety officer (the chief operating officer, if there is no formally designated infection or safety control officer) is the person to approach if an EMT has a question regarding infection control.

REPORTING EXPOSURE

The first question naturally is, What is an occupational exposure? An occupational exposure occurs when an EMT, while in the course of regular and routine duties, comes into contact with a potentially infectious material, such as blood or other body fluids. Contact occurs when the potentially infectious material contacts a mucous membrane, open wound, cut, or laceration or is introduced, by injection, under the skin.

An EMT who believes she has been exposed to a potentially infectious material must seek out medical treatment and follow-up. The first step is usually to notify the infection control officer (safety officer) or supervisor, including date and time of the exposure. The details of the exposure, including the type of exposure (blood or other body fluid), the amount of fluid and possible route of transmission should be conveyed. In most cases, the infection control or safety officer will direct the EMT to see a designated physician immediately. As state laws vary regarding exposure reporting procedures, the EMT should follow state and departmental procedures.

On the basis of the nature of the exposure, the physician may recommend that the EMT initiate treatment to try to prevent or at least lessen the likelihood of becoming ill as a result of the exposure. This type of treatment is called **prophylaxis.** For prophylaxis to be effective, it must begin as soon after the exposure as possible. Some prophylaxis regimens should be started within 1 to 2 hours of the exposure. The sooner it is begun, the better are the chances of avoiding illness. Therefore, all incidents of potential exposure must be reported immediately.

MEDICAL FOLLOW-UP

Follow-up of health care providers who have been exposed to a known or suspected infectious disease can begin any time after treatment has started. Post-exposure follow-up is important because there may need to be a change in treatment regimens as additional information about the exposure or source person becomes available. Post-exposure follow-up includes further testing, evaluation of treatment effectiveness, and counseling.

Specific time frames for post-exposure evaluations are determined by the type of exposure and pathogen. For example, CDC guidelines suggest post-exposure evaluations of persons who have been exposed to HIV to occur within 72 hours of the initial treatment. At that time, individuals are advised to use precautions and avoid blood or tissue donations, breastfeeding, or pregnancy, especially during the first 6 to 12 weeks post-exposure, to prevent a secondary transmission.

Medical follow-up includes monitoring for possible drug toxicities, interactions, reactions, and effectiveness. Additionally, post-exposure adherence to scheduled treatment regimens, effectiveness of treatment, and management of associated symptoms with additional medications or changes in treatments should be evaluated.

Psychological impact of exposures should not be underestimated. Psychological counseling is an essential component of post-exposure management and the overall well-being of the health care provider who has been exposed to an infectious disease.

DISEASE SURVEILLANCE AND NOTIFICATION

The prevention and control of infectious diseases can be accomplished through notification of potential outbreaks to hospitals, public health departments, and other health care agencies. The CDC's National Notifiable Diseases Surveillance System (NNDSS) defines *notifiable disease* as one in which frequent, regular, and timely information regarding individual cases is considered necessary for the prevention and control of the disease.

Surveillance systems established by public health agencies reduce morbidity and mortality and improve health through collection, analysis, and notification of health-related events to hospitals, other health care agencies, and the public. One of the most important public health functions of surveillance systems is outbreak detection.

The Institute of Medicine conducted a workshop in October 2007 which calls for innovative surveillance methods that balance the proven approaches such as diagnosis of infectious illness, a stronger partnership between clinical and prehospital care providers and health departments, and new approaches to disease surveillance.

EMS is emerging as an important link in disease surveillance. The ability to recognize patterns of potential infectious diseases and report to public health agencies and hospitals any clusters of similar symptoms and illnesses is the first step toward early detection of serious outbreaks. Public health

Street Smart

Complete and accurate documentation of every potential occupational exposure is the best guarantee that workers' compensation will protect you if you become ill as a result of the exposure.

agencies are then able to ensure the disease is identified, the exposures are traced, and treatment, quarantine, or other methods are taken to halt and prevent the spread of the disease.

In 1961, the CDC became responsible for the collection and publication of data on nationally notifiable diseases, in collaboration with the Council of State and Territorial Epidemiologists. The data is collected and compiled for publication purposes in the National Notifiable Diseases Surveillance System (NNDSS). The list is revised periodically, as a new pathogen emerges or a disease incident declines.

Mandatory reporting of notifiable diseases is regulated at a state level. All states generally report internationally quarantinable diseases such as cholera, plague, and yellow fever; however, disease outbreaks such as meningitis, mumps, and measles vary from state to state. The *Summary* of notifiable diseases is published weekly and is available on the CDC Web site.

Health care providers in the United States are required to report diseases, illnesses, or outbreaks as defined by local, state, or territorial laws and regulations. Each state has a list of reportable diseases. EMS agencies as health care partners should have knowledge of disease surveillance systems established by local public health agencies.

CONCLUSION

The importance of infection control to the daily practice of an EMT cannot be overemphasized. Education of infectious disease beyond the training received in an EMT class must occur at the agency level. Continuing education should reemphasize the potential hazards and infection control precautions specific to the local community and include practice of skills that protect EMTs from exposures.

EMTs can play an important role in the early detection of an epidemic through understanding of observation of a change in community health pattern, and notification of these changes to hospital or public health officials can be pivotal in early detection of disease outbreaks.

EMTs must know, understand, and continually practice infection control measures outlined in the local protocols and standard operating guidelines.

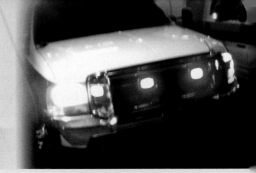

Tim thinks back to the day he answered the call for the car accident in his shorts. He is attending the mandatory class provided by the hospital on infection control and realizing how something as simple as wearing pants could have helped prevent that exposure. After reporting the exposure to his supervisor, there were several forms to fill out, blood tests, and the initial examination by the doctor. He was given medication to take while they waited for the results of the blood tests, to help prevent any disease to which he might have been exposed.

One year later, he is relieved he did not contract any illness from that exposure. Tim learned through his experience that exposure to a possible infectious disease can happen at anytime. There are simple, effective methods to prevent or lessen the transmission of infectious disease that he is relearning today and will be a priority practice each time he is toned out for a person in need.

PURPOSE: To remove any contamination by blood or other bodily fluids from the EMT's hands.

STANDARD PRECAUTIONS:

- ☑ Soap
- ☑ Water
- ☑ Hand brush

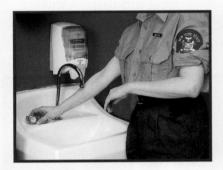

1 The EMT should remove any rings, watch, or other jewelry that could trap contamination.

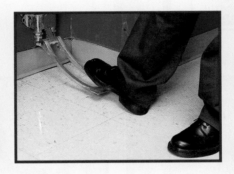

2 A deep basin sink and foot-pedal water faucets are preferable to wash hands. The EMT should adjust the hot and cold water to a comfortable lukewarm temperature.

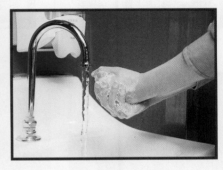

3 The EMT should then wet the hands to the midforearm. After applying a liberal amount of soap, the EMT should wash the hands carefully. The areas between the fingers deserve special attention. A hand brush may be used for contamination that is difficult to remove.

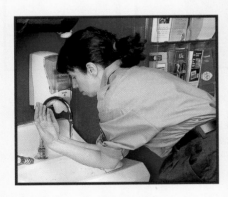

4 The EMT should then thoroughly rinse the hands, allowing the contaminated water to run off the elbow.

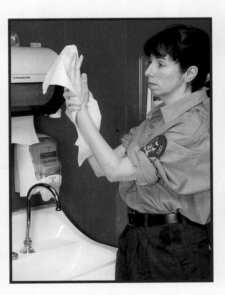

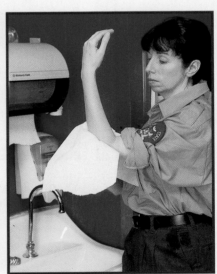

5 The EMT should then turn the water off. Grasping a clean towel, the EMT can turn off the faucet and discard the towel. Using a clean towel, the EMT should dry the hands, starting at the fingers and working toward the elbow.

Skill 8-2 Donning and Removing Personal Protective Equipment (PPE)

PURPOSE: To protect the EMT from blood and other bodily fluids. The task to be performed dictates the appropriate barrier devices to be worn.

STANDARD PRECAUTIONS:

☑ Mask

☑ Goggles

☑ Gown

☑ Nonsterile examination gloves (EMTs with latex sensitivity should wear vinyl gloves)

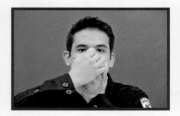 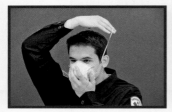 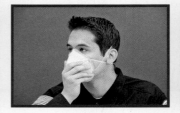 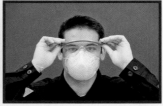

1 The EMT grasps the top ties of the mask and positions the metal strip in the mask over the bridge of the nose.

2 Pull the elastic straps over the head.

3 Grasp and pinch the metal strip around the bridge of the nose.

4 Pick up and apply the protective eyewear.

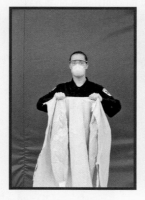 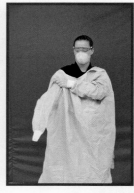 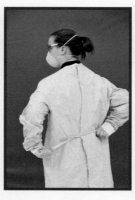 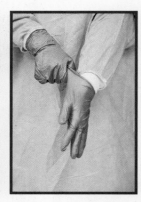 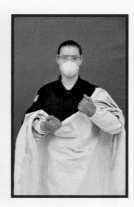

5 The EMT then grasps the gown by the collar and allows it to hang with the inside of the gown toward the EMT.

6 Next, the EMT places her arms in the sleeves.

7 Then the EMT ties the gown behind the neck.

8 Next, the EMT pulls on properly sized examination gloves. Each glove's collar should be over the sleeve of the gown.

9 To remove the PPE, the EMT reverses the order and washes the hands afterward.

PURPOSE: To protect the EMT from blood and bodily fluids.

STANDARD PRECAUTIONS:

☑ Nonsterile gloves
☑ Hazardous waste container

APPLICATION OF NONSTERILE GLOVES:

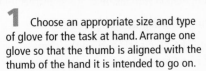 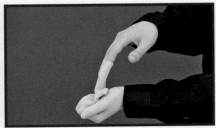 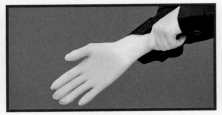

1 Choose an appropriate size and type of glove for the task at hand. Arrange one glove so that the thumb is aligned with the thumb of the hand it is intended to go on.

2 Grasp the front of the cuff with one hand, while inserting the other hand into the glove. Be sure to place each finger within the appropriate finger section. Pull at the cuff to ensure that the glove is completely applied to the hand.

3 Repeat the process for the other hand.

REMOVAL OF CONTAMINATED GLOVES:

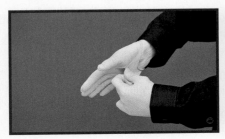 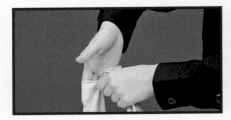 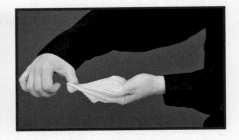

4 Grasp the palm or outside cuff of the left glove with the gloved right hand.

5 Pull the left glove toward the fingertips. The glove should turn inside out as it is removed.

6 Hold the removed glove in the still-gloved right hand. Insert the thumb of the ungloved left hand under the cuff of the right glove, carefully avoiding any contaminated areas. Pull the right glove toward the fingertips, turning it inside out on itself as it is removed. The soiled left glove should remain rolled into a ball in the palm of the right glove after it is removed. The right glove should then be inverted over the left glove and the two gloves balled together and disposed of properly in a red hazard bag. Gloves should never be left on scene. Also, it is dangerous to snap or fling potentially contaminated gloves at any time.

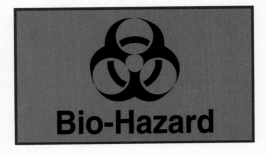

Bio-Hazard

7 Dispose of the gloves in a container clearly marked with the biohazard label and wash hands thoroughly.

Key Concepts Revisited

- Infectious diseases are caused by microorganisms called *pathogens* and can be communicable, or easily transmitted from person to person.

- An EMT's personal safety is one reason infection control is necessary.

- Risk management includes recognition of potential infectious exposures for both EMTs and patients.

- There are common infectious diseases EMTs may routinely encounter.
  - Varicella virus (chicken and shingles)
  - Tuberculosis
  - Hepatitis A
  - Hepatitis B, C, and D
  - Herpes Simplex 1 (oral/cold sores)
  - Herpes Simplex 2 (genital herpes)
  - HIV/AIDS
  - MRSA
  - Meningitis

- Common transmission pathways of infectious diseases are:
  - Contact transmission—direct contact with body substances
  - Airborne transmission—Droplets
  - Vehicle transmission—food, water
  - Vector borne—insects/parasites

- Susceptibility to illness following exposure to infectious diseases depends on the strength of the pathogen and the strength of the individual's immune system.

- Standard precautions and body substance isolation include the use of personal protective equipment (PPE):

  - Gloves
  - Goggles
  - Pocket masks and specialized masks
    - Surgical
    - HEPA
    - Respirators

- Hand washing and immunization are two important elements of infection control procedures.

- EMTs can determine which type of PPE is used on scene based on patient symptoms and "dress up" as additional protective measures are needed.

- The level of decontamination depends on the type of exposure and equipment.
  - Low-level decontamination with hospital-grade disinfectant
  - High-level decontamination by sterilization

- Infection control plans should clearly outline the steps required in the event of an exposure and be readily available to staff at all times.

- Documentation by EMTs has two important components: patient reporting and exposure reporting
  - Exposure reporting should include the time, date, and events of the exposure, potential type of exposurem and what type of PPE was being worn at that time of the exposure.

- EMTs are becoming an important link in public health disease surveillance and notification.

- Medical follow-up following infectious disease exposure important for the:
  - Evaluation of treatment effectiveness
  - Surveillance and tracking of ongoing disease processes
  - Post-exposure prophylaxis treatment, as needed

Review Questions

1. What is infection control?
2. What are the two types of infectious diseases?
3. What are the different modes of disease transmission?
4. What personal measures can be taken to help prevent illness caused by an infectious disease pathogen?

5. What personal protective equipment should an EMT have available to prevent an accidental exposure to an infectious disease?

6. What is meant by the term *standard precautions*?

7. What is an infection control plan, and where can it be found?

8. What elements should be documented when an infectious disease exposure occurs?

9. What is proper medical follow-up for an infectious disease exposure?

10. What is disease surveillance, and what role do EMTs play in it?

Key Terms

Antibodies

Biohazard

Body substance isolation

Carrier

Communicable

Contagious

Decontamination

Direct contact

Immunity

Immunization

Immunocompromised

Indirect contact

Infection control

Infection control officer

Intrinsic

Microorganism

Mucous membrane

Multidrug resistant organism

Pandemic

Personal protective equipment (PPE)

Portal of entry

Prophylaxis

Risk management

Risk profile

Safety officer

Sharps

Sharps container

Standard precautions

Sterilization

Transmission

Vector

Further Study

Centers for Disease Control and Prevention. Immunization of Health-Care Workers: Recommendations of the Advisory Committee on Immunization Practices (ACIP) and the Hospital Infection Control Practices Advisory Committee (HICPAC). *MMWR Morbidity and Mortality Weekly Report,* 1997. *46*(RR-18), 1–42.

Centers for Disease Control and Prevention. Public Health Service Guidelines for the Management of Health-Care Worker Exposures to HIV and Recommendations for Postexposure Prophylaxis. *MMWR Morbidity and Mortality Weekly Report,* 2002a. *47*(RR-7), 1–33.

Centers for Disease Control and Prevention. Recommendations for Follow-up of Health-Care Workers after Occupational Exposure to Hepatitis C Virus. *MMWR Morbidity and Mortality Weekly Report,* 2002b. *50*(RR-11), 1–42.

Occupation Safety and Health Administration. Occupational Exposure to Bloodborne Pathogens (Final Rule No. 29, CFR Part 1910.1030). Washington, DC: U.S. Department of Labor, 1992, July 1.

United States Fire Administration. *Guide to Managing an Emergency Service Infection Control Program.* Emmitsburg, MD: Author, 2004.

UNIT **9** Basic Airway Control

An open and secure airway is vital for adequate breathing and oxygenation. Recognition of airway obstruction, including partial and complete obstruction, is necessary for the EMT to manage the airway and restore adequate ventilation. This unit discusses airway management, recognition of airway compromise, and the skills necessary for the EMT to open an airway and apply the devices used to clear and secure the airway in compromised patients.

Airway management is the single most important skill an EMT can learn to be effective in the overall management of potentially life-threatening illness and injury.

National Education Standard

The Emergency Medical Technician (EMT) will have a fundamental depth, foundational breath of understanding within their scope of practice of airway anatomy, assessment, and techniques of ensuring a patent airway.

Key Concepts

- An open and patent airway is vital for adequate breathing and oxygenation.

- Opening and maintaining a patient airway is the most important lifesaving skill an EMT can learn.

- The sequence for basic airway control—open, assess, suction, and secure—represents one of the most important lifesaving actions EMTs can take.

- Control of the airway essentially involves the realignment of the structures of the upper airway until they create an open passageway for air movement.

- The EMT must place the patient in a position that allows for airway management without causing additional injury in the trauma patient.

- Airway assessment should include a more detailed examination after the airway has been opened to identify and manage any condition that may affect patency.

- Abnormal sounds heard during assessment of the airway, particularly in a patient with an altered mental status, can be important clues to the type of obstruction requiring management.

- An unconscious person cannot clear oral secretions or other foreign matter and may require suctioning.

- Suctioning removes not only fluids but oxygen-laden air and should only be done for 10 to 15 second intervals.

- The single most important aspect of airway control in the field is the continuous maintenance of the manually controlled airway.

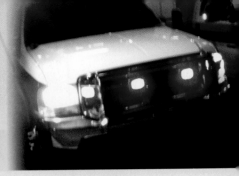

CASE STUDY

It is a little after midnight on New Year's Eve when Debbie and her partner, Eric, are toned out to the local bar for a male not breathing.

On the way to the call, Debbie and Eric discuss what they will need to ensure scene safety, taking into consideration the location and possible involvement of alcohol. Dispatch advises law enforcement is also en route to the same location.

Debbie and Eric run through the list of potential reasons why the patient is not breathing and the equipment they will need to take in with them, including the appropriate PPE of gloves and goggles.

Debbie knows that opening and securing the airway are the first two actions in controlling the airway immediately upon arrival to the patient's side.

When they arrive on scene, they are met by the owner, who leads them to a table at the back of the room. As

they approach, they see an approximately 30-year-old male lying mostly on his side on the floor under the table. Debbie can hear loud, snoring respirations coming from the patient and notices vomit on the front of his shirt.

A distraught female is kneeling next to the patient and tells Debbie his name is Frank. The woman says Frank had gone to the bathroom and after he came back, he sat down in the chair, then suddenly became limp, and began to slide to the floor.

She says she couldn't wake him up and didn't think he was breathing so she told the bartender to call 911.

Critical Thinking Questions

1. Why is Frank snoring?
2. What could the vomit on his shirt implicate?
3. What should be Debbie's first action be?

INTRODUCTION

The ability to open and maintain a patent airway in a patient is the single most important lifesaving skill an Emergency Medical Technician can learn. Remarkably, the most common airway obstruction is created by the patient's own tongue. The most basic airway maneuvers can relieve that obstruction. EMTs, as the largest group of prehospital medical care providers, must be experts at airway control.

The sequence for basic airway control is simple: Open, assess, suction, and secure. This simple order of tasks represents what could be the most important lifesaving actions an EMT can take.

ANATOMY REVIEW

In discussions of the management of a patient's airway, it is useful to have a clear picture of the relevant anatomy. Starting at the lips, the first structures encountered are the teeth. Teeth are usually fairly stable, primarily because they are embedded in bone. Blunt trauma can dislodge the teeth, making them potential airway obstructions. The teeth also have an excellent blood supply and can bleed profusely when disrupted. The loose teeth and blood can obstruct the airway, decreasing or blocking airflow.

The teeth are embedded into two jawbones. The lower jawbone, the *mandible*, serves as the floor of the mouth. Attached to the mandible, at the back of the throat, is the tongue. Therefore, if the mandible is moved, the tongue is also moved. The upper jawbone, or *maxilla*, holds the roof of the mouth, or the hard palate. The palate is the border between the floor of the nose and the roof of the mouth.

Air is most commonly brought into the body through the nose. The nose not only smells aromas in the air, it also adds moisture to the airway and raises the temperature of the air to body temperature. The nose consists of two nostrils that are divided by a septum. A widening of the nostrils from taking in a deep breath is called **nasal flaring.** The nostrils, acting as air intake ports, open larger to take in larger and larger amounts of air. Persistent nasal flaring is a sign of respiratory distress.

The area in the back of the throat, where the oral cavity and the nasal cavity meet, called the **pharynx,** contains several easily identified structures. As seen in Figure 9.1, the most obvious structure is the small piece of flesh that is hanging off the roof of the mouth called the **uvula.** The uvula swings up to help protect the nasal cavity when a swallow occurs. It is also the farthest point that is visible to the EMT without special equipment.

On each side of the back of the throat are two pillars of soft tissue called **tonsils.** These tissues are very fragile, and vigorous suctioning can result in serious bleeding.

The tongue is probably the most important structure in the mouth. The tongue enables us to taste our food when we eat and helps with our speech. The entire surface of the tongue is covered with liquid called **saliva.** Saliva is created by glands lining the mouth. Bacteria and other harmful microorganisms are entrapped in saliva to be swallowed and destroyed in the stomach's acid or

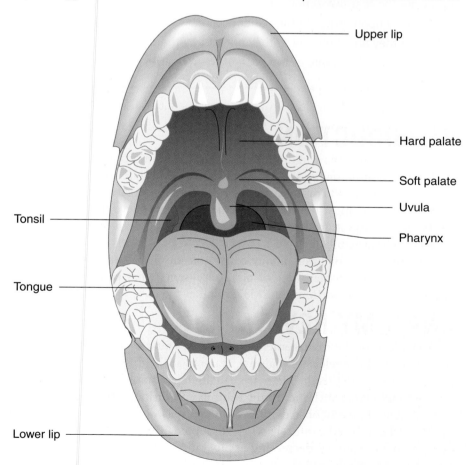

Figure 9.1 Note the various structures in the mouth visible from the front, including the teeth, tonsils, and palate

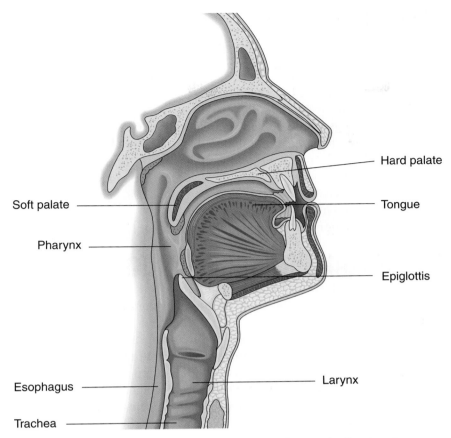

Figure 9.2 Note the relationship of the esophagus to the trachea

"spit" out. This feature of saliva makes the entire interior of the mouth a potential source of infectious body fluids. An EMT working within the mouth (oral cavity) must observe proper standard precautions (body substance isolation).

The tongue is vascular, meaning it has many blood vessels. The source of the blood supply for the tongue comes from under the tongue in an area called the **sublingual** area. Because the area is so rich with blood, medications are often deposited under the tongue to be absorbed into the bloodstream.

In the back of the throat, not visible to the EMT, is the base of the tongue. As seen in Figure 9.2, the base of the tongue is at the top of both the windpipe, called the **trachea,** and the food passage, called the *esophagus.*

The base of the tongue also abuts an important structure called the *epiglottis,* which means "above the glottis." The glottis is the opening to the sound-producing portion of the throat, the voice box or *larynx.* More important, it is the uppermost structure of the lower airway.

To prevent the accidental passage of food into the airway during swallowing, the epiglottis blocks off the trachea. If a food particle enters the trachea, the patient will cough vigorously in an attempt to dislodge it from the airway. This coughing also brings up mucus from the airway called **sputum.**

If a piece of food is too large to be swallowed, it will strike the walls of the back of the throat, and the patient will gag. Stimulation of this protective response, called the **gag reflex,** results in the objects being expelled from the mouth, protecting the airway from blockage by food.

For a more complete review of the structures of the upper airway, please refer to Unit 5.

Pediatric Considerations

The epiglottis in a child is relatively larger and less rigid than that of an adult. As a result, swelling and inflammation can result in a complete blockage of the airway. This condition, called *epiglottitis,* can be life threatening.

The EMT should determine the airway is patent—that is, open and clear—in every patient encountered. The patient who can speak clearly and breathe without excessive noise can be considered to have a patent airway.

PHYSIOLOGY

The human body needs oxygen to allow the cells of the body to produce energy. Without oxygen, the body dies in a process called *shock*. This process is discussed in detail in Unit 11.

The lungs supply the body with oxygen. The lungs get oxygen from the air inhaled into the airway. The airway is a passage starting at the mouth and ending in the lungs. It takes many muscles and nerves to keep the airway open. Whenever a patient cannot maintain this airway as an open passageway, the EMT must be prepared to assist in its maintenance.

Control of the airway essentially involves the realignment of the structures of the upper airway until they create an open passageway for air movement. This movement of air into and out of the lungs is called breathing, or *ventilation*. Ventilation is not possible without a clear airway.

PERSONAL PROTECTIVE EQUIPMENT

An EMT protecting the airway is at an increased risk of exposure to blood, sputum, and saliva. All of these body fluids are potential carriers for infectious disease.

EMTs rarely forget to wear gloves but are often careless in regard to eye protection and masks. A cough is a forceful and sometimes violent exhalation of air. A cough can easily expel microorganism-laden sputum as far as 3 or 4 feet. Some vomiting, called *projectile vomiting*, can go even farther.

When suctioning a patient's airway, or performing any task, the EMT should determine if his eyes and mouth are within 3 to 4 feet of the patient. If they are, those areas are at risk for exposure to sputum, saliva, or vomit. The EMT should always follow standard precautions as appropriate for the situation, as discussed in Unit 8.

THE OPEN AIRWAY

The first question the EMT should ask when assessing a patient is whether an open (patent) passageway for air exists. Because life depends on breathing, and breathing depends on a clear passageway for air movement; the first priority must be to open the air passageway, or **airway.**

The patient with a clear air passage will be able to breathe quietly without any evidence of mechanical obstruction. Air should move into and out of the patient's mouth and nose without any difficulty.

Recognition of a potential airway blockage, or **occlusion,** is of key importance to the EMT. An EMT who cannot recognize an occluded airway will not know to clear the passageway and restore breathing.

Several techniques can be used by the EMT to create a clear air passageway. The method that is used depends on the patient's condition. The patient who has a neck injury will need to have special care taken to avoid any movement of the neck during airway management.

SIGNS OF AN OBSTRUCTED AIRWAY

Loss of consciousness often results in relaxation of the muscles, including the muscles in the airway. The immediate result is that the soft tissues of the throat, and particularly the tongue, collapse into the airway. Therefore, any unconscious patient potentially has an obstructed airway.

The collapse of the pharyngeal soft tissues makes the smooth passage of air more difficult. If the obstruction created by these collapsed tissues is not complete and air is able to get through, the patient may make a

When maintaining a patient's airway for a long period of time, the EMT may become fatigued or inattentive, inadvertently allowing the jaw to slide back and the tongue to partially obstruct the airway. The result is a snoring sound created by air trying to move past the tongue. The EMT must be alert and prevent airway compromise as evidenced by snoring.

characteristic snoring sound as the air pushes past the tongue and pharyngeal tissues. Snoring sounds in the unconscious patient should lead the EMT to check for a partial airway obstruction. The tongue is the single most common cause of airway obstruction in the unconscious patient (Figure 9.3).

If the collapsed pharyngeal tissue, or any other object, has completely occluded the airway, no air movement will occur; therefore, no noise will be present. Breathlessness, or *apnea*, is a potential sign of a completely obstructed airway. A blue discoloration to the skin, called **cyanosis,** is an indication that blood is not getting oxygen, possibly because of an airway obstruction. As demonstrated in Figure 9.4, cyanosis is often most visible in the fingernail beds; along the inner eyelid, called the conjunctiva; and inside the lips. The EMT must be able to quickly recognize the patient with a complete airway obstruction and provide an effective remedy.

PROPER POSITIONING

Often, an unconscious patient is found on the ground or flat on a surface such as a bathroom floor or a bed. If the patient is facedown, or prone, the EMT must decide whether it is necessary to roll the patient over.

The decision to roll the patient onto the back should not be taken lightly. If the patient has a spinal injury, movement must be done with great care to avoid worsening of the injury. This change in position is best done by several EMTs together. The techniques for moving the patient with a possible spine injury are detailed in Unit 35.

If the EMT is alone and the potentially spine-injured patient is in a prone position, the EMT must consider whether the patient has an open airway in that position. If the EMT finds that the patient's airway is open and is not likely to be occluded in that position, then it is advisable to leave the patient in that position until more help arrives.

If the EMT does not suspect a spinal injury, then he may choose to place the patient in a position that allows better airway maintenance. One such position, as seen in Figure 9.5, involves rolling the patient onto the side to allow for easy drainage of oral secretions. This position is known as the *recovery position.*

If the patient is prone and does not have a patent airway, the EMT is forced to act immediately. Unfortunately, most of the airway techniques an EMT can employ require that the patient be lying on the back, or supine.

If the EMT is alone with an unconscious patient who does not have an adequate airway, he must perform a one-person logroll. The one-person logroll is not the preferred method of handling a trauma patient with a potential spinal injury. It should be used only when the risk for death from airway collapse is great.

Once the patient has been placed in a supine position, there are several techniques that the EMT may use to open the airway. The best technique for the situation is decided on the basis of the suspicion, or lack of suspicion, that a spine injury exists.

HEAD-TILT, CHIN-LIFT

The most common airway maneuver used by EMTs is the **head-tilt, chin-lift.** This procedure is reserved for patients for whom trauma, specifically neck injury, has been ruled out. This category would include the patient who is found in bed and a patient who was observed to go unconscious without striking the head when collapsing. The head-tilt, chin-lift is easily done by a single EMT and is detailed in Skill 9-1 at the end of this unit.

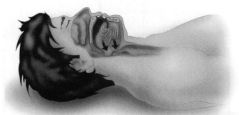

Obstructed airway (tongue against pharynx)

Figure 9.3 The tongue commonly creates an airway obstruction in the supine, unconscious patient

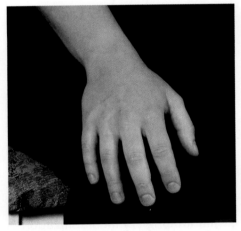

Figure 9.4 Look for cyanosis at the fingernail beds

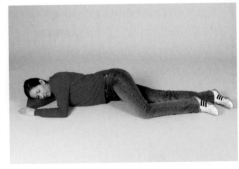

Figure 9.5 The recovery position allows natural drainage of airway secretions

JAW THRUST

Whenever a possible neck injury is suspected, or when the patient's condition is unknown, spinal precautions must be taken. Spinal precautions involve careful attention to stabilization and immobilization of the head, neck, and back to prevent any further injury to the delicate spinal cord. This concept and techniques of spinal immobilization are discussed in Unit 35.

If the patient with a potential neck injury is in need of airway assistance, the EMT should not hesitate to provide it. There are a few special techniques to use when managing the airway of the trauma patient. The first component to trauma airway maintenance involves stabilization of the head and neck. When neck injury is suspected, it is important to minimize any movement.

The usual techniques of airway management would involve too much movement, so a different maneuver is used. This maneuver, the **jaw thrust** maneuver, involves lifting the mandible. Because the tongue is attached to the mandible, lifting the mandible will serve to lift the tongue off the back of the airway. This technique is detailed in Skill 9-2 at the end of this unit.

AIRWAY ASSESSMENT

After the airway has been either opened with one of the techniques discussed or determined to be spontaneously open and patent, a more detailed examination needs to occur. Any condition that may affect the patency of the airway should be found and addressed. The EMT should use a light and look into the patient's mouth for any accumulation of secretions or foreign matter that may cause an airway obstruction. Broken teeth or partial bridges and other dental hardware may occlude the unconscious patient's airway and should be removed.

If the airway is obstructed and simple airway maneuvers such as the head-tilt, chin-lift or jaw thrust do not remedy the problem, then the EMT should consider the possibility of a foreign body airway obstruction. A history of choking will often lead the EMT quickly to this conclusion.

If an airway foreign body is suspected and the patient is unable to speak or breathe, indicating complete airway obstruction, the EMT should perform the maneuvers recommended by the American Heart Association and American Red Cross for management of such a condition. Abdominal thrusts are recommended for the conscious patient with a complete airway obstruction, whereas chest compressions are used in the unconscious victim of a foreign body airway obstruction.

ABNORMAL AIRWAY SOUNDS

Normal breathing through a patent airway should be noiseless and easy. During assessment of the airway, particularly in a patient with an altered mental status, it is important for the EMT to listen for any abnormal sounds. Snoring, as stated previously, occurs when the upper airway is partially obstructed, usually by the tongue or by relaxed muscles and tissues of the pharynx. This type of obstruction can usually be cleared using the head-tilt, chin-lift maneuver or jaw thrust maneuver in the case of a suspected spinal injury.

Crowing is a sound that can occur when the muscles around the larynx spasm. The opening into the trachea narrows and air rushing through the narrowed passage makes the "cawing" sound called crowing.

Significant upper airway obstruction from swelling of the larynx can cause a harsh high-pitched sound heard during inspiration called **stridor.**

Stridor can also sometimes be heard when there is an obstruction from an object, such as food.

Gurgling, a sound like gargling, usually indicates the presence of fluid, such as blood, vomitus, or secretions, in the airway. Gurgling is an indication that immediate suctioning to remove the fluid from the airway may be required.

AIRWAY SUCTIONING

A conscious person may be able to effectively clear oral secretions, but an unconscious person cannot. Saliva and possibly other foreign matter accumulate in the mouth and throat of the unconscious patient. Therefore, every unconscious patient could potentially require suctioning.

EMTs traditionally depend on mechanical suction to clear airways that are filled with vomitus, blood, or other secretions. Unfortunately, the design of mechanical suction devices often does not match the reality of the patient who is vomiting solid materials. In those cases, two fingers must be used to clear out the solid debris first.

These finger sweeps should be done carefully to avoid pushing material farther into the throat. Many EMTs hesitate to place their fingers into the mouth of an unconscious patient, for fear of being accidentally bitten by the patient. An oropharyngeal airway can be placed between the upper and lower molars and held there. The oral airway works very effectively as a bite block to prevent finger injury.

Even if another EMT is using the head-tilt, chin-lift or jaw thrust method to open the airway, it may be necessary to open the patient's mouth even further in order to fully visualize the oropharynx or to introduce the suction catheter tip. To accomplish this, the EMT should use the **cross-fingered technique.**

The cross-fingered technique involves placement of the left hand's forefinger against the lower incisors and thumb against the upper incisors proximal to the midline of the mouth opening. With a scissors like action, the EMT would gently pry the teeth apart and open the mouth even further (Figure 9.6). It should be emphasized that the cross-fingered technique is not a replacement for head-tilt, chin-lift or jaw thrust airway opening techniques but an adjunct technique that improves visualization and control of the airway.

THE SUCTION MACHINE

All suction machines have one quality in common: they are designed to vacuum the debris from a patient's mouth. There are many machines on the market. Each claims to have a special feature that makes it better than all the other machines.

The first category of suction machine, sometimes called an "aspirator," is the manual suction. As the name implies, the power for the suction machine comes from the operator, in this case an EMT. Many models on the market claim rapid evacuation of the fluid and vomit. Many of these machines are portable, making them attractive for the EMT. Clearly, the single largest advantage of the manually powered suction machine is the presence of a dependable power supply, the EMT.

The next category of suction machine is the electric suction unit that may be either vehicle mounted or portable. Some electric suction units run off standard wall current; others are battery dependent. Most can be powered by both. These machines, in many respects, resemble the suction machines in the hospital. One option that can be attractive in certain situations is the ability for electric suction to vary its vacuum power.

Finally, many ambulances are equipped with a suction machine that operates off the power created by either an oxygen device or the electric

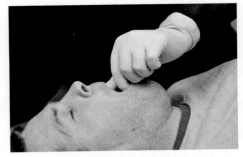

Figure 9.6 The cross-fingered technique can be used to further open the mouth to suction

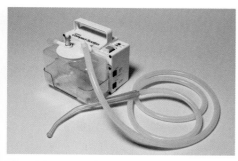

Figure 9.7 The suction machine has several disposable parts, including the suction catheter, the tubing, and the canister

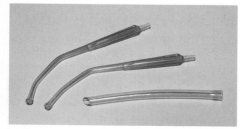

Figure 9.8 Note the relatively large opening at the end of the Yankauer suction catheter compared to the opening of the tonsil tip

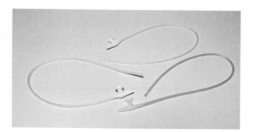

Figure 9.9 Flexible catheters are useful when suctioning through an endotracheal tube

motor. The benefits of this approach include a reliable power source; its main drawback is that a leak anywhere within the system can lessen the suction power.

All suction machines have a collection chamber. Many of these chambers are self-contained and disposable, a feature that decreases the likelihood of accidental spillage. Others require cleaning and decontamination.

Most suction devices have a length of tubing that extends from the collection canister to the suction catheter. This tubing is usually clear plastic and, more important, disposable. The tubing allows the machine to be placed a distance away from the patient. Figure 9.7 highlights the features of a suction machine.

SUCTION TUBING

Suction tubing stretches from the suction machine to the suction catheter and serves as a conduit for the suctioned material to the machine from the patient. Prior to using a suction device, it is customary to bend and occlude the suction tubing to see if adequate suction is being produced by the suction machine. Typically, suction pressures of at least 300 cm H_2O should be produced within 4 seconds of activation (KKK specification 3.12.4).

The EMT should check all connections between the suction machine and suction tubing to ensure a tight fit if the suction machine fails to produce an adequate vacuum. If the problem persists, then the EMT should troubleshoot the suction system and correct any problems before using it on a patient.

THE CATHETER

A variety of suction catheters are available, each designed with a different purpose in mind. The EMT should decide what he needs a suction catheter for and then select the correct catheter for that use.

The tonsil tip catheter is made of a rigid plastic that makes it easy to use even when wearing a pair of gloves. The tip of the catheter is blunted so that when suction is applied, it does not injure soft tissue, such as the tonsils at the back of the throat. The tonsil tip catheter is an excellent choice when used to suction large amounts of saliva or liquid material such as blood.

However, when the EMT needs to suction thick secretions such as blood clots, a **Yankauer** suction catheter with large open tips is more practical. Caution is advised to avoid inadvertently increasing bleeding by injuring soft tissues.

As seen in Figure 9.8, both the tonsil tip and the Yankauer suction tip have a whistle port. If the EMT places his thumb over the whistle port, suction occurs at the distal end of the catheter. Release the thumb and the suction is broken. If the suction catheter does not have a whistle port, the EMT will have to kink the suction tubing in order to control the suction.

Another type of suction catheter used by EMTs is the flexible **French catheter,** sometimes called a "spaghetti" catheter. Most flexible catheters today are disposable clear plastic (Figure 9.9). They are used by EMTs either to suction the external nares of the nose or to suction the opening of a tracheostomy, called a *stoma.* These long, flexible catheters are also used when suctioning through an endotracheal tube.

Often during suctioning, the catheter becomes clogged with debris. An available source of water, such as a container of sterile water, nearby can save time otherwise wasted changing clogged catheters. The EMT simply suctions the water to unclog the catheter until it is clear. It should be noted that an EMT should not pour water into the airway in an attempt to open the airway.

THE PROCEDURE

The EMT must remember that suctioning removes not only fluids but oxygen-laden air as well. Logically, the first step before suctioning is to ensure good oxygenation whenever possible. Occasionally the patient must be suctioned to clear a pathway for the oxygen. Even in those cases, the EMT must keep in mind that the patient may be going without oxygen. Skill 9-3 at the end of this unit lists the steps used in suctioning a patient's airway.

If it is necessary to repeatedly suction, after properly reoxygenating the patient, the catheter should be flushed in water and the procedure repeated as many times as necessary until the airway is cleared.

In some serious trauma cases involving massive facial injuries, an EMT may spend his entire time with the patient suctioning the airway clear of blood. This single task may make the difference between life and death for the patient. Without an airway, there is no breathing; without a breath, there is no life.

SECURING THE AIRWAY

An EMT must maintain a constant vigil of the airway. A moment's inattention can lead to airway collapse. The single most important aspect of airway control in the field is the continuous maintenance of the manually controlled airway. The EMT can augment his efforts at airway control with adjunctive devices. However, these are an accessory to, not a replacement for good manual airway control.

THE OROPHARYNGEAL AIRWAY

An **oropharyngeal airway (OPA),** often referred to as an oral airway, is a disposable molded plastic device designed to help keep the tongue off the roof of the mouth and from falling into the back of the mouth (Figure 9.10). The OPA also creates an artificial channel for the passage of oxygen into the trachea. Additionally it can act as a bite block, preventing the patient from accidentally biting the tongue or the EMT's finger. What it does not do is actually lift the tongue off the back of the throat; only manual control can do that.

There are several types of OPAs; however, all have some sort of flange that rests against the lips and prevents the OPA from accidentally being swallowed. Although some have "channels" to assist the passage of a flexible soft catheter, the use of an OPA for this purpose is not encouraged. Occasionally, the catheter, especially if it is not properly lubricated, becomes lodged and the OPA must be removed.

Whenever an OPA is used to assist with airway control, several cautions must be remembered. It is very common for an OPA to stimulate a gag reflex; therefore, an OPA is used only for unconscious patients who do not have a gag reflex. The EMT must be prepared to immediately remove the OPA if the patient should have a gag reflex to prevent vomiting. Suction must also be ready whenever an OPA is being inserted.

An improperly measured OPA can actually occlude the airway by pushing the tongue into the back of the throat. This problem should be suspected whenever the OPA is seen to advance and then retract with every respiration, in a see-saw type motion. An OPA that is too small will simply be swallowed into the mouth and create an airway obstruction.

It is important to remember to completely suction the mouth before inserting an OPA. If the EMT fails to completely suction the airway, any debris can be pushed farther into the airway and even into the trachea.

The majority of unconscious patients need an OPA to assist with control of the airway. Therefore, every EMT must be skilled at control of the airway and use of the OPA. Skill 9-4 at the end of this unit illustrates the insertion of the OPA.

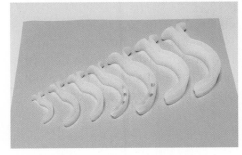

Figure 9.10 The correct OPA must be chosen from the selection available

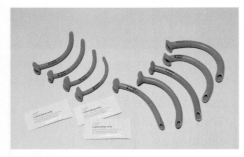

Figure 9.11 NPAs, like OPAs, must be properly fitted to the patient

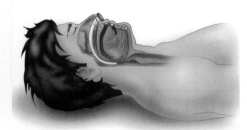

Figure 9.12 In this model, the NPA is clearly behind the tongue in a position where it can help to protect the airway, yet it does not often stimulate a gag reflex

THE NASOPHARYNGEAL AIRWAY

The **nasopharyngeal airway (NPA)**, or nasal airway, is used infrequently in the prehospital setting, yet it is easy to use and provides significant benefits over the oral airway. The NPA is a soft, flexible tube that extends from the external nostril, through the nose, and into the back of the throat. Figure 9.11 shows various NPAs. Because of its unique position in relation to the structures of the airway, the NPA does not induce a gag reflex as frequently as does an OPA (Figure 9.12).

The rigid nature of the OPA makes it the adjunct of choice in the unconscious patient, in whom definitive airway control is needed. However, in cases in which the patient will not tolerate the OPA because of a gag reflex, the airway adjunct of choice is the more flexible nasal airway.

It is impossible to pass an OPA into the mouth of a patient with clenched teeth, as sometimes occurs during seizures. The nasal airway assists in providing a patent airway in those patients during the event and can be easily removed later when the patient's problem has resolved. Skill 9-5 at the end of this unit reviews the procedure for insertion of an NPA.

Use of an NPA should be avoided in patients with known or suspected fracture of the skull or severe facial trauma, such as nasal bone fracture and active nose bleeds.

Once the airway is in place, the entire process taking less than 30 seconds, the patient should be reoxygenated as needed. The NPA still does not substitute for manual control of the airway, and an EMT should maintain the jaw thrust or the head-tilt, chin-lift maneuver as needed.

Safety Tips

The soft tissues within the nose are vascular. Sometimes even slight trauma, such as that involved in placing an NPA, can cause bleeding. Therefore, great care must be exercised to never force an NPA if it does not go in smoothly and easily. The majority of NPA insertions are done without any significant bleeding.

CONCLUSION

Insuring and maintaining an open airway is the first priority in all patient contacts by an EMT. Without a patent airway, the patient has little chance of survival. Fortunately, the manipulation of the airway becomes relatively easy for most EMTs after a little practice.

Practice is the key to gaining mastery of this fundamental skill. The simple mantra of open, assess, suction, and secure will serve the EMT well during airway management.

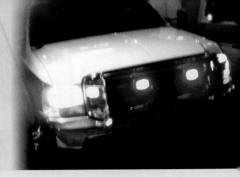

Debbie and Eric logroll Frank onto his back in the supine position after verifying he was assisted to the floor by others at the table when he lost consciousness and did not fall or hit his head. Debbie uses a head-tilt, chin-lift maneuver to open and maintain the airway while Eric suctions any remaining vomit out of Frank's mouth. Frank immediately stops snoring, but does not regain consciousness.

Debbie attempts to insert an oropharyngeal airway but Frank gags even though no vomit is present. Eric inserts a nasopharyngeal airway and places supplemental oxygen by mask on Frank; he is prepared to suction further if needed.

Frank is placed in the ambulance and does not regain consciousness throughout transport, although he does moan and pull away when Debbie pinches the skin on his wrist. Frank's breathing rate is approximate 12 breaths per minute, and he has good chest rise with each breath. His skin is warm, moist, and pink and his pulse is regular at 72 beats per minute.

Debbie continues to monitor Frank's breathing while en route to the hospital and is prepared to suction if needed.

Upon arrival to the hospital, Debbie and Eric help transfer Frank to the cot in the busy emergency department. Debbie reports her assessment findings, treatment initiated, and response to treatment to Sally, RN, at that time. Debbie and Eric clean or properly dispose of all equipment that came in contact with Frank's vomit. They thoroughly clean and restock the ambulance. Debbie and Eric thoroughly wash their hands after removing their gloves and goggles and radio dispatch they are back in service and ready for another call.

Skill 9-1 Head-Tilt, Chin-Lift

PURPOSE: To allow the EMT to open the airway of a nontrauma patient.

STANDARD PRECAUTIONS:

☑ Gloves
☑ Goggles
☑ Mask

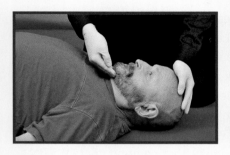 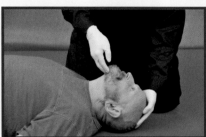 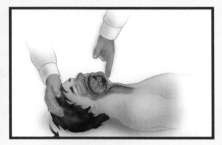

1 After donning the appropriate PPE, the EMT positions himself at the side of the patient's head.

2 The palm of one hand is placed on the patient's forehead, and the fingertips of the other hand on the patient's jaw.

3 The patient's head is tilted back using a firm pressure on the forehead while the jaw is gently lifted up to pull the tongue off the back of the throat. Care should be taken not to push backward on the jaw because doing so will only force the patient's mouth closed.

Skill 9-2 Jaw Thrust Maneuver

PURPOSE: To allow the EMT to open the airway of a nontrauma patient.

STANDARD PRECAUTIONS:

☑ Gloves
☑ Goggles
☑ Mask

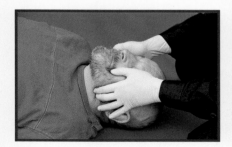 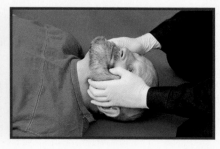 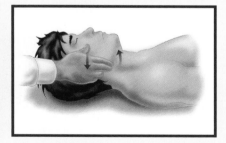

1 After donning appropriate PPE, the EMT should position herself above the patient's head.

2 The EMT places her middle and index fingers on the angles of the patient's jaw and her thumbs on the cheekbones.

3 The middle and index fingers lift the jaw and the tongue up off the back of the throat while avoiding any movement of the neck.

PURPOSE: To clear the airway of secretions that may be preventing air exchange.

STANDARD PRECAUTIONS:

- ☑ Gloves
- ☑ Goggles
- ☑ Mask
- ☑ Suction device (electronic or mechanical)
- ☑ Tubing
- ☑ Catheter
- ☑ Water

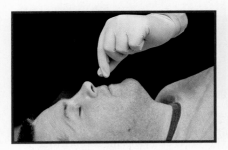

1 One EMT opens and assesses the airway, using the technique appropriate to the patient's situation.

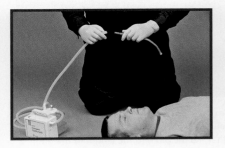

2 Another EMT removes the rigid suction tip from its protective covering, attaches the tip to the tubing, and then the tubing to the intake of the suction machine. Once the equipment is assembled, the EMT tests the machine's suction.

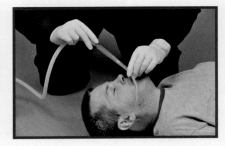

3 One EMT measures the length of the suction tip against the distance from the opening of the mouth to the angle of the jaw.

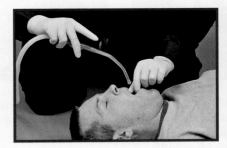

4 The EMT then opens the mouth with the nondominant hand, using a cross-fingered technique. Placing the thumb on the lower teeth and the forefinger on the upper teeth, the EMT holds the teeth apart by a finger-snapping type of motion.

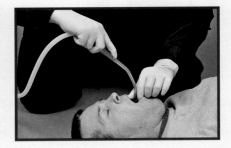

5 The rigid suction tip is then inserted to the depth of the measurement. Suction is applied only as the tip is withdrawn, usually by placing a thumb over a whistle port or releasing the kink of the suction tubing. Repeat suctioning as often as necessary but never for more than 15 seconds. It is important to oxygenate the patient between suction attempts.

PURPOSE: To use a mechanical adjunct to assist the EMT who is manually maintaining the airway.

STANDARD PRECAUTIONS:

☑ Gloves
☑ Goggles
☑ Mask
☑ Assortment of oral airways

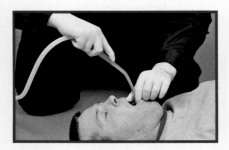

1 First, an EMT must manually open the airway, using the technique appropriate to the patient's condition. The patient's airway should be suctioned as needed.

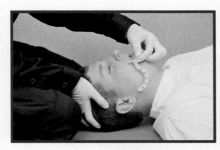

2 The EMT then chooses an oral airway that fits the patient. The length of the oral airway should match the distance from the angle of the jaw to the opening of the mouth.

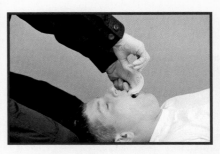

3 Using the cross-fingered technique, the EMT opens the mouth. The EMT begins to insert the airway, curved portion downward, toward the jaw, to about midway.

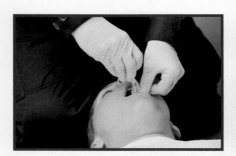

4 The EMT then rotates the oral airway 180 degrees so that the airway naturally follows the curve of the hard palate.

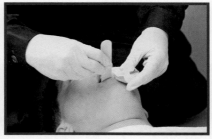

5 Alternatively, the EMT can use a tongue depressor to press the tongue downward and forward. Then an oral airway may be inserted directly into the oral cavity, following the curve of the hard palate.

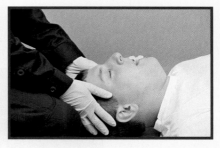

6 The airway is correctly placed when the flange of the airway rests on the patient's teeth.

PURPOSE: To provide an airway for patients who cannot tolerate an oral airway but also cannot protect their own airway.

STANDARD PRECAUTIONS:

☑ Gloves

☑ Goggles

☑ Mask

☑ Assortment of oral airways

☑ Water-soluble lubricant

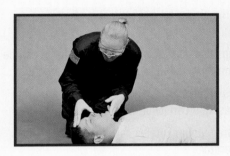

1 The EMT first examines the nostril opening to determine an approximate size of nasal airway that will be needed.

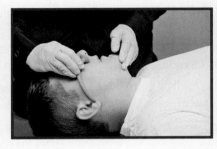

2 The EMT then compares the length of the nasal airway with the distance between the nostril and the tip of the earlobe.

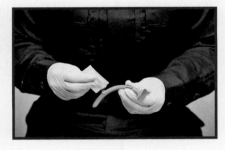

3 The EMT then applies a generous layer of water-soluble lubricant to the length of the nasal airway.

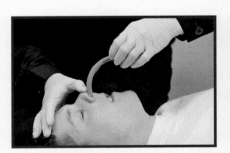

4 The nasal airway is then gently introduced to the nostril. The bevel of the airway should be facing inward toward the nasal septum.

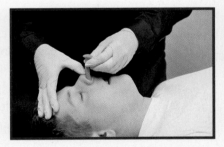

5 A gentle corkscrewing action, back and forth, as the EMT gently pushes straight backward usually allows the nasal airway to be placed.

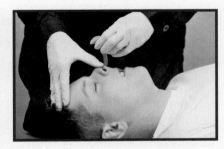

6 If resistance is met, then the nasal airway should be withdrawn and insertion into the other nostril attempted.

Key Concepts Revisited

- An open and patent airway is vital for adequate breathing and oxygenation.

- Opening and maintaining a patient airway is the most important lifesaving skill an EMT can learn.

- The tongue, the most important structure in the mouth, is the most common cause of airway obstruction in the unconscious patient.

- Control of the airway essentially involves the realignment of the structures of the upper airway until they create an open passageway for air movement.

- Quiet, easy movement of air into and out of a patient's mouth and nose is indicative of a patent (open), clear airway.

- Signs of airway obstruction include:
  - Noisy breathing
  - Cyanosis or blue discoloration of the skin
  - Apnea or no breathing

- The EMT must place the patient in a position that allows for airway management:
  - Supine or prone position in patients with spinal injury
  - Logroll to better manage airway
  - Recovery position to drain secretions

- There are several techniques used to open the airway:
  - Head-tilt, chin-lift is most common for patient without trauma.
  - Jaw thrust is used with patients with possible spinal injury.

- Airway assessment should include a more detailed examination after the airway has been opened; any condition that may affect patency should be found and managed.

- Abnormal sounds heard during assessment of the airway, particularly in patients with an altered mental status, can be important clues to the type of obstruction requiring management.
  - Snoring indicates a partially obstructed upper airway, usually by the tongue or relaxed muscles and tissues of the pharynx.
  - Crowing sounds like the "caw" of a crow and occurs when the muscles around the larynx spasm and narrow the opening into the trachea.
  - Stridor is a harsh, high-pitched sound heard during inspiration and indicates a significant upper airway obstruction caused by swelling of the larynx.
  - Gurgling sounds like gargling and usually indicates the presence of fluid in the airway, requiring immediate suctioning.

- An unconscious person cannot clear oral secretions or other foreign matter and may require suctioning.
  - Clearing of the airway by mechanical suction is preferred.
  - Finger sweeps done only to clear visible material can be used when material is too large for suction catheters.

- Suction machines are designed to vacuum debris from the patient's mouth using a variety of methods.
  - Aspirators are manual suction with the power coming from the operator.
  - Electronic suction run off wall current or battery and are usually portable.
  - Suction machines usually mounted in the ambulance run off oxygen or the ambulance-mounted electric motor.

- Suction catheters are available in a variety of designs with a different purpose in mind.
  - Tonsil tip catheter is rigid plastic that is blunted on the end to prevent injury to the soft tissue in the throat, such as the tonsils.
  - Yankauer suction catheters have large open tips more practical for use with thick secretions such as blood clots.
  - French catheter or spaghetti catheter is flexible and used to suction the external nares, opening of a tracheostomy, and through an endotracheal tube.

- Suctioning removes not only fluids but oxygen-laden air and should be accomplished without causing the patient to go without oxygen for an extended period of time.

- The single most important aspect of airway control in the field is the continuous maintenance of the manually controlled airway.

- The oropharyngeal airway and nasopharyngeal airway are two adjunct devices that create an artificial channel for passage of oxygen into the trachea.

- The simple process of airway management can be remembered by: open, assess, suction, and secure.

Review Questions

1. When should a head-tilt, chin-lift maneuver be used to open the airway?
2. When is the jaw thrust preferred over the head-tilt, chin-lift?
3. What does the sound of snoring respirations usually indicate?
4. Gurgling sounds heard when assessing the airway are suggestive of what?
5. What is the most commonly forgotten piece of EMS equipment?
6. What is the danger of suctioning for too long a period of time?
7. How do you measure an oral airway?
8. What is the most significant advantage of a nasal airway over an oral airway?
9. How do you measure a nasal airway?
10. What is the single most important lifesaving skill an EMT can learn?

Key Terms

Airway
Crowing
Cross-fingered technique
Cyanosis
French catheter
Gag reflex
Head-tilt, chin-lift
Jaw thrust
Nasal flaring
Nasopharyngeal airway (NPA)
Occlusion

Oropharyngeal airway (OPA)
Pharynx
Saliva
Sputum
Stridor
Sublingual
Tonsils
Trachea
Uvula
Yankauer

Further Study

American Red Cross. *Cardiopulmonary Resuscitation for the Professional Rescuer.* Washington, DC: Author, (2005).

American Heart Association. *Basic Life Support for Healthcare Providers.* Dallas, TX: Author, 2006.

Scott, A., & Fong, E. *Body Structures and Functions* (10th ed.). Clifton Park, NY: Thomson Delmar Learning, 2003.

UNIT (10) Respiratory Support

After the airway has been opened and assessed for patency, the next step is to establish adequate breathing. The EMT must determine if the rate and volume of air being taken in with each breath is adequate for gas exchange in the alveoli as discussed in Units 5 and 6. This unit will discuss assessment and management of the respiratory system to include the use of supplemental oxygen therapy.

National Education Standards

The Emergency Medical Technician (EMT) will have a fundamental depth and foundational breadth of understanding of the assessment and management of adequate and inadequate respiration and respiratory support, including supplemental oxygen therapy and artificial ventilation.

Key Concepts

- The EMT must assess the efficiency of a patient's ventilation and respiration and support each of these functions when necessary.

- Severe respiratory difficulty and ineffective oxygenation presents as brain dysfunction, including agitation, confusion, and unconsciousness, and requires immediate oxygen therapy.

- The initial steps in the assessment of the respiratory system are look, listen, and feel.

- Patients in respiratory distress are commonly seated forward, hands resting on the knees with chin pointed outward, known as the tripod position.

- Physical findings that can indicate the efficacy of respirations include the respiratory rate, work of breathing, ability to speak normally, and abnormal respiratory noise.

- Oxygen is the most common medication administered by EMTs, who need to be familiar with its indications, contraindications, and methods of administration.

- Humidified oxygen administration can help prevent injury to air passages during long-term oxygen therapy.

- EMTs should be familiar with the parts and functionality of oxygen delivery systems.

- The EMT must be able to determine the appropriate method of artificial ventilation.

- By assisting ventilations, the EMT can avoid periods of hypoxia associated with respiratory failure and respiratory arrest.

- The EMT should be familiar the method of artificial ventilation for patients with surgical airways.

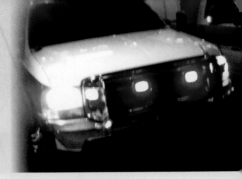

Mrs. Alice sometimes woke up during the night with shortness of breath. If she sits by the open window for a few minutes, her breathing usually gets better and she can go back to bed. Tonight she drifted off to sleep while watching the late shows on TV. It seemed that she had just fallen sleep when she awakes unable to breathe. She goes to the window, but tonight, no matter how far into the fresh air she leans, she cannot get her breath. Mrs. Alice realizes she is not going to get better and pushes the button she wears around her neck to call for help. When the operator comes on the line, Mrs. Alice can barely say: "I can't . . . breathe . . . tonight!" The operator assures Mrs. Alice help is on the way.

Critical Thinking Questions

1. What are the signs of inadequate breathing?

2. How should Mrs. Alice's breathing difficulty be managed?

3. What abnormal breath sounds might be heard in this case?

INTRODUCTION

Even in ancient times, it was known that breathing was associated with life. In 1000 BC, Elijah was reported to have given a breath of air to an apparently dead child and the child arose. The ancient Greeks also understood that breathing was the essence of life. They called it *pneuma*, and they attached great significance to it. It is easy to understand the importance that was placed on this body function. Breathing is a clearly visible sign of life.

Over the centuries, it became known that a patient who had stopped breathing could potentially be revived, or **resuscitated,** with artificial respiration. Early pioneers, such as the Royal Society for the Resuscitation of the Apparently Dead, and, more recently, the American Red Cross and American Heart Association taught these techniques to health care providers as well as the lay public.

Modern techniques of artificial respiration have become a mainstay of EMS. The administration of these lifesaving techniques has been responsible for many favorable outcomes. The public has come to expect that EMTs are experts in the techniques of respiratory support.

BREATHING REVIEWED

Although the act of breathing seems simple, it is actually a fairly complex activity. The lungs, chest muscles, brain, nerves, heart, and blood must all work together to get the right amount of oxygen to the cells of the body.

The oxygen we breathe in comes from the air in our environment. Air consists of 21% oxygen, with the remainder being composed of primarily nitrogen and a little carbon dioxide. As discussed in Unit 6, in certain oxygen-poor environments, such as in confined spaces or at high altitudes, there may not be sufficient oxygen in the air to sustain life indefinitely. In these environments, workers or rescuers would collapse and die without supplemental oxygen.

Although 21% oxygen in the inspired air is sufficient for most people in most circumstances, some illnesses may lead to a need for increased oxygen intake. Certain conditions impair the body's ability to use the inspired oxygen, requiring increased intake to maintain necessary levels of oxygen to the body tissues.

Because oxygen is a necessary fuel for all organ systems, insufficient oxygen supply can lead to system failure. One of the body's responses to hypoxia, the insufficient body stores of oxygen, is to increase the respiratory rate. People with hypoxia will feel as though they need to breathe faster, creating a feeling of shortness of breath.

An increased respiratory rate and feeling of shortness of breath can result in patients exerting more effort to breathe than is normally used. The usual effortless manner of breathing can become labored and require a lot of effort and energy. Severe difficulty with breathing can lead to a failure of the respiratory system as the patient tires of working so hard to breathe. Untreated respiratory failure can lead to death. The EMT must recognize respiratory difficulty before it progresses to respiratory failure and death.

The act of breathing can be divided into two portions, ventilation and respiration. The first part, *ventilation*, refers to the mechanical act of moving air into and out of the lungs. *Respiration* refers to the process of allowing inspired oxygen to get into the bloodstream. Units 5 and 6 discuss the physiology and pathophysiology of ventilation and respiration in greater detail.

The EMT must be able to assess the efficiency of a patient's ventilation and respiration and should be able to support each of these functions if it becomes necessary to do so.

ASSESSMENT OF BREATHING

The initial steps in the assessment of the respiratory system are "look, listen, and feel." Each of these actions will provide the EMT with information to enable appropriate decisions about patient care.

LEVEL OF CONSCIOUSNESS

Immediately upon arrival, the EMT needs to make a rapid determination if the patient is conscious or not. A patient who is awake and talking is obviously conscious. However, even a patient who is seated upright with the eyes open may not be conscious.

To check consciousness of a patient who is not obviously awake, the EMT should first call the patient's name at a normal conversational level. If the patient fails to respond, the EMT should increase the volume of her voice and shout out the patient's name.

If the patient remains unresponsive to loud verbal stimuli, then the EMT should proceed to physical stimuli. Like verbal stimuli, the EMT should escalate her physical stimulus from tapping to a slight pinch of the skin and then proceed to painful stimuli. EMTs commonly use a sternal rub to illicit a response from the patient. The patient's response is noted, using the Alert, Verbal, Pain, Unresponsive (AVPU) scale. Unit 16 covers sternal rub and AVPU scale.

Because oxygen is needed for efficient brain function, patients who have severe respiratory difficulty and are not effectively oxygenating their blood may show evidence of brain dysfunction. A common sign of hypoxia is decreased mental status, which can range from confusion to agitation and combativeness. The patient who shows evidence of respiratory distress and is confused or combative should be considered to be hypoxic. The patient who is not alert or interactive may have severely depressed oxygen levels and must be treated immediately to avoid further decompensation.

QUICK CHECK

If the patient is unconscious, the EMT should perform what is known as a quick check of the respiratory system. This involves the assessment triad of look, listen, and feel. After opening the airway using the techniques outlined in Unit 9, the EMT should look for the chest to rise and fall. This is an indication that air is moving and the patient is actually breathing. Simultaneously, the EMT should position her face close to the patient's mouth and nose to listen and feel for air movement, also indicating the presence of breathing (Figure 10.1). While this respiratory assessment is being done, the EMT can also check for the presence of a carotid pulse at the side of the neck. This quick check takes a mere 15 seconds and is key in the initial assessment of the unconscious patient.

LOOK

Experienced EMTs know that watching the conscious patient for a moment when they initially enter the scene can reveal a great deal about the patient's breathing. The alert, interactive patient who greets the EMT at the door is not quite as distressed as the patient who is slumped in a chair, appears tired, and does not acknowledge the EMT's arrival.

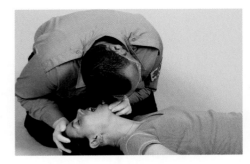

Figure 10.1 The EMT should look, listen, and feel for air movement during the initial assessment of the unconscious patient

Street Smart

The EMT can learn much from observing the patient carefully. If the patient is more comfortable sitting upright in the tripod position at home, the EMT should try to allow a similar position during transport.

BODY POSITION

The position the patient has assumed can be revealing. The patient who is working very hard to breathe will often be in an upright position, leaning slightly forward, supporting himself with his hands against his knees. Although it does not seem comfortable, this position allows the patient to better expand his lungs and draw in more air than if he were leaning back into a chair. This characteristic position is known as the **tripod position** and is usually indicative of significant respiratory distress (Figure 10.2).

SKIN COLOR

A close look at the light-skinned patient may reveal that the skin has a bluish tinge. Blood lacking oxygen gives the skin a dusky, bluish color known as *cyanosis*. The presence of cyanosis tells the EMT that the patient's body is lacking oxygen.

RESPIRATIONS

Remembering that effective ventilation is necessary for adequate respiration, the EMT should observe the patient's efforts at breathing as she approaches. The first obvious quality that would be noted is the rate of breathing, or respiratory rate.

The normal rate of breathing for an adult is between 12 and 20 breaths per minute. Children normally breathe at 15 to 30 times per minute and infants at 20 to 40 times per minute. To count the respiratory rate exactly, the EMT must watch the patient's breathing carefully for 1 minute and count how many breaths are taken. This procedure is detailed in Unit 12. Although an accurate count of respirations is important, initially all the EMT is concerned with is whether the patient's breathing is too fast, too slow, or about normal.

Tachypnea, or rapid breathing, is often associated with shallow breaths, and each breath may not be providing enough air to get deep into the lungs

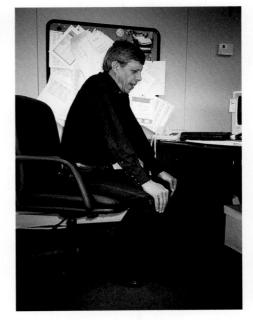

Figure 10.2 Patients with significant respiratory distress may sometimes be found in the tripod position

Cultural Considerations

In darker-complexioned people, cyanosis can be observed at the lips, fingernail beds, or the inside of the eyelids. Often the skin, instead of being bluish, appears paler than usual. Some people may even say that the patient looks gray and ashen.

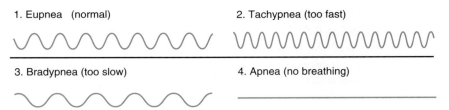

1. Eupnea   (normal)   2. Tachypnea (too fast)

3. Bradypnea (too slow)   4. Apnea (no breathing)

Figure 10.3 Patterns of respiration

where it is needed. The space in the airway above the lungs, including the trachea and larger bronchi, does not have the ability to participate in gas exchange. The air that enters this so-called **dead space** is therefore not used in oxygenation. With very shallow, rapid breathing, much of the inhaled air may stay in the dead space and not be used.

A patient who is breathing too slowly is not moving enough air into and out of the lungs. The air inside the lungs becomes stagnant in between breaths. This condition leads to hypoxia and possibly cyanosis. The patient who is breathing too slowly, regardless of the cause, is experiencing **hypoventilation.** In both cases—breathing too slowly or too rapidly—it may be necessary for the EMT to assist the patient's breathing to allow more effective oxygenation. Patterns of respiration are shown in Figure 10.3.

EFFORT

The next thing the EMT should note is the effort that the patient seems to be expending to breathe. Remembering that normal breathing requires no conscious effort, the EMT should consider any exertion seen with breathing to be abnormal.

Starting at the top of the airway, watch the patient breathe. Is he breathing through the nose or the mouth? In normal breathing, most patients breathe through the nose. When the patient is trying to inhale more air, the nares of the nose can widen to allow increased air entry. This *nasal flaring* permits more air into the nose and is a sign of extra respiratory effort.

A patient's breathing through an open mouth is an indication of **air hunger.** The patient has such a need for air that his body is bypassing the normal safeguards (air filtration and warming) provided by the nose in order to get the volumes of air that it needs. Mouth breathing is usually seen only in patients with respiratory difficulty or in patients with severe nasal congestion.

Pursed lip breathing, as demonstrated in Figure 10.4, is an effort to maintain pressures in the airways during exhalation by keeping the lips half closed and breathing out forcefully against them. This pressure during exhalation is necessary in patients with some chronic lung diseases whose airways can easily collapse. Maintaining a constant airway pressure in this manner keeps airways from collapsing and makes inhalation easier. Although this manner of breathing is characteristic for patients who have chronic lung disease, it can be seen in many patients in respiratory distress.

Normally the primary muscle of respiration is the diaphragm. If the diaphragm alone is unable to provide the ventilation that the body needs, additional muscles are used. Muscles of the neck, chest, and abdomen can act as such **accessory muscles of respiration.**

In the adult, the muscles of the neck and shoulders are useful in lifting the upper ribs and expanding the chest cavity. The muscles of the neck, sometimes called the *strap muscles,* are easily visible when being used to assist respiration. The muscles between the ribs, called the *intercostal muscles,* also

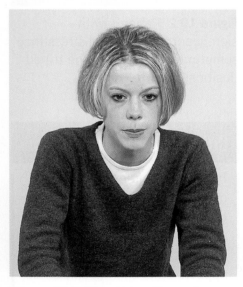

Figure 10.4 Breathing through pursed lips is a sign of respiratory distress

help to expand the chest cavity so that air can be drawn in. The large muscles of the abdomen also contract, decreasing the volume of the abdominal contents and thereby allowing a greater space for the lungs to expand. Use of the abdominal muscles to assist respiration is evident when the abdomen is seen to expand with exhalation instead of inhalation as normally occurs.

When their efforts are combined, the accessory muscles of respiration can greatly assist the patient's breathing, although their use expends a significant amount of energy. The patient using accessory muscles of respiration will quickly tire and progress to respiratory failure.

To properly assess a patient for evidence of accessory muscle use, the EMT may have to remove some of the patient's clothing. Neck muscle use is often evident with clothing on, as seen in Figure 10.5. Intercostal muscle use may be difficult to see, even with clothing removed, owing to increased external musculature and body fat in many adults.

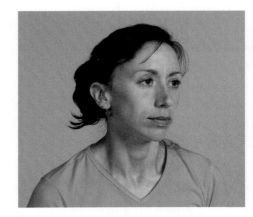

Figure 10.5 The strap muscles in the neck are useful in assisting in respirations in times of distress

Pediatric Considerations

Intercostal muscle use is common in small children with respiratory difficulty. This important physical finding is evidenced by retraction of the skin between the ribs with each breath. Such intercostal retractions obviously are seen only if the shirt is lifted up or removed for the assessment (Figure 10.6).

With increasing distress, a child will often have retraction of the skin above the sternum and even of the sternum itself as every muscle in the child's chest tries to assist with breathing. The finding of sternal retractions is an ominous sign in the child with respiratory distress.

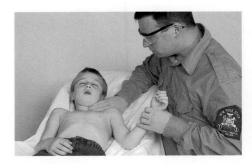

Figure 10.6 Intercostal retractions are a valuable physical finding that are only seen when the patient's shirt is removed

PULSE OXIMETRY

Pulse oximeters are machines that measure the percentage of red blood cells that are saturated with oxygen. The pulse oximeter depends on oxygen-rich blood having a characteristic bright red color and oxygen-poor blood a bluer color. A pulse oximeter is used by many EMTs as an additional tool in the assessment of a patient with respiratory distress (Figure 10.7). The use of the pulse oximeter is detailed in Unit 12.

Well-oxygenated blood has an average oxygen saturation of 96%–100%. Some systems may require that oxygen be administered whenever the oxygen saturation falls below 95%. Local protocols and policies should be followed regarding oxygen administration based on pulse oximetry readings. The patient may be significantly hypoxic when the oxygen saturation falls below 92%. It is important to remember that there are several factors that may impair the accuracy of the pulse oximeter. If the EMT's assessment suggests that the patient is hypoxic, then he should be treated as such, regardless of the reading on the oximeter.

LISTEN

After the EMT has properly identified herself and asks the question, "What is the problem?" it is important to listen carefully not only to what is said but also to how it is said. Patients may complain of "trouble breathing," being "short of breath," or not being able to "catch my breath." Each of these phrases indicates a subjective feeling of respiratory distress. The chief concern should

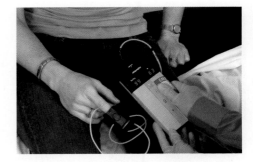

Figure 10.7 A pulse oximeter can be a valuable tool in assessing a patient but must never replace the EMT's own judgment

Although modesty is important to maintain, the EMT must perform an adequate assessment of the patient's work of breathing. Lifting the back of the patient's shirt will often provide a good look at the muscle use while still maintaining modesty of the patient in a public place.

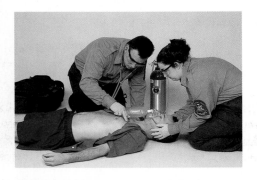

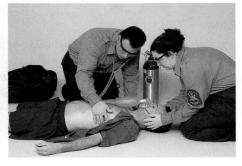

Figure 10.8 Auscultation of lung sounds can reveal important physical findings

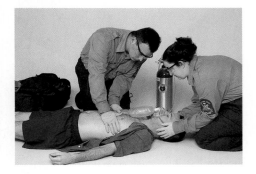

Figure 10.9 Palpation can reveal problems with chest wall expansion and ventilation

be documented, preferably in the patient's own words. A term referring to the feeling or the appearance of respiratory distress is **dyspnea.**

SPEECH

The EMT should note how easily the patient is able to speak. If he is able to speak in full sentences without stopping at every word or two to catch his breath, severe distress is likely not present. However, if the patient answers in short and broken sentences or is able to give only monosyllabic answers, such as "yes," "no," or "OK," severe respiratory distress is present.

This conservation of words is the patient's effort to save breath for living and not speaking. The patient should never be pressed to answer questions more fully in this circumstance. Such pressure leads only to frustration and anger on the part of the patient and generally a worsening of the patient's condition.

OBVIOUS NOISE

As the EMT approaches the patient any noises associated with breathing should be noted. Normal respirations occur without much noticeable noise. Any noise heard should be noted and considered to be a sign of a respiratory problem. As discussed in Unit 9, for example, a snoring sound indicates an upper airway obstruction, often created by the patient's tongue.

BREATH SOUNDS

Finally, the EMT should listen to, or **auscultate**, the patient's lungs. Normal air entry and exit from the chest creates a characteristic sound pattern. This pattern consists of the sound of smooth airflow throughout the chest. Any obstruction to that airflow will create abnormal sounds. The specific sounds associated with different respiratory diseases are discussed in Unit 26.

Auscultation of the lungs should reveal several important pieces of information. Air movement should be evident in both lungs by normal breath sounds heard over both sides of the chest. The absence of breath sounds over an area in which they are expected to be heard indicates lack of air movement in that area. Diminished breath sounds may indicate poor airflow or lung abnormality.

The easiest areas in which to auscultate breath sounds are anteriorly just under each clavicle and laterally, at the nipple line, just below the arm pit. The EMT in Figure 10.8 is demonstrating auscultation of the lungs. When using a stethoscope to auscultate breath sounds, the EMT should place the earpieces forward into the ears, following the natural path of the ear canal. The flat diaphragm at the end of the stethoscope is pressed firmly against the patient's skin, and sounds underneath it will be transmitted through the tubing to the examiner's ears. Use of the stethoscope is addressed in more detail in Unit 12.

FEEL

To conclude the assessment of the respiratory system, the EMT should take a moment to feel, or **palpate,** the chest wall for tenderness, deformity, and equality of movement. This step is useful whenever assessing, in particular, a trauma patient who is short of breath. With the hands under the armpits, the EMT applies a small amount of pressure to the entire rib cage in order to discover any major sources of pain, as is demonstrated in Figure 10.9. The chest assessment of the trauma patient is described in more detail in Unit 36.

OXYGEN THERAPY

Although oxygen is found in the air around us, it is considered a medication and is used in the treatment of many medical conditions. Oxygen is the most common medication administered by the EMT. Therefore, EMTs need to be intimately familiar with its indications, contraindications, and methods of administration.

INDICATIONS

The primary reason, or **indication,** to administer oxygen is to prevent or reverse hypoxia. Physical signs of hypoxia are restlessness, anxiety, confusion, tachypnea or hypoventilation, and tachycardia (rapid heart rate) or bradycardia (slow heart rate). In addition, the presence of cyanosis indicates hypoxia, but the absence of cyanosis does not indicate the opposite.

Although many EMTs do use a pulse oximeter to measure oxygen saturations, this is not a perfect test, and the EMT should always consider all signs and symptoms the patient is exhibiting and rely on their own clinical judgment when it comes to oxygen use. When in doubt, erring on the side of administration is always safe.

In practice, the decision to administer oxygen is based on the patient's chief concern. If the patient complains of feeling short of breath or of having trouble breathing, even if the physical examination does not immediately reveal any reason why the patient should be feeling that way, oxygen should be administered.

Throughout the remainder of this text, the use of oxygen will be discussed as it relates to each medical condition presented. Table 10-1 lists some indications for oxygen administration.

CONTRAINDICATIONS

A **contraindication** is a reason not to use a medication. Although there is no absolute reason not to administer oxygen if there is an indication for it, there are several situations in which it should be used with caution. It is important to remember that oxygen is a drug.

Street Smart

A useful way to quantify a patient's respiratory difficulty is to count the words he is able to speak between breaths. The patient who is initially able to speak five words at a time and progresses to only two words at a time is clearly getting worse, whereas the patient who is able to speak only one word at a time but later is able to speak five words at a time is obviously improving.

Street Smart

The patient with respiratory distress who is quiet is trying to conserve energy. This is a reliable sign of distress. Keep questions brief and to the point, and ask questions that can be answered with a yes or a no.

Table 10-1 Indications for Oxygen Administration

Respiratory distress or failure

Cardiopulmonary arrest

Chest pain

Stroke

Abdominal pain

Hypoperfusion (shock)

Altered mental status

Major Trauma

Severe internal or external bleeding

Exposure to toxins (e.g., carbon dioxide, cyanide)

Near drowning/submersion

Suffocation/foreign body airway obstruction

Drug overdose

Risk for oxygen toxicity, a problem of prolonged oxygen use, is a contraindication to high-concentration oxygen. This most often occurs in premature newborn infants and will rarely affect the EMT.

In the past, EMTs were taught to administer oxygen cautiously to patients with emphysema or chronic obstructive pulmonary disease (COPD). This caution was based on a belief that a small percentage of patients with COPD would actually lose the drive to breathe if given high-flow oxygen. This outcome has been found to occur very rarely, and the EMT should never withhold oxygen from a patient who needs it. The danger of allowing hypoxia to progress is much greater than the small risk of causing respiratory depression in such a patient.

On the other hand, careless administration of oxygen to patients when there is no indication can also have potential complications. It is inconsistent with the standard of care for an EMT to administer 100% oxygen to a patient when the patient's sole concern is ankle pain after twisting his foot. Therefore, the EMT should always know why oxygen is being given. Medical protocols will often guide oxygen administration.

OXYGEN HUMIDIFICATION

Oxygen blowing into the nose or mouth can dry the mucous membranes. For the short period of time involved during most transports, less than 1 hour, this is not a major problem.

However, in the case of a long-distance transport, this drying action can cause significant discomfort and injury to the delicate airway tissues. Instilling moisture, or **humidification,** to the inspired oxygen can help to prevent such injury.

A humidification system can provide sterile, cool moisture to the oxygen being administered. For this mist to actually move through the tubing, the tubing must be of larger diameter than the standard oxygen tubing.

Alternatively, the oxygen reservoir can be removed from the partial nonrebreather mask and nebulizer attached to the bottom of the mask. The oxygen regulator flow should remain the same. Disposable humidifiers are available for one time use (Figure 10.10).

Under no circumstance should an EMT deprive a patient of needed oxygen if humidification is not available, and the EMT should follow local medical protocols. However, the administration of humidification with oxygen is useful and should be considered in patients with croup, asthma, or inhalation burns.

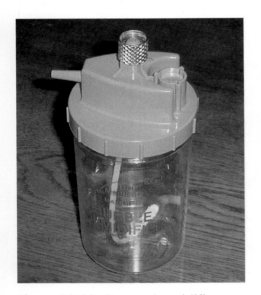

Figure 10.10 Oxygen humidifier

OXYGEN DELIVERY SYSTEMS

EMS providers use two types of oxygen delivery systems, fixed and portable. The fixed systems are found on board the ambulance and operate very much like the wall oxygen in the hospital. The portable systems are easily movable and are designed to be brought to the patient's side.

Although different in size, both systems operate off a tank of compressed gas. Oxygen on the ambulance, **onboard oxygen,** may have 3,000 liters of oxygen, whereas the small handheld portable tank may have only 350 liters. Table 10-2 displays the liter volumes of each size of oxygen tank commonly used by EMTs.

Oxygen tanks hold oxygen under pressure, which is measured in pounds per square inch (psi). By observing the pressure gauge on an oxygen tank, the EMT can determine how much oxygen is in the tank, or "bottle," as it is sometimes called. A tank of any size can generally be filled to about 2,000 pounds per square inch (psi). Many EMTs have the portable tanks refilled before they fall below 200 psi.

Table 10-2 Oxygen Tank Capacity

Use	Size	Capacity (liters)	Factor	6 lpm	10 lpm	10 lpm
Portable	D	300–350	0.16	50 min	35 min	30 min
Portable	E	600	0.28	1¾ hr	1 hr 10 min	1 hr
Onboard	M	3.450	1.37	9½ hr	7 hr	5¾ hr

Note: lpm = liters per minute; hr = hours; min = minutes

At the start of each shift the EMT should make sure the oxygen tanks are full and a backup tank of oxygen is available. This ensures that the EMT will have the oxygen when it is needed. In some cases, such as a long-distance transport or a woodland rescue, it may be necessary to calculate the time the oxygen tank will last. To calculate the time, the EMT would measure the pressure in the tank (seen on the regulator gauge), subtract 200 psi (the safe minimum residual), and multiply that number by the tank factor, seen in Table 10-2. Some departments consider 500 psi as the safe residual. Taking the result, the EMT would then divide that number by the flow rate on the regulator and the subsequent result is the estimated time that the tank will last. Some emergency medical services calculate these values and place them on the inside of the oxygen tank compartment for quick reference.

$$\frac{[\text{Pressure in tank} - 200\ (\text{safe residual})] \times \text{tank factor}}{\text{flow rate}} = \text{tank duration}$$

Example:

$$\frac{(3{,}000\ \text{liters} - 200\ \text{liters}) \times 1.37\ (\text{M})}{15\ \text{lpm}} = 256\ \text{minutes or approximately } 4\tfrac{1}{2}\ \text{hours}$$

ANATOMY OF AN OXYGEN DELIVERY SYSTEM

Each oxygen delivery system has a cylinder that holds oxygen under pressure. If not properly sealed and cared for, this cylinder could leak or rupture. All oxygen tanks therefore undergo regular hydrostatic testing to ensure that they are safe. If the tank is deemed safe, then it is stamped with a time, date, and

Street Smart

One of the worst feelings an EMT can have is to open an oxygen bag and find that the oxygen wrench is missing. If there is no means of opening the tank, the oxygen inside is useless to the EMT. The supply officer should consider purchasing oxygen tanks with a built-in toggle or having a wrench attached to a chain that is secured to the tank.

Street Smart

A new system of oxygen delivery is available using liquid oxygen, or LOX. These systems require that the EMT become familiar with the manufacturer's recommendations before operation. These systems have the advantage of supplying the same amount of oxygen as a standard large tank in about one-third the space.

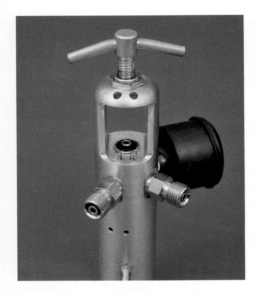

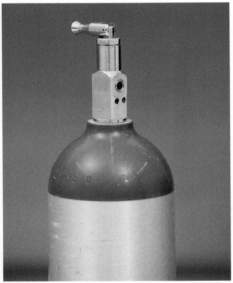

Figure 10.11 The pins of the regulator must exactly match the holes in the tank's stem

symbol indicating the length of time that the tank is considered safe under normal circumstances. Many EMS systems get their oxygen tanks from a distributor and do not have to fill or conduct hydrostatic testing. Other EMS systems use a cascade oxygen system, a method of refilling oxygen tanks by using larger volume oxygen tanks in a series. Other EMS systems are converting to liquid oxygen systems that require very specific refilling procedures; the EMT should refer to the manufacturer instructions. Because EMS often operates under abnormal circumstances, verifying hydrostatic testing has been done is an important safety step.

An oxygen tank is usually turned on or off with either an oxygen wrench or a toggle. If a wrench is used, it is placed on the valve like a key and turned in a counterclockwise direction until all the way on. Many EMTs make a practice of turning an oxygen tank all the way on then turning the valve back one-half turn to ensure that everybody knows that the tank is on.

Oxygen flows out of an oxygen tank through a **regulator,** sometimes called a flowmeter. Safeguards have been put into place to prevent oxygen regulators from accidentally being placed on tanks containing other gases. For one, all oxygen tanks are either painted green or have a green head on the cylinder. In addition, the stems of the tanks are milled with an array of pinholes that will accept only the pins of an oxygen regulator. The National Standard Pin Index System prevents crossover of one type of regulator with another type of tank. Figure 10.11 shows the relationship of an oxygen regulator and the oxygen tank.

Once the regulator has been mated with the proper tank, they are tightened together, usually by way of a T-piece on the yoke of the regulator. Even after the regulator has been tightened to the tank's stem, there is often a leak.

Street Smart

Broken, dried, or even missing washers are the most common reasons oxygen tanks leak. Although these washers are relatively inexpensive, they are one of the most important pieces of the assembly. Without a washer, the oxygen delivery system does not work. Therefore, experienced EMTs always have a couple of extra oxygen washers close at hand.

Safety Tips

The weakest part of every oxygen tank is at the point where the stem is inserted into the top of the tank. If a tank is dropped or falls on its side, the stem can fracture at the neck and the tank could explode.

Therefore, all unsecured oxygen cylinders should be carefully laid down flat. Large oxygen cylinders need to be firmly secured to the wall. It is preferable to secure every oxygen tank to decrease the risk of injury.

All regulators require a washer, an O ring, to prevent these leaks. The washer is often made of plastic, though some are metal with a rubber insert.

The regulator is the active portion of the system. It regulates the amount of oxygen that will flow, usually in liters per minute (lpm). Most modern regulators have a built-in pressure gauge, which tells the EMT the amount of oxygen in the tank and provides a method of controlling the flow rate.

Some regulators control flow using a variable-opening dial; others use a flow gauge that allows the EMT to "dial in" the flow rate. All regulators should be able to reliably produce flow rates from 2 lpm to 15 lpm.

Wall oxygen regulators work on the same principle as those on portable tanks. The Bourdon regulator is a pressure gauge with a needle that indicates the pressure in the tank. It uses the pressure of a column of oxygen against a small ball in a chamber to measure the flow rate while using a constant flow selector valve. Some wall regulators are screwed onto a fitting; others use a quick-release spring mechanism. Oil should never be used at any connection in any part of an oxygen regulator–tank assembly. Figure 10.12 shows a type of wall regulator. Oxygen tank assembly is described in Skill 10-1 at the end of this unit.

OXYGEN DELIVERY DEVICES

A variety of oxygen delivery devices is available on the market. The EMT needs to be primarily familiar with two specific devices, the partial **non-rebreather mask (NRB)** and the **nasal cannula (NC).**

Other types of masks the EMT may encounter in the field include the simple facemask and the Venturi mask. The simple facemask is used when modest amounts of oxygen are desired or the patient needs more oxygen than a nasal cannula can provide. The percentage of oxygen delivered by a simple facemask is a function of the patient's respiratory rate. Alternatively, the Venturi mask is a special mask that is engineered to deliver a specific percentage of oxygen regardless of the patient's respiratory rate. The Venturi mask is used for some patients with lung disease, such as emphysema, who can tolerate neither too much nor too little oxygen. Examples of these devices are shown in Figure 10.13. Table 10-3 lists the oxygen percentages for various flow rates and devices.

THE PARTIAL NON-REBREATHER MASK

The most commonly used oxygen delivery device in the prehospital situation is the partial non-rebreather mask, or NRB. This oxygen delivery device can provide high concentrations of oxygen when the liter flow is greater than 10 lpm. In fact, if the NRB is fit well to the patient's face, oxygen concentration can approach 80% to 95%.

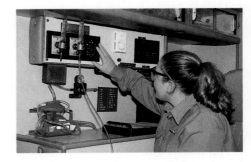

Figure 10.12 Regulators in the ambulance are very similar to the regulators used on the wall in the emergency department

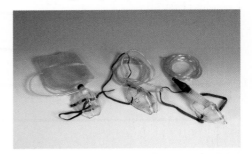

Figure 10.13 Partial non-rebreather mask, simple facemask, and Venturi mask (left to right)

The NRB has a clear plastic mask that is designed to fit snugly over the patient's mouth and nose while a clear plastic bag serves as a reservoir for supplemental oxygen.

In addition, the NRB has a one-way valve that permits oxygen into the mask but does not allow the expired air into the reservoir, thereby preventing the expired air from being breathed again. Oxygen supply tubing provides oxygen directly to the device. Finally, the mask has two exhaust ports, one with a one-way valve, to permit the escape of expired air. This design allows delivery of high-concentration oxygen while preventing rebreathing of exhaled air.

Before applying an NRB to a patient, the EMT must attach the tubing to the oxygen tank, turn on the tank, and allow the oxygen reservoir bag to fill. Filling can be accomplished by placing a clean gloved finger over the delivery

Table 10-3	Oxygen Percentage from Flow Rate at Normal Respiratory Rate (16–20 bpm)			
Liter Flow	Nasal Prongs (Cannula)	Simple Facemask	Venturi Mask	Partial Non-Rebreather Mask
1	24%			
2	28%			
3	32%			
4	36%		28%	
5	40%			
6	44%	40%		60%
10		60%	35%	80%
10				90%
12			60%	>95%

port inside the mask until the bag has filled. The liter flow for an NRB should be between 10 and 15 lpm. Then, the prefilled mask can be placed over the patient's mouth and nose. Secure the nosepiece of the mask to the bridge of the patient's nose snugly and secure the head strap around the patient's head. These two actions provide the closest fit of the mask and prevent accidental dislodgment of the device.

It is important to remember that, although an NRB is capable of delivering high concentrations of oxygen, the gas is not delivered to the patient's lungs unless he is breathing effectively. Without adequate ventilation, the oxygen will not be delivered. The patient who is being given oxygen via an NRB must be continually monitored to ensure that the respiratory status is not changing and another oxygen delivery device is not needed. Application of an NRB is described in Skill 10-2 at the end of this unit.

THE NASAL CANNULA

The nasal cannula (NC) is a flexible plastic device that is composed of two small prongs attached to a length of tubing. The prongs are designed to fit somewhat comfortably into a patient's nose, while the tubing is attached to an oxygen source at relatively low flows. Flow rates for the nasal cannula vary from 1 to 6 lpm. Table 10-4 indicates the oxygen concentration delivered by the NC and NRB at different flow rates.

Because there are not many situations in which the EMT would decide to use low-flow oxygen over high flow, use of an NC by the EMT is generally restricted to patients who are already on low-flow oxygen at home or who absolutely cannot tolerate the NRB. Application of an NC is described in Skill 10-3 at the end of this unit.

TRACHEOSTOMY MASK

A variation of an oxygen facemask is the tracheostomy mask. As the name implies, the "trach mask" fits over tracheostomy opening, called a stoma,

Safety Tips

While a patient is receiving supplemental oxygen, the tubing should never be covered from view. Care should be taken to avoid strapping the tubing under blankets or other items to prevent inadvertent kinking. Such kinking of the tubing may decrease the oxygen flow to the patient.

Table 10-4 Oxygen Concentrations and Flow Rates

Device and Flow Rate (lpm)	Concentration of Oxygen Delivered (in ideal circumstances) (%)
Nasal cannula, 1	24
Nasal cannula, 2	28
Nasal cannula, 3	32
Nasal cannula, 4	36
Nasal cannula, 5	40
Nasal cannula, 6	44
Non-rebreather mask	80–95

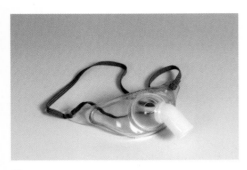

Figure 10.14 The tracheostomy mask is designed to provide high-concentration oxygen to patients with a tracheostomy

and provides oxygen (Figure 10.14). Some trach masks even come with an opening at the front that will permit a flexible French catheter to be used for suctioning.

ARTIFICIAL VENTILATION

If air is not being brought into the lungs through adequate ventilation, then the blood will not become oxygenated. Therefore, the EMT must pay particular attention to the patient's ventilation. It is important to recognize inadequate breathing to choose the appropriate intervention. It is sometimes a difficult decision whether the patient needs to have ventilation assisted or if application of oxygen through one of the previously mentioned methods is all the patient requires to improve oxygenation. If a patient's ventilations are impaired and he requires ventilatory support but is treated only with an oxygen mask, it may mean a difference in that patient's survival. Table 10-5 demonstrates a decision process for assisting ventilations.

If the patient is not breathing at all, then it is quite obvious that air is not getting into the lungs and no oxygenation is occurring. In this situation, the treatment is to immediately provide ventilation for the patient. Providing ventilation to a patient is referred to as **artificial ventilation,** or rescue breathing.

Artificial ventilations literally force air into the patient who is either not breathing adequately or not breathing at all (apneic). Artificial ventilation is referred to as **positive pressure ventilations (PPV)** because air is forced into the patient's lungs. There are numerous methods of providing PPV that require different levels of skill and different equipment. The EMT should be familiar with the different methods that fall within their scope of practice

Table 10-5 Assisted Ventilation Decision Tree		
Assessment	**Respiratory Rate**	**Tidal Volume Conclusion**
Adequate	10–20 bpm	+ Full/equal chest rise = Oxygen by NRB
Inadequate	<8–30>	Shallow/inadequate = Assist Ventilations
Inadequate	10–20 bpm	+ Shallow/inadequate = Assist Ventilations

and apply the appropriate method based on the situation and available resources.

BARRIER DEVICES

To be protected from unnecessary exposure to potentially infectious body fluids, the EMT should use a barrier device when performing artificial ventilation. There are many types of these devices on the market. One such device is shown in Figure 10.15. Each barrier device should have an impervious plastic shield that is accompanied by a ventilation port of some kind.

THE POCKET MASK

When an EMT arrives at the side of a patient who is not breathing and additional help is not immediately available, she should begin artificial ventilation using a **pocket mask**. A pocket mask is a clear plastic dome-shaped tool that is used as a barrier device for artificial ventilation and may also allow supplemental oxygen administration. The side facing the patient usually has a soft air-filled cushion or a shield that is molded to fit the shape of the face, which helps the EMT maintain a tight fit of the mask to the patient's face.

The other side of the mask has a ventilation port. It is designed for the EMT to put her lips around the ventilation port and blow into the mask to deliver ventilation. This port often has a filter device that allows air to go into the patient's mouth and nose but blocks air and other material from coming out of the mask and entering the EMT's mouth.

Many masks also come with an oxygen inlet (Figure 10.16). When oxygen tubing, running from an oxygen source, is attached to the inlet, the percentage of oxygen delivered to the patient increases from the 16% in a typical exhaled breath to about 40% through the use of supplemental oxygen. Whenever possible, a pocket mask should have oxygen attached. The proper use of a pocket mask is described in Skill 10-4 at the end of this unit.

There are several advantages to the mouth-to-mask ventilation method using a pocket mask. The device allows the most effective patient ventilation by the single EMT, using the two-hand technique to achieve a good mask seal around the patient's nose and mouth. As stated previously, the mask eliminates direct contact with the patient's body secretions and the one-way valve at the ventilation port prevents exposure to the patient's exhaled air. Additionally, the mask-to-mouth method can provide more adequate tidal volumes than other one-rescuer methods.

Initial ventilations by the single EMT are generally provided without supplemental oxygen to avoid any delay in beginning ventilation. The 16% oxygen that the EMT can deliver with straight mouth-to-mask ventilation is sufficient for the first minute. When help arrives, supplemental oxygen can be added, or a different device may be used to provide ventilation.

THE BAG-VALVE-MASK

Despite the speed with which it can be set up and its effectiveness in the hands of the single EMT, mouth-to-mask ventilation has several drawbacks. This method of artificial ventilation can become very tiring to the EMT after a relatively short time. Furthermore, the percentage of oxygen provided through a pocket mask, even with supplemental oxygen, is low when compared with the percentage provided by other devices. Therefore, alternative ventilation methods may be more desirable if additional assistance is available.

The **bag-valve-mask (BVM)** is a device used to provide positive pressure ventilations to the nonbreathing patient. The importance of this task is clearly obvious. What may not be as obvious is the practice that is necessary to become

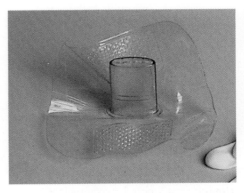

Figure 10.15 Many commercially made face shields can be used as a barrier device during the performance of mouth-to-mouth ventilation

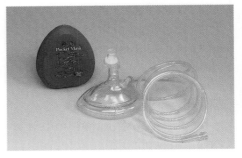

Figure 10.16 Supplemental oxygen has been attached to this pocket mask with oxygen tubing

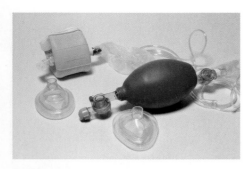

Figure 10.17 The bag-valve-mask device is a useful prehospital tool

proficient with the device and maintain that proficiency through continuous skills practice. The EMT should become well acquainted with all aspects of the BVM and become competent in its use in the classroom before using it in the field. For this reason the anatomy of a BVM is reviewed in depth (Figure 10.17).

ANATOMY OF A BAG-VALVE-MASK

The BVM device originated from the anesthesia bags used in the operating room. The unique feature of the BVM is the self-inflating bag. Originally the bag was made of soft collapsible rubber that filled with a gas, such as oxygen, from a source or tank. This soft texture allowed the operator to have a "feel" of the resistance that was present when ventilating the patient.

Resistance is the firm feel to the bag when it is squeezed to deliver a breath. Resistance to ventilation is the result of chest wall and lung stiffness. A certain amount of stiffness is normal; however, it should not be so great that it is difficult to deliver a breath in normal circumstances. It is important to only use enough volume to cause the chest to rise.

The BVM still has many of the characteristics of the early soft rubber anesthesia bags. Modern bags are self-inflating. This means that once the bag is emptied by delivery of a breath to the patient, it will automatically refill with air when released for the next breath to be delivered.

All bags come with a port for supplemental oxygen. Oxygen tubing is run from either the wall source or a portable oxygen tank to the bag. At the typical rate of oxygen flow, the bag with supplemental oxygen can deliver from 40% to 60% oxygen. This oxygen inlet port is usually found at the back of the bag.

Most BVMs have an attached oxygen reservoir to improve the percentage of oxygen delivered. This reservoir provides a large source of oxygen, which is immediately available, when the bag self-inflates. An oxygen reservoir can allow the EMT to deliver 100% oxygen to the patient. Some reservoirs are corrugated tubes that attach to the rear of the bag. Other reservoirs are collapsible bags that fill with oxygen.

Between the bag and the reservoir, most BVMs have a safety valve. This safety valve permits the bag to reinflate with room air whenever the reservoir is collapsed partially or completely. This feature allows continuous supply of airflow to the bag for delivery to the patient.

The delivery valve is perhaps the most important part of the BVM. Among its several purposes, it first provides a unidirectional flow of gas (oxygen-enriched air) to the patient. The valve is designed to fit all types of ventilating masks and endotracheal tubes that are used to provide direct tracheal ventilation.

When an EMT squeezes the bag, the oxygen-enriched air is forced out the delivery valve and toward the patient. The one-way valve prevents any of the gas from returning into the bag and diluting the mixture.

This one-way valve also blocks any bloody secretions or vomit from entering into the bag. Therefore, the bag and the oxygen reservoir always remain clean on the inside. If vomit should enter the bag-mask assembly, the assembly should be removed from the patient's face, pointed away from others, and quickly and forcibly squeezed to clear it. Under no conditions should the bag-mask assembly be used until the assembly is cleared; the risk of aspiration is too great.

Another unique feature of this valve is that it allows for the air that is exhaled by the patient after each breath to exit the valve through a port. This feature prevents exhaled air from entering the bag and diluting the oxygen-rich air that is stored there for the next ventilation.

The facemask of a BVM is very similar to the pocket mask. In fact, a pocket mask can be used as a facemask during an emergency. The facemask, like the pocket mask, is a clear plastic dome-shaped mask with a soft air-filled cushion.

The clear plastic allows the EMT to monitor the patient's airway for blood or vomit. The mask is applied to the face in the same manner as a pocket mask. The mask seal for a facemask is also important, as was the face seal of a pocket mask. A face mask seal is obtained by first gripping the cushion or seal on the mask and pulling out on both sides and then lying the mask on the face from the bridge of the nose to the cleft of the chin. This maneuver helps to increase surface contact between the mask and face and will help produce a better seal.

Facemasks come in different sizes, including infant, child, and adult sizes. The mask should be fitted to the patient. The correctly fitting facemask should extend from the bridge of the nose to the cleft in the chin while covering both the nose and mouth completely. Various sizes of facemasks should be available to the EMT when preparing to ventilate a patient.

Street Smart

The collapsible reservoir bags have both advantages and disadvantages. On the positive side, these reservoirs visibly expand when filled with oxygen. This expansion is unmistakable evidence that the oxygen source is running. On the negative side, these collapsible reservoirs are usually made of plastic and therefore are easily torn during use, rendering the reservoir useless. Remember to try to keep the reservoir half filled with oxygen at all times.

VENTILATION TECHNIQUE

It is important for the EMT to become proficient in the technique of artificial ventilation. Because the patient's life depends on adequate ventilation and the skill requires practice to perform properly, the EMT should be sure she is adequately practiced in this skill.

For example, some bag-mask assemblies have a adjustable exhalation valve that permits exhaled gases to be directed away from the EMT and crew. Also the mask on most bag-mask assemblies allow the bag to be swiveled to a position that is most convenient and effective for the EMT.

AIR VOLUME

Because all patients are different sizes, not every patient's lungs need the same amount of air delivered when performing artificial ventilation. Care should be taken to deliver a breath to the patient until chest rise is seen. Over-aggressive ventilations can result in distention and even rupture of the lung. Furthermore, excess air with overaggressive ventilation can overflow into the esophagus and stomach. This overflow will result in stomach distention and vomiting. Vomiting in the nonbreathing patient is a serious airway problem and should be avoided at all costs. Alternatively, insufficient delivery of a breath can lead to inadequate ventilation and hypoxia.

The EMT should be familiar with the appropriate rates with which to ventilate adult, pediatric, and infant patients who require manual ventilation. Providing ventilations at a rate lower than what is needed can lead to inadequate oxygen levels and buildup of carbon dioxide in the patient's bloodstream. Conversely, overly rapid ventilations can result in an excessive drop in carbon dioxide levels in the bloodstream. Inappropriately high or low carbon dioxide levels can lead to significant complications of many conditions and should be avoided.

Safety Tips

The EMT should realize that if a BVM is not attached to an oxygen source, the bag will refill with room air. Room air is certainly not as beneficial to the patient as 100% oxygen, which should be delivered via the BVM. The EMT should always ensure that the oxygen source has been turned on and is working properly. Frequently checking the tank capacity is recommended so that when the tank runs low on oxygen, the EMT has a few minutes to find another tank and make the switch.

Street Smart

In the field, the most common reason the EMT will feel resistance to her ventilation of the patient is that the airway has occluded. Be sure the airway is being adequately maintained. Use of an OPA is of critical importance whenever an EMT is assisting with ventilation of an unconscious patient.

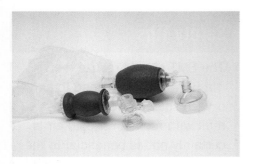

Figure 10.18 There are multiple sizes of bag-valve-mask devices available for the EMT to choose from based on the size of the patient

Pediatric Considerations

Because children have smaller lungs than adults, the EMT must remember that the volume of air that must be delivered for effective ventilation is significantly smaller. Tiny infants may need just a slight puff of air from the BVM. Distending a child's lungs with overaggressive ventilation will result in significant injury and should be avoided. BVM devices come in different sizes (Figure 10.18) to help avoid this type of problem. An infant BVM is much smaller and will deliver a smaller volume of air. It is up to the EMT to choose the properly sized bag for the child and to pay careful attention to each breath delivered to ensure that overventilation does not occur.

It is important to follow the recommended age-appropriate rates and volumes when ventilating patients. More or faster ventilation is not good for patients and may be harmful. Establishing and maintaining an open airway and providing good ventilations with the appropriate rates and tidal volumes using supplemental oxygen are the vital components to artificial ventilations. Age-appropriate rates of ventilation are noted in Table 10-6.

TWO-PERSON VENTILATION

The most effective method of ventilating a nonbreathing patient is to have two EMTs working as a team. The first EMT should be the airway person. The airway person is responsible for maintaining an open airway with either the jaw thrust or the head-tilt, chin-lift method while maintaining a good mask seal. The airway person also watches the airway for blood and vomit or other potentially obstructing materials.

If the airway does become obstructed, the airway person must be prepared to immediately suction. A suction machine should be readily available. Needless to say, the EMT at the airway needs to wear gloves, goggles, and a mask to protect from potentially infectious bodily fluids.

The second EMT becomes the breathing person. The breathing person focuses her attention on properly ventilating the patient by squeezing the bag, with eyes focused on the chest rise while simultaneously looking for abdominal distention.

Obviously, in the cardiac arrest situation, there would be an additional person performing compressions. This circulation person would work with

Table 10-6 Age Appropriate Rates for Manual Ventilation

Age	Normal Rate	Hyperventilation
Adult	10	20
Children	20	30
Infants	25	35

the breathing person to effectively intersperse ventilations with compressions until an advanced airway is in place. Figure 10.19 demonstrates how three EMTs can effectively perform CPR without interfering with one another. Skill 10-5 at the end of this unit describes ventilation with a BVM.

CRICOID PRESSURE

The **Sellick maneuver,** gentle **cricoid pressure,** should be applied to the trachea of the unconscious patient when there are enough EMTs on hand. Cricoid pressure can be used to reduce complications that can occur when positive pressure ventilations are given through a pocket mask, BVM, or other device. Once the airway is protected by an advanced airway, endotracheal tube, or supraglottic airway, the chance of gastric inflation, regurgitation, and aspiration of gastric content is significantly reduced and cricoid pressure is no longer indicated.

The cricoid is a cartilaginous ring that supports and helps hold open the trachea. The cricoid ring is found just below the Adam's apple, or larynx. The EMT using thumb and forefinger, gently but firmly uses backward pressure on the cricoid ring. This action compresses the esophagus, not allowing air to easily enter. Cricoid pressure is being applied to the patient in Figure 10.20.

It is important to remember when an extra pair of hands is not available to perform the Sellick maneuver, slow, sustained ventilations over 1 second, controlling tidal volume, and properly positioning the airway will effectively reduce the incidence of gastric distention.

OXYGEN-POWERED VENTILATION DEVICE

Early EMTs frequently used an oxygen-powered device called the *demand valve.* The demand valve worked simply; the patient could either inspire air or trigger the oxygen valve to come on (hence the name "on demand"), or the EMT could press a trigger and automatically provide oxygen to the patient. The problem with the earlier designed demand valve occurred when the trigger was pressed for too long and the stomach became grossly distended. Whenever the demand valve was used during a cardiac arrest, often the patient's stomach would become distended and the patient would vomit and then aspirate, thereby making a bad situation worse.

With technical improvements to the design of the demand valve, the modern **flow-restricted oxygen-powered ventilation device (FROPVD)** has returned to favored status among many EMTs. Because of the ease of being able to hold a tight mask seal while effectively ventilating the patient, the EMT can single-handedly ventilate the patient with 100% oxygen. Caution is advised, however, because it can still easily overinflate the patient's stomach.

There are big disadvantages to the oxygen-powered ventilation device. Because it delivers oxygen at a high flow rate under high pressure, a special unit must be used on children. Another downside to the FROPVD is that the EMT cannot feel the resistance created by the patient's lungs. Increasing resistance is a clue that something has changed in the patient's lungs. However, this valuable clue is not available when using this device.

SINGLE-PERSON BVM VENTILATION

The EMT who is ventilating a patient alone is doing the work of two EMTs. Frequently, because of poor technique and fatigue, one-person BVM ventilation is far less effective than mouth-to-mask or even FROPVD artificial ventilations.

Because only one hand is available to compress the bag and the other is busy trying to maintain an open airway, insufficient volumes of oxygen are often generated. If the chest does not rise with BVM ventilations, the EMT will need to reevaluate several things. Is the patient's head and chin in the proper position to open the airway? Is the mask sealed onto the face in the proper

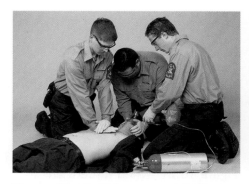

Figure 10.19 This team of EMTs is performing effective CPR

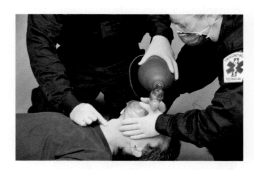

Figure 10.20 Notice that the EMT ventilating the patient is using a free hand to apply some gentle cricoid pressure to the patient

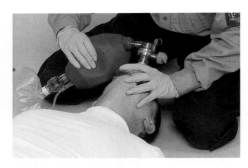

Figure 10.21 When forced, an EMT might have to use a BVM alone. Use the side of the patient's face to compress the bag more completely and help maintain the facemask seal

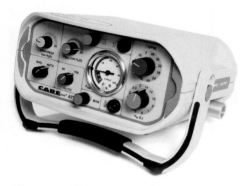

Figure 10.22 Automatic transport ventilator

position? Does the patient have a foreign body airway obstruction? Are all parts of the BVM ventilation system connected and working?

The efficiency of the BVM can be improved by sealing the mask firmly on the face of the patient by pushing down on the mask while pulling up on the mandible to maintain a head-tilt, chin-lift. Using the "E-C" hand-position, thumb and index finger pushing down on the mask while the rest of the fingers of one hand pull up on the mandible, is an effective technique to maintain a mask seal. This technique not only increases the volume delivered but also helps maintain the mask seal (Figure 10.21).

AUTOMATIC TRANSPORT VENTILATORS

The *automatic transport ventilator (ATV)* is another device used for positive pressure ventilation (Figure 10.22). There are several different ATVs currently available. ATVs have been shown to provide and maintain constant rate and tidal volume and as most are oxygen-powered, they provide 100% oxygen during ventilation. Additionally, the ATV is able to deliver lower inspiratory flow rates over longer inspiratory times, making them less likely to cause gastric distention than other ventilation methods, including the BVM, mouth-to-mask, and flow-restricted oxygen-powered ventilation devices.

The use of an ATV enables the EMT to use both hands to hold a good seal on the mask and maintain an open airway position as the device automatically delivers the ventilation. The ATV can be set to provide a specific tidal volume, respiratory rate, and minute volume, with alarms to indicate low pressure if the oxygen tank is low or the device is accidentally disconnected. An additional advantage when using the ATV is that one EMT can hold the mask seal in place with one hand and apply cricoid pressure with the other hand.

Disadvantages associated with the ATV are that they are usually oxygen powered; however, with typical adult ventilation, they only use 5 lpm of oxygen vs. 15 to 25 lpm for a BVM. Once the oxygen supply is gone, the device cannot be used unless it is a device that uses electricity for power. It is always smart to keep a pocket mask or BVM device available as a backup if the ATV can no longer be used. Some ATVs cannot be used in children under 5 years of age. It is important to be familiar with the specific device being used and follow the guidelines set for that specific device. It is important for the EMT to keep in mind that she will not be able to feel lung compliance with an ATV device.

Some ATV devices have a built-in demand valve in case the patient begins to spontaneously breathe on their own. Some of these devices are designed to provide positive end-expiratory pressure (PEEP) or continuous positive airway pressure (CPAP), discussed in Unit 6. ATV use requires special training in the use and specific features of the device.

VENTILATION OF THE BREATHING PATIENT

Many patients with extreme difficulty breathing, inadequate respiratory rate, or inadequate tidal volume must be assisted with a BVM. Although ventilating a breathing patient may feel uncomfortable to the EMT, remember that these patients are breathing ineffectively and delayed assistance may be harmful. Remember, the patient must receive adequate oxygen to have adequate volume for alveolar ventilation, as discussed in previous units.

To review, the patient who may be a candidate for assisted ventilation is usually fatigued to the point of exhaustion or is breathing so rapidly that a sufficient volume of air does not have time to get into the lungs. In both cases, the patient will become cyanotic (blue skin color), tired, and confused. Eventually the patient who is in respiratory failure will cease breathing altogether. By assisting ventilations, the EMT can avoid periods of hypoxia associated with respiratory failure and respiratory arrest.

The patient with severe respiratory difficulty is usually sitting upright and should be allowed to remain so as long as he can support himself. The procedure about to be attempted should be described to the patient in terms that he can understand. For example, "Mr. Jones, I am going to help you breathe using this mask. You will notice that your lungs will feel a little fuller and you should start to feel better."

The EMT should then gently place the BVM over the patient's mouth and let him draw in some oxygen from the bag. Remember that oxygen from a BVM with a reservoir is almost 100%, the percentage that should be administered to any patient in distress. The patient will be able to draw in enough air as long as he is breathing; the BVM acts like a demand valve in these cases.

Carefully watching the patient's respiration, gently collapse the bag as the patient ends an inspiration, thereby filling the lungs. If a little pressure is applied to the bag with the fingertips, the EMT can feel when the patient inspires and should then gently squeeze the bag. These two techniques—gently squeezing the bag while feeling for inspiration and watching the chest rise—should enable the EMT to perfectly time assisted ventilations with the patient's inspiration.

Eventually a regular, often slower, rate will be established. Do not be surprised if the patient stops breathing entirely and allows you to ventilate him. The patient is likely exhausted, and the respite from the work of breathing provides him with a much-needed break. Continue to reassure the patient while constantly monitoring the level of consciousness and the airway.

Many EMTs are somewhat uncomfortable with assisting conscious patients with breathing, but after a few experiences, they realize the incredible difference they have made for these patients.

VENTILATION OF THE SURGICAL AIRWAY

Some patients who have either a long-standing history of lung disease or cancer of the throat undergo a surgical procedure that bypasses the natural airway and creates a new airway. This surgical airway usually consists of an opening to the trachea that is made in the front of the neck. This can allow for easier breathing in the patient who has severe lung disease or diseases of the upper airway.

Although there are several types of surgical airways created for different reasons, the most common surgical airway the EMT will encounter is the **tracheostomy.** A tracheostomy is a hole that is surgically created in the front of the neck that allows air to enter the trachea directly without passing through the mouth and nose. Normally, a rigid plastic tube is left in the hole to protect it from collapse or obstruction. This tube is called a tracheostomy tube. The tracheostomy tube looks just like a very small endotracheal tube. An important feature of interest to EMTs is that the external connection of the tracheostomy tube will fit onto the BVM device connector if ventilation becomes necessary. Figure 10.23 shows how the EMT can easily ventilate these patients.

Ventilation of a patient with a tracheostomy tube is very simple. First, connect the BVM to the 8-mm adapter on the tracheostomy tube and then begin to ventilate, paying special attention to the amount of air being ventilated. Because the mouth, nose, and upper airway are not being filled by this air, less air is needed to ventilate the tracheostomy patient.

Another type of surgical airway involves rerouting the trachea to open at the front of the neck. This type of airway is often used for patients with severe cancers of the upper airway. Initially this opening will be maintained by a tracheostomy tube also, but as time goes on the opening "matures" and will remain open, or patent, without the tracheostomy tube. This opening, called a **stoma,** is now the patient's airway (Figure 10.24).

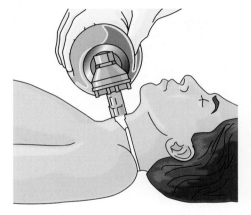

Figure 10.23 The BVM will attach to all standard tracheostomy tubes. Less volume is needed to ventilate the patient, so caution is advised

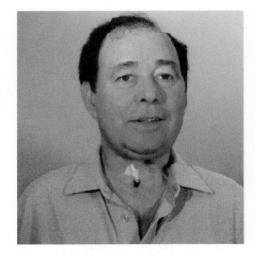

Figure 10.24 The patient with a stoma breathes through a surgically created opening in the anterior neck

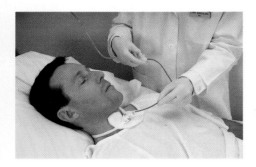

Figure 10.25 Tracheostomy tubes often become clogged with mucus and can be suctioned gently, using a French catheter

Ventilating a stoma at first may seem frightening. The EMT should size the stoma's opening for a properly fitting mask specially designed for tracheostomy ventilation or the EMT can use an infant-sized or small child-sized mask. This mask may be placed over the stoma, and ventilation may proceed as usual.

Because of the lack of adequate humidification normally provided by the nose and mouth, many surgical airway patients develop thick mucus collections around their tracheostomy. These secretions can even obstruct the airway and are called mucous plugs. If such an obstruction prevents the patient from ventilating effectively, the EMT should use a flexible French catheter to suction the tracheostomy. The catheter should be inserted only as far as the EMT can see into the opening. The tracheostomy patient in Figure 10.25 is being suctioned with a flexible catheter. If suctioning is unsuccessful in clearing the airway, then standard obstructed airway procedures should be instituted and the airway reassessed.

Street Smart

Routine airway maneuvers, such as the jaw thrust or the head-tilt, chin-lift, are not necessary when ventilating the tracheostomy tube or stoma. The neck should be maintained in a neutral position, keeping the trachea in a straight line. A folded towel placed under the neck will help to maintain a neutral position while also providing a platform for the EMT to ventilate.

Street Smart

Advances in biomedical technology have reduced the size of bedside ventilators that are seen in a hospital's intensive care unit to ventilators that can be placed on a bedside stand in the home or even on the shelf of an ambulance. Although these machines offer many advantages for long-term ventilation, if the patient goes into respiratory or cardiopulmonary arrest, the ventilation should be removed and the patient manually ventilated with a BVM.

CONCLUSION

Oxygen administration is one of the most commonly used tools of the EMT. Oxygen administration reduces, prevents, or eliminates hypoxia in patients who are having difficulty breathing. Oxygen therapy performed properly can have truly lifesaving results.

Artificial ventilations can be performed on patients whose respirations are too fast or too slow or on patients with normal respiratory rates but inadequate tidal volume. Artificial ventilations are essential in the patient who has stopped breathing altogether. The EMT must also be aware of how to perform oxygen therapy and artificial ventilations on patients with special conditions, such as tracheostomy tubes and stomas.

Careful assessment of the patient and thoughtful decision making regarding oxygen administration and artificial ventilation are tasks with which the EMT should become very comfortable.

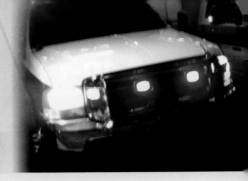

CASE STUDY Continued

Katelyn and her partner arrive on scene to find Mrs. Alice seated in front of the open window in her bedroom in a tripod position, hands supported on her knees, leaning slightly forward toward the window. Katelyn's quick look test tells her Mrs. Alice is using the accessory muscles in her neck and chest to help her breathe. Her nostrils are flaring with each breath, her lips are pursed and slightly blue, and there is a high-pitched noise with each exhalation. Her skin color is pale, warm, and moist, and Katelyn knows from her quick look assessment that Mrs. Alice is in severe respiratory distress and needs immediate intervention.

Katelyn immediately instructs her partner to begin oxygen therapy. Mrs. Alice needs 100% oxygen administered immediately and may need to have her ventilations assisted. A non-rebreather oxygen mask is placed on Mrs. Alice at 15 lpm flow rate as Katelyn continues her assessment. Mrs. Alice is unable to answer questions as she is using all her energy to keep breathing. Katelyn's partner has taken a baseline set of vital signs and reports a pulse of 120 bpm, respirations at 36 and shallow, and a blood pressure of 168/92. Katelyn and her partner immediately get Mrs. Alice ready for transport. Katelyn calls to have an ALS intercept meet them on the way to the hospital.

Once in the ambulance, Katelyn explains to Mrs. Alice that she is breathing too fast and not bringing enough air into her lungs. Katelyn is going to help Mrs. Alice breathe more effectively using a special mask and device that will assist her ventilations. Mrs. Alice weakly nods her head that she understands, and Katelyn begins to assist Mrs. Alice's ventilations using a bag-valve-mask, watching closely to time her ventilations with the patient's inspiration and watching for chest rise.

With Katelyn's assisted ventilations, Mrs. Alice's tidal volume becomes more adequate. Her skin color becomes pink and her breathing becomes easier. Her respiratory rate decreases to 22 with less assistance needed on each breath, and she is no longer using accessory muscles to help her breathe. Katelyn can still hear wheezes with each exhalation and knows the ALS crew that has just arrived will give her medicine to treat the wheezes and Mrs. Alice's breathing will continue to improve. Katelyn gives the ALS crew a full verbal report as they continue on their way to the hospital. As she is relating the improvement in Mrs. Alice's breathing with the assisted ventilations, Mrs. Alice squeezes Katelyn's hand and smiles at her weakly in gratitude for Katelyn's help.

PURPOSE: To permit the EMT to use an oxygen regulator-tank assembly to administer oxygen.

STANDARD PRECAUTIONS:

☑ Oxygen tank
☑ Regulator

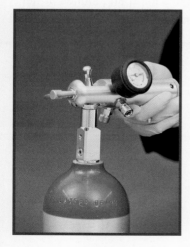

1 The EMT starts by confirming that the tank is an oxygen tank. By convention, all oxygen tanks are standardized with green paint.

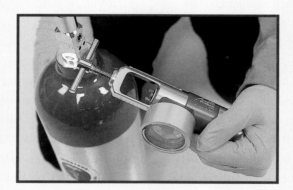

2 The EMT compares the oxygen regulator's pins with the contacts on the oxygen bottle's stem. Again, by convention, oxygen regulators have a specific pin configuration that fits only oxygen bottles.

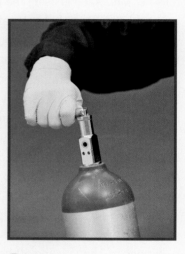

3 Using an oxygen wrench, the EMT mates the key to the latch and quickly opens and closes the oxygen tank. This procedure, called "cracking the tank," blows out any dirt and dust in the outlet.

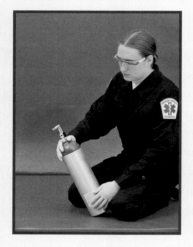

4 The EMT mates the regulator to the oxygen tank, being sure to tightly seal the regulator. A plastic washer is always needed for an airtight fit.

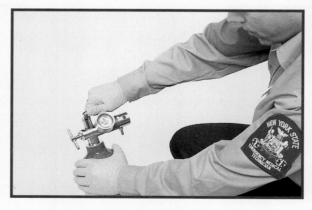

5 The oxygen tank may now be safely opened, and the pressure within the tank noted.

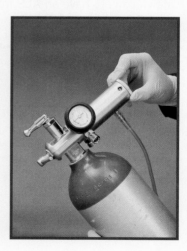

6 To adjust the liter flow rate, the EMT turns the knob in a counterclockwise motion until the correct liter flow appears.

PURPOSE: To permit the EMT to use a non-rebreather oxygen mask to deliver oxygen to a patient.

STANDARD PRECAUTIONS:

☑ Oxygen tank and regulator
☑ Non-rebreather mask
☑ Gloves

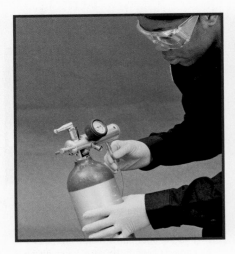

1 First, the EMT must ensure that the oxygen tank and regulator are correctly assembled. The oxygen tank should have sufficient pressure to provide continuous flow.

2 To use the non-rebreather mask, the EMT must attach the oxygen tubing to the regulator and turn on the regulator. As a rule, 10 to 15 liters per minute is sufficient. The regulator should never be turned below 6 liters per minute.

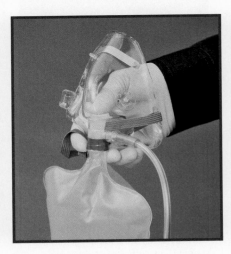

3 The EMT then places her thumb over the valve between the bag and the mask, permitting the bag to fill completely.

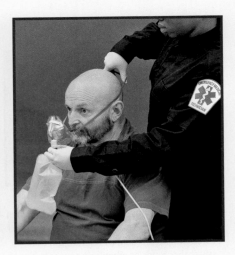

4 Grasping the mask in one hand and the elastic band in the other, the EMT seats the mask firmly on the bridge of the nose and drapes the elastic band around the head. The EMT should form the metal strip around the nose.

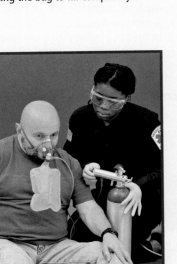

5 The EMT adjusts the liter flow to ensure that the oxygen bag is always filled to about one half.

PURPOSE: To permit the EMT to use a nasal cannula to deliver oxygen to a patient.

STANDARD PRECAUTIONS:

☑ Oxygen tank and regulator
☑ Nasal cannula
☑ Gloves

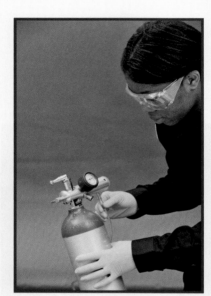

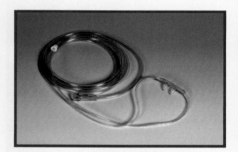

1 The EMT must choose the correct oxygen administration device. A nasal cannula is used when the patient cannot tolerate the non-rebreather mask or when low concentrations of oxygen are required.

2 The EMT must ensure that the oxygen tank and oxygen regulator are correctly assembled. The oxygen tank should show sufficient pressure to provide continuous flow. The oxygen tubing is then attached to the regulator and the regulator is turned on. The regulator should be set from 1 to 6 liters per minute. A nasal cannula should never be used at a higher then 6 lpm flow rate.

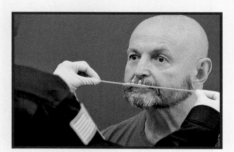

3 The nasal prongs are gently introduced into the nostrils so that they appear to be lying on the floor of the nostril and follow the natural curve of the nose. Some nasal cannula's have a molded lip that should point to the patient's lip.

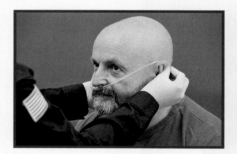

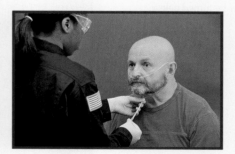

4 The tubing is draped over the ears with the tubing brought back to the front. The nasal cannula should not be draped over the head like a necklace; the danger of injury from strangulation is too great.

5 The tubing should be cinched loosely under the chin with the ring or slider. The EMT then adjusts the liter flow to ensure that the patient is receiving an adequate liter flow.

PURPOSE: To permit the EMT to ventilate the apneic patient while using a barrier device for personal protection.

STANDARD PRECAUTIONS:

- ☑ Pocket mask with oxygen inlet
- ☑ One-way valve
- ☑ Oxygen tubing
- ☑ Oxygen regulator
- ☑ Gloves
- ☑ Goggles

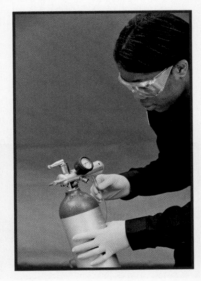

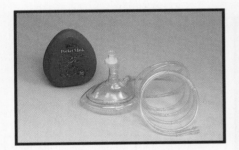

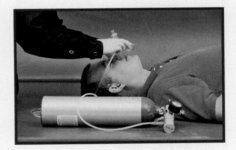

1 The EMT chooses the correct oxygen administration device. A pocket mask with an oxygen outlet is preferred when one EMT must ventilate an apneic patient alone.

2 The EMT must ensure that the oxygen tank and oxygen regulator are correctly assembled. The oxygen tank should have sufficient pressure to provide continuous oxygen flow. The EMT must then attach the oxygen tubing from the pocket mask to the regulator and turn on the regulator. As a rule, 10 to 15 lpm is sufficient.

3 The EMT then places the apex of the mask over the bridge of the nose and lays the mask over the patient's nose and mouth. An oropharyngeal airway (OPA) should already be in place.

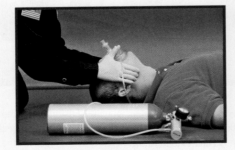

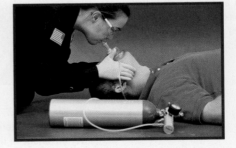

4 The EMT then uses a two-handed grasp around the chimney of the mask while grasping the jaw with the remaining fingers.

5 Tilting the head backward and pulling the jaw upward, the EMT blows into the mask for about 1 1/2 to 2 seconds. The EMT should repeat ventilation every 5 seconds.

PURPOSE: To permit two EMTs to provide positive-pressure ventilation to the apneic patient.

STANDARD PRECAUTIONS:

- ☑ Bag-valve-mask (BVM) assembly
- ☑ Oxygen tubing
- ☑ Oxygen regulator
- ☑ Oxygen tank
- ☑ Gloves
- ☑ Goggles
- ☑ Mask

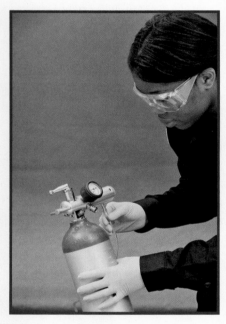

1 The EMT chooses the correct oxygen administration device. A BVM assembly is used when an apneic patient needs to be ventilated by two EMTs. The EMT must ensure that the oxygen tank and oxygen regulator are correctly assembled. The oxygen tank should have sufficient pressure to provide continuous oxygen flow.

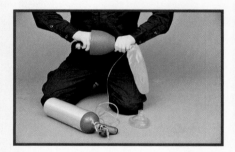

2 The EMT must first attach the oxygen tubing to the regulator and turn on the regulator, filling the reservoir bag. As a rule, 10 to 15 lpm are sufficient.

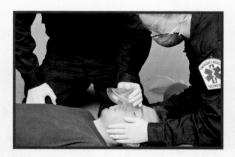

3 Next, the EMT chooses a properly fitting facemask. The facemask should fit securely over the bridge of the nose and extend to the cleft of the chin.

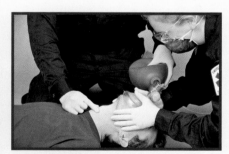

4 Ensuring that the airway is patent and an OPA (oropharyngeal airway) is in place, the EMT places the mask over the apneic patient's face. One EMT holds the mask in place using the two-handed "OK" grasp while another EMT compresses the bag with two hands. The patient should be ventilated every 5 seconds.

Key Concepts Revisited

- The EMT must be able to assess the efficiency of a patient's ventilation and respiration and should be able to support each of these functions if it becomes necessary to do so.
  - Modern techniques of artificial respiration have become a mainstay of EMS.
- The patient who has severe respiratory difficulty and is not effectively oxygenating his blood may show evidence of brain dysfunction such as agitation, confusion, and unconsciousness and requires immediate oxygen therapy.
- The initial steps in the assessment of the respiratory system are the triad assessment of look, listen, and feel.
  - Look for:
    - Body position
      - Tripod position indicative of significant respiratory distress
    - Skin color
    - Respiratory effort, including use of accessory muscles and rate
  - Listen
    - Speech—number of words without being short of breath
    - Abnormal respiratory sounds
      - Wheezes, stridor, snoring, grunting
  - Feel-palpate chest for tenderness, equal rise, and deformity
- Oxygen is the most common medication administered by the EMT. They need to be familiar with its indications, contraindications, and methods of administration.
  - Indications:
    - Physical signs of hypoxia: anxiety, confusion, tachypnea or hypoventilation, tachycardia (rapid heart rate) or bradycardia (slow heart rate), and cyanosis
    - Illness or injury:
      - Respiratory distress or failure, cardiopulmonary arrest, chest pain, stroke, abdominal pain, hypoperfusion (shock), altered mental status, major trauma, severe internal or external bleeding, exposure to toxins (carbon dioxide and cyanide), near drowning/submersion, suffocation, foreign body airway obstruction, drug overdose
  - Contraindications
    - Oxygen toxicity seen in prolonged oxygen use is a contraindication to high-concentration oxygen.

- Humidified oxygen to protect air passages during long-term oxygen therapy.
- There are two types of oxygen delivery systems, fixed and portable, available for EMS use.
  - On board or fixed oxygen tanks; large pressurized tanks that stay on the ambulance
  - Portable, smaller pressurized tanks that can be taken to the patient
- Each oxygen delivery system, fixed or portable, has a cylinder that holds oxygen under pressure, and EMTs should be familiar with the parts and functionality of oxygen delivery systems
- A large number of oxygen delivery devices are available:
  - Partial non-breather mask
  - Nasal cannula
  - Venturi mask
  - Simple face mask
  - Tracheostomy mask
- A patient whose ventilations are impaired or stop requires ventilatory support by artificial ventilation, or air forced into the patient's lungs using a number of methods
  - Barrier devices
    - Pocket mask
  - Bag-valve-mask
- The EMT must be able to determine which method of artificial ventilation should be used for the breathing and nonbreathing patient.
- Adequate artificial ventilation requires skill and practice:
  - Adequate volume and rate of ventilations
  - Two-person bag-valve ventilations
    - Cricoid pressure
  - One-person bag-valve ventilations
  - Flow-restricted oxygen-powered ventilation devices (FROPVD)
  - Automatic transport ventilators (ATV)
- By assisting ventilations, the EMT can avoid periods of hypoxia associated with respiratory failure and respiratory arrest.
- The EMT should be familiar with the method of artificial ventilation for patients with surgical airways:
  - Tracheostomy tubes
  - Stomas

Review Questions

1. What are the signs of hypoxia?
2. What is the triad of assessment of the respiratory system?
3. What are the indications and contraindications of oxygen therapy?
4. Starting at the tank, list all the parts of an oxygen delivery system.
5. What is the minimal acceptable flow rate for a non-rebreather mask? What is the maximal acceptable flow rate for a nasal cannula?
6. When would humidified oxygen therapy be appropriate?
7. What is the preferred method of ventilation when a rescuer is alone?
8. What is the first step in the process of ventilating the breathing patient with a bag-valve-mask?
9. What is the single greatest danger when using a flow-restricted oxygen-powered ventilation device?
10. What two ways can a patient with a tracheostomy be artificially ventilated using a bag-valve ventilation device?

Key Terms

Accessory muscles of respiration
Air hunger
Artificial ventilation
Auscultate
Bag-valve-mask (BVM)
Contraindication
Cricoid pressure
Dead space
Dyspnea
Flow-restricted oxygen-powered ventilation device (FROPVD)
Humidification
Hypoventilation
Indication

Nasal cannula (NC)
Non-rebreather mask (NRB)
Onboard oxygen
Palpate
Pocket mask
Positive pressure ventilations (PPV)
Pursed lip breathing
Regulator
Resuscitated
Sellick maneuver
Stoma
Tachypnea
Tracheostomy
Tripod position

Further Study

Dalton, A. L., Limmer, D., Mistovich, J., & Werman, H. A. *Advanced Medical Life Support* (*3rd ed.*). Upper Saddle River, NJ: Brady/ Pearson Prentice Hall, 2007.

Menegazzi, J. J., & Winslow, H. J. In-Vitro Comparison of Bag-Valve-Mask and the Manually Triggered Oxygen-Powered Breathing Device. *Academic Emergency Medicine*, 1994. *1*(1), 29–33.

Rich, J. M. *SLAM: Street Level Airway Management*. Upper Saddle River, NJ: Pearson Prentice Hall, 2008.

UNIT (11) Circulation and Shock

Cells in the human body require oxygen to function properly. When cells are without oxygen for a period of time, they no longer function properly and eventually die. When many cells in a particular organ die, the organ fails. When several organs in the human body fail, the patient may die.

Oxygen is carried throughout the body in the bloodstream. *Perfusion* is the term describing the distribution of blood, nutrients, and oxygen throughout the body. *Hypoperfusion* refers to inadequate blood flow and oxygenation of body tissues and organs. As stated in Unit 6, poor tissue perfusion with impaired cellular metabolism leads to serious pathophysiological abnormalities.

Extended periods of hypoperfusion will lead to cell death and organ failure. When parts of the body are hypoperfused, it is said to be in **shock.**

National Educational Standards

The Emergency Medical Technician (EMT) will be able to apply a fundamental knowledge of the causes, pathophysiology, and management of shock.

Key Concepts

- Shock occurs when hypoperfusion affects the organs in the body.

- The three basic components of the circulatory system that can affect perfusion are the fluid, the container, and the pump.

- Inadequate pumping of the heart, low fluid volume in the container, and abnormal size of the container can lead to inadequate perfusion and shock.

- Shock progresses through three distinctive phases as the body attempts to maintain homeostasis.

- Signs and symptoms can help the EMT determine which stage of shock the patient is experiencing.

- Signs of compensated shock must be recognized early, and treatment must begin before it progresses into decompensated or irreversible shock.

- Relevant history of the event is vital to assessment for shock and immediate interventions.

- The secondary assessment identifies additional non–life-threatening injuries or conditions.

- The treatment of shock is geared toward restoring oxygenation, ventilation, and circulation.

- Recognition of hypoperfusion (shock) by the EMT is critical in the management of all ill or injured patients.

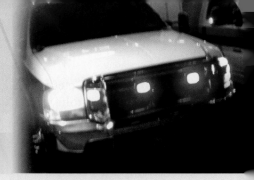

CASE STUDY

Alicia has been an EMT for two weeks. Although she has not had too many calls that seemed serious, she feels she is making a difference. She is discussing her time on the job so far with her partner Jeb when the pagers go off. "Unit 2 from dispatch, you are needed to respond to a motor vehicle crash involving an all terrain vehicle, two injured. Time out 14:05."

Alicia and Jeb immediately head to the ambulance, donning gloves while discussing possible injuries. Alicia knows from her training that significant trauma can be seen when individuals are thrown from an ATV, and she prepares for the patient to have significant injuries, including major bleeding and the potential for shock.

Upon arrival, Alicia is met by a 25-year-old man holding his right arm against his side. He tells Alicia he is okay, but he thinks his friend Joshua is badly hurt. Jeb takes over care of this patient with the help of the Emergency Medical Responders already on scene. Alicia proceeds to the spot where another group of EMRs is working on a second patient. As Alicia approaches, she hears one of the responders say there is deformity and

swelling to the right thigh and deep facial lacerations with major bleeding, and the patient complains of pain in his pelvis when he tries to move.

As Alicia begins her primary assessment, Joshua's friend tells her Joshua was thrown about 10 feet when the ATV hit a fence post, landing on his right side. The ATV then flipped over, landing on his legs and pelvis.

Alicia notices a deep burn to both arms from the exhaust pipe. Joshua is soaking wet from someone hosing off the blood. He is pale, cool, and shaking. Although he is talking and answering questions, his speech sounds a bit slurred to Alicia.

Critical Thinking Questions

1. Is this patient at risk for developing any life-threatening conditions?
2. What signs and symptoms would this patient predictably develop?
3. What treatment and transportation decisions are indicated?

INTRODUCTION

There are many causes of shock, although the end result is similar. It is crucial that the Emergency Medical Technician recognize the early signs of hypoperfusion and be prepared to provide treatment that may help to halt the progression of shock. It is also important to recognize and differentiate between the different etiologies of shock, as there are some specific treatments that may be required for each.

This unit reviews the physiology leading to shock and the body's means of compensating for it. Recognition of compensated shock is stressed as well as the management priorities of the EMT.

PERFUSION

Perfusion is the delivery of oxygenated red blood cells to tissues and organs and the elimination of carbon dioxi de and other waste products of cellular metabolism. All tissues and organs in the human body require constant perfusion to function at their best.

The amount of blood that the heart pumps to the body in 1 minute is called the *cardiac output*. The cardiac output depends on the volume of blood pumped out with each beat, called the **stroke volume,** and the rate at which the heart beats.

The formula for determining cardiac output is CO = SV × HR (CO, cardiac output; SV, stroke volume; HR, heart rate). This formula illustrates how cardiac output can be increased by increasing the heart rate, the stroke volume, or both.

Because the cells, tissues, and organs of the body depend on adequate cardiac output to survive, the body usually regulates stroke volume and heart rate as needed. There are times, however, when such regulation is not possible or not effective in maintaining cardiac output. In these cases, the inadequate cardiac output causes hypoperfusion of body tissues.

HYPOPERFUSION

Hypoperfusion means inadequate circulation of blood, which results in the insufficient supply of oxygen, glucose, and other nutrients to some of the body's cells and an ineffective elimination of carbon dioxide and waste products. The body has some defenses against this condition. Some organs are better equipped to survive temporary decreases in perfusion than others.

The organ in the body most sensitive to decreases in blood and oxygen supply is the brain. After just a few seconds of no blood flow, the brain will cease to function optimally, resulting in loss of consciousness or other signs of neurologic compromise, such as confusion. After 4–6 minutes of hypoperfusion, brain cells are irreversibly damaged.

In contrast, skeletal muscle can survive several hours without adequate perfusion and suffer no permanent consequences. However, when muscles are without adequate oxygen and other nutrients, they do not function optimally. Pain and inability to move the muscle group are common findings in patients with inadequate perfusion to a muscle group.

CAUSES OF HYPOPERFUSION

The three basic components of the circulatory system that affect perfusion are cardiac function, capacity of the vascular system, and circulating blood volume—in other words, the pump, the container, and the fluid. This simple description of cardiovascular anatomy and physiology is useful when identifying the causes of shock.

The EMT must be able to identify the different causes of shock because certain interventions are indicated based on particular conditions. These interventions are discussed in more detail later in this unit. The EMT should attempt to identify the cause, although the initial treatment and transport priorities are similar for all types of shock.

THE FLUID

The fluid of the cardiovascular system is blood. As discussed in Unit 5, blood is made up of several components. The red blood cells carry oxygen; the white blood cells fight infection; the platelets help blood to clot; and the plasma carries all of these cellular components as well as other important clotting factors, immunologic components, and other substances.

When there is not enough fluid (blood) to fill the container (the blood vessels), hypoperfusion will occur. Hypoperfusion may also occur if the blood does not contain enough oxygen-carrying red blood cells. Hypovolemic and hemorrhagic shock are examples of shock resulting from a fluid problem.

Safety Tips

Personal protective equipment, such as gloves, should always be worn when assessing a patient for bleeding. Gowns and eye protection may also be necessary.

HYPOVOLEMIC SHOCK

When body fluids are lost and not adequately replenished, we say that the total body fluid volume is low. A term used to describe this condition of low fluid volume is *hypovolemia.*

A state of hypoperfusion that results from hypovolemia is referred to as **hypovolemic shock.** There are several causes of low fluid volume, such as the loss of body fluid from injury or illness, including plasma loss in burns or excessive diarrhea, vomiting, sweating, or urination causing dehydration.

The most common and more easily recognized cause is the actual loss of blood through external bleeding or hemorrhage, called **hemorrhagic shock.**

The decreased blood volume leads to decreased cardiac filling, reducing both stroke volume and cardiac output. The body will show specific signs and symptoms, depending on the stage of shock. Treatment will be geared toward halting the fluid loss, helping the body to compensate, and replacing lost fluids. The symptoms and treatment of shock will be discussed later in this unit.

THE CONTAINER

Blood vessels have the ability to significantly alter their diameter by contraction or relaxation of smooth muscles within their walls. This ability to alter the flow of blood to a particular area by changing the size of the vessels supplying it is useful in many circumstances.

For example, if an injury is sustained to the radial artery in the wrist, the artery proximal to that can constrict to decrease the blood flow to that injured section of blood vessel, thereby limiting the amount of blood lost. Figure 11.1 illustrates this concept.

The body can cause generalized constriction of blood vessels to decrease the total capacity of the entire vascular system if needed. There are many uses for the body's complex management of vessel size.

This ability to change the size of individual blood vessels and therefore the total capacity of the system can also be harmful in some circumstances, such as when it results in anaphylactic, septic, or neurogenic shock.

ANAPHYLACTIC SHOCK

Anaphylaxis is a condition brought on by exposure to something to which the patient is extremely allergic. Once exposed, the body reacts by releasing several substances into the bloodstream that cause a number of things to happen.

Most commonly, blood vessels close to the skin dilate in small areas, resulting in a pink or red color to areas of skin as the oxygenated (red) blood comes closer to the surface.

In addition, release of certain chemical factors from white blood cells causes leaking of plasma from these blood vessels. This leakage results in swelling, or edema, in the area involved. The area of edema may be localized to patches of skin, as seen in hives (also called *urticaria*), or it may be more extensive. Extensive edema from a severe allergic reaction may cause narrowing of the upper airway causing an obstruction and reduced airflow into the lungs. Bronchioles constrict, and swelling in the lower airways can cause life-threatening breathing difficulty and eventually hypoxia. Figure 11.2 depicts a patient with hives, and Figure 11.3 depicts a patient with severe edema.

Similarly, if dilation of the blood vessels is not strictly localized, as seen in hives, the capacity of the vascular system can be increased. Unfortunately, the volume of blood in the system is not increased proportionately, and as a result, blood pressure decreases, causing hypoperfusion.

A simple way to think about this concept is to imagine a set of pipes that represents the blood vessels. There is only a certain amount of liquid

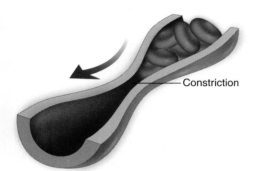

Figure 11.1 Localized arterial constriction can limit blood flow to a particular area if needed

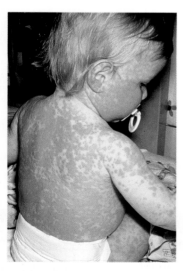

Figure 11.2 This patient is having an allergic reaction as evidenced by generalized hives (Courtesy of Robert A. Silverman, MD, Clinical Associate Professor, Department of Pediatrics, Georgetown University, Georgetown, MD)

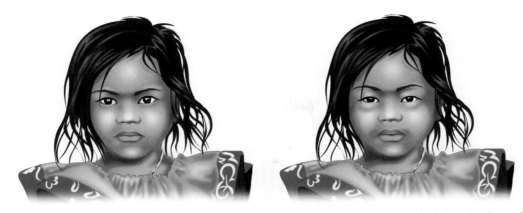

Figure 11.3 An anaphylactic reaction can range from simple hives to severe, life-threatening airway edema and shock

available, therefore if the pipes are replaced with larger pipes without the available liquid increasing, there will be less volume within the pipes. This concept is illustrated in Figure 11.4.

The patient with *anaphylactic shock* will have **urticaria** (hives), airway swelling (evidenced by wheezing or stridor), and hypotension (low blood pressure) as a result of a severe allergic reaction. There is usually a history of a suspicious exposure, such as a bee sting.

The definitive treatment is to stop the reaction and reverse the harmful effects. Epinephrine is a medication that can halt many of the bad effects of a severe allergic reaction, but additional medications are needed to halt the progression of anaphylactic shock. Epinephrine is often prescribed in a pen-style injection to people who have known severe allergic reactions with the potential to result in anaphylactic shock.

SEPTIC SHOCK

Another situation that may lead to generalized blood vessel dilation with a drop in blood pressure and diminished perfusion is a severe infection. Certain types of bacteria can produce toxins that affect the vessels in such a way that they may not appropriately constrict and may become leaky. The resulting hypotension and hypoperfusion is referred to as **septic shock.**

The patient with septic shock may be flushed and warm due to the generally dilated blood vessels and the proximity of the blood to the skin. More often, however, as the condition progresses and volume losses and other chemical factors associated with the infection become more significant, the presentation varies from this description.

The patient with septic shock may have a history that suggests some sort of infection. Definitive treatment lies in the hospital, where a clear diagnosis can be made and antibiotic treatment can be started.

NEUROGENIC SHOCK

One other cause for an inappropriate increase in total vessel capacity is the loss of control of the smooth muscles in the vessel walls. This may occur as a result of a spinal cord injury because the nerves that control the constriction of the vessels come from the spinal cord.

If the nerve connections from the spinal cord to the vessels are interrupted, the vessels no longer have the ability to constrict when appropriate. All of the vessels supplied by the injured nerves will dilate.

This dilation results in a flushed appearance caused by the proximity of the blood to the skin surface as blood is allowed to pool freely in the capillary beds.

Street Smart

Some EMS systems refer to neurogenic shock as "dry shock" because the body is warm and dry below the level of the injury. This characteristic, along with bradycardia, is helpful in distinguishing neurogenic shock from other forms of shock.

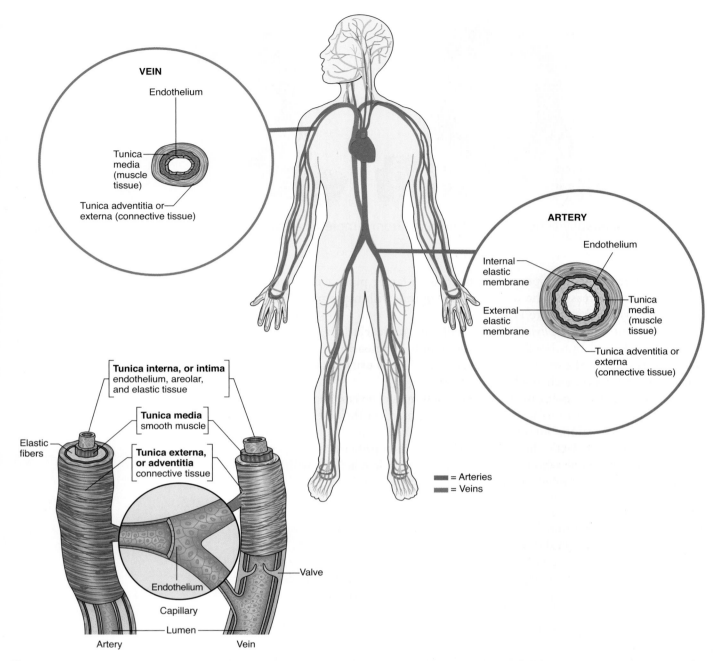

Figure 11.4 Generalized dilation of the blood vessels will cause a decrease in blood pressure as the container becomes too big for the amount of fluid in it

Despite the appearance of adequate perfusion to the skin, other organ systems may not be receiving adequate perfusion owing to low system pressures.

Hypoperfusion resulting from spinal cord injury and disruption of the nerve control to the blood vessels below the level of the injury is called *neurogenic shock.*

Some people refer to neurogenic shock as spinal shock. This is incorrect. Spinal shock is a temporary loss of sensory and motor functions below the level of the injury, which may result in paralysis, bladder and bowel incontinence, and priapism (a painful erection). However, spinal shock does not cause problems with blood pressure or heart rate like the more serious neurogenic shock.

Psychogenic Shock *Psychogenic (vasovagal) shock* is a form of neurogenic shock in which the vagal nerve is stimulated, causing a sudden dilation of the peripheral blood vessels and resulting in a sudden loss of consciousness. Triggers for a vasovagal response are usually intense pain or sudden fright but can include prolonged standing, nausea or vomiting, abdominal straining or "bearing down" (as in defecation), pressing upon certain places on the throat, sinuses, and eyes, and high altitude.

The rapid dilation of blood vessels causes a drop in peripheral vascular resistance; the resulting pooling of blood in the lower extremities causes a decrease in the volume of blood returning to the heart. Cardiac output decreases, blood pressure falls, and bradycardia (slow heart rate) occurs. Perfusion to the brain is decreased, which causes cerebral hypoxia and, ultimately, unconsciousness.

Psychogenic or vasovagal shock usually resolves within a few minutes, when vascular tone returns and the blood vessels constrict to compensate. Treatment is geared toward removing the stimulus that is causing the reaction, such as relieving the pain. Severe forms of vasovagal or neurogenic shock can be treated with intravenous fluids and medications that cause constriction of the blood vessels, resulting in increased cardiac output.

THE PUMP

The final main cause of hypoperfusion is related to inadequate pumping action provided by the heart. If the pump does not have enough power to generate adequate forward flow, the amount of blood pumped (stroke volume) will be smaller, and the smaller volume will result in a lower cardiac output.

CARDIOGENIC SHOCK

If the heart muscle is damaged, as during a heart attack, it does not pump at its full capacity. After a heart attack, if sufficient muscle damage was sustained, the inefficient pumping action of the heart can lead to inadequate perfusion and shock.

Shock that results from inadequate cardiac pumping action is called **cardiogenic shock.** This condition is treated by improving oxygenation and perfusion while addressing the underlying cardiac problem. Patients suffering from cardiogenic shock benefit from timely care and transport to a hospital.

PHYSIOLOGIC RESPONSE TO SHOCK

The human body has an instinct to protect itself from threats to its well-being, working to maintain homeostasis at all times. When faced with hypoperfusion, the body takes compensatory actions to attempt to prevent organ failure and death. These actions can often sustain the body until the source of the shock can be addressed by medical providers.

Shock will progress through three distinctive phases; compensated shock, decompensated (progressive) shock, and irreversible shock.

COMPENSATED SHOCK

When the body recognizes hypoperfusion, it responds in several ways. Compensated shock is the first stage. In compensated shock, perfusion and function are maintained through the use of normal compensatory mechanisms. Some responses are immediately evident to the examining EMT.

Recall that cardiac output is dependent upon both the stroke volume and the heart rate. If perfusion is decreased for any reason, increasing either the volume of blood pumped with each stroke or the heart rate will serve to increase the available blood supply to the body.

Improving the oxygenation of the blood by increased respiratory rate is also a compensatory mechanism. An additional mechanism used in compensation for hypoperfusion is to adjust the blood flow to only the areas that absolutely need it at that time. This adjustment is made by constricting arteriolar circulation at particular places.

The signs of compensatory shock are often subtle and not immediately discernable. As shock progresses through this stage, the signs become more noticeable. The rate and strength of contractions of the heart increase, vaso-constriction occurs, and blood is redirected to the core of the body to maintain perfusion to the vital organs.

The body will preferentially sacrifice perfusion of particular organs to maintain the blood supply to others. This concept is illustrated in Figure 11.5. The patient who exhibits these signs of compensation for hypoperfusion is said to be in **compensated shock.**

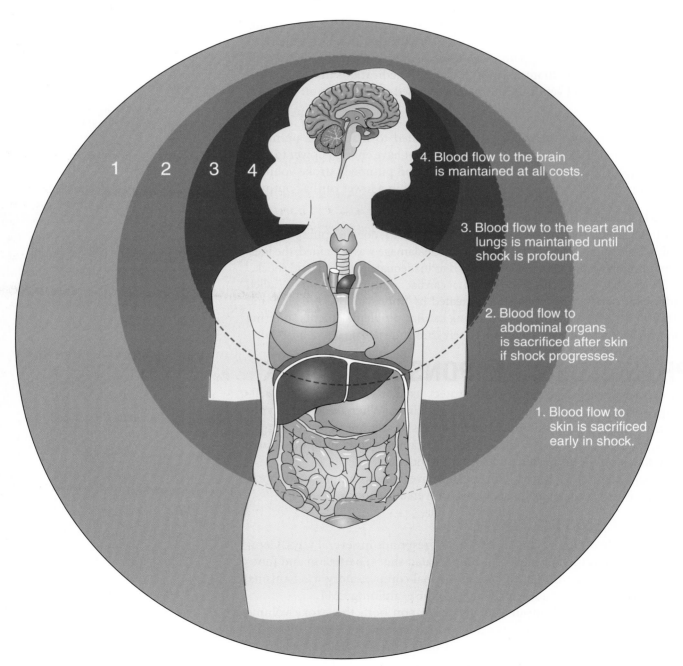

1 2 3 4

4. Blood flow to the brain is maintained at all costs.

3. Blood flow to the heart and lungs is maintained until shock is profound.

2. Blood flow to abdominal organs is sacrificed after skin if shock progresses.

1. Blood flow to skin is sacrificed early in shock.

Figure 11.5 If faced with hypoperfusion, the body will sacrifice the perfusion of particular organs to maintain the blood supply to others

Many older people take multiple medications for different chronic medical problems. Some medications can impede a patient's ability to increase the heart rate, even when an increase is needed, as in shock. Most of these medications are those that are prescribed for control of high blood pressure and other cardiovascular problems.

In addition, the body's ability to compensate for shock may become less effective as it ages. Classic vital signs and physical findings that the EMT can use as warning signs of a serious illness may not be present early on.

Knowing the effects of aging, the EMT must continue to assess for other signs of shock in the elderly patient because the vital signs may not be particularly revealing.

PECKING ORDER OF SHOCK

We can think about the order in which the body will preferentially sacrifice perfusion as a sort of pecking order. The tissues that most easily survive without adequate oxygenation for the longest period of time, and that are the most expendable (the least vital to maintain life), are the first to be cut off.

The skin, soft tissues (e.g., muscles), and bones can function for several hours without oxygen, using anaerobic metabolism. After several hours, damage to tissue becomes evident. When blood supply to the skin is reduced, the light-skinned patient will be pale and cool to the touch, as the warm, red blood is drawn farther from the skin's surface. The peripheral pulses (pedal and radial) will become weaker as further vascular constriction occurs.

As the hypoperfused state progresses, the blood supply to the abdominal organs is then decreased so the remaining blood can be sent to the more vital organs. This change may be evidenced by a feeling of nausea as the stomach loses blood supply. The kidneys also will cease to function optimally, and urine output will greatly diminish (evident if the patient has an indwelling catheter, sometimes seen in nursing home or hospitalized patients). The abdominal organs can tolerate less than 1 hour of decreased blood supply before showing evidence of permanent tissue damage.

If hypoperfusion persists and further shunting of blood supply is needed, some decrease in brain perfusion will occur. This is evidenced by confusion and agitation because the brain does not function well under conditions of poor perfusion. Brain tissue does not tolerate more than 4 minutes of complete lack of blood supply before suffering permanent damage.

In addition to the brain, the organs in the body least tolerant of hypoperfusion are the heart and lungs. The body will attempt in every way to maintain adequate blood and oxygen supply to these organs. If the heart and lungs suffer hypoperfusion, they malfunction in a matter of minutes. When they do, blood pressure falls and decompensation is evident.

SIGNS AND SYMPTOMS OF SHOCK

Knowing how the body compensates for hypoperfusion, the EMT can recognize the extent of a patient's illness by a careful examination. Except in certain cases, such as neurogenic shock, the patient in compensated shock will

Street Smart

Although the vital signs described here are seen in most patients with compensated shock, there are notable exceptions. The patient with neurogenic shock has an interruption in the nerve relays between the spinal cord and the brain. This can result in an inability to generate the classic tachycardia that the EMT may expect to see in shock. With this "relative bradycardia" in the presence of other indicators of shock, the EMT should suspect a spinal cord injury and neurogenic shock.

Street Smart

Pale skin color may be difficult to appreciate in a dark-skinned person. The EMT should look at the patient's nail beds or the mucous membranes of the mouth or eyes. These areas may be pale, indicating possible shock.

be pale, cool, and clammy and will have weakening peripheral pulses. Heart rate will be elevated, as will respiratory rate.

The patient in compensated shock may complain of nausea or may even vomit. An altered mental status in the shock patient is an ominous sign because it indicates poor brain perfusion.

Table 11-1 lists the signs and symptoms of compensated shock with the reason for their presence.

Pediatric Considerations

One physical finding that is particularly useful in children is the perfusion of the skin. This can be measured by using **capillary refill time.** This measurement refers to the time it takes to observe capillary filling (evidenced by return to normal color) at the skin after blanching (loss of color in an area of skin pressed with a finger).

As perfusion decreases to the skin, capillary refill time will become prolonged. Normal capillary refill time is less than 2 seconds. The longer the time necessary for complete refill to occur, the poorer the perfusion to the area.

This sign is a reliable measure of the overall perfusion status in children. For multiple reasons, capillary refill measurement may not always be accurate in adults. The actual technique used to measure capillary refill time is reviewed in Unit 12.

Table 11-1 Signs and Symptoms of Compensated Shock

Sign or Symptom	Reason
Tachycardia	To maintain cardiac output
Tachypnea	To increase oxygenation
Cool, pale skin	Due to shunting of blood to core of body, away from skin*
Nausea	Due to shunting of blood to core of body, away from stomach and other abdominal organs
Thirst	Due to the body's recognition of need for more fluid
Confusion, agitation	Due to poor perfusion of brain

*Patients with spinal shock will have warm and dry skin, an important distinction.

DECOMPENSATED SHOCK

Decompensated shock, also known as progressive shock, occurs when the body's protective, compensatory mechanisms begin to fail and adequate blood pressure to the core organs can no longer be maintained. This low blood pressure (hypotension) indicates the body is no longer able to compensate for the event, and the patient's survival depends on aggressive treatment.

Decompensated shock will lead to multiple organ failure and death of the patient unless the source of the problem is quickly corrected and the hypoperfused state reversed.

The body will continue to try to compensate by further increasing the rate and strength of contractions of the heart (felt as a rapid, bounding pulse) and more profoundly constricting blood vessels to organs, such as the kidneys. As decompensation increases, significant blood pressure drops (<90 mmHg) take place; loss of peripheral pulses occurs; pale, cool, and clammy skin takes on a waxy appearance; and the patient's mental status shows signs of decline such as confusion, slowed speech, listlessness, and eventually unconsciousness.

IRREVERSIBLE SHOCK

Irreversible shock is the third and final stage of shock. When multiple body organs are without oxygen for enough time to cause permanent damage, the patient is unlikely to have a good outcome. Once a patient has been in decompensated shock for a period of time and multiple organs have failed, the patient is said to be in **irreversible shock.** The compensatory mechanisms of the body are exhausted, and the patient begins to fail rapidly. The blood that has been pooled during vasoconstriction has become full of toxic waste products from the cells and capillaries shut off during compensation. This buildup of toxic, stagnant, cold blood is then dumped into the core circulation.

Signs the body has moved into irreversible shock include barely palpable central pulses (carotid and femoral); extremely fast heart rate that begins to slow and eventually stops; rapid, shallow, and inadequate respirations; extremely low blood pressures that eventually no longer register; mottled and cyanotic skin; and unresponsiveness.

Multisystem organ damage may not produce signs and symptoms until several days after the initial injury or illness. Even with treatment, when shock has reached this stage, death will often result.

ASSESSMENT

In assessing a patient, the EMT must be careful to look for the signs of compensated shock. If you don't look for it, you won't find it! It is necessary to begin to treat the patient in shock before she decompensates and becomes hypotensive.

THE SCENE

Before examining any patient, the EMT must ensure his own safety. The safety of the environment must be assessed, and proper personal protective equipment must be used.

As the EMT approaches the patient, he should form a quick general impression of the patient and the scene. What is the scene saying about the potential for shock? What caused the bleeding? Look for blood splatters, pools of blood, or blood-soaked clothing. Is the cause from a traumatic injury such as a penetrating or blunt trauma, or is it from an illness involving extensive fluid loss from diarrhea and vomiting?

On the first look, does the patient appear very sick? Is she pale? Does she appear weak and ill, alert, confused, or unresponsive? The EMT bases his

Pediatric Considerations

Children compensate very well for hypoperfusion. They tend to not show external signs of shock until it is very advanced. Once a child becomes hypotensive, the situation is serious and usually rapidly progresses to an irreversible state. It is imperative that the EMT recognize the signs of compensated shock in the pediatric patient and take appropriate action to prevent decompensation.

immediate priorities in patient care and scene management on this initial impression of the patient.

MENTAL STATUS

The patient's ability to communicate and interact with rescuers is a good indication of brain perfusion. The initial assessment of the patient's level of consciousness is an important piece of information. It is useful to reassess the patient's mental status throughout the incident as a measure of brain functioning.

PRIMARY ASSESSMENT

After the scene and the initial mental status of the patient have been assessed, the next step is the primary assessment of the patient. The primary assessment enables the EMT to identify life-threatening compromise of airway, breathing, and circulation. It is during the primary assessment the first signs of shock may be recognized. Interventions must be taken immediately for any life-threatening injury and illness identified during the primary assessment. The primary assessment is discussed in more detail in Unit 16.

Once the existence or potential for shock has been identified, the next step is to assess the stage or progression of shock. The EMT's first clue to the stage of shock the patient may be in is the level of consciousness the patient exhibits. Is the patient awake and answering question appropriately, or is the patient agitated, confused, and combative? The initial level of consciousness can be determined within a few seconds during first contact with the patient. At the same time the **ABCs** of assessment (airway, breathing, and circulation) can also be assessed. To have adequate oxygenation of the blood, the patient must have an open airway and be ventilating effectively. For this reason airway and breathing management is the primary priority for medical providers at any level.

Once assured that the airway is patent and ventilations are adequate, the EMT should turn his attention to circulation. He should look for signs of hypoperfusion, such as cool and clammy skin, tachycardia, tachypnea, and weak peripheral pulses. Capillary refill can be checked to assess circulation, but it is important to remember that in shock, vasoconstriction to the skin and extremities occurs in the first stage of shock, compensatory. Therefore, capillary refill is not a reliable sign of core organ perfusion in adults. Capillary refill should be considered with other indicators to form an impression of the existence or stage of shock the patient may be experiencing.

As stated previously, it is during the primary assessment that life threats are identified and management begins. The airway must be immediately managed to ensure patency. Oxygenation is maintained through oxygen administration or assisted ventilations in the event of inadequate breathing.

Transport priority decisions should be based on the general impression and primary assessment of the patient's mental status, airway, breathing, and circulation. Patients who are exhibiting signs and symptoms of shock should be transported immediately to the appropriate facility with further assessment and treatment provided in the ambulance. Transport priority decisions should be made immediately following the completion of the primary assessment. The EMT should also consider calling for advanced life support (ALS) if the service is available in the area.

RELEVANT HISTORY

The history of the event and patient is vital to assessing for shock and the prevention of further progression of shock. The history should be relevant to the situation and include information that helps to better identify

Table 11-2 SAMPLE History

S = Signs and symptoms

A = Allergies

M = Medications

P = Past medical history

L = Last oral intake

E = Events leading up to the illness or injury

management priorities. Obtaining a SAMPLE history can provide information to the EMT concerning the patient's current health status and is part of the focused history conducted during the secondary assessment (see Table 11-2).

The mechanism of injury or nature of illness were initially identified during the scene size-up and should be reevaluated at this time. The mechanism of injury is the first relevant indicator of the potential for critical injuries that can cause shock. The more significant the mechanism of injury, the more likely it is that a critical injury exists and the higher the index of suspicion of shock should be.

The relevant history of the present event includes a detailed evaluation of the chief concern, onset or time the event occurred, and a full, clear account of the event, including the signs and symptoms, in chronologic order.

SECONDARY ASSESSMENT

The secondary assessment, usually conducted on the way to the hospital, includes the physical examination, baseline vital signs, and focused history. It is used to identify any additional injuries or conditions that are not life threatening. Further management will be determined based on the information gathered from the physical exam. During the secondary assessment, the head-to-toe physical exam is conducted for the unstable trauma or medical patient, or a more focused physical exam can be conducted on the stable trauma or medical patient. Baseline vital signs should be obtained and a focused history should be taken if the patient is conscious.

PHYSICAL EXAMINATION

The physical exam is conducted to identify injuries or serious signs of illness not immediately seen during the primary assessment. This is especially important when a patient is showing signs of shock without a corresponding injury or illness. The physical exam will be discussed in more detail in Unit 19.

BASELINE VITAL SIGNS

The EMT should obtain an initial heart rate, respiratory rate, blood pressure, and pulse oximetry value as well as note the skin temperature, condition, and color. It is important to be complete in this assessment and to continue to reassess the patient for any change during the course of treatment and transport. These procedures are detailed in Unit 12.

ORTHOSTATIC VITAL SIGNS

If a patient's blood volume is low and she stands up suddenly, blood will pool in the legs and the blood pressure will fall. The result is that the brain is temporarily deprived of oxygen. The patient may complain of feeling dizzy or may even pass out. This change in blood pressure associated with a change in position, or posture, is called **postural hypotension.**

The EMT can test for postural hypotension by checking the patient's vital signs in the supine position, having the patient stand up, and rechecking the vital signs in the standing position. Dizziness, a rise in heart rate of more than 20 beats per minute, and a fall in blood pressure of more than 20 mmHg is referred to as a positive **tilt test.** This may be indicative of volume loss. This process of measuring the vital signs in two different positions is called taking **orthostatic vital signs.** Skill 11-1 at the end of this unit describes this process.

When taking orthostatic vital signs, the EMT should be prepared for the patient to become dizzy or even lose consciousness. If this should happen, lay the patient on the stretcher and assume that the tilt test is positive.

Orthostatic vital signs are useful for determining borderline shock patients. This procedure is not used on any patient with suspected spinal injury or whose initial vital signs indicate shock.

FOCUSED HISTORY

A focused history identifies the patient's current health status. A current health status can be gathered through a SAMPLE history and provides important information about the patient's health that could affect how the patient's body will compensate for shock.

The SAMPLE history can be conducted while en route to the hospital when the patient is conscious. The EMT will need to attempt to get as much of the history from a family member or bystanders prior to leaving the scene when the patient is unresponsive. History taking should not delay assessment, treatment of life threats, or transport of critically ill or injured patients. Table 11-2 briefly defines the acronym SAMPLE, and the SAMPLE history is explained in more detail in Unit 18.

REASSESSMENT

Patient assessment is an ongoing process used to identify changes in the patient's condition. The primary assessment is performed to identify and manage life-threatening injuries or illnesses. Repeating the primary assessment is the main component of the ongoing assessment. The primary assessment in particular and vital signs should be reassessed every 5 minutes in the unstable patient and every 15 minutes in a stable patient. Deterioration of mental status and changes in the airway, breathing, and circulation, especially a drop in blood pressure, are indicators of progression of shock. Improvement in the findings of the initial primary assessment and vitals signs indicate current management of the patient is working.

MANAGEMENT OF HYPOPERFUSION

The treatment of shock is geared toward restoring adequate oxygenation, ventilation, and circulation. Specific interventions such as epinephrine may be useful in selected situations such as anaphylactic shock. However, the majority of patients with signs of hypoperfusion have conditions that are not definitively treated by BLS (basic life support) techniques. The EMT must maximize the perfusion while rapidly transporting the patient to a hospital, where definitive treatment may be available.

Shock resuscitation should be guided by the answers to four specific questions:

- What is causing this patient to show signs of shock?
- What type treatment should be used for the type of shock the patient appears to be experiencing?
- To which facility should the patient be transported to receive definitive care for shock?
- What can be done for the patient during transport to slow or stop the progression of shock?

OXYGEN

After securing the airway and assisting with ventilations as needed, the EMT should apply supplemental oxygen. The patient in shock is suffering from a lack of sufficient oxygen delivery to the tissues. Regardless of the etiology, increasing the oxygen content of the blood is useful to the tissues.

When the amount of oxygen in the blood is increased, there is more of a chance that some of that oxygen will get to the affected tissues and organs. It is always appropriate to administer 100% oxygen to the patient in any stage of shock.

CONTROL BLEEDING

If the patient is suffering from hemorrhagic shock, the EMT should locate the source of the bleeding and, if external, should control it in whatever way possible. Controlling bleeding should slow down the progression of shock. Techniques used in bleeding control are presented in Unit 37.

PATIENT POSITIONING

The best position for the patient in shock is in a supine position. Patients in hemorrhagic shock are already vasoconstricted through normal compensatory mechanisms, meaning the blood from the lower extremities is not available to provide the movement of blood up to the core organs.

Modified Trendelenburg is a position that was once believed to improve circulation and perfusion to the core organs by elevating the patient's legs above the heart. However, recent studies have shown that this position allows the organs in the abdomen to move up against the diaphragm, impeding the movement of the diaphragm and compromising ventilation and oxygenation. Therefore, Trendelenburg is no longer the recommended position for patients showing signs of shock.

MAST/PASG

The **pneumatic anti-shock garment (PASG)**, also called **military anti-shock trousers (MAST)**, is a device that also may serve to slow the progression of shock in certain circumstances. A balloon-like set of pants is applied to the patient's lower body and then inflated. The device is separated into three individual sections (abdomen, right leg, left leg) that may be inflated individually.

INDICATIONS

According to the medical literature, MAST/PASG has been shown to be useful for patients who have severe hypotension (systolic blood pressure less than 50 mmHg) or patients who are hypotensive (systolic blood pressure less than 110 mmHg) due to severe pelvic injuries. In these patients, the pressure exerted by the inflated pants may serve to limit bleeding within the pelvis, thereby improving the blood supply to the upper body and the vital organs.

Street Smart

If MAST/PASG is used in patients with lower extremity fractures, there is an increased rate of complications with the fractures due to the increased pressures. For this reason, MAST/PASG use is discouraged in the treatment of lower extremity fractures alone.

CONTRAINDICATIONS

MAST/PASG can create complications. It creates an increased pressure within the thorax and may potentially worsen thoracic injuries, if present.

Use of MAST/PASG is not advised, or is absolutely contraindicated, when the patient has a penetrating thoracic injury or pulmonary edema. The increased thoracic pressure may worsen these conditions.

RELATIVE CONTRAINDICATIONS

Relative contraindications to the use of MAST/PASG include pregnancy, penetrating object, and evisceration. The abdominal section of MAST/PASG is not inflated on an obviously pregnant woman to avoid fetal injury.

The abdominal section should also not be inflated if there is a penetrating injury to the abdomen in which bowel is showing through. The medical term for this condition is **evisceration.**

The EMT should never remove a penetrating foreign body from a patient's body and so will not be able to apply MAST/PASG over a body part that has a penetrating foreign body in it.

MAST/PASG APPLICATION

When considering application of MAST/PASG, the EMT must perform an initial assessment (including listening to lung sounds) and obtain an initial set of vital signs. If there are indications for use of MAST/PASG and there are no contraindications, the patient must then be fully exposed. A brief exam of the abdomen and lower extremities before covering them with MAST/PASG is useful because once the trousers have been applied, these areas will be covered and inaccessible to the examiner.

Several techniques are commonly used to apply the trousers; any one of them may be used. The goal is to apply the device quickly with minimal movement of the patient.

Figures 11.6 and 11.7 demonstrate two methods of MAST/PASG application for the supine patient. The first is the trouser method—as in putting on a pair of pants, one leg on, then the other. Finally, the entire garment is pulled up to the bottom of the lower ribs.

Alternatively, the garment may be situated on a backboard and the patient placed on top of MAST/PASG during immobilization. This method, the wrapper method, is useful when legs may have fractures or the pelvis is unstable.

Regardless of the method of application, the trousers should be snugly fit to the patient using the Velcro attachments. Once the trousers have been fully applied, the air pump should be attached and the hoses opened for filling.

The EMT then must use the foot pump to inflate MAST/PASG. Inflation takes several minutes and may be done in the ambulance during transport. The MAST/PASG device is completely inflated when a pressure gauge attached to the device reads approximately 106 mmHg or the pop-off valve releases.

Once inflation is complete, the hoses should be turned so that air cannot escape. The patient must then be reassessed for the ABCs and vital signs. As with any procedure, MAST/PASG application should be practiced until the provider is comfortable with the process.

MAST/PASG REMOVAL

MAST/PASG should never be deflated by the EMT or in the field. There is a specific procedure followed in deflation that involves adequate intravenous access and fluids to maintain blood pressure.

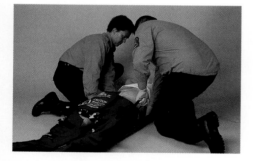

Figure 11.6 The trouser method for MAST/PASG application

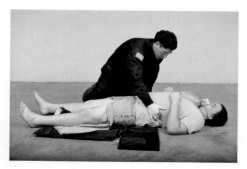

Figure 11.7 The wrapper method for MAST/PASG application

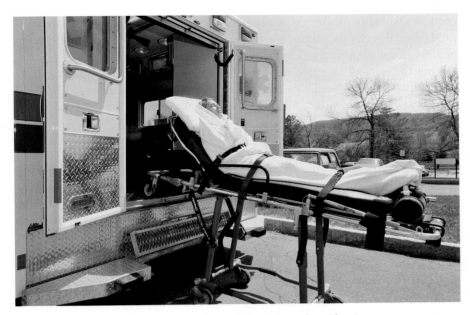

Figure 11.8 It is important to keep the injured patient warm

Physicians in emergency departments should be familiar with the procedure involving slow deflation of the device with frequent blood pressure monitoring, not allowing the blood pressure to fall more than 5 mmHg at a time. This is often a gradual process and should not be attempted outside the hospital unless specifically directed by a physician.

REDUCE HEAT LOSS

The body's heat regulation may be impaired, especially in the patient experiencing a decreased blood flow. Heat loss may be minimized or avoided by preventing prolonged exposure of the patient. Once an assessment has been accomplished, the patient should be covered with blankets (Figure 11.8). Care should be taken to remove the patient from cold, wet surfaces and to remove wet clothing from the patient.

TRANSPORT

After assessing a hypoperfused patient and beginning appropriate BLS treatment, the EMT must decide what mode of transportation is most appropriate. The decision-making process that goes into determining whether a patient should be transported by ground ambulance or by helicopter is discussed in a later unit.

During transport, it is imperative that the EMT reassess the patient at frequent intervals. The patient with signs of hypoperfusion should be constantly observed, with vital signs monitored at least every 5 minutes. Changes in mental status or vital signs should be recorded carefully and reported to the destination facility.

ALS INTERCEPT

Some patients will need therapies that are beyond the scope of practice for the EMT. Some of these therapies, such as medication administration and IV therapy, can be initiated by properly trained advanced life support (ALS) personnel.

The hypoperfused patient requires ALS modalities. If the EMT is practicing in a system that has access to ALS personnel, he must decide whether to request assistance at the scene, meet with an ALS team en route to the hospital or go directly to a hospital for such treatment. Transport directly to the nearest hospital should be considered if an ALS intervention would prolong getting the patient to more definitive care. The need for ALS interventions is addressed throughout this text as each condition is discussed. The EMT should always be familiar with and follow local protocols.

DESTINATION DETERMINATION

It is important for the EMT to be aware of the general capabilities of the surrounding medical facilities in order to decide to which hospital the patient should be transported. In general, the patient in shock should go to the closest hospital. However, trauma patients often are diverted to a specialty center. Examples of specialty centers include trauma centers, burn centers, pediatric hospitals, stroke centers, cardiac care centers, and even hyperbaric chambers. Local protocols will govern these issues.

CONCLUSION

Shock is a state of hypoperfusion in which the body tissues are not receiving an adequate supply of oxygenated blood. The patient in shock will show classic signs and symptoms that, if unrecognized and untreated, will lead to death.

The EMT should be knowledgeable about the different etiologies of shock and must be able to recognize and identify signs of compensated and decompensated shock.

Regardless of the cause of the hypoperfused state, the initial treatment consists of maintenance of an adequate airway and ventilations, with oxygen administration and circulatory support if necessary. Recognition of hypoperfusion by the EMT is critical in the management of the ill or injured patient.

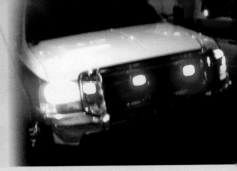

As Alicia approaches she hears the patient repeatedly saying "it hurts" in a slurred voice. Alicia asks his name and age, and he tells her his name is Scott and he is 22 years old. Scott then immediately goes back to repeatedly saying "it hurts." Alicia begins her primary assessment and determines his airway is patent with rapid, shallow breathing at approximately 28 breaths a minute. Alicia can feel a rapid radial pulse at a rate of 120 beats per minute, and his skin is pale, cool, and wet from being washed by a hose. Scott is trembling and says he is cold.

Alicia determines he is in compensated shock at this time and needs to be transported immediately with further treatment taking place en route. The emergency medical responders have already initiated oxygen therapy by mask at 15 lpm.

Because there is evidence of major trauma, Alicia advises the emergency medical responders on scene that there is a need for full spinal precautions as they assist her in splinting Scott's right thigh and packaging him for immediate transport to the trauma center 20 miles away. Alicia further asks for an advance life support intercept. Alicia knows Scott needs IV fluids to replace the blood lost from internal bleeding taking place in his right thigh.

Once Scott is packaged and placed in the warmed ambulance, Alicia notices Jeb is there to assist her because a second ambulance has arrived and taken over care of his patient. Alicia instructs Jeb to carefully remove Scott's wet clothing, ensuring his privacy and covering him quickly with dry blankets as she performs a rapid trauma assessment.

Alicia notices there is not active bleeding from Scott's nose and there are no lacerations to his face. As Alicia palpates Scott's pelvis, she does not notice any instability and Scott denies pain in his pelvis but continues to complain of pain in his upper right thigh. Alicia rechecks the pulses in his extremities and is able to palpate weak radial and distal pulses, including the right foot. Alicia covers the burns on Scott's arms with a dry dressing while Jeb obtains a set of vital signs.

Jeb informs Alicia that Scott's blood pressure is 100/60 mmHg, pulse is 130 bpm, and respirations have decreased to 28 per minute with deeper breaths. Scott's skin is pale, cool, and clammy. Alicia knows that Scott's vital signs indicate he is still compensating for the internal bleeding, but that further intervention is needed to keep him from moving into decompensated shock. She asks the driver to radio the ALS unit to determine how close they are to intercept and is told they should be there within 5 minutes. Alicia asks the driver to start driving toward the ALS unit and the trauma center.

Alicia performs an ongoing assessment while en route, which reveals improvement in respiratory rate but no other changes in Scott's condition. As the ALS crew arrives and assists with care of the patient, they tell Alicia and Jeb they did a good job of recognizing and treating the initial signs of shock and their treatments aided in keeping the shock from progressing until more advance care could be rendered.

Later that evening, Alicia calls the hospital and is told Scott had a fracture to his right femur, second-degree burns to the front of both arms, and a fractured nose. He is resting comfortably at this time, after having his fractured leg repaired, and he asked the nurses to thank Alicia and Jeb when they talk to the EMTs.

As Alicia and Jeb discuss the call, they agree that their rapid recognition and field treatment of Scott's early signs of shock prevented the shock from progressing. Alicia and Jeb's actions gave Scott the opportunity for a quick, full recovery from his injuries.

PURPOSE: To obtain a baseline set of vital signs lying and standing for assessment and comparison.

STANDARD PRECAUTIONS:

☑ Stethoscope
☑ Blood pressure cuff
☑ Watch with second hand
☑ Gloves

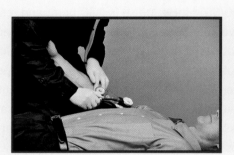

1 Obtain a full set of vital signs from the lying patient.

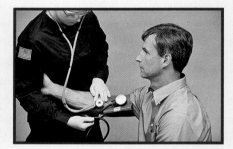

2 Assist the patient to a sitting position with an assistant behind the patient for support when possible and reassess vital sign.

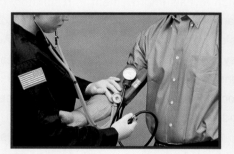

3 Assist the patient to a standing position with an assistant behind the patient for support if available. Reassess vital signs.

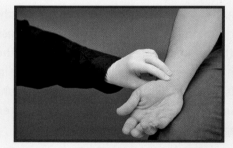

4 Compare vital signs lying, sitting, and standing.

Key Concepts Revisited

- Hypoperfusion or shock is the state the body is in when hypoperfusion affects certain systems and organs.

- The inadequate cardiac output causes hypoperfusion of body tissues.

- The three basic components of the circulatory system that can affect perfusion are:
  - The fluid (blood)
  - The container (blood vessels)
  - The pump (heart)

- Low fluid volume in the container can lead to hypoperfusion and shock:
  - Hypovolemic shock
  - Hemorrhagic shock

- The ability to change the size of individual blood vessels and size of the container is affected by certain types of shock:
  - Anaphylactic shock
  - Septic shock
  - Neurogenic shock
    - Psychogenic shock

- Inadequate pumping of the heart can lead to inadequate perfusion and shock, referred to as *Cardiogenic Shock.*

- Shock will progress through three distinctive phases as the body attempts maintain homeostasis:
  - Compensated shock
  - Decompensated or progressive shock
  - Irreversible shock

- The body will sacrifice perfusion to the tissues least vital in maintaining life first, a sort of pecking order to preserve life.
  - Skin, soft tissues (muscles), and bones can function for several hours without oxygen, using anaerobic metabolism.

- Signs and symptoms of shock can help the EMT determine which stage of shock the patient is experiencing.

- Signs of compensated shock must be recognized early, beginning at the scene with an assessment of mental status and the primary assessment, to begin treatment before the shock progresses into decompensated or irreversible shock.

- Relevant history of the event is vital to assessment for shock and immediate interventions:
  - Mechanism of injury or nature of illness
  - Chief concern
  - Onset or time of the event

- The secondary assessment is used to identify any additional non–life-threatening injuries or conditions and includes:
  - Physical exam
  - Baseline vital signs
  - Focused history

- Reassessment of the primary assessment is important to identify any changes in the patient's condition and the effectiveness of ongoing treatments.

- The treatment of shock is geared toward restoring oxygenation, ventilation, and circulation.
  - Oxygenation
  - Control bleeding
  - Patient positioning
  - MAST/PASG
  - Reduction of heat loss

- The mode of transport as well as the destination should be determined after the primary assessment and reevaluated during transport of the patient.

- The hypoperfused patient often requires treatments beyond the scope of the EMT, and an ALS intercept is warranted.

- The destination of transport should be based on the local capabilities of the surrounding medical facilities or the need for specialized trauma center.

- Recognition of hypoperfusion (shock) by the EMT is critical in the management of all ill or injured patients.

Review Questions

1. What is shock?
2. What three components of the circulatory system affect perfusion?
3. List six types of shock.
4. What are the three phases of shock?
5. List the signs and symptoms of compensated shock.
6. What is the "pecking order" of shock?
7. What is irreversible shock?
8. What are the steps of assessment of the patient in shock?
9. List appropriate steps in management of the patient with signs and symptoms of shock.
10. Describe the indications for MAST/PASG use.
11. List the absolute and relative contraindications for MAST/PASG use.
12. What transport decisions need to be made for a patient in shock?

Key Terms

ABCs
Anaphylaxis
Capillary refill time
Cardiogenic shock
Compensated shock
Decompensated shock
Evisceration
Hemorrhagic shock
Hypovolemic shock
Irreversible shock

Military anti-shock trousers (MAST)
Orthostatic vital signs
Pneumatic anti-shock garment (PASG)
Postural hypotension
Septic shock
Shock
Stroke volume
Tilt test
Urticaria

Further Study

Cayten, C. G., Berendt, B. M., Byrne, D. W., et al. A Study of Pneumatic Anti-Shock Garments in Severely Hypotensive Trauma Patients. *Journal of Trauma*, 1993. *34*, 728–735.

Dalton, A. L., Limmer, D., Mistovich, J., & Werman, H. A. *Advanced Medical Life Support* (3rd ed.). Upper Saddle River, NJ: Brady/Pearson Prentice Hall, 2007.

Domeier, R. M., O'Connor, R. E., Delbridge, T. R., & Hunt, R. C. Use of the Pneumatic Anti-Shock Garment (PASG). National Association of EMS Physicians. *Prehospital Emergency Care*, 1997. *1*(1), 32–35.

Emergency Cardiac Care Committee and Subcommittee, American Heart Association. Guidelines for Cardiopulmonary Resuscitation and Emergency Cardiac Care, 2005.

Mattox, K. L., Bickell, W., Pepe, P. E., Burch, J., & Feliciano, D. Prospective MAST Study in 911 Patients. *Journal of Trauma*, 1989. 29(8), 1104–1111.

O'Connor, R. E., & Domeier, R. M. An Evaluation of the Pneumatic Anti-Shock Garment (PASG) in Various Clinical Settings. *Prehospital Emergency Care*, 1997. *1*(1), 36–44.

UNIT (12) Baseline Vital Signs

The EMT will learn many skills necessary for the assessment and management of patients. One skill that will be used in every patient encounter is obtaining the patient's vital signs. Baseline vitals signs are the initial measurements of signs that give clues to what is happening inside the body. Correctly measuring and interpreting the patient's vital signs are essential to correctly assessing for and managing illness or injury, monitoring the effectiveness of treatments, and providing vital information to the next provider in the continuum of patient care.

National Education Standard

The Emergency Medical Technician (EMT) will have a fundamental depth and foundational breadth of understanding and skill for obtaining baseline vital signs, including obtaining and using information from patient monitoring devices.

Key Concepts

- The most frequently used skill of an EMT is obtaining and monitoring the patient's vital signs.

- Baseline vital signs obtained at the onset of care enable the EMT to quickly recognize and react to changes in the patient's condition.

- Baseline vital signs are the measurement of how core systems of the body, respiratory and circulatory, are functioning.

- Knowledge of the normal rate and quality of respirations is essential to recognize and manage conditions affecting the respiratory system.

- Knowledge of the normal rate and quality of the pulse is essential to recognize and manage conditions affecting the circulatory system.

- Blood pressure can be assessed through auscultation or palpation and is a measure of how effectively the heart is functioning.

- Changes in the rate and/or quality of the pulse can be an important indicator of serious conditions or injuries.

- The skin signs can be a rough indicator of a patient's circulatory status.

- Capillary refill is an additional tool that can be used along with the other baseline vital signs in assessing the adequacy of perfusion.

- An essential part of every neurologic exam is checking the pupil size and response to light.

- The pulse oximeter can be an additional tool used in determining the effectiveness of breathing and perfusion.

- Accurately reassessing, reporting, and recording the baseline vital signs is essential to appropriate patient management and the continuum of patient care.

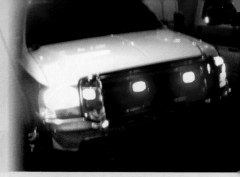

CASE STUDY

Kasey has been an EMT for several years and today is working with Sally, a newly graduated EMT on her first shift. Shortly after completing the equipment checks for the day, they are dispatched for a 46-year-old male having trouble breathing.

Upon entering the patient's house and noting no safety hazards, Kasey notices the patient is sitting on his couch, leaning forward with his hands on his knees. He looks pale with blueness around his mouth, and his skin appears wet. Kasey introduces herself and Sally, asking his name as she reaches for his wrist to check his pulse. Kasey notices his pulse is difficult to feel, his skin feels very warm, and his breathing seems to be too fast.

The patient tells her his name is Mr. Young, and he has been having an asthma attack for more than 2 hours, even after using his inhaler. Kasey notices that Mr. Young can only say two words at a time before needing to stop and take a breath.

Critical Thinking Questions

1. What is abnormal about this patient's skin condition?
2. What is normal or abnormal about this patient's pulse?
3. What further assessment of this patient's breathing and circulatory status needs to be conducted?

INTRODUCTION

During the course of training, the EMT will learn many skills. Those used most frequently will be obtaining and monitoring the patient's vital signs.

The vital signs such as respiratory rate, heart rate, blood pressure, skin parameters, and pulse oximetry provide a great deal of information about the patient's physical condition and present state of health. Examination of the pupils can also provide valuable information. Monitoring these vital signs over time allows the EMT to identify acute changes in the patient's status.

BASELINE VITAL SIGNS

After the primary assessment and management of the airway, breathing, and circulation, the EMT must take the time to quantify actual vital signs. The first measurement of vital signs is sometimes referred to as **baseline vital signs.**

These numbers serve as the initial measurement of a patient's physical condition against which subsequent readings, or values, are compared. It is important to obtain an accurate baseline set of vital signs at the onset of care so that any changes can be recognized early and acted upon quickly.

Time should be spent during EMT training practicing measuring vital signs. This unit discusses each of the vital signs in detail, reviews normal and abnormal values, and describes how to measure each of them appropriately.

RESPIRATION

Many parts of an EMT's assessment of a patient are accomplished through observation. As the EMT approaches the patient and begins the initial assessment, several aspects of breathing should be noted. The patient's breathing can first be assessed by observing the rise and fall of the patient's chest.

RESPIRATORY RATE

First, how quickly does the patient appear to be breathing? Does the patient's breathing seem very fast or particularly slow? To determine the appropriateness of the respiratory rate, the EMT must be familiar with normal respiratory rates.

To determine the exact respiratory rate, the EMT must observe the patient's breathing and count the number of breaths taken in 1 minute. Each breath consists of an **inspiration** (breathing in) and an **exhalation** (breathing out). This breathing rate is then reported as the number of breaths per minute.

Often, it is easier and more convenient to shorten the time necessary to obtain such a respiratory rate. It is acceptable to count the number of breaths taken for 30 seconds then multiply by 2 to equal the number of breaths taken in 1 minute. The EMT should avoid shortening the measurement time any more than this to avoid inaccuracy.

Adult respiratory rates under 10 or greater than 30 are of concern and may require immediate intervention. It is important to obtain an accurate respiratory rate; therefore, if the patient's breathing is irregular, the EMT should count the respirations for a full minute to avoid obtaining an inaccurate respiratory rate. Table 12-1 shows normal respiratory rates for people of different ages.

RESPIRATORY QUALITY

In addition to counting the respiratory rate, the EMT should note the quality of the respiration. She should observe for depth, regularity, and any unusual noise or effort.

Normal breathing quality is of a moderate depth (chest rise is visible), regular (approximately one breath every 3–5 seconds for an adult), and quiet. Any unusual effort or noise, indicating that the patient may be struggling for breath, should be noted.

LABORED BREATHING

The EMT can describe a patient's breathing as being labored if there is any apparent unusual effort or noise during the respiratory cycle. Patients who are having difficulty breathing for any reason may appear uncomfortable and may show classic signs of increased respiratory effort or difficulty.

Pediatric Considerations

Nasal flaring is commonly seen in infants and small children who are having respiratory difficulty. An EMT seeing nasal flaring in a child should be concerned. Respiratory failure is often the cause of death for infants and children, and nasal flaring is one of the first signs of respiratory difficulty. Figure 12.1 illustrates such a finding.

Table 12-1 Normal Respiratory Rates, by Age	
Age	**Normal Respiratory Rate (breaths/minute)**
Adult	12–20
Adolescent (11–14 yr)	12–20
School-aged child (6–12 yr)	15–30
Preschool-aged child (1–5 yr)	20–30
Infant (1 mo–1 yr)	20–40
Newborn (0–1 mo)	30–50

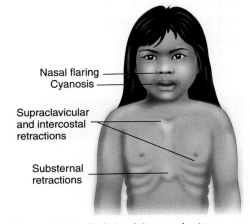

Nasal flaring
Cyanosis
Supraclavicular and intercostal retractions
Substernal retractions

Figure 12.1 Child with respiratory distress using accessory muscles

It is important that the EMT avoid telling the patient that she is counting the respiratory rate. The patient may become self-conscious about his breathing and alter his breathing pattern if he is aware that the EMT is counting his respirations.

It is often useful to count the respiratory rate while holding the patient's wrist on the patient's abdomen, acting as if the pulse is being counted. This method provides a distraction to the patient and allows the EMT to count a more accurate respiratory rate. Figure 12.2 shows the assessment of respirations.

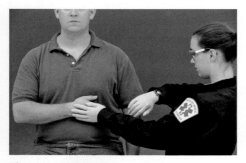

Figure 12.2 EMT assessing respirations

It will be necessary to look under the patient's clothing to observe some signs of respiratory difficulty. Attempting to maintain some modesty is always appropriate.

The prominent use of additional muscles to breathe is a sign of increased respiratory difficulty. The muscles of the chest and neck are thought of as accessory muscles of respiration and normally work together with the diaphragm to create smooth inspiration and exhalation.

When breathing becomes more difficult, these muscles work harder. Increased use of chest and neck muscles is sometimes referred to as **accessory muscle use.** Increased effort is also evidenced by nasal flaring as the patient tries to get as much air in as possible during inspiration. Nasal flaring is the wide opening of the nostrils with each breath.

The patient who is having difficulty breathing may also have abnormal noises during breathing. When air flows through a narrowed upper airway, such as in a common pediatric illness called croup or with any upper airway obstruction, a harsh sound can be heard on inspiration. This sound is called *stridor.*

Another sound created by an upper airway obstruction, often because the tongue falls back in the throat of an unconscious patient and partially occludes it, is **snoring.** The patient who is snoring could potentially occlude his airway and therefore needs a manual airway maneuver, such as the jaw thrust, to open his airway to relieve the partial obstruction created by the tongue.

A **gurgling** sound may be heard if liquid material is in the upper airway. This sound should immediately indicate to the EMT that suctioning is necessary to clear the patient's airway. If the airway is not suctioned, then the patient risks aspirating, or inhaling the liquid into his lungs. Aspiration is a leading cause of pneumonia.

Immediately after suctioning an airway, the EMT should consider whether the patient would benefit from the insertion of an oral airway to help keep the airway open.

Wheezing is a high-pitched sound that is more typical of lower airway obstruction, as seen with foreign body obstruction deeper in the chest or with the disease asthma. It is most commonly heard on expiration but may also be heard during inspiration. The EMT should listen for wheezing at the top of the patient's lungs, near the clavicles, or collarbones, as well as at the base of the lungs, below the scapulas, or shoulder blades, in order to describe the extent of the wheezing throughout the entire lung.

A **grunting** sound can also be heard in patients who are working very hard to breathe. This sound is indicative of extreme effort being exerted and should not be ignored. Frequently, small children and infants will continuously grunt when they are having trouble breathing. Grunting is an important physical finding that must be noted.

It is standard practice to mention any changes from a normal respiratory pattern when describing respirations during a report of vital signs. The combination of the respiratory rate, the quality of breathing (including additional breath sounds), and any patterns of breathing provides an excellent description of the patient's respiratory status.

PULSE

The pulse is the pressure generated by the contraction of the left ventricle of the heart. The pulse is a measure of the rate, strength, and regularity of the contraction of the heart and the volume of blood the heart is pumping out to the body. A patient's pulse can give the EMT information about the severity of the patient's illness or injury. Following these values over time allows the EMT to also note any change in the patient's condition or overall health.

A pulse can be measured at any point where an artery comes close to the skin, allowing the examiner to feel the pressure of the blood as it is pumped through the artery. Central pulse sites are at the carotid and femoral artery, and peripheral pulse sites are the radial, brachial, posterior tibial (medial aspect of the ankle), and the dorsalis pedis (on top of the foot on the great toe side). The most common sites for a pulse check in an adult are over the radial, femoral, and carotid arteries. Figure 12.3A–D illustrates where these common pulse points are found.

The radial pulse is the most commonly assessed pulse site in patients age 1 year and up. Brachial pulses are checked in infants less than 1 year old. When a pulse cannot be felt at a peripheral site, such as the radial pulse site, the EMT should then assess for a pulse at the carotid site. It is important to not press too hard when assessing the carotid pulse, and never check the carotid pulse on both sides of the neck at the same time, because these actions could occlude blood flow to the brain.

PULSE RATE

As with respiration, to recognize the appropriateness of a particular heart rate, the EMT must be familiar with normal heart rates. Table 12-2 lists normal heart rate ranges for different age-groups.

To measure the patient's pulse rate, the EMT must choose a pulse site, most commonly the radial pulse at the wrist. This pulse can be found by placing the pads of two fingers on the wrist, just below the base of the thumb. Figure 12.3A demonstrates this position. Once the pulse is felt, the EMT should count the number of pulse beats felt in 30 seconds, and then multiply this number by 2 to calculate the beats per minute. It is important to note that any patient who is very cold may have a slow pulse. The cold patient's pulse should be checked for 1 full minute (see Skill 12-1 at the end of this unit).

PULSE QUALITY

In addition to counting the pulse rate, the EMT should note the strength and regularity of the pulse beat. Common terms used to describe the strength of a pulse are *strong* and *bounding*. A strong pulse is full and normally strong; however, a bounding pulse is abnormally strong. A pulse that is *weak* doesn't feel full and may be difficult to find and feel. A weak pulse is also often a rapid pulse. A weak, rapid pulse is referred to as a *thready* pulse. A pulse can also be

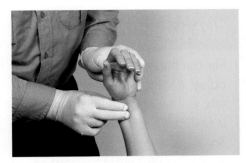

A.

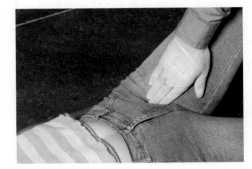

B.

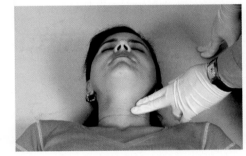

C.

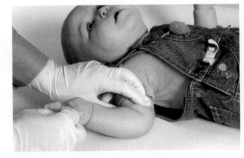

D.

Figure 12.3 Pulse points: A. Radial B. Femoral C. Carotid D. Brachial

Table 12-2 Normal Pulse Rates, by Age

Age	Pulse Rate (beats per minute)
Adult	60–100
Adolescent (11–14 yr)	60–105
School-aged child (6–12 yr)	70–110
Preschool-aged child (1–5 yr)	80–120
Infant (1 mo–1 yr)	90–140
Newborn (0–1 mo)	120–160

For the patient with an irregular pulse, a more accurate heart rate will be obtained if the pulse is counted for 1 full minute. An irregular pulse can be an indication of a potential cardiac abnormality. It is important that an EMT report if a pulse is regular or irregular and consider whether advanced life support is needed. In some cases, the patient will tell the EMT that he normally has an irregular pulse. The EMT should always remember to ask the patient if he normally has an irregular pulse or has been told his heart "skips beats."

Pediatric Considerations

Although blood pressure cuffs can be purchased in sizes appropriate for tiny infants, the general assessment of the infant and small child is much more valuable than obtaining a blood pressure reading. Blood pressures are often not obtained for children under the age of 3.

Table 12-3 Normal Blood Pressures

Age	Systolic (mmHg)	Diastolic (mmHg)
Adults	90–150	60–90
Children	Approx. 80 + [2 × age (in years) for children over 1 yr]	Approx. 2/3 systolic

described as *regular* if the beats seem to be spaced evenly. If the beats seem to occur in no regular pattern, the pulse is described as *irregular*.

BLOOD PRESSURE

The blood pressure is the measure of the pressure of the blood against the artery walls each time the left ventricle contracts, ejecting blood into the systemic circulation. Blood pressure is measured using a special tool called a **sphygmomanometer,** or blood pressure cuff, and a stethoscope.

Blood pressure is reported in two numbers. The first, or top, number is called the **systolic** pressure. *Systole* means contraction. This number refers to the pressure in the arteries during the contraction phase of the heart. This is the highest pressure created when the heart pumps blood out of the ventricles and into the circulation.

The lower number in the blood pressure is the **diastolic** pressure. *Diastole* means relaxation. The diastolic pressure refers to the pressure in the artery during the relaxation phase, immediately after a pulse. The diastolic pressure may be thought of as the resistance that the heart must pump against with each contraction. Table 12-3 shows normal blood pressure values.

The blood pressure is measured by inflating the sphygmomanometer around the patient's arm and measuring the pressure at both the contraction (systole) and relaxation (diastole) phases. There are two common methods of measuring the pressure: auscultation and palpation. Auscultation means listening, and palpation means feeling. Auscultation provides more accurate and more complete information than palpation and is generally preferred in most circumstances.

CUFF APPLICATION

Before measuring a patient's blood pressure, the EMT should select the proper size cuff. A properly fit blood pressure cuff should cover two-thirds of the upper arm, elbow to shoulder.

The Velcro attachments should securely close the cuff around the arm. Blood pressure cuffs come in several sizes. If an improper size is used, the numbers obtained will be inaccurate and misleading.

Once the proper size cuff is chosen, it should be applied to the patient's bare upper arm. If clothing is present, either remove it or roll the sleeve up to expose the upper arm. Be careful not to allow the rolled sleeve to form a constricting band around the upper arm, potentially making the blood pressure inaccurate by inhibiting blood flow to the arm.

MEASUREMENT BY AUSCULTATION

The most complete method of blood pressure measurement is by auscultation. To measure blood pressure by auscultation, the EMT should apply the cuff and then find the brachial pulse. This pulse is usually found toward the medial part of the **antecubital fossa,** the space opposite the elbow on the front of the arm.

The blood pressure cuff is inflated until the radial pulse is no longer felt, then inflated no more than 20 mmHg higher. Place the stethoscope in the ears with the earpiece facing forward and place the bell of the stethoscope on the area of the brachial pulse. Slowly release the pressure in the cuff, allowing the cuff to deflate.

The EMT should listen for the sound of the pulse, which can sound like a dull thud or swooshing. When the return of pulse is first heard, the number on the dial should be read. This is the systolic blood pressure.

The EMT should continue to listen while releasing the pressure in the cuff until the audible pulse disappears. When it does, the EMT notes the number on the dial at the last beat. This number is the diastolic pressure. The blood pressure is then reported as systolic pressure over diastolic pressure. Skill 12-2 at the end of the unit illustrates this procedure.

The **pulse pressure** is the difference between the systolic blood pressure and diastolic blood pressure and can only be obtained when using the auscultation method of blood pressure measurement. If the patient's blood pressure is 120/80, the pulse pressure is 40 mmHg (120 − 80 = 40 mmHg). The pulse pressure can be an important indicator of some conditions or injuries. Patients with head injuries may have widened pulse pressures (pulse pressure greater than 50% of the systolic blood pressure). A narrow pulse pressure (pulse pressure less then 25% of the systolic blood pressure) may be seen in shock and other conditions discussed later in this book.

Abnormal pulse pressures and trend changes in pulse pressure should be monitored and reported to emergency department staff so they can determine changes that may be occurring with blood pressure. Abnormal or changing trends of pulse pressures can be an important element in diagnosing life-threatening conditions.

MEASUREMENT BY PALPATION

In some circumstances, an EMT may not be able to hear the blood pressure because of interference from other noises. Examples of noisy interference include road noise while en route to the hospital, vibrations from a helicopter during flight, and noisy machinery in an industrial setting. In these cases, the blood pressure may be estimated by the palpation method, illustrated in Skill 12-3 at the end of this unit. Palpated blood pressures are merely an estimate, and blood pressures by palpation are often lower than those obtained by auscultation. Any blood pressure obtained by palpation should be confirmed with a standard auscultated blood pressure as soon as possible.

Blood pressures by palpation are accomplished by palpating the return of the radial pulse during deflation of the cuff and noting that number on the blood pressure gauge as the systolic pressure. Because a stethoscope is not used, the loss of the pulse cannot be heard and the diastolic pressure is therefore not available. This blood pressure is reported as the systolic number over palpation, as in "one-twenty by palpation" or "120/P."

Street Smart

New technology has brought with it automatic blood pressure cuffs, sometimes called a *noninvasive blood pressure monitor* (NIBP). Many EMS systems are using this tool, particularly on patient transfers. Every time an NIBP is used, a manual blood pressure should be taken first to compare with the NIBP reading to ensure that cuff placement is correct and the readings are dependable.

Street Smart

In the past the presence of a radial or carotid pulse was assumed to mean that the patient had a certain blood pressure. Current research has rejected that notion. It is more accurate to assume that the patient with a strong radial pulse has an adequate blood pressure, while a patient without a radial pulse may have a low blood pressure. No further assumptions about the blood pressure can be made without measurement by the EMT.

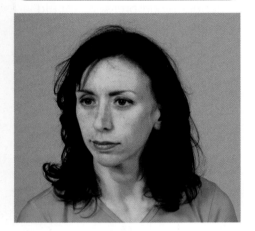

Figure 12.4 Note the pallor, a sign of shock

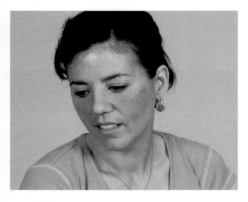

Figure 12.5 A flush can occur from embarrassment or disease

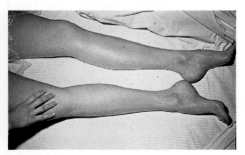

Figure 12.6 Jaundiced skin can be caused by liver disease

SKIN SIGNS

The appearance and condition of the skin can tell the EMT a lot about the patient's circulatory status. For this reason, it is crucial that the EMT pay attention to skin signs when measuring vital signs. Together with the heart rate and blood pressure, skin condition can clue the EMT in to potentially serious circulatory problems.

SKIN COLOR

The patient's skin color can be initially assessed when the EMT sees the patient for the first time. Skin color is a direct measurement of the adequacy of blood supply and oxygenation to the skin and a sign of how well the respiratory and circulatory systems are functioning. The patient's skin color should be further evaluated by assessing the nail beds, oral mucosa, or conjunctiva (the pink underside of the eyelid). Normally, these areas will have a healthy pink color from good blood flow, or perfusion.

If blood supply is decreased, as in hypoperfusion, the light-skinned patient's skin will become pale. The patient's skin is sometimes described as looking pallid or having a **pallor** (a deficiency of color). A dark-skinned patient will show a lighter complexion as well. This change has been described as looking dusky or gray. Figure 12.4 shows an example of pallor.

If a state of poor oxygenation exists, a bluish discoloration, or cyanosis, may be present. Peripheral cyanosis, a bluish hue to the fingertips, may also represent poor circulation. Central cyanosis, a bluish hue to the lips or inner eyelids, is a sign of hypoxia, or lack of oxygen in the blood.

Other skin colors may give the EMT clues about underlying disease states. **Mottling,** a color similar to cyanosis but in a blotchy pattern, may be seen in shock. A flushed red appearance to the skin may indicate a sunburn, heat exposure, or serious carbon monoxide poisoning; flushed red skin is considered a late sign in carbon monoxide poisoning. A yellow appearance, called **jaundice,** may indicate liver disease. Figures 12.5 and 12.6 show examples of these skin colors.

SKIN TEMPERATURE AND MOISTURE

A healthy person normally has warm, dry skin. It is important to actually measure the relative skin temperature with your hand on a central part of the patient's body. Measuring temperature peripherally—at the hands, for example—may be misleading if the temperature at the scene is at an extreme of hot or cold.

To measure temperature, partially remove a glove and place the bare skin from the back of the hand against the patient's bare skin on either the forehead or the abdomen.

The skin temperature should be described as hot, warm, cool, or cold. A patient with a fever or exposure to heat would usually be called *hot to the touch.* Cool to the touch could be a sign of inadequate circulation (shock) or exposure to cold. *Cold to the touch* usually indicates exposure to extreme cold.

Changes in skin temperature or skin that has differing temperatures in various parts of the body can be a significant sign. For example, if the patient has normal skin temperature overall, but the skin is hot in one specific area, that could be a sign of infection in that area.

Moisture on the surface of the skin may represent normal sweating if the patient is in a hot environment. Moist or sweaty skin may also represent a nervous system reaction to a stressful situation, shock (hypoperfusion), poisoning, or a cardiac or diabetic emergency. *Cool and clammy* skin is different from hot and sweaty skin and usually indicates that the patient has a circulatory problem. Skin that is abnormally dry may be an indicator of severe dehydration or spinal injury.

CAPILLARY REFILL

Capillary refill is the time it takes for the capillaries to fill back up with blood after they have been compressed. It is a more reliable sign in infants and children than in adults, who may suffer from a disease process, take certain medications, or generally have poor circulation, all of which affect perfusion in the capillaries. It is important to keep in mind that capillary refill in adults and older children can be influenced by a cold environment, certain preexisting conditions, and certain medications; therefore, it should be only one piece of the overall assessment picture. The presence of good capillary refill in an adult is a good sign. However, poor capillary refill in an adult may be the result of other factors and not a sign of poor perfusion. In short, poor capillary refill in adults is an unreliable sign.

Capillary refill is an additional tool that may be useful in assessing the adequacy of circulation and perfusion. Recall that early in a state of hypoperfusion, or shock, the body preferentially shunts blood away from the skin to compensate for poor circulation, and the skin is therefore not supplied with blood. This important bodily response allows continued perfusion of important central body organs when the blood supply is limited. We can see evidence of this selective shunting of blood away from the skin by assessing the time it takes for the blood to return to the skin when the skin is compressed. This measurement is called *capillary refill time.*

The capillaries of a healthy individual have a constant supply of oxygenated blood. If the blood were pushed out of a capillary bed, by external pressure on the area, the area would become pale.

The normal response of the skin is to rapidly refill those capillaries with blood, and the skin becomes pink again. This capillary refill normally occurs in less than 2 seconds. The EMT can test capillary refill by compressing and releasing the fingertip of the individual or the skin of the forearm of an infant or child.

If more than 2 seconds elapse before the capillary bed refills and the area becomes pink, the individual's skin can be said to be hypoperfused, which may indicate the presence of shock.

Capillary refill by itself is not a specific indicator of shock, especially in the adult. Therefore, it is important to include all the skin and vital signs together with capillary refill to get a more accurate indicator of early shock.

PUPILS

It has been said that the eyes are the windows to the soul. For the EMT, the eyes are the windows to the brain and how well it is functioning. An essential part of every neurologic exam includes checking the pupil's response to light.

The **pupil** is the black part in the center of the eye. It is usually round and changes size in reaction to changing light conditions. The EMT should check this response during each measurement of the vital signs and note any changes. A change in pupillary reaction may mean the patient's neurologic status, or brain function, is improving or deteriorating.

When checking pupil response, the EMT should shield the patient's eyes from the room light, or turn down the lights and then use a handheld penlight to assess size, shape, and reaction. Figure 12.7 shows pupils being assessed using a penlight.

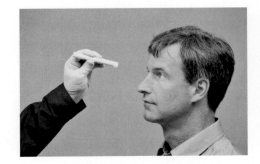

Figure 12.7 Pupils being assessed using an penlight

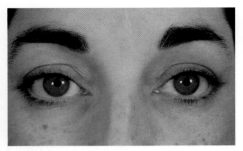

A.

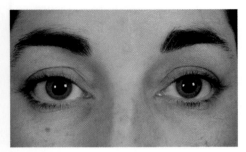

B.

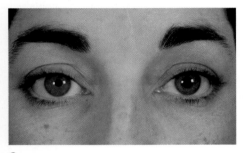

C.

Figure 12.8 A. Constricted pupils B. Dilated pupils C. Unequal pupils (anisocoria)

SIZE AND SHAPE

Pupil diameter can be described using exact millimeters, ranging from 2 mm to 8 mm. Some providers may prefer to use less precise terms, such as *dilated,* meaning large, or *constricted,* meaning small. Figure 12.8A shows constricted pupils and Figure 12.8B shows dilated pupils.

Dilated pupils can be an indicator of drug use such as amphetamines, cocaine, and LSD and are often seen in cardiac arrest, whereas constricted pupils can be indicators of a central nervous system disorder or narcotic drug use.

Table 12-4 lists some terms used to describe pupils. The pupil of the eye is normally round. The two pupils are usually the same size. They tend to react together when one is exposed to light. This is called a **consensual response.**

If the pupils are not of equal size, this condition is termed **anisocoria.** Figure 12.8C shows a patient with anisocoria. Some people naturally have this condition; however, it can also be a sign of serious eye or brain injury. Unequal pupils can be seen in stroke, head injury, patients who use medicated eye drops to dilate their pupils, and individuals who have an artificial eye.

REACTIVITY

When the eye is exposed to light, the normal response of the pupil is to constrict rather briskly. When the light is removed, the pupil should dilate just as quickly. If this response occurs, the pupil is considered normal and reactive. If no response to light is seen, the pupil is considered nonreactive or a fixed pupil. One

Table 12-4	Descriptive Terms for Pupils
Pinpoint	Tiny pupils, usually smaller than 2 mm diameter
Constricted	Small, usually 2–3 mm
Midposition	Medium-sized, usually 4–5 mm
Dilated	Large, usually 6–8 mm
Blown	Huge, usually greater than 8 mm

or both pupils can become fixed and dilated with severe hypoxia or extremely inadequate perfusion to the brain, as seen in cardiac arrest and severe head injuries. If the pupil responds slowly, the pupil is described as being sluggish. Sluggish pupils can be an indicator of hypoxia, drug overdose, or poor perfusion.

When an EMT shines a light into a patient's eyes, she should observe the size, shape, and reactivity of the pupil. Often the normal response is described with an acronym: PERRL. **PERRL** stands for pupils equal, round, and reactive to light.

Some neurologic or brain injuries and injuries directly to the eye will alter this normal reaction. It is important that the EMT note the pupil response with each set of vital signs to recognize any changes from the initial baseline exam.

PULSE OXIMETRY

At times it may be useful to quantify the effectiveness of a patient's breathing. The EMT can count the breaths per minute and describe the quality of the breathing effort. These observations tell a great deal about the effectiveness of the patient's respirations.

An additional tool that can be useful to determine how effectively a patient is breathing is the **pulse oximeter.** The pulse oximeter is a noninvasive machine that indirectly measures the amount of oxygenated blood in a patient's circulatory system. It can be a useful tool in detecting hypoxia.

The pulse oximeter uses an infrared light to estimate the percent of blood that appears to be oxygenated in the capillaries. The pulse oximeter relies on the difference in appearance of blood cells that are bound to oxygen (hemoglobin) and those that are not bound to oxygen, to make this determination. The normal percent of blood that is saturated by oxygen is 96% to 100%.

If the respirations are effective, the blood will be well oxygenated and the pulse oximetry reading will be normal. Less than 96% indicates that the blood may not be adequately oxygenated and that there may be problems with breathing or circulation. Below 90% is considered to be a serious problem in oxygenation.

These numbers are described as percent saturated. If the device reads "97," this reading would be described as "97 percent saturated" and would be considered within the normal oxygen saturation range.

The pulse oximeter should not be used to determine whether a patient needs oxygen. The EMT should base oxygen administration upon the patient concern, assessment of the patient's respiratory rate and tidal volume, and assessment of the patient's overall condition. If the EMT decides that the patient needs oxygen on the basis of the patient's presenting problem and physical exam, it should be given. Measuring the pulse oximetry should not delay oxygen administration when assessment of the airway, breathing, and circulation indicate signs of compromise or hypoxia.

The pulse oximeter can be used to judge the effectiveness of the EMT's treatment. If oxygen has been applied and the pulse oximeter reading is dropping, the EMT should rapidly reassess the patient's status and need for further interventions, such as bag-valve-mask ventilation, or an adjustment to the current treatment, such as increasing the amount of oxygen being applied.

For the machine to accurately determine the percent of saturated blood, it must "see" an adequate sample of capillary blood. For various reasons, an adequate sample is not always available. For example, if the patient has heavy nail polish, the device may not be able to sense accurately through the polish. The nail polish must be removed, usually with acetone or nail polish remover,

Street Smart

Bright overhead lights can interfere with a pulse oximeter. If an EMT is having difficulty obtaining a pulse oximeter reading in a bright environment, she should try putting a washcloth over the finger probe to block out some of the environmental light.

Street Smart

It is important to remember that the pulse oximeter is merely a machine that is to be used in conjunction with the EMT's clinical judgment. If an EMT suspects that a patient is in need of oxygen for any reason, regardless of the pulse oximeter reading, she should provide it.

Cigarette smoke has carbon monoxide in the inhaled smoke and that carbon monoxide interferes with pulse oximeter. For this reason a pulse oximeter reading for cigarette smokers will indicate oxygen saturations that are higher than the true oxygen saturation level.

in order to get an accurate reading. Artificial nails cannot be removed and may also interfere in the pulse oximeter accurately reading oxygen saturation. An alternate method such as a probe that can be used on the ear lobe or taking a reading of a toe may be used in these cases.

If the patient does not have adequate blood flow to the finger on which the device is placed, an adequate sample will not be seen. For example, while a blood pressure is being taken, the pulse oximeter reading may become low temporarily.

Many devices have an indicator light, or a lighted meter, to tell the EMT that an adequate sample has been "seen" and that the number given is accurate. It is recommended that the EMT use a pulse oximeter that indicates when the reading is adequate. A lighted bar meter or a green or yellow light indicator visually confirms that the sample is adequate and reliable.

Oxygen should never be withheld from a patient who needs it because of a normal pulse oximetry reading. There are certain situations in which the pulse oximetry may be normal, but the patient is in need of supplemental oxygen.

One such example is carbon monoxide poisoning. The carbon monoxide binds to the hemoglobin, causing the pulse oximeter to "see" completely saturated hemoglobin (100% saturation). This device cannot distinguish between oxygen and other molecules attached to the hemoglobin and will read a normal saturation despite a lack of oxygen.

REASSESSMENT OF THE BASELINE VITAL SIGNS

An EMT will often care for a patient over an extended period of time. During that time it is important that the EMT be aware of any change in the patient's condition. Changes can be determined only if the EMT repeatedly reassesses the patient.

It is imperative that the EMT repeat the assessment of vital signs frequently during care for any emergency patient. If the patient's initial vital signs were within normal range and the patient seems stable, the vital signs should be repeated every 10–15 minutes to assess for changes.

If the patient is unstable or had abnormal vital signs at the first check, the EMT should repeat the vital signs at least every 5 minutes.

If a medication is administered to the patient, the EMT should repeat the vital signs within 5 minutes after administering any medication, including oxygen.

All measurements of vital signs should be carefully documented, with the time that they were obtained noted on the record. Noting changes in any vital sign and passing that information on to the hospital providers are crucial and will help them understand the changes in the patient's condition.

CONCLUSION

The EMT is responsible for gathering certain baseline information on every patient she encounters. This information consists of repeated vital sign measurements throughout the period the EMT is responsible for the patient's care.

The EMT must be well practiced at assessing respiration, pulse, blood pressure, pupils, skin condition, and pulse oximetry. Familiarity with normal values for each of these parameters is important if the EMT is expected to identify abnormal vital signs.

Ongoing assessment is useful in recognizing any changes, positive or negative, in the patient's condition and enables the EMT to adjust treatments to improve the patient's response and overall condition.

The EMT must accurately reassess, record, and report the baseline vital signs and any changes in the patient's condition to the hospital staff to ensure the accurate and effective continuum of care the patient receives throughout the prehospital and hospital health care encounter.

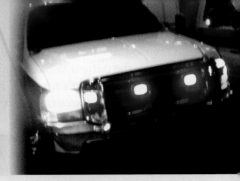

Kasey knows Mr. Young's skin signs—cyanosis around his mouth, skin warm to the touch, and sweating—are signs of a serious illness. She will need to obtain a full set of baseline vital signs to help discern what is the best treatment for the patient.

Kasey tells Sally to get a baseline set of vital signs while she applies high-concentration oxygen by face mask. Mr. Young's respiratory status is labored with use of accessory muscles, cyanosis around the lips, and sitting in a position to aid his respirations. Kasey knows all these signs together tell her to not wait to apply oxygen to take a pulse oximeter reading.

Sally takes a set of baseline vital signs and reports Mr. Young's respirations are at 32 and labored, with wheezing noises on exhalation; pulse is 126 and bounding; blood pressure is 148/90 mmHg; skin is flushed, warm, and wet, with cyanosis around the mouth; pupils are round, equal, and reacting to light; and the pulse oximeter reading is 89%.

Kasey knows Mr. Young needs a special medicine to open up his lower airway and help him breathe. His vital signs are indicating he has been working hard to breathe

for an extended period of time and his body is beginning to tire out. Mr. Young needs immediate treatment for his asthma before he goes into respiratory arrest.

Kasey and Sally immediately load Mr. Young in the ambulance and request an ALS service to intercept with them between Mr. Young's residence and the nearest hospital. Kasey tells Sally to reassess the vitals signs after 5 minutes. Sally reports the pulse oximeter has improved to 92%. Mr. Young is still using accessory muscles to help him breathe and wheezes are still present, but his respirations have decreased to 28 a minute. His pulse is 110 and strong; blood pressure is 140/88 mmHg; and skin is moist, pink, and warm with the cyanosis no longer present around his mouth.

As Kasey turns patient care over to the ALS crew on intercept, she includes the baseline vitals signs and the current vital signs in her report. Kasey knows the reassessment of Mr. Young's vital signs show some improvement with the oxygen administration; however, Mr. Young is still at risk for respiratory arrest and very much in need of the medications offered by the ALS provider.

Skill 12-1 Measurement of Radial and Carotid Pulse

PURPOSE: To obtain a baseline pulse rate for assessment and comparison.

STANDARD PRECAUTIONS:

- ☑ Watch/clock with second hand
- ☑ Patient care report and pen
- ☑ Gloves

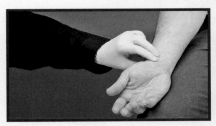

1 The EMT finds the radial pulse on the anterior surface of the distal forearm, proximal to the thumb. The EMT notes the quality and regularity of the pulse as weak or strong, regular, or irregular.

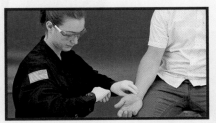

2 The EMT counts the number of pulse beats felt over a 30-second period and multiplies this number by 2 to obtain beats per minute. (If the pulse is irregular, then the EMT counts for 1 minute.)

When a radial pulse cannot be palpated, the EMT should check for a central pulse such as the carotid.

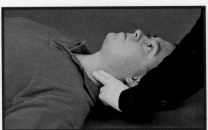

3 Using two fingers, locate the larynx (Adam's apple), then slide the fingers to one side, stopping in the groove between the larynx and large neck muscles. Feel for the pulse but do not compress the artery. Do not use the thumb or rest your hand across the throat.

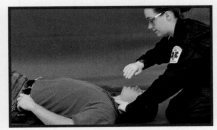

4 The EMT counts the number of pulse beats felt over a 30-second period and multiplies this number by 2 to obtain beats per minute. (If the pulse is irregular, then the EMT counts for 1 minute.)

	TIME	RESP	PULSE	B.P.	LEVEL OF CONSCIOUSNESS	GCS	R	PUPILS	L	SKIN
V I T A L S I G N S	1 0 1 5	Rate: ☐ Regular ☐ Shallow ☐ Labored	Rate: 70 ☑ Regular ☐ Irregular		☐ Alert ☐ Voice ☐ Pain ☐ Unresp.		☐ ☐ ☐ ☐	Normal Dilated Constricted Sluggish No-Reaction	☐ ☐ ☐ ☐	☐ Unremarkable ☐ Cool ☐ Pale ☒ Warm ☐ Cyanotic ☐ Moist ☐ Flushed ☒ Dry ☐ Jaundiced
		Rate: ☐ Regular ☐ Shallow ☐ Labored	Rate: ☐ Regular ☐ Irregular		☐ Alert ☐ Voice ☐ Pain ☐ Unresp.		☐ ☐ ☐ ☐	Normal Dilated Constricted Sluggish No-Reaction	☐ ☐ ☐ ☐	☐ Unremarkable ☐ Cool ☐ Pale ☐ Warm ☐ Cyanotic ☐ Moist ☐ Flushed ☐ Dry ☐ Jaundiced
		Rate: ☐ Regular ☐ Shallow ☐ Labored	Rate: ☐ Regular ☐ Irregular		☐ Alert ☐ Voice ☐ Pain ☐ Unresp.		☐ ☐ ☐ ☐	Normal Dilated Constricted Sluggish No-Reaction	☐ ☐ ☐ ☐	☐ Unremarkable ☐ Cool ☐ Pale ☐ Warm ☐ Cyanotic ☐ Moist ☐ Flushed ☐ Dry ☐ Jaundiced

5 Record the quality and regularity of the pulse rate and the condition of the skin.

PURPOSE: To obtain a baseline blood pressure for assessment and comparison.

STANDARD PRECAUTIONS:

☑ Stethoscope

☑ Properly sized blood pressure cuff

☑ Gloves

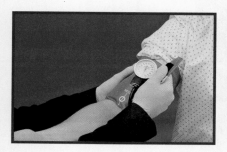

1 The EMT places the blood pressure cuff around the patient's upper arm snugly. The cuff should cover more than half but less than two thirds of the length of the upper arm.

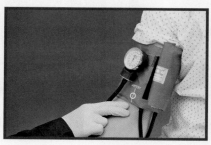

2 The EMT then finds the brachial pulse. The brachial pulse is usually found on the medial side of the elbow.

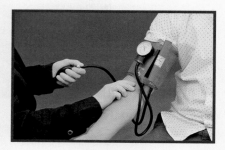

3 Next, the EMT closes the valve on the cuff and inflates the cuff until the brachial pulse is no longer felt, then continues inflating for 20 mmHg higher.

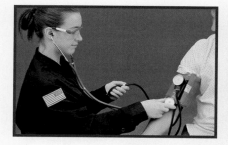

4 Then the EMT places the head of the stethoscope on the brachial pulse and the ear tips in the ears.

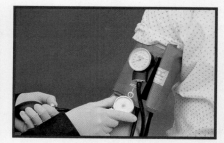

5 Slowly deflate the blood pressure cuff, at about 12 mmHg per second, using the relief valve next to the bulb.

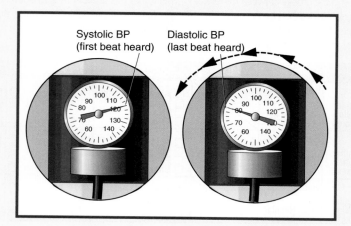

Systolic BP (first beat heard)

Diastolic BP (last beat heard)

6 Note the systolic and the diastolic pressures.

PURPOSE: To obtain a baseline blood pressure for assessment and comparison.

STANDARD PRECAUTIONS:

☑ Properly sized blood pressure cuff

☑ Gloves

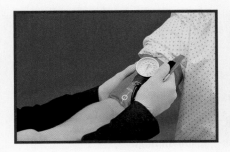

1 The EMT places the blood pressure cuff around the patient's upper arm snugly. The cuff should cover more than half but less than two thirds of the length of the upper arm.

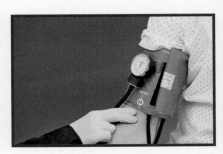

2 The EMT then finds the brachial pulse. The brachial pulse is usually found on the medial side of the elbow.

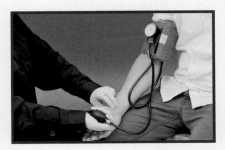

3 Next, the EMT closes the valve on the cuff and inflates the cuff until the brachial pulse is no longer felt, then continues inflating for 20 mmHg higher.

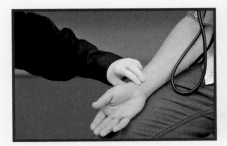

4 The EMT places her fingertips over the radial pulse.

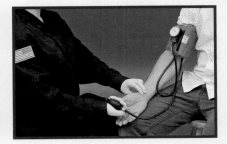

5 The EMT slowly deflates the blood pressure cuff and notes the pressure on the valve at the time she feels the return of the radial pulse.

Key Concepts Revisited

- The most frequently used skill an EMT will use is obtaining and monitoring the patient's vital signs.

- Baseline vital signs obtained at the onset of care enable the EMT to quickly recognize and react to changes in the patient's condition.

- Baseline vital signs are the measurement of how core systems of the body, the respiratory and circulatory systems, are functioning and include measurement of:
  - Respiration
  - Heart
  - Blood pressure
  - Skin signs
  - Pupils
  - Pulse oximetry

- Measuring the effectiveness of the patient's breathing includes:
  - Respiratory rate (number of breaths taken in 1 minute)
  - Respiratory quality (depth of breaths, use of accessory muscles, and respiratory sounds)

- Measuring the pulse, where an artery comes close to the skin, includes assessing:
  - The pulse rate (number of beats of the heart in 1 minute)
  - The pulse quality (strength and regularity)
    - Strong or bounding
    - Weak and thready
    - Regular or irregular

- Blood pressure can be assessed through auscultation or palpation and is a measure of how effectively the heart is functioning.
  - Systolic (top number) measures the pressure in the arteries when the heart contracts.
  - Diastolic (bottom number) measures the pressure in the artery when the heart is in the relaxation phase.
    - Measurement by auscultation is the most complete method of blood pressure measurement and involves measuring both the systolic and diastolic blood pressures.
    - Measurement by palpation is an estimate of the systolic blood pressure.

- Changes in normal pulse pressure can be an important indicator of some serious conditions or injuries.
  - Narrow pulse pressure is pulse pressure less than 25 percent of the systolic blood pressure.
  - Widened pulse pressure is greater than 50% over the systolic pulse pressure.

- The skin signs can be the first indicator of a patient's circulatory status and include:
  - Skin color
    - Pallor—pale or blanched of color
    - Cyanosis—bluish-tint
    - Mottling—blotchy dust-tint or marbled
    - Jaundice—yellowish tinge
  - Skin temperature
    - Hot, warm, cool, or cold
  - Skin moisture
    - Moist or clammy
    - Sweaty or diaphoretic
    - Dry

- Capillary refill is an additional tool that can be used in accord with the other baseline vital signs in assessing the adequacy of perfusion.

- An essential part of every neurologic exam is checking the pupils:
  - Pupil size includes dilated (large), constricted (small), pinpoint (tiny), and blown (huge).
    - Pupils are usually round and equal although a percentage of the population have unequal pupils, called anisocoria.
  - Pupils' reactivity to light include:
    - PERRL: pupils equal, round, reactive to light
    - Nonreactive or fixed
    - Sluggish
    - Fixed
    - Dilated

- The pulse oximeter can be an additional tool used in determining the effectiveness of breathing and perfusion.
  - Measures the percent of blood that appears to be oxygenated
  - Less accurate in adults and older children

- Disease
- Cold
- Medications
- Accurate in infants and small children

- Accurately reassessing, reporting, and recording the baseline vital signs are essential to appropriate patient management and the continuum of patient care.

Review Questions

1. Define baseline vital signs.
2. Why are baseline vital signs important to measure?
3. What are the normal respiratory rate and quality for adults and children of different ages?
4. Define what is meant by the quality and quantity of the pulse.
5. What are the normal pulse rate and quality for adults and children of different ages?
6. What are the two methods of assessing blood pressure?
7. Define systolic and diastolic blood pressure.
8. What is *pulse pressure*, and why is it important?
9. Why should the EMT assess pupils?
10. What are the methods of assessing skin color, temperature, and condition?
11. How is capillary refill measured?
12. How is oxygen saturation in the blood measured using a pulse oximeter?
13. Why is it important to accurately reassess, report, and record the baseline vital signs?

Key Terms

Accessory muscle use
Anisocoria
Antecubital fossa
Baseline vital signs
Consensual response
Diastolic
Exhalation
Grunting
Gurgling
Inspiration
Jaundice

Mottling
Pallor
PERRL
Pulse pressure
Pulse oximeter
Pupil
Snoring
Sphygmomanometer
Systolic
Wheezing

Further Study

Dalton, A. L., D. Limmer, J. Mistovich, and H. A. Werman. *Advanced Medical Life Support.* 3d ed. Upper Saddle River, NJ: Brady/ Pearson Prentice Hall, 2007.

DeLaune, S., and P. Ladner. *Fundamentals of Nursing: Standards & Practice.* 2d ed. Clifton Park, NY: Thomson Delmar Learning, 2002.

Estes, M. E. Z. *Health Assessment and Physical Examination.* 2d ed. Clifton Park, NY: Thomson Delmar Learning, 2002.

Lindh, W., C. Tamparo, M. Pooler, and J. Cerrato. *Comprehensive Medical Assisting.* 2d ed. Clifton Park, NY: Thomson Delmar Learning, 2002.

UNIT (13) Basic Pharmacology

The EMT will encounter patients who require medication. The EMT may be responsible for administering a medication carried in the ambulance or assisting patients with administration of their own prescribed medication for a specific illness. It is the EMT's responsibility to be knowledgeable in basic information about commonly encountered medicines and proper administration procedures, thereby avoiding improper use and potentially life-threatening consequences for the patient.

National Education Standards

Emergency Medical Technicians (EMTs) will be able to apply fundamental understanding of the medications they may assist/administer to a patient. The EMT will have a fundamental depth and foundational breadth, within the scope of practice of the EMT, on how to assist with or administer medications to a patient.

Key Concepts

- The EMT should be knowledgeable in basic principles of pharmacology of commonly encountered medications and their administration.

- The EMT should be familiar with the two most commonly used names for medications: generic and trade or brand name.

- The dose of a drug is the amount of the drug that should be administered to achieve the desired effect.

- The route of administration of a drug affects how quickly the drug enters the patient's circulation and is absorbed by the body.

- The EMT should be familiar with the various forms of medication commonly prescribed.

- The "five rights" of drug administration verify if the medication is safe and appropriate for the situation.

- The EMT must be familiar with the many routes of drug administration.

- The exact name of the medication, dose, and route should be carefully documented, as well as the time it was administered and by whom.

- The EMT may be required to assist the patient in administering medications specifically prescribed for the patient by a physician.

- The EMT must understand some basic principles of pharmacology to ensure correct administration of medications in the prehospital setting.

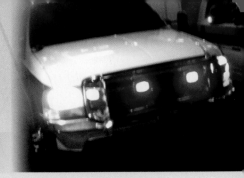

CASE STUDY

Bill is an EMT who volunteers on his local ambulance service for special events that require the presence of an ambulance. Today Bill and his fellow volunteers are standing by during the Figure 8 car races when the pagers go off for a "man not acting right" in the grandstands, possible diabetic. Upon arrival at the grandstand on the other side of the racetrack, Bill and his crew see an approximately 40-year-old male seated on the steps going into the grandstand. A small group of people are standing nearby talking to him. He appears to not be paying attention but occasionally looks around as if he's unsure where he is.

As Bill approaches, a female from the group tells him her name is Kathy and she is Jason's wife. Kathy informs Bill that Jason is a newly diagnosed diabetic, and she

thinks he forgot to eat after taking his insulin a little over an hour earlier. Kathy states that Jason suddenly began acting confused, almost dazed, about 15 minutes ago. She tried to get him to the concession stand for food when he suddenly sat down and refused to go any farther, arguing that they would miss the "horse races."

Critical Thinking Questions

1. What are indications for administration of oral glucose?

2. What are contraindications for administration of oral glucose?

3. What is the best route of administration of oral glucose?

INTRODUCTION

The study of medications and their interactions is called **pharmacology.** This chapter provides the information that an EMT will need to safely administer or assist the patient in administering medications that may be encountered by the EMT during an emergency.

PRINCIPLES OF PHARMACOLOGY

The EMT will encounter medications quite often throughout his career. Among the basic principles of pharmacology the EMT needs to understand are some basic terms used when discussing medications, the variety of forms of medication, and the various routes of administration.

MEDICATION TERMINOLOGY

Pharmacology, like all medical practice, involves terms that must be learned so that the EMT can clearly communicate with patients and other medical professionals. It is important for the EMT to be familiar with a few key pharmacological terms when caring for patients requiring medications.

DRUG NAMES

Medication terminology can seem complex and difficult to remember, and the EMT may wonder why he needs to be familiar with the different names a medication or drug can have. It is important for the EMT to be familiar with all the information about a medication, including the different names of medications commonly encountered in the field. It is especially vital to know the names of medications approved for use by the EMT.

While a medication is being developed, it can have up to four names: chemical, generic, trade, and official. The EMS should be familiar with the two most commonly used names once a drug is through development: generic and trade or brand name. No single person can be expected to remember every name of every medication. Even physicians carry pocket reference books to look up medications. It may be helpful for the EMT to also carry a similar handbook that includes some basic medication information for prehospital use.

GENERIC

The name a medication is given when it is developed will appear in a governmental publication listing all drugs in the United States, called *U.S. Pharmacopoeia*. This initial name is often a short form of the chemical name and is referred to as the **generic name.** The generic name is often longer and more difficult to pronounce than the more commonly known names given to the medications later when they are marketed by different companies.

TRADE

The brand name that is given to a medication by the manufacturer is called the **trade name.** The trade name is often shorter and easier to pronounce than the initial generic name. This trade name is used in marketing a medication. Because some medications are manufactured by several different companies, one medication may be given several different trade names. This multitude of names may seem confusing, but the EMT can refer to a drug handbook to cross-reference trade name and generic name, and to find medication information. For this reason, some health care providers choose to learn and remember the generic names for the most common medications. Table 13-1 lists some common medications by both their generic and trade names.

DRUG ACTIONS

The **action** of a drug is the effect the drug will have on the body. The **mechanism of action** is how a drug works on the body to get the intended response, called the **therapeutic effect.** Administration of a drug should be based on the action, therapeutic effect, and mechanism of action. As an example, aspirin is given to patients experiencing chest pain or discomfort. The action of aspirin is that it prevents platelets in the blood from sticking together and forming a blood clot. Therefore, giving aspirin can help prevent clot formation or keep

Table 13-1 Common Medications by Generic and Trade Names

Generic Name	Trade Name
acetaminophen	Tylenol
ibuprofen	Motrin, Advil
albuterol	Ventolin, Proventil
pseudoephedrine	Sudafed
diphenhydramine	Benadryl

a clot, the most common cause of acute myocardial infarction, from getting bigger. The EMT must be familiar with the action of a medication given to know what to expect once the medication has been administered.

INDICATION

The reason for giving a medication is called the *indication*. The indication to give a drug is most commonly based on the signs, symptoms, or specific condition that needs to be relieved. To administer a medication properly, an EMT must know its most common indications.

A common example of an indication for a medication is the use of acetaminophen for fever. Indications for specific medications used by the EMT are covered in detail later in this unit.

CONTRAINDICATION

There are certain circumstances in which a particular medication should not be administered because it may cause more harm than good. In other cases, a medication should not be given because the action of the drug would not improve the patient's condition. These instances are considered *contraindications*.

A good example of a contraindication is an allergy to the medication. If a patient states he is allergic to penicillin, then penicillin is contraindicated for that patient. An allergy to a medication is always a contraindication to that medication. In some cases the patient or the EMT may be uncertain whether a patient truly has an allergy to a medication or has experienced an unpleasant side effect. It is best to err on the side of caution and not administer the drug if there is doubt. The best approach in those cases would be for the EMT to contact medical control for further instructions and guidance.

SIDE EFFECTS

The EMT should also know the side effects of a medication. A **side effect** is usually an unintended and often undesired effect that occurs in addition to the intended desired effect. It may be unpleasant or harmful to the patient but is not an allergic reaction to the drug. A side effect can also be an unintended effect that is discovered to have benefit in treating another condition. As an example, the drug nitroglycerin, discussed in more detail later in this unit, has a side effect of lowering blood pressure; as a result, nitroglycerin is sometimes administered to patients experiencing a hypertensive (high blood pressure) crisis.

An example of an unintended side effect is the administration of nitroglycerin to a patient complaining of chest pain. Nitroglycerin is intended to open up the blood vessels supplying the heart, increasing oxygen delivery to the heart muscle and decreasing chest pain. The side effect of nitroglycerin can be a fall in blood pressure, sometimes quite significantly. This fall in blood pressure is not the intended action of the medication, although it is expected once the EMT learns the profile of the drug.

Not everyone who uses a medication experiences every reported side effect; therefore, not every patient who receives nitroglycerin will experience a decrease in blood pressure. If a patient's blood pressure falls after nitroglycerin administration, the EMT should be prepared for it and ready to effectively manage the situation.

It is useful for the EMT to be aware of potential side effects from medications that may be encountered during patient care so he can be ready to deal with their consequences.

DOSE

The **dose** of a drug is simply how much of the medication should be administered to achieve the desired effect. The dose of a medication is often based on the weight and sometimes the age of the patient. It is important to know and distinguish the differences in the dosages of medications given to adults from those given to children and infants. An inadequate amount of a drug may have no effect; however, if the dose is increased or given all at once instead of over a period of time, it could cause serious side effects for the patient.

ROUTE

The **route** of administration of a drug affects how quickly the drug enters the patient's circulation and is absorbed by the body. The routes most commonly used for drug administration include the **enteral** (ingested) medications (sublingual and oral) and **parenteral** (inhalation and injection). The routes of drug administration will be discussed in more detail later in this unit.

PRESCRIBING INFORMATION

When prescribing medications, physicians use several common abbreviations to instruct the patient on how to take the medicine (Figure 13.1). These abbreviations are helpful for the EMT to know and are listed in Table 13-2 just as they may be found on prescription labels.

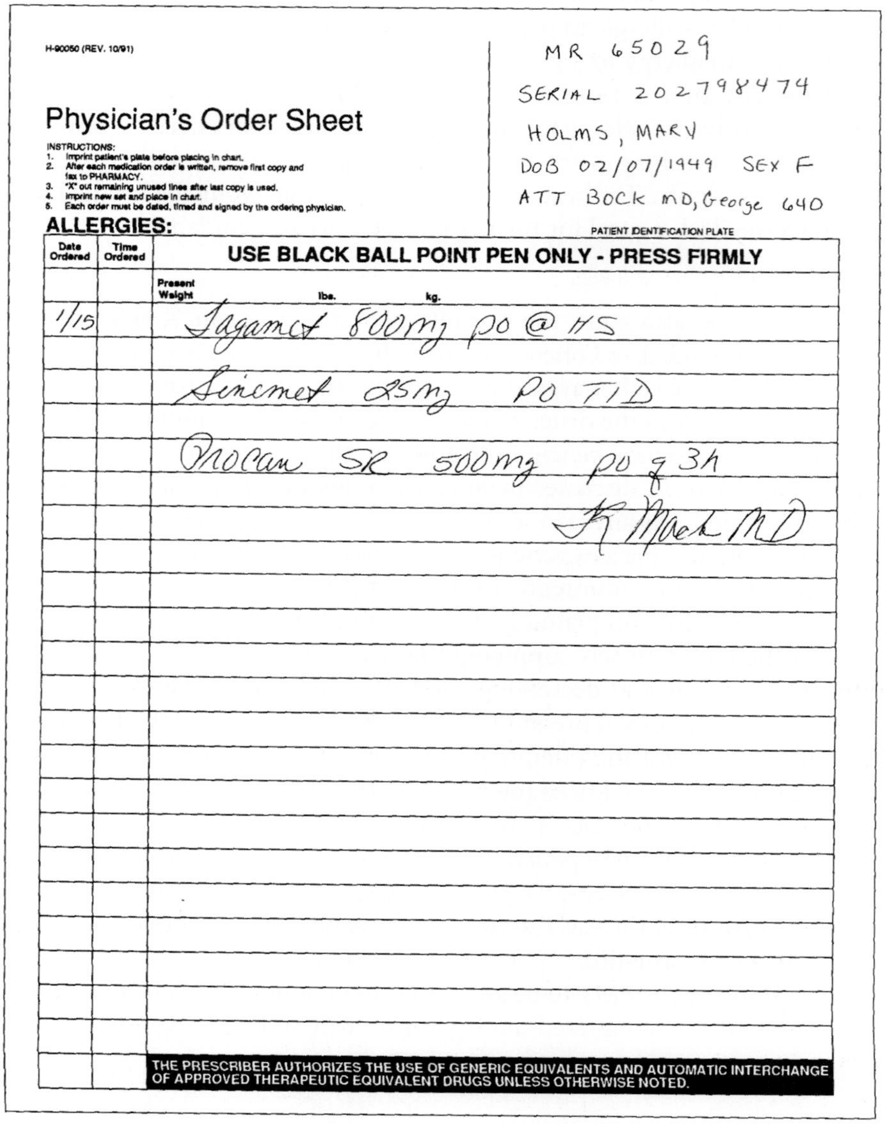
H-90050 (REV. 10/91)

Physician's Order Sheet

INSTRUCTIONS:
1. Imprint patient's plate before placing in chart.
2. After each medication order is written, remove first copy and fax to PHARMACY.
3. "X" out remaining unused lines after last copy is used.
4. Imprint new set and place in chart.
5. Each order must be dated, timed and signed by the ordering physician.

ALLERGIES:

MR 65029
SERIAL 202798474
HOLMS, MARY
DOB 02/07/1949 SEX F
ATT BOCK MD, George 640
PATIENT IDENTIFICATION PLATE

Date Ordered	Time Ordered	USE BLACK BALL POINT PEN ONLY - PRESS FIRMLY
		Present Weight lbs. kg.
1/15		Tagamet 800mg po @ HS
		Sinemet 25mg PO TID
		Procan SR 500mg po q 3h
		K Mack MD

THE PRESCRIBER AUTHORIZES THE USE OF GENERIC EQUIVALENTS AND AUTOMATIC INTERCHANGE OF APPROVED THERAPEUTIC EQUIVALENT DRUGS UNLESS OTHERWISE NOTED.

Figure 13.1 The EMT should be able to recognize the abbreviations commonly used to describe medication dosing

Table 13-2 Common Prescribing Abbreviations

Abbreviation	Meaning
bid	Twice daily
IM	Intramuscularly
IV	Intravenously
PO	By mouth
PR	Per rectum
prn	As needed
qid	Four times daily
SC	Subcutaneously
SL	Sublingually
tid	Three times daily

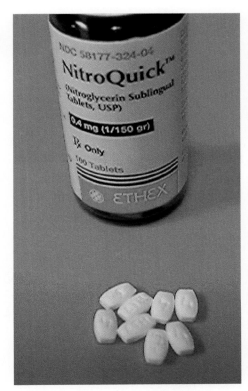

Figure 13.2 Some medications are produced as a powder and are compressed into tablet shape for administration

FORMS OF MEDICATIONS

Medications come in many different physical forms. Some may be liquids, others may be solid tablets or powders, and some may be in gas form. The EMT should be familiar with all the possible medication forms encountered during patient care.

COMPRESSED POWDERS AND TABLETS

Some medications are produced as a powder and are easily compressed into a tablet shape for ease of measurement and administration. Tablets are usually placed in the mouth to be either swallowed or dissolved and absorbed. Nitroglycerin is an example of a tablet meant to be placed under the tongue to dissolve (Figure 13.2).

Certain medications must be inhaled into the lungs to act directly on the airways. These medicines may be in a powdered form. Inhalers used by patients with chronic respiratory problems may contain powdered medications that are aerosolized to be inhaled directly into the airways, or they may be a dry powder delivered through a special inhaler that releases the powder when the patient inhales quickly. Figure 13.3 shows a dry powder inhaler.

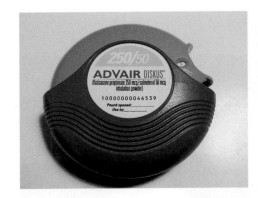

Figure 13.3 Dry powder inhaler (Photo courtesy of Brooke Wilson)

LIQUIDS

Medications such as epinephrine come in a liquid form that must be injected into a muscle to be absorbed and be effective (Figure 13.4).

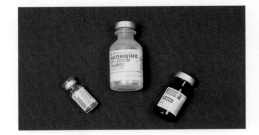

Figure 13.4 Medications may come in a liquid meant for injection

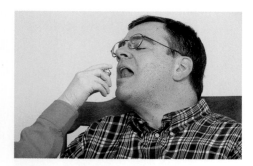

Figure 13.5 The EMT will assist a patient to take nitroglycerin in either tablet or spray form

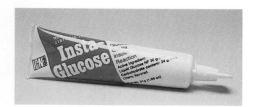

Figure 13.6 Oral glucose is a medication that is commonly marketed in a gel form for ease of administration

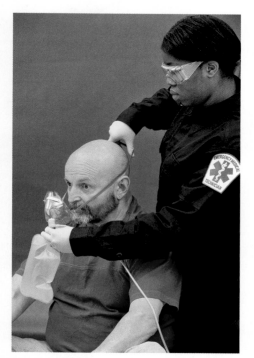

Figure 13.7 The EMT commonly administers oxygen

Some medications are in a liquid form that can be absorbed under the tongue into the many blood vessels located there. *Sublingual* is a term used to describe the space under the tongue. Nitroglycerin also comes in a liquid form (spray) for placement under the tongue (Figure 13.5).

GELS

Oral glucose is an example of a medication commonly formed as a gel for ease of administration and absorption (Figure 13.6). Gel medications are most often designed to be administered orally because they can be easily absorbed through the well-vascularized mucous membranes of the mouth.

Safety Tips

If an EMT is using medications in a liquid form for injection, he must be familiar with the proper handling of needles. Every health care provider must abide by important safety rules when handling needles to avoid inadvertent injury. Great care should always be taken to properly handle and dispose of sharp instruments such as needles. Unit 11 reviews these principles.

Street Smart

Gel medications are often quite temperature sensitive. A very warm environment may cause the gel to melt, resulting in easy spilling of the medication. Similarly, a very cold environment may cause the gel to harden. Frozen glucose gel is hard to get out of its container and does no good for the patient. Medications should be stored in a climate-controlled environment.

SUSPENSIONS

Some medications are initially in a powder form, but to make them more palatable to the patient, they are suspended, or mixed, in a liquid. This powder suspended in a liquid is referred to as a **suspension** taken orally by patients once it has been mixed.

GASES

An example of a medication in a gas form is oxygen. Special administration systems are often required to administer a gas to a patient while avoiding excess leakage into the environment, where it can be inhaled by the health care providers. Most often, a pressurized tank will be attached to a mask, which can then be applied to the patient's face (Figure 13.7).

AEROSOLS

Liquid medications may also be inhaled and absorbed directly into the airways. Examples of inhaled liquid medicines are bronchodilators, medications often used for asthma.

These liquids can be placed in a device that will be attached to an air source and aerosolized into the air so that the liquid is broken up into tiny particles and can easily be inhaled. This device is called a **nebulizer** and is commonly used by asthma patients (Figure 13.8).

MEDICATION ADMINISTRATION PROCEDURE

Before administering medications, the EMT must assess the patient and determine whether a medication is appropriate for the given condition. It is imperative for the EMT to thoroughly assess the patient and the need for the medication as well as the presence of any allergies to medications. After medication administration, the EMT also must continually reassess the patient to see whether the drug had its desired effect or any unwanted side effects.

PATIENT ASSESSMENT

The EMT should accomplish a complete patient assessment as appropriate for the individual patient. The assessment should include the primary assessment followed by the secondary assessment, including the physical examination, a focused history, and vital sign measurements. A complete medication history is needed if a medication is to be administered. A complete medication history should include current prescriptions, over-the-counter medications, and herbal or homeopathic medications the patient is taking, along with information about any allergies to medications.

THE "FIVE RIGHTS" OF DRUG ADMINISTRATION

The EMT must address a standard set of questions each time a medication is administered, no matter how routine it may seem. These questions address whether the medication is safe and appropriate for the given situation (Figure 13.9).

Street Smart

Just as patients sometimes carry medications without prescription labels on them, some people also tend to carry medicines not in their original containers. If a medication is not in its labeled container and the EMT cannot be sure of what the drug actually is, it should not be administered. The potential for significant harm exists if an inappropriate medication is inadvertently given to a patient.

THE RIGHT PATIENT

The EMT must determine whether the medication in question is indicated for that particular patient. If it is a prescribed medicine, does the prescription label have that patient's name on it? The EMT should never administer medication that belongs to someone other than the patient.

If the medication does not have a prescription label on it, the EMT must use his judgment to determine whether the drug is actually prescribed to the patient. If there is any question about who is actually prescribed the medicine, the EMT should speak with a medical control physician for

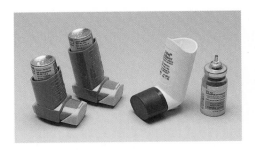

Figure 13.8 A metered dose inhaler (MDI) allows aerosolization of a liquid medication for inhalation

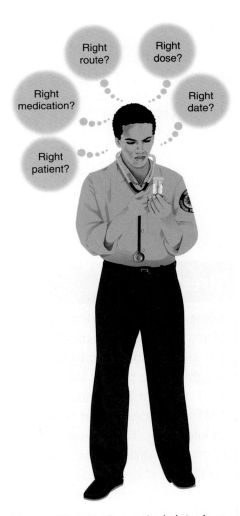

Figure 13.9 Before administering medication, the EMT must ensure the right patient, medication, route, dose, and date

advice on the situation. When in doubt, the safest course is to withhold the medication.

THE RIGHT MEDICATION

In addition to ensuring that the medication in question belongs to the patient, the EMT must be certain that it is the right drug for the patient's current problem. The name of the drug should be clearly labeled on the packaging. Many elderly patients will put pills in a container organized by the day and time they should be taken. Additionally, patients may have several different medications in the same container. If the medication is not clearly labeled, it should not be administered to the patent.

THE RIGHT ROUTE

Once the EMT is certain of the right patient and the right drug, the right route of administration must be determined. Most prescription labels will state which route (e.g., oral, intramuscular) should be used. If a medication is administered by the wrong route, the result may be detrimental to the patient or have no effect on the condition being treated. For example, nitroglycerin works quickly by being absorbed by the mucous membranes under the tongue. If the patient swallows the nitro tablet, the desired immediate effect on the patient's condition will not occur.

If any doubt exists, the EMT should ask the patient how she normally takes the medicine. If asking the patient does not clear things up, the EMT should speak with a medical control physician. The use of online medical control is discussed in detail in Units 21 and 23.

Street Smart

Some medications, such as prescribed inhalers and nitroglycerin, are frequently carried around by the patient and may not have a prescription label on the medication itself. Often, the prescription label was placed by the pharmacist on the cardboard box in which the drug was initially dispensed.

The box is inconvenient to carry around, so the patient will usually take the inhaler or bottle of medicine out of the box and carry it individually. An EMT is left to wonder whether the prescription belongs to the patient or to someone else.

A good rule of thumb is to trust the patient in this matter. If she claims that the medication is her own, it is usually safe to believe her. Of course, if there is any question in the EMT's mind, the drug should not be given.

Street Smart

Some medications are dosed in terms of a unit of medication per kilogram of patient body weight. If the patient tells the EMT a weight in pounds, the EMT must convert that figure to kilograms. This conversion is made by dividing the number of pounds by 2.2. This calculation provides the number of kilograms of body weight. For example, 110 lb equals 50 kg ($110 \div 2.2 = 50$).

THE RIGHT DOSE

Medications are prescribed in a particular dose, or amount. When administering a medication, the EMT must be certain that the correct dose is given. Underdosing a patient will result in the medication having little effect. Giving a patient too much, or an overdose, of the drug may result in serious harm. It is important to remember once a medication has been given, it cannot be taken back. The label of a prescribed medication will specify how many tablets, sprays, or units of a drug to use. The EMT must understand the difference in dosing for pediatric and adult patients.

If administering a medication such as oxygen, oral glucose, or activated charcoal, the EMT should follow local protocols. The usual doses of medications the EMT will commonly use will be reviewed.

THE RIGHT DATE

When medications are made, they are not guaranteed to remain in the same form, or at the same strength, over an indefinite period of time. Usually, the manufacturer will guarantee the medication to be safe and effective for a certain period of time after its production. Beyond this guaranteed time frame, the medication may be less potent or may even degenerate into a potentially harmful compound.

All medications have what is known as the **expiration date.** This date identifies the length of time that a medication remains effective. Medications should never be used past their expiration date.

The EMT must always check the date on any medication to ensure that it has not expired. An expired medication should never be administered.

ROUTES OF ADMINISTRATION

Just as there are many forms of medication, there are many ways to administer these drugs. The EMT must be familiar with the many routes of drug administration.

INHALATION

Liquid, powdered, or gaseous medicines may be inhaled into the lungs, where they will come into direct contact with airways. Most often, these medicines are meant to act on the airways directly; therefore, applying them directly makes sense. The patient usually must be conscious and breathing for inhaled medications to be effective. The EMT may be asked to assist ventilations using a bag-valve-mask device that advanced life support (ALS) providers use to administer an inhaled medication, such as a bronchodilator. The EMT will learn to assist a patient in taking specific previously prescribed inhaled medicines.

SUBLINGUAL

The space under the tongue has many blood vessels very close to the surface. If a medication is allowed to dissolve in this sublingual space, it will be well absorbed into these blood vessels. The patient must be alert for medication to be administered through this route. Medications administered orally or sublingually to a patient who is unresponsive or not alert could become an airway obstruction. Sublingual administration is an effective route for medicines that require rapid absorption, such as nitroglycerin.

INJECTION

Some medications are not effective unless they are injected with a needle directly into or very near a blood vessel. There are several means of injecting liquid medicines.

SUBCUTANEOUS

Injecting the medicine just under the skin in the subcutaneous tissue allows the medicine to be gradually absorbed into a blood vessel (Figure 13.10). This subcutaneous space is made up of fat and tiny blood vessels, and the medicine will be slowly absorbed into the tiny blood vessels. Insulin, a medicine used by diabetic patients, must be injected subcutaneously.

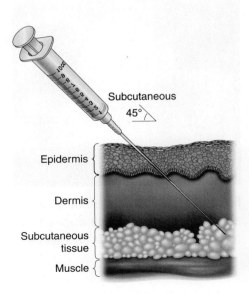

Figure 13.10 The subcutaneous space is just under the skin

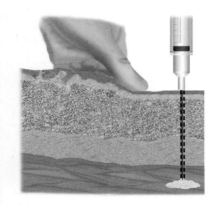

Figure 13.11 Epinephrine is commonly administered into the intramuscular space in an emergency

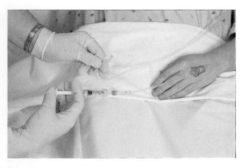

Figure 13.12 Advanced-level providers can access the intravenous space to directly administer medications into the bloodstream

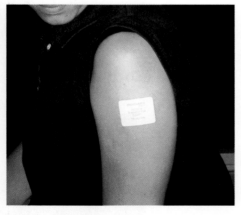

Figure 13.13 A transdermal patch allows medication to be applied topically to the skin for absorption

INTRAMUSCULAR

If the medicine must be delivered closer to a larger blood vessel, but it is not desirable to inject it directly into a vessel, the medicine may be administered into a muscle, or **intramuscularly** (Figure 13.11).

Medicines such as epinephrine may be given in this manner because it is desirable to have fairly rapid absorption into the bloodstream, but direct intravenous injection may be potentially harmful.

INTRAVENOUS

If a medication is injected directly into a blood vessel, it is being given **intravenously.** Medication injected intravenously has a rapid onset. This route will not be used by the EMT-Basic but is used regularly by more advanced-level providers to administer medications directly into the bloodstream (Figure 13.12).

ORAL

Perhaps the most familiar route of medication administration is by direct oral consumption. When a medication is swallowed, it is being given by the **oral** route. Most medicines are prescribed for oral use. Although the EMT will not often have occasion to administer a drug orally, an example of an orally administered drug is aspirin. The patient must be alert and conscious for any medication that is administered by mouth.

TOPICAL

It is sometimes desirable to allow a medication to be absorbed slowly and gradually. Some medications can be made into a paste or gel-like material that can be applied to the skin under a patch of waterproof material (Figure 13.13). This method of drug administration is called **topical.**

This topical application of a medication is a way to allow slow absorption through the skin over time. Nitroglycerin is made in the form of a topical patch, as are some medications for chronic pain. EMTs will not administer medications topically; however, the EMT may encounter patients who have a chronic condition that is being treated with medication patches.

MEDICAL CONTROL

There is perhaps no place in the EMT's practice in which it is more necessary to have physician input than in the administration of medications. Medications are prescribed by a licensed physician or by the physician's designee. When the EMT administers a medication, he is acting as the designee and therefore must follow the physician's instructions in this matter. The EMT should be familiar with and follow local protocols on administration or assisted administration of medications.

OFF-LINE MEDICAL CONTROL

It is important for a physician to have input in the preparation of protocols as well as in the quality review of instances of medication administration. Off-line medical controls are written (standing) order or protocol for the EMT to follow if the physician is not available for direct communication. Off-line medical control is of key importance in the EMT's practice.

STANDING ORDERS AND PROTOCOLS

When instructions for caring for particular types of patients are written down and made into a policy, they are referred to as *protocols*. Protocols that allow medication administration or procedures to be done in certain circumstances are known as *standing orders*.

An EMT does not have to contact medical control to perform procedures allowed under standing orders. Of course, if there is ever a question about the appropriateness of the procedure or medication administration, the EMT should discuss it with medical control.

ON-LINE MEDICAL CONTROL

An EMT's direct communication with a medical control physician during the course of caring for a patient is referred to as *on-line medical control*. Local protocols require on-line medical control in specific situations. The EMT should be familiar with local protocols and requirements for contacting medical control.

When an on-line medical control physician orders the administration of a medication, it is the EMTs responsibility to verify the order prior to administration to reduce the chances of the inappropriate administration or administration of the wrong drug. The EMT should verify the order by repeating the name and dose of the drug and the route of administration back to the ordering physician. If there is confusion over any part of the order, the EMT must clarify with on-line medical control prior to administering the medication.

In many situations, the EMT must use his clinical judgment when a patient's condition changes before the medication ordered is administered. As an example, a patient who is confused or incoherent but awake and showing the signs and symptoms of low blood glucose would usually be treated with oral glucose gel. The EMT obtains an order by on-line medical control to administer oral glucose; however, before the medication can be administered, the patient becomes unconscious. In this case, the EMT should not administer the oral glucose, because medications should not be given by mouth to an unconscious patient. The EMT should contact medical control, advise the physician of the change in patient condition, and ask if there are any further orders from medical direction for care of the patient.

REASSESSMENT

After any intervention has been provided to a patient, including medication administration, the EMT must perform a thorough reassessment. A reassessment should be done and documented within 5 minutes after the medication has been given. The reassessment findings should be recorded. The primary assessment should quickly be reviewed, and then the relevant parts of the focused exam should be reviewed. The patient should be questioned about any changes in symptoms, and a complete set of vital signs should be obtained. The results of the reassessment should be noted, with special attention to any changes.

DOCUMENTATION

As with any other aspect of patient care, when it comes to medication administration, it is not over until the paperwork is done. It is critically important that the EMT completely document the patient interaction.

Documentation should include the findings on the patient assessment and the history that led the EMT to administer a medication. The EMT should carefully consider local protocols when deciding to administer a medication for a particular problem.

The exact name of the medication, dose, and route should be carefully documented, as well as the time it was administered and by whom.

The symptoms and signs that led the EMT to administer the medication should be addressed in the reassessment. Any contact with medical control should be accurately documented in the Prehospital Care Report as well. Figure 13.14 illustrates the appropriate documentation of nitroglycerin administration.

Safety Tips

Because the medication on a topical patch is absorbed through the skin, the EMT should handle these patches only while wearing gloves to avoid any absorption of the drug into his body.

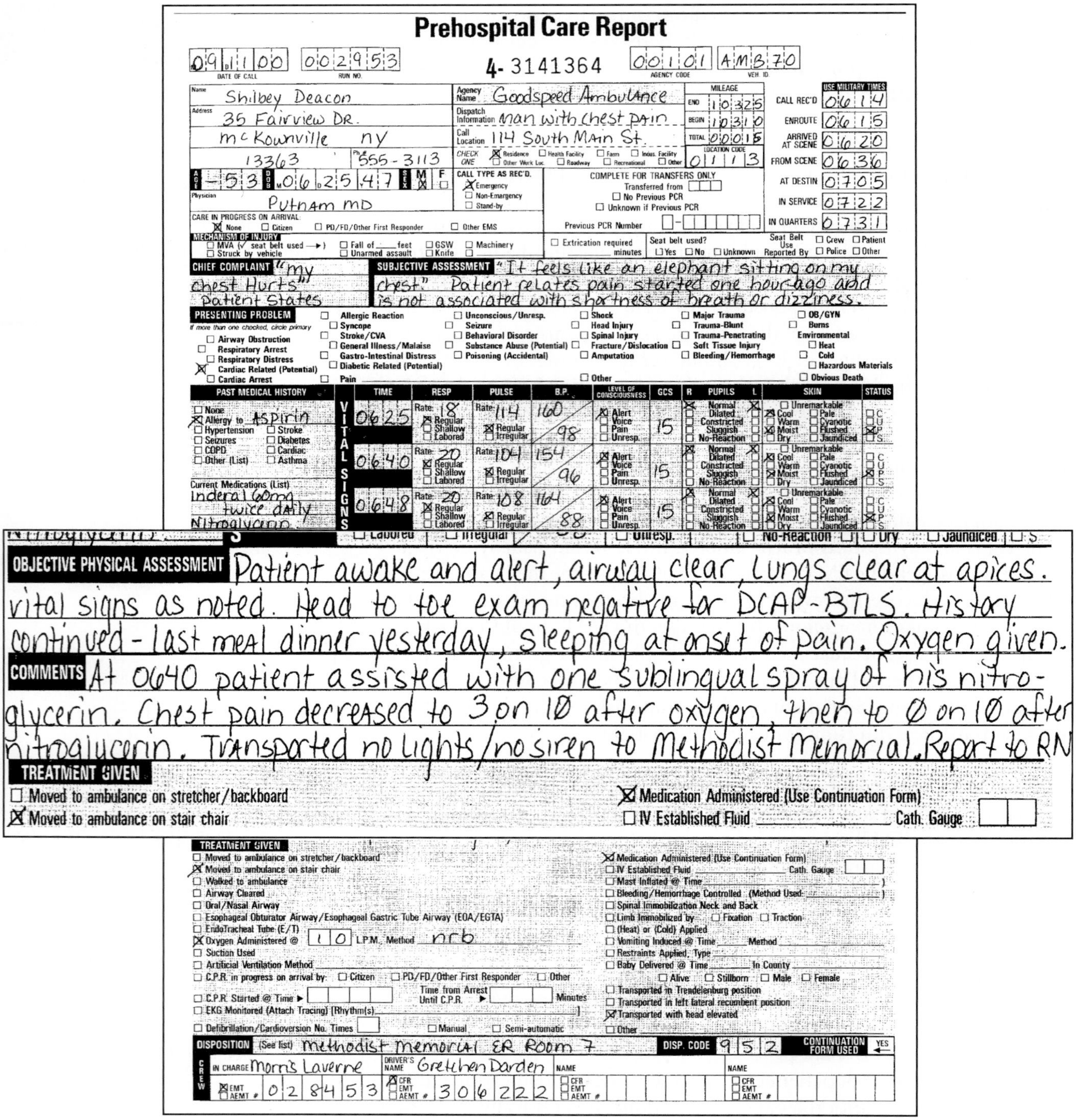

Prehospital Care Report

`[0 9 1 1 0 0]` DATE OF CALL `[0 0 2 9 5 3]` RUN NO.   **4- 3141364**   `[0 0 1 0 1]` AGENCY CODE `[A M B 7 0]` VEH. ID.

Name **Shilbey Deacon**	Agency Name **Goodspeed Ambulance**
Address **35 Fairview Dr.**	Dispatch Information **man with chest pain**
mcKownville ny	Call Location **114 South Main St**
13363 Ph **555-3113**	

MILEAGE: END `[1 0 3 2 5]` BEGIN `[1 0 3 1 0]` TOTAL `[0 0 0 0 1 5]`

USE MILITARY TIMES:
CALL REC'D `[0 6 1 4]`
ENROUTE `[0 6 1 5]`
ARRIVED AT SCENE `[0 6 2 0]`
FROM SCENE `[0 6 3 0]`
AT DESTIN `[0 7 0 5]`
IN SERVICE `[0 7 2 2]`
IN QUARTERS `[0 7 3 1]`

CHECK ONE: ☒ Residence ☐ Health Facility ☐ Farm ☐ Indus. Facility
☐ Other Work Loc. ☐ Roadway ☐ Recreational ☐ Other

LOCATION CODE `[0 1 1 3]`

AGE `[5 3]` DOB `[0 6 2 5 4 7]` ☒ M ☐ F

Physician **Putnam MD**

CALL TYPE AS REC'D.: ☒ Emergency ☐ Non-Emergency ☐ Stand-by

COMPLETE FOR TRANSFERS ONLY: Transferred from ☐ ☐ ☐
☐ No Previous PCR ☐ Unknown if Previous PCR
Previous PCR Number `[ - ]`

CARE IN PROGRESS ON ARRIVAL: ☒ None ☐ Citizen ☐ PD/FD/Other First Responder ☐ Other EMS

MECHANISM OF INJURY: ☐ MVA (√ seat belt used →) ☐ Fall of ___ feet ☐ GSW ☐ Machinery ☐ Extrication required Seat belt used? ☐ Yes ☐ No ☐ Unknown Reported By Seat Belt Use ☐ Crew ☐ Patient ☐ Police ☐ Other
☐ Struck by vehicle ☐ Unarmed assault ☐ Knife minutes

CHIEF COMPLAINT "my chest Hurts" Patient States

SUBJECTIVE ASSESSMENT "It feels like an elephant sitting on my chest" Patient relates pain started one hour ago and is not associated with shortness of breath or dizziness.

PRESENTING PROBLEM (If more than one checked, circle primary)
☐ Allergic Reaction ☐ Unconscious/Unresp. ☐ Shock ☐ Major Trauma ☐ OB/GYN
☐ Airway Obstruction ☐ Syncope ☐ Seizure ☐ Head Injury ☐ Trauma-Blunt ☐ Burns
☐ Respiratory Arrest ☐ Stroke/CVA ☐ Behavioral Disorder ☐ Spinal Injury ☐ Trauma-Penetrating Environmental
☐ Respiratory Distress ☐ General Illness/Malaise ☐ Substance Abuse (Potential) ☐ Fracture/Dislocation ☐ Soft Tissue Injury ☐ Heat
☒ Cardiac Related (Potential) ☐ Gastro-Intestinal Distress ☐ Poisoning (Accidental) ☐ Amputation ☐ Bleeding/Hemorrhage ☐ Cold
☐ Cardiac Arrest ☐ Diabetic Related (Potential) ☐ Pain ☐ Other ☐ Hazardous Materials ☐ Obvious Death

PAST MEDICAL HISTORY
☐ None
☒ Allergy to **Aspirin**
☐ Hypertension ☐ Stroke
☐ Seizures ☐ Diabetes
☐ COPD ☐ Cardiac
☐ Other (List) ☐ Asthma

Current Medications (List)
Inderal 60mg twice daily
Nitroglycerin

VITAL SIGNS	TIME	RESP	PULSE	B.P.	LEVEL OF CONSCIOUSNESS	GCS	R PUPILS L	SKIN	STATUS
	0625	Rate: 18 ☒Regular ☐Shallow ☐Labored	Rate: 114 ☒Regular ☐Irregular	160 / 98	☒Alert ☐Voice ☐Pain ☐Unresp.	15	Normal/Dilated/Constricted/Sluggish/No-Reaction	☐Cool ☒Warm ☒Moist ☐Dry / ☐Unremarkable ☐Pale ☐Cyanotic ☐Flushed ☐Jaundiced	☐C ☐U ☒P ☐S
	0640	Rate: 20 ☒Regular ☐Shallow ☐Labored	Rate: 104 ☒Regular ☐Irregular	154 / 96	☒Alert ☐Voice ☐Pain ☐Unresp.	15	Normal/Dilated/Constricted/Sluggish/No-Reaction	☐Cool ☒Warm ☒Moist ☐Dry / ☐Unremarkable ☐Pale ☐Cyanotic ☐Flushed ☐Jaundiced	☐C ☐U ☒P ☐S
	0648	Rate: 20 ☒Regular ☐Shallow ☐Labored	Rate: 108 ☒Regular ☐Irregular	164 / 88	☒Alert ☐Voice ☐Pain ☐Unresp.	15	Normal/Dilated/Constricted/Sluggish/No-Reaction	☐Cool ☒Warm ☒Moist ☐Dry / ☐Unremarkable ☐Pale ☐Cyanotic ☐Flushed ☐Jaundiced	☐C ☐U ☒P ☐S

OBJECTIVE PHYSICAL ASSESSMENT Patient awake and alert, airway clear, Lungs clear at apices. vital signs as noted. Head to toe exam negative for DCAP-BTLS. History continued - last meal dinner yesterday, sleeping at onset of pain. Oxygen given.

COMMENTS At 0640 patient assisted with one sublingual spray of his nitroglycerin. Chest pain decreased to 3 on 10 after oxygen, then to Ø on 10 after nitroglucerin. Transported no lights/no siren to Methodist Memorial. Report to RN

TREATMENT GIVEN
☐ Moved to ambulance on stretcher/backboard
☒ Moved to ambulance on stair chair
☒ Medication Administered (Use Continuation Form)
☐ IV Established Fluid Cath. Gauge ☐ ☐

TREATMENT GIVEN
☐ Moved to ambulance on stretcher/backboard
☒ Moved to ambulance on stair chair
☐ Walked to ambulance
☐ Airway Cleared
☐ Oral/Nasal Airway
☐ Esophageal Obturator Airway/Esophageal Gastric Tube Airway (EOA/EGTA)
☐ EndoTracheal Tube (E/T)
☒ Oxygen Administered @ `[1 0]` L.P.M. Method **nrb**
☐ Suction Used
☐ Artificial Ventilation Method
☐ C.P.R. in progress on arrival by: ☐ Citizen ☐ PD/FD/Other First Responder ☐ Other
☐ C.P.R. Started @ Time ► Time from Arrest Until C.P.R. ___ Minutes
☐ EKG Monitored (Attach Tracing) (Rhythm(s))
☐ Defibrillation/Cardioversion No. Times ___ ☐ Manual ☐ Semi-automatic

☒ Medication Administered (Use Continuation Form)
☐ IV Established Fluid Cath. Gauge ☐ ☐
☐ Mast Inflated @ Time ___
☐ Bleeding/Hemorrhage Controlled (Method Used ___)
☐ Spinal Immobilization Neck and Back
☐ Limb Immobilized by ☐ Fixation ☐ Traction
☐ (Heat) or (Cold) Applied
☐ Vomiting Induced @ Time ___ Method ___
☐ Restraints Applied, Type ___
☐ Baby Delivered @ Time ___ ☐ In County
  ☐ Alive ☐ Stillborn ☐ Male ☐ Female
☐ Transported in Trendelenburg position
☐ Transported in left lateral recumbent position
☒ Transported with head elevated
☐ Other

DISPOSITION (See list) **Methodist Memorial ER Room 7** DISP. CODE `[9 5 2]` CONTINUATION FORM USED ☐ YES

CREW: IN CHARGE **Morris Laverne** ☒EMT # `[0 2 8 4 5 3]` ☐AEMT DRIVER'S NAME **Gretchen Darden** ☒CFR EMT # `[3 0 6 2 2 2]` ☐AEMT NAME ☐CFR ☐EMT ☐AEMT # NAME ☐CFR ☐EMT ☐AEMT #

Figure 13.14 It is imperative for medication administration to be thoroughly documented

ADMINISTERED AND ASSISTED MEDICATIONS

There are two types of medications an EMT will handle in the prehospital setting. The first are medications the EMT carries on the ambulance and administers to a patient based on the indications presented by the patient. These are not medications that have been specifically prescribed for the patient by a physician. The second are those medications that an EMT may assist a patient in taking and are medications that have been prescribed for the patient.

ADMINISTERED EMERGENCY MEDICATIONS

In the first category, the EMT bases the administration of specific medications on the indications and local protocols or orders from medical control. These medications are stocked and carried in the ambulance. Examples of these medications are oxygen, oral glucose, and in some areas epinephrine or albuterol. Some agencies may include other medications on this list. As usual, the EMT should be familiar with local protocols.

OXYGEN

Oxygen is a colorless gas the body needs in adequate amounts to function normally. It is used to produce energy by all of the tissues of the body. Oxygen is found in the ambient air taken into the body through respiration at a concentration of 21%. Without appropriate amounts of oxygen, systems of the body begin to fail. When the body is not receiving adequate oxygen, common signs and symptoms will appear, indicating a need for supplemental or replacement oxygen administration.

An EMT should administer oxygen to any patient who complains of respiratory difficulty or has any potentially cardiac-related concern. Patients who show evidence of poor oxygen supply to the brain, as seen in stroke patients, seizure patients, or patients with an altered mental status, would also benefit from oxygen administration. Patients suspected to be in shock should be given oxygen to try to increase the oxygen content of the blood. Each of these conditions will be discussed in detail later in this text.

ADMINISTRATION PROCEDURE—OXYGEN

As discussed in Unit 10, oxygen may be administered in a variety of ways depending on the patient's condition. If the patient is not breathing, the oxygen must be administered with positive pressure ventilations as given by a bag-valve-mask, pocket mask, oxygen-powered ventilation device, or transport ventilation device.

If the patient is ventilating adequately on her own, the EMT should apply supplemental oxygen to allow the patient to breathe in a higher concentration of oxygen than is in the ambient air. A non-rebreather mask is the most appropriate device used to administer high-concentration oxygen to a patient in need of this medication. If the patient does not tolerate this mask or does not need such a high concentration of oxygen, a nasal cannula may be used.

ASPIRIN

After calling 9-1-1, in the case of a suspected heart attack, the American Heart Association recommends that patients who are able should take aspirin. Aspirin prevents the platelets in the blood from sticking together and forming blood clots or can help to prevent a clot from becoming larger. Aspirin, given early, has been shown to significantly improve the patient's chances of survival from an acute coronary event, such as acute myocardial infarction. Some EMS systems permit an EMT to either administer aspirin to a patient with symptoms of an acute coronary event or to assist the patient with self-administration of aspirin.

Aspirin should not be given to a patient with active bleeding or to those with a bleeding disorder such as hemophilia. Similarly, aspirin should not be given to patients who are allergic to aspirin or who have aspirin-induced asthma.

Aspirin is usually given in doses from 81 milligrams (mg) to 325 mg immediately following the onset of symptoms associated with an acute coronary event. Often one to four chewable baby aspirins or one adult aspirin is administered.

Pediatric Considerations

Young children often will not tolerate having a mask applied to their face. If an EMT wants to supply a small child with supplemental oxygen and the child will not allow a non-rebreather mask to be placed on her face, the EMT may choose to administer oxygen through a method called blow-by.

This is a technique whereby oxygen tubing or a pediatric oxygen mask is placed near the patient's mouth and nose and high-flow oxygen is delivered into the air directly in front of the face. In this position, the child will breathe in a higher concentration of oxygen than is in regular room air, although not as high as with the non-rebreather mask. Asking the parent to hold the oxygen source is usually helpful because the child may not feel as threatened with a parent nearby.

In some cases, the patient may already take aspirin daily as part of a medical regimen to prevent an acute coronary event. Those patients may take another dose of aspirin without risk of harm.

ORAL GLUCOSE

Glucose is a substance used by the body for fuel. All the body organs, especially the brain, depend on this important carbohydrate for energy. The body regulates the blood glucose levels carefully with special hormones.

Insulin is a hormone that helps the body use glucose effectively. Because insulin assists the body in using glucose, it lowers the blood glucose level. Most people have the ability to release glucose from stored supplies if the blood level gets too low. People with a condition called diabetes may not be able to do this.

People with diabetes take medicines, such as insulin, that help them use their glucose and keep the blood level balanced. Sometimes their glucose level gets out of balance and becomes either too high or too low. A person with very low blood glucose levels, called *hypoglycemia*, will show some specific signs and symptoms that indicate the need for oral glucose administration. Signs and symptoms of hypoglycemia include shakiness, tremulousness, tachycardia, moist skin, dizziness, and confusion. If hypoglycemia is allowed to progress to the point where the glucose levels are so low that the brain no longer has enough fuel to function, the patient may become unconscious or may suffer a seizure.

If an EMT is treating a patient who has these symptoms and a low blood glucose level is suspected, oral glucose is indicated. When oral glucose is administered to a patient with low blood glucose, the glucose level in the blood will rise and the patient's symptoms should rapidly resolve.

Oral glucose administration should only be administered to a patient capable of swallowing the gel-like material. If the patient is unconscious or otherwise unable to swallow, it is dangerous to put any substance in her mouth because it may create an airway obstruction or be aspirated into the lungs.

If the EMT is unable to administer oral glucose but believes the patient suffers from hypoglycemia, he must make every effort to intercept with an advanced-level provider who can give glucose intravenously. If a hospital is closer than the advanced life support (ALS) intercept, then the EMT should bring the patient immediately to the closest hospital.

ADMINISTRATION PROCEDURE—ORAL GLUCOSE

Once the EMT has determined that it is safe to administer oral glucose, the next step is to check the "five rights" as discussed earlier, then open the medication container. The patient will often be able to hold the tube of glucose on her own and suck the sweet gel out. The EMT may have to help by squeezing small amounts of the glucose material into the patient's mouth (Figure 13.15).

If at any time the EMT becomes concerned that the patient is not swallowing effectively or the patency of the airway becomes questionable, he should immediately stop administration of the medication and suction out any remaining material.

When documenting oral glucose administration, as with any medication administration, the EMT should take care to note the patient's condition before and after its administration.

Even if the patient's condition has completely resolved after oral glucose administration, the patient should be evaluated by a physician. If the patient resists being transported, the EMT should contact a medical control physician, explain the situation, and ask for instruction.

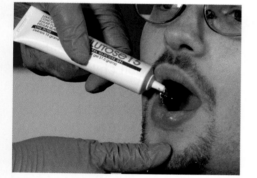

Figure 13.15 Oral glucose is given to the conscious patient suffering a diabetic emergency

Street Smart

A good rule of thumb in oral glucose administration is that if the patient is awake and swallowing her own secretions, she can safely be given oral glucose. If she is not awake or is drooling profusely, then it is not safe to give anything by mouth for fear the patient may aspirate the glucose into the lungs.

ASSISTED EMERGENCY MEDICATIONS

The second type of medication the EMT must be familiar with are those that they may help a patient use that have been specifically prescribed for that patient by a physician. The EMT should confirm that the medication has been prescribed for that patient to treat the exact symptom or disease process that seems to be affecting the patient when the EMT is asked to help administer the medication.

The EMT is relying on the fact that the patient has been diagnosed by a physician with a condition that could benefit from the medication in question. Perhaps more importantly, the physician has determined that the risk to using the medication for that patient is low. An EMT does not have the training or licensure to allow diagnosis of diseases or assessment of the risk for administering controlled substances to individuals.

DEFINITIONS

Several terms in this text may be difficult to define in a universal way and should probably be left up to local and state agencies to define. EMTs should clarify in their own region what specifically is expected of them when dealing with prescribed medications. Local protocols should provide this clarification.

One of the terms that may differ in interpretation from state to state is *assist*. What exactly does allowing an EMT to assist a patient in taking her own medication mean? Each locale must decide and clarify in its protocols whether an EMT may hand the patient the medication, help the patient place her hand to her mouth to take the drug, or simply give the patient the substance if she is unable to take it herself. The definition of assist must be clear to every EMT.

INHALED BRONCHODILATORS

Many patients with lung diseases such as asthma, emphysema, and bronchitis use inhaled medications to help keep the airways open and ease their breathing. These medications, called **bronchodilators,** dilate or increase the diameter of the bronchioles, increasing airflow through the airway and into the alveoli in the lungs. Inhaled bronchodilators may come in the form of a metered dose inhaler. Patients may use other medicines in an inhaled form. However, only the bronchodilators will be quickly helpful to patients with constricted airways.

An example of a commonly used bronchodilator is albuterol (trade names Proventil and Ventolin), but there are certainly more. The EMT should review local protocols regarding which specific medications are approved for EMT assistance.

Metered dose inhalers (MDI) are handheld devices that carry a form of medication that may be aerosolized upon discharge of the inhaler device. The device expels a specific amount of medication with each puff; therefore, these types of medicines are often dosed in numbers of puffs rather than in milligrams.

This aerosolized medication can then be inhaled by the patient, allowing the medication to directly contact the constricted airways. It is this direct contact that allows this medication to exert immediate effects of relaxing the constricted airways. Figure 13.16 illustrates how these devices work to get medication into the airways.

If local protocols allow, the EMT may assist a patient to use a prescribed bronchodilator inhaler if the patient complains of shortness of breath and has been prescribed that specific medication for such a concern. After administration of this medication, the EMT should reassess the patient and document any changes in condition, concern, or vital signs.

Street Smart

Many patients using an inhaler will not wait 1 full minute between puffs. Taking a second puff too soon will not result in optimal relief and should be discouraged. It is useful for the EMT to carefully instruct the patient to use the inhaler properly to get the most benefit from the medication.

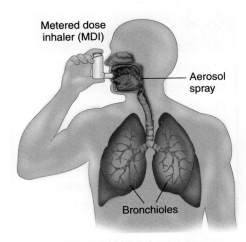

Figure 13.16 The metered dose inhaler aerosolizes medication for inhalation directly into the airways

Children (and some adults) may use a device called a *spacer* between the inhaler and their mouth to assist in coordination (Figure 13.17). This device reduces the coordination of breathing necessary to effectively administer the medication. The EMT should definitely use this device if it is available with the inhaler.

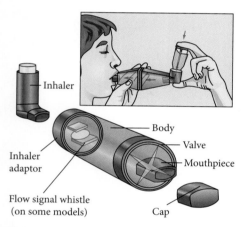

Inhaler

Body

Valve

Inhaler adaptor

Mouthpiece

Flow signal whistle (on some models)

Cap

Figure 13.17 A spacer is a device that is commonly used in conjunction with an inhaler, especially by children

In some areas, an EMT may be trained to administer albuterol by a nebulizer in specific circumstances. This may be useful if a patient is unable to cooperate enough for coordination of the metered dose inhaler. Further training should be provided to the EMT who will be administering albuterol by nebulizer.

ADMINISTRATION PROCEDURE

If the EMT is to assist a patient in using an inhaler, he must be familiar with the administration procedure. However, it is important for the EMT to complete the primary assessment before assisting the patient with any medications. When the patient has a decreased level of consciousness and cannot operate the inhaler with assistance or if the patient requires ventilatory assistance, the EMT should not attempt to administer the metered dose inhaler, because the medication would not be effective.

Once it has been decided that a metered dose inhaler is needed, the EMT should confirm the "five rights" as previously discussed and then prepare the inhaler for use. An inhaler comes with a cover over the mouthpiece that must be removed. The container must be shaken several times to suspend the medication inside it.

If the patient has allowed an oxygen mask, it should first be removed from the patient's face and the patient should be instructed to exhale, then inhale deeply. As the patient begins to inhale, the inhaler device should be held up to the mouth and a puff should be administered during the inhalation. The patient should continue the inhalation as long as possible and then should hold her breath as long as possible. This procedure allows a maximal amount of medication to enter the lungs and settle into the smaller airways, where it will have the greatest effect.

After holding her breath for a few seconds, the patient should be instructed to breathe normally for a minute while oxygen is reapplied. After 1 minute, the procedure is repeated a second time to administer a second puff of medication. The typical dose is two puffs. This skill can be reviewed in Skill 13-1 at the end of this chapter.

NITROGLYCERIN

Nitroglycerin is a medication that dilates, or opens, blood vessels. It specifically dilates the blood vessels that supply the heart with oxygenated blood, the coronary arteries. Widening these narrowed vessels during a possible heart attack may reduce or alleviate chest pain.

Sudden narrowing or blockage of a coronary artery will cause decreased blood supply to the heart. This decreased blood supply causes pain as the heart is without oxygen for a short period of time. Pain as a result of such lack of blood supply to the heart is known as *angina*. The details of cardiac disease will be discussed in detail in Unit 25.

The action of nitroglycerin is the vasodilation of narrowed coronary arteries, which reduces the workload on the heart by improving blood flow to the heart. This in turn improves oxygenation of the heart muscle and decreases or relieves the symptoms of angina (Figure 13.18). This medication is an important adjunct to the EMT's care of the heart attack victim.

Unfortunately, the use of nitroglycerin can produce an untoward side effect. As it dilates the coronary arteries, it also dilates many other vessels in the body, resulting in a fall in blood pressure. Sometimes this drop in blood pressure is insignificant; at other times it can be extremely serious. Whether any one patient will experience a drop in blood pressure cannot be predicted, so the EMT should be prepared for hypotension in any patient being given nitroglycerin.

The EMT should not assist a patient in taking nitroglycerin if the patient has a low blood pressure at the time of assessment. Local protocols will dictate what constitutes a low blood pressure, but many locales require a patient to have a minimal systolic blood pressure of 100 or 120 mmHg for nitroglycerin to be considered.

Some regions will not permit nitroglycerin administration without intravenous access having been established. This practice is to allow for rapid fluid administration in the event of a significant drop in blood pressure. If the EMT practices in a system that requires intravenous access prior to nitroglycerin administration, ALS intervention should be requested immediately if administration of nitroglycerin is indicated.

Another bothersome side effect that nitroglycerin commonly has is that of headache. This effect is also thought to be related to dilation of blood vessels in the head. This side effect is rarely serious and can be relieved with a dose of acetaminophen (Tylenol) or other mild analgesic by emergency department staff once the patient arrives at the hospital.

Nitroglycerin is administered in the form of a small tablet under the tongue, or via a spray sublingually. The dose of a single tablet is 0.4 mg and can be repeated every 5 minutes if the chest pain continues, as long as the blood pressure remains high enough to allow repeated administration. Usually, no more than three doses are used without consultation with a doctor.

The EMT must thoroughly assess the patient before medication administration and then reassess 2 to 5 minutes after the medication is given. Any changes in condition, symptoms, or vital signs should be recorded.

Local protocols may differ significantly in the regulations and requirements for nitroglycerin administration by the EMT. It is the responsibility of the EMT to be familiar with local protocols. If there is ever any question about the administration of nitroglycerin, as with any medication, the EMT should contact medical control for direction.

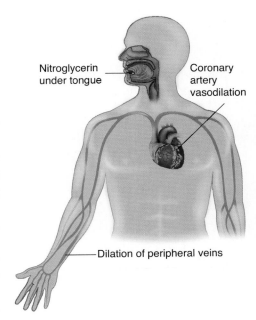

Figure 13.18 Nitroglycerin dilates blood vessels

Safety Tips

Knowing that hypotension can occur after administration of nitroglycerin, the street-smart EMT will ensure that the patient is seated or in the semi-Fowler position on the stretcher before helping her take this medication. In this position, if the patient's blood pressure should fall significantly, she is less likely to become dizzy or to fall down. Having her seated or reclining will protect the patient from being injured and will save the EMT the work of having to pick her up! In this situation, as in many faced by the EMT, it pays to be prepared for the worst possibility.

Street Smart

Nitroglycerin has a limited "shelf life." Light, heat, and especially moisture can "denature" nitroglycerin; to denature a drug is to render it impotent and therefore ineffective. An opened container of nitroglycerin tablets may only be potent for as little as 30 days. If the patient has self-administered nitroglycerin that is outdated or stored in packaging other than the original packaging, it may not be potent and therefore may not relieve the patient's symptoms.

Safety Tips

Nitroglycerin comes in many forms such as tablets, metered dose sprays, slow release patches, or paste that is meant to absorb through the skin slowly. Because of the potential for nitroglycerin to absorb through the skin, the EMT should always wear gloves when handling this medication to avoid unnecessary exposure and potential side effects.

Patients who call an ambulance and who require nitroglycerin may be suffering from a life-threatening condition. The EMT should never delay transport to administer nitroglycerin and should always attempt to intercept with an ALS agency if it is available so that advanced-level treatment may be given to the patient.

ADMINISTRATION PROCEDURE—NITROGLYCERIN

When assisting a patient to take nitroglycerin, the EMT must ensure that several steps have first been accomplished. A primary assessment should have been completed, including initiation of oxygen as appropriate. The focused history, including all the patient's medications and allergies, and physical examination should be completed. Transport decisions should be made and ALS intervention requested if available.

The patient suffering from cardiac chest pain requires timely transport to an appropriate hospital with an ALS intercept along the way if it does not delay arrival at the hospital. The EMT should consider nitroglycerin administration to the patient who is having chest pain that is believed to be cardiac in nature and who has been prescribed nitroglycerin.

The EMT should never assist a patient to use someone else's prescription for nitroglycerin. An EMT does not have sufficient training or licensure to diagnose cardiac disease or to prescribe medications for it. There are significant risks to using nitroglycerin inappropriately.

After completing the assessment, the EMT should be sure that the patient is comfortably seated or reclined, preferably on the stretcher. The "five rights" should be confirmed and the patient's systolic blood pressure is at least 100 mmHg (or whatever minimum number is dictated by local protocols). The EMT should then assist the patient in taking nitroglycerin according to local protocols.

After the medication has been administered, the EMT should carefully recheck the patient's vital signs and ask whether the discomfort has subsided Medical control is an important resource in assisting the EMT in making a wise treatment plan for the cardiac patient.

EPINEPHRINE

Epinephrine is a medication that dilates the airways and constricts the blood vessels. It is used commonly for an anaphylactic reaction to an allergen. Anaphylaxis can cause airway swelling, bronchoconstriction, dilation of blood vessels with hypotension, and hives, as discussed in Unit 11. This type of allergic reaction can come on within minutes; therefore, speed of administration of this medication is crucial.

Epinephrine is an effective antidote for this severe allergic reaction and is often prescribed to patients in the form of an easily used EpiPen, or auto-injector, for intramuscular injection. The EMT should become familiar with this single-dose preloaded syringe to assist the patients in its use should the need arise.

As do many medications, epinephrine has many potentially significant side effects. In addition to its beneficial effects of bronchodilation and vasoconstriction, epinephrine can cause a significant rise in heart rate. In addition, the heart is forced to work much harder after epinephrine administration. These effects will likely cause the patient to feel as if her heart is pounding very quickly and may cause some tremulousness. These are the same effects as seen when epinephrine is secreted by the body itself during a fight-or-flight response (Figure 13.19).

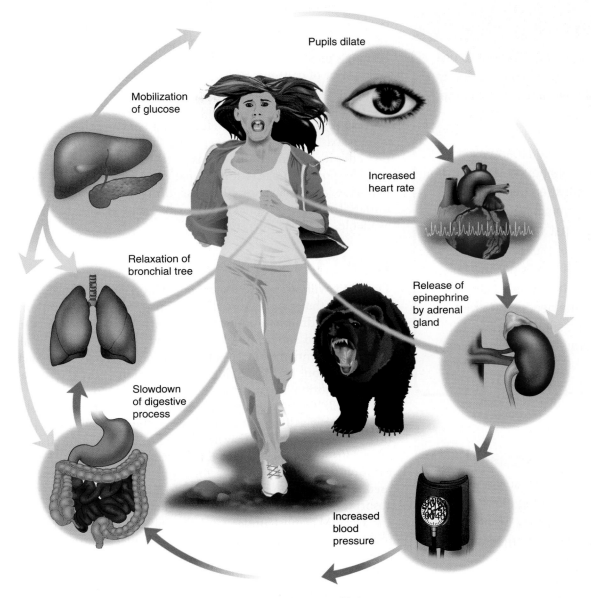

Figure 13.19 Epinephrine administration mimics the fight-or-flight response

Potential severe side effects are associated with epinephrine. Epinephrine should be used with particular caution in older patients with underlying cardiac disease. There must be clear indications for its use, and local protocols must be followed.

Under no circumstances should an EMT assist someone to use an epinephrine injector that has not been prescribed to the person by a physician unless doing so is specifically allowed by local protocol. A medical control physician can help determine whether the helpful effects of the drug are worth the potential risks of its use. If any question arises, medical control should be consulted immediately.

ADMINISTRATION PROCEDURE—EPINEPHRINE

The primary assessment of the anaphylactic patient must be done quickly and must include administration of high-flow oxygen. If it is determined that a prescribed epinephrine injector is indicated and it is present on the scene, the EMT should assist the patient to use it (Figure 13.20).

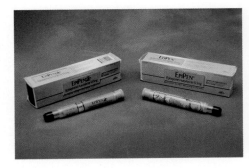

Figure 13.20 Epinephrine may be packaged in a preloaded syringe for ease of administration

When assisting a patient to use an epinephrine auto-injector, the EMT should take care to properly handle and dispose of the needle. Proper disposal includes placement into an approved sharps container, as discussed in Unit 8. Most epinephrine auto-injectors have a safety function that will withdraw the needle after the drug has been injected. If this is not the case, the EMT should never attempt to force the needle to retract. He should simply dispose of the entire unit in an appropriate manner.

Children are also susceptible to life-threatening allergic reactions and may be prescribed epinephrine auto-injectors. The pediatric dose is smaller than the adult dose, often 0.3 mg, and will be indicated on the injector device. EpiPen Jr. is a common trade name for the pediatric dose of the medication.

The most common site for injection of this medication is the thigh because it is the largest muscle that is easily accessible to a patient who is self-administering the medication. If possible, the side of the leg should be bared, although most of the auto-injectors are designed to be able to go through a single layer of clothing. Skill 13-2 at the end of this chapter depicts this procedure in detail.

As with any other medication administration, the EMT should take care to reassess the patient and carefully document any changes. The patient with anaphylaxis who receives epinephrine should begin to improve within minutes after its administration if it is going to be effective.

The potential exists for the patient to decompensate, even after epinephrine administration. Because of this possibility, the EMT should initiate transport as quickly as possible and arrange for ALS intercept, if available.

CONCLUSION

The EMT will often care for patients who have potentially life-threatening conditions that may require the administration of medication. The goal of medication administration is to improve patients' conditions and gain relief from pain and suffering. Administration of medication can also be harmful, even potentially fatal, if administered incorrectly. Incorrect medication administrations include giving the medication to the wrong patient, for the wrong condition, in the wrong dose, and by the wrong route.

The EMT must know some basic principles of pharmacology to ensure he is correctly assisting or administering medications in the prehospital setting. Medications EMTs may administer or assist in administering can come in various forms such as tablet, powder, liquid, or gas. The route of administration will be based on the form of the medications and how rapid the medication needs to be absorbed. Injected medications have the most rapid absorption, while oral medications will take longer to absorb.

The EMT must understand the indications, contraindications, doses, routes of administration, and potential side effects and actions of any medication he plans to administer. The "five rights" of medication administration—right patient, right medication, right route, right dose, and right date—must be used to confirm each medication before it is given.

EMTs must be thoroughly familiar with the medications they are responsible for carrying and administering, such as oxygen, oral glucose, and aspirin. In addition, they must be familiar with a few prescribed medications for patients who have serious medical problems and may require assistance in administration. These medications include bronchodilator inhalers, nitroglycerin, and epinephrine auto-injectors.

Each EMT must be responsible for knowing the local regulations pertaining to the common use of the medications discussed in this chapter and the protocols governing their use. These protocols may differ significantly from one locale to another. The involvement of medical control physicians in the administration of medications by the EMT is often helpful and may be required by local protocols.

All medication administrations must be followed by reassessment and documentation of the effect of the medication and if there are any changes in the patient's condition.

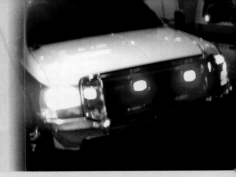

CASE STUDY Continued

Bill quickly performs his primary assessment, obtains baseline vital signs, and performs a thorough medication history with the assistance of Kathy. Jason is able to tell Bill his name, but is not able to correctly state the day, place, or events. Bill establishes that oral glucose is indicated based on his patient assessment, signs and symptoms, and Jason's medical history of new-onset diabetes and insulin use.

Following local protocols and the standing orders for glucose administration, Bill reviews the "five rights" of medication administration, verifying he has the right patient: Jason; right medication: glucose; right route: oral; right dose: up to one single tube of glucose; and the right date: glucose expires in 8/2012.

Bill opens the tube of glucose and explains to Jason how he will squirt this in Jason's mouth. Bill further instructs Jason to swallow the gel as it is being squeezed into his mouth in small amounts.

Bill administers two thirds of the tube of glucose before Jason tells him to stop. Bill documents the administration of the glucose, making sure to include the name of the medication, date, time, dose, and name of the patient.

Jason states he cannot remember what has happened; however, he is able to answer all questions appropriately now. Jason's wife explains he had started acting funny, like he does when his blood sugar gets too low, so she called the ambulance.

After completing a reassessment of the primary assessment and vital signs, Bill determines the glucose has raised Jason's low blood sugar. He explains to Jason that although he feels completely normal right now, it is very important for him to be evaluated by a physician in case his blood sugar should drop again.

Jason agrees to be transported to the local hospital for further evaluation for his low blood sugar.

Skill 13-1 Assistance with a Metered Dose Inhaler

PURPOSE: To assist the patient with the use of a prescribed metered dose inhaler.

STANDARD PRECAUTIONS:

☑ Appropriate prescribed metered dose inhaler

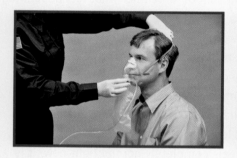

1 The EMT assesses the patient and applies oxygen as appropriate.

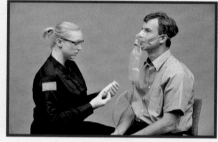

2 The EMT next confirms that the inhaler is the patient's prescribed inhaler and checks the expiration date.

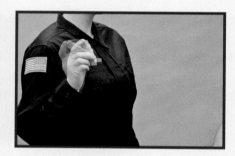

3 The EMT vigorously shakes the inhaler and removes the mouthpiece.

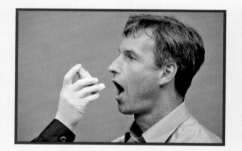

4 After removing the oxygen mask, the EMT asks the patient to exhale, then inhale slowly and deeply, as the EMT depresses the inhaler for one puff.

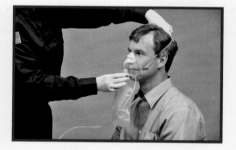

5 The EMT removes the inhaler from the patient's mouth and reapplies oxygen while instructing the patient to continue to hold his breath for several seconds. The EMT then reevaluates the patient and considers whether a second dose of medicine is needed.

PURPOSE: To assist the patient in administration of prescribed epinephrine, using the auto-injector.

STANDARD PRECAUTIONS:

☑ Oxygen
☑ Prescribed epinephrine auto-injector
☑ Scissors
☑ Sharps container

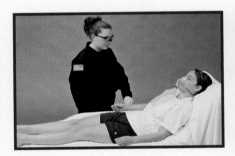

1 The EMT assesses the patient and applies oxygen as appropriate.

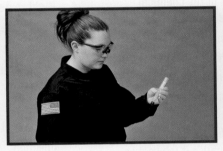

2 The EMT confirms that the auto-injector is the patient's prescribed auto-injector and checks the expiration date.

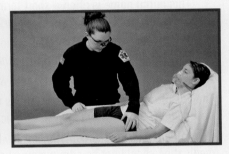

3 The EMT bares the patient's lateral thigh (using scissors to cut away clothing if necessary) and then removes the safety cap on the auto-injector.

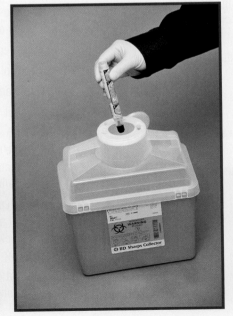

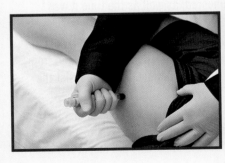

4 Pressing the auto-injector firmly against the patient's lateral thigh, midway between the knee and the hip, the EMT allows about 10 seconds for the medication administration.

5 The EMT removes the auto-injector and properly disposes of the auto-injector in a sharps container at the patient's side.

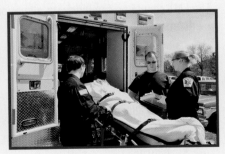

6 The EMT reassesses the patient and initiates transport as soon as possible. The EMT should arrange for an ALS intercept, if possible.

Key Concepts Revisited

- The EMT should be knowledgeable in basic principles of pharmacology of commonly encountered medications and their administration.

- The EMT should be familiar with a few key pharmacological terms to be able to communicate effectively with patients and other health care professionals.

- The EMT should be familiar with the two most commonly used names for medications: generic and trade or brand name.
  - This initial name is often a short form of the chemical name and is referred to as the *generic name.*
  - The brand name given to a medication by the manufacturer is called the *trade name.*

- The action of a drug is the effect the drug will have on the body.

- The indication or reason to give a drug is most commonly based on the signs, symptoms, or specific condition.

- Contraindications are circumstances in which a particular medication should not be administered because it may cause more harm than good.

- A side effect can be an undesired or unintentional effect that occurs in addition to the intended desired effect.

- The dose of a drug is the amount of the drug that should be administered to achieve the desired effect.

- The route of administration of a drug is significant for how quickly the drug enters the patient's circulation or is absorbed by the body.
  - Sublingual or oral medications are administered through the enteral or ingested route.
  - Inhaled and injected medications are administered through the parenteral route.

- EMTs should be familiar with the common abbreviations physicians use when prescribing medications.

- The EMT should be familiar with all various forms of medications:
  - Compressed powders and tablets
  - Liquid
    - Gel
    - Suspension
  - Gases
    - Aerosols

- The patient must be thoroughly assessed before the EMT can make the right decision on the appropriate medication to be administered for the given condition.

- A medication history must include current prescriptions, over-the-counter medications, and herbal or homeopathic medications the patient is taking and any allergies to medications.

- The "five rights" of drug administration verify if the medication is safe and appropriate for the situation:
  - Right patient
  - Right medication
  - Right route
  - Right dose
  - Right time

- The EMT must be familiar with the various routes of drug administration:
  - Inhalation
  - Sublingual
  - Injection
  - Subcutaneous
  - Intramuscular
  - Intravenous
  - Oral
  - Topical

- The EMT should be familiar with and follow local policies on administration or assisted administration of medications:
  - Off-line medical control
    - Protocols or written orders
  - On-line medical control

- A reassessment should be done and documented within 5 minutes after the medication has been given.

- The exact name of the medication, dose, and route should be carefully documented, as well as the time it was administered and by whom.

- There are two types of medications EMTs will handle in the prehospital setting: medications administered from ambulance stock and medications they will assist the patient in taking.

- The administration of specific medications must be based on the indications and local protocols or direct orders from medical control. These medications are stocked and carried in the ambulance:
  - Aspirin
  - Oxygen
  - Oral glucose

- The EMT may be required to assist the patient in administering medications specifically prescribed for the patient by a physician.
  - Inhaled bronchodilators
  - Nitroglycerin
  - Epinephrine auto-injectors (EpiPen)

- The EMT must understand some basic principles of pharmacology to ensure correct administration of medications in the prehospital setting.

Key Terms

Action
Bronchodilator
Dose
Enteral
Epinephrine
Expiration date
Generic name
Intramuscular
Intravenous
Mechanism of action
Metered dose inhaler

Nebulizer
Nitroglycerin
Oral
Parenteral
Pharmacology
Route
Side effect
Suspension
Therapeutic effect
Topical
Trade name

Review Questions

1. Why must an EMT understand principles of basic pharmacology?
2. What is the difference between the generic name and the trade name for medications?
3. Why is it important to know the indications and contraindications of medications?
4. List the different forms in which medications may come.
5. What routes of medication administration will be used by the EMT most often?
6. Review the "five rights" that must be verified before drug administration.
7. What should be reassessed after drug administration and why?
8. Explain how drug administration is documented.
9. What are the common drugs an EMT carries and administers in the prehospital setting?
10. What is the difference between an EMT administering a drug and assisting a patient to take a previously prescribed medication?
11. What are the common medications an EMT could be requested to assist a patient in administering?
12. What role does medical control play in the administration of medication by an EMT?

Further Study

Beck, R. K. *Pharmacology for the EMS Provider.* Clifton Park, NY: Thomson Delmar Learning, 2003.

Beck, R. K. *Drug Reference for EMS Providers.* Clifton Park, NY: Clifton Park, Thomson Delmar Learning, 2002.

Gonsoulin, S., & W. Raynovich. *Prehospital Drug Therapy.* Philadelphia: Mosby, 2000.

Packaging, lifting, and carrying patients is necessary on every EMS call. Whether the plan is to "scoop and run" or to "load and go," the mission has remained the same for EMS: the safe transportation of the patient to definitive medical care.

> ## National Education Standard
> The Emergency Medical Technician (EMT) should have a fundamental depth and foundational breadth of knowledge on lifting and moving patients and the prevention of work-related injuries.

Key Concepts

- Principles of back care are important to overall back health of the EMT.

- Proper body mechanics can help the EMT prevent back injuries.

- Guidelines for safe reaching can help the EMT prevent back injuries.

- Guidelines for safe lifting of patients can help the EMT prevent back injuries.

- Guidelines for safe carrying equipment can help the EMT prevent back injuries.

- Many methods of emergency drags can be used by the EMT to remove a patient from immediate danger.

- Many methods of emergency carries can be used by the EMT to expeditiously move a patient from one area to another.

- The EMT's proper use of patient-carrying devices can help ensure a safe and orderly transfer of the patient from the field to the ambulance.

- Proper patient packaging provides warmth as well as security for the patient during transport.

- Following proper procedures permits the safe transfer of the patient from stretcher to gurney by the EMT.

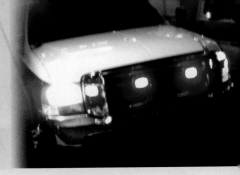

CASE STUDY

Sean climbs into the rig, turns to Aimee, and says, "The call is for a woman who has fallen down a flight of stairs." Aimee thinks to herself, "This ought to be easy enough. She is at the bottom of the stairs. We will logroll her onto the backboard, load her onto the stretcher, and transport her after assessing her for injuries."

While en route, the radio chirps and the fire department's emergency medical responder comes on the air advising all responding units that the patient has fallen down into the basement of the house and that the stairs are broken. Furthermore, the patient weighs more than 400 pounds.

The EMS supervisor comes on the air and requests heavy rescue, including the rope rescue team, the bariatric ambulance, and additional manpower to respond to the scene.

Aimee reflects on the situation and wonders, "How are we going to care for this poor woman?" She thinks, more importantly, "How are we going to get her out of the basement?" Most basements only have one staircase and small 1 foot by 2 foot windows for ventilation.

Then it occurs to Aimee that the building may not be structurally sound. This call suddenly becomes a lot more difficult, and they aren't even on scene yet.

Critical Thinking Questions

1. What challenges does moving this patient present?
2. How can the EMTs get this patient out of the basement?
3. Why did the supervisor call for rope rescue?
4. Why did the supervisor call for the bariatric ambulance?

INTRODUCTION

Although lifting and carrying a patient may seem routine, there are many decisions an Emergency Medical Technician (EMT) makes regarding lifting and carrying that can have a dramatic impact on the patient and the EMT.

By choosing the wrong lifting technique, an EMT can get hurt. If an EMT uses a carrying device improperly, the patient can be dropped to the ground and sustain injuries.

As more EMTs sustain work-related back injuries, EMS leaders are becoming increasingly attentive to the manner in which EMTs lift and carry. Back braces, reengineered carrying devices, and back care programs are becoming more commonplace. The key to a long career in EMS hinges on proper lifting and carrying of patients and equipment.

BACK INJURIES

The scenario is all too common: an EMT lifts someone or something, thinking that the task can be done easily, and disaster strikes. A back injury occurs. A **back injury** is any injury of the muscles, tendons, or ligaments that support the torso and spine. A back injury may occur that could take the EMT out of work, perhaps permanently. Every EMT needs to know how to prevent back injuries.

ANATOMY REVIEW

Back injuries are actually injuries of the spine's ligaments and tendons or the muscles adjacent to the spine that support the torso, or both. The spine carries the weight of the upper body and anything carried by the person. This

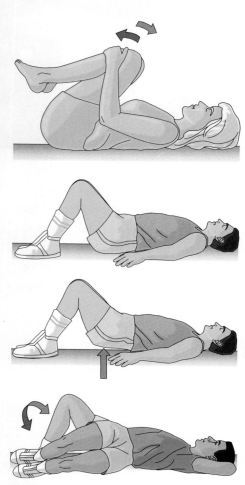

Figure 14.1 Back exercises reduce the chance that an EMT will suffer a back injury

weight is primarily borne by the lumbar section of the spinal column. The lumbar spine is the location of about 85% of all back injuries.

The spine is not rigid as are some other bony structures in the body. The spinal column is a series of bone segments, called *vertebrae,* that are stacked one on top of the other. This arrangement gives the spine an ability to bend and flex as well as to hold great weight.

Although the flexible nature of the spinal column allows the person to bend and move easily, these movements require a great deal of balance and muscle coordination. The spine is supported by a large number of muscles and ligaments to help with support and balance.

Between the vertebrae are soft discs that act as shock absorbers. These discs help the spine absorb pounding and vibrations. They occasionally deteriorate, are crushed, or move and slip out of place. In any case of crushed, deteriorated, or slipped disc, the result can be severe back pain.

The lower back, and the lumbar spine in particular, can be injured by strains or sprains of the muscles, by destruction or movement of intervertebral discs, or by fractures to the lumbar vertebrae themselves. These injuries are often the result of careless lifting and carrying.

BACK CARE

EMTs regularly lift and carry patients and equipment. Therefore, it is important that an EMT keep his back strong and healthy. The key to a strong back is regular exercise. Exercise strengthens the back muscles and prepares them for the hard work ahead. Regular back exercises along with practice in proper lifting techniques and use of certain lift assist devices are part of a program of **back care.** Good back care is essential for long-term survival of the EMT in EMS.

Companies, particularly health care organizations, have experienced the benefits of back care programs. Some companies encourage participation or provide for employee exercise programs to strengthen their backs. Others encourage the practice of tai chi or weight training. Exercise has benefits for employer and employee alike. Figure 14.1 shows a number of lower back exercises that will help improve the EMT's back strength.

An EMT's back must be strong, flexible, and able to withstand the demands of bending and twisting that are required of it. The most frequent source of back injury is twisting while lifting an object.

To prevent these injuries, every EMT should take a few minutes at the start of every tour of duty to warm up the lower back. These exercises seldom take more than 10 minutes to perform and can help prevent a lower back injury.

BACK EXERCISES

A variety of simple back exercises can help the EMT maintain flexibility and strength as well as reduce the incidence of injury. However, an EMT should never exercise an injured back nor exercise the back to the point of pain. The old adage "no pain, no gain" does not apply to preventing back injuries. Exercising during injury only leads to more injury.

The following back exercises are simple, easy to do, and can be done while on the job. A good habit is to perform this routine first thing in the morning before the vehicle equipment check. To begin the first exercise, the EMT should stand and grasp her hands above the head with palms facing upward. Now, the EMT should try to stretch her arms upward as far as possible. It is important to breathe normally during this exercise and not to arch the lower back. Once in position, the EMT should hold the position for a 10- or 15-second count. This exercise, called the tall stretch, helps to exercise the upper back.

For the next upper back exercise, the EMT, while in a standing position with knees slightly bent and hips directly over the feet, should reach out with outstretched hands that are shoulder width apart. With her hands placed on a countertop, the EMT then bends down at the hips until she feels a gentle stretch and holds that position for a count of 10 or 15. This exercise can be repeated three times.

The next exercise stretches the lower back and is called the standing lower back stretch. Again the EMT assumes a standing position with hips directly over the feet and places her hands on her hips at the back, as if to support the lower back. The EMT then gently arches the back backward, against the palms of her hands, and holds that position for a count of 10 or 15. This exercise can also be repeated several times.

The last exercise, illustrated in Figure 14.1, requires that the EMT lie on a firm surface. Called the tuck stretch, the EMT lays his head flat on the ground and pulls his knees toward the chest while pushing the lower back against the ground. Once in position the EMT should hold the position for a count of 10 or 15 and then relax. A variation of this exercise includes placing the feet flat on the ground and lifting just the lower back or rolling the hips back and forth in a gentle rocking motion.

KNOW YOUR LIMITS

The EMT should take a moment whenever she is about to lift a patient and ask herself two important questions: (1) Is there enough help to lift this patient? (2) Is the right equipment being used?

The answers to these questions will affect the patient, the EMT, and the EMS agency. Failure to answer the questions correctly can mean further injury for the patient, injury and disability for the EMT, and unnecessary expenses for the EMS agency.

IS THERE ENOUGH HELP?

The typical functional job description for an EMT states that the EMT must be able to lift and carry 125 to 150 pounds. Essentially, when two EMS providers respond to a call, they should be able to safely lift and carry the average patient without difficulty.

Additional assistance should be requested for any patient who weighs more than 250 pounds. It may be possible for EMTs to lift a heavy patient, but it is not necessarily wise to do so.

The EMT should factor in the weight of the stretcher as well as any equipment that is being carried. These items can quickly add another 50 pounds.

Patients over 300 pounds present a special challenge to the EMT. Careful planning and additional resources are often needed to ensure that the EMT can safely move the patient without danger to herself or her crew.

WHAT IS THE "RIGHT STUFF"?

There are many methods of carrying a patient, as well as adjunctive equipment to assist the EMT in the carry. Careful consideration of the problem at hand and the method that will be used to perform the carry improves the likelihood that the EMT will perform a safe carry.

Like an Olympic athlete, the well-trained EMT mentally visualizes the carry. She then considers what equipment she could use to improve her performance. For example, it is much easier to carry a person down a flight of stairs in a stairchair than on a stretcher, and it is easier to take the stretcher down an elevator than carry the person down the stairs in a stairchair.

SAFETY FIRST

Orthopedic back supports, or back braces, are wide cloth belts that wrap around the torso to provide support to the lumbar area. Orthopedic back supports are designed to support the lower back and prevent injuries. Whenever a heavy patient is carried, a back support should be worn.

Unfortunately, back supports are frequently misused and can be harmful if not used correctly. A supporting brace should not be worn at all times. If the brace is worn tightly for long periods, the brace may actually weaken the back muscles.

Most braces are intended to be worn loosely around the waist then tightened up with a belt, or some other means, when needed just before lifting a heavy object. A back brace helps to support the lumbar spine under extraordinary circumstances.

Back support braces come in different sizes. A properly fitted brace will perform as it was designed, as a back support. Some back support braces have foam padding built into the belt to provide warmth as well as support.

FOOTWEAR

Proper footwear is also important. Closed-toed shoes are required for the EMT to prevent accidental exposure to blood if blood should drip on them. Closed-toed shoes also prevent injuries if the EMT should stub her toe. But an EMT's boots are more than just footwear. Boots serve as the foundation for lifting and carrying as well as protection for toes and feet.

The soles of the boots should be nonskid, preferably with a traction lug sole to prevent slipping. The boots should preferably be mid-calf boots. Mid-calf boots provide additional ankle support. This added support is important when the EMT is carrying a patient across uneven terrain and can help prevent twisted ankles. In a sense the mid-calf boot works like a back brace but for the ankle (Figure 14.2).

SLIPPERY SURFACES

Experienced EMTs know that the combination of rubber fire boots and antifreeze on a roadway is a formula for disaster. The image of an EMT going head over heels might appear comical, but the injuries sustained are no laughing matter.

Some firefighters involved in EMS wear mid-calf boots, or even duty shoes, instead of fire boots when on EMS duty. Experienced emergency responders may come equipped with cat litter or some other similar absorbent to spread over an antifreeze spill to provide traction and prevent an accident. Often it is the duty of the safety officer to ensure that slip hazards are identified and eliminated where possible.

BODY MECHANICS

Body mechanics is the proper or most efficient way to perform physical activities that are safe and energy conserving and help prevent the physical strains that may cause injury. The primary goal of understanding proper body mechanics is to learn how to lift and carry without injury to the spine. Awareness of common mistakes and principles of body mechanics can help the EMT achieve this goal. Table 14-1 lists the principles of good body mechanics.

REACHING

Whether the EMT is reaching for a piece of equipment or to grasp a wrist for a pulse, there are several fundamental rules for reaching.

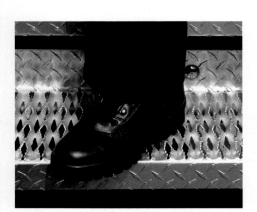

Figure 14.2 Proper footwear is an important part of maintaining the health and physical fitness of the EMT

Street Smart

After having a stretcher roll over her toes a couple of times, the experienced EMT buys boots that have a reinforced toe, maybe even a steel toe. Typically, toes are not broken, but the pain and discomfort that can be avoided make the extra money spent on safety boots worth every penny.

Table 14-1 Principles of Good Body Mechanics

1. Keep feet apart about shoulder width.
2. Keep chin up and back straight when lifting.
3. Bend at the knees and not at the back.
4. Keep objects close to your body.
5. Do not twist your body when lifting or carrying.
6. Exhale when lifting.
7. Lift with the legs and not with the back.
8. Push or pull instead of lifting.
9. Never reach more than 18 inches away from the body.
10. Avoid fast, jerking motions when lifting.

First, the EMT should never lean backward to reach for a piece of equipment. Neither should an EMT twist her back to reach a piece of equipment. Twisting and arching the back backward can lead to injury.

Instead, the EMT should pivot on her heels and face the object for which she is reaching. While facing the object and keeping the back straight, the EMT can reach to grasp the object.

The EMT should never reach more than 18 inches away from the body to grasp an object. That's about the length of the arm from elbow to hand. In addition, the elbows should not leave the side of the body. Equipment that is not readily accessible in this manner should be rearranged.

If the object is heavy, more than 10 pounds, the EMT should bend at the knees, while keeping the back straight, and lift the object to her. Again, the elbows should be close to the body but never farther out than the knees.

LIFTING

When lifting an object off the ground, the EMT should carry the load as close to the body as possible. A straight back, with good vertical spinal alignment, will place the weight of the load on the pelvis and strong leg muscles while taking the weight off the lower back.

POWER LIFT

Whenever a person or heavy object is lifted, the EMT should use a **power lift.** This technique, sometimes called the *squat lift,* uses the stronger muscles of the legs instead of the weaker muscles of the lower back. The power lift is useful when lifting baskets or stretchers or even when moving heavy furniture out of the way to gain access to the patient.

An EMT first stands within 6 inches of the object to be lifted. The closer the body's center of gravity is to the object, the more powerful the lift. Notice how an Olympic power lifter will place his feet under the bar before lifting. As the lift is accomplished, the bar moves parallel to and next to the center of mass. The EMT should use the image of an Olympic power lifter when she is performing this lift.

The EMT's feet are the foundation of the lift. One slip of a foot spells disaster for both the EMT and the patient. Good footwear, discussed previously, is imperative. A comfortable stance, with the feet evenly placed, is important. Finally, the EMT's feet should be flat on the ground, with the soles of the boots making firm contact with the surface.

POWER GRIP

When preparing to perform a power lift, the EMT squats to reach the item to be lifted, such as a backboard. The EMT should obtain a firm grasp, usually palms up. The palms-up grasp, sometimes called the **power grip,** uses the most powerful muscles of the forearm. The amount that can be lifted is limited only by the strength of the grip.

The EMT's arm should be locked out, meaning that the elbows are straight and the arm is one long rigid structure. This maneuver ensures that the EMT is using her back and legs to lift rather than her weaker arm muscles.

On signal, usually from the EMT at the head, two EMTs should slowly lift together. The lift should never be jerky or so fast that it jars the patient. The lift is complete when, and only when, the EMT is in an upright position and the weight is being suspended directly in front of her.

Skill 14-1 at the end of this unit shows an EMT lifting a backboard, demonstrating proper technique. Notice that the back is straight. He has knelt down to the load. He has not bent down. He carefully secures his hand grasp on the litter grips. His arms are straight, and his elbows are locked out. He then crouches to a squatting position. The load is very close to the center of his body, the center of his mass.

He is lifting using the strong muscles of his thighs and not the weaker muscles of his lower back. As he is lifting, the EMT is slowly exhaling forcefully. Forceful exhalation while lifting helps him tighten his abdominal muscles and further support his lower back.

The lift should occur in one fluid motion, smoothly and without hesitation. Note that the elbows are never beyond the knees. If the EMT has to turn, to transfer the patient, for example, he will shuffle his feet sideways rather than twist his back.

CARRYING

Radios, jump kits, suction units, backboards, and oxygen bottles are some of the most common equipment an EMT carries every day. Improved technologies, such as automatic external defibrillators (AEDs), have resulted in more equipment for an EMT to carry to a scene. Sometimes, the EMT feels more like a pack mule than a health care provider.

Whenever possible, a bag or case should be carried by a shoulder strap that is slung over the shoulder. This method of carrying tends to keep the weight of the object close to the body.

The EMT in Figure 14.3 is carrying two jump kits. Note that his back is straight and that he has a balanced load—that is, one kit in each arm. When he arrives at the patient's side, he bends his knees and slips the bag straps off his shoulders, to release the load, while using the handles to gently place the bags on the ground.

PUSHING AND PULLING

Whenever possible, an EMT should try to push an object rather than pull it. The muscles of the body are more adept at pushing than pulling. Trying to pull patients out of cars and other confined spaces has resulted in back injuries for many EMTs.

By following a few simple rules when pushing and pulling objects, listed in Table 14-2, the EMT can avoid back injuries and enjoy a long career in EMS.

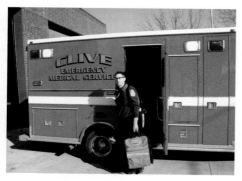

Figure 14.3 Keeping his back straight, the EMT balances his load by carrying equipment on each side of his body (Courtesy of Clive Fire Department, Clive, IA)

Table 14-2 Lifting and Pulling Guidelines

1. Avoid pulling objects. Push objects whenever possible.
2. Keep the back straight when moving an object, either by pushing or by pulling.
3. Push while standing and walking only if the object is at waist height.
4. If the object is below the waist, either kneel or use a rope or similar device to extend the arm's reach.
5. Try to keep your elbows bent and close to your sides while pushing.

PLANNING A MOVE

The EMT should always have a plan for how she wants to move a patient. Even in an emergency, there are several methods of quickly moving a patient. The advantage to having a plan is that the patient can be moved quickly, without further injury, while the safety of the EMT is not compromised.

First, survey the scene and determine the priorities. The means to move someone at a house call is different from the means to remove someone from a motor vehicle collision (MVC). The scene often dictates the best means of carry.

What is the patient's priority? Is it a life-or-death emergency? If the patient is high priority, then time is of the essence and only a few carries are useful. If the patient is low priority, then more time can be taken to safely move the patient.

What are the resources at hand? The EMT carefully assesses the amount of "muscle" that will be needed. Calling for help from the middle of the staircase is a little too late.

Next the EMT should communicate the plan of carry to everyone involved. Sometimes a more experienced EMT may have an alternative approach that saves time or energy. However, once the decision has been made on how to carry the patient, it is important that everyone stick to the plan.

During a carry, the person at the head of the patient typically makes the calls for when to lift, turn, and move. When loading the stretcher into the ambulance the EMT is usually on the patient's left side, closest to the bench seat, and the driver or another EMT is on patient's right side, closest to the driver's side. These basic understandings improve efficiency and help to prevent people from having to go around one another.

The heaviest end of a stretcher is the top half, where the torso lies. Typically, when a heavy person is being carried, the strongest EMT takes the head. When the patient is being brought down a flight of stairs, the situation is reversed, and the strongest person should be at the feet.

Whenever a carry is being planned, the most important point for the EMT to remember is to know his personal limits. Stopping a carry to rest the back or relax the fingers can prevent fatigue. Every EMT wants to get the job done. However, no EMT wants to get hurt or to cause further injury to the patient while getting the job done.

CIVILIAN ASSISTANCE

Most EMS agencies do not permit the assistance of civilians with a carry as a matter of policy. An EMT who is injured during a carry can receive medical care under workers' compensation and disability, but civilians who help and get hurt are left to depend on their own health insurance. A back injury can be a lifelong affliction, so to ask a family member, or any civilian, to help may be exposing the person to unnecessary injury, long-term medical care, and perhaps no chance of recovering related costs.

OBESE PATIENTS

Overweight or obese patients provide the EMT a unique transportation challenge. Most standard EMS carrying devices are not designed to carry the additional weight of these patients. For example, a typical backboard may be rated for only 300 pounds maximum. Loading a heavier patient onto these backboards risks breaking the backboard and potentially dropping the patient. Every EMS system should make arrangements, also known as preplan, that includes both manpower and equipment, to be able to provide care and transportation to these patients.

EMERGENCY MOVES

In some situations, the patient needs to be moved immediately, as in during a fire or flood. It is considered an **emergency move** when the risk for serious injury, or even death, outweighs the risk for harm that might occur from hastily moving the patient.

In those emergencies, the EMT should first consider whether she is prepared and capable of entering the scene and removing the patient. In a fire, for example, does the EMT have proper firefighting turnout gear and self-contained breathing apparatus (SCBA)? If not, then the EMT should not enter the scene. The first priority for every EMT is personal safety.

In the case in which the EMT can reasonably enter the scene safely and rapidly remove the patient, she should attempt to do so. Table 14-3 lists the several reasons that a patient should be removed quickly using an emergency move technique.

CAR FIRES AND EXTRICATION

Although car fires do occur, the number of fires that occur in MVCs is extremely small, as little as 1%. Patients in MVCs should be properly assessed for spinal injury before a decision is made to remove them. The danger of

---

Table 14-3 Reasons for an Emergency Move

- Presence of fire or immediate danger of fire
- Rapidly rising flood waters
- Oncoming train
- Explosions or immediate danger of explosions
- Potential for structural collapse
- Gathering hostile crowd
- Gunfire in the vicinity
- Access to another more seriously injured patient is blocked by the patient

---

creating permanent paralysis from aggravating a cervical spine injury is greater than the theoretical danger of the patient suffering burns in an automobile fire that does not exist. A rule of thumb is that the patient should remain in the car unless smoke is clearly visible. Consult the fire officer on scene for guidance in such matters.

EMERGENCY DRAGS

When the situation is critical and time is of the essence, the EMT cannot afford to wait for additional support. She must act quickly and efficiently. In these cases, she should perform an emergency drag. When an EMT, using a minimum of supplies, grabs a patient and hauls him to safety, she is performing an **emergency drag.**

CLOTHING DRAG

The easiest emergency drag to perform is the clothing drag. As shown in Skill 14-2 at the end of the unit, a **clothing drag** is performed when the patient's shirt collar or a handful of clothing is grabbed from behind the neck and used as a purchase point on which to pull the patient. Using two hands, the EMT walks backward while dragging the patient along with him. The patient's head remains cradled between the rescuer's forearms.

ARM DRAG

If a good handhold on the clothing cannot be obtained, then the EMT can try an arm drag. During an **arm pull,** the EMT, as seen in Skill 14-3 at the end of the unit, grasps the wrists of the patient, pulls her arms to her chest, and drags her by the arms. The arm drag can be very effective provided the patient can hold her head up. If the patient is unconscious, do not use the arm drag. The head of an unconscious patient may fall forward, blocking the patient's airway, or fall backward, injuring the head and neck.

First, the EMT must partially prop the patient up to a semi-reclined position, holding the patient upright against his knee. The EMT then slips each of his arms under the patient's shoulders. Grasping the patient's right wrist with the left hand and the patient's left wrist with the right hand, and crossing them over the patient's chest, the EMT has a tight grasp of the patient. The EMT squats and then stands erect, walking backward to safety.

BLANKET DRAG

If the patient is large or the EMT is having trouble dragging the patient, a blanket can be an invaluable tool. For a **blanket drag** the EMT logrolls the patient onto a blanket, sheet, or drape, then grasps a handful of blanket and drags the patient to safety.

The EMT should quickly straighten the patient's legs, place his forearm along the patient's spine while cradling the patient's head in the palm of the hand. Using the other arm, the EMT should reach under the patient's arm and grasp the patient by the shirt or chest, then carefully roll the patient over onto her back, trying to move the patient as a unit.

Once the patient is supine, the EMT rolls up the edges of the blanket to form a horseshoe-shaped collar. The patient's head, now partially supported by the blanket, is protected from striking the floor. The patient can now be dragged, using a blanket drag, across the floor quickly.

A distinct advantage of the blanket drag is that when other help arrives, there are many readily available handholds to help with the drag; with enough hands, the body can even be lifted and carried. Skill 14-4 at the end of the unit demonstrates the blanket drag.

FIREFIGHTER'S DRAG

All of the preceding drags require that the EMT drag the patient backward. These drags are effective when the patient has to be moved only a few yards. However, these drags are physically exhausting for a single EMT to perform. The **firefighter's drag** uses a simple cotton triangular bandage, called a cravat, tied around the patient's wrists to make the work of dragging the patient much easier.

The EMT uses the cravat to secure the patient's wrists together. A hitch over each wrist and then a knot will securely tie the wrists together. With the hands securely fastened together, the wrists are draped over the neck and shoulders of the EMT while the EMT is on hands and knees. The patient is then dragged under the EMT. The EMT can still look forward and see where he is going, as shown in Skill 14-5 at the end of the unit. The patient is also protected from any falling debris by the body of the EMT.

EMERGENCY CARRY

Drags can only be used to move the patient a few yards. Longer distances are physically exhausting. If the patient must be moved in an emergency over a greater distance, a technique called an **emergency carry** should be used. If the EMT has the strength or the patient is small enough, it may be easier to just pick up the patient and carry her. Such a carry, although more difficult to perform than a drag, will result in the patient's being moved farther from the danger more quickly.

RESCUER ASSIST

The simplest, and least taxing, carry is the rescuer assist. A **rescuer assist** is used when the patient is able to walk and an EMT is available to assist the patient with walking. The patient slings his arm over the EMTs shoulder and grasps the EMT for support. The EMT then grasps the patient's wrist. Next the EMT grasps around the patient's thorax, partially supporting the patient's weight while assisting the patient to the standing position. While the EMT supports the patient with the rescuer assist, the patient is using the rescuer like a crutch.

The distinct advantage of a rescuer assist is that if the patient suddenly becomes weak, the EMT can drag the upright person to safety. This rescue move is used by soldiers to assist exhausted or "walking wounded" comrades. Skill 14-6 at the end of the unit demonstrates the techniques used.

Note that, if necessary, the EMT can let go of the wrist and waist and the patient can be lowered flat onto the ground. Also, if another rescuer suddenly becomes available, he can take the patient's other side and assist the first rescuer.

PACK STRAP CARRY

If during an assist, a walking patient becomes weak or even loses consciousness, the EMT can quickly change from a walking assist to a pack strap carry. As the name implies, the **pack strap carry** uses the patient's arms draped over the shoulders as straps to lift the patient onto the EMT's back.

When converting from the rescuer assist to the pack strap carry, the EMT simply lets go of the arm under the patient's shoulder, steps in front of the patient, reaches back, and grabs the now hanging arm by the wrist. Once the EMT has a firm grasp of the wrist, the EMT pulls both arms forward while he is bending over. When the pack strap carry is done correctly, as shown in Skill 14-7, the patient's weight should be on the EMT's back and the patient's feet should be off the ground. This technique is hard on the EMT's back and

Street Smart

Securing a patient's wrists together whenever the patient is being moved is so common that many EMTs keep a cravat in the pocket of their coat or cargo pants. Practice tying someone's wrists together until it becomes second nature.

should be done only in an emergency when no other means of transport are feasible.

CRADLE CARRY

A **cradle carry** simply has the EMT carry the patient like a mother would carry a child in her arms. If the patient is a child, often the EMT can pick the patient directly into in her arms. If the patient is a little larger, like a small adult, someone may need to help lift the patient into the EMT's outstretched arms. Skill 14-8 at the end of the unit demonstrates this cradle carry technique. This technique permits the EMT to quickly move the patient to safe ground. But it also places a great deal of stress on the EMT's back. Only small adults or a child should be picked up and carried in this manner, provided the EMT has the physical capacity to do so.

FIREFIGHTER'S CARRY

If the patient is unconscious and needs to be moved quickly from the scene, the firefighter's carry remains one of the most effective carries.

The **firefighter's carry** is a series of carefully planned maneuvers whereby the patient eventually ends up on the EMT's back. Unfortunately, although it is effective, it is also difficult to master and takes a great deal of practice to perform correctly. Skill 14-9 at the end of the unit shows the series of maneuvers that must be performed to properly execute the firefighter's carry.

The patient must start supine in front of the EMT. The patient's knees must be flexed. Flexing the patient's knees is accomplished by pushing the patient's feet backward toward the body using the EMT's feet. Locking the patient's feet down by stepping on the toes with the tip of the EMT's boots, the EMT reaches forward and grasps both of the patient's wrists.

The next step is critical and must be done in one fluid motion. A moment's hesitation and the EMT could drop the patient. The patient is quickly moved to a near-standing position by being pulled upward to her feet. At the same time, the EMT ducks under the patient and then drops a shoulder down under the patient and into the patient's abdomen (center of gravity).

When the patient is squared over the EMT's back, the EMT stands up. Putting his arm between the patient's legs and coming around the front of the knee, the EMT grasps the arm that is dangling in front. Locking his hand and arm around the patient's wrist and leg effectively fixes the patient onto the EMT's shoulders. The EMT now has one hand free to open doors or carry bags. The bulk of the patient's weight is over the EMT's shoulders and is easier to carry.

SEAT CARRY

The **seat carry** requires a cooperative patient and two EMTs who lock their arms to form a seat. With the seat carry, the two EMTs form a seat by grasping wrists, as demonstrated in Skill 14-10 at the end of the unit. With arms locked out at the elbows, the two EMTs drop to opposite knees and the patient sits.

The patient can now place her arms around the shoulders of the two EMTs for balance. Standing upright, the two EMTs are able to walk while carrying the patient.

Note that the patient must remain capable of assisting with the carry. This carry is very useful if the patient has a leg or foot injury and is unable to walk.

CHAIR CARRY

Carrying a person by the wrists or clothing can be very difficult at times. When there are two EMTs, and time permits, transferring a patient to a carrying device, such as a backboard or a stairchair (a specially designed chair for carrying patients down stairs) can be very helpful. If no such devices are available or time is of the essence and the patient needs to be moved quickly, any standard kitchen chair can be used for a chair carry.

A **chair carry** provides the EMT with a solid object to grip to safely lift and move the patient. Initially the EMT may be seated in the chair or the patient could be supine. If the patient is supine, then lift the patient's legs and lay the chair down and slide it in under the patient's buttocks. While grasping the patient's waistband, advance the chair until the patient appears to be sitting in the chair, flat on his back. Now lift the chair to the normal seated position, as shown in Skill 14-11 at the end of the unit.

If the patient is unable to assist the EMT with sitting in the chair, a cravat secured to the chair can be wrapped around the chest. One EMT turns and, facing forward, grasps the legs of the chair. The other EMT grabs the back of the chair.

Together, on the call of the EMT at the head, the two EMTs lift the chair and proceed to walk out of the room. Skill 14-11 at the end of the unit demonstrates how two EMTs perform the chair carry. Although this carry is useful for the debilitated patient, it should not be used with unconscious patients.

NON-URGENT MOVES

Most of the time patients are not in immediate life-threatening danger and thus their movement is not urgent. When an EMT takes the time to carefully prepare for the carry, it is a low-priority or urgent but not emergency move. The patient's safety and comfort, as well as the safety of the entire prehospital team, are the EMT's primary concerns. A number of devices and methods can be used to safely move a patient from the scene, to an ambulance cot, and then to the hospital gurney.

However, one misstep can turn a simple lift-and-carry into a disaster. Without coordination of all team members, a fall may occur that could injure the patient, the crew, or the EMT. A few simple rules, agreed to ahead of time, can prevent tragedy from striking.

Almost by convention, the EMT at the head of the patient or to the patient's left side is in charge. That EMT decides when to lift, when to turn, or when to stop.

It is expected that the team's leader will exercise command by giving specific orders, such as, "Turn on three—three, two, one, lift."

To be understood, orders must be loud and clear. There is no room for confusion or misunderstanding. The EMT should state the objective clearly and ensure that all members of the team, even if it is just one more EMT, understand.

By agreeing to these simple rules of lifting and moving, the EMTs can ensure that the patient's transport will be uneventful and the EMTs can decrease their risk of back injury.

EXTREMITY LIFT

The extremity lift is perhaps one of the most commonly used lifts in EMS. It is used to transfer a patient from a bed to a stretcher or from the floor to a stretcher. It cannot be used to transfer a trauma patient to or from a stretcher because the extremity lift does not protect the spine.

As the name implies, the **extremity lift,** uses the patient's extremities, such as the ankles and wrists, as purchase points to grasp the patient and lift. The first EMT comes from behind the patient and slips her hands under the patient's arms. The first EMT then grasps the opposite wrist of the patient from her own. It is helpful if the second EMT grasps the patient's wrists and brings them to within reach of the first EMT.

The second EMT then slips his hands under the patient's knees or grasps the ankles by the pant leg. If the patient must be carried any distance, then the second EMT kneels between the patient's knees and grasps each knee with his hands. While facing forward, he stands up while lifting the patient and then walks. Skill 14-12 at the end of the unit demonstrates this useful technique.

DIRECT LIFT

When the patient needs to be moved from the floor to a bed or to a stretcher, and only one side of the patient is accessible, the EMTs can try a direct lift. The **direct lift** uses several EMTs who grasp the patient like a bundle and carry the patient close to their chests. It takes disciplined teamwork to perform a direct ground lift correctly. The direct ground lift does not protect the spine during movement and therefore is not used for trauma patients.

The two or, preferably, three EMTs line up next to the patient. All three kneel with one knee down and one knee up. The EMT at the patient's head cradles the patient's head and neck with his hand. The same EMT slides his arm under the patient's shoulders.

The second EMT slides one hand under the lumbar section of the patient's back, in the hollow of the back, and the other hand under the patient's buttocks. The third EMT slides one hand in the hollow under the back of the knees and the other hand under the patient's ankles.

On command, all three EMTs lift the patient, as a unit, to their knees. The patient should be resting comfortably, with arms crossed upon the chest, perhaps secured with a cravat, in the arms of the three EMTs. Skill 14-13 at the end of this unit demonstrates the position in which the patient should be resting.

If the patient needs to be moved only a foot or so—to an awaiting stretcher, for example—then all three EMTs, on command, lean forward while dropping the raised knee to the ground.

If the patient needs to be moved a greater distance—across a room, for example—then all three EMTs, on command, roll the patient toward their chests. This technique keeps the patient's weight centered over the EMTs' center of gravity and helps prevent back injuries. The three EMTs then stand and walk, in unison, lock-step fashion, to the stretcher or bed.

SCOOP STRETCHER

The **orthopedic "scoop" stretcher** is a lightweight aluminum carrying device. Originally the "Robinson" orthopedic stretcher was used for supine patients with spine injuries, but it fell out of favor as the device of choice with the advent of backboards.

The orthopedic stretcher was designed to fit into tight spaces, where both sides of the patient could be reached. Places an orthopedic stretcher can be useful is when a patient falls and breaks a hip in the bathroom or next to the bed in a small bedroom.

The orthopedic stretcher is meant to be broken into two halves, using the releases at both ends. Each half of this split stretcher is then slipped under the patient. When the patient is firmly on the orthopedic stretcher, the orthopedic stretcher is reconstructed. In effect, the patient is scooped up by the two halves of the orthopedic stretcher. This is why the orthopedic stretcher got the nickname *scoop stretcher*.

Although the operation of the scoop stretcher, demonstrated in Skill 14-13 at the end of the unit, appears easy, the EMT must be cautious. Often the

Street Smart

Current models of stairchairs offer the advantages of rollers or slides that decrease the lifting and carrying required by the EMT. Whenever they are available the EMT should consider taking advantage of these labor-saving devices, which also help to reduce the danger of back injury.

patient's clothing, floor coverings, and even the patient himself, are pinched by the scoop stretcher.

The scoop stretcher has a void in the middle and therefore does not support the spine directly. For this reason, the scoop stretcher is currently used as a temporary transfer device while a patient is moved to a backboard for routine spinal immobilization.

Scoop stretchers are designed to be narrow and are made of rigid tubular aluminum, which adds strength to the frame. Some design features make the scoop stretcher ideal for transfers out of cramped quarters, confined spaces, or narrow hallways. For example, if a sailor became ill and had to be carried out through narrow ship corridors, the scoop stretcher would be useful.

STAIRCHAIR

Occasionally a patient will not tolerate lying flat on a litter, scoop stretcher, or Reeves stretcher. Most such patients have some difficulty breathing while lying flat. The solution is simple: Use the chair carry described earlier. Manufacturers of patient-carrying devices have taken the simple chair carry to its logical conclusion. By adding seat belts for the patient and handles for the EMT to a sturdy aluminum-framed chair, they created the **stairchair.**

The stairchair is frequently used in the city or anywhere there are narrow hallways and flights of stairs. It requires two EMTs to move the patient. Skill 14-14 at the end of this unit demonstrates this maneuver. Some stairchairs are lightweight and compact, requiring the EMT to carry the patient. Others are designed with rub bars and wheels. The rub bars permit the stairchair to be slid from step to step down a flight of stairs. The wheels permit the stairchair to be used like a wheelchair, rolling the patient down hallways, and to the ambulance.

The wise EMT buckles the patient's arms inside the straps of the stairchair or other device. Securing the arms prevents the patient from reaching out and grabbing a rail suddenly. The wise EMT also tells the patient to keep his hands inside the blankets and explains why. A few moments reassuring the patient may prevent a disastrous fall due to the patient's suddenly flailing and grabbing, throwing the EMTs off balance.

STAIR CARRY

Stair carries, using a stairchair or other carrying device, can be very dangerous. The EMT must concentrate on both balancing and carrying the load as well as stepping from step to step without the benefit of seeing where she is stepping.

Note the EMT in Figure 14.4 at the bottom of the stairs. Her hand is on the small of the back of the EMT at the feet, providing a little reassurance as well as some immediate support should the EMT walking backward stumble and fall. It is important that the EMT does not grab the belt. With the hand on the belt, the hand can become trapped; if someone stumbles, then everyone falls.

Figure 14.4 A hand in the small of the back reminds the EMT that there is help if needed

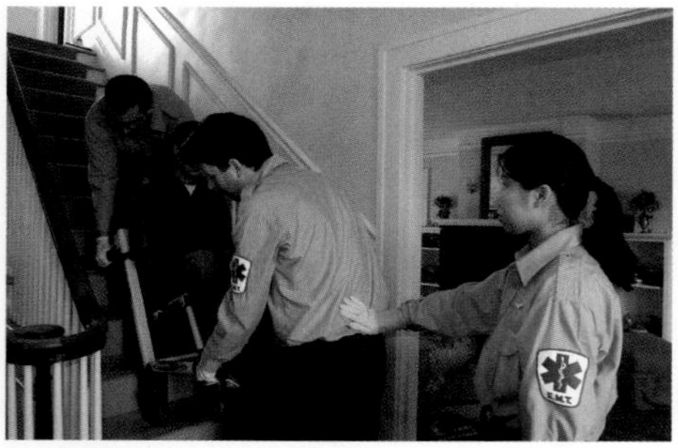

With each step, the EMT guiding the crew should be calling out the steps until the EMT carrying the patient reaches bottom—for example, "Step, another step, three steps left."

Often the EMT carrying the patient has a difficult time seeing the steps and feels for them with his foot first, then places it flat when he is sure it is on a firm surface. A little reassurance by the guide EMT can be comforting and help ensure patient safety.

The patient should always be carried down the stairs feet first for a number of reasons. One of the most important reasons is to keep the patient from feeling as if she is falling.

Whenever an EMT is carrying a patient down stairs, it is important that he keep his back straight and bend at the hips and knees. The stairchair or stretcher needs to be carried as close to the body as is practical. The entire sequence is shown in Skill 14-14 at the end of the unit.

OFF-ROAD STRETCHERS

Walking across uneven terrain and rough ground while carrying a patient can be dangerous. To help the EMT with these carries, special off-road stretchers have been developed. The use of special off-road stretchers decreases the hazard that uneven surfaces pose to the EMT and the patient.

BASKET STRETCHER

A **basket stretcher,** as the name implies, is a rigid litter designed to carry a patient; litters are generally made of canvas. The original basket stretcher, designed by Charles Stokes, was made of chicken wire stretched over a rigid steel metal frame. It was designed to carry a patient in the basket, hanging from a cable, between ships during World War II. Basket "Stokes" stretchers were made available to fire rescue after the war by Civil Defense and have seen active use ever since.

Modern basket stretchers are made of fiberglass-plastic composites to withstand rugged use. The earlier wire baskets were difficult to use in wilderness situations because they tended to get caught on tree branches and did not protect the patient. The full fiberglass shell of a modern basket avoids this problem.

Furthermore, a modern basket can be pulled across snow and ice much as a sled would be. However, in defense of the wire basket, other similar plastic shell baskets are heavier to carry. For this reason, many rope rescue experts still prefer the lighter wire baskets.

FLEXIBLE STRETCHER

A modern cousin of the basket stretcher is the flexible stretcher. An example of a flexible stretcher is a SKED. These plastic stretchers are lightweight and can be rolled up. In use, the flexible stretcher wraps around the patient, like a cocoon, and becomes rigid. Because of its small size, it is useful in confined-space rescues and cave rescues.

Moreover, because it is lightweight, it has seen extensive service in wilderness and rope rescues. The U.S. military uses the SKED flexible stretcher in many of its tactical rescue operations.

All baskets have multiple handholds for convenience. Some manufacturers have even attached a tubular metal rail around the top of the basket. This permits a limitless number of handholds. In all cases, these handholds serve as both a grab point for rescuers and a point of fixation for straps or webbing.

For protection, the patient in a basket stretcher must be securely strapped in. While the patient is being carried over rough terrain, he might be tipped over accidentally and may even be dropped. The patient can be securely anchored to the basket using a length of webbing, looped like a shoestring, between handholds.

Another device commonly used in transporting a patient out of a house is the **Reeves stretcher.** This flexible stretcher was designed by a Philadelphia police officer named Reeves and a tent maker named Smith.

The problem they had was carrying patients out of the two- and three-story walk-ups in the city. Using a little imagination, they created a flexible stretcher that worked something like the corsets commonly worn at the time.

The Reeves stretcher has long, thin slats that run lengthwise down the stretcher. These slats are sewn into a canvas litter. The result is that the Reeves

Street Smart

A common problem with carrying a patient on a Reeves flexible stretcher is that the patient's feet rub against the pant legs of the EMT. To prevent this problem, the EMT places the patient on the Reeves flexible stretcher with about a foot of material left below the feet. When the patient is lifted, the extra material folds over the feet and protects the EMT's pants.

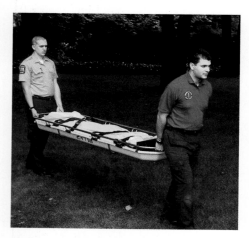

Figure 14.5 The end-to-end stretcher carry can be used to carry patients long distances

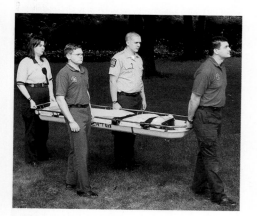

Figure 14.6 The diamond stretcher carry is used to transport patients over uneven terrain

can be rolled up and carried under the arm. Yet, when a patient is placed on top of the Reeves the slats create a rigid surface to carry the patient.

Handholds for carrying are provided at each corner and on the sides of the Reeves. The patient is usually rolled to one side, the Reeves is slid under the patient, then the patient is rolled to the other side, and the Reeves is pulled through. Three straps, sewn into the stretcher, secure the patient.

OFF-ROAD CARRY

There are a number of methods of carrying a stretcher off-road. Some are more suited to short hauls, whereas others are more suited to long wilderness carries.

Each carry is also dependent on the number of providers available. Whereas four people can carry a stretcher, it may be preferable to let two carry the stretcher if the hallway, or trail, is narrow. Rescuer fatigue, the patient's weight, and the distance to be covered must all be factored into the decision of which carry is to be used.

END-TO-END CARRY

Since early history, wounded soldiers have been removed from the battlefield to an aid station or field hospital by fellow soldiers, paramedics, or corpsmen using a portable stretcher called a *litter*.

The U.S. Army litters were typically made of sturdy canvas and two rigid poles. Some of these portable litters even had legs that could be used to convert the litter to a temporary bed when needed. A quick emergency litter can be rigged up using two pike poles and a woolen blanket.

Usually only two EMTs are available to carry the patient. In those cases, each EMT grabs the end of the litter and lifts at each end, a procedure called an **end-to-end stretcher carry** (Figure 14.5). If any amount of distance needs to be covered, the two EMTs need to be facing the same direction. Careful observation of army medics evacuating a wounded soldier will reveal that no one is walking backward. Both carriers face forward because the danger of tripping is greater when walking backward.

However, if the ground is level and the patient is being moved only a few feet, then the two EMTs can face one another during the carry. If the carry is more than 20 feet, then both EMTs should be facing forward.

DIAMOND CARRY

If the trip is more than a dozen or so feet and the ground is uneven, then it is not safe for two people to carry a patient. It is important that all sides of the litter, basket, or backboard be supported.

A **diamond carry** has an EMT at each end and each side of the stretcher to provide maximum stability. As described earlier, the first two EMTs each take an end of the carrying device, facing each other. The next two EMTs take a position at each side of the carrying device. All EMTs are now in a position for a diamond stretcher carry (Figure 14.6).

On the signal of the EMT at the head, the four EMTs lift together. All of the EMTs should be using a power grip and be performing a power lift. The lift should be steady and even.

Once all EMTs are fully erect and comfortable with their stance, the EMT at the patient's feet turns around and face forward, in the direction of travel. Notice that the EMT at the head of the patient is facing the patient. He is monitoring the patient's condition—mental status, airway, and so on—while carrying the patient.

Now the team is ready to move, again on the signal of the EMT at the head. Once the team has arrived at the destination, the procedure is reversed. The patient has now been moved safely and effectively.

FOUR CORNERS CARRY

Very similar to the diamond carry is the four corners carry (Figure 14.7). With a **four corners carry**, an EMT takes each of four corners of the stretcher. The four corners carry is useful when carrying a basket or similar device over a great distance: for example, for several miles out of the backcountry. As many as six or even eight EMTs can be involved in this carry. Therefore, it is a useful carry for extremely heavy patients or for a combination of patients and heavy equipment.

Each EMT grabs either the corner of the basket or somewhere in the middle, and they all face one another. It is preferable to pair EMTs across from each other according to height and strength. This arrangement works to even the load when it is carried and to create a balance.

On the signal of an EMT at the head, everyone squats, and then they all lift together. After the team has adjusted its stance and is ready, the team turns together in the same direction. This means that only one hand is in contact with the basket. It is important to remember to lift with the legs and not with the back.

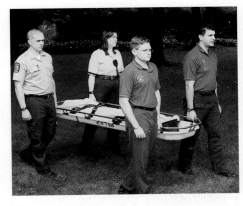

Figure 14.7 The four corners carry is used to transport patients over long distances and rough terrain

THE USE OF SLINGS

It is tiring to carry a patient on a litter or in a basket with one hand. The body has a tendency to twist to one side, and the uneven load forces the muscles of the back to compensate to keep the back straight. Loops of webbing called slings are used to help even the load and relieve the back.

The **stringer**, as demonstrated in Skill 14-15 at the end of this unit, is a nylon webbing loop tied in a half-hitch through the handhold or rail. It is then slung over the shoulder to the opposite hand. After the load is lifted, the EMT grasps the sling, or stringer, and pulls down. Pulling down on the stringer uses the shoulders as a fulcrum and helps to balance the load.

CATERPILLAR PASS

In the course of moving a patient, many obstacles may get in the way. A common obstacle is the guardrail along the roadside. The EMT must be careful not to drop the patient while overcoming the obstacle.

The best way to overcome an obstacle is to pass the patient hand over hand over the obstacle to waiting EMTs on the other side. This maneuver is called the **caterpillar pass.**

Stopping in front of the obstacle, the EMTs turn and face each other, firmly grasping the backboard or basket with two hands. Two or more EMTs line up on the other side. The backboard or basket is now handed over, hand over hand, to the EMTs on the other side.

The key is to have all EMTs standing still. No feet should be moving. If the obstacle is a low embankment, in which case establishing a rope system would be time consuming or unnecessary, then a human chain is created up the embankment. Skill 14-16 shows a group of EMTs working together using the caterpillar pass to carry a patient up the embankment.

When the EMTs become fatigued, they use the caterpillar pass to hand off the patient to other EMTs. Two EMTs, who may have been ahead clearing the path, stop at the front of the basket. The team turns and grabs the basket with two hands.

The two fresh EMTs replace the two EMTs at the head. The two EMTs at the head slide down to the middle, and the two EMTs in the middle replace the two EMTs at the end. The last two EMTs are now relieved of duty and typically take a position in front of the team as scouts.

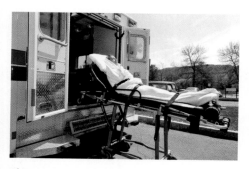

Figure 14.8 The patient must be safely secured to the stretcher before transportation can begin

PACKAGING THE PATIENT

Trundle, gurney, stretcher, and cot—these are all names for the portable rolling bed in an ambulance. Yet, the ambulance cot is more than just a conveyance. It is part of the plan of treatment. Older litters provide only one position, flat. Modern ambulance cots may be adjusted to different positions according to the patient's needs.

Ambulance cots usually have linens that provide comfort and warmth to the patient. These linens are called **bedrolls** and are wrapped around the patient as he is prepared for transportation. The EMTs in Skill 14-17 at the end of the unit are demonstrating one method of making a bedroll and how to wrap the patient in the bedroll.

A large percentage of body heat is lost from the head and neck. To conserve this heat and to make the patient more comfortable, the EMT should wrap the head with the bedroll's collar. Loss of body heat can lead to a condition called *hypothermia*. Hypothermia is an especially serious problem for trauma patients.

POSITIONING

If the patient's feet are up, more blood goes to the brain; if the head is up, the patient breathes more easily. The EMT must make a conscious decision every time she places a patient on a stretcher about which position is best for the patient. That decision must be medically motivated.

An EMT can transport a patient on a stretcher in one of five common positions. The patient may be transported flat either in the supine (i.e., face up) position or prone (i.e., face down) position.

The other two positions are variations of sitting upright. The patient can either sit semi-reclined (referred to as *semi-Fowler's*) or bolt upright (high-Fowler's). Fowler's positions are intended to allow the patient's abdominal muscles to relax so that they can breathe easier. Fowler's position also allows the lungs to hang, or be suspended, making ventilation easier.

The final position, Trendelenburg, is supine with the feet elevated. This position, also called the *shock position,* was originally intended to allow blood from the feet to flow to the torso during shock. This theory is now in dispute. However, some patients with abdominal pain and low blood pressure, who cannot tolerate sitting upright for fear of passing out, may feel better in Trendelenburg position as long as the position does not compromise respiratory effort.

STRAPPING

To prevent the patient from being thrown from the ambulance cot during sudden stops, the EMT must secure her to the cot. Usually seat-belt–style straps are used, just like the type used on a backboard. Figure 14.8 shows a patient properly secured to the ambulance cot.

The first strap secures the upper torso. If it is cold outside, the patient's arms are bundled inside the blankets and both arms and chest are strapped in. Otherwise, most patients prefer to have their arms outside the strap. Leaving the strap under the arms and over the chest allows the EMT to take blood pressures and pulses more easily.

The middle strap is usually adjusted over the pelvis, as a seat belt would be. It is important to place the middle strap over the bony pelvis. If the seat belt is riding higher on the abdomen and the ambulance is struck from behind, the patient may experience internal damage to abdominal organs because of the whiplash effect.

The final strap is across the legs, usually at or about the knees. Often equipment, such as an oxygen tank, is secured with this strap as well. It should be emphasized that whenever a hard object is placed against soft tissue and then securely strapped in place, there is a potential that the object will hurt the patient. A pad, such as a small pillow, should be placed over the patient's knees to prevent this discomfort.

TRANSFERRING TO THE AMBULANCE

Ambulance cots come with wheels for a reason. Ambulance cots are usually rolled to their destination. However, whenever an ambulance stretcher is in the high position, which is usually waist height for most EMTs, the center of gravity for the stretcher is elevated and the stretcher can tip over. Although large wheels and a large base provide some stabilization, all ambulance cots are prone to tipping, especially when going around corners.

For this reason, many rescue squads and ambulance companies have policies that state that "loaded" cots must be in the low position every time the patient is moved. In every case in which the ground is rough or uneven, an EMT should be on each side of the cot to protect the patient from a fall.

LOADING THE AMBULANCE

How an EMT loads an ambulance cot depends on the ambulance manufacturer's recommendations. Nevertheless, the principles of lifting remain the same. The EMT must have his feet firmly planted and his back straight, lifting with the legs and not the back, using a power grip and lifting as a team member (Figure 14.9).

The hardware placed on the floor of the ambulance is designed to hold the ambulance cot in place in case of a collision (Figure 14.10). These pieces of hardware are subject to some of the most grueling conditions of any equipment on board an ambulance. Consider the fact that the ambulance cot is the single most used piece of equipment aboard any ambulance. For this reason

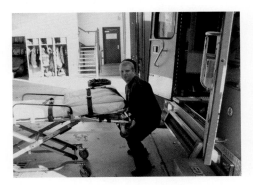

Figure 14.9 With knees bent and back straight, heavy equipment can be lifted and carried safely (Courtesy of Clive Fire Department, Clive, IA)

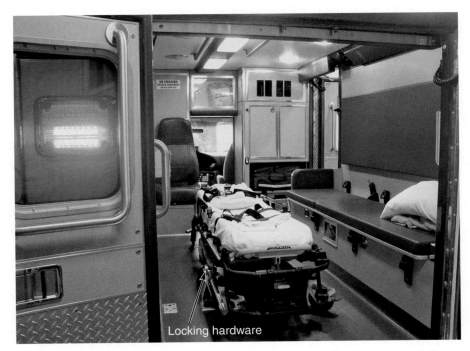

Locking hardware

Figure 14.10 Ensure that the ambulance cot has firmly engaged the locking hardware (Courtesy of Henry County Health Center EMS, Mt. Pleasant, IA)

alone, ambulance cots need to be inspected daily and given regular preventive maintenance.

TRANSFERRING TO THE HOSPITAL BED

Arriving at the hospital, the crew unloads the ambulance cot, following good back care practices, and proceeds to roll the patient into the hospital. Some patients, when lying flat and moving backward, complain of feeling nauseated. As a matter of practice, most EMTs roll the cot feet first. As noted earlier, many EMTs leave the cot in the low position, decreasing the likelihood that the cot will tip over.

The first person the crew is likely to encounter is the triage nurse. He will assign a room and even may be the nurse who will be taking the report. Occasionally, the patient is transferred from the ambulance cot to a hospital wheelchair. The extremity lift is very effective in those cases. Be sure the wheels on the wheelchair are locked before moving the patient over.

Once the patient's room has been found, the EMTs will prepare to transfer the patient over to the hospital gurney. Be sure the wheels of the hospital gurney are in the locked position. Leave the hospital gurney flat. It is easier to transfer a patient to a flat surface than it is to an incline. Once the patient is on the hospital gurney, the head can be elevated as needed.

A number of transfer devices can be used to move a patient from the ambulance cot to the hospital gurney. By far the most common device used to transfer patients is the backboard.

Get the two stretchers as close to each other as possible. Be sure to lower any side rails that would interfere with the transfer. Next, release the ambulance cot straps but not the backboard straps. Check the backboard straps, and make sure they are secure. Often, straps are loosened during transport to access arms for blood pressures and the like.

One EMT takes a position on each end of the backboard, and they move the patient over as a unit, on the signal of the EMT at the head. If the patient is heavy, consider either having two EMTs on each end or lifting the patient and having a third EMT switch the two stretchers.

CARRY TRANSFER

Occasionally a cubicle, at a doctor's office or a clinic, is too narrow to accept the crew, the ambulance cot, and the gurney. In those cases, the ambulance cot is placed against an adjunct wall and the crew performs a direct carry, or a carry transfer, from the ambulance cot to the gurney. At the end of this unit, Skill 14-18 shows the position of the two stretchers.

The EMT should take the time to plan this move. Standing in the middle of the room holding a patient in midair and then realizing that the stretcher is positioned incorrectly (i.e., the patient's head is at the foot of the stretcher) can be embarrassing.

DRAW SHEET TRANSFER

For many decades, nurses have used draw sheets to transfer or "draw" a patient from one bed to another or from hospital bed to gurney. A draw sheet is either a regular sheet folded over in half or sturdy linen of equal length and width. The advantage is that a patient can be pulled across from bed to bed with ease.

Many EMTs use the draw sheet transfer technique for transferring patients from the ambulance cot to the hospital gurney. With the two stretchers next to each other, and with side rails down, each EMT grabs a side of the cot's linen. If the patient is heavy, the EMT may have to climb onto the hospital gurney; remember to lock the gurney's wheels.

Each EMT grabs a handful of sheet and rolls it into a stiff collar. Taking a moment, each EMT pulls against the other. This pulling performs two functions. First, it checks the integrity of the sheet; if it is going to tear, it may do so now. Second, it ensures that all the slack has been taken out from under the patient. Skill 14-19 at the end of the unit shows how the patient is transferred in an almost hammock-like affair.

EMTs are cautioned that it is very easy to overextend their backs in these cases, with resultant injury. If in doubt, consider alternatives such as the transfer board, discussed next.

TRANSFER BOARD

In response to the alarming rise in back injuries, many hospitals have purchased transfer boards. **Transfer boards,** also called *slide boards,* act as a smooth surface on which to slide the patient from one stretcher to another. Some newer-model hospital gurneys have a transfer board built into the frame.

The transfer board simply reduces the friction, and therefore the work, between the patient and the stretcher. With the hospital gurney slightly lower than the ambulance cot, the patient is pulled across using the draw sheet technique.

New technology has also created what are called **slippery sheets.** Like a satin sheet, these specially coated sheets reduce friction between the patient and the bed and allow for an easier transfer.

Safety Tips

Restless patients can easily fall from stretchers if preventive action is not taken. A fall can be prevented if the side rails are in the upright position whenever someone is not at the bedside. The EMT should never leave a patient's bedside without first putting up the side rails. A patient's falling out of bed translates to broken hips or other injuries, angry family members, and maybe even a claim of negligence. Prevent a patient from sustaining a preventable injury by always double-checking before leaving the room to be sure that the side rails are up. Then document that the side rails were up on the prehospital care report.

CONCLUSION

Without exception, every EMS call involves lifts, carries, and/or transfers. That means every EMS call holds the potential for a back injury or worse. Unfortunately, transfers are so commonplace that the EMT may forget to practice good back care principles; in those instances, injuries can occur.

Exercise, use of braces, and proper lifting techniques can help prevent back injuries. Most importantly, every EMT should know her limits. An EMT should never be afraid to ask for lifting assistance.

Every back injury means pain and suffering for the EMT as well as another provider potentially lost to EMS.

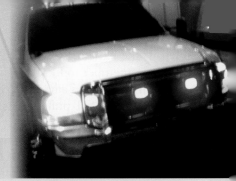

CASE STUDY Continued

Aimee is impressed. The fire department has managed to get the patient out of the basement using something called a Z rig, lots of rope, and a basket. Carrying the patient requires six firefighters who use slings to carry the patient to the stretcher.

While Aimee continues to take care of the patient, the second crew, with the bariatric ambulance, uses the electric winch and ramps to help load the patient into the ambulance for transport. Jumping in the side door Aimee prepares to transfer the patient to the on-board oxygen. And she reminds herself to call ahead to the hospital to advise the staff there of the patient's status and to ask for help when they arrive.

Skill 14-1 Proper Lifting Techniques

PURPOSE: To allow the EMT to lift objects without causing back injury.

STANDARD PRECAUTIONS:

- ☑ Appropriate personal protective equipment
- ☑ Appropriate back support
- ☑ Proper footwear
- ☑ Adequate numbers of trained assistants

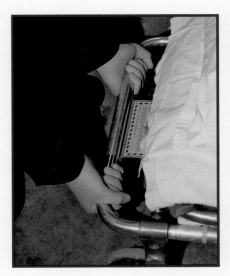

1 The EMT positions his feet about shoulder length apart, facing forward.

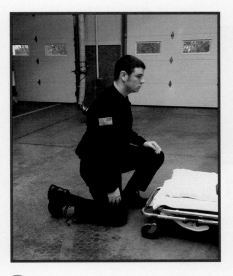

2 The EMT lowers his body by bending at the knees, one knee down, keeping the back straight.

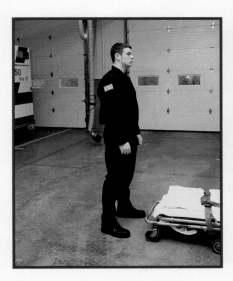

3 The EMT grasps the object with both hands, palms upward (power grip), then lifts evenly and smoothly.

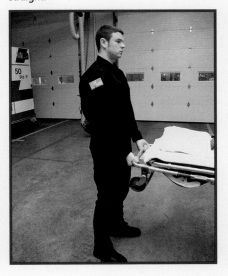

4 With arms locked out straight, the EMT stands fully upright.

PURPOSE: To permit the EMT to drag the patient to safety using the patient's clothing.

STANDARD PRECAUTIONS:

☑ Appropriate personal protective equipment

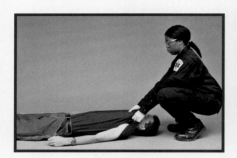

1 The EMT grasps the patient's clothing at the collar, while cradling the patient's head on his forearms.

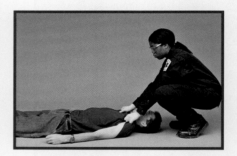

2 Crouching down, with back straight, the EMT walks backward.

PURPOSE: To permit the EMT to drag the patient to safety using the extremities.

STANDARD PRECAUTIONS:

☑ **Appropriate personal protective equipment**

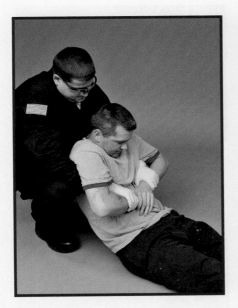

1 Kneeling down, the EMT slides his arms under the patient's arms and grasps the wrists across the chest.

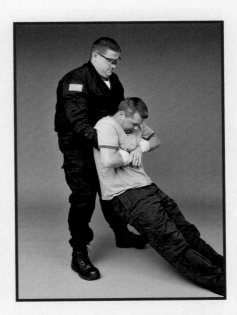

2 Standing up, the EMT walks backward.

PURPOSE: To permit the EMT to drag the patient to safety using a blanket.

STANDARD PRECAUTIONS:

☑ Appropriate personal protective equipment

☑ Blanket, tarp, drapes, or similar covering

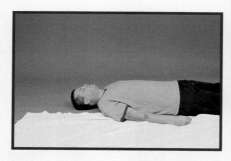

1 Place the blanket along the long axis of the body, leaving about a foot of material at the head.

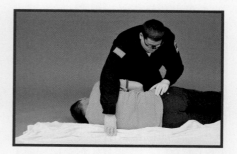

2 Logroll the patient onto the blanket, pulling the blanket underneath the patient.

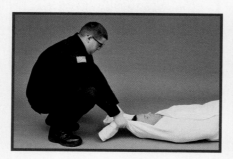

3 Wrap the patient with the blanket, protecting the patient.

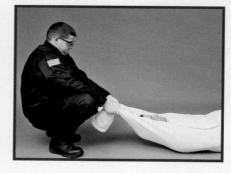

4 Roll up the excess material at the head and grasp the roll.

PURPOSE: To permit the EMT to drag the patient to safety while still looking forward.

STANDARD PRECAUTIONS:

☑ Appropriate personal protective equipment

☑ Triangular bandage

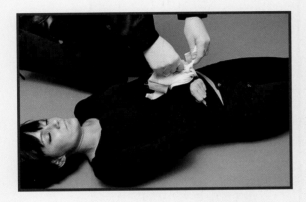

1 Using the triangular bandage, folded into a cravat, the EMT secures the patient's wrists together.

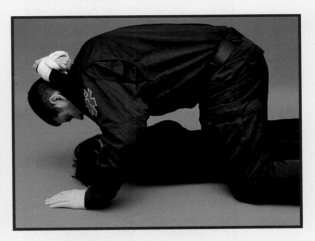

2 While on all fours, the EMT drapes the tied hands over his shoulders and drags the patient underneath him.

PURPOSE: To permit the EMT to assist the walking, but injured, patient to safety.

☑ Appropriate personal protective equipment

STANDARD PRECAUTIONS:

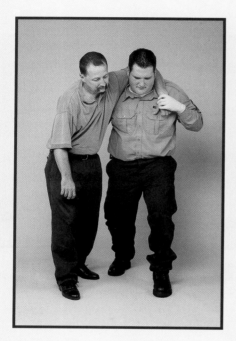

1 The EMT crouches to the patient's level and swings one arm over the EMT's shoulders.

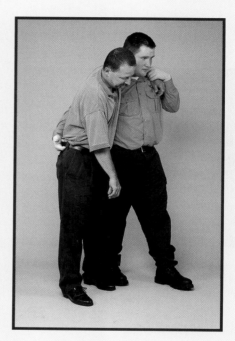

2 With one hand grasping the patient's beltline and another grasping the patient's wrist, the EMT stands and assists the patient with walking.

PURPOSE: To permit the EMT to carry an injured person on his back to safety.

☑ Appropriate personal protective equipment

STANDARD PRECAUTIONS:

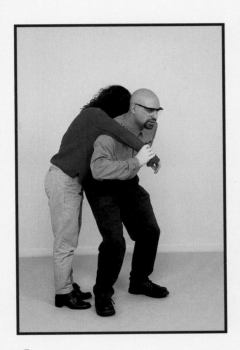

1 Crouching in front of the seated patient, the EMT grasps the patient's wrists and then pivots on his heels, draping the patient's arms over his shoulders in the process.

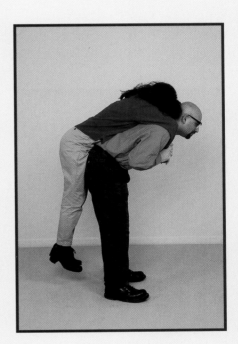

2 The EMT then stands, hoisting the patient onto his shoulders and off her feet. (This carry is also useful if the patient who is being assisted suddenly tires and needs to be carried. The EMT simply releases the belt and steps in front of the patient, grasping the free hand and placing it over his shoulders.)

PURPOSE: To permit the EMT to carry a nonambulatory or unconscious patient to safety.

STANDARD PRECAUTIONS:

☑ Appropriate personal protective equipment

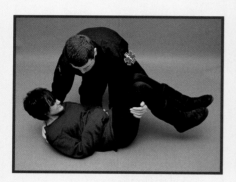

1 The EMT first kneels next to the supine patient, placing one hand under the shoulders and the other hand under the knees.

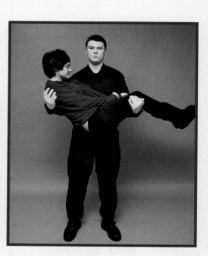

2 The EMT then stands, keeping the patient's body close to his.

PURPOSE: To permit the EMT to carry an unconscious patient quickly to safety.

STANDARD PRECAUTIONS:

☑ **Appropriate personal protective equipment**

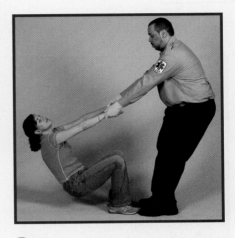

1 The EMT starts by standing toe to toe with the supine patient. Crouching down, he grabs the patient's wrists and proceeds to roll the patient to a seated position.

2 Without stopping, the EMT then pulls the patient as nearly erect as possible.

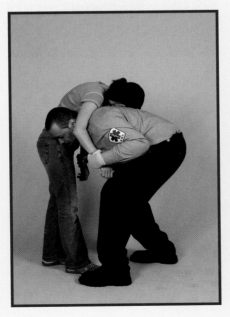

3 Quickly crouching again, the EMT places his shoulder into the patient's abdomen, while simultaneously standing.

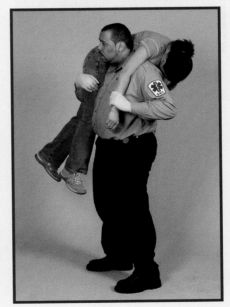

4 The EMT then puts one arm through the patient's legs and grasps the patient's hand with his free hand. (Another EMT may help hoist the patient up onto the shoulders of the EMT. The second EMT waits until the patient is up and over the first EMT's shoulders, then, grasping the patient's knee, helps hoist the patient.)

PURPOSE: To permit two EMTs to assist an injured, but conscious, patient to safety.

STANDARD PRECAUTIONS:

☑ Appropriate personal protective equipment

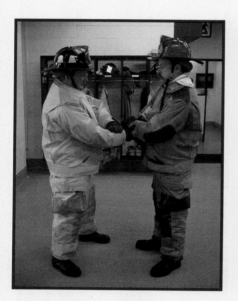

1 The two EMTs clasp arms. Each EMT grasps the other EMT at the elbow as shown here.

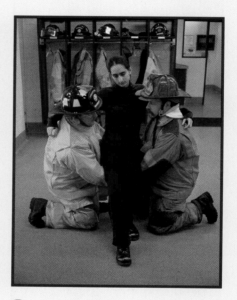

2 With one pair of arms high, the patient sits back into the seat that has been created. The EMTs then stand together, at the same time.

PURPOSE: To permit two EMTs to safely move a conscious patient, using a chair as a carrying device.

STANDARD PRECAUTIONS:

☑ Appropriate personal protective equipment

☑ Hardback chair

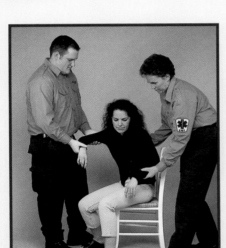

1 The patient is assisted to sitting in the chair.

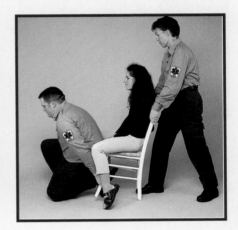

2 One EMT kneels in front of the chair, facing forward and between the patient's legs. He reaches back and grasps the legs of the chair.

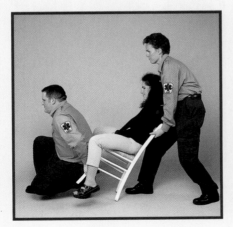

3 The second EMT, at the back of the chair, grasps the uprights of the chair and leans the chair backward.

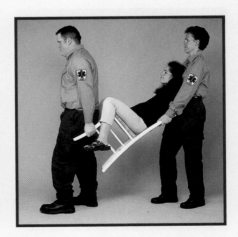

4 Simultaneously, the two EMTs lift the patient up and proceed to walk forward together.

PURPOSE: To permit two EMTs to lift a patient onto a carrying device.

☑ Appropriate personal protective equipment

STANDARD PRECAUTIONS:

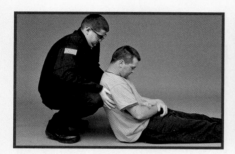

1 The first EMT kneels behind the patient and helps the patient up to a sitting position. The patient can be rested against the EMT's knee for a moment.

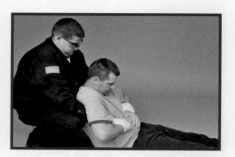

2 The EMT then reaches under the patient's arms and grasps the patient's wrists, pulling them against the patient's chest tightly.

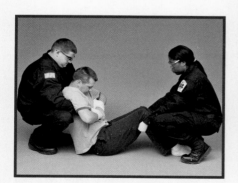

3 The second EMT then crouches. Reaching down on each side, the EMT grasps under the patient's knees. (In some cases, it may be more convenient to crouch beside the patient's knees and hook arms under the patient's knees.)

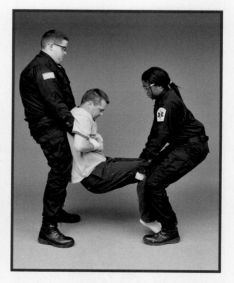

4 Simultaneously, the two EMTs stand with the patient and walk forward together.

PURPOSE: To move a patient from a narrow space or with a minimum of movement onto a backboard or stretcher.

STANDARD PRECAUTIONS:

☑ Appropriate personal protective equipment

☑ Orthopedic stretcher

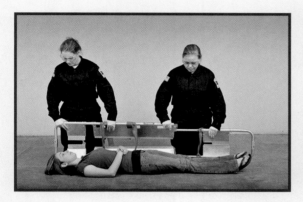

1 EMTs next to the patient estimate the need for equipment adjustment.

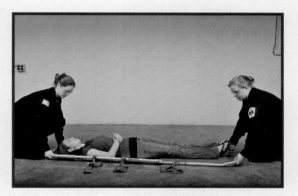

2 The EMT places the two halves of the orthopedic stretcher on each side of the patient and adjusts to the appropriate length for the patient.

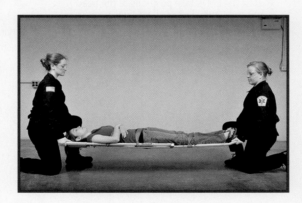

3 The patient is logrolled onto the orthopedic stretcher and secured with straps.

PURPOSE: To carry a patient down, or up, a flight of stairs.

STANDARD PRECAUTIONS:

☑ Appropriate personal protective equipment

☑ Stair chair

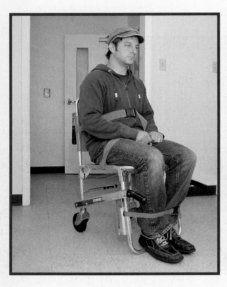

1 The patient is secured to the stairchair.

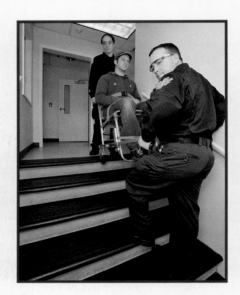

2 The EMTs take positions at the head and foot of the stairchair and lift the patient, extending hand rails as needed.

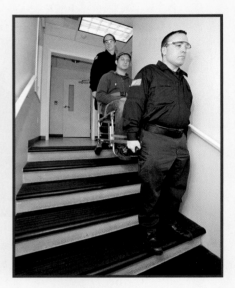

3 The EMT guiding the foot of the stairchair can face toward or away from the patient while carrying the patient down the stairs.

PURPOSE: To aid the EMT who is carrying a stretcher a distance.

STANDARD PRECAUTIONS:

☑ Appropriate personal protective equipment

☑ Loop of webbing, approximately 6 feet long

☑ Stretcher

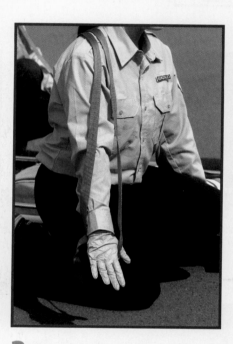

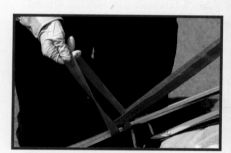

1 The EMT places the webbing under the bar, or under the handhold, and loops it back through itself, in effect creating a half-hitch.

2 The EMT then kneels next to the stretcher and slips the loop of webbing over his shoulder, being sure that the webbing knot is not on the shoulder.

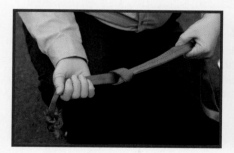

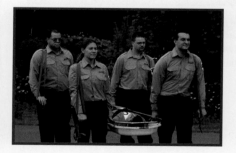

3 Then the EMT slips his opposite hand inside the loop. It may be necessary to shorten the length of the loop by tying a knot in the webbing.

4 Once standing, the EMT adjusts the loop over his shoulders. One hand should be carrying the stretcher, and the other hand should be exerting downward force on the loop, in effect balancing the load.

PURPOSE: To permit the EMT to move the patient on a stretcher or litter over an obstacle.

STANDARD PRECAUTIONS:

☑ Appropriate personal protective equipment

☑ Stretcher or litter

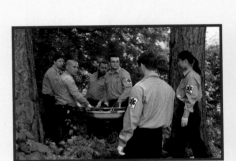

1 Coming to the obstacle, all EMTs stop and turn toward each other.

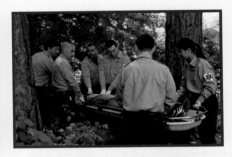

2 Two EMTs go around or over the obstacle and take a position across from the litter. The front of the litter is then handed to them across the object.

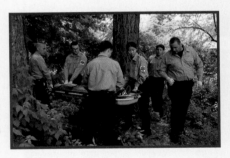

3 As the litter is passed forward, the two EMTs in the rear move forward to take position beyond the obstacle.

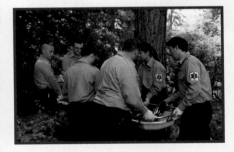

4 All EMTs remain standing with feet firmly planted as the litter is passed. Once the litter is beyond and clear of the obstacle, all EMTs turn and face forward. The EMTs may then move forward together as a unit.

PURPOSE: To allow the EMT to provide warmth and comfort to the patient.

STANDARD PRECAUTIONS:

☑ Appropriate personal protective equipment

☑ Stretcher, blanket, sheet, pillow, pillowcase

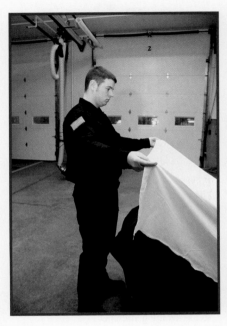

1 The first EMT centers the blanket on the stretcher and then places the sheet on top of that.

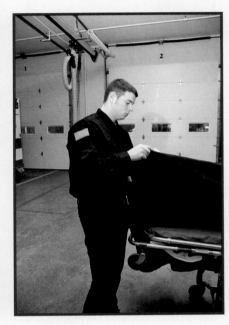

2 The first and second EMT grasp one half of the linen and fold it in half, creating a collar. Then they do the same with the other side. To open the bedroll, the EMTs simply grasp the collar and unfold the edges.

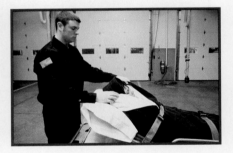

3 With the patient lying supine, the EMTs can fold the upper edge over the patient's head, then secure the edge with the lower edge. The pillow should then be placed behind the head, outside the linen.

PURPOSE: To permit the EMT to move the patient from one stretcher to another stretcher.

STANDARD PRECAUTIONS:

☑ Appropriate personal protective equipment

☑ Two stretchers, gurneys

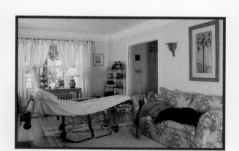

1 The first stretcher is placed with the patient's head at the foot of the other stretcher at a 90-degree angle.

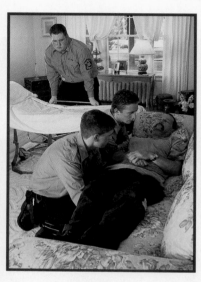

2 The two EMTs stand on the side of the patient, and the first EMT places one arm under the patient's head and neck and the other arm under the shoulders. The second EMT places his arms under the patient's lower back and buttocks.

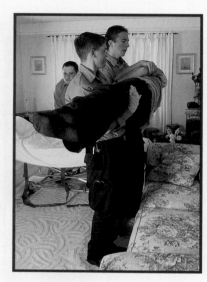

3 Simultaneously, the two EMTs hoist the patient to their chest. Shuffling sideways, the two EMTs move the patient to the awaiting stretcher.

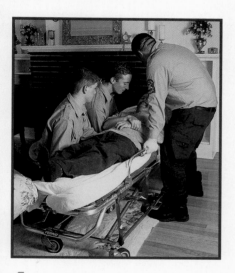

4 The patient is then gently laid onto the awaiting stretcher. The EMT should be sure that all stretcher straps are attached before moving the patient.

PURPOSE: To allow a patient to be moved from stretcher to hospital gurney.

STANDARD PRECAUTIONS:

☑ Appropriate personal protective equipment

☑ Two stretchers, draw sheet or bed linen

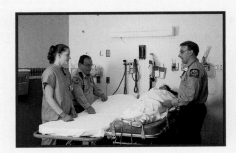

1 The two stretchers are placed side by side. The EMT should be sure that the stretcher brakes are engaged before moving the patient. Any side rails present will have to be lowered.

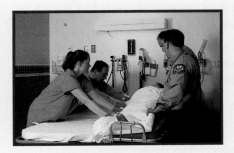

2 Two EMTs are on the one open side of both stretchers. Rolling the edge of the draw sheet or bed linen into a collar, the EMTs grab a firm purchase. (It is a good practice to have the two teams of EMTs pull vigorously against each other to test the strength of the sheet.)

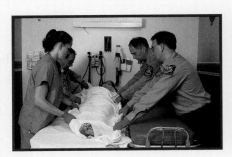

3 Simultaneously, the four EMTs slide the patient from one stretcher to the other in one fluid motion.

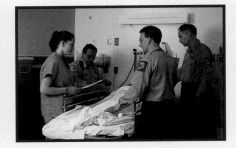

4 Once the patient is on the new stretcher, the side rails should be replaced.

Key Concepts Revisited

- Back care is an important aspect of an EMT's overall back health.

- Use of proper body mechanics during lifting can help reduce back injuries.

- Use of safe reaching techniques can help reduce the risk for the EMT sustaining a back injury.

- Use of safe lifting techniques can help reduce the risk for the EMT sustaining a back injury.

- Use of safe carrying techniques can help reduce the risk for the EMT sustaining a back injury.

- Emergency drags are limited to special circumstances in which the patient's life is in danger because these maneuvers put the EMT at greater risk for back injury.

- Emergency carries are usually limited to special circumstances where the patient needs to be moved expeditiously because they place the EMT at greater risk for back injury.

- The proper use of patient-carrying devices can help promote a safe and orderly transfer of the patient from the field to the ambulance while decreasing the risk for a back injury for the EMT.

- Proper packaging of the patient is therapeutic, providing warmth, and demonstrates compassionate care.

- Safe transfer of the patient from ambulance stretcher to the gurney helps prevent injury to both the EMT and the patient.

Review Questions

1. What is proper back care?
2. What are the proper body mechanics that an EMT should observe?
3. What safety precautions should an EMT observe before lifting?
4. What are the guidelines for lifting?
5. Why would an emergency move be necessary?
6. What are the four emergency drags?
7. What are the six emergency carries?
8. How does an EMT lift a patient from the ground to the stretcher?
9. What precautions must be taken when carrying a patient down a flight of stairs?
10. What are the safe transferring techniques EMTs use at the hospital?

Key Terms

Arm pull

Back care

Back injury

Basket stretcher

Bedrolls

Blanket drag

Body mechanics

Caterpillar pass

Chair carry

Clothing drag

Cradle carry

Diamond carry

Direct lift

Emergency carry

Emergency drag

Emergency move

End-to-end stretcher carry
Extremity lift
Firefighter's carry
Firefighter's drag
Four corners carry
Orthopedic back supports
Orthopedic "scoop" stretcher
Pack strap carry
Power grip

Power lift
Reeves stretcher
Rescuer assist
Seat carry
Slippery sheets
Stairchair
Stringer
Transfer boards

Further Study

American Academy of Orthopaedic Surgeons. *You Are the EMT: Lifting and Moving,* videocassette. Sudbury, MA: Jones and Bartlett, 1999.

Friese, Greg. "EMS Teamwork Lifting and Injury Prevention." Research Review, MERGINET.com, March 2005. http://www.merginet.com/index.cfm?searched=/operations/field/liftstrength.cfm

U.S. Fire Administration and Federal Emergency Management Agency. *EMS Safety: Techniques and Applications* (Publication No. FA-144). Emmitsburg, MD: USFA Publications, 1994.

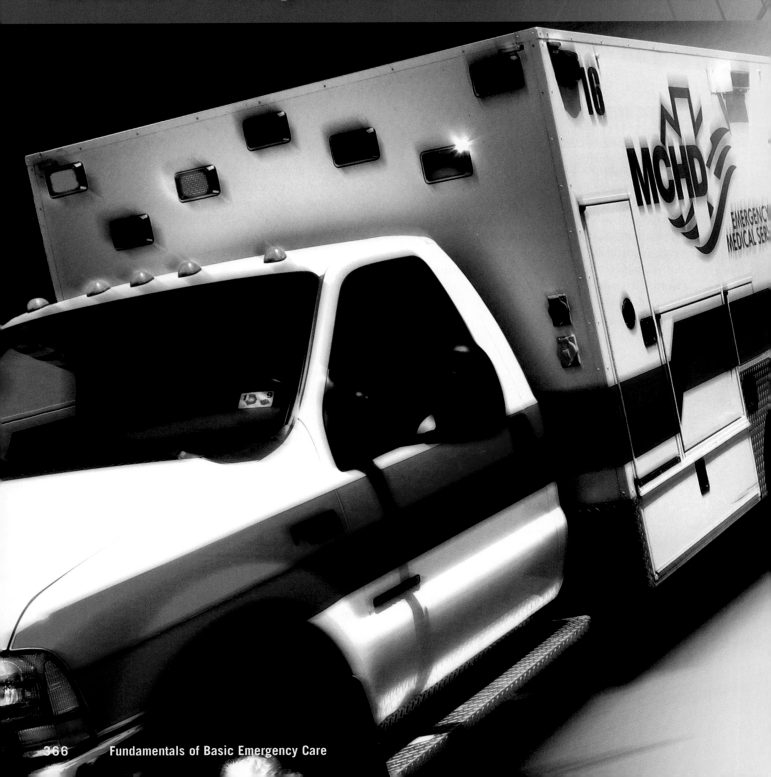

CHAPTER 4

General Principles of Patient Assessment

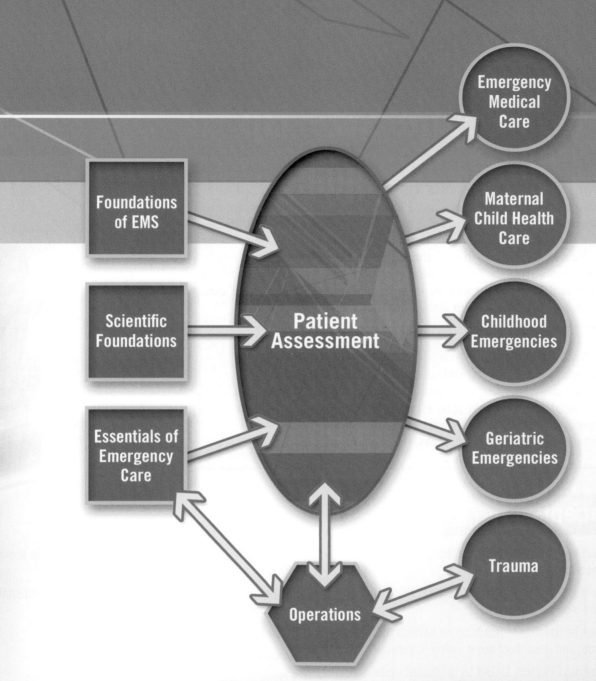

Foundations of EMS

Scientific Foundations

Essentials of Emergency Care

Patient Assessment

Operations

Emergency Medical Care

Maternal Child Health Care

Childhood Emergencies

Geriatric Emergencies

Trauma

General Principles of Patient Assessment

Before an EMT can apply the new skills he has acquired, he must learn how to assess a patient and determine what help is needed.

The EMT must quickly make an assessment, decide what needs to be done, and then prioritize care so that the patient receives the maximum benefit from on-scene care without needless delay to definitive treatment.

The EMT must also be vigilant, constantly assessing and reassessing, looking for those changes that may signal deterioration in the patient's condition and intervene before the patient suffers further harm, or even death.

This chapter begins with the primary assessment, including the scene size-up, and takes the EMT through the entire patient contact, ending with the ongoing assessment.

UNIT (15) Scene Size-Up

Many Emergency Medical Technicians (EMTs) will admit they were attracted to the field of Emergency Medical Services because of how exciting the profession appears to be. Obviously, no one joins EMS expecting to get hurt. Unfortunately, injuries—including preventable injuries—do occur. By the very nature of the environment, EMTs work in situations in which the weather can be hazardous, the scene can be chaotic, and emotions run high. Determining that the scene is as safe as possible before entering it is the first and most important step toward good patient care. After all, EMTs cannot help the patient if they themselves are hurt.

National Education Standards

The Emergency Medical Technician (EMT) will have a fundamental depth and foundational breadth of understanding and application of scene management, including the impact of the environment on patient care, addressing scene hazards including violence, the need for additional or specialized resources, standard precautions, scene stabilization, security, and effectively handling multiple patient situations.

Key Concepts

- The EMT must be knowledgeable in methods of protection against foreseeable injury.

- The first job of EMTs on any scene is to protect themselves, their partners, and the patient.

- The EMT must be trained to identify scene hazards, mitigate those hazards, and implement scene safety in general.

- The assessment of hazards should be conducted while approaching the scene.

- The scene size-up is the first step in patient assessment.

- The EMT must be able to identify hazards on any type of emergency call.

- Hazards at house calls can vary and are often not anticipated by EMTs.

- EMTs are at high risk for injury from the hazards at motor vehicle collision scenes.

- The EMT must be alert for numerous hazards at crime scenes.

- Risk management on emergency responses provides protection from hazards and controls the scene.

- Motor vehicle collision scene management is vital to scene safety.

- The number of patients determines the need for additional resources.

- Patients should be protected from scene hazards.

- Bystanders should be protected from scene hazards.

- A correctly completed scene size-up can protect EMTs, patients, and the public from avoidable dangers.

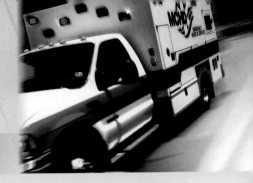

CASE STUDY

Kayla and Jan are dispatched to a woman not feeling well. Kayla recognizes the address from previous calls and explains to Jan that they will need to conduct a thorough scene size-up before entering the residence because Mrs. Smith has a tendency to acquire pets. As they approach the house, Jan notices there are numerous dogs in the yard. The front door to the house is inside the fence. Kayla contacts dispatch to inquire if there is anyone with Mrs. Smith to control the dogs and let them in the house. When dispatch advises that Mrs. Smith's son is present but doesn't feel he can control the dogs on his own, Kayla requests animal control be called. Kayla explains to Jan that a couple of EMTs have been bitten by Mrs. Smith's dogs in the past. They cannot enter the house until the dogs have been controlled.

Critical Thinking Questions

1. Why is a scene size-up important?
2. What steps can be taken to control the scene?
3. What hazards might be present at trauma or medical calls?

INTRODUCTION

Unit 4 stressed the importance of personal well-being and a healthy lifestyle in reducing the chances of injury or illness. This unit examines the protective behaviors an EMT should practice while on scene. Please read this unit carefully. The life you save may be your own!

HISTORY OF SAFETY IN EMS

EMTs have always faced hazards while providing patient care. Extremes of weather, hazardous road conditions, and infectious diseases are just a few of the more common hazards EMTs routinely face.

In the early years of EMS, not much attention was given to responder safety and injury prevention. In 1973, the federal report *America Burning* drew attention to the growing problem of on-the-job injury in the fire and emergency services. National groups, such as the National Fire Protection Association (NFPA), started to publish recommendations and standards for safe emergency operations. Yet many of these recommendations and standards were not actively pursued by many fire and EMS agencies.

The complacency of fire and emergency services toward safety standards, particularly related to infectious disease, all changed on March 6, 1992, when the federal Occupational Safety and Health Administration (OSHA) issued the blood-borne pathogens rule, OSHA 1910.1030 (29 CFR 1910.1030). The blood-borne pathogens rule simply says that EMS agencies are responsible for the safety of their employee-members. It further states that the government can enforce that responsibility.

With that single regulation, the federal government assumed a prominent role in EMS safety. The intent of the rule was to eliminate or reduce the incidence of EMS workers' exposure to blood-borne pathogens. It also had the effect of shaking up the emergency services community and awakening emergency responders to these serious safety concerns. Table 15-1 reviews

Table 15-1 Rules, Regulations, and Standards That Affect EMS

1. Occupational Safety and Health Administration (OSHA) Regulations
   1910.10.146, *Confined Spaces*
   - Outlines training and precautions, including a permit, required to enter confined spaces
   1910.134, *Respiratory Protection*
   - Provides guidelines for use of respiratory masks, fit testing, and physical performance requirements
   1910.120, *Hazardous Waste Operations and Emergency Response*
   - Also known as HAZWOPER, establishes requirements for hazardous materials awareness for all emergency responders
   1910.1030, *Occupational Exposure to Bloodborne Pathogens*
   - Requires emergency responders be protected from blood-borne pathogens; includes training mandates as well as exposure procedures

2. National Fire Protection Association (NFPA) Standards NFPA 473, *Competencies for EMS Personnel Responding to Hazardous Materials Incidents*
   - Establishes standards for emergency responders to hazardous materials incidents
   NFPA 1500, *Fire Department Occupational Safety and Health Program*
   - Establishes standards and guidelines for fire service health programs
   NFPA 1521, *Fire Department Safety Officer*
   - Establishes standards for the safety officer, outlining duties and responsibilities
   NFPA 1561, *Fire Department Incident Management System*
   - Establishes standards for a common approach to public safety incidents for the fire service
   NFPA 1581, *Fire Department Infection Control*
   - Establishes standards for infection control programs and departmental guidelines
   NFPA 1582, *Fire Department Medical Requirements for Fire Fighters*
   - Establishes standards for physical requirements, including immunizations, for firefighters
   NFPA 1999, *Protective Clothing for Emergency Medical Operations*
   - Establishes standards for protective clothing, including protection against infectious materials

3. Infection Control Guidelines from the Centers for Disease Control and Prevention (CDC)
   - Provides guidelines for prevention of transmission of human immunodeficiency virus

4. Ryan White Comprehensive AIDS Resource Emergency Act of 1990
   - Requires the creation of a designated officer as well as disease-reporting requirements

5. Environmental Protection Agency (EPA)
   40 CFR 311, *Hazardous Materials Response*
   - Establishes requirements for responders to hazardous materials incidents

a number of important regulations and standards that have had a dramatic impact on emergency services nationwide.

In response to this challenge, EMS and the fire service have institutionalized safety practices and distributed standard operating guidelines and are starting to employ safety officers.

These safety officers are charged with upholding applicable federal and state law as well as departmental regulations. This duty includes training EMTs and firefighters about safe practices. On the scene of a major incident, the safety officer performs as a member of the incident management's command staff.

Today's workforce issues in EMS place safety as the top priority, and ongoing studies are examining how to improve the safety of ambulances as well as the EMTs who staff them. EMTs cannot afford to ignore the risks associated with their profession. They must be knowledgeable in methods of protection against foreseeable injury and illness. They must be trained to identify scene hazards, mitigate those hazards, and implement scene safety in general. Whenever an EMT is responding to an EMS call, the first question the EMT must answer is, "Is the scene safe?"

SCENE APPROACH

When EMTs approach a scene, they should all think the same thought: "Is the scene safe?" Only when the EMT has assessed the scene for hazards and has controlled those hazards can a decision be made on how to care for the patient. Scene safety should be thought of as the first step in performing patient care.

Careful attention to the scene approach, assessment, and hazard control helps to ensure the safety of the EMT and the patient. Eventually the EMT will automatically integrate the process of approach, assessment, and control into practice as they gain experience.

DISPATCH INFORMATION

The first source of information about scene hazards is information provided by the communications center. The dispatch information will sometimes differ from the findings upon arrival because the dispatcher is relying on the 911 caller to provide the pertinent information. Emotional response to the event, language barriers, and confusion on the part of the caller can contribute to some information not being conveyed to the dispatcher. The EMT should always assume the information from dispatch is accurate and begin his scene preplanning based on that information.

The dispatch information may describe the mechanism of injury or the nature of illness. The nature of the call, medical or trauma, must be confirmed on arrival.

Listening carefully to the dispatch of other emergency services can also provide the EMT with additional information regarding on-scene hazards. For example, if a police unit is dispatched for a fight in progress, the EMT might conclude that there is violence on scene and weapons may be present.

When a rescue unit is requested by the first arriving law enforcement units, the EMT can conclude that patients might be entrapped. If multiple emergency services are responding to the same accident, then perhaps there are several cars and multiple patients involved. Dispatch can sometimes also give the approximate number of patients and the need for additional resources based on the type of incident.

All this information should help the EMT to form a mental picture of the scene and the hazards that might exist.

PREARRIVAL INSTRUCTIONS

The dispatch information provided by the emergency medical dispatcher, or communications specialist (COMSPEC), contains an abundance of clues regarding the character of the scene. By paying careful attention to the details of the initial dispatch report and prearrival instructions, the EMT can get an early idea—a "heads-up"—on what may be encountered.

Table 15-2 lists some of the information that the communications specialist may have available. Most communications centers are electronically linked to an array of computers and information sources. The communications center can advise on weather information, minute-to-minute road conditions, global positioning coordinates, and a "history" of prior calls at the same location. The EMT should use all the information the communications center has available at the time of dispatch to be prepared for all potential scene situations.

Street Smart

A senior EMT will often sense that something is "just not right," take in all the information on the scene, compare it to a past experience, and come to a subconscious conclusion that danger is present. This so-called intuition is often the result of right-brain thinking, and all of this information processing is often accomplished in a matter of seconds. Whenever a senior EMT has a "gut instinct" that the scene is not safe, listen!

Table 15-2 Dispatcher Information
1. Nature of emergency—medical versus trauma
2. Patient's level of consciousness
3. Patient's breathing
4. Potentially life-threatening conditions
5. Violence on scene—police en route or on scene
6. Fire or smoke condition reported
7. Special equipment needed— rescue/extrication
8. Special rescue—for example, confined space, hazardous materials
9. Traffic conditions—fastest route and traffic delays
10. Other responding emergency vehicles

PERSONAL PROTECTIVE EQUIPMENT

The EMT should don the minimum (gloves) personal protective equipment (PPE) while en route to the scene based on dispatch information. The type and amount of PPE needed is determined by the nature of the call. Medical calls may require gloves, goggles, and a mask. A trauma call may require the EMT to wear a complete set of turnout gear, including a helmet with an eye shield, a rescue coat, heavy-duty gloves, and a specific type of boots.

The dispatch information provides clues to the nature of the call and therefore the PPE that will be needed. Review Unit 8 for more information on a symptom-based approach to PPE for medical calls.

SCENE STAGING

After careful consideration of the dispatch information, the EMT prepares physically by donning gloves and mentally by imagining how the scene may appear upon arrival.

It is important that the EMT does not hastily enter the scene. It is better to proceed slowly into a scene, making assessments for hazards, than to pull into a dangerous situation and try to make a hasty retreat.

Some situations call for the EMT to place the emergency vehicle a safe distance from the scene. This allows the EMT to observe the scene first (Figure 15.1) and keep the equipment available from a safe distance. Stopping the emergency vehicle a safe distance from the scene is called **staging.**

Staging serves two purposes. First, it may keep the EMT out of harm's way. The best defense against hazards such as explosions, gunfire, and hazardous materials exposure is distance.

Second, it gives the EMT time to assess the scene from the relative safety of the vehicle. Staging should be a part of the routine response to all calls and particularly any hazardous calls.

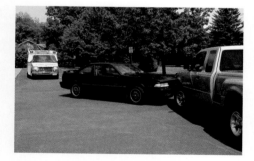

Figure 15.1 Parking the ambulance away from the scene provides safety for the EMT and the crew while allowing for an assessment of hazards and needed resources

SCENE SIZE-UP

The EMT must perform a scene size-up on every call. A **size-up** is the process of observing a scene and making judgments about the equipment, resources, and personnel that will be needed to stabilize the scene or provide additional or advanced patient care.

The scene size-up should begin with the prearrival instructions, at which point the EMT started to visualize the scene in his mind. The size-up continues when EMS arrives and begins the scene assessment to identify potential hazards, to determine what led the EMS to be called to the scene, and to assess all other factors, including any unusual characteristics of the scene not previously relayed by dispatch.

The on-scene size-up consists of several parts that are done in sequence and eventually become second nature to the EMT. It is important the EMT remembers there could be circumstances that may require flexibility to perform certain elements of the scene size-up as they become available.

The EMT must be concerned with the entire scene and what hazards may be present. If the scene is determined to be safe and stable, the EMT then either begins treatment on scene or proceeds to move the patient to safety. Scene safety is an ongoing process; if the scene becomes unstable, the EMT must remove the patient quickly or retreat until the scene can be made safe once again. The EMT must remember his first duty is to his own safety and then the patient's. The patient will not benefit if the EMT is injured and unable to help.

The EMT then determines the nature of the illness (NOI) for a medical patient or the mechanism of injury (MOI) for a trauma patient. In some situations, the MOI or NOI cannot be determined without further assessment.

The EMT should determine the number of patients and call for whatever additional resources are needed to help stabilize the scene or treat additional patients. When requesting additional resources, the EMT should call in an initial report to the dispatch center. The **initial report** establishes that EMS is on scene and in the process of controlling the scene. It also typically describes the scene. Finally, any other resources such as additional EMT units, law enforcement, fire departments, power companies, or hazardous material units that may be needed are requested at the end of the initial report.

SCENE SAFETY

Why is the scene size-up important? The EMT must evaluate the scene for any physical or environmental hazards prior to entering the scene. When the scene is determined to be safe, the EMT can then proceed into the scene to begin assessment of the patient.

If the scene is unstable, the EMT must make the determination, "What can be done to make the scene stable?" If the EMTs do not have the ability to stabilize the scene while keeping themselves and the patient safe, then they must not enter the scene.

It is natural for a new EMT to become distracted by the excitement of an emergency scene. Rolled-over cars, burned patients, and gunshot wounds can distract the EMT from seeing potentially life-threatening hazards that are always present on scene. These scenes also contain some serious hazards to the EMT. The standardized size-up approach ensures that the EMT does not fail to identify the danger present before rendering care. To avoid this situation, and to improve the chances of survival, the EMT should take a careful approach and *stop, look, and listen* before entering the scene.

Stop the ambulance several hundred feet from the scene and visually scan not only the scene but areas around the scene. The EMT should look for hazards, such as downed power lines, signs of a crime, potential hiding spots for criminals, and the size of any crowd that may be present. These are just a few examples of potential hazards to the EMT.

An EMT can use a pair of binoculars to extend sight and improve vision of the scene (Figure 15.2). Binoculars can be an invaluable tool, especially when dealing with a potential toxic or hazardous material incident; they should be readily available in the front compartment of every emergency vehicle.

The EMT should also listen to the sounds of the environment. The sounds of breaking glass and gunfire are clearly signs of danger ahead. The sound of thunder may indicate the approach of a potentially severe or hazardous electrical storm.

Perhaps more alarming than gunshots or shouting is the complete absence of sound. When first arriving on scene, to a house call, for example, the EMT would expect to see a light on the porch or someone at the door waving them down. If the house is dark and the scene is quiet, there are two possibilities. One, the EMT has simply responded to the wrong address. Or, two, the EMT could be walking into an ambush situation. The EMT should first call to confirm the address, then if the address is confirmed, request law enforcement to the scene.

Scene assessment and safety require the EMT to be a leader and take control of the scene, even if that means not approaching the patient or allowing others to approach the patient when indications of an unsafe scene exist. This can be a difficult position; however, the safety and care of the patient begins with the safety or stabilization of the scene and the emergency responders.

GLOBAL ASSESSMENT

Once the EMT has performed an overall scene assessment, taken actions to reduce or eliminate hazards and safety issues, determined the number of patients and appropriately requested additional resources, the next step is to stop and make a global assessment. A **global assessment** involves the EMT taking in all the information gathered, including the dispatch information and scene size-up, into consideration and then determining an initial action plan.

This process of assessment and evaluation of information is turned into action as the EMT gives the initial report and proceeds either to care for the first patient or to establish EMS command.

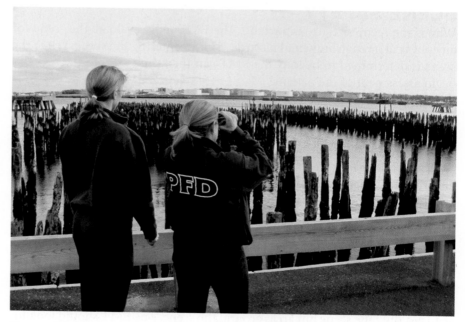

Figure 15.2 Binoculars can extend an EMT's field of vision, helping to identify hazards earlier (Courtesy of Larry Torrey & MEDCU, Portland, ME)

IDENTIFYING HAZARDOUS CONDITIONS

The EMT must be able to identify hazards on all calls. Safety is everyone's job. As an example, take the case of a single patient with a gunshot wound. If law enforcement officers are on hand, creating a perimeter with a safe zone, and the scene is quiet, the EMT might decide to do lifesaving treatments on scene, such as airway control.

However, if a hostile crowd has gathered at the perimeter, the EMT may decide to quickly move the patient to the relative safety of the ambulance or to "scoop and run" with the patient, rather than risk an exposure to violence on the street. There have been cases in which EMTs were trying to save a gunshot wound victim, only to have a gang member reach over the EMT's shoulder and shoot the patient again!

These illustrations represent the same situation, the same mechanism of injury, but different on-scene hazards. The patient's condition was not different. It was the hazards that created a unique environment.

RISK FACTORS

A *risk,* by definition, is an exposure to a hazard that could lead to injury. EMS is a risky business, and injuries do occur, but many hazards are predictable, and therefore many risks are preventable.

Certain risks are common and predictable, becoming an almost routine response by EMTs. For example, broken glass would be a typical hazard found on the scene of many motor vehicle collisions, and every EMT knows specialized equipment such as heavy gloves or a reflective vest when responding to a motor vehicle collision are protective measures that should be automatically taken.

Predictable risks, those seen commonly at certain scenes, can be grouped together and called **risk factors.** Table 15-3 lists risk factors common to two typical EMS calls, motor vehicle collisions and house calls.

HIGH INDEX OF SUSPICION

A **high index of suspicion** describes a way of thinking. This term describes the viewpoint an EMT should always take when approaching any scene. When a medical provider is given specific information about a condition, he should have a high index of suspicion that other complications extenuating from that condition may be present.

For example, an EMT may have a high index of suspicion that a patient with chest pain may also have shortness of breath. If the EMT is told that the call is a motor vehicle collision, he should have a high index of suspicion that broken glass, spilled fuel, and blocked traffic may be present at the scene.

The EMT should carefully consider what hazards could be present and verify whether the hazard is in fact present. Any EMT who approaches a scene unaware of or, worse, ignoring the potential existence of scene hazards, risks endangering themselves, their crew, and the patient. The EMT will likely overlook hazards if he does not anticipate and look for them. Making the connection between what is seen and the danger present is the key to rescuer survival.

INFORMATION OVERLOAD

Too much information about the condition of the scene and scene hazards can lead the EMT to feel frustrated from *information overload.* Information overload can lead to inaction or, worse, inappropriate action. How is an EMT expected to sift through the incredible amount of information that is present on scene?

Table 15-3 Risk Factors

Motor Vehicle Collisions

1. Oncoming traffic
2. Passing traffic
3. Spilled fuels—rear
4. Spilled antifreeze—front
5. Wires down
6. Utility pole suspended
7. Smoke from vehicle
8. Fire visible
9. Surface—slope or uneven
10. Broken glass
11. Loaded bumpers

House Calls

1. Animals
2. Damaged stairs
3. Loose rugs
4. Poor lighting

First, learning the components of a scene size-up from an experienced EMT helps a less experienced EMT feel more comfortable and able to appropriately prioritize the pertinent information. A mentor should discuss what is seen and the danger it presents so the EMT can see and understand the situation as it presents.

The EMT should maintain a high index of suspicion on every call, regardless of experience. Using the same reasoning as the bank robber Willie Sutton, who is quoted as saying he robbed banks "because that is where the money is," EMTs should look for specific hazards where they are most likely to be. For example, flammable liquids flow and are likely to be found under a vehicle or in a low depression, while smoke rises and would most likely be seen in the sky. EMTs must use their training, experience, intelligence, and a high index of suspicion to ascertain hazards up, down, and at eye level.

HAZARDS AT A HOUSE CALL

Residential or house calls are the most common calls to which an EMT responds, and hazards may range from poor lighting to house pets. In many cases, the patient or the patient's family has a pet in the house. Pets can range from the common house cat to the exotic boa constrictor. Many of these animals, under the right conditions, can pose a danger to the EMT.

Among the most common animals an EMT will encounter on scenes are dogs. Dogs, both large and small, can be a formidable obstacle, especially when the animal thinks that it is protecting its fallen master (Figure 15.3). In most cases, it is a good idea to insist that the dog be shut in another room before attending the patient.

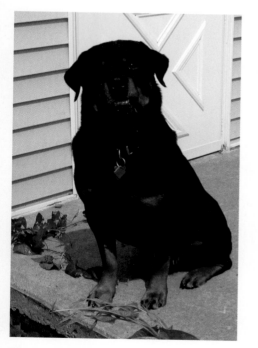

Figure 15.3 Dogs represent a real and common hazard to EMTs

The EMT should be cautious around dogs, especially a mother dog with pups or a dog that is feeding; at these times the dog is likely to be more aggressive. If the dog should run toward the EMT, the EMT should remain motionless, with hands down by his side, and should always avoid eye contact with the dog because the animal may see this as a threat. The EMT should never run or scream because the dog's natural instincts are to chase anyone running away. If the dog knocks the EMT down, the best action is to roll into a ball and keep quiet; the dog will quickly lose interest and disengage from the attack.

Another threat to the EMT's safety is poor lighting. Poorly lit hallways and entranceways obscure trip hazards. The EMT risks slipping and falling on loose floorboards or throw rugs. The use of a flashlight to illuminate the doorway or hallway can help prevent fall hazards.

Physical hazards to the EMT can often be identified and dealt with accordingly. It is the unseen, or unsuspected, hazard that can be the most dangerous. Family members who initially welcomed the EMT and ushered the EMT into the house can suddenly change their attitude and pose a formidable risk. It is imperative for EMTs to always be prepared for a potentially changing scene environment. The dynamics of scene assessment must continue throughout the call, and the need for vigilance does not end with patient contact.

As a matter of practice, an EMT will always try to keep the pathway to the nearest door clear, permitting a quick exit if needed. Most EMS services have crews with a minimum of two EMTs. While one EMT's attention is focused on the patient, the other EMT is observing the scene, including family members, for any sign of danger. This practice of "watching your partner's back" is an example of a safe practice that is easily employed by EMTs.

As the EMT enters a room, he should conduct a visual sweep of the room for any deadly weapons or potentially dangerous instruments. A **deadly weapon** is any device that, by its nature, is intended to cause death. Knives, rifles, and shotguns are examples of deadly weapons. EMTs usually do not have any difficulty identifying a deadly weapon. However, EMTs frequently fail to identify dangerous instruments. **Dangerous instruments** are things capable of producing death or serious bodily injury when used in certain circumstances. For example, a pair of sewing scissors or a broken whiskey bottle can be used as a dangerous instrument.

Stairs can also represent a serious hazard to the EMT. Loose boards and broken handrails can cause an EMT to lose his equilibrium and fall. Many EMTs lean against the inside wall when carrying a patient down the stairs rather than trust the handrail.

HAZARDS AT A MOTOR VEHICLE COLLISION

The scene of a motor vehicle collision can be one of the most dangerous scenes in which an EMT works. Flammable liquids, slippery antifreeze, sharp glass, and jagged metal edges are some of the more common hazards caused by the collision that an EMT will encounter. Snowy, icy roads and sharply curving roads are hazards that may also present at the scenes of motor vehicle collisions.

When a semi-truck is involved in a motor vehicle collision, look at the truck carefully. Are fumes visible? If fumes are visible, are the fumes white, like steam, or tinged with color? Do the fumes stream skyward, or do they hug the ground?

Are there any diamond-shaped hazardous materials placards on the side of the truck? What is the name of the carrier? Gasoline company trucks usually transport gasoline.

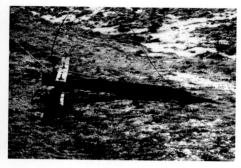

Figure 15.4 Downed power lines pose a serious threat to the EMT

These are all signs of a potential toxic environment caused by a hazardous materials spill. More information on hazardous materials identification and the EMT's response to hazardous materials is provided in Unit 50.

DOWNED POWER LINES

When a vehicle strikes a utility pole, it can bring electrically charged wires down. The EMT should look for downed power lines on the scene of any motor vehicle collision (Figure 15.4). Smoldering grass fires, so-called hot spots, or clearly visible sparks flying are indications of a downed power line. The EMT must treat all downed lines as potentially dangerous, even if they suspect they are telephone or television cable lines.

It is important for an EMT to look up for downed power lines. Disrupted power lines can be found either sagging dangerously low, but not touching the ground, or with one end dangling over the EMT's head. If the EMT's head should come into contact with the line, his body would complete the circuit and he could be electrocuted.

The EMT should never assume that a downed power line that seems safe will remain safe. Power is routinely interrupted by squirrels and other animals. When these interruptions occur, the power company reroutes electricity through other paths in the power grid to bypass the short in the line and restore electricity to the affected customers.

A downed power line is not safe until the power company physically removes or otherwise isolates the power line. All downed lines should be assumed to be energized, and therefore dangerous, until proved otherwise.

New housing developments routinely bury unsightly power lines underground to obscure them from view. The only sign that a power line may be buried is the aboveground splice box or a transformer. These splice boxes and transformers are often hidden in the shrubbery. When a car comes crashing across someone's lawn and through the shrubs, the car can come to rest on one of these boxes and become energized. It is important to look both under the car and over the top of the car for power lines.

If downed power lines are visible on scene, do not approach the scene. Park the ambulance at least one full span of wires away from the pole with the downed wires. Use the public address (PA) system in the ambulance to warn the occupants of the motor vehicle to stay in the car. They are safer inside the car. Down power lines lying on the ground, especially on a wet surface, can energize a large area of the scene.

Also, warn curious onlookers to stay away from the vehicles, again using the PA system. After warning the vehicle occupants and onlookers, call for the power company or fire department to come to the scene. Some areas require a fire engine to respond on all motor vehicle collisions or downed power line calls. It is always a good idea to verify they are en route to the scene if the ambulance arrives and finds any of the previously mentioned hazards. As always, follow local protocols and operating guidelines.

TOXIC SUBSTANCES

The EMT may be called to a scene where a toxic substance exists. A **toxic substance** is any substances that is poisonous to the human body. As previously discussed, a tanker truck hauling hazardous material may be involved in a motor vehicle crash in which the tanker is ruptured, spilling the contents. It will be relatively easy for the EMT to know there is obvious hazard present based on dispatch information, visualization of the spill, and the identification marking on the side of the truck. Hazardous material spills will be discussed in more detail in Unit 50.

Street Smart

A car may strike a telephone pole so hard that it shears the pole from its foundation. The only thing holding the pole upright is the power lines. Unsuspecting EMTs may be hurt if the wires snap and the pole drops. All broken poles should be treated with the same respect as a downed power line.

Toxic substances are not always easily identified and may be so subtle the caller does not even recognize their existence. An example of a toxic substance and low-oxygen environment that is hazardous to an EMT is carbon monoxide. The EMT may be called to a residence for a patient feeling nauseous, dizzy, and weak with a headache. The patient may not realize she is being exposed to a toxic gas that has been replacing the oxygen in the air and her lungs; therefore, she would not think to alert dispatch or EMS of the presence of this toxic gas.

The EMT needs to use good scene assessment skills and a high index of suspicion to determine the presence of many toxic gases based on the clues the environment, patient, and scene is providing.

Scenes that involve obvious spills, leaks, or a fire easily alert the EMT to the potential for a hazardous toxic substance or low oxygen environment requiring specialized resources. Other scenes, such as confined spaces, are sometimes not recognized as hazardous environments until the EMT has become a victim himself. Extreme caution should always be used when an EMS team is called to the scene where a patient may be in a confined space such as caves, wells, manholes, sewers, closed garages, and other spaces where the limited area may have created low oxygen or toxic air environments. EMTs should not enter these scenes unless they have the specialized training and equipment to keep them safe.

One important clue that there may be a toxic environment is if there are multiple patients with similar symptoms in the same area or home. If the EMT responds where all the occupants, including the pets, are exhibiting the same or similar signs and symptoms, assume the environment is toxic. If encountering this scenario in the winter months, the EMT should suspect carbon monoxide poisoning due to a faulty furnace or gas water heater and inadequate ventilation.

CRIME SCENES

The EMS profession often works with other public safety partners such as fire and law enforcement and will be called to treat patients who have been involved in a crime, whether as the victim, a bystander, or the individual suspected of committing the crime. Crime scenes require special considerations on the part of the EMT, including preserving evidence on the scene; however, the number one priority is personal safety of the EMT.

Scene size-up is vitally important when approaching a crime scene. If EMS is dispatched to the scene of a crime, never enter the scene until law enforcement is present and has secured the scene.

There will be times when EMS is dispatched to a scene where no crime was reported by the caller, but during the scene size-up, the EMT suspects a crime has taken place. An example is being called to a bar for an injured person. The EMT should have a high index of suspicion that the injury may have been caused in a fight, even if the dispatch information doesn't state a fight has taken place. Remember, the dispatchers are relaying information they have gathered from the caller. Often the caller does not want law enforcement to respond and therefore does not indicate the true cause of the injury.

The EMT must always be alert to potential danger when called to an area known for having a high incidence of crime, regardless of the nature of the call. In these instances, always verify with the dispatcher that law enforcement is also en route to the area or request law enforcement if they have not been dispatched.

Street Smart

Downed power lines create a "field" of energy around the point where they contact the ground. When the unsuspecting EMT approaches the scene, he will feel a kind of tingling sensation in his legs. The tingling sensation indicates that the EMT has entered an electric field.

Once an EMT realizes that he has entered the energy field of a downed power line, the worst thing he can do is turn and run. Lifting one leg and then placing it down creates a pathway, or a circuit, for the electricity to travel.

Instead, the EMT should stand completely still until the power is turned off. If standing still is not practical, then the EMT has two choices. He can either "shuffle" off the scene, keeping his feet and knees in contact at all times, or can "hop" off the scene, again with both feet together. Shuffling and hopping prevent a circuit from being created and injury from occurring.

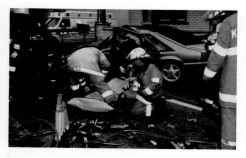

Figure 15.5 Risk management is a team effort requiring the cooperation of many public safety agencies

RISK MITIGATION

Whenever a hazard has been identified, during any part of a call, the EMT must act to protect himself and his partner, the public, and the patient, in that order, from bodily harm and risk for injury. The process of identifying hazards and ensuring protection is called **risk mitigation.**

Even though a patient has gotten into a dangerous situation, it does not automatically mean the EMTs must endanger themselves to rescue the person. The EMT's first duty is to protect himself. The courts have upheld that although an EMT cannot simply refuse to act, he can refuse to enter an inherently dangerous situation. The EMT must act to try to mitigate the danger and make it safe to provide care. However, until that danger has been reduced to an acceptable risk, or eliminated, the EMT should not enter the scene (Figure 15.5).

CRIME SCENE MANAGEMENT

Once a crime scene has been secured by law enforcement and the EMT is allowed to approach, the scene must be continually assessed for other hazards that may still exist, such as a toxic environment, animals, or emotional bystanders or family members. All scenes have the potential to become dangerous at any time; however, the emotion and violence usually associated with a crime scene highly increase the potential for danger.

When approaching a high crime area, turn off the lights and sirens before arriving in the area. Lights and sirens can sometimes increase the danger by drawing attention to a situation and attracting a crowd. Again, if the area is known as a high crime area, do not enter until law enforcement arrives. If possible, park two or three houses away from the residence. The scene can be observed from a distance and enable the EMT to form a safe plan of approach and, more importantly, retreat if the need arises.

If the call is to a known crime scene involving a shooting, the ambulance should be positioned outside the **killing zone,** the area controlled by hostile gun fire. The killing zone can be subject to change depending on where the gun fire is coming from and the mobility of the person or persons with the guns. The EMTs must be prepared to move themselves and the ambulance to a safe zone at any time.

Invariably a crowd will form at the scene, drawn by the excitement of law enforcement, EMS, or fire department personnel present at a crime scene. If the crowd has already formed prior to arrival, the EMT should study the crowd. The size of the crowd is important to note; however, the mood of the crowd is by far more relevant to gauge. Is the crowd angry at the situation? Are they hostile to the presence of EMS or law enforcement? Is the scene chaotic or hysterical? Do not enter scenes where a crowd is unsecured and angry. Do not allow the crowd to pull you into the chaos, and always be prepared to retreat until the crowd has been controlled. It is a good idea to move the patient to the more controlled and safe environment of the ambulance, away from the crowd as quickly as possible.

Once the scene has been controlled and the EMT is allowed to more fully enter the scene to begin patient management, it is important to remember to be alert to any possibility there could still be elements that may present a danger. Again, the EMT must always be prepared to retreat, even when it may feel that you are not doing your duty to the patient. Protecting yourself and your partner will always remain your top priority, even as you approach the patient and begin patient assessment and management.

While approaching the patient, always scan the area around the scene, noting possible places someone could be concealed. Hold a flashlight down next to the body, but use it to illuminate and scan the area for movement as you

Table 15-4 Crime Scene Procedures for EMS

- Limit the number of responders that enter the scene to only what is needed for patient care and to keep watch on the scene's safety.
- Be prepared for the possibility the patient may also be the individual who committed the crime. Make sure there are no weapons or potential weapons the patient could suddenly grab.
- Take care to not disturb evidence, such as foot prints, broken glass, or any items that look out of place.
- Do not touch anything that is not needed in treating the patient.
- Always wear gloves to avoid leaving your fingerprints at the scene.
- Keep any clothing that is removed from the patient. Additionally, when cutting through clothing, try to avoid cutting through what could be a bullet hole or knife slash.
- Document everything about the scene thoroughly, including who was at the scene upon arrival and any individual items from the scene that were turned over to law enforcement personnel.

approach the house. Assess the situation closely before entering the house, leave the door open, and always keep the path between you and the door clear. It is imperative to always be prepared for the scene where a crime has or may have been committed and that may continue to pose some danger to the EMT.

Preservation of the crime scene should be attempted within the best ability of the EMT as long as it does not keep the EMT from protecting himself or the patient. EMTs should follow a few key procedures when entering and working within a known or suspected crime scene. Table 15-4 lists procedures that should be followed when entering or working where a crime may have taken place.

It is important to remember the primary job of EMTs on any scene is to protect themselves and their partners and to provide medical assistance to the patient. It is not the EMT's job to solve the crime. Law enforcement will be aided through preservation of evidence and thorough documentation of the incident, including recording anything found on the patient while rendering care.

MOTOR VEHICLE COLLISION SCENE MANAGEMENT

The single largest danger to the EMT at the scene of a motor vehicle collision is not on scene when he arrives! The danger is traffic. Every year, passing motorists strike and kill law enforcement officers, firefighters, and EMTs while they are performing their duty.

Careless drivers, sometimes referred to as *rubberneckers,* focus on the carnage of twisted metal and bleeding patients and fail to notice the people working around the scene trying to rescue those patients. The use of effective warning devices and proper vehicle placement can reduce the chance of an EMT being struck by passing motorists.

VEHICLE PLACEMENT

EMTs can use several tactics to improve the odds of survival and protect themselves and the patient on the scene of a motor vehicle collision.

Law enforcement officers position their patrol vehicles purposefully when they make a vehicle stop, using the vehicle as a physical barrier. What the law enforcement officer has created, in effect, is a **safety corridor** between the patrol car and the stopped vehicle. Figure 15.6 demonstrates the effect of positioning the emergency vehicle at the roadside of a scene to create a safe zone from within which the EMT can work more safely.

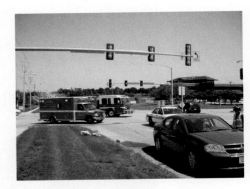

Figure 15.6 The EMS vehicle can be used as a physical barrier, creating a safety corridor in front of it (Courtesy of Clive Fire Department, Clive, IA)

An important decision an EMT must make is how close to park the vehicle to the scene. How close the emergency vehicle should be placed to the scene depends on several factors:

- The types of vehicles on the road
- The average speed of the traffic on the road
- The type and weight of the emergency vehicle

As an example, depicted in Figure 15.7, let's say the roadway is an interstate, and the vehicles range from personal cars to tractor-trailers. Remember that the emergency vehicle is serving as a barricade. The object of a barricade is to either stop or slow another vehicle from coming down on the EMTs or at least to allow them enough time to escape when the vehicle strikes the ambulance.

How far back an ambulance should be positioned on a busy interstate, where vehicles are driving by at 60 to 70 miles per hour (mph), depends on how far a tractor-trailer can push an ambulance. The EMT should consider placing the ambulance at least 30 yards, or about three roadside markers, from the scene.

Compare that first example to the scene of a motor vehicle collision within a small village. Local traffic is light, and the posted speed limit is 30 mph. This scene presents a different picture than the previous scenario. The degree of danger may be less, but danger still exists. In all cases, the minimum safe distance to position an emergency response vehicle is about 50 feet.

WARNING LIGHTS

The emergency warning lights are a valuable tool for safety. Arguments flourish about what is the best array of emergency lights. Some prefer beacons because they strike overhead power lines and reflect back to oncoming drivers. Others prefer strobe lights that emit a powerful glow visible for miles.

The color of emergency lights has also been a matter of debate. Some states have adopted blue lights for all emergency vehicles; others have red lights. Some studies have indicated that blue lights are more visible after dark than red lights. However, the most visible color at night is yellow light. Recently, the federal ambulance specifications have required the presence of one rearward-facing yellow light on all ambulances. Yellow lights have been generally accepted as "warning lights" by the public.

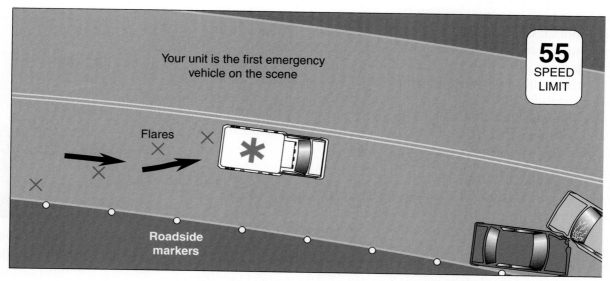

Figure 15.7 The EMS vehicle should be at least three roadside markers away from the scene on a controlled-access highway

There is one point of agreement among emergency responders. Emergency lights are an important part of scene safety. The EMT should turn them on and leave them on whenever an emergency vehicle is on scene.

The best situation for an EMT is one in which other responders have already shut down the closest lane prior to arrival on scene (Figure 15.8). From a safety standpoint, the safest place for an ambulance is ahead of the collision site. The EMT can pull the emergency vehicle ahead of the others and leave the emergency lights flashing.

Typically, traffic is backed up behind the collision site. If the ambulance is in front of the scene, then it is not blocked by traffic and has a clear exit to the hospital. Whenever possible, the EMT should position the ambulance facing the direction of travel to the appropriate hospital.

If the patient is seriously injured, rapid transportation to a trauma center may be needed. Precious time can be lost trying to make a three-point turn on a narrow roadway.

ROAD FLARES

Flares are commonly used by EMTs as a traffic warning device. Portable and highly visible both day and night, flares can also be very dangerous. By following a few simple rules, the EMT can safely use flares.

A lit flare is actually burning metal and when lit, flares tend to sputter and throw sparks in every direction. EMTs must be wearing minimum PPE of firefighter-grade gloves and protective eyewear prior to lighting a flare. These sparks from the flares can cause serious burns to the unprotected EMT. If available, the EMT should also wear a turnout coat, or similar flame-resistant coat. This will protect him from burns to the forearms. Sparks can fly into the eyes of the EMT as well and lead to permanent blindness. Eye protection, safety glasses, or a helmet shield must be worn by an EMT who is lighting a road flare.

To light the flare, the EMT removes the striker from the head of the flare. Firmly grasping the shaft of the flare about 6 inches from the head with one hand, the EMT lights the flare by placing the striker on the head, or igniter, of the flare and firmly striking the flare, with the striker, away from the body. Sometimes it takes several hits before ignition occurs. Always follow the manufacturer's instructions to light flares properly.

Once the flare is ignited, either stand the flare up with wire legs or use the spike to stick it into the ground. Use caution whenever spiking a flare, because falling embers can severely burn the EMT. Skill 15-1 at the end of this unit describes the procedure for lighting a road flare.

The position and pattern of flare distribution will determine the effectiveness of the flare as a warning device. The farthest flare should be placed so that the oncoming driver can see the flare, react, and bring the vehicle to a stop, if needed, before entering the scene.

To estimate where the first flare should be placed, take the posted speed limit, convert it to feet, and then multiply by 4. If the posted speed is over 50 mph, add 100 feet to the total. This figure is the number of feet away from the scene that the first flare should be dropped. Table 15-5 lists the suggested distance from the first flare to the scene according to the posted speed.

The distribution of the flares is also very important. On a straight road, the EMT would calculate the distance needed to the first flare, as shown in Table 15-5, and then place the first flare there.

If the crash scene is on a curve, then the EMT must add the radius of the curve to the total distance calculated. Finding the radius sounds difficult, but it really is not that hard. The EMT simply calculates the distance from the

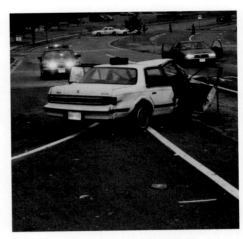

Figure 15.8 Police officers will often secure the scene of a motor vehicle collision before EMS arrives (Courtesy of Craig Smith)

Street Smart

Often drivers approaching the scene of a collision come from around a curve on the road or from the top of a hill and therefore cannot see the flashing hazard lights of the emergency vehicles. In those cases, the EMT should use safety devices, such as flares or cones, to enhance scene visibility.

The EMT should select the surface on which to place the flare with care. Telephone poles can ignite from the heat of a flare. Dried underbrush will act like kindling and start a grass fire. Fumes from spilled fuels are frequently heavier than air and, when carried to the flare, can ignite. Spilled gasoline has been known to run downhill to a lit flare, ignite, and follow the stream back to the automobile.

An EMT always surveys the surroundings before placing a flare on the ground to ensure the safety of everyone on scene.

bottom of the curve to the top of the curve and then adds that to the distance given in Table 15-5.

The same theory is applied for collisions that have occurred in a hollow or even a ravine off road. The EMT would add the distance from the bottom of the hill to the top of the hill to the distance given in Table 15-5.

If the crash is a head-on collision in the middle of the roadway, then flares must be placed both in front of and behind the site, effectively isolating the scene. If the road is a two-lane road, it is often safer to close the road and reroute traffic around the scene.

After determining the number and placement of the flares, the EMT should walk to the farthest point first, making sure to always face traffic and walk on the shoulder of the road.

Starting at the farthest point, the EMT would proceed to "drop flares" every 50 feet or so, as the situation dictates. While walking along the shoulder of the road, the EMT should never have his back to the oncoming traffic.

Figure 15.9 demonstrates the proper distribution, as well as the order of flare placement, for crash scenes on straight roads, curves, and hollows. Note that flares should never be placed closer than 100 feet to any spilled fuels.

Even with safety precautions and the proper use of flares, the danger of fire and explosion still exists. For this reason, many EMS agencies are using electric or battery-operated hazard lights instead of flares. These hazard lights are an excellent alternative to flares. EMS agencies that have EMTs who may have little or no experience using flares should consider using electric hazard lights instead of flares.

During daylight hours, traffic cones provide an excellent alternative to flares as well. Used by highway construction crews for years, these cones provide a highly visible and generally recognized hazard warning device.

Highway traffic cones also make a loud noise when they are struck, alerting the driver to the hazard ahead. Finally, traffic cones are reusable and therefore are a cost-effective traffic warning device.

Table 15-5 Flare Distances

Speed Limit (mph)	Conversion to Feet	Distance of First Flare (feet)
30	30	120
40	40	160
45	45	180
50	50	200
55	55 (+100)	320
60	60 (+100)	340
65	65 (+100)	360

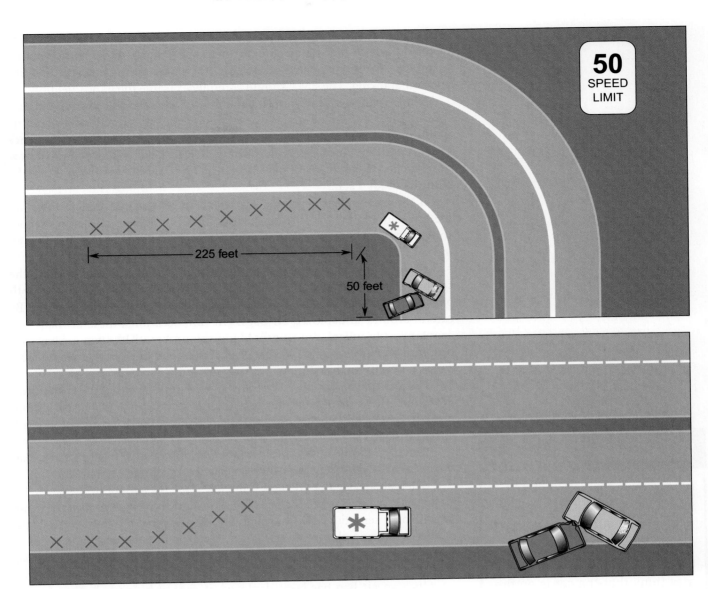

Figure 15.9 Proper vehicle positioning ensures better response

DAMAGE SURVEY

Starting at the driver's side, the EMT starts a clockwise walk around the car. If the driver or passengers are conscious, the EMT should call out to them to stay seated and not to move. When the walk is completed, the EMT should be at the driver's-side door.

The EMT starts by looking at the front bumpers to see if there are **loaded bumpers.** A bumper becomes loaded when the shock absorbers behind the bumper are compressed but not allowed to release. The energy is stored in the bumper, and the now-loaded bumper can suddenly release, injuring nearby rescuers. EMTs should always keep several feet between themselves and a loaded bumper.

The EMT should look for damage to the bumper as well. Current bumpers are designed to absorb a low-speed impact, preventing damage to the car. If the bumper and the fender behind the bumper are severely damaged, then the EMT can assume that the car was moving faster than 10 mph.

The fenders of modern cars are also designed to absorb energy by deforming in **crumple zones.** Any car with a crumpled fender can be assumed to have been in a moderate-speed collision.

A crack at the base of the windshield indicates that a great deal of force traveled through the engine compartment and into the passenger compartment. The front windshield is designed to withstand a great deal of force without cracking. The EMT should carefully examine the windshield.

While examining the windshield, the EMT should look for a small fracture in the glass, called a star. A star indicates that something struck the windshield at one specific point. The object could have been the patient's head. A starred windshield could be equated to head and neck injuries for the unbelted driver or front passenger. The EMT should always examine the windshield for a star.

If the mechanism of injury is a lateral-impact motor vehicle collision, the EMT should be focusing on the amount of intrusion into the passenger compartment. If it is greater than 12 inches, then the EMT should have a high index of suspicion that the occupants may have serious injuries.

Looking into the passenger compartment, the EMT should see if the car has air bags and whether they are deployed. Many vehicles have both passenger-side and lateral-side air bags as well as the driver-side air bags. Be careful around undeployed air bags. On rare occasions, these air bags will spontaneously inflate, injuring EMTs in the process. Although air bags are ordinarily very safe, some EMS agencies choose to disarm or even remove air bags to prevent further injury.

The fact that an air bag has deployed does not mean that the patient was protected. Air bags are most effective against frontal impacts. The forces that result from a lateral or rotational impact may throw the driver out of the path of the air bag.

The EMT should always lift up and look under the air bag to see whether the patient's body struck the steering wheel hard enough to bend it.

When an air bag does deploy, it literally slaps the patient in the face. This violent action can leave a mild superficial burn, and the patient may complain of a burning sensation. This burning sensation is generally short-lived. If the patient is wearing glasses, the glasses may fragment and cause lacerations as well. The patient's face should be examined for injuries following an air bag deployment.

Once an air bag has been deployed, it cannot be reused. Therefore, if the car is struck from behind after striking another car in front, the air bag will not protect the driver. These so-called *double taps* occur most often on congested city streets or in limited-visibility conditions such as fog or rain. Drivers in cars with a double tap should be assessed for both frontal and rear impact injuries. Table 15-6 summarizes what an EMT should assess on a vehicle involved in a motor vehicle collision.

VEHICLE STABILIZATION

All motor vehicles involved in a collision should initially be assumed to be unstable. Even cars that are on all four tires have been known to roll or shift. Any vehicle that is not on all four wheels must be stabilized with wood blocks or cribbing, or both, before any EMT enters the vehicle to perform patient care.

An EMT should never enter a vehicle that is not stable. Instead, the EMT must take immediate action to either stabilize the vehicle, if trained to do so, or to call for resources, such as fire rescue.

Fortunately, most motor vehicles can be made safe with a few simple actions. These actions, taken by the first EMT on scene, can remarkably improve EMT safety and decrease the risk of further patient injury. Every EMT should make these actions a routine part of initial entry into a car involved in a collision.

Street Smart

Air bags are covered in starch, which helps the air bag deploy more evenly. After the air bag does deploy, a cloud of smoke may be visible. Some occupants may think that the car is on fire. The explosive charge to inflate the air bag is contained and self-limiting. Danger of fire from an air bag is almost nonexistent.

Table 15-6 Assessment of Vehicle Damage

Damage to Vehicle	Point of Patient Impact
Star on windshield	Forehead
Rearview mirror broken	Forehead
Air bag deployed	Face or torso
Locked seat belt	Torso
Steering wheel bent	Torso
Broken headrest	Head
Broken dashboard	Knees
Broken or bent pedals	Feet or legs
Seat broken off pedestal	Body
Side-door intrusion	Body, same side

First, the EMT should take the car with automatic transmission out of drive. This step seems obvious, but most drivers do not stop and think to take their car out of gear after a collision. Whenever a car's automatic transmission is still engaged, the car can move and the EMT is at risk for personal injury.

Next, the EMT should turn the car's engine off. A car that is still running is energized and capable of moving. In some circumstances, such as very cold weather, it may seem reasonable to leave the car running with the goal of preventing hypothermia. However, a misplaced elbow or knee while moving the patient could shift the car into drive. It is always safer for everyone to turn the car off.

Before turning off the car, be sure that if the car has power windows or door locks that they are left open. Also, check the seat to see whether it is electric. The EMT may want to move the seat backward before turning the car off for easier patient extrication, but he should manually stabilize the patient's head before moving the seat.

The EMT should immediately engage the parking brake. Severe damage to the car's engine may disrupt the hydraulic lines to the power brakes, allowing the car to roll. Applying the mechanical parking brake greatly enhances the margin of safety for the EMT.

Finally, the EMT should block the wheels. Some EMS agencies, as a matter of practice, automatically place a wedge, or chock, behind two wheels on opposite sides of the car. Using a chock prevents the vehicle from rolling even if both braking systems have failed.

If the car is still unstable, it may be necessary for properly trained personnel to isolate the wheels from the frame of the car by using special cribbing called **step blocks.** Step blocks are designed to be placed under the frame of the vehicle to lift it off its wheels.

When cribbing is needed to stabilize a car, the EMT should consider requesting heavy rescue units or fire service assistance. Skill 15-2 at the end of this unit describes vehicle stabilization.

NUMBER OF PATIENTS

There can be more than one patient on any call; however, on the scene of a motor vehicle accident, there frequently is more than one patient. When more than one patient is present, the EMT must decide who will get treatment first and who will wait for additional responders. In short, the patients must be sorted according to the severity of their injuries.

This decision-making process requires a special approach called **triage.** Triage should take only a few minutes and can potentially save more lives than an approach that assesses one patient at a time. Triage is discussed in more detail in Unit 49.

Triage is a part of the incident management system (IMS). The IMS is an effective means of caring for multiple patients. The IMS is discussed in fuller detail in Unit 49.

The entire IMS depends on the first-arriving EMT or emergency services worker to establish that there are multiple patients. It is important for the EMT to determine the number of patients during the scene size-up and to call for additional resources during the initial report. Calling for additional personnel and equipment immediately to care for the additional patients prevents unnecessary delays in transportation or care.

If the EMT runs up to the first patient encountered and begins to render care, other patients who may have more serious injuries could die needlessly.

PROTECTING THE PATIENT

Protection of the patient is an important element of the scene size-up. As stated previously, the EMT's first duty is safety for himself, then for his partner, and then for the patient. If there are hazards to EMS on scene, it stands to reason those same hazards are dangerous for the patient.

EMTs will respond to accidents and medical emergencies that occur in public places and in various types of weather. Crowd control can be an issue of safety for everyone on scene. In addition, the EMT should always remember the importance of protecting the patient's privacy from a curious public. Exposing the patient to look for injuries or further assess vitals signs can be uncomfortable in a public place. The patient is in a high stress situation with strong emotions that may be difficult to control. The EMT must do all he can to protect the privacy of the patient when removing clothing or asking personal questions that are necessary to assess and manage the patient.

A victim of a trauma or medical emergency is experiencing emotions that are sometimes uncontrolled due to the increased stress of the incident. The EMT can either increase or decrease the stress the patient is feeling by his behavior. Speaking in a calm, quiet voice while reassuring the patient can help to calm the patient and keep the situation from getting out of control.

Emergencies can and do take place in all environments. Some emergencies are the direct result of the environment and will be discussed in detail in Unit 39, Environmental Emergencies. Adverse weather can create hazards for both the rescuer and the patient. Elements of weather such as extreme cold can cause a secondary illness or injury that can place the patient into a critical health situation. For example, an elderly patient falls outside on an icy sidewalk, fracturing a hip and unable to get back into the house, she lies outside until a neighbor finds her. The patient can become hypothermic from both the cold atmosphere and lying on the icy sidewalk. It will be important to get the patient onto a backboard and off the icy ground immediately to prevent further heat loss and make her more comfortable. Once on the backboard, the patient can be moved into the warm ambulance, protected from further exposure to the cold.

There are many things the EMT can do to protect patients and make them more comfortable. If it is raining at the scene, cover the patient's head while moving her to the ambulance. Shade the patient's face from bright sunlight while completing your assessment.

Protecting patients will make them more comfortable physically and emotionally. These often-simple acts of courtesy also show respect and care for the patient. A calm, reasonably comfortable patient will allow the EMT to more easily complete the patient assessment and management of the emergency.

PROTECTING THE PUBLIC

The EMT can use flares to establish a **perimeter** or safety zone in which to work in the midst of motor vehicle traffic. This is also one aspect of public safety. The EMT must be concerned about pedestrian traffic and protecting bystanders from the hazards discussed previously. Motor vehicle collisions tend to draw the attention of people, especially children.

High-speed, limited-access highways usually have wire fences along the roadside to prevent pedestrians from wandering onto the highway. Local roads and secondary roads usually do not have fences. The EMT on scene should make some effort to protect pedestrians. Ensuring pedestrian safety usually involves enlisting the aid of law enforcement officers.

Medical emergencies can also draw crowds. The neighbors are concerned about what may be happening in their neighborhood or to a friend. Although they are usually well meaning, their presence can create an unsafe environment. The best way to protect bystanders on any scene is to keep them from getting too close to the scene.

CONCLUSION

All EMTs approach a scene in a similar manner and ask themselves the same questions: Am I safe? Is the scene safe? What is the nature of the call? How many patients do I have? What other resources do I need?

The answers will vary from scene to scene, but the questions remain the same. EMTs should be asking themselves these questions when approaching any emergency scene. For the experienced provider, these questions have become second nature and the first action at every scene.

The most important person on any EMS call is the EMT. There is nothing more disturbing than to hear an EMT was seriously injured or killed because he or she did not follow a few simple guidelines of protection from avoidable hazards on the scene. By completing the scene size-up correctly, the EMT can protect himself, his partner, the patient, and even the public from avoidable danger and provide patient care in a safe environment with the appropriate resources available.

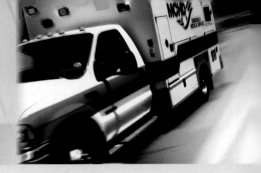

CASE STUDY Continued

Kayla backs the ambulance into Mrs. Smith's driveway and instructs Jan not to enter the fenced-in yard until animal control arrives. Kayla walks the perimeter of the house, looking carefully for any additional hazards and a back entrance that may be available for use.

Mrs. Smith's son, Kyle, opens the front door, asking if they are going to come in and help his mother. Kayla verifies there is only one patient and explains to Kyle they cannot enter the scene until they can confirm it is safe and the dogs are under control. She asks if it would be possible to use a back entrance. Kyle states the back door is blocked by cat cages, and it would take too much time to try to move them all.

Animal control and local law enforcement arrive as Kayla is getting more information about Mrs. Smith's condition. She is told Mrs. Smith has been feeling short of breath for the past 3 hours, and her inhaler is not helping. Mrs. Smith has a history of asthma. When Kyle

arrived to check on her today, she was having a very hard time breathing. When he checked the inhaler she was using, he found that was out of date and she did not have a new one.

Animal control and law enforcement block the dogs from reaching the front door, allowing Kayla and Jan to enter the house. Kyle states he has locked the inside pets in a bedroom. Kayla and Jan carefully continue to assess for more hazards as they approach Mrs. Smith who is seated in the living room. Kayla takes note of a small dog sitting on Mrs. Smith's lap and asks Kyle to remove the dog, knowing that even the nicest animal can become aggressive when seeking to protect its master.

Jan and Kayla begin their patient assessment, placing oxygen on Mrs. Smith and moving her to the ambulance for transport to the hospital. Mrs. Smith is anxious about her pets, and Kayla reassures her they are being taken care of by her son and animal control.

PURPOSE: To protect the EMT from injury while lighting a road flare.

STANDARD PRECAUTIONS:

☑ Road flare
☑ Helmet with eye shield
☑ Gloves
☑ Turnout coat

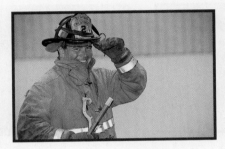

1 The EMT first puts on eye protection and gloves, minimally. It is preferable for the EMT to wear a turnout coat as well.

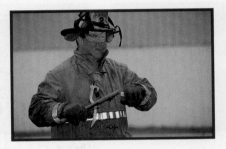

2 The EMT holds the flare 6 inches below the head and then removes the striker from the end of the flare.

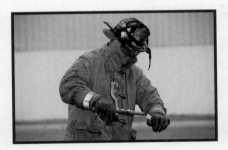

3 The EMT then briskly strikes the striker against the flare's igniter while aiming it away from his body.

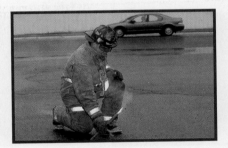

4 The EMT then keeps the lit flare away from his body and places it on the ground.

PURPOSE: To protect the EMT from hazards created as the result of a motor vehicle collision.

STANDARD PRECAUTIONS:

☑ Flashlight
☑ Turnout coat
☑ Helmet

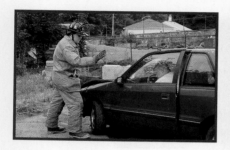

1 The first EMT circles the car, starting from the driver's side. The EMT advises the patient to sit still for a minute. The EMT is checking for vehicle damage.

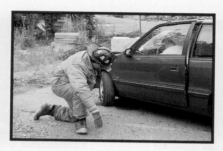

2 The second EMT circles the car from the opposite side. The EMT is checking for hazards above and beneath the car.

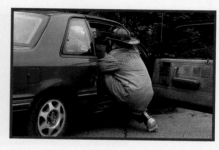

3 After the second EMT calls "all clear," the first EMT enters the passenger side and stabilizes the patient's head.

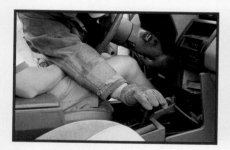

4 The second EMT then reaches in and checks to see that the car is in park.

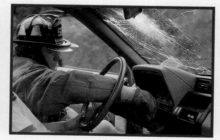

5 After checking for electric locks, windows, and seats, the EMT confirms that the car is turned off.

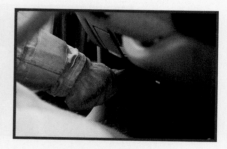

6 Finally, the EMT confirms that the car's emergency brake is engaged.

Key Concepts Revisited

- The EMT must be knowledgeable in methods of protection against foreseeable injury.
- The first job of EMTs on any scene is to protect themselves, their partners, and the patient.
- The EMT must be trained to identify scene hazards, mitigate those hazards, and implement scene safety in general.
- The assessment and control of hazard while approaching the scene includes:
  - Dispatch information
  - Prearrival instructions
  - PPE requirements
  - Scene staging
- The scene size-up includes:
  - Scene safety, number of patients, mechanism of injury or nature of illness, and need for additional resources.
    - Global assessment of information gathered in the scene size-up.
- The EMT must be able to identify hazards on any type of emergency call.
  - Risk factors are predictable risks commonly seen at certain types of scenes.
  - A high index of suspicion prompts attention to additional scene hazards.
  - Information overload can lead to confusion and inaction.
- Hazards at house calls can include:
  - Animals, emotional reactions by patients and/or other household members, toxic substances, furniture, and other structures in the house.
- Hazards at motor vehicle collisions include:
  - Traffic
  - Downed power lines
  - Toxic or hazardous materials

- Environmental concerns (weather)
  - Bystanders
- Crime scene hazards include:
  - Violent individuals
  - Weapons
- Risk management on emergency responses include:
  - Crime scene management
    - Law enforcement involvement
    - Preservation of evidence
    - Ambulance staging
    - Crowd control
  - Motor vehicle collision scene management includes
    - Vehicle staging
    - Warning lights
    - Flares
    - Traffic cones
    - Damage survey
  - Vehicle stabilization
    - Blocks or cribbing
- The number of patients determines
  - Need for additional resources
- Patient must be protected from scene hazards:
  - Weather
  - Bystanders
- Bystanders are protected from scene hazards:
  - Crowd control
  - Limited scene access
- A correctly completed scene size-up can protect EMTs, patients, and the public from avoidable dangers.

Review Questions

1. What regulatory agencies have established safety rules for EMS?
2. What is the first step in patient assessment?
3. What information can be obtained from the prearrival instructions?
4. What is the importance of staging to an EMT's safety?
5. What risk factors exist on the scene of a medical emergency? Of a trauma emergency?
6. What additional resources could be called to manage risks at a motor vehicle collision?
7. How should the EMT approach a crime scene?
8. What toxic substances might be present at a medical emergency?
9. Whose safety comes first?
10. What can the EMT do to protect the patient?
11. How would an EMT protect the public from becoming injured?
12. What are the minimal actions an EMT should take to stabilize a motor vehicle?

Key Terms

Crumple zone
Dangerous instrument
Deadly weapon
Global assessment
High index of suspicion
Initial report
Killing zone
Loaded bumper
Perimeter

Risk factors
Risk mitigation
Safety corridor
Size-up
Staging
Step blocks
Toxic substance
Triage

Further Study

Elling, B., & K. Elling. *Principles of Patient Assessment in EMS.* Clifton Park, NY: Thomson Delmar Learning, 2002.

Haskell, G. H., and R. C. Krause. *EMT-Basic, Pearls of Wisdom.* 2d ed. Boston: Jones and Bartlett, 2007.

Krebs, D. *When Violence Erupts: A Survival Guide for Emergency Responders.* Boston: Jones and Bartlett, 2002.

UNIT (16) Primary Assessment

It is important for the EMT to develop a systematic approach to patient assessment and to routinely perform that assessment the same way every time. Of course, it will vary slightly depending upon patient situations, but the order of the assessment and the priorities must always remain the same. If assessments are done systematically, the EMT will be less likely to leave something out or to forget to assess something.

Every patient an EMT encounters will be different in some way from all the others. Many may have similar concerns, but each patient must be evaluated thoroughly by the EMT. This unit covers the recommended method of the primary assessment of patients.

Units 17 through 20 discuss further assessment techniques for both medical and trauma patients.

National Education Standard
The Emergency Medical Technician (EMT) shall have a fundamental depth and breadth of understanding to perform a primary assessment for all patient situations, which includes determining an initial general impression, level of consciousness, assessment of the ABCs, identifying life threats, assessment of vital functions, and integration of treatment/procedures needed to preserve life.

Key Concepts

- The primary assessment follows specific steps for the detection and immediate intervention of life-threatening conditions.

- The primary assessment will be conducted on all patients, whether critical or non-critical.

- The primary assessment is a rapid, systematic assessment of the most vital functions of the human body: the airway, breathing, and circulatory status.

- The ABCs are the highest priorities in emergency care.

- The general impression is formed after looking at the patient and determining how ill or injured the patient appears to be.

- The patient's general mental status or state of consciousness can be quickly assessed using the AVPU mnemonic.

- The EMT can confirm the patency of the airway in the awake and alert patient by observing the patient's effort to breathe and speak.

- To determine the presence of breathing, the EMT should lean over the patient and look, listen, and feel for air movement.

- The C of the primary assessment involves assessment and support of the circulatory system.

- Capillary refill should be measured as an indicator of peripheral blood flow in children and infants.

- Prioritizing patient treatment and transport must take place immediately after the primary assessment of mental status, airway, breathing, and circulation has been completed.

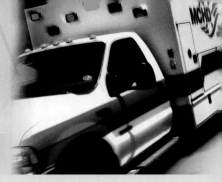

CASE STUDY

After Tillie determines the scene is safe, she enters the kitchen and observes Mrs. Scott seated at the table. Mrs. Scott is a 62-year-old female who appears pale, sweaty, and anxious. She is leaning forward with her hands rubbing her jaw, complaining of a very bad toothache on both sides of her mouth. She states it began while she was doing her morning exercises and nothing she has done, including brushing her teeth, has helped.

Critical Thinking Questions

1. What is your initial general impression of Mrs. Scott?
2. Is she showing signs of a life-threatening illness?
3. What treatments, if any, will Mrs. Scott need immediately?

INTRODUCTION

After the scene has been determined to be safe, the EMT approaches the patient to begin her evaluation and treatment plan. The primary assessment begins while approaching the patient, determining whether the patient is suffering from an injury or illness. The primary assessment follows specific steps for the detection and immediate intervention of life-threatening conditions. The primary assessment will be conducted on all patients, whether critical or non-critical.

THE PRIMARY ASSESSMENT

Assessment priorities on every patient are to find and treat any life-threatening problems first. The assessment that is done first to find such life threats is called the **primary assessment.** The primary assessment is a rapid, systematic assessment of the most vital functions of the human body: the airway, breathing, and circulatory status.

The purpose of the primary assessment is to allow the EMT to rapidly find and treat any immediate life-threatening problems, such as an occluded airway. During the primary assessment, life-threatening problems are managed as they are found. In contrast, less urgent problems will be managed at the completion of the appropriate secondary assessments.

Because every patient has the potential to have a life-threatening problem, every patient the EMT encounters will get a primary assessment upon first encounter. We will discuss how the primary assessments differ according to the patient's status.

STEPS OF THE PRIMARY ASSESSMENT

You will recall from Unit 15 that the first thing an EMT must do while approaching a scene is to perform a scene size-up and ensure that it is safe to approach the patient. The EMT should also be using the appropriate personal protective equipment that is expected for the situation. Once the scene has been deemed safe, the next step is to make contact with the patient and begin the primary assessment.

The mnemonic used to remember the essential parts of the primary assessment is ABC: airway, breathing, and circulation. The **ABCs** are highest priorities in emergency care. While approaching the patient, the EMT begins assessment of the ABCs by noting the patient's general appearance and mental status.

GENERAL IMPRESSION

While approaching a patient, the EMT should be assessing the scene for clues as to the mechanism of injury or nature of the illness. If the person is a trauma patient, does the mechanism suggest spinal injury? Is the patient in a position that will require the EMT to move him into a position that allows proper assessment of the airway and breathing?

The EMT should then observe the patient; general age and gender of the patient may influence assessment and treatment plans. If the patient is conscious, try to determine the patient's chief concern; in other words, why did they call EMS?

A **general impression** of the patient's status can be formed in the first 15 seconds of observation. As the EMT becomes more experienced, forming the general impression through observation becomes second nature. The EMT should ask several questions while forming the general impression:

- Does the patient appear to be awake?
- Does the patient appear to be very ill or in pain?
- Does the problem seem to be related to a medical illness or to a traumatic injury?

The general impression begins as the EMT is walking across the room, onto the scene, toward the patient. Based on observation the EMT must decide how quickly and how urgently she must act in managing the patient.

The general impression is often referred to as the *look test*. That is, when you first look at the patient, does he look sick? Does the patient have a significant traumatic injury, or is he showing signs of shock? This impression should stimulate the EMT and her crew into moving more quickly to assess and manage this patient.

MENTAL STATUS

As the EMT approaches the patient, the general state of consciousness should be easily noted. Does the patient seem to be awake? The patient's general mental status or state of consciousness can be quickly assessed using the AVPU mnemonic.

The abbreviation **AVPU** is often used in determining and reporting the patient's level of consciousness. A stands for Alert; V stands for responsive to Verbal stimulation (Voice); P stands for responsive to Pain; and U stands for Unresponsive.

ALERT

If the EMT observes that the patient's eyes are open and he seems aware of the crew as they approach, the patient is considered to be **alert.** This can be further qualified as the EMT speaks with the patient by determining whether the patient is oriented or not. Three common questions to test orientation are related to person, place, and time. Table 16-1 lists examples of questions the EMT might ask to determine orientation.

If the patient correctly answers each of these questions, he is determined to be alert and oriented to person, place, and time. Sometimes this status is abbreviated as "A/OX3," or "alert and oriented times three," referring to person, place, and time.

Table 16-1	Questions to Determine Orientation

Person: What is your name?

Place: Where are you right now?

Time: Can you tell me the time of day? What day is it today?

If the patient is unable to answer any of these questions, he is said to be disoriented. If the patient knows his name but not the place or time, the patient is said to be oriented to person but not to place or time. It is useful to specify to which question the patient is oriented and to which he is disoriented so that a reevaluation by health care providers who assume care for the patient later can assess for improvement or decline in the patient's orientation.

RESPONSIVE TO VOICE

If the patient does not seem to be awake as the EMT approaches, the EMT should attempt to arouse the patient first by speaking. Asking "Are you all right?" or using the patient's name in a firm voice is a good way to perform verbal stimulation. If the patient opens his eyes when spoken to but closes his eyes again when not spoken to, he is considered to be **responsive to voice.**

If a normal tone of voice does not arouse the patient, then a louder tone may be used. If this arouses the patient, we say the patient is responsive to loud verbal stimuli. The difference between the "alert" and the "responsive to voice" categories is that the alert patient does not require verbal stimuli to stay awake and interactive. When not being spoken to, the V patient closes his eyes and withdraws from interaction.

Pediatric Considerations

When assessing infants and small children who don't speak or are not old enough to know where they are or what the day is, the EMT cannot use the same criteria as she does for adults. If a child is awake, the EMT should observe how the child interacts with the parents or caregiver.

If the child is awake and clinging to the caregiver, looking around at things going on in the immediate environment, and acting in a manner appropriate for a child of that age, we refer to the child as being awake and appropriate, rather than oriented.

RESPONSIVE TO PAIN

If the patient does not respond to loud verbal stimuli, the next most appropriate action would be to attempt to awaken him with physical stimuli. A firm tap on the shoulder is a good way to start. If this awakens the patient, the terminology used is "responds to physical stimuli." If this does not awaken the patient, a more noxious physical stimulus must be used.

A common maneuver used by EMS providers in this situation is the **sternal rub** (Figure 16.1). The knuckles of the EMT's hand are rubbed against the

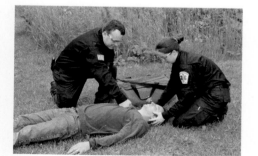

Figure 16.1 Use a sternal rub to check for a patient's response to a painful stimulus

patient's sternum firmly in an attempt to arouse the patient. Another method of central painful stimulation is the trapezius pinch. The EMT pinches the muscle that extends from the neck to the shoulder and squeezes the muscle.

Other methods of painful stimulus involve the extremities and are called *peripheral painful stimuli.* Applying pressure to the cuticle of the nail bed, pinching the web between the thumb and index finger or pinching a finger, toe, hand, or foot are all examples of peripheral painful stimuli.

If any of these stimuli arouse the patient, we say that the patient is **responsive to painful stimuli.** The EMT should describe what the patient's response to this stimulus was.

UNRESPONSIVE

If no response is elicited by verbal or painful stimuli, the patient is truly **unresponsive.** An unresponsive patient usually does not have a gag or cough reflex and therefore has an inability to protect his airway. The tongue and epiglottis are not controlled and can block the airway, requiring that the airway be opened and maintained manually, as discussed in Unit 9. The unresponsive patient is very ill and requires rapid interventions.

AIRWAY

Once the general impression has been formed and the level of consciousness determined, the EMT must address the state of the patient's airway. If the patient is awake and alert, the airway is likely being maintained without difficulty. The EMT can confirm the patency of the airway in the awake and alert patient by observing the patient's effort to breathe and speak. If the patient is speaking and seems to be moving air in and out without difficulty, then the airway is considered open, or patent.

If the patient is awake but cannot speak or is showing signs of an inability to move air in and out, the EMT must further assess the airway. Drooling is a sign that the patient is having difficulty with his airway. Normally, a person can swallow his own saliva. If an airway obstruction is present, the saliva may not be able to get by the obstruction to be swallowed. This means that air may not be able to get by either.

If the patient is not awake, then the EMT must be immediately concerned about the status of the airway. The airway will not be maintained by the patient and remain clear of saliva and debris as the patient becomes less responsive.

The EMT should use a methodical process of assessing and managing a patient's airway. The order in which actions are taken is "open, assess, suction, secure" (Figure 16.2). Such airway assessment and management techniques are discussed in detail in Unit 9 and should be reviewed.

Once the EMT has assessed and appropriately secured the airway, she can move on to the next step in the assessment.

BREATHING

After ensuring the airway is open and secure, the EMT turns her attention to the patient's breathing.

The EMT begins the breathing assessment by determining whether the patient is breathing at all. To determine the presence of breathing, the EMT should lean over the patient and look, listen, and feel for air movement. She should look for chest rise, listen for air coming from the mouth and nose, and feel for the air against her cheek.

If the patient is not breathing, then appropriate actions must be taken to establish effective ventilations as described in Unit 24.

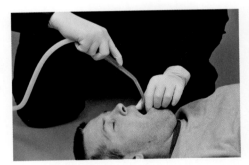

Figure 16.2 Open, assess, suction, and secure the airway

If the patient is breathing, the EMT should assess the adequacy of breathing by determining a respiratory rate. If the patient's respiratory rate is between 10 and 24 and appears to be adequate in volume, then supplemental oxygen should be administered by means of a non-rebreather mask.

If the patient is breathing, but the breathing is too fast or too slow (>24 or <8) and of inadequate depth or requires marked effort, then the EMT should assist the patient's ventilations using a bag-valve-mask with 100% oxygen.

All patients who are not completely awake and oriented should be given high-concentration supplemental oxygen via non-rebreather mask.

Patients who are awake and oriented may also require oxygen, depending on the presenting medical condition. Concerns such as chest or abdominal pain, difficulty breathing, or any signs or symptoms of shock are indications for high-flow oxygen by non-rebreather mask. The use of oxygen in the management of specific complaints will be addressed throughout the book.

After assessing the presence and the adequacy of breathing, the EMT must assess for potential problems with breathing. This assessment involves a careful examination of the patient's chest for any injuries that may cause problems with adequate respirations. Again, the EMT should look, listen, and feel.

LOOK

The patient's chest should be exposed sufficiently to inspect for any obvious wounds or uneven breathing. Open chest wounds, such as stabs or gunshot wounds, create problems with effective breathing because they allow air into the chest via the wound, and air in the chest can impede adequate lung expansion. These types of open chest wounds are called **sucking chest wounds.** Normal negative intrathoracic pressure pulls air into the chest through the wound and can make bubbling or sucking sounds. The appropriate immediate action for the EMT to take is to cover the open wound with an occlusive dressing that does not allow air to pass through. Management of such chest injuries is described in more detail in Unit 36.

The chest should be evaluated for equal and adequate chest movement. Poor chest movement such as one side of the chest moving in the opposite direction with respirations (paradoxical movement) as seen with a flail segment is an indication of inadequate tidal volume. Additionally, a patient with shallow respirations is not taking in enough air with each breath and may also have inadequate tidal volume.

Abnormal respiratory rates such as **bradypnea** (too slow) or *tachypnea* (too fast) may result in inadequate minute volume as discussed in Unit 6. When a patient has abnormal respiratory rates, his mental status must be evaluated along with other signs of hypoxia to determine if this slower or faster respiratory rate is adequate or inadequate.

While looking at the chest for equal chest rise and respiratory rate, check for additional signs of inadequate breathing such as the use of accessory muscles. Is the chest sinking in between the intercostal spaces (between the ribs), the suprasternal notch (above the sternum), or supraclavicular spaces (above the clavicles)? Is there excessive abdominal use, nasal flaring, or use of the neck muscles on inhalation?

The EMT must also note the skin signs to help determine adequacy of breathing with the presence of any of the previously described signs. The presence of cyanosis around the nose, lips, and fingernail beds and pale, cool, clammy skin are signs of inadequate oxygenation.

LISTEN

While looking at the chest, the EMT should place her ear near the nostrils and listen for air movement. Little air movement felt with each breath indicates inadequate breathing. No movement of the chest, along with no air being heard or felt, is called *apnea*. The patient who is apneic requires immediate intervention with artificial ventilations.

The EMT should then use a stethoscope to evaluate the effectiveness of air movement by listening to the chest wall. The best place to listen is just below the clavicles and at their midpoint. This location will allow the EMT to hear the air movement into the lung on that side. Listening to both sides will allow the EMT to assess for equality of the breath sounds.

Figure 16.3 shows the proper position to auscultate, or listen to, lung sounds during the primary assessment. The clear sound of air moving in and out should be heard. If air movement is diminished when compared with the other side, or if it is not heard at all, the patient may have a serious injury. The EMT should take steps to rapidly transport the patient to the most appropriate hospital. If an advanced life support (ALS) intercept is available, it should also be arranged. It is important for the EMT to note any abnormal sounds when listening to the lung sounds. These abnormal lung sounds may fall into several categories, which are described in Table 16-2.

FEEL

Finally, the EMT should quickly feel for any deformity or instability within the chest by using both hands to press on both sides of the chest wall and the sternum. Any point of tenderness on the chest wall suggests a rib fracture. A rib fracture should not be ignored because it could eventually puncture a lung.

Evidence of subcutaneous air, or **crepitus,** should be noted. Crepitus is the sensation of air under the skin that feels like bubble wrap popping under the fingertips. This indicates a potentially serious chest injury in which air is escaping the lung into the chest cavity.

Only after completing the assessment of the breathing and managing any life threats in that step can the EMT move on to circulation in the primary assessment.

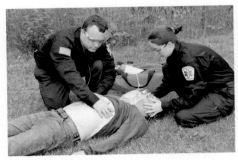

Figure 16.3 Look, listen, and feel for breathing

Table 16-2 Abnormal Lung Sounds	
Sound	**Potential Diagnosis**
Absent	Complete airway obstruction
Diminished (volume of sound)	Collapsed lung (pneumothorax)
Wheezing (whistling sound)	Air moving through narrowed lower airways (asthma or partial airway obstruction)
Crackles (or rales)	Fluid in smaller airways (heart failure)
Rhonchi (rumbling sound)	Fluid in larger airways (bronchitis)

CIRCULATION

Once the airway and breathing have been assessed and managed appropriately, the EMT must then direct her attention to the C of the primary assessment. This involves assessment and support of the circulatory system.

ASSESS FOR A PULSE

The first step in assessing the circulatory status is to check for a pulse. It is useful to check the radial pulse first. If a radial pulse is present, the EMT can assume that the patient has enough blood pressure to supply blood to that peripheral site. In addition to noting whether the pulse is present, the EMT should note its strength, rate, and regularity.

If a radial pulse is not present in either wrist, the EMT should move directly to the carotid pulse. If the carotid pulse is present but the radial pulse was not, the EMT should assume that the blood pressure is quite low. If a carotid pulse is not present after a 5- to 10-second pulse check, the EMT should begin external chest compressions.

ASSESS FOR BLEEDING

After assessing for the presence of a pulse, the EMT should quickly assess the patient for evidence of any condition that may compromise the circulatory system. Massive bleeding may cause a patient to go into shock and die. The EMT must assess the patient for evidence of life-threatening hemorrhage.

External hemorrhage can be easily found by swiping gloved hands under each part of the patient's body and checking the hands to see whether any blood was recovered from that area. Any areas of active bleeding should be immediately assessed more carefully.

If the amount of bleeding seems small and not life threatening, the EMT should leave that wound to be addressed at a later point in the assessment. If the amount of bleeding appears large and potentially life-threatening, the EMT should immediately control the bleeding by applying direct pressure to the wound, usually with a gloved hand. This pressure should be initiated immediately when extensive bleeding is found.

After assessing for gross external hemorrhage, the EMT should assess the patient for hidden, or occult, bleeding. This type of bleeding can be determined by assessing the patient for signs of hypoperfusion.

At this point, the EMT has already assessed mental status, respiratory rate, and heart rate. The next part of the assessment should involve checking the skin signs, including temperature, condition, and color.

The details of how to check skin temperature and condition can be reviewed in Unit 12. Pale, cool, and clammy skin along with rapid breathing and a rapid pulse are signs of shock and should be identified quickly during the initial assessment.

CIRCULATORY SUPPORT

When signs of inadequate circulation are present, the EMT must immediately initiate treatment to support circulation. If signs of circulation are absent, CPR should be immediately initiated. If severe bleeding is present, it must be immediately controlled. If indications are present for use of MAST/PASG (military anti-shock trousers/pneumatic anti-shock garment; MAST/PASG local protocols will vary), then it should be applied immediately.

Only after completing the assessment of the circulatory status and addressing any life threats in those steps can the EMT move forward in the assessment process.

DETERMINE PATIENT PRIORITY

Once the primary assessment of mental status, airway, breathing, and circulation has been completed, the EMT must make a decision about the priority of the patient. On the basis of the findings in the primary assessment, the EMT must decide if the patient has any life-threatening problems that require immediate, rapid transport to the hospital or if the focused physical exam and history should be completed on scene prior to transport. Additionally, the EMT must determine the need for an ALS intercept or aeromedical transport at this time.

Certain conditions are considered to be life-threatening emergencies or potentially life-threatening emergencies. At the end of the primary assessment, the EMT must determine whether any of these conditions exist. Table 16-3 lists findings during the primary assessment that should be considered potentially life-threatening. Patients with these findings should be identified as high-priority patients in need of rapid transport and ALS assistance.

HIGH PRIORITY

If a patient is identified as a high-priority patient, he must be appropriately packaged and loaded into the ambulance for transport to the closest appropriate hospital. Sometimes the phrase "load and go" is used to describe the actions needed when a high-priority patient has been identified. Most patients in this category require an ALS intercept if one is available. Local protocols will dictate which hospital to take the patient to and when ALS should be called.

High-priority patients are considered unstable or potentially unstable. Their conditions are critical or are extremely serious with the potential to become critical. The best treatment for these patients is to get them to the definitive care provided by advanced life support providers or hospitals.

High-priority transport does not mean additional assessment will not take place, it simply determines where that assessment will be taking place—on scene or in the ambulance on the way to the hospital.

Table 16-3 Life-Threatening Physical Assessment Findings

Poor general impression

Unresponsive

Decreased level of responsiveness

Responsive but not following commands

Difficulty breathing

Shock (evidence of hypoperfusion)

Complicated childbirth

Chest pain

Uncontrolled bleeding

Severe pain anywhere

LOW PRIORITY

A patient identified as stable is considered a low-priority patient who does not have any immediate life-threatening problems. The EMT should continue with the assessment of the patient on scene unless it is unsafe to do so. The next step in patient assessment will depend on the type of problem, medical or trauma. Although scene time is not extended beyond that necessary to complete the relevant assessment, a phrase that is sometimes used to describe the disposition of the low-priority patient is "stay and play," indicating that immediate rapid transport is not necessary.

In the next phase of patient assessment, the secondary assessment, the EMT focuses on the patient's presenting problem or concern and assesses the particular areas that are involved. Further history is elicited on the basis of the type of presenting problem. Units 18 through 20 describe these assessment techniques. Skill 16-1 at the end of this unit describes the procedure for the primary assessment.

CONCLUSION

The primary assessment is the first step of patient assessment and must be completed by the EMT on every patient to expediently find and address life-threatening problems.

A general impression helps guide the EMT to prioritize the care that must be initiated during the primary assessment. The patient's mental status is assessed so that any changes may be noted during later assessments.

Airway, breathing, and circulation are quickly evaluated during the primary assessment with any life-threatening problems addressed as they are found. At the completion of the primary assessment, the EMT will determine if the patient is stable, unstable, or potentially unstable and assign a priority to the patient that will guide transport decisions and the location where further assessments and care will be conducted.

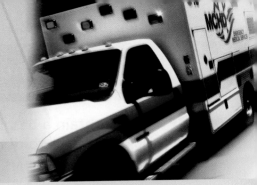

CASE STUDY Continued

Tillie's general impression of Mrs. Scott is that she is awake, alert, and oriented. Her mental status is normal at this time; however, she looks very ill, with pale, sweaty skin and anxious, rapid breathing. She appears to be very uncomfortable, rubbing her jaws with both hands and stating the ache in her jaws has been getting steadily worse for the past hour.

Tillie's primary assessment shows Mrs. Scott's airway to be open and patent. She is breathing rapidly with equal chest rise and adequate depth. Mrs. Scott has a respiratory rate of 22 with clear breath sounds on both sides. Mrs. Scott is moving air adequately in and out. Tillie directs her partner to apply oxygen by non-rebreather mask at a rate of 15 lpm.

Mrs. Scott's radial pulse is weak and rapid at a rate of 120, and Tillie further notes Mrs. Scott's pale, moist skin also feels cool to touch.

Tillie knows from experience that Mrs. Scott is showing the signs and symptoms often seen in women having heart attacks. Tillie determines Mrs. Scott is seriously ill and unstable at this time; therefore, she is a high-priority transport.

Tillie requests immediate transport with an ALS intercept while en route to the hospital. Tillie conducts the remainder of the patient assessment in the ambulance while en route to meet with the ALS intercept.

PURPOSE: To obtain a baseline examination for assessment and comparison as well as to detect and treat life-threatening injuries.

STANDARD PRECAUTIONS:

☑ Personal protective equipment

☑ Stethoscope

☑ Scissors

☑ Airway management equipment

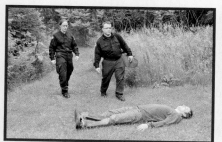

1 Survey the scene for safety hazards as well as any potential mechanism of injury. Don needed personal protective equipment.

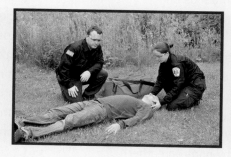

2 Form a general impression of the scene upon approaching the patient. Is it trauma or medical in nature?

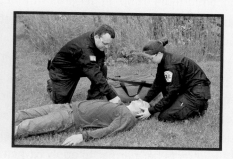

3 Determine the patient's mental status on an AVPU scale. If the scene is trauma in nature, a second EMT should immediately take responsibility for head stabilization.

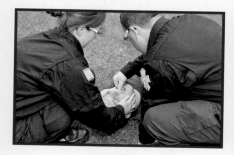

4 Assess and manage the airway as needed.

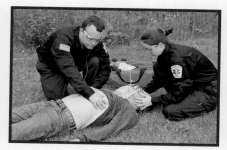

5 Assess and manage breathing.

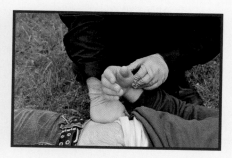

6 Assess and manage circulation. If the patient is a high-priority patient, he should be transported immediately.

Key Concepts Revisited

- The primary assessment follows specific steps for the detection and immediate intervention of life-threatening conditions.

- The primary assessment will be conducted on all patients whether critical or non-critical.

- The primary assessment is a rapid, systematic assessment of the most vital functions of the human body: the airway, breathing, and circulatory status.

- The ABCs are the highest priorities in emergency care:
  - Airway
  - Breathing
  - Circulation

- The general impression is formed after looking at the patient and determining how ill or injured the patient appears to be.

- The patient's general mental status or state of consciousness can be quickly assessed using the AVPU mnemonic:
  - Alert
  - Responsive to voice
  - Responsive to pain
  - Unresponsive

- The EMT can confirm the patency of the airway in the awake and alert patient by observing the patient's effort to breathe and speak.

- To determine the presence of breathing, the EMT should lean over the patient and look, listen, and feel for air movement.
  - Look equal and adequate chest movement.
  - Listen for equal and clear air movement in and out of the lungs.
  - Feel for warm, moist breath on the cheek while listening and looking at the chest.

- The C of the primary assessment involves assessment and support of the circulatory system:
  - Assess for a pulse (radial in adults, brachial in infants).
  - Assess and manage bleeding.
  - Measure capillary refill as an indicator of peripheral blood flow in children and infants.

- Prioritizing patient treatment and transport must take place immediately after the primary assessment of mental status, airway, breathing, and circulation has been completed.
  - High-priority patients are considered unstable or potentially unstable.
  - Low-priority patients are stable patients who do not have any immediate life-threatening problems.

Review Questions

1. What is the purpose of a primary assessment?
2. What observations of the patient are used in forming a general impression?
3. How is a patient's mental status assessed?
4. What are the steps in assessing the airway?
5. How do you determine a patient is breathing?
6. How would you care for a patient who is not adequately breathing?
7. What method is best used in obtaining a pulse in an adult, a child, and an infant patient?
8. Why do you assess for external and internal bleeding?
9. Why is it important to prioritize patient care and transport?
10. What is the difference between a high-priority and low-priority patient?

Key Terms

Alert

AVPU

Bradypnea

Crepitus

General impression

Primary assessment

Responsive to painful stimuli

Responsive to voice

Sternal rub

Sucking chest wound

Unresponsive

Further Study

Dalton, A. L., D. Limmer, J. J. Mistovich, and H. A. Werman. *Advanced Medical Life Support.* Upper Saddle River, NJ: Brady/Prentice Hall, 2006.

Elling, B., & K. Elling. *Principles of Patient Assessment in EMS.* Clifton Park, NY: Thomson Delmar Learning, 2002.

UNIT (17) Therapeutic Communications

Emergency Medical Services is first and foremost a people business. Taking care of people takes more than machines and high technology. It takes compassion and a human touch. That human touch can be best illustrated through therapeutic communication. This unit will investigate the complexities of therapeutic communication.

National Education Standard

The Emergency Medical Technician (EMT) shall apply a fundamental depth and foundational breadth of the principles of communicating with patients in a manner that achieves a positive relationship.

Key Concepts

- The process of communication is central to an EMT's assessment.

- Good interviewing techniques are critical for the EMT's success in obtaining an accurate history.

- The EMT should learn means to improve communication with the patient to improve the quality of history taking.

- Culture can have a significant influence on communication and can make history taking more difficult.

- An EMT should avoid several common mistakes in communication.

- An EMT should avoid several common obstructions to communication.

- Communicating with frightened, aggressive, and depressed patients can be a challenge for the EMT.

- Communicating with pediatric patients can be a challenge for the EMT.

- The process of communicating the news of death to family requires a focused approach and compassion.

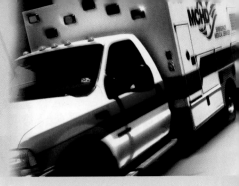

CASE STUDY

Eric is excited about his new job. Growing up in rural Montana, he always dreamed of working in the "big city," but there is so much to learn about EMS and so many different people in the city. Eric remembers his last call. He and his partner, Aaron, were sent to care for a sick Muslim woman. Aaron thought it was better that Eric take care of her, because he is Jewish. But the communication problems had less to do with religion than gender, and the call seemed to go bad from the beginning. Now he is being dispatched to Chinatown. Eric realizes that he knows less about Chinese-Americans than he does about Arab-Americans. He gets a sick feeling in the pit of his stomach as he thinks about the challenge of communicating in an emergency situation with people of diverse cultures. Arriving on scene Eric is greeted at the door by an elderly woman who smiles but obviously does not understand what is being asked of her. She leads them into a back bedroom where a younger woman, who speaks English, starts to tell them about her sick father.

Critical Thinking Questions

1. What are the obstacles to communication here?
2. What could Eric do to overcome these obstacles?
3. What are some other situations in which communication can be difficult?

INTRODUCTION

Communication is the exchange of information between two or more people, which would seem simple enough. However, communication is a complex process that has many potential obstacles. In the case of the EMT, the purpose of the communication, the exchange of information, is to facilitate medical care. The information exchanged is crucial to patient care; therefore, the EMT must be familiar with and overcome obstacles to communication to be a good medical communicator and an effective EMT.

Key to being a good medical communicator is compassion and respect for the patient. Demonstrations of compassion through communication can have a positive effect on the patient's health. These communications are called **therapeutic communications.**

PROCESS OF COMMUNICATION

A conversation starts with an idea or a question. For communication to occur, the idea must be conveyed from the person with the idea or question to another person who understands and responds to the idea or question. Communication may be spoken (verbal communication) or written (documentation). This unit focuses on verbal communication.

THE SENDER

Communication for an EMT has two purposes. The first is the collection of medical information for purposes of assessing and treating the patient. The second is as a means to offer comfort and solace to the patient.

The latter purpose speaks to the human condition. While pain and suffering is bad, suffering alone can be worse. Suffering with another, be it family or a compassionate person such as an EMT, seemingly makes the pain more bearable. Expressions of compassion expressed through the assessment of the patient are comforting.

The former purpose, the collection of information as part of a medical assessment, relies on accurate information. To obtain this information, the EMT must have good communication skills. The process of good communication starts with forming the question—that is, the message—and transmitting that message. Then, the patient must understand the question and respond in kind to the message. These four steps are called encoding, transmission, decoding, and feedback.

ENCODING

The medical care of a patient is based on history and a physical assessment. To obtain the patient's history, the EMT must ask a series of pointed questions intended to get to the core of the matter. The conversation starts with the patient's chief concern. The chief concern helps direct the conversation. For example, an EMT would not question an 85-year-old woman with a chief concern of chest pain about her obstetric history. Instead, the EMT should think the problem is of a cardiac origin and start a line of questioning that focuses on cardiac disease.

The EMT should adhere to the adage to "think before you speak" and carefully choose his words before speaking. At best, poorly chosen words may hamper communication. At worst, they may insult the patient or elicit the wrong information.

Words also have meaning for the patient beyond those that the EMT might understand because the meaning of some words is based on individual life experience. These **trigger words** remind the patient of a painful past experience and, in turn, stimulate a sympathetic fight-or-flight response. This physiologic response is evidenced by sweating, pallor, tachycardia, and pupil dilation. Even the use of the word *pain* should be avoided. Almost everyone has memories of some painful event in their past and will correspondingly react to the word. Instead of using the word *pain,* the EMT should consider if the same message can be conveyed using the word *discomfort* or *ache.*

The EMT starts the conversation, after introductions, by asking for the patient's chief concern through an offer of help. Asking a patient what is bothering her tends to illicit a different response from the patient than opening the conversation with a different question, "How can I help you?" The second implies a willingness to assist the patient. The EMT in Figure 17.1 is starting a conversation with a patient by introducing herself.

MEDICALESE

Learning to be an EMT involves learning a new language, the language of medicine, or **medicalese.** Medicalese encompasses unique medical terms and phrases, the terminology used in the practice of medicine (Figure 17.2). Terms like *AMI,* for acute myocardial infarction, soon become common in the conversation of an EMT.

However, many patients do not have the benefit of medical training, and these terms are foreign to them. To help the patient understand, the EMT must be skilled in the ability to use a medical term and then translate it into simple lay terms so that the patient can understand. For example, the EMT might tell the patient he suspects she is having an AMI, or in lay terms, a heart attack. Restating the message by using simpler terms will improve communication and increase the chance the patient will understand the message.

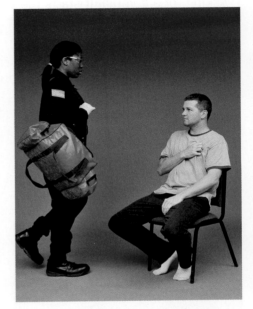

Figure 17.1 A proper introduction sets the stage for good communication

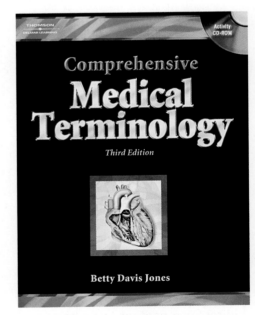

Figure 17.2 A medical terminology textbook is one source of medicalese

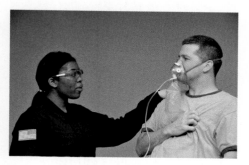

Figure 17.3 Kneeling in front of the patient, at eye level, conveys a positive message to the patient

TRANSMISSION

After the message, be it question or statement, is formulated in the EMT's mind, it must be transmitted. Many factors may affect the quality of transmission, collectively called **interference.** Examples of interference could be other providers talking to the patient simultaneously. Patients, particularly children, often have a difficult time focusing on more than one conversation, and thus some of the information in one conversation is lost to another.

During a crisis a person's focus is generally narrowed, a function of the sympathetic nervous system's fight-or-flight response. For that reason it is important that only one person speak to the patient at a time. In fact, the practice of one EMT taking charge of speaking and listening to the patient improves communication.

Another example of interference is ambient noise. Noise in the environment, such as idling diesel trucks or another person yelling, can obscure the message that an EMT is trying to deliver. In those instances it may be prudent to move the patient to a quiet location, such as the back of the ambulance.

The way the message is delivered can also have an impact on its reception. Changes in pitch, volume, and cadence of the voice, collectively called **intonation,** can alter a message. A mother calling a child to come inside can modulate her message to convey urgency. The mother may repeat the same words several times, each with a different level of urgency, to get across several different messages.

UNSPOKEN MESSAGE

Experts in communication contend that the majority of a message is conveyed through unspoken means rather than through spoken words. The unspoken message is called **body language,** that combination of posture, gestures, eye contact, head movement, and facial expression that conveys attitude and intent.

A mime is a classic example of how a message can be transmitted without the use of words. Similarly, the EMT standing over a patient, clinched fists on hips, with a frown on the forehead, glaring at a patient is transmitting a menacing message, even if the words sound kind.

To convey a more positive message through body language, the EMT should squat, on the balls of the feet, to the patient's eye level (Figure 17.3). The EMT should exhibit genuine concern through the softening of facial expressions as he directly faces the patient. **Blading** the patient, a defensive sideways stance that minimizes body exposure, sends the message to the patient that the EMT is concerned about attack and may convey—or invite—aggression.

Similarly, the EMT should keep his hands at his sides and in plain view. An arm crossed over the chest is an example of closed body language. Closed body language suggests that the person is not open to conversation.

Eye contact can also convey compassion. If the EMT is "looking through" the patient—that is, focused on a far distant object or not focused on the patient at all—the message is that the EMT is bored or disinterested. This may stop the communication.

RECEIVER

The message is meant for the receiver—in this case, the patient. To receive the message, the ear must function and the brain must receive the message. Patients who are deaf or hearing impaired may not hear the message. This obstacle to communications is discussed in more detail later in this unit.

There are a number of reasons why the brain may not receive the message. For the brain to function, it needs oxygen, glucose, and perfusion. If the patient is hypoxic, then the patient may not be able to receive the message. If the patient is hypoglycemic, or suffering from low blood sugar, then the patient may not be able to receive the message. Hypoperfusion, as evidenced by a low blood pressure or hypotension, also may prevent the patient from receiving the message.

Severe injuries can also **interfere** with communication between the EMT and patient. The patient tends to focus her attention on the painful injury to the exclusion of everything and everyone else. Examples of these **distracting painful injuries** include long bone fractures, such as a severe hand injury as shown in Figure 17.4, or burns. It will take extra effort on the part of the EMT to get the patient to listen to the message rather than focus on the injury.

DECODING

Once the receiver, the patient, has been given the message from the sender, the EMT, then the brain has to process the message to have meaning. That complex function of processing the message is performed by the brain.

Words in the spoken message are actually symbols. These symbols are interpreted by the brain based on a combination of life experience and intelligence. Intelligence is a function of an individual's physical makeup—his or her physiology and native faculties. Intelligence includes the person's ability to reason and to use language to communicate. Some patients have limited intelligence. This limited intelligence may be due to a variety of issues, such as fetal alcohol syndrome, congenital abnormalities like Down syndrome, birth anoxia, malnutrition, failure to thrive, and poisoning, to name a few.

On the other hand, life experience is, in part, a function of education. Obviously, a young child would have limited life experience, limited exposure to words, and thus a limited vocabulary. However, communication problems stemming from illiteracy are not limited to young children. **Illiteracy** is the inability to read, write, or understand the spoken word. Adult illiteracy in the United States is low, less than 1% nationwide, but in some regions the rate is much higher. High percentages of high school dropouts in urban centers and a large population of undocumented aliens in an area can increase illiteracy.

It is important that the EMT anticipate that some patients may be illiterate. These patients may be embarrassed by their illiteracy, and some have developed elaborate ploys to prevent detection. Chief among these ploys is silence. These patients may simply nod their head in agreement and appear to be listening carefully. Feedback from the patient is the only means that the EMT has to ensure that the message sent is understood.

FEEDBACK

Feedback is a return conversation that helps the EMT ensure that the message sent was correctly understood by the patient. The patient's failure to understand the message, barring physical or psychological reasons previously discussed, is called *miscommunication*. Miscommunication can be summed up best in the statement, "I know what you heard, but that's not what I said."

One of the more common reasons for miscommunication is human nature. The average person can hear and understand approximately 500 words per minute. But the average person can only speak about 125 to 150 words a minute. As a result the patient is not listening about two-thirds of the time. During these gaps the patient's mind is either thinking about what is being said, and often rushing to judgment, or thinking about something else, such as how they feel.

The only way the EMT can be sure that the message was understood is to listen to the response. However, keep in mind that the EMT is human, too,

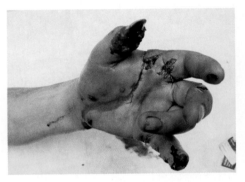

Figure 17.4 A painful injury can distract the patient from the conversation (Courtesy of Larry Torrey, RN, Portland, ME)

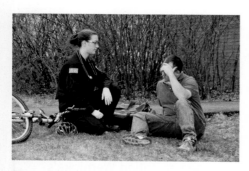

Figure 17.5 Active listening involves giving the patient your undivided attention

and must resist the urge to let his mind wander. Instead, he must listen carefully. Careful listening, or **active listening,** is an effort to listen for the meaning in a patient's statements. The active listener allows the patient to complete a statement, without interruption. An active listener acknowledges the patient's statements by nodding agreement or uttering encouraging phrases, such as "go ahead," that do not interrupt the patient. An active listener may also rephrase and repeat the patient's message back to the patient to ensure that he has understood it correctly. The EMT in Figure 17.5 is involved in active listening.

The active listener is listening for more than the spoken word. He is also listening to the message behind the message, or the hidden message. For example, cracks in a person's voice or pressured speech may indicate that the patient is not being truthful. Similarly, carefully prepared answers may not be truthful.

The active listener takes into account the patient's body language. A grimaced facial expression even as the patient insists "I'm fine" may indicate that the patient is in pain and is being stoic.

Finally, the active listener compares earlier statements to what is being said now. Any inconsistencies in statements should be clarified or possibly viewed as an indication of conflict. There are a number of techniques, which will be discussed shortly, that can help the EMT be a better active listener and communicator.

INTERVIEWING TECHNIQUES

To facilitate good communication, the EMT should practice proven interviewing techniques. These interviewing techniques can be summed up as the three Ps of proper manners, positioning, and privacy.

An EMT should always introduce himself by name and title. While some agencies and individuals prefer to not use a last name during introductions, it may be an agency policy or state regulation that the EMT use his full name; the EMT should verify this with local officials.

If the patient is older than the EMT, then it is proper to refer to the patient as Mr., Ms., or Mrs. with their last name, unless the patient requests that the EMT use a different form of address. For example, the EMT might say, "Good evening, Mrs. Robinson, my name is Benjamin and I am an EMT." If the patient is younger than or the same age as the EMT, it is acceptable to refer to the patient by first name. This behavior helps to establish the patient's trust in the EMT.

An EMT may overhear someone refer to a patient as "Honey" or "Sweetheart." These terms of endearment should be reserved for family members only. The use of these terms by the EMT suggests a level of familiarity that the EMT does not have and depersonalizes the patient. Therefore, EMTs should avoid using these terms, which might be considered demeaning.

When making an introduction, the EMT should be at eye level with the patient. Standing over patients is a position of dominance and immediately diminishes the patients' sense of themselves, making them feel vulnerable and even defenseless. Positioning himself at eye level with a patient helps to show the EMT's warmth and compassion.

The EMT should be aware that distance between the EMT and the patient also has an impact on the interview. People generally have four spaces, in concentric circles, around them. The largest space, the public space, is six or more feet around the patient. This space generally cannot be violated by any stranger without causing the patient some concern. Entry into this space may generate the fight-or-flight response in some people. The next space is considered the social space. This is the distance that an average conversation is held. People are generally not permitted into a person's personal space without permission. The next space is personal space. This space, within two feet of the patient, generally makes the patient feel vulnerable. The last space, the intimate space, can, as the name suggests, involve touch. Intimate space is so close that most people only allow a few close people into that space. Figure 17.6 illustrates these distances.

The EMT must eventually be permitted into the intimate space of the patient and that takes a lot of trust from the patient. The EMT must earn the patient's trust. In the beginning, the EMT should make no assumptions about the patient's trust and start the interview, kneeling on the balls of the feet, from within the social space. The EMT should then look for signs, such as an outstretched arm, that permits the EMT into the patient's personal and, ultimately, intimate space.

A final aspect of effective interviewing is that the EMT should attempt to have any conversations about the patient's medical history in private. Privacy helps to decrease interference such as loud noises from obstructing communication. Privacy also helps to ensure that the patient will be more forthcoming and honest to the EMT. Taking the extra effort to ensure privacy helps establish the EMT's genuineness and sincerity.

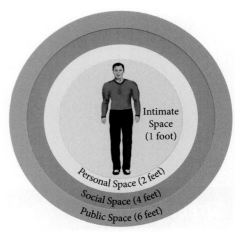

Figure 17.6 There are four spaces around a person; public, social, personal, and intimate

After establishing the three Ps, the EMT should use the following techniques to improve communication. The first is to ask open-ended questions. **Open-ended questions** are questions that cannot be answered with simple yes or no. Open-ended questions require the patient to be more expressive.

Many EMTs take notes while interviewing a patient. Note taking is acceptable but should not be taken at the expense of the interview. Instead the EMT should take notes after the patient is finished with a statement. Some EMTs prefer not to take notes. Understanding the complexity of a patient's history, it is hard to imagine that anyone can accurately remember all of the information provided during a patient interview. Sparingly taking notes, writing down the highlights of the conversation, is probably better than taking no notes at all.

The EMT should not be afraid to use silence as a technique. In a rush to give the EMT an answer, the patient may not have provided the best answer. Permitting a moment of silence can allow the patient time to rephrase and restate the answer, improving the quality of the answer in the process.

Another interviewing technique is sharing observations. Sharing an observation helps to connect the EMT to the patient. For example, the statement "You appear to be in discomfort" not only demonstrates the EMT's empathy but opens the door for a conversation about the patient's pain.

Similarly the EMT can acknowledge the patient's emotional statements. An acknowledgement such as "I understand that you don't feel well" shows that the EMT has empathy for the patient's condition and may encourage the patient to share her feelings.

The EMT can also choose to use the technique of reflection in which the EMT takes the patient's own words and repeats them, usually in a more concise statement. For example, the patient who has expressed frustration over her pain management and has offered a lengthy medical history may be encouraged to offer more information with the statement, "So you feel that nothing is helping you with the pain?"

When the message is unclear, the EMT may ask for clarification. Typically the patient restates the answer in other words that provide the EMT more insight into the patient's condition.

All of these techniques, silence, sharing observations, acknowledgement, reflection, and clarification, are intended to encourage patients to talk about their illness or injury. To help make the history succinct and accurate, the EMT may choose summarization. Summarization is a technique that not

Table 17-1 Interview Techniques
1. Intentional silence
2. Shared observations
3. Acknowledged feelings
4. Clarifying statements
5. Reflection
6. Summarization

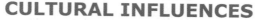

Street Smart

On occasion the EMT may be able to influence the patient's behaviors in the future because the patient's mind is receptive to suggestion today. This is referred to as a **teachable moment**. Teachable moments are unplanned and unpredictable, but there is a time when the patient is open to suggestion. By capitalizing on the teachable moment, such as encouraging a teenager to wear a seatbelt after a motor vehicle collision, the EMT can prevent future injuries.

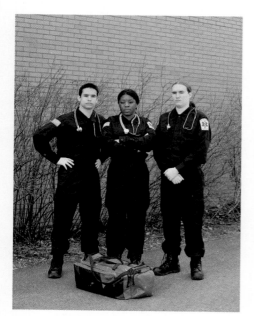

Figure 17.7 EMS is becoming multiethnic and cross-cultural

only provides an intellectual break—that is, an opportunity to reflect upon what has been said—but can be used to signal a change of approach, typically from history gathering to physical examination. A report to the physician at the bedside would be an example of summarization, and the patient should be provided with the same report. This helps to prevent contradictions at the hospital as well as solidifying what the EMT understands about the patient's condition. Table 17-1 lists these effective interviewing techniques.

Some EMT may consider the use of confrontation to help open the dialogue. This is a potentially dangerous technique that may have the unintended effect of halting the patient's attempts to communicate. With minimal information about the patient and her circumstances, the EMT is well advised to avoid confrontation as an interviewing technique.

While an EMT must be very aware of personal space, at the right time a simple touch can be reassuring to a patient who feels alone and vulnerable. Holding a patient's hand, for example, offers the patient reassurance and demonstrates the EMT's compassion. Compassionate touch should used when circumstances deem it appropriate.

CULTURAL INFLUENCES

In the 1990s, 75% of the population of the United States consisted of Euro-Americans; by 2020, that rate will drop to approximately 53%. This changing demographic is a result of the nation's increasing cultural diversity. The U.S. population now consists of almost every cultural and ethnic group found in the world.

To be effective an EMT must attain **cultural competency.** Cultural competency is the ability to understand, respect, and positively interact with—and in the case of an EMT, care for—persons of many cultures. This requires the EMT to learn about the culture of others. Most people have a natural bias toward their own culture, called **ethnocentrism.** In other words, most people tend to think that their culture is superior or more desirable. To become culturally competent, the EMT must learn about other cultures and accept that people, while their cultures may be different, are not inferior or less desirable in any way. Figure 17.7 shows a multiethnic, cross-cultural team of EMTs.

Culture is a system of symbols, icons, and activities that are important to a group of people. A person's culture includes customary beliefs, shared attitudes, and common beliefs that a person shares with the community and that have been acquired during a lifetime of contact. Culture includes one's manners and dress.

Influences that affect one's culture are race, religion, nationality, and ethnicity. Other influences that affect one's culture might be socioeconomic status, sexual preference, marital status, and even one's occupation.

MISTAKES IN COMMUNICATION

While learning the skill of communications is often a function of trial and error, there are three common mistakes in communication to avoid. These mistakes in communication can be summed up by the three Cs; clichés, criticism, and contradiction.

With good intention, the EMT may use a trite phrase such as "everything will be alright." These phrases are not only meaningless—the EMT has no control over the patient's destiny—they offer false reassurance. This false reassurance can damage the EMT's credibility if the patient's condition should worsen.

Likewise the EMT should not criticize the patient. This criticism can be very subtle, in the form of "why" questions. For example, a vulnerable patient might find a question such as "Why did you do that?" to be harsh and judgmental. The EMT would be better served to rephrase the question in a way that does not seem to target the patient's motives or intelligence.

Finally, the EMT should not contradict the patient. While this may sound like common sense, statements such as "You shouldn't feel that way" may be intended to reassure or comfort but instead challenge the patient's dignity and may be met with resistance. Such statements usually stem from the EMT's own life experience with illness or pain. But patients' responses to pain or illness are based on their individual life experiences. Empathy is a more effective response than the EMT attempting to apply his own perspectives and life experience.

On occasion an EMT might feel compelled to offer the patient medical advice, especially if the patient asks the EMT's opinion. While it may be flattering to think that the patient holds the EMT in high regard, the EMT should resist the temptation to offer advice. Statements giving advice usually start with "If I were you…" in an effort to make it sound as if the EMT is not giving advice. The patient should instead be directed to a physician for any medical advice.

The EMT should also avoid the use of leading questions. Leading questions are those questions that suggest an answer. A classic example of a leading question is, "Have you stopped beating your wife?" There is no satisfactory answer to the question. To say yes would imply the person beat his wife in the past; to say no implies continued guilt. Leading questions also have a tendency to be closed-ended questions, which can be answered with a yes or no. Instead of a closed-ended question, the EMT should rephrase the question to be an open-ended question. For example, instead of asking "Are you in less discomfort now?" the EMT could ask "How are you feeling now?"

OBSTRUCTIONS TO COMMUNICATION

Sometimes the patient unwittingly provides an obstruction to communication by using psychological defense mechanisms, such as those listed in Table 17-2. Patients may use psychological defense mechanisms to protect themselves from painful or unpleasant feelings, but these behaviors interfere with clear communication. The EMT should keep in mind that patients use defense mechanisms to protect themselves; thus, in many cases, confronting patients about these behaviors in the field and attempting to make them face their problems are inappropriate responses and may even be dangerous. Instead, the EMT should seek to understand the source of these behaviors and accept the patient as being human. Many patients will be anxious,

Street Smart

On occasion a patient may use the time with an EMT to complain about other EMTs or other health care providers. The EMT should avoid becoming defensive and try to refocus the patient on the present, without denying or acknowledging past misconduct by others.

Table 17-2 Psychological Defense Behaviors

1. Projection
2. Questioning
3. Repression
4. Rationalization
5. Suppression
6. Threatening behaviors

nervous, and unpredictable. They can even become violent. These defense mechanisms can be remembered by the mnemonic PQRST.

Projection involves one person attributing her thoughts or feelings to another. For example, an uncooperative patient, unwilling to admit she is being difficult, might claim that the EMT was "not very nice." Persons who are paranoid or antisocial commonly use this defense mechanism.

Some patients manifest their insecurity by asking questions—sometimes many questions. These questions may border on the absurd and demonstrate the patient's fear or apprehension. Patience and a calm demeanor are the most effective means of dealing with this defense mechanism.

For some patients the situation is too difficult to cope with, psychologically speaking, and they react by eliminating all thoughts of the event from their mind. **Repression** is not a conscious effort on the part of the patient, but a subconscious response. By putting all memories or thoughts of the painful event out of the mind, the patient subconsciously spares herself from the trauma. Patients who are repressing events, such as murder, may appear to be amnesic. Amnesia can be caused by traumatic brain injury; therefore, the EMT should first consider the possibility of a medical source for the amnesia before assuming it is repression.

Some patients develop logical explanations to events to avoid dealing with painful emotions. These **rationalizations** serve to protect the patient, psychologically speaking. For example, a drunk driver hears that he may have killed another driver and then finds out the other driver wasn't wearing a seatbelt; the drunk driver might rationalize the severity of his behavior by saying that the other driver would have lived if he had worn his seatbelt.

Like repression, **suppression** involves putting a painful event out of one's mind. Unlike repression, suppression is a conscious and voluntary act. In other words, the person makes a choice to not think about it. The statement "I don't want to talk about it" indicates suppression.

Sometimes people act in a threatening manner for no apparent reason. In order to avoid painful emotions with another, a patient might transfer his anger to the EMT. This reaction, called **displacement,** may be observed during a domestic disturbance. The EMT, being an unwitting victim, is attacked, either verbally or physically, rather than the spouse. The attacker deflects his anger, knowing that attacking the spouse would result in an arrest for domestic violence. The attacker gets to vent his feelings without risking arrest. These situations are complex and dangerous, and personal safety should be the EMT's first concern.

FRIGHTENED OR AGITATED PATIENT

Fear is a response to a perceived threat to life or limb. The emotional response is accompanied by a physical response from the sympathetic nervous system—that is, the fight-or-flight response. The patient has pallor and pupils are dilated. The patient's pulse and blood pressure are elevated. These physical responses are short lived and, given time, the excited or frightened patient will return to normal.

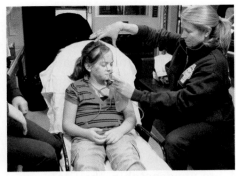

Figure 17.8 Treatment such as oxygen administration is less stressful when the EMT communicates with the patient (Courtesy of Larry Torrey, RN, Portland, ME)

However, on occasion and for reasons that have not been fully explained, some patients remain agitated or frightened. They may be apprehensive about the care being received or hypercritical of the care being provided. It seems that nothing can satisfy these patients. In general, they are uncooperative with care, seeking to either control the care provided or refusing care offered.

The EMT should try to recognize that these behaviors are based in fear and not react as if the behaviors are criticisms of themselves or their care. The EMT should try to work with the patient to find an acceptable treatment plan with which the patient feels safe (Figure 17.8). This can be accomplished by offering alternatives. For example, if the patient refuses an oxygen mask, then the EMT may offer a nasal cannula instead. The EMT should never offer alternatives that are unacceptable. For example, an agitated patient who is hypoxic should not be offered the opportunity to refuse care.

AGGRESSIVE OR VIOLENT PATIENT

Like the frightened or agitated patient, the behaviors of the aggressive or violent patient are based in fear. Initially an aggressive patient may appear calm, but the EMT should be alert for signs of escalating violence. Early signs of violence include the use of vulgarities, sometimes to excess. After exhibiting aggressive verbal behavior, the patient may escalate to subtle physical violence, such as pinching, scratching, or abrupt exaggerated movements. Other signs of the potential for violence include a clenched jaw or fists, narrowed eyes, and tensed muscles.

As with the agitated patient, the EMT should accept the patient but not the behavior. Establishing boundaries can sometimes be helpful. For example, sometimes an elderly demented patient will pinch the EMT. The EMT should quietly but firmly explain that pinching is not permitted. No threats should be made about what will happen if the patient pinches again, but the EMT should consider a response such as soft restraints.

In every instance the EMT's safety is the first priority, and the EMT may need to choose a tactical withdrawal, returning to the patient's side only when the scene is safe.

It is important to document the patient's behaviors. In some cases the patient may have a problem with impulse control and be in need of anger management therapy.

SEXUALLY AGGRESSIVE PATIENT

Some patients may show an inappropriate sexual interest in the EMT. Examples of this interest include inappropriate touching or sexual innuendo. When a patient misbehaves sexually, the EMT must take immediate action to terminate the behavior.

First the EMT should understand that the behavior may be the result of fear and feelings of insecurity. The patient is making an effort, though inappropriate, to be liked. The patient needs reassurance that she will be treated well and she does not have to fear the EMT.

Next the EMT needs to establish clear boundaries. This is done by reinforcing the professional relationship that the EMT has with the patient and explaining that such behaviors are not acceptable.

The elderly demented patient and the intoxicated patient both suffer from disinhibition, the lack of inhibitions, and they may "act out" in inappropriate ways. While these behaviors are unacceptable, the EMT must understand that it is the "disease talking" and must not permit personal feelings from interrupting patient care.

Any sexual conduct with a patient is inappropriate, both ethically and legally, and interferes with the therapeutic relationship. The patient should always be treated with objectivity and respect.

DEPRESSED PATIENT

Everyone can feel depressed at one time or another. These isolated episodes of depression, called situational depression, are usually due to life-altering events such as the death of a loved one or loss of job. Situational depression is normal and lasts for a few days or weeks.

A major depression goes on for several months, and the person becomes dysfunctional, unable to complete activities of daily living. Major depression is not normal and is considered a psychiatric emergency. EMS is often called to the scene of a depressed person who is a danger to herself or others.

As with the angry patient, the EMT should accept the patient but not the behavior. The EMT should try to stress to the patient that he will provide a safe environment and that the patient will not be harmed.

The EMT should document any statements that indicate that the patient feels helpless or hopeless. Feelings of helplessness and hopelessness are common in depressed patients.

SPECIAL CASE: SUICIDAL PATIENT

Suicide can result from depression. It tends to occur in the very young, ages 15 to 24, and the very old, those greater than age 65. Suicide is more common among males; in the case of adolescents, the ratio of male suicide victims to females is 5:1.

Patient statements such as "I am useless," which indicates a lack of self-worth, or "I wonder what it would be like to be dead" should alert the EMT to the potential for suicide. Other warning signs of suicide include previous suicide attempts and a history of major depression.

When confronted with a suicidal patient with a weapon, the EMT's first thought should be personal safety. In those cases a tactical withdrawal is appropriate until the scene is safe and weapons have been secured.

When caring for a patient who may have attempted suicide, the EMT should listen carefully to the patient and document her responses. It is acceptable to ask the patient if she meant to kill herself. Asking the question does not put the idea in the patient's mind. The EMT should try to understand the patient, and while not accepting the behavior, try to support the patient and show empathy, if appropriate.

HEARING IMPAIRED

Communications with the deaf and hearing impaired is a challenge. In some cases the patient has partial hearing. Patients who are hard of hearing (HOH) depend on hearing aids to function. If the patient appears to be straining to hear, the EMT should look to see if the patient has a behind the ear (BTE) or an in the ear (ITE) hearing aid and then speak to that side of the patient, as the EMT in Figure 17.9 is doing. The EMT should avoid the temptation to shout. Patients who are hard of hearing often have loss a range of hearing and can understand parts of speech at a normal conversational volume. Therefore, the EMT should speak in a normal tone and volume of speech. If the patient has lost all hearing, then no amount of volume will overcome the deafness.

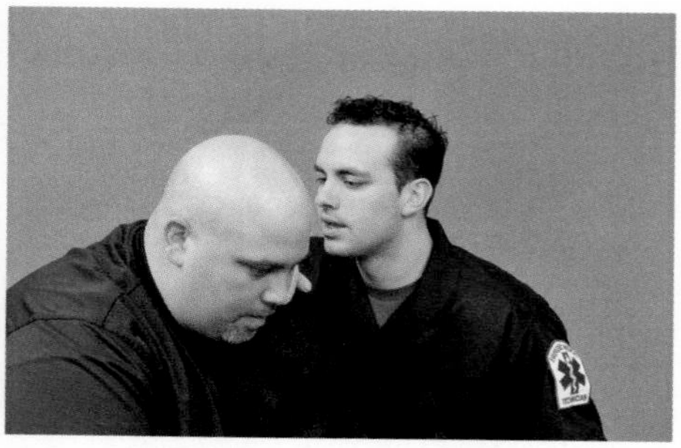

In some cases, a deaf or hearing impaired individual may have learned to communicate with the hearing population by reading lips. A few simple rules will help the patient understand the EMT. First, the EMT should sit

Figure 17.9 Speak into the ear that has the hearing aid

directly at eye level and across from the patient. The EMT should avoid back-lighting that silhouettes the face and makes the lips hard to see. Next the EMT should speak slowly and articulate words carefully. The EMT should avoid slang words such as nope or yeah and instead use standard English. To ensure that the communication is complete, the EMT should ask the patient to acknowledge what was said.

Some patients may attempt to use American Sign Language, a series of hand gestures and movements that convey words. This form of communication is useful if the EMT understands it or can communicate through a family member or friend with the patient. Otherwise, the EMT may need to resort to sign boards or offer a simple pen and paper.

PEDIATRICS

Young patients pose special communication challenges for the EMT. To communicate effectively, the EMT must adjust the approach to the child according to the child's developmental age.

Infants are completely dependent on their parents. Therefore when caring for an infant, the EMT should speak directly to the parent and use the child's name. While the EMT may be able to hold the infant, it is sometimes best to assess the infant while she is being held by a parent.

Conversely, communicating with preschool-aged children may be complicated by their independent nature. These children see the world only in terms of how it affects them. The EMT should kneel in front of the child and attempt a dialogue. These children think in concrete terms, so the EMT's questions should be concrete. Any questions about past medical history should be directed to the caregiver while the EMT is still engaged with the child. It is important to give these preschool-aged children positive reinforcement for good behaviors, such as cooperation. A stuffed animal can help gain the toddler's cooperation.

School-aged children are more sophisticated and more likely to interact with the EMT. The EMT should keep questions simple and instructions short. School-aged children want to be seen as cooperative in most cases, as shown in Figure 17.10.

For the adolescent, privacy is important. The adolescent may not be willing to communicate if a parent is present. History gathering and other communication should be performed in private, and the patient's modesty should be respected at all times. Treating an adolescent with respect and dignity often results in cooperation.

DEATH AND DYING

Perhaps one of the most difficult jobs an EMT may have is delivering bad news to a family. With an increasing number of terminations of cardiac arrest in the field, an EMT may be called on to provide the family with a death notification. At other times, an EMT may be required to inform the family of the death of a loved one when resuscitation is medically futile.

Breaking the bad news can be less traumatic if the EMT follows a few basic rules. First, the EMT should choose a place that is quiet and private. This affords the family the chance to grieve without fear of embarrassment.

After introducing himself, the EMT should address the closest relative. In some cases the family spokesperson is not the eldest. The EMT should attempt to identify who is the family spokesperson.

Speaking directly to and at eye level with the primary survivor, the EMT should first briefly summarize the event and actions in a few sentences. After

Street Smart

Some patients with a hearing impairment have working dogs. These working dogs listen for and protect their masters; they are the ears of their masters. It is inappropriate to touch or pet a working dog without the master's permission. In many EMS systems, guide/working dogs are permitted to travel with their master in the ambulance.

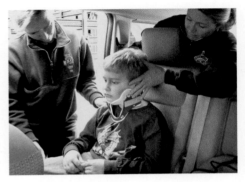

Figure 17.10 Communication with the child enables the EMT to gain the child's cooperation (Courtesy of Larry Torrey, RN, Portland, ME)

the summary, the EMT should make the statement, or declaration, using the words dead or has died. The declaration should be spoken slowly and clearly. The declaration should be direct and without ambiguity. Euphemisms for death, such as "He passed away", can be confusing to the family. The EMT may elect to offer his sincere sympathy.

After delivering the news, the EMT should wait a respectful period of time, usually 5 to 10 minutes, before speaking to the family again. The EMT may wish to use that time to help prepare the body. Following local protocols, the EMT may wish to cover the body with a clean sheet, leaving the face and arms exposed. The EMT may also want to place a box of tissues near the patient's side.

The EMT should also be prepared in case of a medical emergency involving another family member or friend of the family. The stress of losing a loved one can precipitate an acute illness or exacerbate a pre-existing condition.

Finally, the EMT should inform the family of the local protocols and procedures used when a patient is either found dead or dies during EMS care. It may be helpful to have clergy present during this time.

Some cultures have particular death rituals that an EMT might want to be aware of when delivering a death notification. It is important that an EMT remain nonjudgmental about these behaviors, particularly psychosomatic expressions of grief, and continue to provide comfort to the family.

The following is a brief overview of the death rituals of some minority groups in the United States. However, because a person or family belongs to an ethnic group does not mean that they will necessarily practice the death rituals of that group. And in some cases, the individuals may have mixed cultural influences.

After notifying an African-Americans family of death, the EMT may witness open expressions of grief and loud calling out to the deceased. In some cases a family member may suddenly collapse, or "fall out." These episodes are a psychic response to the trauma. The EMT may also notice some members of the patient's family speaking incoherently. This speech, called "speaking in tongues," is personal and limited in duration.

Families of an Arabian heritage may request time alone with the body. It is customary for the family to wash the deceased's body three times and shroud it in white. The EMT should sensitive to Muslim traditions. Muslim men should be handled by and cared for by other Muslim men. It should be noted that while most Arabs are Muslim, not all Muslims are Arab. Finally, the family may wish the bed or the body be turned to face the east and Mecca.

The Chinese view death as a part of life and have a strong belief in the afterlife. The EMT may witness a stoic acceptance of death and the importance of respect for the elderly. Because the Chinese practice many religions, including Islam, Catholicism, Buddhism, and Taoism, it is difficult to generalize about their death rituals. Instead, the EMT should follow the instructions of the eldest family member.

While many Euro-Americans consider themselves Christian or come from a Christian background, the death rituals are varied. Because circumstances can vary, the EMT generally delivers the information to the primary survivor. This individual will provide the EMT with direction and guidance regarding the family.

Jews, including American Jews, have codified death rituals. These practices include having the closest relative close the eyes and mouth of the deceased and place a sheet across the face. Ultra-Orthodox Jews may wish the deceased body to be placed on the floor with the feet toward the door and a candle placed at the head. The body of the deceased is never left alone.

Mexican-American families often have extended family involvement at the scene. The men may approach death stoically, while the women are more demonstrative. Some women may experience "ataque de nervios," or an attack of nerves. An attack of nerves is seizure-like hypermotor activity that is self-limited and not dangerous. The family may also insist on the use of candles in the room with the deceased.

Americans of Puerto Rican heritage usually prefer that the EMT speak with the head of the family, usually an eldest daughter or son. Once the message has been delivered, the family will prefer that clergy be present and that the extended family be allowed to view the body.

CONCLUSION

Good EMS care is often based on effective communication between the EMT and the patient. By understanding the principles of communication and the potential obstacles to communication, the EMT can improve the quality of the conversation. Practicing cultural tolerance, respect for all persons, and compassion for the patient, the EMT can engage the patient in therapeutic communication.

Street Smart

The death of a patient is hard on everyone, including members of the EMS team. The EMT should observe fellow providers for signs of stress and consider a critical incident stress debriefing, especially in cases of pediatric death or particularly gruesome deaths.

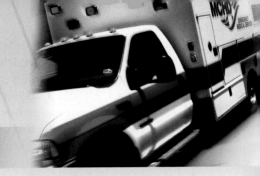

CASE STUDY Continued

After the call Eric decides to cancel his plans to go to the movies. On the advice of his partner Aaron, Eric is going to the local mosque to meet with the Imam.

Aaron tells him it is his responsibility to learn about his "communities of interest" and learn the customs of those he is going to serve.

Key Concepts Revisited

- The process of communication between a sender and receiver includes encoding, transmission, decoding, and feedback.

- Mistakes in communication include use of clichès, criticism, and contradiction.

- Obstructions to communication include fear, aggression, sexual innuendo, hearing impairment, and depression.

- Psychological defense mechanisms that can impair communication include projection, repression, rationalization, suppression, and threatening behaviors.

- Communications with pediatric patients must be adjusted to their developmental age.

- Delivery of a death notification must include cultural sensitivity.

Review Questions

1. What are the four parts of communication?
2. What is medicalese?
3. What is body language?
4. What are some examples of distracting painful injuries that could interfere with communication?
5. What is active listening?

6. What is an open-ended question?
7. What is cultural competency?
8. What influences affect a person's culture?
9. Name the five defense mechanisms.
10. Describe how an EMT can help a hearing impaired person lip-read in communicating with the EMT.

Key Terms

Active listening
Blading
Body language
Cultural competency
Culture
Displacement

Distracting painful injury
Ethnocentrism
Feedback
Illiteracy
Interference
Intonation

Medicalese
Open-ended questions
Projection
Rationalization
Repression

Suppression
Teachable moment
Therapeutic communication
Trigger words

Further Study

Purnell, Larry D., and Betty J. Paulanka. *Guide to Culturally Competent Health Care*. Philadelphia: F. A. Davis, 2005.

Taparo, Carol T., and Wilburta Lindh. *Therapeutic Communications for Health Professionals*. 2d ed. Clifton Park, NY: Thomson Delmar Learning, 2000.

UNIT (18) History Taking

Patient assessment is a systematic approach to gathering the vital information needed to provide the best possible patient care. A component of patient assessment that follows the initial scene size-up, primary assessment, and baseline vital signs is taking a patient history. The patient's history includes information on past medical conditions and injuries as well as investigating current medical conditions and events leading up to the need for EMS. The information gathered through the process of taking a thorough history can be a vital component to the overall assessment.

Key Concepts

- Information gathered through the assessment process of taking a thorough history can be vital to ongoing patient care.

- A complete patient history that includes the history of the present illness or injury will allow the EMT to find conditions that may not have been apparent during the primary assessment.

- Collecting or gathering pertinent history requires the EMT to consider several factors, including the age, race, and gender of the patient.

- The content of the history must be documented and include correct dates and times of previous and current treatments.

- The components of history taking should help the patient feel comfortable with the process.

- History taking techniques include a professional, compassionate demeanor and making the patient comfortable.

- The EMT should develop a standardized approach to history taking.

- SAMPLE history is the patient's pertinent individual information.

- OPQRST is a detailed evaluation of the current illness.

- The patient may be experiencing associated signs and symptoms or concerns directly related to the present illness.

- Pertinent negatives can provide important clues to the present condition.

- The EMT may have to ask the patient questions involving sensitive topics.

- The EMT may experience special challenges in history taking.

- Family and friends can be an additional resource for history gathering when the patient is unable to provide the pertinent information.

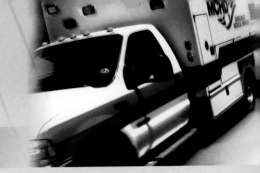

CASE STUDY

Tillie completes her primary assessment of Mrs. Scott in the kitchen, while her partner Ben takes Mrs. Scott's baseline vital signs. Tillie determines that Mrs. Scott appears very ill. Tillie requests an ALS intercept and determines this is a high-priority patient in need of immediate transport. Ben gathers Mrs. Scott's current medication bottles from Mr. Scott to take with them to the hospital.

While en route to the hospital Tillie begins gathering information from Mrs. Scott that could be passed on to the doctor. Tillie knows a number of illnesses may be affecting Mrs. Scott, and she needs more information to determine if she is providing the correct treatment or what

other treatments Mrs. Scott may need from the ALS crew. Tillie begins gathering information by evaluating Mrs. Scott's chief concern.

Critical Thinking Questions

1. What questions should Tillie ask to learn about Mrs. Scott's present illness?

2. Why are Mrs. Scott's current medications significant?

3. What methods should be used to gather the pertinent information used in determining the appropriate treatment?

INTRODUCTION

The objective of the primary assessment is to find and treat life-threatening injuries. The patient who is seriously ill or injured is then immediately transported. Once the primary assessment is completed, with any life-threatening condition managed, the EMT should continue her assessment by gathering as much **patient history** as possible. The patient's history is a more in-depth investigation of the details of the present illness or injury, including the patient's pertinent past medical history and current health status. There will be times, however, when assessment and treatment of the critical patient goes no further than maintaining an open airway or performing cardiopulmonary resuscitation (CPR). Even at those times, getting as much information about the history of the event or the patient from bystanders or family can make a difference in patient care down the line.

When no life-threatening conditions are detected in the primary assessment, the EMT should take some time gathering a thorough history on scene, using the resources of the family members present when the patient is unable to communicate.

Taking a complete patient history that includes the history of the present illness or injury allows the EMT to find conditions that may not have been apparent during the primary assessment. These conditions are usually minor; however, they may need stabilization before transportation.

This unit discusses the components of a patient history and techniques the EMT can use to develop a standardized approach to history taking

EVENT HISTORY

In most cases, the EMT determines that the patient's injuries are traumatic due to the presence of a mechanism of injury. For example, when a patient in a motor vehicle collision (MVC) complains of forearm pain and has an obvious swollen deformity of the forearm, then the assumption is that the patient suffered a broken arm as a result of the MVC.

Sometimes the mechanism of injury is not apparent. Take the case of the unconscious woman who is found sitting in her car, which is against a guardrail on the side of a rural road just past a bridge. There is minimal damage to the fender of her car and no other vehicle is present. Is the woman unconscious because she collided with the guardrail? If there is doubt whether the patient has a medical condition or traumatic injury, it is safest to assume the unconscious patient is suffering from a traumatic injury. If the patient is conscious and able to answer questions, investigating the present condition through history taking is appropriate.

Following the initial scene size-up, which includes a consideration of the mechanism of injury or nature of illness, and the primary assessment for life-threatening injuries, the EMT should make a determination if the patient is high priority or low priority. This decision is important to determining the next step.

If the patient is high priority, then efforts should be made to immediately package and transport the patient before proceeding with history taking and the secondary assessment. In some cases, with sufficient personnel, the EMT may be able to gather pertinent history from bystanders and family or friends of the patient while preparing the patient for transport.

Alternatively, if the patient is low priority, the EMT may elect to gather the patient's history and conduct the secondary assessment while on scene.

HISTORY COLLECTION

Collecting or gathering pertinent history requires the EMT to consider several factors and components of history taking. A pertinent history can be associated with or is relevant to the management of the patient's current condition. Who is providing the information, the patient, a friend, family member, or another health care provider? If the patient is conscious and responsive, he is usually the best source to provide accurate information. If the information is coming from someone else, how accurate and reliable is the information? The information the EMT receives from friends and family can be variable, depending on how close of a relationship they have with the patient. Therefore, it is important to document the source of information.

Data that must be included in every history is the age and gender of the patient. The content of the history must be documented and include correct dates and times of previous and current treatments.

COMPONENTS OF PATIENT HISTORY

Patient history is important to gather because it will direct assessment of the medical patient and help in the development of treatment plans for both medical and trauma patients. In the case of the trauma patient who is unresponsive, the primary assessment with management of life-threatening conditions is the first step, followed by a rapid physical assessment that identifies additional injuries that may be contributing to the patient's unresponsiveness. Physical examination is discussed in more detail in Unit 19. In the responsive patient, the patient history should be gathered and include the chief concern, history of present illness or injury, pertinent past medical history, and current health status.

In the responsive medical patient, gathering the patient's history will focus the physical exam during the secondary assessment on the area of concern. In other words, a patient who is complaining of abdominal pain will not require the EMT to spend a lot of time examining the head. It will guide the EMT to focus her exam to the area of concern and body systems that may indicate the cause of the abdominal pain.

CHIEF CONCERN

The **chief concern** is typically the reason EMS was called and the first verbal clue from the patient for why the ambulance was called. The chief concern should be further investigated, as it is not always the reason the patient called EMS "today." For example, the EMT may have been called for a patient with pain in his lower legs. After the EMT arrives and begins the patient interview, the patient tells her he has had some pain and numbness in his lower legs for the past several years. Therefore, the chief concern needs to be investigated further to determine why the patient felt the need to call for an ambulance *today*. What has changed or made the pain more severe today?

The chief concern is usually associated with pain or discomfort and a feeling that is not normal for the patient. It may be a sudden dysfunction, such as an inability to walk or stand or move a part of the body. When the chief concern is documented, the EMT should describe the chief concern using the patient's own words. The chief concern can be further defined when documenting the history of the present illness and result of the secondary survey. There will be times when the patient complains of multiple symptoms and past medical conditions. The EMT needs to investigate, sometimes using pertinent negatives (discussed later in this unit), to discern which concern and symptom are the cause for today's request for assistance.

The chief concern is not a condition. In other words, if the patient has a history of bone cancer, the chief concern should not be documented as "Patient complains of bone cancer." The patient is living with bone cancer every day; the EMT needs to establish why he felt the need to call an ambulance today. The patient's chief concern should be associated to a concern, sign, or symptom, such as increased pain or a fracture from the weakened bone.

The unresponsive patient or patient with an altered mental status obviously cannot state his chief concern for the EMT. In these cases, family members can help provide a more complete and, perhaps more importantly, objective history, such as the patient's history of drug or alcohol use. It is also important for the EMT to not become so focused on the stated chief concern that other signs or symptoms are missed, however minor they may seem. Other concerns that may appear minor may actually be more important than the original concern.

HISTORY OF PRESENT ILLNESS

The history of the present illness consists of the detailed evaluation of the chief concern and should provide a full, clear, chronological account of the signs and symptoms. The history of the present illness will include determining the onset of signs and symptoms, what might make the conditions better or worse, how severe the pain is, what the pain feels like, if the pain is stationary or moves to other parts of the body, and how long the sign and symptoms have been occurring.

PAST MEDICAL HISTORY

Pertinent information to the current condition or medical event can be gathered from the patient's past medical history. It is important to guide the questioning to establish the information that is pertinent to this event and filter the information that is not relevant at this time for this condition. The information that is gathered should involve past medical issues, trauma, or surgical events that may be associated to what the patient is experiencing now. As an example, a patient experiencing abdominal pain should be asked if he has ever experienced this pain before or ever had surgery for an abdominal condition.

Checking for medical identification tags can provide past history information if an unresponsive patient is unable to disclose this information.

CURRENT HEALTH STATUS

The current health status of the patient can be especially important to how well the patient responds to treatment or how well the patient can compensate for the current illness. The current health status focuses on the patient's present health, current treatments, and medication use pertinent to the current medical event. The environmental condition where the patient lives is also pertinent to the patient's current health status.

INDIVIDUAL FACTORS

The patient's current health status includes several elements or **individual factors,** along with the patient's current allergies and medication use. Does the patient use tobacco, alcohol, drugs, or other recreational substances? How is the patient's diet? Does the patient's living environment pose any special concerns, such as numerous animals in the house or unusual heat or cold? Are hazardous living conditions present? Does the patient need safety measures in and out of the house, such as hand rails or ramps?

TECHNIQUES

The EMT should employ certain techniques when taking a patient history. The first step is to make the patient as comfortable as possible. The appearance of the EMT will have a direct effect on how comfortable a patient will be in allowing the EMT to conduct the assessment and treatment. Patients will not answer questions if they do not trust the individual asking the questions. The EMT should always present a clean and neat appearance of professionalism at all times. It is also important to be aware of body language. The EMT who exhibits a confident, calm, compassionate demeanor will put the patient and patient's family at ease, calming and comforting the patient immediately (Figure 18.1).

The EMT should try to ensure the patient is in an environment that is quiet enough for the patient to hear the questions and for the EMT to hear the patient's answers. Anxiety is normal when an individual is not feeling well or is injured. Keep the patient calm and reassured. It may be difficult to remember all the details of the patient's history, but asking the patient to keep repeating answers increases anxiety and may cause the patient to feel the EMT is not being attentive. The EMT should be actively listening to the patient's responses and take notes of the important details pertinent to the patient's current condition.

STANDARDIZED APPROACH

Developing a standardized approach to history taking and using that approach each time a patient history is taken helps avoid the loss of potentially vital information. A thorough history involves details of the present illness and past pertinent health history. This standardized approach can be accomplished through use of the SAMPLE and OPQRST mnemonics.

SAMPLE HISTORY

The **SAMPLE history** is the information focused on the patient's past and current health. The SAMPLE history is used to systematically seek and document information of the patient's past health conditions and ongoing treatments and the current chief concern. The use of the mnemonic helps the

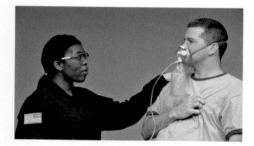

Figure 18.1 The EMT should always exhibit a confident, calm, and compassionate demeanor while actively listening to the patient during history taking

Table 18-1 SAMPLE History

S—Signs and symptoms

A—Allergies

M—Medications

P—Pertinent past medical history

L—Last meal or drink

E—Events leading up to the present illness or injury

EMT remember the questions designed to seek out pertinent information concerning the patient's past medical history, medications, allergies, signs and symptoms, last meal, and events leading to the current event. Table 18-1 lists the components of the SAMPLE history.

SIGNS AND SYMPTOMS

The chief concern is the reason EMS was called and is almost always based on the signs or symptoms the patient is experiencing. *Signs* are what the EMT can see is happening, such as diaphoresis (sweating) or pale or cyanotic skin. *Symptoms* are what the patient is feeling, such as pain, shortness of breath, or even a vague feeling of "something is wrong." Signs and symptoms will be further defined through the OPQRST assessment.

ALLERGIES

It is important to ask if the patient is allergic to anything, particularly medications. Allergies may be the cause of the signs and symptoms the patient is experiencing. Additionally, it is important to discern allergies in the event the patient will be given a medication during treatment. Allergies to medications are the primary information the EMT is seeking; however, it is also important to ask if the patient has any environmental allergies if he is exhibiting certain signs or symptoms. As an example, a patient who is experiencing shortness of breath and complaining of tightness in his chest after working in the yard may have been stung by a bee or wasp and his symptoms are due to an allergy to the venom.

MEDICATIONS

When asking the patient what medications he may be taking, it is important to ask for both prescription and nonprescription medications. It does not always occur to patients to think of over-the-counter medications, vitamins, and homeopathic or herbal mixtures as the type of medications they are being asked to list. Also ask if the patient is compliant, or taking his medications as he has been directed to take them. This can be an important clue to the reason for the patient's current condition, such as a patient having a seizure. If the patient has not been taking his anti-seizure medicine as prescribed, this could be the cause for sudden seizure activity.

The interaction of certain medications with other medications that may be administered in an emergency or hospital setting make finding, documenting, and reporting the patient's current medication use vital information. As an example, a patient having chest pain is commonly administered nitroglycerin. Viagra, a prescription medication commonly used for pulmonary hypertension and erectile dysfunction, and nitroglycerin both lower blood pressure.

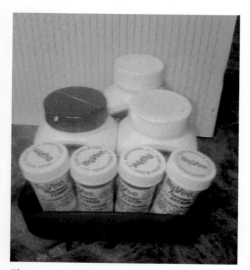

Figure 18.2 Medication bottles should be packaged and transported with the patient when possible

When nitroglycerin is administered to a patient who has recently taken Viagra, a dangerous and sometimes fatal drop in blood pressure can occur.

It is also important to ask the patient if he has taken any recreational (street) drugs. The EMT should advise the patient of the importance of being truthful about drug use and assure him the information is needed in determining the appropriate treatment for his condition. It is sometimes helpful to explain to the patient that any information he provides to the EMT is protected by patient privacy and confidentiality laws. The EMT cannot share that information with law enforcement or anyone else without the patient's permission.

Finally, ask the patient if he has taken medications that may belong to a spouse, parent, or sibling. Family members sometimes share medications, such as nitroglycerin. This can often be seen with the elderly who are on fixed incomes and taking numerous medications. They attempt to save money by filling a prescription for the same medication, not realizing or understanding the dosages are specific to the individual. Another common occurrence is that a well-meaning family member previously prescribed medication for symptoms similar to those of the patient shares that medication with the patient.

Documentation of the patient's medications and the dose of those medications is crucial. It is often easier, especially in the case of numerous medications, to gather all the patient's medications and transport them to the hospital with the patient (Figure 18.2).

PERTINENT PAST MEDIAL HISTORY

Pertinent past medical history is relevant information concerning past illness or injuries the patient has experienced that are pertinent to the current condition. Pertinent past medical history may include past medical problems or surgeries, physicians the patient sees on a regular basis for the current concern, and the patient's social history. The patient's family history may also be relevant in certain circumstances.

PREEXISTING

Ask the patient about any preexisting medical problems, including current illnesses such as heart disease, respiratory problems, hypertension (high blood pressure), diabetes, or stroke. It is also important to ask about any past surgeries that are pertinent to those past medical problems or the current concern. An example of pertinent past surgeries would be the patient who is experiencing chest pain and has undergone a coronary artery bypass graft (CABG), more commonly referred to by patients as *bypass surgery*. Information concerning past surgeries such as bypass surgery can be pertinent information concerning the severity of the past condition.

PHYSICIAN

The physician the patient sees on a regular basis for current conditions can be helpful information to the receiving hospital. If the patient is seeing a regular physician and a specialty physician, the information each of them can provide together or individually concerning the patient's status at the most recent visit can help establish any new changes in the condition.

FAMILY HISTORY

The patient's past family history is important in certain circumstances. A family history of heart disease is relevant and important information when the patient is young and complaining of typical cardiac symptoms. In this instance, the family history of cardiac disease demonstrates the patient has a higher degree for risk for a cardiac event.

The family history is also important in certain cultures, because there are specific conditions, such as sickle cell disease seen in African-Americans, that could be relevant to the patient's concern. In the case of infectious disease transmission, the patient's family history becomes extremely important, as well as in conditions such as tuberculosis (TB) or meningitis.

SOCIAL HISTORY

The environment in which the patient lives, including housing environment, occupation, economic status, travel history, and high-risk behaviors, make up the patient's **social history.** Patients who have an inadequate income may not purchase needed medications such as insulin or respiratory medications. The elderly often choose to buy their medications instead of food and thereby suffer malnutrition and vitamin deficiencies. Exposure to chemicals or other occupational substances and/or circumstances of the patient's living conditions, such as exposure to extreme heat or cold, may provide clues to certain disease etiologies.

Recent travel can be extremely important because public health in some countries is not as good as public health in the United States. The patient may have been exposed to infectious diseases, insects, animals, or other environmental elements that could cause an illness. Malaria is an example of a disease spread by infected mosquitoes that is widespread in subtropical and tropical countries. Another travel-related condition is deep vein thrombosis (DVT), or blood clots believed to originate in the legs due to a decrease in circulation from sitting for long periods of time, as on long air flights. Information about the patient's recent travel can be pertinent if the patient is complaining of leg pain or sudden onset of shortness of breath with no other history following an extended flight.

LAST ORAL INTAKE

What the patient has eaten or had to drink can be a significant clue to what is causing certain conditions. The diabetic patient who has taken insulin and then becomes busy and doesn't eat is likely to have a hypoglycemic event. Or, if the patient is experiencing signs of an allergic reaction, he may have eaten something without knowing he was allergic to it. What the patient last ate provides important clues to what may be causing the symptoms. It is also important for the hospital to know when the patient last ate in the event that surgery or other procedure is required.

EVENTS LEADING UP TO THE EVENT

The EMT should determine what the patient was doing or feeling prior to the onset of the illness or injury. Was the patient with chest pain engaged in strenuous physical activity when the chest pain began? Did the patient who had a seizure experience an "aura," a feeling or other indication he was about to have a seizure? The events leading up to the current illness or injury can be important pieces of information in patient management.

HISTORY OF PRESENT ILLNESS

The first step in investigating the history of the present illness is to evaluate the chief concern in more depth. The EMT can ask specific, open-ended questions to gather the information needed to help determine the condition the patient is suffering from and how best to manage that condition in the field. The mnemonic **OPQRST** can help the EMT place the questions in a systematic order that, when used consistently each time a patient history is taken, will ensure no essential information is missed. Table 18-2 summarizes the OPQRST history.

Geriatric Considerations

The elderly can be highly susceptible to heat- or cold-related illness due to medications and physiology changes in temperature regulation. Additionally, elderly patients living on a fixed income may not have an air conditioner, putting them at a higher risk for a serious heat-related illness.

Table 18-2 Components of the OPQRST History

O—Onset
P—Palliative/provocative/position
Q—Quality
R—Radiation
S—Severity
T—Time/duration

ONSET/SETTING

Onset is the time the chief concern began. The EMT should specifically ask the patient for the date, day, and time the chief concern began. It is also important to determine if the onset was gradual or sudden.

The EMT should determine the setting the patient was in at the time of onset. What was the patient doing when the pain or dysfunction began? What the patient was doing can have significant meaning to the concern. For example, the patient is complaining of a sudden onset of chest pain. The patient was shoveling snow when the chest pain began, an indication the pain started with exertion. The fact the pain started while the patient was involved in physical exertion is significant in evaluating chest pain. If the patient states he was simply sitting in a chair watching the ballgame on TV, the absence of physical exertion is also significant.

It is important to determine if the symptoms have ever occurred before, and if so, how often and how long ago the patient last experienced these same symptoms. Additionally, if the patient has experienced these symptoms previously, did he see a physician? What was the diagnosis and what treatment did the patient receive at that time? How has the symptom progressed? Is it worse, better, or unchanged since its onset?

PALLIATION/PROVOCATION/POSITION

The EMT should establish whether there is anything that makes the symptom worse or better. **Palliation** or alleviation of symptoms can be determined by asking the patient, "Does anything make the symptoms better?" This can include the patient's position. If the patient is experiencing shortness of breath, the EMT should take note of the position the patient is in when she arrives. If the patient is semireclining and is then assisted to sit more upright, did that move in position make the symptom better? If the patient has medications for chronic breathing problems, did taking that medication make the symptoms better for a time or not at all?

Provocation or aggravation of the symptom is simply what makes it worse. If the patient experiencing shortness of breath is seated upright and the patient is placed in a supine position, does lying flat cause breathing to become more labored?

Establishing what makes the patient's symptoms better, worse, or unchanged is useful in both ruling out certain conditions and developing an effective treatment plan.

QUALITY

Every individual has a different perception of pain. There are several commonly used descriptions of the quality or type of pain the patient is experiencing. The patient who is experiencing chest pain may describe the pain as tearing, sharp or knifelike, dull, heavy, crushing, or tight. A patient may describe abdominal pain as more of a cramp or generalized body pain as "achy." The EMT should get the patient to describe the pain in his own words. It is important to report and document the patient's exact words in describing the pain or discomfort.

RADIATION/LOCATION

Where the patient's discomfort or pain is located must be determined, followed by an evaluation of whether the pain radiates (moves) or is stationary. Ask the patient to point to where the pain is located using one finger. This establishes a point of reference for the pain and narrows the area of pain to a more specific starting point.

Once the point of reference or starting point for the pain or discomfort has been established, ask the patient if that pain moves, or radiates, to any other location. As an example, the patient states he is having chest pain and indicates the very center of his chest (the sternum) when asked to point to where the pain is located. The next question the EMT should ask is if that pain moves or goes anywhere else other than the chest. Patients may experience what is called *referred pain*, so it is important to establish all locations of pain, beginning with the pain's point of origin. **Referred pain** occurs in another area of the body that is not directly associated with the body system affected by the condition causing the pain. For example, a patient who has experienced a hip injury may experience pain in his knee, or liver disease may cause the patient to experience pain in his right shoulder.

SEVERITY

Severity can be assessed by asking, "How bad is the pain, discomfort, or difficulty?" Again, individuals have differing perceptions of pain; including the severity of pain. Therefore, the assessment for pain severity is subjective. Using a scale gives the patient a guide in rating pain and helps the patient express how badly he is hurting. The most commonly used rating scale is 0 to 10, with 10 being the worst pain the patient has ever experienced; however, others use a 0 to 5 scale, with 5 being the worst pain the patient has ever experienced. Regardless of which scale is used, the EMT should try to get the patient to rate the severity of his pain using a pain scale.

When asking the patient to rate pain or discomfort using a pain scale, it may be necessary to give the patient a reference point for the severity of his pain. For example, the EMT may ask "on a scale of 0 to 10, with 10 being the worst pain you have ever experienced, how would you rate the pain or discomfort you are feeling right now?"

Even giving patients a reference point, they will sometimes not be able to rate their pain using the scale. This can be especially true with the elderly and young children. At these times, using objective observation can be more reliable for establishing a pain level. A patient who is experiencing severe abdominal pain may be lying on his side, knees drawn up to his chest, and his arms wrapped around his abdomen, moaning. This position may indicate the patient is experiencing pain at a higher severity level such as 8 to10. The patient complaining of abdominal pain who is seated, conversing easily and lightly rubbing his abdomen when asked to rate his pain is most likely experiencing pain more on lower severity level such as the 0 to 4 range on the pain scale. When the patient points directly to his pain with one finger, this may indicate pain at a moderate level, perhaps in the 5 to 7 range on the pain scale.

It is also important to note the patients' facial expressions, such as grimacing, and other objective indicators of pain severity, such as moaning,

Street Smart

A patient sometimes will deny having what he perceives as "pain." If the patient denies having pain but continues to look uncomfortable, ask the patient if he is experiencing any discomfort and to describe what that "discomfort" feels like. Oftentimes patients deny chest pain but describe a heaviness or discomfort in their chest.

groaning, crying, slow movements, irritability, and constantly shifting positions. All of these signs can indicate a level of severity for the patient's pain or discomfort. The patient holding himself in a position called *self-splinting*—supporting the area of pain with his body position—is a good indicator of a potentially serious injury and moderate to severe pain.

Communication barriers, such as language barriers or the patient's inability to speak due to a stroke or other previous history, as well as the age of the patient (children, infants, and the elderly) create challenges in establishing the severity of pain using a standard pain scale. There are other pain assessment scales that can be used to assess the amount of pain the patient is experiencing when a standard 0 to 10 scale is not practical (see Figure 18.3A). The **Wong-Baker FACES scale** is a card that uses faces to indicate pain levels. The faces on the Wong-Baker FACES scale show varying facial expressions from smiles to grimacing to crying, to indicate a pain level the patient may be experiencing (see Figure 18.3B). The Wong-Baker FACES scale is used primarily for children over 3 years of age; however, it is also a good resource tool for individuals who do not speak the language of the health care provider, the elderly who cannot qualify their pain easily, or who may have lost their ability to speak.

The FLACC behavioral scale was designed for assessment of pain in children under 5 years of age. This scale assesses the patient's Face, Legs, Activity, Cry, and Consolability to measure the level of pain the patient is experiencing.

Finally, the EMT can carry a simple card with descriptor words for the patient to use to measure his pain level. This can be especially helpful for elderly patients who sometimes have a difficult time using the 0 to 10 scale. The descriptor card gives the patient parameters to qualify his pain using the following descriptors: no pain, mild, discomforting, distressing, horrible, and

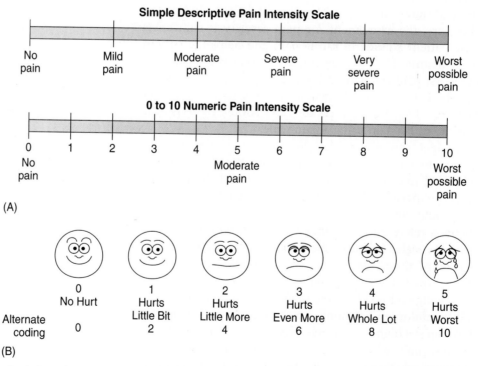

Figure 18.3 The pain intensity scale. (*From* Acute Pain Management: Operative or Medical Procedures and Trauma. Clinical Practice Guideline *(AHCPR Publication No. 92-0032), by the Acute Pain Management Guideline Panel, 1992, Rockville, MD. Agency for Health Care Policy and Research.* B. Wong-Bake FACES Pain Rating Scale. (*From Hockenberry, M, Wilson, D., Winklestein, M.: Wong's* Essential of Pediatric Nursing, *7th ed., St Louis, MO, 2005, p.663. Copyrighted by Mosby, Inc. Reprinted by permission*)

excruciating. The EMT should show the card to the patient and have him indicate the word that best describes his pain and then document the level of pain from 0 to 5 based on the descriptor word the patient selects.

Regardless of the method of measurement, it is important for the EMT to establish the patient's pain level, reassess the level of pain throughout treatment and transport, and report and document the initial pain level and any changes to that pain level.

TIME/DURATION

The time element of the OPQRST mnemonic is sometimes confused with the O, or onset assessment. Time is how long the symptoms have been present. If a patient has been experiencing leg pain for three days, why did they call for an ambulance today? The EMT asks, "How long have you been experiencing this pain or discomfort?" If the patient indicates he has experienced this symptom in the past, the EMT should ask, "How long did the pain last when you have experienced it in the past?" It is also important to note if the pain is constant or intermittent—that is, if it comes and goes.

ASSOCIATED SIGNS AND SYMPTOMS/ PERTINENT NEGATIVES

The patient may be experiencing signs and symptoms or concerns that can be associated to the present illness. Investigating for associated conditions usually requires direct questioning by the EMT to find concerns that are directly associated with the condition or chief concern. For example, is a patient who is experiencing chest pain also experiencing shortness of breath, nausea, and/ or weakness? The EMT often has to ask direct questions to ascertain associated conditions.

If the patient says no to direct questions concerning associated signs and symptoms such as "Are you having difficulty breathing?" or "Are you sick to your stomach?" this denial is called a pertinent negative. **Pertinent negatives,** when the patient denies the specific signs and symptoms, should be documented and reported to the receiving hospitals. A useful method of documenting pertinent negatives is for the EMT to report "the patient denies associated shortness of breath, nausea, or vomiting."

SENSITIVE TOPICS

The EMT may need to ask questions the patient may not want to answer. As previously discussed, the use of alcohol or recreational drugs is among the sensitive topics the EMT may have to address with the patient. Additionally, the EMT may need to confront the patient about his condition or history to get the answers needed to provide the appropriate care. Asking the patient about his or her sexual history is uncomfortable for both the patient and the EMT, but it is necessary in dealing with certain concerns of pain. For example, a female of child-bearing age complaining of lower abdominal or pelvic pain should be asked if she is sexually active.

When patients have been physically or sexually abused, they are often uncomfortable and even fearful of discussing the event. The EMT should employ all the techniques previously discussed to put the patient at ease as much as possible. The single most important thing the EMT can do in the case of physical or sexual abuse is to be professional and show a caring and sensitive understanding for the patient's emotional state. The EMT must never appear judgmental of the patient or the person accused of the abuse if he is still present on scene. Be conscious of the tone of voice and words used when asking the patient to relate the events leading up to his present illness or injury.

Showing respect for the patient and his privacy will go a long way to developing a positive rapport with the patient and may help him be comfortable with answering even the most sensitive of topics.

CHALLENGES

The EMT will encounter challenges in history taking many times throughout her career. The silent patient can sometimes be more challenging than a patient who talks excessively throughout the interview process. Silence can be uncomfortable for both the EMT and the patient. The silence may be due to the patient's inability to verbally communicate, or it could be a response resulting from the patient's perception of a lack of sensitivity on the part of the EMT. When dealing with the silent patient, the EMT must be attuned to any nonverbal communication that may provide clues to the patient's chief concern.

Overly talkative patients should be allowed to talk unrestrained for the first few minutes. This can aid the patient in releasing some of the stress and anxiety he may be feeling. However, the EMT must take and maintain control of the interview. One method of controlling the overly talkative patient is by summarizing frequently what the patient is saying. This method will help the patient stay on track in relating information that is pertinent to the current condition.

Anxiety, anger, and hostility are all natural reactions to stressful situations the EMT may encounter in patients. Anger over the situation may be displaced and projected on the EMS provider. Again, be sensitive to nonverbal clues and do not take the patient's anger or hostility personally or get angry in return. Offer patients who are anxious, angry, and hostile reassurance and understanding of the situation and emotions they are feeling. Like angry and hostile patients, the crying patient may provide valuable information and require the EMT to be sympathetic and understanding of their emotions.

Intoxicated patients can present a variety of challenges to the EMT. Certain behaviors associated with intoxication can make conducting the history interview frustrating for both the EMT and the patient. The best method of controlling the situation and gaining cooperation from the intoxicated patient is by not challenging him but accepting the information he is giving and filtering the pertinent facts from the information. Telling the intoxicated patient to lower his voice or trapping him in small areas in an attempt to control him may aggravate the situation. Treat the intoxicated patient with respect and dignity despite his intoxicated state.

Patients with confusing behavior or history may suffer from mental illness, delirium, or dementia. Additionally, the EMT should be alert for signs of depression. The EMT should not be judgmental; instead, she must be willing to listen to the patient who is showing signs and symptoms of depression, mental illness, delirium, or dementia.

The EMT may encounter individuals with limited cognitive abilities, hearing problems, and visual impairment, or there may be a language barrier. Do not overlook the ability of individuals with limited cognitive abilities to provide adequate information concerning their history and present illness; however, be alert for omissions. Individuals who have hearing problems can write questions and answers on paper. When approaching individuals with visual impairments, make sure to announce your presence and give clear, careful explanations throughout the assessment process. The EMT-patient language barrier can create unique situations for the patient and EMT attempting to use hand gestures and loud speech to communicate. To ensure there is no misunderstanding about what is being communicated, take every step to find a translator. This can be family or friends who are bilingual and present on the scene.

Family and friends are the next best resource for gathering a patient history when the patient is unable to answer questions. At times a third party can provide clarification of the situation from an objective view. Review Unit 17 for more specific methods and techniques of communication.

CONCLUSION

The EMT should develop a systematic approach to history taking that includes the use of SAMPLE and OPQRST. SAMPLE history includes the patient's signs and symptoms, allergies, current medications, past pertinent history, last oral intake, and events leading up to the current conditions. OPQRST can be used to evaluate the present illness, including the time of onset, palliative or provocative factors, the quality of pain or discomfort, the location and radiation of the pain, its severity, and the length of time the signs or symptoms have been present.

Showing respect and compassion for all patients will help the EMT to collect and report the vital information concerning the patient and current condition to provide the appropriate patient care in the prehospital setting and throughout the continuum of the patient's treatment.

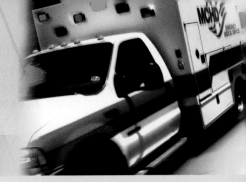

CASE STUDY Continued

While en route to the hospital, Tillie begins gathering Mrs. Scott's history, beginning with her chief concern. Mrs. Scott states she called the ambulance because of the pain in her jaw that started while she was pulling weeds in her flower garden. She thought she had perhaps been clenching her jaw too tightly as she tends to do when pulling weeds, but the pain did not go away when she relaxed her jaw. She came into the house and called the ambulance when the pain kept getting worse instead of better.

Tillie asks Mrs. Scott questions using the SAMPLE and OPQRST mnemonics to guide her and documents Mrs. Scott's answers for the ALS crew they will be meeting en route.

Mrs. Scott states she has pain in her jaw and felt nauseous when the pain got really bad. She denies any allergies and states she is on medication to relieve anxiety and to prevent blood clots she has a history of occasionally getting in her legs. She had last seen her family doctor three weeks ago for another blood clot, but that has been gone for over a week. She had last eaten breakfast 5 hours ago and that she was bent over weeding her flower beds when the pain started.

Mrs. Scott states this all started about an hour ago, and nothing makes the pain better or worse. She describes the pain as a bad ache, like a horrible toothache involving all her teeth. She rates the pain at a 10 on the 0 to 10 scale. Mrs. Scott states the pain does not go anywhere other than her jaw, and the pain has been going on for more than 1 hour without relief.

Tillie reports all her findings, including the history gathered from Mrs. Scott, as she turns over patient care to the ALS crew that has just arrived. Mrs. Scott reports to the paramedics that her pain had improved with the oxygen Tillie had begun in the house, rating her pain at a 7 on the 0 to 10 pain scale at this time.

Key Concepts Revisited

- Information gathered through the assessment process of taking a thorough history can be vital to ongoing patient care.

- A complete patient history that includes the history of the present illness or injury will allow the EMT to find conditions that may not have been apparent during the primary assessment.

- Collecting or gathering pertinent history requires the EMT to consider several factors, including the age, race, and gender of the patient.

- The content of the history must be documented and include correct dates and times of previous and current treatments.

- Components of a patient history include:
  - The chief concern, or primary reason for the call
  - History of the present illness
  - Detailed evaluation of the chief concern
  - Past medical history
  - Current health status
  - Individual factors

- History taking techniques include a professional, compassionate demeanor and making the patient comfortable.

- A standardized approach to history taking includes the use of the SAMPLE and OPQRST mnemonics.
  - SAMPLE history is the patient's pertinent individual information, including:
    - Signs and symptoms
    - Allergies
    - Medications
    - Past medical history
    - Last oral intake
    - Events leading up to the current situation
  - OPQRST is a detailed evaluation of the current illness, including
    - Onset
    - Provocation/palliation/positioning
    - Quality of discomfort

- Radiation
  - Severity
  - Time (duration of signs and symptoms)
- The patient may be experiencing associated signs and symptoms or concerns directly related to the present illness.
- Pertinent negatives are the denial of specific signs and can provide important clues to the present condition.
- The EMT may have to ask the patient questions involving sensitive topics:
  - Alcohol and drug use
  - Physical abuse and violence
  - Sexual history
- The EMT may experience special challenges in history taking, including:
  - Silent or overly talkative patients
  - Patients with multiple symptoms
  - Anxious patients
  - Angry and hostile patients
  - Intoxicated patients
  - Crying patients
  - Depressed patients
  - Patients with confusing behavior, histories, or limited cognitive abilities
  - EMT-patient language barriers
  - Patients with hearing problems or visual impairment
- Family and friends can be an additional resource for history gathering when the patient is unable to provide the pertinent information.

Review Questions

1. When should a patient history be conducted?
2. Why is a complete patient history important?
3. What components are involved in a patient history?
4. What two types of communication will the EMT use?
5. What is the primary technique the EMT should use for successful history taking?
6. Explain the components of the SAMPLE history.
7. What is the purpose of the SAMPLE history?
8. What does the mnemonic OPQRST stand for?
9. What is the purpose of OPQRST assessment?
10. What special history taking challenges may the EMT encounter?

Key Terms

Chief concern
Individual factors
OPQRST
Palliation
Patient history

Pertinent negatives
Pertinent past medical history
Provocation
Referred pain

SAMPLE history
Social history
Wong-Baker FACES scale

Further Study

Bickley, L. S., and P. G. Szilaqyi. *Bates' Guide to Physical Examination and History Taking.* 9th ed. Hagerstown, MD: Lippincott Williams & Wilkins, 2007.

Dalton, A. L., D. Limmer, J. J. Mistovich, and H. A. Werman. *Advanced Medical Life Support.* Upper Saddle River, NJ: Brady/Prentice Hall, 2007.

Kraytman, M., L. M. Tierney, and M. Hendersen. *The Complete Patient History.* 3d ed. Columbus, OH: Lange/McGraw-Hill, 2007.

Tierney, L. M., and M. Hendersen. *The Patient History: Evidence Based Approach.* Columbus, OH: Lange/McGraw-Hill, 2004.

UNIT (19) Secondary Assessment

The purpose of the primary assessment is the identification and management of life-threatening problems in patients. Once this has been completed, the Emergency Medical Technician (EMT) moves on to the next phases of patient assessment: baseline vital signs, history taking, and the secondary assessment.

The secondary assessment is the physical examination conducted to further evaluate the presence of additional injuries or the depth of an illness not addressed in the primary assessment.

National Education Standards

The Emergency Medical Technician (EMT) shall demonstrate a fundamental depth and foundational breadth of understanding and techniques to perform a physical examination of the patient accessing all anatomical regions and body systems.

Key Concepts

- The detailed physical examination is a patient-specific, injury-specific examination.

- The history will be used to guide the physical examination in the medical patient.

- The physical examination is a complete head-to-toe examination of all body regions in the trauma patient.

- A serious mechanism of injury will create a high index of suspicion that a serious hidden injury may exist.

- The techniques used during the physical assessment are inspection (look), palpation (feel), and auscultation (listen) of the body's systems and regions.

- EMT professionalism and respect for the patient's privacy must be maintained throughout the physical examination.

- The categories of the physical exam include assessment of mental status, a general survey, and the detailed physical examination of all body regions and systems.

- The objective of the detailed physical examination is to discover conditions or injuries that were not uncovered during the primary assessment.

- The detailed physical examination should not be performed on scene, except if transport to the hospital cannot immediately take place.

- The detailed physical examination measures the effectiveness of prehospital treatments that were initiated early on in the assessment.

- The detailed physical exam is a systematic head-to-toe physical examination.

- The DCAP-BTLS initials are the types of underlying serious injuries the EMT should look for during the detailed physical exam.

- The detailed physical examination should be followed up with a full set of vital signs.

- The physical examination may uncover further injuries or conditions that may or may not be life threatening.

Gary and his partner Larry are dispatched to an unconscious male, unknown cause. Upon arrival, Gary finds an approximately 35-year-old male lying on the ground of the soccer field, surrounded by his teammates. Assessing scene safety as they approach the patient, Larry asks the bystanders to move out of the area of the patient and enlists the help of one of the players in moving them away. One individual approaches Gary and explains that the patient, Liam, was hit directly in the face with the kicked soccer ball. He seemed to be okay, but suddenly fell forward, striking his head on the post of the goal. The teammate states that Liam has not moved or opened his eyes since it happened approximately 10 minutes ago.

Gary performs a primary assessment and a quick general physical survey for any obvious injuries, noting swelling to the forehead and what appears to be blood in the corner of Liam's mouth. Liam groans in response to painful stimuli as Gary pinches the muscles of his shoulder. Gary determines Liam is a priority patient and requires immediate transport and ALS intercept.

Critical Thinking Questions

1. What is the next step in assessing the unresponsive patient?

2. How can Gary determine if Liam's condition is due to trauma or a medical condition?

3. What information will Gary look for during the detailed physical examination?

INTRODUCTION

The secondary assessment will be performed on all patients; however, the order of the exam and the extent of the physical examination depends primarily on the responsiveness of the patient. When dealing with a stable medical patient, the baseline vital signs and history taking components of patient assessment will take place prior to the physical examination. Additionally, the physical examination of the responsive medical patient will focus on the area of chief concern. In other words, the patient with a chief concern of abdominal pain does not necessarily require a thorough head-to-toe examination, but a physical examination focusing mostly on the abdomen and body systems that affect abdominal pain.

The unresponsive medical and trauma patient will benefit from a more rapid physical examination of the entire body immediately following the primary assessment and baseline vital signs measurements. The rapid physical examination in the unresponsive patient is required to gather important clues as to why the patient is unresponsive. If family members or bystanders are present, a quick history of the event can be gathered while the physical examination is being conducted.

The detailed physical examination is a patient-specific, injury-specific examination. It is patient specific because it is typically used for patients who are unconscious or who have a decreased level of consciousness. It is injury specific because it is performed on all patients who have endured a significant mechanism of injury or who have sustained significant injuries. This unit reviews the detailed physical examination during secondary assessment in depth.

HISTORY

It is very important to identify and examine the mechanism of injury for the trauma patient. The medical patient has an illness that progressed in some way to result in a call for emergency care and transport. It is important to remember the unresponsive patient may have had a medical event that resulted in a trauma. As the EMT considers the mechanism of injury, he should keep in mind the possibility that a medical condition may also exist.

The EMT can determine the progression of the physical examination by obtaining a history in the responsive, stable patient, as discussed in Unit 18. The history provides the information needed to prioritize the care of the medical patient.

PHYSICAL EXAMINATION APPROACH

In the assessment of the medical patient, the EMT will use the history to guide the physical examination. The physical examination findings will often confirm the suspicions the EMT formed on the basis of the history. For example, a patient who gives the history of extensive vomiting and diarrhea for several days will likely be severely dehydrated and may even be in hypovolemic shock. Physical examination may reveal evidence of dehydration and shock.

In the trauma patient, the physical examination will be a complete head-to-toe examination of all body regions. A rapid physical examination, consisting of quickly scanning and palpating the body may be required in the unresponsive trauma patient immediately following the assessment and management of the airway, breathing, and circulation during the primary survey. The detailed head-to-toe examination will still be performed on the unresponsive trauma patient if possible and will be discussed later in this unit.

RECONSIDER THE MECHANISM OF INJURY

Obvious serious injuries are usually discovered and treated during the primary assessment. In many trauma cases, it is not what can be seen that may kill the patient in the end but what cannot be seen. Therefore, an EMT needs to reconsider the mechanism of injury and ask, "In the worst case scenario, what injuries could this patient have?"

A serious mechanism of injury creates a high index of suspicion that a serious hidden injury may exist. The American College of Surgeons Committee on Trauma has developed a list of mechanisms that can produce serious injury. This list is summarized in Table 19-1. The amount of force involved in each of these types of incidents is often associated with serious injury, even without obvious initial physical findings.

The mechanism of injury for a trauma patient can be thought of as the history of the present illness (HPI), which is often obtained for the medical patient (refer to Unit 18). The EMT should gather as many details as possible regarding the mechanism of injury.

Any of the events listed in Table 19-1 fit the category of a serious mechanism of injury; however, this list is not exhaustive. Experience with trauma often teaches EMTs that a seemingly minor mechanism can have a major impact, especially in certain patient populations. Elderly patients and patients with chronic illness are often highly susceptible to serious injury even with a minor mechanism. Such patient factors must be considered when determining the risk for injury from a particular mechanism.

Other factors of the mechanism of injury and scene observations may indicate the need for a thorough physical examination. An example is the patient who was not wearing a seat belt at the time of a crash who may have

Table 19-1 Serious Trauma by Mechanism

1. Falls of 20 feet or more
2. Crash speed 20 mph or greater
3. Twenty inches of front-end impact damage
4. Twelve inches of side-impact damage from same side
5. Twenty inches of side-impact damage from opposite side
6. Death of another occupant in automobile
7. Ejection from a motor vehicle
8. Rollover MVC with unrestrained patient
9. Pedestrian struck by a vehicle at 20 mph or greater

bounced around within the vehicle. A bent steering wheel may be an indication that the patient's chest was injured on impact. These patients may appear stable initially, but they may have internal injuries that can cause deterioration. These patients should have a complete physical assessment to detect any additional serious injuries not found during the primary assessment.

Unconsciousness after trauma implies serious injury that has altered perfusion to the brain. After completion of the primary assessment and management of immediately life-threatening problems, all unconscious trauma patients and those suffering from multiple injuries should have a rapid general survey for other significant injuries, followed by a complete physical examination after they have been stabilized. Patients who have suffered multiple obvious traumatic injuries may also have significant internal injuries, placing them at a higher risk for developing shock. The rapid general assessment and more detailed physical exam should be performed while en route to the closest appropriate hospital. If transportation is not immediately available, the assessment and exam can be done on scene.

BASIC ASSUMPTIONS

When caring for injured patients in the prehospital environment, the EMT is forced to make several assumptions. Because the diagnostic capabilities of the EMT in the field are somewhat limited, injuries often are assumed to be present if there is suspicion based on the mechanism of the injury. This assumption may result in overtreatment of patients but will avoid the disaster of undertreatment with a bad outcome. This concept of presumed injury based on mechanism applies to any injuries suspected in the field. If an EMT suspects the possibility of an injury, the patient should be treated for that suspected injury. This practice will make it less likely that the EMT will miss an injury that may cause harm to the patient.

This assumption of injury is crucial in the situation of spinal injury. A patient who has sustained any significant force applied to the body has the potential to have an injury to the cervical spine. As will be discussed in detail in Unit 35, any movement of the patient's head or neck in the presence of certain types of spinal injuries can result in worsening of the injury. Spinal cord injuries carry with them a high rate of morbidity and mortality.

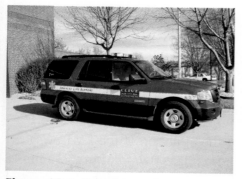

Figure 19.1 Consider advanced life support backup for a seriously injured patient (Courtesy of Clive Fire Department, Clive, IA)

It is best to assume that the patient who has sustained a significant mechanism of injury has a spinal injury and to treat that patient presumptively by stabilizing the head and neck to avoid any movement and potential of worsening a less-than-obvious injury.

ALS BACKUP

Advanced life support (ALS) personnel (i.e., EMT–Intermediates or Paramedics) should be called to the scene or should be asked to intercept the ambulance while it is en route to the closest appropriate hospital on all patients with a serious mechanism of injury or who have experienced what appears to be a minor mechanism of injury with evidence of significant injury (Figure 19.1). These patients may have vital signs that are unstable or a significant presenting injury following physical examination or a confounding medical condition that is revealed during history taking. These three factors—unstable vital signs, significant physical injuries, or a significant past medical history—are reasons to call for ALS backup during the secondary assessment (see Table 19-2).

PHYSICAL EXAMINATION TECHNIQUES

The techniques used during the physical examination follow the "look, listen, and feel" process employed in other components of patient assessment. The EMT inspects (looks at), palpates (feels), and auscultates (listens to) the patient's body and body systems. Equipment that will be required during the physical examination includes a stethoscope, blood pressure cuff, and pulse oximeter for measurement of baseline vital signs and a pen light for assessment of the patient's pupil response. Review Unit 12 on baseline vital signs.

The patient's height and weight should also be assessed. Height and weight measurements will be approximate unless the patient can provide this current information. Weight is used in determining drug dosages for many medications, particularly for children. Additionally, height and weight are both important assessments in the treatment of children and infants. If the patient, or parent in the case of a pediatric patient, cannot provide this information, the EMT should estimate the weight and height to the best of his ability.

GENERAL APPROACH

The professionalism and compassion of the EMT as he approaches the patient to conduct the physical examination is of the utmost importance. Patients are understandably anxious and apprehensive when illness or injury occurs. Most patients feel vulnerable and exposed when presented with the need for a physical examination, causing an even higher level of apprehension and anxiety. The EMT must maintain professionalism throughout the physical examination, respecting the patient's privacy and displaying compassion for the patient's situation.

The EMT explains the reason and need for the physical examination to conscious patients and obtains their consent. He describes what the physical exam will entail before beginning and explain his actions each time he moves to a new area of the body. Some people do not like to be touched and may refuse to allow the EMT to palpate their body for tenderness or deformity. In these cases, the EMT should explain the importance of being able to feel for injuries that are not always obvious; however, he must respect the mentally

TABLE 19-2 When to Call for ALS Backup

Unstable Vital Signs (Adult)

Glasgow Coma Scale <14

Respiratory rate <10 or >29

Systolic blood pressure <90

Revised trauma score <11

Significant Injury

Open or depressed skull fracture

Flail chest

Pelvic fractures

Paralysis

Two or more proximal long bone fractures

Amputation proximal to the wrist and ankle

Penetrating wounds of the head, chest, abdomen, or pelvis and
of the extremity proximal to the knee or elbow

Major burns

Trauma with burns

Significant Past Medical History

Age <5 or >55

Cardiac disease

Respiratory disease

Diabetes

Pregnancy

Immunosuppressed

   AIDS patient

   Leukemia patient

   Cancer patient undergoing chemotherapy

Bleeding disorders

   Hemophilia

Anticoagulant medication

   Heparin

   Lovenox

   Coumadin

   Plavix

competent patient's right to refuse. If a patient refuses to allow any or all parts of the physical examination, the EMT should thoroughly document the patient's refusal, in the patient's own words.

The EMT exercises a relationship similar to the physician-patient relationship when the physician is performing an examination in the clinic or hospital setting.

The relationship between the EMT and the patient is based on trust and respect. It is an EMT's duty to gain the patient's trust and maintain respect for the patient. For this reason, every EMT should exercise the following principles whenever performing a physical examination:

1. Be polite. Introduce yourself by giving the patient your name and title and refer to the patient by social title, such as Mr. or Ms. Jones. Using the patient's first name is appropriate only if the patient is of similar age or younger; otherwise, using the patient's first name may be construed as impolite. Consider asking the patient how she would prefer to be addressed. A patient should never be called "honey" or "bud" or other such terms.

2. Offer explanations. A patient has a right to know what an EMT is going to do. The EMT should use common courtesy by explaining to the patient how and why she will be assessed for further injuries.

3. Maintain the patient's privacy. If a patient is awake or is in a public place, the EMT should endeavor to unclothe the patient only when necessary and only those portions of the body that need assessment. Once the assessment is complete, the patient should be covered.

4. Make eye contact. Eye contact, in most cases, demonstrates the EMT's caring attitude. Always make an effort to reestablish eye contact after assessing each portion of the body.

5. Be honest. A medical emergency is, by definition, a crisis for the patient. The patient is fearful about pain or suffering. An EMT's honesty will help comfort the patient and alleviate the anxiety the patient is experiencing. As far as is practical, an EMT should always speak honestly about matters that the EMT knows—for example, that the oxygen should help make the patient feel better.

6. Focus the patient's attention. In times of crisis, patients have a tendency to focus on one person, to see one individual as the healer. It is important for the EMT to provide that focus. Although several EMTs may be treating a patient, only one should be performing the assessment and giving verbal instructions to the crew.

CATEGORIES OF THE PHYSICAL EXAM

The categories of the physical exam include assessment of the patient's mental status, a general survey to detect any obvious signs or symptoms of the patient's condition, and the detailed physical examination of the anatomic regions and body systems.

The patient's mental status was initially assessed during the primary assessment for consciousness and response to stimuli. The secondary mental status assessment further explores the level of orientation and alertness of the patient.

A general physical survey consists of a quickly conducted inspection of the patient to detect any obvious signs of injury or illness that can be seen. The patient may have obvious bruising or deformities in the case of trauma. The patient in shock may appear pale and diaphoretic. The initial inspection component of the physical exam completed through a general physical survey can direct a more focused examination on the unresponsive patient. The general survey may have been quickly conducted immediately following the primary assessment or as the baseline vital signs were being measured.

The detailed physical examination includes a combination of inspection, auscultation, and palpation of all body regions and their underlying systems. It includes all anatomic structures of the body, musculoskeletal function, vascular function in the extremities, and a neurologic exam.

MENTAL STATUS

The patient's baseline mental status was assessed during the primary assessment using the AVPU scale. Review the details of the AVPU assessment in Unit 16. Mental impairment is an indicator of a pathology involving the brain. Illness, or injury causing intracranial bleeding, stroke, infections, seizures, and hypoxia can all cause changes in normal mental status. Altered mental status will be discussed in more detail in Unit 27.

During the secondary assessment, prior to the detailed physical exam, the EMT should reassess the mental status in more detail. In addition to the level of consciousness the patient is exhibiting, observe the patient's position and motor behavior. Are her movements appropriate and purposeful? Is the patient able to locate pain? Is her movement appropriately away from the pain, or does she move into the painful stimuli?

What are the patient's facial expressions, speech and language patterns, and mood? The patient's facial expression provides many clues to the situation and the pain or discomfort the patient is feeling. Is she angry or fearful? Does she show emotion or is her affect flat, showing no reaction or emotion at all? The patient's speech and language pattern can provide valuable clues. The patient who is speaking rapidly and excitedly could be suffering from anxiety, or if she is speaking rapidly with random thought, without pause, she could be showing signs of a deeper mental illness. The patient who is speaking slowly, with slurred speech, may be confused and attempting to think of the appropriate words, or may know what she wants to say, but be unable to appropriately or clearly state it. Inappropriate speech may be a sign of conditions such as head injury, stroke, or drug use.

The patient's mood should be part of your scene size-up as you approach the patient. The patient showing intense emotion, such as angry or hysterical behavior, could present a hazard at any time if she is unable to control her emotions. Additionally, the patient who has suicidal ideation poses a danger to everyone on the scene. These patients are often severely depressed and may actually resent anyone's attempt to keep them from "ending it all." The EMT must be prepared to keep himself, his partner, and any other people on scene safe, even if it means leaving the scene and the patient if she becomes violent and threatening.

How are the patient's thought processes? Is she answering questions appropriately, with logic and organized thoughts, or is she having unusual and unpleasant thoughts? Is the patient hearing unusual sounds, ringing in the ears, or voices speaking to her? Is she seeing things that are not there? The patient with irrational thoughts may also pose a danger to the EMT as well as to herself.

Finally, reassess the patient's orientation to person, place, and time. A patient who was alert and oriented during the primary assessment who is now oriented to only person and place is showing a deterioration in mentation. This deterioration is often a serious sign that her condition is worsening.

DETAILED PHYSICAL EXAMINATION

The primary objective of the detailed physical examination is to discover conditions or injuries that may not have been uncovered during the primary assessment, general physical survey, and history taking of the conscious patient. Because it is a more extensive assessment that takes time to complete, a detailed physical examination should not be performed on scene, except if transport to the hospital is not yet available.

The goal of an EMT in completing a detailed physical exam is to uncover those signs of injury or illness that could be treated while en route to the hospital. The fact that the detailed physical examination must be conducted during transport substantially limits the length of time available to complete it. Nevertheless, it may take an EMT 10 minutes to properly complete a detailed physical examination.

A detailed physical examination is always performed after the primary assessment on the unresponsive trauma patient. A focused physical examination should be performed on all medical patients following the baseline vital signs and history taking. The detailed physical examination measures the effectiveness of prehospital treatments that were initiated early on in the assessment. In addition, further attention is paid to details of the physical exam that were not addressed in the previous assessments.

Changes in a patient's condition, especially deterioration, may require the EMT to rethink decisions. Should the patient's priority be upgraded? Would the patient benefit from the assistance of an ALS unit if one has not already been requested? Is the destination hospital still appropriate, or should the patient be diverted to a specialized trauma center? These decisions are based on changes in the patient's condition that are often noted during the detailed physical exam.

The detailed physical exam is a systematic head-to-toe physical examination. All patients who may have further injury that was not uncovered by the primary assessment should be given a detailed physical examination. This category includes any trauma patient who had a significant mechanism of injury or who shows signs of serious or multiple injuries. The detailed physical exam should be performed during transport to the hospital only if enough personnel are present and time permits. Ongoing treatment of life-threatening conditions may preclude the completion of this examination.

The detailed physical examination need not be done on trauma patients with an isolated injury. Performing a detailed patient assessment on these patients would be too intrusive and therefore inappropriate.

STEPS IN THE DETAILED PHYSICAL EXAMINATION

The detailed physical examination will detect the elements of the mnemonic DCAP-BTLS, used to describe the signs of injury that should be sought. The DCAP-BTLS initials stand for the types of underlying serious injuries the EMT should look for during the detailed physical exam. Table 19-3 lists the initials and their meanings. However, additional special elements to the detailed physical examination will be discussed as each body section is addressed.

HEAD

Beginning at the head, the EMT should carefully palpate the entire skull (see Skill 19-1 at the end of this unit). Starting at the rear of the skull, in the occipital area, the EMT should look and feel for DCAP-BTLS. Even small external

Street Smart

A professional attitude, coupled with the seclusion of the ambulance compartment, is usually enough to convince the patient to agree to a detailed physical examination.

Table 19-3 DCAP-BTLS

Term	Meaning	Lay Term
Deformity	Distorted, unnatural	Looks funny
Contusion	Injury where the skin is not broken	Bruise
Abrasion	Scraping away the top layer of skin	Skinned knee
Puncture	A wound that pierces the skin	Knife wound
Burns	Tissue injury due to heat or chemical	Burns
Tenderness	Pain when pressure is applied	Tender, sore
Laceration	Torn skin	Cut
Swelling	Abnormal enlargement	Swollen

injuries may indicate the possibility of serious internal head injury and should be carefully noted. Inspect and palpate the head and scalp for deformities (depressions), lacerations, abrasions, hematomas (swelling), bruising, and punctures. Keep in mind the patient who has been immobilized will have limited access to the head depending on the immobilization device.

Carefully remove any glass shards that might cause injury. Use a penlight to improve your vision. If a spot of blood is found, take a piece of gauze and blot the area gently. Is a small laceration causing the bleeding? This detailed exam of the head can reveal signs of injury that may be important in the care of the patient.

EARS

Next, the EMT should examine the ears for deformities, contusions, abrasions, punctures, burns, lacerations, or swelling. Using a penlight, look into the ears for the presence of any drainage. Clear fluid from the ear may be *cerebrospinal fluid (CSF)* (Figure 19.2). This is the nutrient-rich fluid that bathes and protects the brain and spinal cord. Because this clear fluid comes from inside the skull, the presence of CSF in the ears indicates a skull fracture. Never attempt to stop the flow of CSF because doing so can result in increased pressure inside the skull. The EMT can use clean gauze to absorb the fluid that is leaking. Unit 34 discusses skull fractures in more detail.

Certain types of skull fractures can create characteristic physical findings. The EMT should carefully look for these findings and report them to hospital staff if found. Bruising behind the ears, called **Battle's sign,** can indicate a fracture to the base of the skull. This condition will be discussed further in Unit 34.

EYES

Moving toward the front of the skull and the face, the EMT should take time to thoroughly examine the patient's eyes. Although trauma to the eyes may not be life threatening, it can have a lifelong impact on the patient. It is useful to compare one eye with the other to look for differences while checking for DCAP-BTLS.

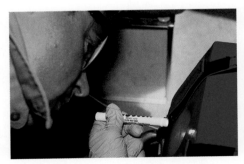

Figure 19.2 Clear fluid from the ear could be cerebrospinal fluid (CSF)

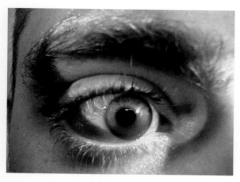

Figure 19.3 Blood in the front of the eye is called a hyphema (Courtesy of Kevin Reilly, MD, Albany Medical Center, Albany, NY)

Street Smart

What if the eye does not react and the patient has not experienced any head trauma? Ask the patient if she has a prosthetic eye; they are more common than one might expect.

In addition to the usual signs of injury, the EMT should look for several findings that may be specifically sought out in the eye examination. Discoloration such as bruising around the eye should be noted. Bruising around the eyes is sometimes called **raccoon's eyes** and may be indicative of a fracture to the base of the skull.

During the eye examination, the pupils should be carefully assessed for size, shape, and reaction to light. Any inequality, irregular shape, or lack of constriction to light may indicate serious eye or brain injury and should be carefully noted. Unit 12 discusses the examination of the pupils in detail.

Any foreign material, such as dirt or glass, should be brushed away from the eyes if possible. If this material does not easily brush away, the EMT should leave it alone and allow the hospital staff to remove any objects that are stuck in the eye.

Injuries to the eye can result in bleeding both outside and inside the eye. Accumulation of blood inside the eye can sometimes be seen as haziness in the front of the eye. This haziness may settle out into a layer of blood that is visible in the front of the eye. The term for blood that has accumulated inside the eye is **hyphema** (see Figure 19.3).

Occasionally, an EMT will observe a pupil that is irregularly shaped. This irregularity is often the result of surgery to remove abnormal growths in the front of the eye, called *cataracts*. The irregularly shaped pupil resulting from surgery may not react to light.

If the pupils of the eye are equal in size, round, and react to bright light by constricting bilaterally, then EMTs will document PERRL. PERRL means the Pupils are Equal, Round, and Reactive to Light.

If the patient is wearing contact lenses and has sustained a burn to the eye, particularly if a chemical is involved, remove the contact lens to allow for adequate flushing and to prevent the chemical from being trapped underneath the lens.

The sclera (white) of the eye should be checked for color changes. A yellow sclerae could indicate a problem with the liver. The color of the conjunctiva of the eye should be checked by pulling the bottom eyelid down slightly. The conjunctiva will appear red when the eye is irritated. Eyes that appear sunken into the eye socket may indicate dehydration, and the conjunctiva may appear pale in the patient showing signs of poor perfusion as seen in shock.

FACE

Moving away from the eyes, the EMT should carefully assess the rest of the face. Careful inspection and palpation of each of the bony prominences in the face will reveal any evidence of DCAP-BTLS. If the patient is unable to bring her teeth together in alignment, there may be a fractured or dislocated lower jaw (mandible). A fracture or dislocation to the upper or lower jaw can be of concern in maintaining a patent airway.

The patient should be able to smile or display a symmetrical expression unless she has sustained a previous injury that prevents symmetrical movement, such as a stroke. Additionally, take note of the patient's expression. Is it appropriate for the situation?

The face should also be inspected for soot or singed or burnt eyebrows, nasal hairs, beard, or hair. Patients who have signs of burns or extreme heat to the face may have sustained burns to their upper airway. Burns to the upper airway often cause swelling, and the airway can become completely occluded at the level of the larynx.

NOSE

The EMT should turn his attention to the nose next. Inspection and palpation for DCAP-BTLS should reveal any injuries. Injuries to the nose may not in and of themselves be life threatening, but they may have implications for the EMT. A painful, swollen, and deformed nose may be broken. Excessive bleeding may result if a nasopharyngeal airway is inserted into a broken nose.

To assess for any bleeding or drainage, the EMT can use a penlight to look into the nares. Blood running down the back of the throat may nauseate the patient and cause vomiting. Always be prepared to suction the airway when bleeding or vomiting is present from an injury to the nose.

Any clear fluid running from the nose should be reported immediately. It may only be mucus, but it can also be CSF. Any CSF draining from the nose indicates that a serious head injury may have occurred.

MOUTH

The mouth is the beginning of the airway. Injury to the mouth can create a potential airway problem. Careful inspection for signs of injury to the inside or outside of the mouth should be performed. Assessment for DCAP-BTLS will reveal such injuries.

In addition, the EMT should examine the inside of the mouth carefully because anything that is in the mouth could block the airway. The stability of the teeth should be assessed by gently pressing on them with a gloved finger. Broken pieces of teeth and any other foreign object should be immediately removed from the mouth to prevent aspiration. Any secretions or bleeding should be immediately suctioned.

If a bleeding source can be identified, direct pressure on the site may help to slow the bleeding, decreasing the potential for an airway problem. Lacerations to the cheek can be controlled by direct pressure applied to both the inside and the outside of the mouth.

Is the tongue swollen, or are the surrounding tissues reddened or otherwise discolored? Swelling in the mouth—from burns, for example—can mean swelling in the lower airway as well. Continued swelling can lead to a complete airway obstruction. A hoarse voice after airway injury is one sign of lower airway swelling and should be considered a true emergency.

What about dentures or other oral hardware? If a piece of a dental appliance is loose in the mouth, then it should be removed and stored safely in a cup. If the dentures are intact, then leave them in place. The dentures serve as a platform for a mask seal if the patient needs to be ventilated.

The tongue is very vascular, and even a minor injury to the tongue can cause excessive bleeding. The tongue should be inspected for any lacerations or swelling, both of which could indicate the patient has had a seizure. What color is the tongue? A pale tongue may indicate the patient is going into shock. Cyanosis of the mucosa indicates inadequate oxygenation, and burns or extremely white patches to the tongue could be a sign the patient has ingested a chemical poison.

Take note of any odors such as alcohol. The smell of alcohol could indicate the patient has been drinking, or it could indicate another condition. Alcoholics drink many substances in desperation if they do not have alcohol available. This can include hair spray, rubbing alcohol, cleaners, or cough syrup. Children may accidently ingest cleaners. A fruity breath odor may indicate the patient is a diabetic, experiencing an unusually high blood sugar level.

Street Smart

If for some reason the EMT removes a bridge or a denture, it should be carefully stored in a plastic denture cup or similar device, and the cup should be turned over to the nurse in the emergency department or to family members. The whereabouts of the cup should be clearly documented.

NECK

Moving down to the neck, the EMT should gently palpate the anterior soft tissues. When injured, these tissues can quickly swell and threaten the airway. Careful inspection for DCAP-BTLS should reveal evidence of injury. An open wound to the neck must be covered immediately with an occlusive dressing to prevent an air embolus forming from air being sucked into the large vein of the neck.

Does the neck appear large or swollen? Air trapped under the skin or blood collection in the tissue of the neck can cause swelling and asymmetrical appearance to the neck. The vessels within the neck are great (large) vessels and bleeding from an injury to any of these vessels can cause severe bleeding. The presence of a hematoma (swelling of blood) can create an airway obstruction by compressing the trachea. Air that has become trapped under the skin can be palpated, and crackling can be heard. This is a sign of subcutaneous emphysema, which means air under the skin and is an indicator of trauma to the airway, respiratory tract, lungs, or esophagus.

The jugular veins are the large veins on each side of the neck. The patient's carotid pulses should be assessed, and the jugular veins should be inspected for distention (Figure 19.4). Jugular vein distention (JVD) is a sign of several potentially life-threatening conditions.

When assessing the anterior neck, the EMT should identify the position of the trachea. It is normally easily palpated anteriorly at the base of the neck right in the midline. A displaced trachea is a sign of increased pressure in the chest.

Excessive neck muscle use is a sign of severe respiratory distress. When assessing the neck, check for excessive muscle use as well as other signs of respiratory distress and inadequate breathing that may not have been present when the primary assessment was completed.

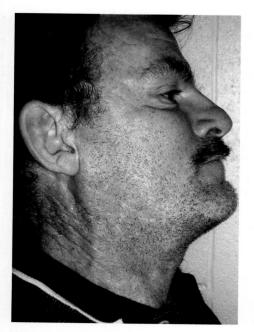

Figure 19.4 Jugular venous distention can be an indicator of several serious conditions, including serious internal chest injuries

Safety Tips

Rigid cervical immobilization devices are often placed on the patient quickly, sometimes before a complete neck assessment has been performed. Most cervical immobilization devices have holes in the front or sides, or both, to allow for examination after placement. If these spaces do not allow the necessary examination and the EMT must open the collar anteriorly, he must be sure to maintain adequate cervical spine immobilization during this assessment. A second EMT manually holding cervical spine stabilization is appropriate in this case.

If it is not absolutely necessary to the care of the patient, the cervical collar should not be removed once it has been applied. Keeping it in place reminds the patient she should not move her head or neck, thus avoiding any further injury of a potentially unstable neck.

CHEST

In the detailed physical examination, the chest should be exposed appropriately for inspection and thoroughly examined using the look, listen, and feel methodology. The EMT should examine the entire chest wall, front and back. DCAP-BTLS should be sought during this assessment. How is the shape and symmetry of the chest? Check the armpits and under the breasts for wounds, as small punctures can easily hide in these places.

Take a moment to watch the patient breathe. Is the breathing comfortable and effective? Does the patient have a "catch" when asked to breathe deeply? This could be a sign of a broken rib because deep inspiration will cause pain. Shallow breathing can also mean that there are rib fractures.

Watch for use of intercostal muscles or interspace retractions, both signs of respiratory distress.

Using a stethoscope, the EMT should reassess the same four areas on the anterior chest, as demonstrated in Skill 19-1 at the end of this unit. It is important to keep the "scope on the skin" to avoid extraneous sound.

The EMT should also listen to the posterior lung fields, if possible. Sliding the stethoscope between the patient and the backboard, the EMT should attempt to listen at the apices by placing the head of the stethoscope at the top of the shoulder blades. The EMT can slide the stethoscope in laterally behind the patient to better assess the base of the lung. While assessing breathing, what sounds are being heard in the lung fields? Is the patient wheezing, which indicates a serious constriction in the lower airways? Absence of breath sounds on one side is an indication of a serious lung injury and potentially life-threatening condition, requiring immediate intervention and ALS intervention.

A patient can fracture a rib without creating a deformity; this is called a nondisplaced rib fracture. These fractures can be discovered only by running your fingers over the bones until the patient complains of tenderness in one particular area.

Starting at the sternum, the EMT should place his forearm flat against the sternum and press firmly but gently downward. In this way, fractures of the sternum, or the rib attachments to the sternum, can be detected. Gentle palpation of the ribs anteriorly from top to bottom should reveal any areas of tenderness or deformity, as well as any crepitus.

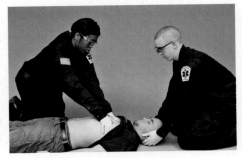

Figure 19.5 Gentle chest compression will reveal rib fractures

If an area of tenderness or bony crepitus is found, the EMT should take care not to cause further pain or injury by repeated palpation of the area. Finding no tenderness, the EMT should gently, but firmly, compress the rib cage (Figure 19.5). Any crepitus or paradoxical motion of a section of rib cage should be noted.

Starting at the top of the sternum, the EMT should run his fingers along the clavicles, feeling for deformity as well as tenderness. Once both hands are on the shoulders, the EMT should gently squeeze the shoulders together to see whether the shoulder girdle is intact.

If the patient is not immobilized or showing signs of a spinal injury, assess the posterior chest for injuries. Listen to lung sounds in the posterior lung fields at that time. If the patient does have a suspected spinal injury and has already been secured on the backboard, do not move the patient to examine the posterior thorax.

ABDOMEN AND PELVIS

Before starting the examination of the abdomen and pelvis, explain to the patient what is about to happen. The look, listen, and feel methodology works well for an abdominal assessment. The abdomen needs to be exposed appropriately for inspection, with the patient lying flat, if possible. Look for any injuries as evidenced by DCAP-BTLS. Identify landmarks, such as the umbilicus and the margins of the ribs. Assess for any distention, which may indicate bleeding internally. Bruising around the umbilicus is an indicator of possible significant bleeding in the abdomen and is a very late sign. Patients with bruising around the umbilicus from internal bleeding may also be showing signs of decompensated shock.

Note the presence of urinary incontinence. Injuries to the spine can cause the patient to lose control of her bladder. Local trauma to the bladder, such as a penetrating knife wound, can also cause incontinence. Finally, certain medical conditions, such as seizures, can lead to incontinence.

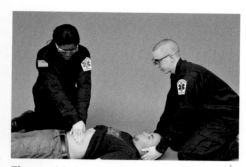

Figure 19.6 Careful examination of the abdomen will reveal tenderness

Always document the presence of urine on clothing. Frequently, clothing is cut away from the patient and discarded. After that, it may be impossible to know whether the patient was incontinent on scene unless the EMT documents it.

Listen to what the patient tells you. Where is the pain? Does one area of the abdomen hurt more than another? Palpate all four quadrants of the anterior abdomen gently (Figure 19.6) using the pads of the fingers and one hand on top of the other. Does the abdomen feel firm or soft when palpated? A firm, tender abdomen indicates the natural muscular guarding of an injury. Such guarding is suspicious for abdominal bleeding.

Have the patient point to the area of pain with one figure. If the patient indicates a specific area of pain, begin palpation of the abdomen in the quadrant or area furthest from that point of pain. If necessary, palpate the area of pain last; however, if the patient has shown signs of tenderness and guarding on previous physical exams, then it is unnecessary to reassess the areas. Little more can be gained from the information, and the unnecessary creation of pain is cruel. If an object is impaled in the abdomen, do not remove it. If one of the abdominal organs is protruding from an open abdominal wound, do not attempt to push the organ back into the abdomen. Cover the organ with a sterile moist dressing and occlusive dressing, and transport immediately. Treatment of abdominal wounds will be addressed in more detail in Unit 36.

If a pulsating mass is present in the abdomen, do not palpate the mass. A pulsating mass in the abdomen may be a weakened, bulging area of the abdominal aorta. This is a life-threatening condition, and immediate transport is warranted if not already in progress.

When palpating the abdomen of an unresponsive patient, take note of the patient's body movements and facial expressions that may indicate a response to pain on palpation. Additionally, the type of body movement in response to palpation may be significant. Did the patient flex or extend their extremities or move away from or toward the pain? These are responses in the unresponsive patient that should be documented and reported to the receiving facility or ALS crew.

The final step of the detailed physical examination of the abdomen involves compression and flexion of the pelvis. Injury to the pelvis can cause serious and potentially life-threatening bleeding. The pelvic area should be exposed to inspect for injuries that can be visualized: obvious deformities, contusions, abrasions, punctures, burns, lacerations, or swelling. The external genitalia should be assessed for signs of trauma or bleeding and signs of loss of bladder control or priapism, persistent erection of the penis that may indicate a possible spinal cord injury. Keep in mind the patient may be more uncomfortable with this area of the physical exam. Ensure the patient's privacy and expose only what is needed to conduct your exam, while explaining what you are doing and why it is necessary.

When examining the pelvis, gently compress downward on the iliac wings, watching the patient's face for signs of discomfort. Pressing inward on the hips will help to discover a hip fracture. Finally, gently press downward on the pubis to stress the bony pelvic ring (see Figure 19.7A-C). Tenderness during any part of this exam indicates possible fracture. If pelvic pain is present, a gentle palpation of the area should be performed to assess the area of tenderness.

Compression and flexion is not indicated for the patient in whom a pelvic injury is already suspected.

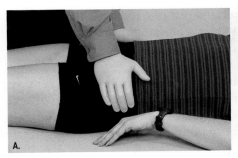
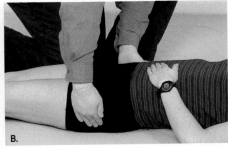
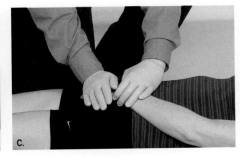

Figure 19.7 A. Gentle pressure downward on the iliac wings may reveal fractures and sites of patient discomfort in the pelvic area B. Gentle pressure inward on the hips may reveal a hip fracture C. Gentle downward pressure on the pubis will reveal pelvic fractures

EXTREMITIES

The detailed physical examination for the limbs looks for injuries that are not life or limb threatening, such as superficial wounds. As with all areas of the detailed physical examination, to perform an appropriate inspection, the extremities will need to be exposed. If an injury is known to be present, cut the clothing away from the extremity.

Starting with a visual inspection, the EMT should look for any evidence of injury in the presence of DCAP-BTLS. In the medical patient, look for swelling in the ankles and feet that may indicate the patient is experiencing cardiac insufficiency.

Each limb should be separately examined, carefully and firmly palpating along the length of each bone. Take time to discover any localized tenderness that might indicate an injury of the bone underneath. A nondisplaced bone fracture will be straight, and the bone may even support some weight. Treat any bone pain as if it were a fracture, until an x-ray proves otherwise. Management of bony injuries is described in Unit 38.

Most extremities are quite symmetrical in appearance, so comparing one extremity to the other make it possible to see differences in size and coloration. In the medical patient, assess for equal strength and sensation in the extremities. If one extremity is weaker or has less sensation than the other, this may be a sign of neurologic impairment.

Every examination of the extremities includes a reassessment for pulses, movement, and sensation (PMS). Each peripheral pulse should be checked (pedal and radial pulses) and compared from side to side. An absent pulse on one side indicates injury to that extremity. The patient's ability to move an extremity should be tested. To assess for movement in the hands, the EMT should ask the patient to grasp his index finger and squeeze. He should be assessing the equality of the grasp as well as the strength.

To assess for movement in the feet, the EMT should ask the patient to flex and extend her feet, as shown in Figure 19.8. Ask the patient to "point your toes to your nose and then press on the gas." This instruction encourages the patient to fully extend and flex both feet. No further movement should be requested of the patient with multiple injuries to avoid aggravating any existing injuries. Finally, the sensation in each extremity is checked by gentle squeezing a toe or finger.

BACK AND BUTTOCKS

The patient's back and buttocks can hide many wounds such as lacerations or exit wounds from a gunshot or lightning injury. While maintaining continuous manual stabilization of the head, preferably with a cervical

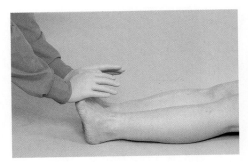

Figure 19.8 Flexion and extension of the toes can test the strength of the lower extremities

collar in place, the EMT should carefully examine the back and buttocks for injury. Any deformity, contusion, abrasion, punctures, burns, tenderness, lacerations, or swelling should be carefully examined and noted in the patient's report.

Common examples of back injuries include stab wounds in the upper back from an overhead knife and abrasions caused by the road surface after the patient has been ejected from a vehicle. A common example of a buttock wound would be a partial avulsion of the buttocks following a motorcycle collision.

VITAL SIGNS REVISITED

The detailed physical examination should be followed with a full set of vital signs. This set of vital signs should then be compared with the baseline set, and any changes should be noted. A rising heart rate could be a sign of shock. An increasing respiratory rate may indicate worsening chest injuries. Any significant changes in vital signs should be reported to the hospital staff.

Vital signs in the unresponsive or unstable patient should be reassessed every 5 minutes. The new EMT may be asked to monitor serial vitals signs every few minutes in a major trauma call, reporting them out loud to the rest of the crew. The stable, conscious patient should have vital signs reassessed every 15 minutes. If the patient is being treated for life-threatening conditions, vital signs may not be possible to monitor. It is important to remember ongoing care for life-threatening conditions will always take precedence over the physical exam and vital signs measurements.

CONCLUSION

The detailed physical examination is a comprehensive head-to-toe examination of the patient, looking more specifically for injuries that need to be addressed. The problems found during the secondary assessment may not be conditions the EMT will be able to treat. Internal damage to organs such as the lungs, heart, and brain or conditions such as a drug overdose require direct definitive care by a physician.

The physical examination will alert the EMT to potential injuries or conditions not found during the primary assessment that may be life threatening and in need of rapid transport or non–life-threatening conditions that can be stabilized in the field. Regardless of whether the findings are life threatening or not, they should be documented and reported to the next level health care provider assuming the patient's care.

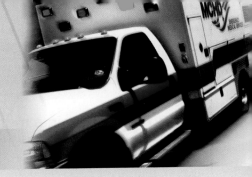

CASE STUDY Continued

En route to the hospital, Liam has regained consciousness but continues to be confused and unable to answer questions appropriately. He has been placed on oxygen by non-rebreather mask at 15 lpm and has been packaged using full spinal immobilization. Larry had obtained a set of baseline vital signs showing a blood pressure of 110/60, pulse of 90, and respirations of 16.

Gary begins a detailed physical examination after his primary assessment showed no obvious injuries with the exception of the hematoma on Liam's forehead and abrasions to his tongue. Liam's teammates denied any knowledge of Liam having a seizure history when asked prior to transport.

The only additional information Gary found during the detailed physical examination was a medic alert necklace stating Liam had a history of seizures and non–insulin dependent diabetes.

Upon arrival of the ALS unit called to intercept for an unresponsive patient, Gary gives a report, including all findings of the primary and secondary assessments and the information gathered during the focused physical exam.

PURPOSE: To obtain a more thorough physical examination of injuries to a trauma patient; usually performed en route to the hospital.

STANDARD PRECAUTIONS:

☑ Penlight

☑ Stethoscope

☑ Blood pressure cuff

☑ Scissors

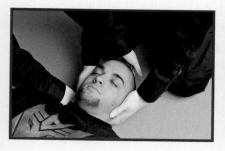

1 The EMT starts at the top of the head and assesses the scalp and the face for DCAP-BTLS. Next, the ears, nose, and throat are assessed, noting any bleeding or drainage of fluids as well as jugular venous distention or displacement of the trachea.

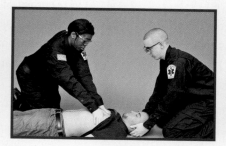

2 Then the EMT proceeds to looking, listening, and feeling the chest wall for injury, including crepitus and paradoxical motion.

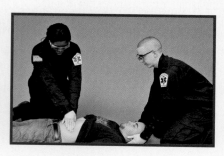

3 Turning next to the abdomen and the pelvis, the EMT assesses for DCAP-BTLS. Assessment of the pelvis should include gentle pressure inward on the hips to check for hip fracture.

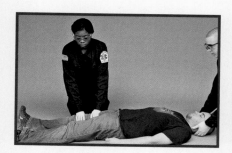

4 Then the extremities are assessed for pulses, movement, and sensation as well as DCAP-BTLS.

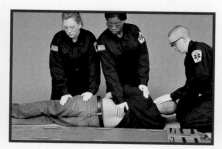

5 The patient's posterior is assessed during the logroll onto the long spine board.

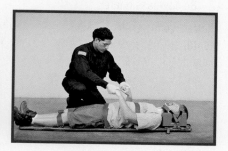

6 The patient is then secured to the long spine board, and vital signs and motor sensation are reassessed.

Key Concepts Revisited

- The detailed physical examination is a patient-specific, injury-specific examination.

- The history will be used to guide the physical examination in the medical patient.

- The physical examination is a complete head-to-toe examination of all body regions in the trauma patient and a focused physical examination to the affected area of the medical patient.

- A serious mechanism of injury will create a high index of suspicion that a serious hidden injury may exist.

- The techniques used during the physical assessment are:
  - Inspection (look)
  - Palpation (feel)
  - Auscultation (listen)

- Professionalism must be maintained throughout the physical examination.
  - Be polite.
  - Give explanations.
  - Maintain patient privacy.
  - Make eye contact.
  - Be honest.
  - Focus the patient's attention.
  - Be compassionate.

- The categories of the physical exam include assessment of mental status, a general survey, and the detailed physical examination of the body regions and systems:
  - The head
  - The ears
  - The nose
  - The neck
  - The chest
  - The abdomen and pelvis
  - The extremities
  - The back and buttocks

- The objective of the detailed physical examination is to discover conditions or injuries not uncovered during the primary assessment.

- The detailed physical examination measures the effectiveness of prehospital treatments that were initiated early on in the assessment.

- The detailed physical exam is a systematic head-to-toe physical examination.

- DCAP-BTLS refers to the types of underlying serious injuries the EMT should look for during the detailed physical exam.
  - Deformities
  - Contusions
  - Abrasions
  - Punctures/penetrations
  - Burns
  - Tenderness
  - Lacerations
  - Swelling

- The detailed physical examination should be followed up with a full set of vital signs that are compared to the baseline vital signs to determine the progression of the patient's condition.

- The physical examination may uncover further injuries or conditions that may be life threatening and in need of rapid transport or non–life-threatening conditions that can be stabilized in the field.

Review Questions

1. Who should always receive a detailed physical examination?

2. What three methods of assessment will the EMT use during the detailed physical examination?

3. What is the primary objective of the detailed physical examination?

4. To what types of injuries does the abbreviation DCAP-BTLS refer?

5. What additional points of examination beyond DCAP-BTLS should be assessed?

6. What all should be examined when assessing the patient's pelvic region and why?

Key Terms

Battle's sign
hyphema
raccoon's eyes

Further Study

Bickley, L. S., and P. G. Szilaqyi. *Bates' Guide to Physical Examination and History Taking.* 9th ed. Hagerstown, MD: Lippincott Williams & Wilkins, 2007.

Dalton, A. L., D. Limmer, J. J. Mistovich, and H. A. Werman. *Advanced Medical Life Support.* Upper Saddle River, NJ: Brady/ Prentice Hall, 2007.

National Association of Emergency Medical Technicians. *PHTLS: Basic and Advanced Prehospital Trauma Life Support.* 6th ed. Clinton, MS: Mosby, 2007.

UNIT (20) Reassessment

In the days of the hearse ambulance, an attendant would sit in a small seat next to the door. During transport to the hospital, there was not enough room to do much with the patient. Simple airway management was difficult, and effective cardiopulmonary resuscitation (CPR) was almost impossible.

Today, prehospital care has evolved to a point where we are able to continue to provide care to patients in the back of the ambulance during transport to the hospital. Sometimes this transport time can be lengthy. No matter how long it is, the Emergency Medical Technician (EMT) is responsible for observing and caring for that patient until patient care is turned over to the next level of care, whether that is an advanced life support (ALS) intercept or arrival at the hospital.

National Education Standard

The Emergency Medical Technician (EMT) shall have a fundamental depth and foundational breadth of understanding and ability to perform a reassessment for all patient situations at the appropriate time.

Key Concepts

- The purpose of reassessment is to identify any significant changes.

- The ongoing assessment consists of repeating the primary assessment, vital signs, chief concern, and secondary assessment.

- The first step of the reassessment is to repeat the ABCs and mental status of the primary assessment.

- The destination decision may change during transport based on reassessment findings.

- Vitals signs repeated in reassessment should be compared to baseline vital signs.

- Reaffirming a patient's history improves the reliability of that history.

- Reassessment of the secondary assessment can expose injury indicators.

- Interventions must be reevaluated following the reassessment and adjusted accordingly.

- The priority level of the patient will determine the frequency of reassessment.

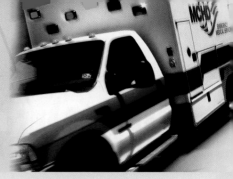

CASE STUDY

While en route to meet the ALS crew, Tillie has completed her primary assessment, baseline vital signs, history taking, and a physical examination that focused on Mrs. Scott's chief concern. Mrs. Scott has high flow oxygen by non-rebreather mask. Mrs. Scott seems to be less anxious than just prior to transport, and the crew tries to reassure her that everything that can be done for her is being done and that she will be at the hospital shortly. Mrs. Scott seems relieved that she is on the way to the hospital and is pleased she is in good hands.

Critical Thinking Questions

1. What is the next step in Tillie's care of Mrs. Scott?
2. How will Tillie be able to determine if the oxygen is helping?
3. How will Tillie determine if Mrs. Scott needs any further or different treatments?

INTRODUCTION

Patients who require ambulance transport are at risk for having an unstable, or changing, medical condition. It is therefore critical that the EMT continue to observe the patient and assess for any changes during transport. This unit discusses and emphasizes the importance of continuous reassessment.

REASSESSMENT

Once the patient has been thoroughly assessed through the primary assessment, a transport decision has been made, and history taking, baseline vital signs, and secondary assessments have been completed, the next step is to reassess the prior findings and vital signs.

The purpose of reassessment is to identify any significant changes in the patient's condition that need immediate attention. During the reassessment, the EMT evaluates the effectiveness of medical care by comparing baseline vital signs and assessment findings with repeat assessments that are done periodically during transport. The reassessment is conducted at intervals after the history taking and physical examination of the trauma or medical patient.

COMPONENTS OF REASSESSMENT

The ongoing assessment consists of repeating the primary assessment and vital signs and monitoring the chief concern and any areas that were previously of concern. Interventions such as oxygen, a splint, or bleeding control should be reassessed to see whether the patient is improving as a result of implementation. Any changes should be managed and documented.

THE PRIMARY ASSESSMENT REPEATED

The first step of the reassessment is to repeat the primary assessment. The patient's condition will dictate whether this step will take more than a moment. An EMT should take the time to carefully reassess the ABCs of the primary assessment in the seriously injured patient.

MENTAL STATUS

During the reassessment, the EMT reevaluates the patient's mental status. AVPU (alert, voice, pain, unresponsive) is the method that will be used to do this reassessment, just as it was in the primary assessment. Mental status changes may occur gradually but may have devastating consequences if not recognized and quickly acted upon by the EMT.

AIRWAY

The patient's airway is critical. The EMT must maintain a constant vigil over the airway, making sure that it remains open and clear (Figure 20.1). If the patient is unconscious, the EMT should continue to manually maintain the airway with an adjunct oropharyngeal airway or nasopharyngeal airway in place. If the EMT is tiring, he should switch roles with his partner.

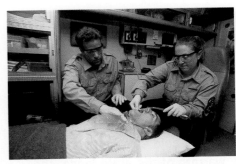

Figure 20.1 Some treatments must be repeated while en route

BREATHING

Although a patient may have been breathing adequately while on scene, the patient's condition may worsen and cause respiratory decompensation. Adequacy of breathing should be reevaluated by reassessing both the breathing rate and effort. Oxygen via a non-rebreather mask may not be enough. The EMT may have to ventilate the patient who is no longer able to breathe effectively on his own.

Oxygen is probably one of the most commonly administered treatments in Emergency Medical Services (EMS). Once the oxygen has been given to a patient, its effectiveness must be evaluated. Did the oxygen relieve the patient's pain or make him feel better? If not, why not? A common problem is that the oxygen tubing becomes kinked under linen or the patient. The EMT should always leave oxygen tubing in plain view on top of the linen.

Oxygen in a tank is limited. Failure to notice an empty oxygen tank could force the patient to rebreathe his own exhaled air, because he is no longer getting the supplemental oxygen he requires. Oxygen tanks, both on board and portable, need to be checked frequently. Some EMTs check the tank whenever they take a set of vital signs.

The pulse oximeter can aid the EMT in assessment of the patient's breathing. Constant readings confirm the EMT's assessment findings (Figure 20.2). It is important to remember that the pulse oximeter reading is a supplement to, not a replacement for, a good assessment of the patient's respiratory effort.

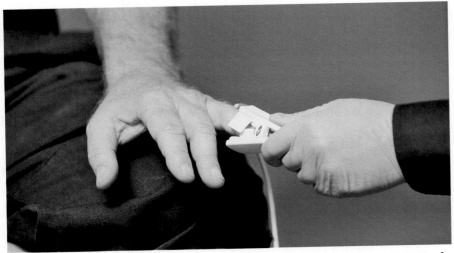

Figure 20.2 The pulse oximeter provides continuous reassessment of oxygenation

During cold weather, the body shunts blood away from the skin and into the body's core. When the injured patient is moved from a cold environment to the warmth of the ambulance, the process reverses.

The result is that wounds that were relatively bloodless out in the cold may suddenly begin to bleed profusely in the back of the ambulance.

Many EMTs place the pulse oximeter on the patient in the ambulance to monitor oxygen saturation throughout transport.

CIRCULATION

Vigorous external bleeding would have been controlled on the scene. Less obvious, slowly bleeding wounds also need attention. During reassessment, the EMT should turn her attention to ensuring that all bleeding has been addressed and remains controlled. That includes reassessing any external bleeding that was discovered and initially managed on the scene.

An EMT can assess and control external bleeding, but she cannot control internal bleeding directly. A high index of suspicion based on the mechanism of injury would make an EMT suspect that the patient may be bleeding internally.

Constant reassessment of indicators of perfusion, such as central and distal pulses as well as skin temperature and color, gives an EMT a clue about the presence of internal bleeding.

REEVALUATE PATIENT PRIORITY

Occasionally, patients deteriorate while en route to the hospital. Rarely does a high-priority patient recover sufficiently to be considered low priority. The EMT should always be prepared to upgrade the patient's priority on the basis of the most current assessment findings.

If the hospital has been notified of an impending arrival and the patient's condition changes, the EMT should reestablish contact. Early notification of patient changes permits the emergency department to properly prepare.

If a patient is deteriorating, an ALS intercept should be arranged if it is possible. Often, a patient who suddenly becomes unmanageable for an EMT can be successfully stabilized by a paramedic (Figure 20.3).

DESTINATION

If the patient's condition changes, the appropriate facility the patient is being transported to may also have to change. This decision should be based on knowledge of local resources and regional transportation protocols.

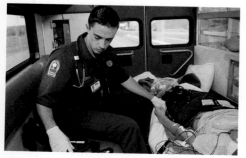

Figure 20.3 Patients do deteriorate, and advanced life support can help

REASSESS VITAL SIGNS

Baseline vitals signs, the first set of vital signs taken following the primary assessment, need to be reassessed following the secondary assessment. Each set of vital signs taken following the baseline vital signs establish whether there has been any change in the patient's condition. Repeat vital signs, including measurement of the pulse, respirations, blood pressure, pupils, and skin signs, are good indicators of whether current treatments are working or if the EMT needs to adjust her treatment plan.

Every patient, regardless of circumstances, should have at least two full sets of vital signs obtained, assessed, and recorded.

REPEAT HISTORY

People, in general, do not always think clearly when they are under stress. When the patient was giving a historical account of his illness on scene, distractions may have confused him. In the relative calm of the back of an ambulance and away from distractions, the patient may give a more accurate account of his injury or illness (Figure 20.4).

Reinvestigate the patient's chief concern. Has the chief concern changed? Is the patient experiencing increased pain or discomfort, has it remained the same, or has it gotten better? The EMT should ask the patient if there

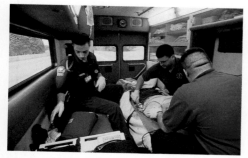

Figure 20.4 A repeated history improves reliability

are any new concerns or something he did not feel previously but is now experiencing.

Reaffirming a patient's history improves the reliability of that history. A reliable history gives the EMT confidence that the treatments being administered are correct. Perhaps more important, new historical findings, like new physical findings, give the EMT an opportunity to adjust treatments and patient priorities.

REPEAT SECONDARY ASSESSMENT

Physical findings, such as bruising and swelling, take time to develop. Bruises across the abdomen from a seat belt may not appear for 20–30 minutes.

The EMT should reassess the patient using DCAP-BTLS previously assessed during the initial detailed physical exam, especially if the transporting time is extended. Comparisons should be made between on-scene assessment findings and the reassessment.

It is best if the EMT who did the primary assessment also does the reassessment. It is impossible to determine whether a leg is more swollen if there was no baseline for comparison. Only the first EMT would have that information.

CHECK INTERVENTIONS

After completing the reassessment, the EMT should check all treatments in progress and adjust them as needed. "Is it working?" is the central question on the EMT's mind.

Previously applied dressings should be examined to ensure proper placement and adequate bleeding control. Splints that were applied for suspected broken bones should be assessed and readjusted as needed for patient comfort. Additionally, pulses in the fractured extremities need to be reassessed to ensure the splint has not impaired circulation. As you will learn in Unit 41, when splints are applied, it is important to assess the distal pulse, motor function, and sensation frequently. This process is repeated during reassessments.

If the EMT assisted the patient in taking previously prescribed medications as allowed by local protocols, the effects of these medications should also be reassessed. For example, if an inhaler was used for the asthma patient with difficulty breathing, the EMT should carefully reassess the breathing and determine the effectiveness of the medication.

NOTE CHANGES

All changes in the patient's condition from the time on the scene and while en route must be noted. Observant EMTs may notice that these changes represent a pattern. For example, pale, cool, and clammy skin, with steadily dropping blood pressures and increasing pulse rates, is indicative of progressing shock.

Reassessments will reveal these patterns, or **trends.** Such trends, either positive or negative, should be reported and recorded.

FREQUENCY OF REASSESSMENT

The frequency with which these repeated assessments are performed is determined by the priority of the patient. If the patient is considered to be a high-priority patient, it is appropriate to continually monitor the ABCs and recheck vital signs every 5 minutes.

Patients who are not considered high priority should be reassessed every 10–15 minutes during transport to find any changes in condition. Table 20-1 provides a list of suggested patient classifications based on patient problem. Remember that if a patient deteriorates, the priority may change from a low priority to a high priority and the issues involved in the transport as well as the frequency of repeated assessments must be readdressed.

Table 20-1 Patient Classification Guidelines

High priority:	Cardiac or respiratory arrest
	Ventilations require assistance
	Severe upper airway difficulties
	Serious chest trauma
	Decompensated shock
	Decreasing level of consciousness
	Uncontrollable external hemorrhage
	Penetrating injury to head, neck, chest, abdomen, pelvis
Low priority:	Early signs of compensated shock
	Kinematics or injuries suggest hidden injury
	Major isolated injury
	Minor isolated injuries
	Uncomplicated extremity injury

It is important that the EMT use these frequent reassessments to note any trending, or changes over time, in the patient's condition. The EMT should carefully document any changes in condition or any trends noted during transport. Passing this information along to hospital staff upon arrival will also help them to better care for the patient.

Skill 20-1 at the end of this unit describes the ongoing assessment.

CONCLUSION

Once an EMT has assessed a patient, she must continue to reassess in regular intervals to notice any trends or changes over time. These repeated assessments should continue during the entire time that the EMT is caring for the patient.

Reassessment is of key importance in caring for emergency patients, who may have changes in condition over time and need different treatment because of these changes. It is the responsibility of the EMT to recognize these changes and take appropriate action.

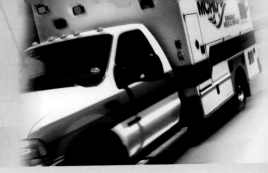

CASE STUDY Continued

Tillie begins repeating the primary assessment, determining that Mrs. Scott's airway is patent, she is breathing adequately, and her pulse is still present but weak. Mrs. Scott states she is less anxious, and during the reassessment of her medical history, she reveals she has experienced these same symptoms a week before, but not as bad. She further states her mother died of a heart attack when she was 62.

Mrs. Scott states the pain is better and now rates it a 4 on a scale of 0 to 10. She reaffirms the pain is an ache in her jaw and now feels like it may also move down into her neck off and on.

Tillie determines the treatment of oxygen and emotional support are helping Mrs. Scott at this time. Tillie documents all the findings of her reassessment and provides a complete report of all assessments, reassessments, and treatments to the paramedic assuming Mrs. Scott's care.

PURPOSE: To continue to monitor the patient for assessment and comparison with baseline examinations.

STANDARD PRECAUTIONS:

☑ Penlight
☑ Stethoscope
☑ Blood pressure cuff

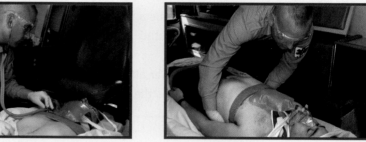

1 While en route to the hospital, the EMT repeats the primary assessment, reassessing the patient's mental status using the AVPU scale and monitoring the airway.

2 The patient's breathing must be reassessed for rate and quality, and lung sounds must be monitored.

3 The EMT then reassesses the patient's circulatory status, including skin temperature, and notes any additional bleeding.

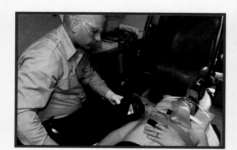 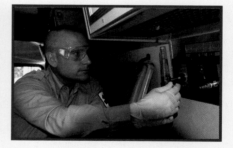

4 After mentally reviewing the patient's priorities, the EMT reassesses the vital signs and repeats a physical examination as needed.

5 The EMT rechecks the interventions, such as oxygen regulator flow rate.

Key Concepts Revisited

- The purpose of reassessment is to identify any significant changes.

- The ongoing assessment consists of repeating the primary assessment, vital signs, chief concern, and secondary assessment.

- The first step of the reassessment is to repeat the ABCs and mental status of the primary assessment.
  - Airway
  - Breathing
  - Circulation

- Mental status is reassessed using the AVPU scale:
  - Alert
  - Responsive to verbal/voice
  - Responsive to painful stimuli
  - Unresponsive

- The destination decision may change during transport based on reassessment findings.

- Vital signs repeated in reassessment should be compared to baseline vital signs.

- Reaffirming a patient's history improves the reliability of that history
  - SAMPLE history
  - OPQRST history

- Reassessment of the secondary assessment can expose injury indicators.

- Interventions must be reevaluated following the reassessment and adjusted accordingly.

- The priority level of the patient will determine the frequency of reassessment.
  - For high-priority patients, reassess every 5 minutes.
  - For low-priority patients, reassess every 10–15 minutes.

Review Questions

1. What is the purpose of the reassessment?
2. What about the patient's mental status should the EMT reassess?
3. What does an EMT reevaluate in breathing?
4. Why does an EMT reevaluate in circulation?
5. What is meant by the term *trend?*
6. How often does a low-priority patient need reevaluation?
7. How often does a high-priority patient need reevaluation?
8. How many times is the primary assessment completed and documented on any patient?
9. How many sets of vital signs should an EMT obtain on any patient?
10. On what should the decision to change destination hospitals be based?

Key Terms

Trends

Further Study

Elling, B., and K. Elling. *Principles of Patient Assessment in EMS.* Clifton Park, NY: Thomson Delmar Learning, 2002.

UNIT (21) EMS System Communication

After World War II, radios made their way into civilian emergency services, in large part owing to efforts of the Civil Defense. The result was a more rapid dispatch and arrival of lifesaving aid units.

In the past, the public thought of Emergency Medical Technicians (EMTs) as ambulance drivers. Similarly, EMTs think of the professional **communications specialist (COMSPEC)** as the dispatcher. Modern telecommunications has evolved into a complex field involving not only radios but also computers, digital technology, and even satellite linkups.

EMS system communications is a partnership requiring the EMT to understand the workings of radio and paging systems, the role of the COMSPEC, and the appropriate communications methods when transferring patient care.

Typically, a health care provider will transfer patient care to another health care provider and give a verbal report. The verbal report summarizes the patient's condition for the new provider. The acceptance of the report represents the willingness of the other party to accept the patient. The failure of an EMT to give a report about a patient to the next health care provider could be construed as abandonment.

Beyond the medical-legal justification, giving a patient report offers two health care professionals an opportunity to focus on one patient and exchange observations, records, and physical findings regarding that patient.

National Education Standard

The Emergency Medical Technician (EMT) will demonstrate a simple depth and breadth of understanding of the function of the EMS communications system, team communications and dynamics, and the ability to communicate with other health care professionals.

Key Concepts

- All EMS communication is done via the emergency services communications system.

- Definitive patient care begins with effective communications between the public, emergency services personnel, and hospital staff.

- The role of the communications specialist is to coordinate all aspects of an emergency response.

- The core of most modern emergency service communications systems is the two-way radio system.

- A communications system is made up of base radios, mobile radios, portable radios, repeaters, digital radio equipment, telephones, cellular phones, and satellite telephones.

- The Federal Communications Commission is responsible for allocating radio frequencies, licensing base stations, issuing call signs, and monitoring radio operations.

- FCC designated a specific group, or band, of radio frequencies for use by EMS providers.

- The dispatch frequency is reserved for communications between EMS units in the field and the communications center.

- The use of basic radio procedures begins with familiarity with the function of radio.

- Proper radio procedure begins with the "you first then me" approach.

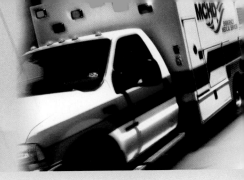

CASE STUDY

An elderly male who lives alone has fallen down the stairs, injuring his hip. Mr. Kase wears a Lifeline button around his neck and is able to notify the local hospital he cannot get up or get to the telephone to call for help. The hospital notifies the communications center an ambulance is needed at 100 Christopher Road for a man who has fallen, possible hip injury.

Kent is completing his equipment check on squad 81-40 when the tones go off:

"Squad 81-40 from Dispatch—you are needed at 100 Christopher Road, for an elderly male who has fallen, possible hip injury. Time out 07:00."

"Dispatch-squad 81-40—acknowledges, 100 Christopher Road for elderly male who has fallen, possible hip injury. Squad 81-40 is en route to scene."

Dispatch replies, "Squad 81-40 en route—07:02."

Upon arrival Kent's partner radios the communications center they are on scene, and dispatch acknowledges squad 81-40 is on scene at 07:12.

Critical Thinking Questions

1. What types of communication system might be used throughout the progression of this call?

2. What role does the communications center play in patient care?

3. What method should the EMT use to communicate information concerning the patient to the receiving facility?

Key Concepts Continued

- The dispatcher should be aware of the location of each in-service unit.

- Medical control consultation and the prehospital radio report are the two most common communications conducted with the hospital.

- Medical control consultation is conducted when on-line medical direction is needed.

- The prehospital radio report alerts the hospital of impending arrival of a patient and a brief description of the patient's concern.

- The verbal report is an expanded radio report an EMT will give to another health care provider who is taking over.

- The verbal report effectively tells the right person, at the right place, at the right time about the patient.

- Interpersonal communication is part speech and part body language.

- Communications barriers can prevent the right information from being communicated and understood.

- Avoid communication barriers through the stop, look, and listen technique.

- EMS system communication use is an everyday part of the EMT's responsibility.

INTRODUCTION

Before the advent of modern radio and paging systems, rescue squads were typically summoned by a telephone operator who called a designated telephone, often called the "hot line," to alert the squad of a call for Emergency Medical Services (EMS). The rescue squad member who received the notification would then call the next crew member. Precious minutes were lost trying to round up the crew.

Radio and paging equipment and systems have evolved to a point at which a much more efficient means of notification, dispatch, and communication between health care partners is available.

Although the EMT's knowledge need not be as extensive as that of a communications specialist, he must have a basic understanding of communications systems and how to operate them. The EMT must then be able to appropriately communicate his findings and treatments to another health care provider who is assuming ongoing care of the patient.

Restrictions on radio time, conditions on scene, and the presence of family members near the radio all may prevent the EMT from fully relating the patient's condition to the medical control physician. The face-to-face verbal report is the opportunity an EMT has to tell the whole story.

This unit discusses the components of EMS system communications and the verbal patient report required in the continuum of patient care.

COMMUNICATIONS SYSTEMS

Modern communications systems are made up of many pieces of equipment and as many equipment operators. The public accesses emergency services through a central point, usually by dialing 9-1-1 on a telephone. The information is recorded by a communications specialist, who then dispatches the closest, most appropriate emergency crews to the scene to render aid and assistance. Finally, the patient is transported to the hospital, and the hospital is alerted to the patient's condition and urgency. All of the notifications that are necessary throughout this process are done via the emergency services communications system.

Effective communications between the public, emergency services personnel, and hospital staff is necessary to rapidly access, treat, and transport the patient to definitive care. For some medical conditions, every second counts. Modern communications systems facilitate the rapid treatment and transport of a critically ill or injured patient to the hospital.

COMMUNICATIONS SPECIALIST

The communications specialist is a person who has been trained to facilitate communications between the public, emergency service personnel, and in some cases, hospital staff. These professionals help to coordinate all aspects of an emergency response through the use of radios, computers, and telephones. Table 21-1 lists some of the roles of communications specialists and the pieces of the communications system that facilitate their job.

Through a guided interview with the caller, the communications specialist determines the number and types of units needed for any given emergency. By using predetermined protocols and a knowledge of the location and capabilities of each unit within the region, the communications specialist can dispatch the closest appropriate units with the safest priority for the situation (Figure 21.1).

Radio dispatch of emergency units is often done through the use of a CAD, or computer-aided dispatch system. This computerized program, together with a status management system, helps the communications specialist to track each of the units that are in service. Such organization also helps maintain efficiency and allows effective networking of resources when needed.

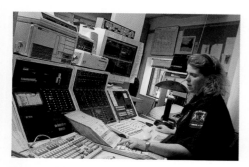

Figure 21.1 Predetermined protocols, such as those outlined on these dispatch cards, facilitate safe dispatch of emergency units to a medical emergency

Table 21-1 Roles of Communications Specialists

Role	System Support
Telephone interrogation	9-1-1 telephone systems
Triage	Emergency medical dispatch
Radio dispatch	Computer-aided dispatch
Logistics coordination	System status management
Resource networking	Public safety critical incident management
Prearrival instructions	Emergency medical dispatch

One of the other important jobs of the communications specialist is to provide prearrival instructions. Even under the best conditions, EMS may take several minutes to arrive on the scene. Simple first-aid instructions given to a bystander or family member can mean the difference between life and death.

SYSTEM COMPONENTS

The core of most modern emergency service communications systems is the two-way radio. The **two-way radio** is a wireless electronic device that permits the transmission of messages to distant radio receivers as well as receipt of signals from those distant radios.

BASE STATIONS

The original radio transmitters were large, cumbersome base stations that used large amounts of electricity to transmit a signal. Modern base station radios have evolved into powerful compact base units capable of fitting under a desk (Figure 21.2). The **base station** radio is a large, powerful radio that is located at a stationary site such as a dispatch center.

Radio signals are created in the base station and transmitted from a radio tower via an antenna. The antenna of a receiving radio unit converts the signal back into sound and the message is heard.

Radio signals travel in concentric arcs emanating straight out from the source. Therefore, the distance a radio signal can travel is influenced by many factors. Dense foliage or large buildings can either block or absorb some of the radio signal, thereby decreasing the distance the signal will travel (Figure 21.3).

The most important barrier to a long-distance radio signal is the curvature of the earth. More powerful radios, their strength measured in watts, are often used to overcome the impact of the earth's curvature, allowing farther transmission of a radio signal. Tall radio towers place the antenna high above the ground, allowing farther transmission of signal. Therefore, many radio towers are located on the top of a mountain or tall building.

An airplane flying at 38,000 feet can use a very low-powered radio and still transmit over hundreds of miles. Why? Because the airplane acts like a 38,000-foot-tall antenna!

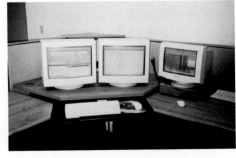

Figure 21.2 A fixed radio communication point is called a base station

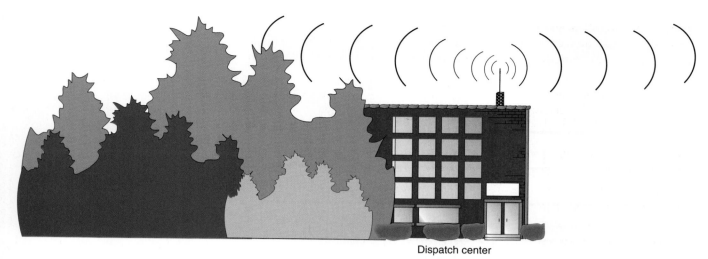

Figure 21.3 Foliage and buildings can dampen the radio wave coming from an antenna

MOBILE RADIOS

A radio that is mounted inside a vehicle is referred to as a **mobile radio.** Most mobile radios transmit at a lower power than base stations, typically 20 to 50 watts. Therefore, the typical transmission range will be less than that of the more powerful radios. Over average terrain, a mobile radio may transmit 10 to 15 miles.

The advent of the mobile radio allowed emergency service units to be dispatched from the streets. This advancement in radio technology permitted communications between a central dispatch point, or a communications center, and mobile EMS units.

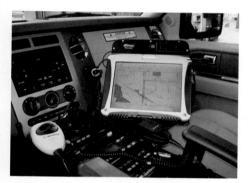

Figure 21.4 Modern EMS command/control is accomplished via the mobile radio (Courtesy of Clive Fire Department, Clive, IA)

Most EMS units have a mobile radio mounted inside the vehicle, in the trunk or a compartment, while the radio head is mounted in the driver's compartment. The **radio head** includes the microphone and volume and channel controls (Figure 21.4). This allows the operator to choose radio channels, control volume, and transmit messages.

In situations in which there is a great deal of interference from buildings or a long distance between the mobile radio and base station, a repeater is used. A **repeater** is a radio receiver/transmitter that picks up the signal from a mobile radio transmitter and increases, or boosts, the signal to the base station receiver (Figure 21.5).

PORTABLE RADIOS

The portable radio revolutionized emergency services at every level. The portable radio provides two-way communication that allows an EMT at the patient's side to request additional resources, consult with a physician, or

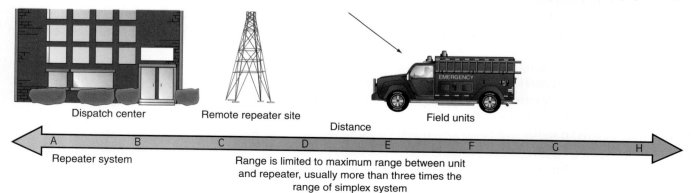

Dispatch center   Remote repeater site   Field units

Distance

A   B   C   D   E   F   G   H

Repeater system   Range is limited to maximum range between unit and repeater, usually more than three times the range of simplex system

Figure 21.5 Repeaters are used to transmit messages over distances

slow (downgrade) responding units (Figure 21.6). More importantly, if an EMT discovers a dangerous situation, the portable radio provides immediate access to law enforcement or other resources and the ability to warn others of danger. This advantage cannot be overemphasized.

These **portable radios** are small and transmit with less power than a larger radio. The power output of 1 to 5 watts limits their range.

RADIO ARRAY

The first portable radios permitted one-way communication. These portable radios, called **simplex** radios, could either receive or transmit but could not do both at the same time. The handset looks like a telephone handset (Figure 21.7), with a button in the cradle. By pushing the button and speaking into the microphone, the EMT could transmit a message.

The problem with a simplex radio was that the receiver had to wait until the transmitter was finished before she could speak. Simplex radios evolved into **duplex** radios, which allowed the EMT to both speak and listen at the same time, like a telephone.

In the early days of EMS, paramedics used an electrocardiogram (ECG) machine to obtain an electrocardiographic tracing and then transmit that to a hospital base station for a physician to interpret. This process was called **telemetry.** Telemetry made it necessary for radios to be able to transmit and receive spoken messages as well as complex data. These multiple-channel radios were called **multiplex radios.** As paramedics became proficient at interpreting ECGs in the field, the use of multiplex radios became less common.

RADIO FREQUENCIES

Radio waves, a part of the electromagnetic spectrum, are used to transmit messages from one point to another. Each radio wave has a length and a height. Early radios were primarily amplitude modulation (AM) radios. Modern radios are frequency modulation (FM) radios. These FM radios alter or modulate the speed, or frequency, of the radio waves. These frequencies are measured in megahertz (MHz).

There are as many radio frequencies in the radio spectrum as there are colors in a rainbow, which is a spectrum of light. These ranges of radio frequencies are divided into **VHF,** for very high frequency, and **UHF,** or ultrahigh frequency.

Communication by radio has become increasingly popular with the government, businesses, and even the public. The result has been that often many users are sharing radio frequencies. Although considerate use of a radio frequency, or channel, should allow for multiple users, problems can arise.

Channel crowding has become such a problem that some services use channel guards. **Channel guards,** sometimes called *private lines* (PLs), prevent extraneous interference by blocking radio transmissions from outside the base station.

THE FEDERAL COMMUNICATIONS COMMISSION

In an effort to prevent problems and maintain some control of the radio airwaves, Congress established the **Federal Communications Commission (FCC).** The FCC is charged with allocating radio frequencies, licensing base stations, issuing call signs, and monitoring radio operations. A **call sign** is a group of letters or numbers, or both, that is assigned to a particular group using a frequency.

In 1974, the FCC set a specific group, or band, of radio frequencies aside for use by EMS providers. From 460 MHz to 470 MHz is restricted to EMS

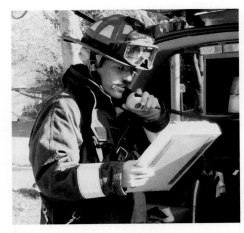

Figure 21.6 Portable radios provide added safety and quick access to resources (Courtesy of Clive Fire Department, Clive, IA)

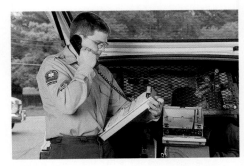

Figure 21.7 The push-to-talk feature is a feature of a simplex radio

Although radio technology has made great advances, occasionally a radio system will fail. Lightning strikes, battery failure, and computer freezes are some of the problems that can cripple a radio communications system. Consequently, there should always be a backup plan. Many EMS systems use cellular telephones as a backup system, if not a first route of communication. This prevents problems when communications fail and ensures the safety of the public.

providers only. These 10 frequencies, called **Med channels,** are frequently used by paramedics and EMTs to speak to medical control physicians and receiving hospitals. In a given region, certain frequencies may be dedicated to a particular purpose or facility.

In 1993, the FCC set the 220-MHz band aside for EMS. Despite these two restricted-access bands, EMS still does not have enough channels (frequencies) to operate without occasionally experiencing channel crowding.

RADIO CHANNELS

Once an emergency call is received, it is transmitted to the appropriate EMS units. The dispatch frequency is reserved for communications between EMS units in the field and the communications center.

During a multiple-casualty incident, or when several EMS calls are occurring simultaneously, frivolous radio chatter may prevent much-needed resources from being dispatched. When communications between EMS units and other emergency services must occur on scene, all on-scene units should select a designated incident or operations channel. An operations channel is a channel that is kept free for nondispatch-related radio traffic. The use of such a channel permits efficient scene coordination without interfering with system management.

Many communities have a predesignated tactical frequency, such as 155.715, that all EMS units switch to when they arrive on scene. This kind of preplanning decreases scene confusion and keeps essential radio channels open for emergency radio traffic.

Hospital communications is usually done on another frequency entirely than used for dispatch or on-scene operations. This frequency, like one of the Med channels discussed earlier, permits privacy and no interruptions. Because of the nature of these communications, many Med channels are recorded.

COMPUTERS AND RADIOS

Computers are used to sort through the incoming messages and allow priority messages to be transmitted on any available frequency while diverting or delaying lower-priority messages to an available channel. The use of computers to assist radios allows for truncated frequencies, so-called **trunked lines.** The newer 800-MHz radios, along with computers, are frequently used by municipalities for these trunked lines.

TELEPHONES

Telephones are a vital link between the public and emergency services. Although 9-1-1 has become the most used system for the public to access emergency services, some communities still use other means, such as longer telephone numbers, while they work toward that goal.

Telephones also serve as a link between the EMT and the communications center and the EMT and the hospital. To ensure that the EMT can reach either the communications center or the base hospital, EMS agencies may install separate dedicated telephone lines (Figure 21.8). These limited-access phone lines are often used by medical control physicians to give EMTs medical orders and may be recorded.

CELLULAR PHONES

Cellular telephones are actually low-powered duplex radios that communicate with a series of interconnected radio repeaters. This series of repeaters creates a grid, within which there are cells that permit the EMT to roam around inside the grid and still transmit.

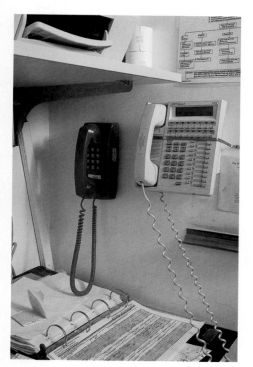

Figure 21.8 Dedicated hot lines ensure EMTs have unimpeded access to the physician

Although commercial cellular services usually charge for the service, calls to 9-1-1 from cellular phones are not charged. This is a valuable public service.

When a patient calls 9-1-1 on a telephone, in many cases the exact location of the telephone is displayed in the communications center. Cell phones, on the other hand, are mobile and therefore the communications center does not know the location of the phone. That means that the caller must describe his location exactly (Figure 21.9). Technology is currently in place in many localities to allow tracking of the location of a cellular phone for emergency purposes.

Some EMS services are using cellular phones as their primary means of communication when giving reports to the receiving hospital and requesting orders from medical control. Cellular phones are easy to use and maintain, and they provide better patient privacy than standard radio communication. The disadvantages of cellular phones are areas where there is no reception for a specific carrier and the likelihood that the cell phone network will be overwhelmed during a mass-casualty disaster.

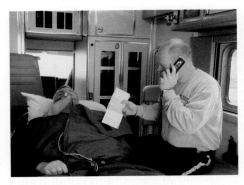

Figure 21.9 It is sometimes difficult to pinpoint the location of a cellular call

DIGITAL TECHNOLOGY

Digital technology uses an encoder to convert sound waves (messages) into digitally coded signals and then transmits them at a high rate of speed. The receiver uses a decoder that recognizes and responds only to those specific codes to reconstruct the signal into a readable form. This technology can be used for written, verbal, or electronic data. Using this technology, base stations and mobile devices can operate on the same broadcast frequencies. This enables more information to be transmitted in various forms over frequencies that may already be somewhat crowded. The fax and an ECG transmitted over a telephone line are examples of the use of digital technology (Figure 21.10).

SATELLITE PHONES

Using a series of low-earth-orbiting satellites, communication is now possible in areas where cellular service may be poor or nonexistent. These satellite phones transmit their digital signal to a satellite, called an uplink, and the satellite retransmits the signal down to a waiting receiver, called a downlink. The use of satellite phones permits radio communications in areas where traditional communication is limited by rough terrain, such as mountainous areas, or great distance, such as ships at sea.

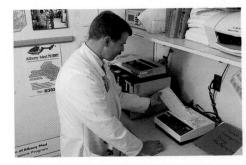

Figure 21.10 Digital technology offers new opportunities for EMS

BASIC RADIO OPERATION

There are many types of radio design. The EMT should take a moment, preferably before the radio is needed, to examine the radio. Where is the power switch? Where is the volume control? Adjust the volume to a comfortable level. Test the radio briefly.

When it comes to using a radio, it is important that the EMT be brief and concise. Careful consideration of the message before transmitting prevents the EMT from rambling in a disjointed fashion. The message should be thought out and then delivered.

Before pressing the transmit button, wait for several seconds to be sure that no other radio traffic is present. If the air is clear, then proceed to transmit. Hold the microphone about 2 inches from the mouth. Speak clearly and slowly in a normal conversational tone (Figure 21.11). If the EMT must raise his voice to hear himself speak, then he should consider rolling up the window or moving to another location to transmit.

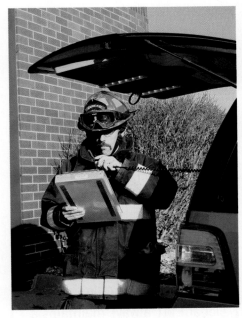

Figure 21.11 Press to talk, wait 2 seconds, and speak slowly and clearly (Courtesy of Clive Fire Department, Clive, IA)

RADIO PROCEDURES

When an EMT is attempting to call another party, a "you first then me" approach should be used. First identify the other unit or person to be called. Then identify yourself by unit identifier—for example, "EMS command, this is squad 11, requesting instructions."

When speaking to other units, use plain English. In the past, when radios were not as dependable, transmissions were made shorter by using special codes. These codes varied from community to community. Because of the confusion sometimes created and with the availability of higher-quality radios, radio transmissions can and should be made in plain English.

Profanity is not tolerated on the radio under any circumstance. The FCC monitors transmissions and will investigate concerns of profanity. The FCC is empowered to suspend or cancel a radio operator's license for use of profanity over the air.

It is not necessary to say "please" or "thank you" over the air. These amenities are implicit in a professional radio transmission. Avoid using slang or meaningless phrases such as "be advised." Instead, conserve valuable air time.

If a long transmission is necessary, stop every 30 seconds to permit other EMTs an opportunity to interrupt the transmission. This practice ensures that air time is available in case of emergency. It also encourages EMTs to be brief and to the point.

STANDARD RADIO TERMINOLOGY

If the EMT needs to pause the conversation and wishes the other party to stay near the radio, the commonly used phrase is to ask the party to **stand by.** This request means that the EMT will return to the radio shortly.

Whenever an EMT is answering a yes or no question over the radio, he uses the terms *affirmative* or *negative.* Short answers such as yes and no are frequently not heard or may be misunderstood.

When the EMT is done with a statement, the word "over" is commonly used. This indicates to the other party that the line is now open for her to speak.

When the EMT is completely done with his radio transmission, he should clear the air, typically by stating his identifier and saying the word "clear"—for example, "This is Ambulance 2-4 clearing Med channel 1." Other users who are listening now know that the frequency is available for their use.

When giving a number over the radio, the EMT should say each number individually. For example, the number 15 may sound like 50. Saying "one-five" leaves little room for doubt.

INITIAL RADIO COMMUNICATIONS

During the course of daily operation, EMTs will have many opportunities to use the radio to keep the communications center apprised of their status. The dispatcher should always be made aware of the location of each in-service unit to ensure the most appropriate units are dispatched to calls.

During the course of an emergency call, the EMT should continue to apprise the dispatch center of the status of the call. Table 21-2 lists the common times the EMT would update the dispatch center. The needs of each emergency system are different, and the EMT should follow local protocols regarding notifications.

HOSPITAL COMMUNICATIONS

There are two common reasons for an EMT to use a radio to call the emergency department. The first reason is to contact medical direction regarding the patient's condition and request or obtain orders the physician may have

Table 21-2 Notification Points During an Emergency Call

Event	Example of Transmission
Call received	"Dispatcher, Ambulance one received the information."
En route to scene	"Ambulance one is en route to 123 Main Street."
Arriving on scene	"Ambulance one is arriving at 123 Main Street."
Request additional resources when needed	"Dispatcher, send an ALS unit to 123 Main Street."
En route to hospital	"Ambulance one is en route to Memorial Hospital."
Hospital communications	As in Table 21-3
Arrival at hospital	"Ambulance one has arrived at Memorial Hospital."
Return to service	"Ambulance one is back in service, returning to quarters."
Arrival at quarters	"Ambulance one is back in quarters."

regarding patient care. This kind of radio report is understandably longer and more detailed than many other radio transmissions. This type of communication may be referred to as a *consultation*.

MEDICAL DIRECTION CONSULTATION

Most of an EMT's instructions for medical care are written in a set of orders called *protocols*. Protocols offer a standardized approach to caring for a typical patient. Some patients are not typical. In those cases, a consultation with a medical control physician is appropriate. The EMT is asking for on-line medical direction.

Several goals can be accomplished by calling for medical control. First, the doctor is alerted to the impending arrival of a complex patient. Second, the doctor will have advanced knowledge of the patient's condition and can more adequately prepare. Finally, the doctor can give patient-specific medical orders that may ease the patient's concern or improve his condition.

It is important that the EMT give a complete and accurate report to the doctor. For the EMT to be effective, the doctor needs the information she would get if she were physically with the patient. The EMT is the instrument the doctor can use in the field.

Table 21-3 details all the elements of a medical consultation report. Note that there are many similar elements in the prehospital radio report and the full medical consultation report. It is good practice to have a novice EMT practice several prehospital radio reports before trying the first medical consultation report.

All radio reports commence with the standard introduction—that is, hailing the hospital and providing the EMS unit identification. The EMT then proceeds with the patient's demographics: age, sex, and private physician.

The report of the patient's mental status and chief concern are the same as in the prehospital radio report, but more information is provided to the physician in the remainder of the medical consultation report.

Table 21-3 Elements of a Radio Report

Item of Information	Prehospital Radio Report	Consultation Report
Unit ID	X	X
Level of provider		X
Patient's age and sex	X	X
Chief concern	X	X
Brief history of present illness		X
Relevant past illnesses		X
Mental status	X	X
Vital signs	X	X
Pertinent findings on physical exam		X
Treatments in progress	X	X
Patient's response to care provided		X
Estimated time of arrival	X	X

The EMT should expand on the history of the present illness, following the SAMPLE format as discussed in Unit 18. It is important that the physician hear the patient's entire pertinent past medical history as well as any allergies and prescription medications the patient currently takes.

After describing the pertinent physical findings from the detailed physical examination, using the DCAP-BTLS format discussed in Unit 19, the EMT should give both the baseline and the most current set of vital signs.

Any treatments the EMT has instituted should be reported as well as the patient's response to those treatments; for example, "The patient was placed on high-flow oxygen and says it gave him some relief from his chest pain." End every report with the expected time of arrival (ETA). Then ask the physician whether she has any questions or needs further information.

ACCEPTING A MEDICAL ORDER

When a medical control doctor gives an order, it is important for the EMT to understand the order clearly. Several procedures decrease the likelihood of errors.

The EMT must be sure the information provided to medical direction has been communicated clearly and accurately and the orders given back to the EMT have been understood completely.

The EMT should use a technique of echoing what medical control communicates. For example, the physician gives the order. The EMT then repeats the order back and asks to have the read-back confirmed as correct. The physician then confirms the read-back. Notice that there are a minimum of three communications before an EMT accepts the order. This method of echoing should also be used when medical direction orders an EMT not to do a procedure normally performed for the concern being treated.

In some systems, another EMT has to hear the order as well. Some radios have a speaker option that facilitates this process. In other cases, the EMT hands the radio or telephone to another EMT.

If unsure of the order, for whatever reason, the EMT should question the order. Repeat the report, or portions of it, if it appears that the physician did not understand the situation and ask the physician if there are any further questions.

PREHOSPITAL RADIO REPORT

The other reason to make a radio call is to alert the emergency department of the patient's impending arrival. This is the most common type of report. Medical orders are not being requested, nor are they expected. This report should be concise. Typically, this report can be given in less than 30 seconds. The person who takes this report then advises the attending physician, the triage nurse, the charge nurse, and other personnel of the situation. In this case, many important emergency team members may need to be prepared for the patient.

The elements of a complete report are listed in Table 21-3. Some elements are not needed in the brief initial notification report but may be required if the EMT is looking for medical consultation. These are indicated in Table 21-3. First, contact with the emergency department has to be made. The EMT should follow local protocols regarding how to initiate radio contact with the emergency department.

Once contact has been confirmed, the EMT should start by repeating the EMS unit identifier—for example, "Bay State ED, this is Ambulance one." Once the hospital acknowledges the transmission, begin the report. These first few words should be thought of as a standard introduction. It sets up both the speaker and the listener for the report to follow.

It is traditional among medical professionals to identify the age and sex of the patient at the beginning of the report—for example, "We have a 45-year-old male."

Some EMS systems add the patient's estimated weight. Other systems include the name of the patient's personal physician. If the age is unknown, then an estimate is usually given—for example, "We have an approximately 45-year-old male patient of Dr. Putnam."

The patient's chief concern lends a great deal of insight into the patient's problems. A patient's chief concern should be stated in the patient's own words, and in a single sentence.

The key to the patient's overall condition is mental status. Regardless of the cause, an unconscious patient is seriously ill and considered urgent. Typical descriptions of a patient's mental status include "awake and alert," "conscious but confused," or "unconscious." The EMT uses the AVPU (alert, voice, pain, unresponsive) scale when choosing a description.

Next, the EMT proceeds to the most recent set of vital signs. Minimally, this should include the patient's respiratory rate, pulse rate, blood pressure, and skin signs. Major treatments that have been provided should also be relayed. Finally, give the hospital an estimated time of arrival. Simply stated, "Our ETA is 5 minutes" allows the emergency department to adjust to the incoming workload. Patients may be either transferred or discharged to prepare a room for the incoming patient.

Street Smart

It may be helpful for the EMT to have a radio call form completed that contains those elements listed in Table 21-3. Using this form as a tool, the EMT would then have the information readily available to give in a concise radio report.

Street Smart

Some EMTs have a fear of the radio. The thought of speaking to a physician or a nurse is intimidating to them. The best way to get over this fear is through frequent practice.

Start by giving another EMT report, after the call. First, write the report down on a sheet of paper. Then read the report aloud like a movie script. Start by giving short alert reports, and then work up to a medical control report.

THE VERBAL REPORT

The **verbal report** is an expanded radio report an EMT gives to another health care provider who is taking over or joining the patient's care. Using the same information that was provided in the radio report, the EMT describes any changes in the patient's condition and provides a set of the most current vital signs.

The verbal report may be the single most important activity the EMT performs for a patient, especially for the patient who is unable to speak for herself. The key to effective communication is to tell the right person, at the right place, at the right time about the patient.

THE RIGHT PERSON

Tell the right person the patient's story. This may seem like common sense, but many EMTs have wasted a great deal of time telling the wrong person the patient's information.

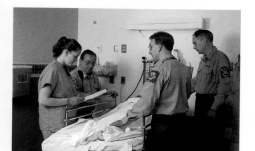

Figure 21.12 Most patient reports are received by a registered nurse at the bedside

A verbal report should be given to a nurse or physician at the bedside (Figure 21.12). Giving the report to the nurse is appropriate because the nurse will be coordinating the patient's care while she is in the hospital.

There are times when the patient's condition needs to be reported directly to the doctor. Whenever the patient's condition warrants immediate attention to prevent loss of life, then a doctor needs to be notified.

THE RIGHT PLACE

Consideration should be given to where the report is given. Family members and friends are often standing outside in the hall. These well-meaning people are listening for some hopeful news about the patient's condition.

Because they are not the intended audience and may not be knowledgeable about medical terminology, these people may misinterpret what they hear. In addition, the EMT must always remember that every patient has a right to **confidentiality.** The EMT must ensure that private medical information is provided only to those health care providers who will be caring for the patient. The EMT should take measures to ensure that nonprivileged personnel cannot overhear the report. Failure on the part of the EMT to notice that others are listening may be embarrassing or, worse, a breach of the patient's rights (Figure 21.13).

Most health care providers would prefer to get the patient's history directly from the patient, provided the patient is awake and alert. In those cases, the EMT should provide the health care provider pertinent information about the patient that the patient would not know. For example, the mechanism of injury, the significance of impact, and the patient's vital signs should be reported.

Common courtesy dictates that whenever a question can be answered by the patient, she should answer the question. The EMT should never give a report by talking over the patient. Ignoring the patient's attempt to answer questions and tell her story is discourteous and unprofessional. Always encourage the patient to enter the conversation at the appropriate time.

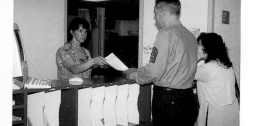

Figure 21.13 Caution should be exercised about what is said about the patient. The patient's condition should not be discussed with bystanders

THE RIGHT TIME

Although every patient is important, there are patient priorities, as discussed in Unit 16. The patient with a painful, swollen deformity on the hallway stretcher will have to wait while the busy emergency physician treats the patient in cardiac arrest in the trauma room.

The EMT should consider the patient's urgency before insisting on being heard by emergency department personnel. This simple courtesy improves relationships and ultimately speeds patient care.

INTERPERSONAL COMMUNICATION

Interpersonal communication is part speech and, in larger part, body language. Eye contact, gestures, and posture all communicate a message. Poor eye contact, for example, may indicate that the EMT lacks interest in the patient. This is not the message an EMT wants to convey to another health care professional.

Whenever an EMT gives a verbal report, the EMT should stand straight, look the other person in the eye, and give a clear report of the patient's condition. Facial expressions, tone of voice, and a quick response to questions convey the impression that the EMT is a caring professional.

COMMUNICATION BARRIERS

Communication barriers include language barriers, competing activities, and the ineffective delivery of the message or report.

"I know that's what you heard, but that's not what I said." This statement could be made by many EMTs. Some health care providers may rush to judgment because of personal bias, emotions, or beliefs, after listening to an EMT's report. A problem arises when those providers do not understand the patient's problems.

To prevent premature evaluation of a patient's problems, an EMT should try to give a complete report. If giving a complete report is not possible, then the EMT should focus the report on the most important aspects of the patient's condition.

If the message is not getting across to the other individual, the EMT should try a technique that communications specialists use called **repetitive persistence.** While remaining calm and in control, the EMT simply repeats the message until he is sure the message has been understood.

Communication is a two-way street. The EMT may also fail to understand the questions that are asked of him. To prevent this failure to communicate, simply stop, look, and listen. Stop whatever it is you are doing. Look at the person who is speaking to you. Listen to the person, giving him your undivided attention. Review Unit 17 detailing therapeutic communication.

CONCLUSION

EMS system communication use is an everyday part of the EMT's responsibility. It is important to understand the basic concepts behind radio operation and when to use each form of communication device. Part of the job with which every EMT must be familiar is proper radio terminology and etiquette. The key elements of communication during an emergency call, including hospital notification, should be practiced by the new EMT.

The purpose of a patient report is to communicate urgent patient information to someone who can do something. Therefore, careful attention to the right person, place, and time will increase the impact of an EMT's patient report.

The EMT should take the time to stop, look, and listen to the person who is asking questions. The EMT may be the only person who can answer these questions, and the answers are essential to patient care. Failures of communication can be costly in terms of money, time, and more importantly, lives.

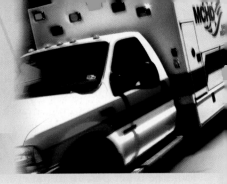

CASE STUDY Continued

Kent and his partner assess and package Mr. Kase, immobilizing his hips before beginning transport to the hospital. Kent's partner radios the communications center they are en route to the hospital. Dispatch acknowledges en route to hospital 07:25.

While en route, Kent calls the hospital by cellular phone and gives a brief verbal patient report, stating Mr. Kase's age and gender, physician, chief concern, pertinent past medical history, vital signs, treatments, and estimated time of arrival in 10 minutes. The hospital acknowledges Kent's report and advises they will receive a room assignment upon arrival.

As they pull into the hospital, Kent's partner radios the communication center they have arrived at their destination. Dispatch acknowledges arrived at hospital 07:40. Kent turns Mr. Kase over to the ED staff with a verbal report given at that time. Kent then writes a patient care report (PCR), leaving a copy with the nurse who has assumed Mr. Kase's care.

As Kent and his partner return to service, they notify the communication's center squad 81-40 has completed assignment and is available for service. Dispatch acknowledges: "Squad 81-40, back in service, 08:15."

Key Concepts Revisited

- All EMS communication is done via the emergency services communications system.

- Definitive patient care begins with effective communication between the public, emergency services personnel, and hospital staff.

- The role of the communications specialist is to coordinate all aspects of an emergency response.

- The core of most modern emergency service communications systems is the two-way radio system.

- A communications system comprises:
  - Base radios
  - Mobile radios
  - Portable radios
  - Repeaters
  - Digital radio equipment
  - Computers and radios
  - Telephones
  - Cellular phones
  - Satellite telephones

- The Federal Communications Commission is responsible for
  - Allocation of radio frequencies
  - Licensing
  - Issuing call signs
  - Monitoring radio operations

- The FCC has designated a specific group, or band, of radio frequencies for use by EMS providers.
  - Med channels used by hospitals and EMS
  - 220-MHz band set aside for EMS
  - Radio channels specific to EMS system communications

- The dispatch frequency is reserved for communications between EMS units in the field and the communications center.

- The use of basic radio procedures begins with familiarity with the function of radio.
  - Proper radio procedure begins with the "you first then me" approach.
  - Do not use unnecessary communications, courtesy is assumed.

- The dispatcher should be aware of the location of each in-service unit.

- Medical control consultation and the prehospital radio report are the two most common communications conducted with the hospital.

- Medical control consultation is conducted when on-line medical direction is needed.
  - Repeat orders back for clarification.
  - Have repeated order confirmed.
  - Do not complete an order not completely understood.
- The prehospital radio report alerts the hospital of impending arrival of a patient and a brief description of the patient's concern.
- The verbal report is an expanded radio report an EMT will give to another health care provider who is taking over.
- The verbal report effectively describes the patient to:
  - The right person,
  - At the right place,
  - At the right time.
- Interpersonal communication is comprised of both speech and body language.
- Communications barriers can prevent the right information from being communicated and understood.
- Avoid communication barriers through the stop, look, and listen technique.
- EMS system communication use is an everyday part of the EMT's responsibility.

Review Questions

1. What are the roles of communications specialists?
2. What are the components of a typical radio system?
3. What is the role of the Federal Communications Commission?
4. How has modern technology advanced communications?
5. What are the basic radio procedures for initiating and terminating a radio call?
6. What are the elements of a medical direction consultation report?
7. What are the elements of a prehospital radio report?
8. When is radio communication generally conducted during an emergency call?
9. What is the importance of a verbal report?
10. What are the three "rights" of effective communication?
11. What are the barriers to effective communication?
12. How can EMTs overcome communications barriers?

Key Terms

Base station
Call sign
Channel guard
Communications specialist (COMSPEC)
Confidentiality
Duplex
Federal Communications Commission (FCC)
Med channels
Mobile radio
Multiplex radio
Portable radio

Radio head
Repeater
Repetitive persistence
Simplex
Stand by
Telemetry
Trunked line
Two-way radio
UHF
Verbal report
VHF

UNIT (22) Medical Terminology

Medicine is full of terms and abbreviations for terms. To communicate clearly with other EMTs and health care providers, the EMT needs to know how to use proper medical terminology. By examining common grammatical rules to see how words can be broken down to their simple meanings, terms can be understood and used in verbal reports and patient care records.

National Education Standard

The Emergency Medical Technician (EMT) shall be able to use a foundational knowledge of anatomical and medical terms and abbreviations in written and oral communication with colleagues and other health care professionals.

Key Concepts

- All medical terms can be broken down into their fundamental parts for easier comprehension.

- Root words within medical terminology convey the main meaning or idea of the term.

- Prefixes and suffixes complement a root word's meaning.

- Proper pronunciation of many difficult medical terms requires practice and perfect articulation.

- The correct spelling of medical terminology is important because it reflects on the EMT and EMS.

- Standard abbreviations can be helpful in communicating a message, provided that they are used correctly.

- Medical terms are used to describe many facets of medicine, including topographic anatomy, patient condition, diseases, and syndromes.

"What, the. . .?" Dean thinks as he watches the front door close. Dean and his partner have been dispatched to meet with a homecare health aide who is caring for an elderly male in his 80s. When they arrive, the aide explains that the patient, Mr. Washington, had been running a fever of unknown origin and his private physician asked that he be transported immediately to the hospital for evaluation. Then the aide briskly turns around and leaves, shouting over her shoulder that she has other clients to see and wishes them good luck. All she leaves in Dean's hands are some rather cryptic handwritten notes using a whole bunch of terms that he doesn't understand.

Dean thinks to himself, "This stuff looks Greek to me." Underneath the aide's notes are three pages of medical documentation. Most of it uses medical terms and abbreviations that Dean has never seen before. Dean is starting to get a little more than agitated. His partner is not trained as an EMT and was only recently cleared as a driver. So he won't be any help trying to sort through all this paperwork.

Dean just wants to understand the patient's previous conditions so that he can relate to the patient. Dean understands that a knowledge of the patient's past medical history, as well as the history of the present illness, will help him be better prepared in case an emergency should arise.

To worsen the situation, it quickly becomes apparent to Dean that Mr. Washington suffers from dementia and will be unable to answer his questions coherently. In other words, the patient will be no help to Dean as he tries to understand his medical condition. With all this, Dean elects to package the patient as quickly as possible and transport Mr. Washington to the hospital, hoping the hospital staff can make some sense of the notes and paperwork.

Critical Thinking Questions

1. Why is documentation important?
2. What are the obstacles to communication?
3. Why does this EMT need to know about the patient's history of present illness and past medical history?

INTRODUCTION

While reading a patient's chart from a nursing home transfer or overhearing a conversation between a physician and a paramedic, the EMT may come across or hear many unfamiliar terms and wonder what they mean. These medical terms may appear difficult to learn and even more difficult to pronounce. The EMT might even think she needs to learn a whole new language. That would be correct. The language of medicine is called *medicalese*, first discussed in Unit 17. By understanding a few rules of medical terminology, the EMT can quickly decipher a term's meaning. At first the EMT will learn a few key terms; over time, her vocabulary will expand and she will likely become fluent in medicalese. This chapter is an overview of terms and abbreviations commonly used by EMTs and all medical professionals.

ANATOMY OF MEDICAL TERMINOLOGY

By following several basic rules, the EMT can understand and learn medical terminology. First, most medical terms consist of four parts, the root word(s), a prefix and/or a suffix, and a combining form. A combining form is not used in every case; nor are prefixes or suffixes. These parts can be thought of as the building blocks of medical terminology. To read and understand a term, the EMT need only dissect the term into its various parts, interpret each part, and form an understanding of the meaning of the entire word.

READING MEDICAL TERMINOLOGY

When both a suffix and a prefix are used in a word, the suffix is read first, then the root, and then the prefix (read last, middle, and first part). For example, the term *hypoglycemia* has "gly" as its root, which refers to glucose. But to read this term correctly, first read the suffix, "emia", referring to blood, then "gly," and then "hypo," meaning low. Together the term means blood with sugar low, or low blood sugar.

All medical terms are read backward—that is, from right to left. This concept is difficult for most people, who have been educated to read from left to right. It takes practice to become proficient at deciphering medical terminology right to left. With a little practice, the EMT rapidly becomes proficient at learning the meaning of these terms and can incorporate them into the documentation and communication.

ROOT WORDS

A **root word,** sometimes called the *stem,* relates to the main idea and serves as the foundation of the word. A root word often describes the organ involved or the key symptom. For example, "cardi/o" means the heart. Learning root words means memorizing these words. Fortunately, using prefixes and/or suffixes, many terms are built from a relative handful of root words. Prefixes and/or suffixes build on a root word to give it a more specific meaning. Some terms use a combining form, described later, to connect several root words. For example electrocardiogram (ECG), pronounced (ee – lek – troh – CAR – dee – oh – gram) is divided into three roots, "electro" for electrical, "cardi/o" meaning heart, and "gram" for record. An ECG is a recording of the heart electricity. Table 22-1 lists some common root words used in medical terminology.

Table 22-1 Common Word Roots Used in Medical Terms

Root	Meaning	Root	Meaning	Root	Meaning
Arthr/o-	Joint	Hem/o-	Blood	Path/o-	Disease
Card/o-	Heart	Hepat/o-	Liver	Ped/o-	Children
Cephal/o-	Head	Ile/o-	Small intestine	Ren/o-	Kidneys
Cerebr/o-	Cerebrum	Nephr/o-	Kidneys	Splen/o-	Spleen
Enter/o-	Intestines	Neur/o-	Nerves	Thromb/o-	Clot
Gastr/o-	Stomach	Oste/o-	Bone	Trach/o-	Trachea

Table 22-2 Partial List of Medical Prefixes

Prefix	Meaning	Prefix	Meaning	Prefix	Meaning
a/-	"without"	hydro/-	"water"	patho/-	"suffering"
ab/-	"from," "away from"	hypo/-	"beneath," "low"	phlebo/-	"vein"
ad/-	"toward"	macro/-	"large," "long"	pneumo/-	"air"
ambi/-	"both"	mega/-	"great"	poly/-	"many"
dia/-	"throughout"	micro/-	"small"	pro/-	"before"
entero/-	"within"	neo/-	"new"	tachy/-	"rapid"
hetero/-	"different"	orth/-	"straight"	trans/-	"across"
homo/-	"same"	osteo/-	"bone"		
hyper/-	"beyond," "high"	oto/-	"ear"		

MEDICAL PREFIX

When a **prefix** complements a root, it is placed at the beginning of the root and adds meaning to the word. Take, for example, the word *pericardium* (per – ih – CAR – dee – um). The root, on the right, is "cardi," meaning heart. The prefix, "peri," means around, so the term pericardium would mean "around the heart." Table 22-2 shows prefixes commonly used in medical terminology.

PREFIXES DESCRIBING COLOR

Some prefixes describe color. For example, *cyanosis* (sigh – ah – NO – sis) means "blue – condition." It describes the skin color of oxygen-deprived, or hypoxic (high – pox – ick) patients. Table 22-3 lists some common prefixes for basic colors.

PREFIXES DESCRIBING POSITION

Some prefixes refer to the position of something in relation to something else. For example, a shoulder dislocation (diss – loh – KAY – shun) would mean a shoulder apart from the bone socket. Table 22-4 provides a partial list of common prefixes used to describe position.

NUMERICAL PREFIXES

Some prefixes are used to describe a number, not as an integer like one, two, three, but as a description. For example, the word *hemiplegia* means "half paralyzed." Table 22-5 lists some common prefixes that mean numbers.

MEDICAL SUFFIX

A **suffix** complements a root when it is placed behind the root and changes the meaning of the term. Using the term, *myocarditis* (my- oh – car – DYE – tis), for example, and reading from right to left, the term "-i" means inflammation,

Table 22-3 Prefixes of Color

Alb/-	"White"
Chlor/-	"Green"
Cyan/-	"Blue"
Rube/-	"Red"
Glauco/-	"Grey"
Leuk/-	"White"
Melan/-	"Black"

Table 22-4 Prefixes of Position

Ad/-	"toward"	Epi/-	"upon"	Posto/-	"after"
Ante/-	"in front"	Later/-	"side"	Pre/-	"in front"
Anti/-	"against"	Eco/-	"out"	Pro/-	"in front"
Apo/-	"separate"	Endo/-	"in"	Re/-	"again"
Circum/-	"around"	Exo/-	"out"	Retro/-	"backward"
Contra/-	"against"	Intra/-	"within"	Trans/-	"through"
Dia/-	"through"	Inter/-	"in between"	Ventro/-	"in front"
Dis/-	"apart"	Opistho/-	"backward"		
Dorso/-	"back"	Peri/-	"around"		

Table 22-5 Prefixes of Numbers

Aniso/-	"unequal"	Iso/-	"equal"	Oligo/-	"few"
Bi/-	"two"	Macro/-	"large"	Pan/-	"all"
Diplo/-	"double"	Mega/-	"large"	Poly/-	"many"
Hemi/-	"half"	Micro/-	"small"	Prim/-	"first"
Hyper/-	"above"	Milli/-	"one thousandth"	Prot/-	"first"
Hypo/-	"below"	Mono/-	"single"		
In/-	"none"	Multi/-	"many"		

the term "cardi-" means heart, and the prefix "myo" means muscle. The term *myocarditis* means an inflammation of the cardiac muscle. Table 22-6 shows some common suffixes used in medical terminology.

MEDICAL CONDITIONS AND SURGICAL SUFFIXES

Many medical diagnostic procedures and surgical operations have a medical term. These terms are used to vividly describe the procedure or operation with a minimum of words. For medical documentation, brevity is important, and these terms are descriptive with a conservation of words. Table 22-7 and Table 22-8 list some of the common medical and surgical procedures.

MEDICAL INSTRUMENT SUFFIXES

Similarly medical terms are used to describe medical instruments and surgical tools. Table 22-9 lists some suffixes used to describe medical instruments.

Table 22-6 Partial List of Common Suffixes for Diagnosis

Suffix	Meaning	Used	Pronunciation	Meaning
-algia	Pain	Neuralgia	noo – RAL – jee – ah	Nerve Pain
-al	Pertains to	Spinal	SPY – n – all	Spine
-emia	Blood	Anemia	an – NEE – mee – ah	Without Blood
-ic	Pertains to	Pelvic	pell – vik	Pertains to Pelvis
-itis	Inflamed	Pharyngitis	fair – in – JYE – tis	Sore Throat
-phasia	Speech	Aphasia	ah – FAY – zee – ah	Without Speech
-plegia	Paralysis	Hemiplegia	hem – ee – PLEE – jee – ah	Half paralyzed

Table 22-7 Surgical Suffixes

Suffix	Meaning	Used	Pronunciation	Meaning
-ectomy	Removal	Appendectomy	ap –PEN – deck – toe –me	Remove Appendix
-centesis	Drain	Pericardiocentesis	car – dee – oh – sen – TEE – sis	Drain around Heart
-ize	To Make	Anesthetize	an – ess – THEE – ties	Without Feeling
-lysis	Divide	Fibrinolysis	fih – BRIN – o – lye –sis	Divide Clot
-plasty	Repair	Angioplasty	an – jee – o – plas – tee	Repair Artery
-stomy	Opening	Tracheostomy	TRAY – kee – os – to – mee	Hole in Throat

Table 22-8 Medical Suffixes

Suffix	Meaning	Used	Pronunciation	Meaning
-iac	Afflicted	Hemophiliac	hee – moh – FILL – i – ack	Blood Disorder
-ism	Condition	Alcoholism	al – CO – hall – is – em	Alcohol Disease
-ist	Expert	Cardiologist	car – dee – ALL – oh – jist	Heart Doctor

Table 22-9 Diagnostic Suffixes for Medical Instruments

Suffix	Meaning	Used	Pronunciation	Meaning
-gram	Record	Electrocardiogram	ee – lek – troh – CAR – dee – oh – gram	ECG
-meter	Measuring	Capnometer	cap – NO – me – ter	Measures CO_2
-scope	Instrument	Laryngoscope	lair – in – JYE – scope	Throat Tool

COMBINING FORMS

A **combining form** is used when two or more roots are placed together. These root words must be separated by a vowel. These are basic rules of the Greek and Latin languages. Physicians often use these combining forms to explain a complex process. For example, the term *cardiomyopathy* has as its roots "cardi-," meaning heart; "my," meaning muscle; and "patho," meaning disease. The letter O separates the roots cardi, my, and path. Cardiomyopathy, reading from right to left, means disease of the muscle of the heart.

Sometimes two root terms are used and a combining vowel must be used to make the two root terms distinguishable but connected. Typically the letter "o" is used. For example, cardi – o – logy is the study of the heart.

However, if the root word ends with a vowel, then it is unnecessary to use a combining vowel. For example, combining cyst- with -itis would be cystitis, not cystoitis. Table 22-10 shows some common examples of combining terms.

PLURAL FORMS

When more than one thing is being described by the EMT, a **plural form** is needed. To establish a plural meaning from a singular word, the EMT only needs to apply a few rules. For example, if the singular word ends with "ax," then remove the "ax" and replace it with "aces" to make the meaning of the word plural. Table 22-11 shows the rules for making plural forms.

PRONUNCIATION

Mispronunciation of a medical term makes the EMT appear uneducated, and patients may question her competency. Proper pronunciation of medical terms is important to learn. Proper pronunciation of medical terms is key to the patient's understanding as well as effective communication with fellow health care providers. While verbalizing these terms may seem difficult, dissection of the term to its constituent parts (root, suffix, and prefix), and careful articulation will likely produce satisfactory results.

Often other medical professionals will help to correct errors in inflection or in pronunciation. By repeating the corrected pronunciation, the EMT helps to commit the term to memory. Furthermore, computer-assisted pronunciation guides for medical terminology are available. A computer with a speaker is all that is needed to hear the medical term spoken. Finally, almost all medical schools, nursing schools, and allied health schools offer courses in medical terminology, usually at a modest cost.

As with all languages, there are some regional dialects that make the same word sound different. Whenever there is a question, the term should be spelled out. This is particularly important in radio communication, where

Table 22-10 Examples of Combining Terms

Suffix	Meaning	Used	Pronunciation	Meaning
-edema	Swelling	Laryngoedema	lah – ring – go – e – dem – a	Swollen Throat
-ist	Practitioner	Hemotologist	hee – mah – TALL – oh – jist	Blood Doctor
-lysis	Divide	Hemolysis	hee – MALL – ih – sis	Blood Dissolved
-megaly	Enlarged	Cardiomegaly	car – dee – oh – meg – a – le	Enlarged Heart
-oma	Tumor	Carcinoma	kar – sin – NOH – mah	Cancer Growth
-pnea	Breathing	Orthopnea	or – THOP – nee – ah	Short of Breath
-pathy	Disease	Neuropathy	ner – OP – Po – thee	Nerve Disease
-rrhage	Burst	Hemorrhage	HEM – rij	Bleeding
-rrhea	Discharge	Otorrhea	oh – toh – REE – ah	Ear Discharge
-scopy	Visualize	Bronchoscopy	brong – KOSS – koh – pee	Throat Inspect
-spasm	Contraction	Bronchospasm	brong – koh – spa – sim	Bronchi Contraction
-stomy	Surgical Hole	Tracheostomy	tray – KEE – os – to – me	Hole in Neck

Table 22-11 Making Plural Forms of Terms

Singular Form		Plural Form	
-a		add	-e
-ax	drop -ax	add	-aces
-en	drop -en	add	-ina
-is	drop -is	add	-es
-ix	drop -ix	add	-ices
-sis	drop -sis	add	-ses
-um	drop -um	add	-a
-us	drop -us	add	-i
-x	drop -x	add	-es
-y	drop -y	add	-ies

Street Smart

While speaking medicalese is an expectation between medical professionals, it is unwise and inappropriate to use medical terminology with a patient. The EMT must be adept at translating a medical term and explaining it in plain English to the patient.

two words with a similar pronunciation can have very different meanings (e.g., hypo and hyper).

SPELLING

Correct spelling of medical terms is important for several reasons. First, the prehospital patient care record is read by other health care professionals. Misspelled words are confusing and tend to reflect poorly on the EMT. In addition, the patient care record may be used for purposes of revenue recovery. Medical coders, people who use numeric identification of medical conditions for purposes of billing insurance companies, may not correctly code a condition if the condition is misspelled. Finally, the patient care report may be used in a court of law. It is a problem when an attorney cannot understand what the EMT has written. It can be embarrassing when an attorney points out misspelling in a court of law, in front of a jury, suggesting the EMT is amateurish, unqualified, or incompetent.

It is not enough to try to phonetically spell out a word. Many medical terms have similar sounding components but are spelled differently. Spelling them correctly can be difficult, especially if the EMT hears the word spoken and then must spell it. For example, the "si" sound can be spelled with "psy," as in psychiatry, "sy" as in symptom, or "cy" as in cystitis. To avoid errors and confusion, the term should be spelled correctly. When in doubt, the EMT should consult a medical dictionary for the correct spelling. Small, pocket-sized medical spellers are available, as well as medical spellers for pocket computers.

TOPOGRAPHIC ANATOMY

Medical terminology includes a number of positional and directional terms. These terms direct an EMT to an area of the body or the organs involved. To serve as a reference, the body is divided into three planes. The frontal plane divides the body in half, front from back. The sagittal plane divides the body from left to right and the transverse plane divides the body into upper and lower. With these reference points in place, the EMT can more accurately describe a specific location on the body using topographic anatomy.

In every case the assumption is that the patient is standing in the standard anatomical position—that is, the patient is standing upright, eyes forward, hands to the side, with the palms of the hand forward and feet together. Table 22-12 lists the body's cavities. Table 22-13 lists some of the more common directional terms used in topographic anatomy. Tables 22-14, 22-15, and 22-16 present terms introduced in Unit 5 and reviewed here.

Table 22-12 Body Cavities

Term	Pronunciation
Abdominal	ab – DOM – ih – nal
Cranial	KRAY – nee – al
Pelvic	PELL – vik
Spinal	SPY – in – al
Thoracic	tho – Rass – ic

Table 22-13 Directional Terms

Term	Plane	Relation	Description
Caudal	Transverse	Inferior	Toward the feet
Cephalic	Transverse	Superior	Toward the head
Dorsal	Frontal	Inferior	Toward the back
Ventral	Frontal	Anterior	Toward the front

Table 22-14 Relational Terms

Term	Description
Apex	Top of the pyramid
Base	Bottom of the pyramid
Distal	Away from the structure
Lateral	To the side of the structure
Medial	Toward the structure
Deep	Away from the surface
Superficial	Toward the surface

Table 22-15 Terms Describing Patient Positions

Term	Description
Prone	Lying on belly
Supine	Lying on back
Left Lateral	Lying on left side
Fowlers	Sitting upright
Trendelenburg	Supine with legs elevated
Sims	Knee to chest

Table 22-16 Terms Describing Movement

Term	Description	Term	Description
Abduction	Away from midline	Extension	Straightening
Adduction	Toward the midline	Flexion	Bending
Circumduction	Circular motion	Inversion	Turn inward
Dorsiflexion	Backward	Pronation	Turn downward
Eversion	Turn outward	Supination	Turn upward

ABBREVIATIONS

The reason for abbreviations is brevity, meaning short and concise, and EMTs strive to be short and concise in their patient care reports (PCRs). The correct use of abbreviations can help with that process, provided that the meaning of the communication is not lost in the process. Problems can occur when an abbreviation stands for two different things. For example, the abbreviation "Ca" can mean both calcium and cancer.

Universality is another problem. Universality means that everyone knows the meaning of the abbreviation. Emergency physicians, critical care nurses, allied health care professionals, EMS managers, EMS educators, and attorneys are just a few of the people who may read a PCR. Without a common understanding, abbreviations can become meaningless to the reader, and the PCR loses its potency as a tool for communication. For this reason many EMTs use a regionally accepted list of abbreviations or refer to the list of accepted abbreviations that exist at the hospital; hospitals often have a posted list of accepted abbreviations.

Abbreviations can sometimes lead to miscommunication. As a result of common medical errors, some abbreviations are no longer accepted. For example, the abbreviation for morphine sulfate is MSO_4. Unfortunately, the abbreviation MSO_4 may be confused with $MgSO_4$, which is magnesium sulfate. For this reason clinicians, including EMTs, should spell out the abbreviation MSO_4 as morphine to decrease confusion and prevent errors.

To help head off miscommunication, many EMS agencies have a list of accepted abbreviations. This list is usually gleaned from a similar list of abbreviations used by health care professionals at the local hospital(s). Table 22-17 is one example of an accepted abbreviation list, *provided for illustrative purposes only*. EMTs should obtain and use a similar list.

Street Smart

Whenever there is a possibility that an abbreviation might be unclear to another health care provider, the word should be spelled out. The maxim is "when in doubt, spell it out."

Table 22-17 List of Common Abbreviations

ā	before	A fib	atrial fibrillation
AAA	abdominal aortic aneurysm	AIDS	acquired immune deficiency syndrome
AAL	anterior axillary line	ALS	advanced life support
AB	abortion	AMA	against medical advice
ABCs	airway, breathing, circulation	AMI	acute myocardial infarction
Abd	abdominal	AMS	altered mental status
ACLS	advanced cardiac life support	A/O	alert and oriented
ADL	activities of daily living	A/P	anterior - posterior
AED	automatic external defibrillator	ASA	aspirin

Table 22-17 List of Common Abbreviations (continued)

ATV	automatic transport ventilator		CPR	cardiopulmonary resuscitation
AV	atrio-ventricular		CSF	cerebrospinal fluid
BAC	blood alcohol content		CSM	circulatory/sensory/motor function
BG	blood glucose		CT	computerized tomography
BLS	basic life support		CVA	cerebral vascular accident
BM	bowel movement		D5W	5% dextrose in sterile water
BP	blood pressure		d/c	discontinue
BPM	beats per minute		DKA	diabetic ketoacidosis
BVM	bag valve mask		DM	diabetes mellitus
/c̄	with		DOA	dead on arrival
C	Celcius/centigrade		DOB	date of birth
Ca	cancer		DOE	dyspnea on exertion
CABG	coronary artery bypass graft		DTs	delirium tremens
CAD	coronary artery disease		Dr.	doctor
c/c	chief concern		Dx	diagnosis
cc	cubic centimeters		ECG	electrocardiogram
CHF	congestive heart failure		EID	esophageal intubation detector
CNS	central nervous system		EJV	external jugular vein
c/o	complained of		EMD	emergency medical dispatch
CO	carbon monoxide		EMT	Emergency Medical Technician
CO_2	carbon dioxide		EMS	Emergency Medical Service
COPD	chronic obstructive pulmonary disease		EPI	epinephrine
CP	chest pain		Eq	equivalents

(continued)

Table 22-17 List of Common Abbreviations *(continued)*

ET	endotracheal tube	ICU	intensive care unit
ETA	estimated time of arrival	IDDM	insulin dependent diabetes mellitus
EtOH	ethyl alcohol	IM	intramuscular
°F	Fahrenheit	IO	intraosseous
FU	follow up	IV	intravenous
FUO	fever of unknown origin	IVP	IV push (medication)
Fx	fracture	JVD	jugular venous distention
GCS	Glascow Coma Score	KED	Kendrick Extrication Device
GI	gastrointestinal	Kg	Kilogram
GSW	gunshot wound	KVO	keep vein open
gtt	drops	L	liter
GU	genitourinary	Lac	laceration
GYN	gynecologic	LLQ	left lower quadrant
Hr	hour	LMP	last menstrual period
HBO	hyperberic oxygen	LPN	licensed practical nurse
HBV	hepatitis B virus	LOC	loss of consciousness
HIV	human immunodeficiency virus	LR	lactated ringers solution
h/o	history of	LUQ	left upper quadrant
HPI	history of the present illness	MCI	multiple casualty incident
HTN	hypertension	MCL	modified chest lead
Hx	history	MD	physician
ICP	intracranial pressure	mEq	milliequivalents

Table 22-17 List of Common Abbreviations *(continued)*

mg	milligram		OTC	over-the-counter
MI	myocardial infarction		oz	ounce
mL	milliliter		P	pulse
mm	millimeter		P	after
mmHg	millimeter mercury		PA	physician assistant
MVC	motor vehicle collision		PAC	premature atrial contraction
N/A	not applicable		PAT	paroxysmal atrial tachycardia
NAD	no apparent distress		PCN	penicillin
NG	nasogastric		PE	physical exam
NKA	no known allergies		PERRL	pupils equal, round and reactive to light
NPA	nasal pharyngeal airway		PIAA	personal injury auto accident
NPO	nothing by mouth (nil per os)		PID	pelvic inflammatory disease
NRB	non-rebreather face mask		PJC	premature junctional contraction
NS	normal saline		PMH	past medical history
NSR	normal sinus rhythm		PND	paroxysmal nocturnal dyspnea
NTG	nitroglycerin		PO	by mouth
N/V	nausea and vomiting		Pm	as needed
O_2	oxygen		Pt	patient
OB/GYN	obstetrics/gynecology		PVC	premature ventricular contraction
OD	overdose		Q	every
OPA	oral pharyngeal airway		Qh	every hour
OR	operating room		Qid	four times a day

(continued)

Table 22-17 List of Common Abbreviations *(continued)*

RLQ	right lower quadrant		TIA	transient ischemic attack
RMA	refused medical assistance		Tid	three times a day
RN	registered nurse		TKO	to keep open
ROM	range of motion		TOT	turned over to
RUQ	right upper quadrant		Tx	treatment
r/o	rule out		URI	upper respiratory infection
RR	respiratory rate		UTI	urinary tract infection
Rx	prescription or treatment		VD	venereal disease
S	without		VS	vital signs
SIDS	sudden infant death syndrome		VF/VFib	ventricular fibrillation
SE	sublingual		VT	ventricular tachycardia
SOB	shortness of breath		w/	with
SQ/SC	subcutaneous		WNL	within normal limits
SSCP	substernal chest pain		w/o	without
STD	sexually transmitted disease		y/o	year old
STAT	immediately		xport	transport
TB	tuberculosis			

MEDICAL SYMBOLS

Table 22-18 lists some symbols commonly used by EMTs. Although these symbols are useful in many instances, there may be some cases in which using the symbol is more confusing than spelling out its meaning. In such instances, it is better to opt for clarity and spell out the meaning of the symbol.

DOCUMENTING NUMBERS

In some cases confusion occurs when numbers are read. To simplify documentation and to prevent errors, there are several simple rules for recording numbers. Whole numbers are always documented as whole numbers, such as 1 or 2, and are never followed by a decimal point and zero, such as 1.0, which might be mistaken for 10.

Similarly, decimal fractions are always preceded by a zero. For example one half is documented as 0.5. Reading .5 (read as point five) might be confused with 5, and an error might be made.

If the number is both whole and fraction, such as 1.5, an effort should be made to round the number to a whole number; rules of rounding make the number go to the higher number if the fraction is five or more. For example, 1.5 would be documented as 2. However, if the number must include the fraction for accuracy, then the EMT should consider spelling it out, such as one point five. Or the EMT could exaggerate the decimal point for legibility.

CONCLUSION

Abbreviations and medical terminology used inappropriately serve only to confuse the message. The EMT should never be afraid to refer to a medical dictionary or speller, or ask another health care provider how to pronounce or spell a word. Ultimately if the EMT cannot spell or speak the term, the idea she is trying to impart should be conveyed in simpler terms. But the EMT should go back and try to learn that term later.

Medical terminology is a part of the language of medicine. Understanding and using these terms correctly aids in communication with other medical professionals. The EMT should learn how to write and speak that language. With practice and careful use, the EMT can learn medicalese and become fluent with fellow health care professionals.

Table 22-18 Approved Symbols

Symbol	Meaning
+○	Female
←○	Male
=	Equal
+	Positive
−	Negative
>	Increase
<	Decrease
△	Change
R	Right
L	Left
×	Times or multiply

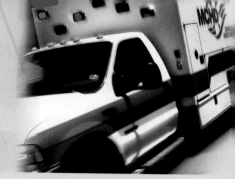

CASE STUDY Continued

When Dean arrives at the hospital, he explains the situation to the nurse. Sensing the opportunity for a "teachable moment," the nurse elects to take 5 minutes to review the chart with Dean.

First she translates the patient's medical conditions into plain English and encourages Dean to write this information in his notepad for future reference. Then she explains some of the abbreviations to Dean. But before

Dean can write them down, she hands him a copy of the hospital's accepted abbreviations from the policy and procedures manual.

Dean carefully folds the abbreviations, places them inside his pocket notepad, and thanks the nurse for her understanding and assistance. Leaving the emergency department, Dean thinks to himself, "This is a good day. I learned something new today."

Key Concepts Revisited

- The parts of medical terms include the root, prefix, suffix, and combining form.
- Medical terms are generally read from right to left.
- Prefixes and suffixes complement a root word's meaning.
- Proper pronunciation requires practice and perfect articulation.

- Correct spelling of medical terminology improves the quality of medical records.
- The use of standard abbreviations is acceptable provided everyone knows the abbreviations.
- Medical terms are used to describe many facets of medicine, including topographic anatomy.

Review Questions

1. What are the four basic parts of a medical term?
2. How are medical terms generally read?
3. What is a root word?
4. What is a prefix?
5. What is a suffix?
6. What is a combining form?
7. What is the purpose of the plural form of a term?
8. How can an EMT learn proper pronunciation of a medical term?
9. Where can an EMT check the spelling of a medical term?
10. Where can an EMT get a list of commonly accepted abbreviations?

Key Terms

Combining form
Plural form
Prefix

Root word
Suffix

Further Study

Jones, Betty. *Delmar's Comprehensive Medical Terminology: A Competency Based Approach.* Clifton Park, NY: Thomson Delmar Learning, 1999.

MedicineNet.com: Medical Dictionary, http://www.medterms.com/script/main/hp.asp

MediLexicon: Medical Dictionary, Medical Terminology: http://www.medilexicon.com/medicaldictionary.php

Nagel, K. R. "Prohibited Abbreviations." *American Journal of Health-System Pharmacy* 62, no. 15 (2005): 1559.

UNIT (23) Documentation

"The job isn't over until the paperwork is done." State and federal regulations, insurance carriers, and the courts all demand complete and accurate documentation. Complete and accurate documentation of medical care is a fundamental function of every health care professional, including the Emergency Medical Technician (EMT).

An EMT, as a part of the medical team, is held to the same documentation standards as any other health care provider. The **patient care report (PCR)** must include the history of the patient's illness, the findings of the physical examination, the treatments rendered, and any difficulties or complications that were encountered in the course of patient care.

National Education Standard

The Emergency Medical Technician (EMT) will display a fundamental depth and foundational breadth of understanding in the principles of medical documentation and ability of report writing.

Key Concepts

- Complete and accurate documentation of medical care is a fundamental function of the EMT.

- The function of the prehospital PCR is documentation of the patient's condition and prehospital treatments.

- The PCR is a legal document.

- State and federal governments have established minimum data sets for patient care documentation.

- Documentation can be in written or electronic forms, using a variety of formats.

- The EMT can use certain principles of documentation to ensure complete, accurate, and timely patient care record keeping.

- The standards of documentation communicate the patient's condition to other health care providers accurately and legibly.

- The EMT must not attempt to omit or alter facts in documentation to cover up an error.

- A special report form is used for documentation of incidents such as crew injuries or equipment problems.

- The EMT must document the patient's decision to refuse treatment and transport very carefully.

- The PCR is the EMT's primary record of patient care.

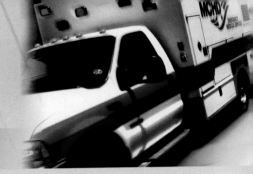

CASE STUDY

Mr. Thominnson has called for EMS only a couple of times since moving in to the retirement village. He has a history of emphysema, chronic back pain, and arthritis. Today Mr. Thominnson doesn't have the strength to get from his bed to the bathroom without having to stop and rest every couple of steps. He called EMS because he needs assistance getting to the bathroom.

Upon arrival Casey finds Mr. Thominnson seated on the side of his bed, leaning slightly forward. He states he just doesn't have the energy to get to the bathroom today. He denies any increased respiratory problems, although he is using accessory muscles to help him breathe. Casey suggests Mr. Thominnson be evaluated for his increased

weakness and he agrees, after they assist him to the bathroom.

After transporting Mr. Thominnson to the hospital, Casey sits down to complete her report of the run.

Critical Thinking Questions

1. What essential elements should be included in the patient care report?
2. What format could be used to organize the information?
3. What are some important documentation standards?

INTRODUCTION

An EMT must document patient care as carefully as a physician must. Documentation is vital to the continuum of patient care as well as collecting important data to be used in improving prehospital treatments and system development and billing for EMS services. The patient care report (PCR) is a legal document that could be used in court proceedings to prove the patient was provided the standard of care by the EMT, as discussed in Unit 3. This unit details the elements and characteristics of prehospital documentation and the professional patient care report.

THE RECORD

Over the decades, each health care profession, from medicine to nursing to physical therapy, developed a method of documentation specific to its specialty. Because of the wide variety of reporting styles, it was often difficult to follow the patient's condition from one record to another.

In the 1970s, Dr. Lawrence Weed of the University of Vermont created a system called problem-oriented medical record-keeping (POMR) as a universal standard of documentation for all health care professionals. POMR quickly gained acceptance in the medical community.

A problem or diagnosis list is used as an index, and all patient care records are entered under a problem that the patient experiences. This method of record keeping, POMR, is ideal for Emergency Medical Services (EMS).

The patient's chief concern (CC) is the basis for all care rendered by the EMT. Using the CC, the doctor can link the PCR to a tentative diagnosis in the emergency department. Then the EMT's PCR is attached to a diagnostic group or problem list within the medical record for all health care providers to review.

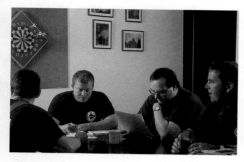

Figure 23.1 PCRs are used for quality improvement purposes

FUNCTIONS OF THE RECORD

The prehospital PCR is an important part of a complete medical record. It is a record of the patient's condition and the treatment that took place before the patient's arrival at the emergency department.

The PCR can speak for the patient when the patient cannot speak for himself, as when the patient is unconscious, long after the EMT has left the hospital. The PCR can also describe the scene in which the patient was found. The EMT is the eye of the physician in the field. The EMT may be the only health care professional who saw the mechanism of injury and can describe it.

QUALITY IMPROVEMENT

The PCR is more than just a part of the patient record. The PCR is also used for administrative purposes. Most EMS agencies use the PCR as part of their continuous quality improvement (CQI) process.

EMTs, in a process called *peer review,* take all the PCRs on a subject, such as motor vehicle collisions, and review the PCRs for accuracy and compliance with medical protocols (Figure 23.1). If a problem is consistently identified in the PCRs, then educational sessions can be created to address the problem.

Specific PCRs may be singled out for call review. These PCRs present an unusual circumstance that deserves special consideration. These designated PCRs, called **sentinel PCR**s, are reviewed by the medical director or a risk management group (Figure 23.2).

RESEARCH

Scientific research is relatively new in EMS but vitally important to determining the best evidence-based prehospital patient treatments. Using the experience of other EMTs, as documented on the PCR, researchers strive to improve the practice of EMTs by identifying what works and what does not. Research has helped identify treatments that were not effective in the field and are therefore no longer used. Similarly, collection of data from the PCR can lead to support of a particular practice or suggest ways to improve patient care. Research is a part of every profession's development.

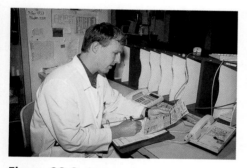

Figure 23.2 An emergency physician should review sentinel PCRs

ADMINISTRATIVE PURPOSES

The PCR fulfills many administrative purposes that are not directly tied to patient care. For example, to bill a patient for the services rendered, the business office will minimally need the patient's name, address, date of birth, and Social Security number.

The PCR also contains information for other reports. Some EMS agencies routinely track figures such as response, on scene, or transport times. Additionally, service and individual statistics can be tracked and actions taken to improve outcomes. For example, a BLS service may set a measurable outcome of oxygen administration to patients with chest pain 100% of the time. Through statistical tracking of oxygen administration during encounters with patients with chest pain, skills maintenance programs can be developed to help providers who fall under that 100% goal improve chest pain care. This information is usually found on a PCR.

LEGAL DOCUMENT

The PCR is also a legal document. As such, it is used in a court of law to show the events surrounding an illness or injury. When called to court to testify, the EMT who completed the report is often questioned closely about the details of an injury or illness as well as about the care he provided (Figure 23.3).

Documentation of the emergency medical care provided, the status of the patient on arrival at the scene, and any changes upon arrival at the receiving

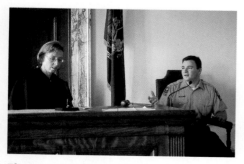

Figure 23.3 The PCR is the EMT's written record of care

facility should be written clearly and include both subjective and objective information.

A legal case may not reach the courts for months or even years. The EMT must depend on the written record, the PCR, to refresh a memory regarding the circumstances surrounding the call. Therefore, it is in an EMT's best interest to document carefully the entire patient encounter.

MINIMUM DATA SETS

The amount of information an EMT could record on a PCR is almost endless. Recording all the possible information is often wasteful in terms of time and utility. Every PCR requires a minimum amount of information to prevent EMTs from sacrificing accuracy for brevity. These specific bits of information are called the **minimum data set.** Minimum data set information can be divided into two sections: patient information and administrative information.

State and federal governments have established certain minimum data sets for EMS agencies in an effort to standardize the information collected on PCRs. Standardization enables EMS administrators to create uniform reports of EMS activity across a state or across the country. The U.S. Department of Transportation, in which EMS is housed on the federal level, has established specific information to be documented on all PCRs. The elements of the DOT minimum data set are outlined in the following section.

ADMINISTRATIVE INFORMATION

For administrative purposes, it is important to have the patient's name, date of birth, address, and other such demographic information. This information will be used in billing and patient tracking.

The timeline of the response is also part of this data set. The timeline includes the initial 911 call or when the incident was reported to the communications center, time the unit was notified or dispatched, time of arrival to the scene and patient's side, time the unit left the scene, time of arrival at destination or ALS intercept, and the time patient care is transferred to another individual. It is important that the times are accurate between entities; therefore, the EMS services and communications center should have synchronous clocks. The EMT should check and synchronize the clocks on equipment that displays and records time, such as ECG monitors.

PATIENT INFORMATION

Patient information gathered by the EMT must be documented clearly in the patient care report. The minimum data set for patient information includes the patient's chief concern; level of consciousness or mental status (AVPU); and skin signs, including color, temperature, and perfusion, using capillary refill in children. The patient's systolic blood pressure is acceptable in some services, while others require an auscultated blood pressure documenting both the systolic and diastolic pressures. The patient's pulse and respiratory rate and quality are all part of the minimum data set.

Some services may require the patient's history, current medications, and allergies as part of their minimum data set. It is important to know and follow local protocols and guidelines in documentation.

DOCUMENTATION FORMAT

Somehow the patient information has to get onto the PCR. How that information is recorded is partly a function of the form. PCR forms can be written forms, generally categorized as either open format or closed format.

Street Smart

Accurate documentation of time is important on the PCR. Often, the time on the EMT's watch doesn't exactly match that on the dispatcher's desk. Every effort should be made to synchronize timepieces or, at least, work consistently from one clock so that documentation of time on a PCR is accurate.

The format becoming more common in practice is the ePCR, or electronic patient care report. The advantages and disadvantages to both types of PCRs are discussed in the following sections.

WRITTEN PCRS

A closed-format PCR uses either checklists or bubble blanks for patient information (Figure 23.4). This format is useful for recording a large quantity of the same or similar information, such as run numbers and times.

Closed PCRs can also be read directly by a computer, using optical character recognition (OCR) technology. This enables EMS administrators to obtain large amounts of data quickly and accurately.

A disadvantage of the closed format is that little space is provided for any distinctive information regarding the patient. The alternative form developed, using an open format, provides plenty of space for a narrative account of the patient's care.

Resembling a blank sheet of paper, the open PCR gives the EMT space to write his observations in longhand. The open form provides the EMT the opportunity to individualize the patient record. However, it does not provide the EMT the structure in which to organize his thoughts. The following section describes several commonly accepted arrangements that an EMT can use to organize the narrative.

Each format, open and closed, has advantages, but each also is insufficient for effective documentation. For this reason, most PCRs are a hybrid of the two formats, taking the best from each for an efficient, comprehensive record-keeping system (Figure 23.5).

SOAP CHARTING

All essential elements of the PCR can be summed up in the acronym SOAP. Subjective, objective, assessment, and plan are the components of the SOAP format.

SUBJECTIVE

The S in SOAP stands for **subjective information,** or the information that the patient, a family member, or a bystander tells the EMT (Figure 23.6). This is information the patient senses or feels. If the patient is describing how she feels, then the information is called a *symptom* and is considered subjective information.

OBJECTIVE

Objective information, the O in SOAP, is knowledge that the EMT obtains through his own senses. For example, the EMT measures the patient's pulse. The rate of that pulse is called a *sign* and is considered objective information (Figure 23.7). Heart rates, respiratory rates, and blood pressure, as well as skin signs of temperature, color, and quality, are called the *vital signs*.

ASSESSMENT

The EMT uses both subjective and objective information to form an assessment, the A in SOAP, of the patient's problem. For example, for a patient whose subjective chief concern is "I can't breathe" and whose respiratory rate is 30 times a minute, an EMT would make the assessment that the patient is short of breath.

PLAN

The EMT would apply oxygen to the patient who is assessed as being short of breath. This is part of the plan (the P in SOAP) of treatment for the patient.

Many EMS systems find the SOAP method of charting satisfactory. Others have felt that additional elements of the record, particular for EMS needs, should be included in the charting method for EMTs.

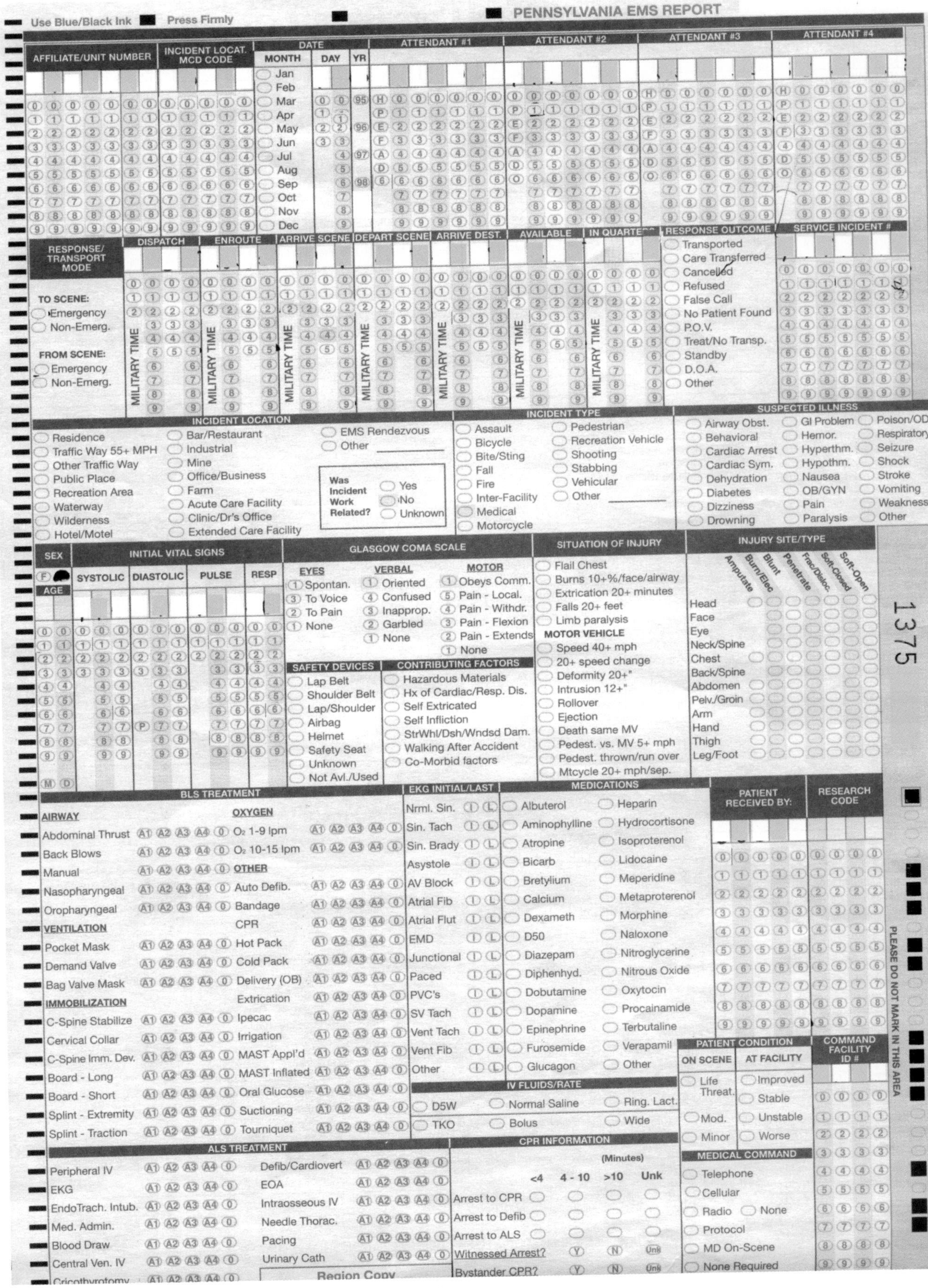

Figure 23.4 An example of a closed-format patient care report (PCR)

Prehospital Care Report

| M | D | Y | | RUN NO. | | 4- 3421055 | | AGENCY CODE | | VEH. ID. | |

DATE OF CALL

Name

Address

Ph #

| A G E | | D O B | M | D | Y | S E X | M | F |

Physician

CARE IN PROGRESS ON ARRIVAL:
☐ None ☐ Citizen ☐ PD/FD/Other First Responder ☐ Other EMS

MECHANISM OF INJURY
☐ MVA (✓ seat belt used →) ☐ Fall of ___ feet ☐ GSW ☐ Machinery
☐ Struck by vehicle ☐ Unarmed assault ☐ Knife ☐ ___

Agency Name

Dispatch Information

Call Location

CHECK ONE ☐ Residence ☐ Health Facility ☐ Farm ☐ Indus. Facility
☐ Other Work Loc. ☐ Roadway ☐ Recreational ☐ Other

CALL TYPE AS REC'D.
☐ Emergency
☐ Non-Emergency
☐ Stand-by

MILEAGE
END
BEGIN
TOTAL
LOCATION CODE

COMPLETE FOR TRANSFERS ONLY
Transferred from ☐☐☐
☐ No Previous PCR
☐ Unknown if Previous PCR
Previous PCR Number ___ - _____

☐ Extrication required ___ minutes

Seat belt used? ☐ Yes ☐ No ☐ Unknown

Seat Belt Use Reported By ☐ Crew ☐ Patient ☐ Police ☐ Other

USE MILITARY TIMES
CALL REC'D
ENROUTE
ARRIVED AT SCENE
FROM SCENE
AT DESTIN
IN SERVICE
IN QUARTERS

CHIEF COMPLAINT | **SUBJECTIVE ASSESSMENT**

PRESENTING PROBLEM
If more than one checked, circle primary

☐ Airway Obstruction
☐ Respiratory Arrest
☐ Respiratory Distress
☐ Cardiac Related (Potential)
☐ Cardiac Arrest

☐ Allergic Reaction
☐ Syncope
☐ Stroke/CVA
☐ General Illness/Malaise
☐ Gastro-Intestinal Distress
☐ Diabetic Related (Potential)
☐ Pain _____

☐ Unconscious/Unresp.
☐ Seizure
☐ Behavioral Disorder
☐ Substance Abuse (Potential)
☐ Poisoning (Accidental)

☐ Shock
☐ Head Injury
☐ Spinal Injury
☐ Fracture/Dislocation
☐ Amputation

☐ Other _____

☐ Major Trauma
☐ Trauma-Blunt
☐ Trauma-Penetrating
☐ Soft Tissue Injury
☐ Bleeding/Hemorrhage

☐ OB/GYN
☐ Burns
Environmental
☐ Heat
☐ Cold
☐ Hazardous Materials
☐ Obvious Death

PAST MEDICAL HISTORY	V I T A L S I G N S	TIME	RESP	PULSE	B.P.	LEVEL OF CONSCIOUSNESS	GCS	R	PUPILS	L	SKIN	STATUS
☐ None ☐ Allergy to ___ ☐ Hypertension ☐ Stroke ☐ Seizures ☐ Diabetes ☐ COPD ☐ Cardiac ☐ Other (List) ☐ Asthma			Rate: ☐ Regular ☐ Shallow ☐ Labored	Rate: ☐ Regular ☐ Irregular		☐ Alert ☐ Voice ☐ Pain ☐ Unresp.			Normal Dilated Constricted Sluggish No-Reaction		☐ Unremarkable ☐ Cool ☐ Pale ☐ Warm ☐ Cyanotic ☐ Moist ☐ Flushed ☐ Dry ☐ Jaundiced	☐ C ☐ U ☐ P ☐ S
Current Medications (List)			Rate: ☐ Regular ☐ Shallow ☐ Labored	Rate: ☐ Regular ☐ Irregular		☐ Alert ☐ Voice ☐ Pain ☐ Unresp.			Normal Dilated Constricted Sluggish No-Reaction		☐ Unremarkable ☐ Cool ☐ Pale ☐ Warm ☐ Cyanotic ☐ Moist ☐ Flushed ☐ Dry ☐ Jaundiced	☐ C ☐ U ☐ P ☐ S
			Rate: ☐ Regular ☐ Shallow ☐ Labored	Rate: ☐ Regular ☐ Irregular		☐ Alert ☐ Voice ☐ Pain ☐ Unresp.			Normal Dilated Constricted Sluggish No-Reaction		☐ Unremarkable ☐ Cool ☐ Pale ☐ Warm ☐ Cyanotic ☐ Moist ☐ Flushed ☐ Dry ☐ Jaundiced	☐ C ☐ U ☐ P ☐ S

OBJECTIVE PHYSICAL ASSESSMENT

COMMENTS

TREATMENT GIVEN

☐ Moved to ambulance on stretcher/backboard
☐ Moved to ambulance on stair chair
☐ Walked to ambulance
☐ Airway Cleared
☐ Oral/Nasal Airway
☐ Esophageal Obturator Airway/Esophageal Gastric Tube Airway (EOA/EGTA)
☐ EndoTracheal Tube (E/T)
☐ Oxygen Administered @ ___ L.P.M., Method _____
☐ Suction Used
☐ Artificial Ventilation Method _____
☐ C.P.R. in progress on arrival by: ☐ Citizen ☐ PD/FD/Other First Responder ☐ Other
☐ C.P.R. Started @ Time ▶ ___
Time from Arrest Until C.P.R. ▶ ___ Minutes
☐ EKG Monitored (Attach Tracing) [Rhythm(s) _____]
☐ Defibrillation/Cardioversion No. Times ___ ☐ Manual ☐ Semi-automatic

☐ Medication Administered (Use Continuation Form)
☐ IV Established Fluid _____ Cath. Gauge ___
☐ Mast Inflated @ Time _____)
☐ Bleeding/Hemorrhage Controlled (Method Used: _____)
☐ Spinal Immobilization Neck and Back
☐ Limb Immobilized by ☐ Fixation ☐ Traction
☐ (Heat) or (Cold) Applied
☐ Vomiting Induced @ Time ___ Method _____
☐ Restraints Applied, Type _____
☐ Baby Delivered @ Time ___ In County _____
    ☐ Alive ☐ Stillborn ☐ Male ☐ Female
☐ Transported in Trendelenburg position
☐ Transported in left lateral recumbent position
☐ Transported with head elevated
☐ Other _____

DISPOSITION (See list) | **DISP. CODE** | **CONTINUATION FORM USED** YES

C R E W	IN CHARGE	DRIVER'S NAME	NAME	NAME
	☐ EMT ☐ AEMT #	☐ CFR ☐ EMT ☐ AEMT #	☐ CFR ☐ EMT ☐ AEMT #	☐ CFR ☐ EMT ☐ AEMT #

© COPYRIGHT 1986 NEW YORK STATE DEPARTMENT OF HEALTH

AGENCY COPY/WHITE   RESEARCH COPY/YELLOW   HOSPITAL PATIENT RECORD COPY/PINK

EMS 100 (11/86) provided by NYS-EMS PROGRAM
DOH 3283 (6/94)

Figure 23.5 An example of a hybrid form PCR
(Reprinted with permission of the New York State Department of Health)

SOAPIE (subjective, objective, assessment, plan, intervention, evaluation), CHART (chief concern, history, assessment, Rx-treatment, transport), and **CHEATED** (chief concern, history, examination, assessment, treatment, evaluation, disposition) represent three examples of expanded charting methods. All of these methods, and many others, still include the fundamental elements contained within SOAP as their basis. Unless the local EMS agency requires a specific charting method, EMTs should find a method of charting that is complete and with which they are comfortable. Using the same method of charting every time is the best way to develop complete documentation.

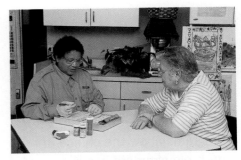

Figure 23.6 The patient's history of present illness is subjective

CHEATED

One of the more EMS-specific charting methods uses the acronym CHEATED. Table 23-1 lists the components of this charting method. Starting with the initial contact with the patient, the CHEATED method continues with documenting care to the emergency department.

CHIEF CONCERN

The C in CHEATED refers to the patient's chief concern. As far as is practical, the patient's chief concern should be written in the patient's own words. If the patient is unconscious, then the statement of a family member or bystander should be used.

HISTORY

The H in CHEATED refers to history. The first history is the history of the present illness (HPI). Some EMTs refer to this as the nature of the illness (NOI). In the case of trauma, the mechanism of injury (MOI) is described.

The patient's past medical history (PMH) also needs to be included. The use of the acronym SAMPLE ensures that the EMT will get the minimum history needed.

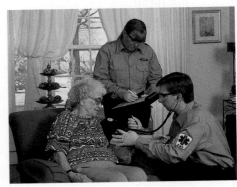

Figure 23.7 The EMT's physical examination is objective

EXAMINATION

The E in CHEATED refers to the physical *examination*. Starting with the primary assessment, the EMT would continue by documenting any physical examination that is performed either prior to or during the secondary assessment.

ASSESSMENT

Then the EMT is asked to make an assessment (the A in CHEATED) of the patient's situation. This assessment is the basis for the patient's treatment. The assessment is one of the titles under the EMT's protocols.

TREATMENT

The EMT would then proceed to document the patient's treatment (the T in CHEATED). Typically at this point the patient is either en route to the hospital or being packaged for transportation. Part of the continuum of care an EMT provides is frequent reassessment of the patient.

EVALUATION

Both patient improvement and deterioration are noted in the evaluation (the E in CHEATED) portion of the patient care report. The patient's response to prehospital treatments helps guide the physician's decision regarding which hospital treatments to proceed with.

DISPOSITION

Patient care is transferred to another health care professional upon arrival at the emergency department or intercept with an ALS unit. The disposition of the patient (the D in CHEATED) is a matter of both medical and legal

Table 23-1 Cheated	
C =	Chief concern
H =	History
E =	Examination
A =	Assessment
T =	Treatment
E =	Evaluation
D =	Disposition

concern. Patients may be transferred only to another health care provider capable of continuing patient care.

The patient's condition as well as treatments in progress should also be documented. If family members are present, their presence should also be noted. Any personal property of the patient that is given to emergency department staff, for example, canes and dentures, should be documented.

ELECTRONIC PCRs

Electronic PCRs, or ePCRs, are computerized reports using software developed for the specific purpose of prehospital documentation. The software can vary, with most programs formatted to use both on-screen check boxes and narratives (Figure 23.8).

The advantages of the ePCR are a consistent method of documentation that is used by everyone in the service. In other words, all documentation is completed in the same method and format by each individual in the service.

Additionally, computerized systems allow for more storage of information, are more legible formats than handwritten reports, and are efficient for services to store, retrieve, and use the data collected by the EMT. EMS can track skills, equipment, inventory control, personnel, e-mail, and payroll. As more advances are made in ePCR programs, the ability to link to computer-aided dispatch (CAD) and hospital systems has improved information sharing vitally important to the patient's continuum of care.

The required reporting of data points contained within the minimum data sets to the state or federal government can be accomplished as the report is being completed. This real-time reporting allows for greater proficiency in gathering the data needed for system development and research in EMS.

Finally, the ePCR system provides a clear, clean, and concise document because it can check spelling, use of appropriate abbreviations, and typewritten narratives that are professional and accurate. Quality assurance and quality improvement programs can be more readily facilitated, in some cases through a component of the ePCR alerting EMTs if required elements are missing in reports.

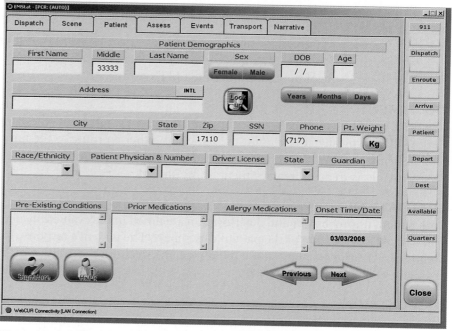

Figure 23.8 Electronic PCR (Courtesy of Med Media, Inc.)

PRINCIPLES OF DOCUMENTATION

Documenting care may seem complicated, but remembering a few general principles can make the EMT's job easier. To begin, the PCR is no place for personal opinions or bias. Record all observations objectively. It is important to document what the patient says but document only those statements that help bring the patient's condition to light for the physician.

Document all the care that was provided. In legal circles there is a saying, "If it wasn't written, it didn't happen." A failure to document care gives an opportunity for a lawyer to convince a jury that proper care may not have been given.

PCRs must be submitted promptly. Most EMTs complete their PCRs in the emergency department, at the point of transferring patient care. In those rare cases in which a PCR is not completed before the EMT leaves the emergency department, a copy should be faxed, via a secure line, as soon as possible (Figure 23.9).

When disseminating PCRs, care must be used in handling any information about the patient to ensure patient privacy and confidentiality is not compromised. Patient confidentiality is a legal right of the patient, the EMT is expected to ensure that this right is protected. Information documented in the PCR is considered confidential and cannot be legally shared with anyone not providing direct patient care without the patient's permission. Review Unit 3 for more specific details on HIPAA and patient confidentiality.

It is always best to follow service guidelines or local protocols concerning the sharing of patient information and PCRs.

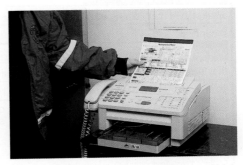

Figure 23.9 Always promptly submit or fax a PCR to the emergency department

DOCUMENTATION STANDARDS

To ensure uniformity in reporting and simplicity in data retrieval, many EMS organizations and agencies have adopted documentation standards for their EMTs. These documentation standards are often very similar to the documentation standards required by the federal Center for Medicare and Medicaid.

STANDARDIZED ABBREVIATIONS AND SYMBOLS

When it comes to shortening paperwork by using abbreviations, EMTs are some of the most imaginative people alive. However, it must be remembered that the primary purpose of documentation is to communicate the patient's condition to other health care providers, so they must be able to read and understand the patient's record.

Although abbreviations may decrease documentation time, they occasionally increase confusion. For example, the abbreviation Dx may mean discharge to an EMT but could mean diagnosis to a doctor or even defendant to a lawyer. It is important for the EMT to use accurate abbreviations if they are used at all.

ERRORS AND CORRECTIONS

In the course of documenting patient care, errors will occur. Sometimes they are spelling errors or errors in order. Regardless, the EMT should make one single cross-out over the error and then initial the cross-out.

Use of white correction fluid or vigorous blackout only creates a question in the mind of the reader, including attorneys, as to what was originally written. Leave no room for guessing on the part of others. A clean, simple cross-out shows there is nothing to hide (Figure 23.10).

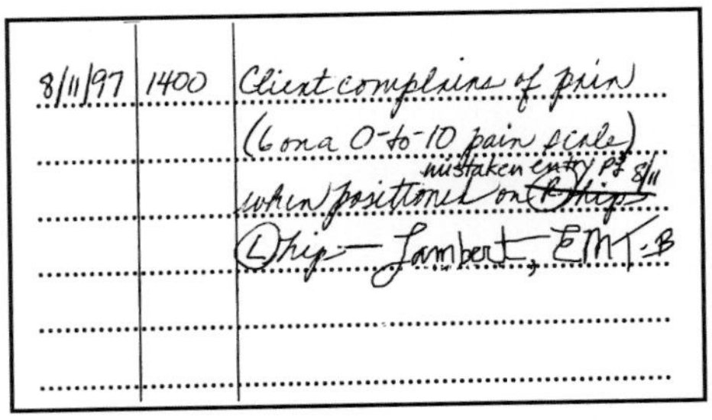

After the PCR is completely written, always initial the last sentence. This indicates that this was the last point of documentation. It is assumed that the date on the PCR is the date the PCR was written. However, some EMS agencies require the EMT to write his initials, date, and time at the end of the document as well (Figure 23.11).

Figure 23.10 Cross out errors with one single line, then initial

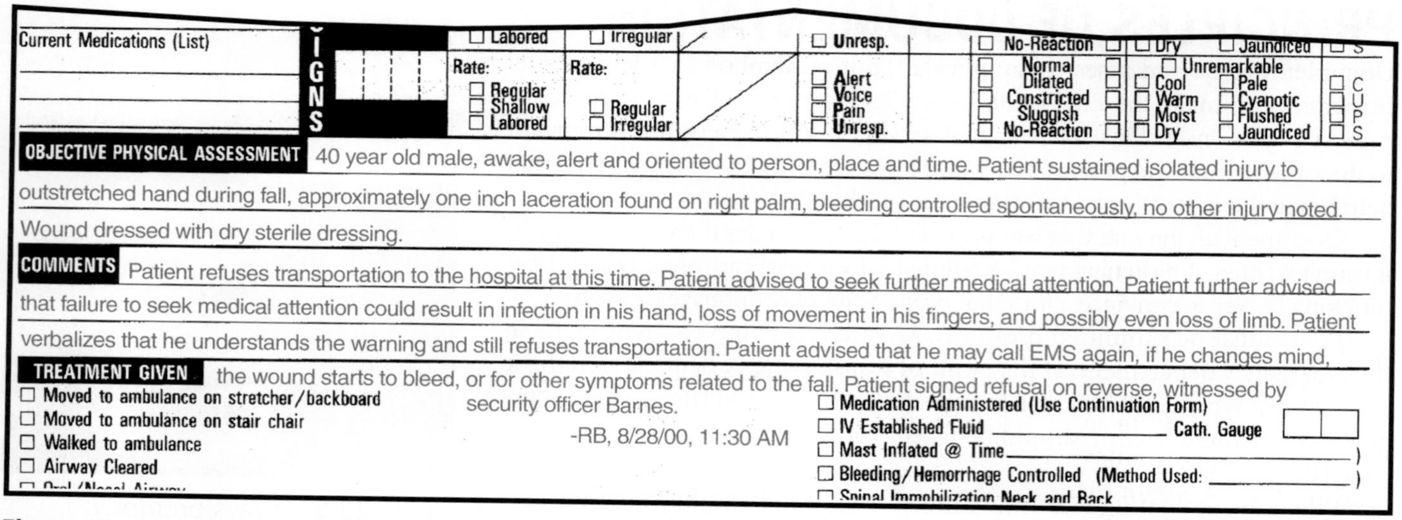

Current Medications (List)	S I G N S		□ Labored	□ Irregular		□ Unresp.		□ No-Reaction		□ Dry	□ Jaundiced	□ S
			Rate: □ Regular □ Shallow □ Labored	Rate: □ Regular □ Irregular		□ Alert □ Voice □ Pain □ Unresp.		□ Normal □ Dilated □ Constricted □ Sluggish □ No-Reaction		□ Unremarkable □ Cool □ Warm □ Moist □ Dry	□ Pale □ Cyanotic □ Flushed □ Jaundiced	□ C □ U □ P □ S

OBJECTIVE PHYSICAL ASSESSMENT 40 year old male, awake, alert and oriented to person, place and time. Patient sustained isolated injury to outstretched hand during fall, approximately one inch laceration found on right palm, bleeding controlled spontaneously, no other injury noted. Wound dressed with dry sterile dressing.

COMMENTS Patient refuses transportation to the hospital at this time. Patient advised to seek further medical attention. Patient further advised that failure to seek medical attention could result in infection in his hand, loss of movement in his fingers, and possibly even loss of limb. Patient verbalizes that he understands the warning and still refuses transportation. Patient advised that he may call EMS again, if he changes mind,

TREATMENT GIVEN the wound starts to bleed, or for other symptoms related to the fall. Patient signed refusal on reverse, witnessed by security officer Barnes.

- □ Moved to ambulance on stretcher/backboard
- □ Moved to ambulance on stair chair
- □ Walked to ambulance
- □ Airway Cleared
- □ Oral/Nasal Airway

-RB, 8/28/00, 11:30 AM

- □ Medication Administered (Use Continuation Form)
- □ IV Established Fluid _____ Cath. Gauge ___
- □ Mast Inflated @ Time_____)
- □ Bleeding/Hemorrhage Controlled (Method Used: _____)
- □ Spinal Immobilization Neck and Back

Figure 23.11 Complete the PCR with your initials, time, and date

Sometimes after a PCR has been completed, the EMT wishes to add to the record. The EMT can reopen the documentation either by adding to the existing record and then adding initials, time, and date to the last entry or, preferably, by adding to the record another sheet that reflects the new date and time.

FALSIFICATION ISSUES

The PCR is intended to be a complete, thorough, and accurate record of the entire patient encounter by the EMT. Mistakes during the patient encounter can and do occasionally occur and must be documented accurately and completely in the PCR. When mistakes occur the EMT may be tempted to omit or even falsify the PCR.

Inaccurate and false information must never occur in documentation. The EMT must not attempt to omit or alter facts to cover up an error of omission or treatment. When an error of omission or commission occurs, the EMT should document what did or did not happen and what steps were taken (if any) to correct the situation.

Falsification of patient data will compromise patient care and could ultimately compromise the patient's outcome. The vitals signs documented must have been actually taken. If placing the patient on oxygen was overlooked, the PCR should not state oxygen was administered. If oxygen was initially overlooked but was administered at a later time in patient care, the time of oxygen administration should be accurately documented. It is important to remember other health care providers taking over the care of the patient rely on the accuracy of the information given them by the EMT in the continuum of care.

In many states, falsification of documentation by EMTs can lead to suspension or revocation of their certification or license. Falsifying documentation could also potentially lead to criminal charges in some cases.

LEGIBILITY

Illegible documentation helps no one. It is important for the EMT to write clearly. Most EMS agencies still prefer that PCRs be written in black ink. In the past, old records would be placed on microfilm for storage. Blue ink does not show up well on microfilm or on photocopies. PCRs are photocopied for many reasons.

SPECIAL INCIDENT REPORTS

Equipment failure and personal injuries to the crew occasionally occur, but do these incidents belong on the PCR? No, these extraordinary situations should be documented in a special incident report. A **special incident report** has been designated for documentation of specific incidents such as crew injuries or equipment problems (Figure 23.12).

Most EMS agencies have guidelines for when a critical or special incident report should be generated. Some general guidelines are listed here. The EMT should be aware of the reporting guidelines in his agency.

INJURY TO THE EMT

If an EMT is injured while on duty, the injury needs to be reported immediately to his supervisor and by completing a special incident report. The special incident report may serve as the basis for a claim under the workers' compensation system or disability insurance.

INFECTIOUS DISEASE EXPOSURE

Whenever an EMT may have had a potential infectious disease exposure, a special incident report should be completed and returned to the designated infection control officer. The Federal Occupational Safety and Health Administration (OSHA) has established strict guidelines regarding the reporting and management of potential infectious disease exposure. Always follow local protocols for reporting potential infectious disease exposure.

EQUIPMENT FAILURE

Any time equipment fails to operate properly while on an EMS call, the failure should be reported. One reason is to ensure that the equipment is removed from service until it has been properly repaired. Faulty equipment presents a hazard to other patients and EMTs.

All reports of equipment failure should be directed to the attention of a supervisor. In some instances, these reports will be entered as evidence in a court trial. The supervisor should review the report for accuracy.

In the eyes of a jury, it is more acceptable to have had a piece of equipment fail and be repaired than to ignore the failure. Table 23-2 lists several common conditions or problems that should be reported to an EMT's supervisor or chief officer.

Table 23-2 Problems That Should Be Reported

Confrontations on the scene with the family or public

Confrontations with police or firefighters

Confrontations with hospital personnel

Perceived malpractice by another EMT

Equipment failure

Infectious disease or other hazardous exposure

Lost patient property, such as dentures or glasses

Collision involving an emergency response vehicle

INCIDENT REPORT

CASE NUMBER	DUTY STATION	FDS NUMBER

ADDRESS		

CITY	STATE	ZIP CODE

DATE OF REPORT	DATE OF INCIDENT

TYPE OF INCIDENT

Initial ☐   Follow-up ☐

	YES	NO
1. Employee Injury	☐	☐
2. Patient Injury	☐	☐
3. Visitor Injury	☐	☐
4. Medical Device Injury	☐	☐
5. Property Damage	☐	☐
6. Hazardous Condition	☐	☐

SEVERITY

☐ 1. Fatal
☐ 2. Hospitalized
☐ 3. Ambulatory
☐ 4. No Treatment

LOST TIME *(days)* _____

DISABILITY

☐ 1. Temporary
☐ 2. Partial Permanent
☐ 3. Full Permanent
☐ 4. None

SERIOUS INCIDENT TYPE
(Check one)

☐ 1. Fatal
☐ 2. More than 3 injured
☐ 3. Property damaged $25,000.
☐ 4. Aircraft
☐ 5. Radiation Release
☐ 6. Biological Release

EXAMINED BY PRIMARY CARE PROVIDER ☐ YES ☐ NO	MEDICAL EXPENSE INCURRED: ☐ YES ☐ NO	ESTIMATED COST: $ _____

INVESTIGATION CONDUCTED BY:	PHONE NUMBER ( )

INDIVIDUAL INVOLVED

NAME	TORT POSSIBLE ☐ YES ☐ NO

SOCIAL SECURITY NUMBER	DATE OF BIRTH	SEX ☐ MALE ☐ FEMALE

ADDRESS		

CITY	STATE	ZIP CODE

PHONE NUMBER ( )	TIME OF INCIDENT

EMPLOYEE

JOB TITLE	OWCP FORM FILED ☐ YES ☐ NO

PERSONNEL STATUS - CO, GS, WG, TRIBAL, VOLUNTEER, OTHER	GRADE LEVEL / STEP

NUMBER OF DEPENDENTS *(Spouse and Children under 18)*	SUPERVISOR'S NAME

WORK PHONE NUMBER ( )	SHIFT ONE, TWO, OR THREE ☐ 1 ☐ 2 ☐ 3	TIME ON DUTY BEFORE INCIDENT

PATIENT

DATE OF ADMISSION	DEPARTMENT	DEPARTMENT PHONE NUMBER ( )	CHART NUMBER

DIAGNOSIS ON ADMISSION	MEDICAL DEVICE RELATED ☐ YES ☐ NO

CONDITION BEFORE INCIDENT	

MEDICATIONS ADMINISTERED ☐ YES ☐ NO	TYPE OF MEDICATION

COMMENTS

VISITOR

PURPOSE OF VISIT

EF

Figure 23.12 Special incident report

INCIDENT REPORT

PROPERTY

OWNER	PRIVATE PROPERTY ☐ YES ☐ NO

ADDRESS

CITY	STATE	ZIP CODE

PROPERTY MANAGEMENT NOTIFIED ☐ YES ☐ NO	DATE	NATURE AND EXTENT OF DAMAGE
ESTIMATED REPAIR / REPLACEMENT $ _____	GOVERNMENT VEHICLE INVOLVED ☐ YES ☐ NO	REGISTRATION / TAG NUMBER

NARRATIVE

Give a factual description of incident, location, and other important specifics (i.e. body part(s), other individual involved, etc.)

FACILITY NAME: _____   DEPARTMENT: _____

DESCRIPTION:

DIAGRAM OF INCIDENT

CODING SECTION

INCIDENT LOCATION CODE:	DESCRIPTION:
OSHA TYPE CODE:	IHS TYPE CODE:
OHSA SOURCE CODE:	ICD NATURE CODE:
OCCUPATION CODE: ___ ___ ___ — ___ ___ ___ ___	ICD EXTERNAL CAUSE CODE:
OWCP AGENCY CODE:	

SIGNATURE AND TITLE OF REPORTING EMPLOYEE	DATE	PHONE ( )
SIGNATURE AND TITLE OF REVIEWING OFFICIAL	DATE	PHONE ( )
SIGNATURE AND TITLE OF CODING OFFICIAL	DATE	PHONE ( )

The information collected on this form is to be utilized in compliance with the Privacy Act of 1974.

Figure 23.12 Special incident report (*continued*)

CRIME SCENE

There are times when an EMT comes across what appears to be criminal activity. In all cases, patient care is the EMT's first responsibility. When the call is completed, however, the EMT may have other responsibilities.

In most states, EMTs are required to report suspected child abuse. It is important that an EMT comply with the law in those cases because failure to report them may result in civil or criminal liability.

In all states, it is within the scope of an EMT's practice to report suspected child abuse to a licensed physician or registered nurse. As *mandated reporters,* physicians and nurses must then investigate the concern further. In some instances, the involvement of the physician or nurse may relieve the EMT of further responsibility.

Elder abuse has become an increasingly common occurrence. As in child abuse, an EMT's responsibility to report suspected elder abuse is a function of state and local laws.

Every EMS agency should have a procedure in writing to deal with these all-too-common events. In all cases, the advice of a competent lawyer should be sought.

An EMT may be called upon to offer written testimony, called an **affidavit,** regarding anything seen or heard when on an EMS call. Or he may be called upon to testify in court (Figure 23.13). Frequently, this request is made days, weeks, or even months after the call has occurred.

It is a good practice to write a special incident report for these types of calls. In the future, the EMT may refer to the special incident report for clarification of forgotten details regarding the call.

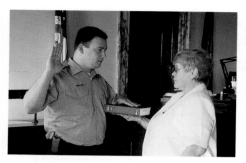

Figure 23.13 EMTs may be asked to testify in court about criminal activity

MULTIPLE-CASUALTY INCIDENT (MCI)

When there are several patients, from half a dozen to a hundred or more, it is impractical to complete a PCR for each patient. Writing a PCR for each patient would slow patient care. When there is not enough time to complete a full patient report, the EMT can use special documentation records called **triage tags** as an initial report; however, a full report will need to be completed later.

These triage tags, shown in Figure 23.14, provide enough space to write a patient's name and address, vital signs, and a few other pertinent facts. The number on each tag is used to track the patient. Other logs and records used by EMS command personnel will also track these patients using that identification number. More details regarding the triage tag systems as well as other logs are provided in Unit 49.

The standard for completing a patient care form is not usually the same as the form used for typical EMS calls. Local protocols or MCI plans have specific guidelines for patient reports. The EMT should be knowledgeable about documentation of patient care during a multi-casualty incident.

PATIENT REFUSAL DOCUMENTATION

A patient's refusal to accept either care or transportation runs counter to an EMT's expectation of the patient. When an EMT is called to a scene, there is an expectation of the patient to be cooperative and accept the care offered. In cases in which the patient does refuse care or transportation, the EMT needs to carefully examine the patient's reason.

The details of who can reasonably refuse care and the legal ramifications surrounding such a refusal are detailed in Unit 3. The EMT must document the patient's decision in this situation very carefully.

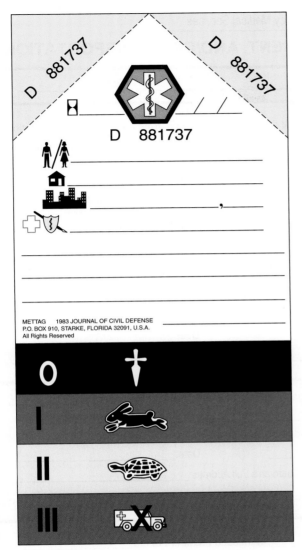

Green (bottom strip):
    Symbol: Ambulance–crossed out
    Meaning: No hospital treatment needed; first aid only
Yellow (second strip from bottom):
    Symbol: Turtle
    Meaning: Nonurgent; hospital care
Red (third strip from bottom):
    Symbol: Rabbit
    Meaning: Urgent; hospital care
Black (fourth strip from bottom):
    Symbol: Cross/dagger
    Meaning: Dead or unsalvageable; no CPR

Figure 23.14 Triage tags are used to document care of multiple patients (Courtesy of American Civil Defense Association)

When all efforts at swaying the patient have failed, most EMS systems have a **patient refusal form** for the patient to sign (Figure 23.15).

Several antecedent conditions are required before a patient refusal can be said to be valid. These are listed in Table 23-3 and must be documented carefully on the refusal form.

Because of the high litigation potential associated with refusals, many EMS systems require that an EMS supervisor be consulted before the patient refuses. In other systems, medical control has decided that contact must be made with an emergency department physician to discuss the case and possibly talk to the patient prior to accepting the patient's refusal.

In every case, a witness should attest that the patient refused care without threat or duress. This witness should be able to testify that the patient was given a medical warning and that the patient understood this warning. Other EMTs may not be considered good witnesses. Choose family members or noninvolved parties, such as police officers or bystanders, whenever possible.

REFUSAL OF MEDICAL CARE, TREATMENT, AND/OR TRANSPORTATION

PCR Number: _____ **Date:** _____ **Time:** _____

PATIENT: I understand that competent persons maintain the right to refuse medical care, treatment and/or transportation.

I, _____, hereby acknowledge that I have been advised by members of

the _____ [AGENCY], that they recommend that I receive medical care, treatment

and/or transportation to a hospital emergency department for further evaluation by a physician.

I further understand that I may refuse medical care, treatment and/or transportation, but do so at my own risk.
I do not have any known physical or mental condition that would prohibit me from making an informed, competent, and intelligent decision to refuse the medical care, treatment and/or transportation that has been offered and recommended.

THE RISK ASSOCIATED WITH REFUSAL MAY INCLUDE POSSIBLE LOSS OF LIMB OR LIFE

I HAVE ALSO BEEN ADVISED THAT IF I DEVELOP ANY MEDICAL COMPLAINTS OR SYMPTOMS, I SHOULD IMMEDIATELY CONTACT AN AMBULANCE, HOSPITAL EMERGENCY DEPARTMENT, OR MY PHYSICIAN.

I hereby release _____ [AGENCY], its officers, agents, personnel, and employees from any and all claims, causes of action or injuries, of whatsoever kind or nature, arising out of or in connection with my refusal of medical care, treatment and/or transportation.

Patient's Signature: _____   Date: _____

Patient's Name (print): _____   Patient's Age: ____   Patient refused signature: _____

FOR MINORS OR PERSONS WHO HAVE GUARDIANS: I am the patient's legal guardian. My relationship to the patient is _____.
I am hereby acting on behalf of the patient, _____ [PATIENT'S NAME]. I have
read the above information and refuse medical care, treatment and/or transportation on behalf of the patient.

Guardian's Signature: _____   Date: _____

Guardian's Name (print): _____   Guardian's Full Address: _____

_____

WITNESS: I, _____, witnessed members of the _____

_____ [AGENCY] recommend to the patient medical care, treatment, and/or transportation to a hospital emergency department for further evaluation and attention. I further witnessed the above-named patient (or patient's guardian) decline such medical care, treatment, and/or transportation.

Witness Signature: _____   Date: _____

Witness Name (print): _____   Witness' Full Address: _____

Occupation: _____   _____

EMS PROVIDER: I, _____ [EMS PROVIDER], have offered and recommended to

_____ [PATIENT'S NAME OR GUARDIAN'S NAME], emergency medical care and treatment, including transportation to a hospital. The patient (or patient's guardian) has refused my recommendation for medical care, treatment, and/or transportation. I have fully explained the reasons for medical care, treatment, and/or transportation to the patient (or patient's guardian). I have also explained this form to the patient (or patient's guardian) and have requested that he/she personally read it. The patient (or patient's guardian) has expressed to me an understanding of the information contained herein and did not have any questions regarding the content of this form. The patient (or patient's guardian) did not appear to me to be suffering from any illness or injury nor any condition that would affect his/her ability to refuse medical care, treatment, and/or transportation. The patient (or patient's guardian) is alert and oriented to person, place, time, and situation.

EMS Provider Signature: _____   Date: _____

Provider Certification Level / NYS ID Number: _____

Police Officer's Name: _____   Police Agency Present: NO_____ YES_____

Police Agency Name: _____

Figure 23.15 Many EMS agencies use a separate patient refusal form
(Courtesy of Rensselar County Emergency Medical Services)

Table 23-3 Conditions for Patient Refusal of Care

Patient is older than 18 or is an emancipated minor.

Patient is not obviously intoxicated by alcohol or drugs.

Patient understands potential medical condition and consequences of refusal of care.

Patient is provided with other reasonable options and is given instructions to seek further medical care.

Standardizing the documentation of a refusal of medical assistance (RMA) is important. Some agencies use a standardized form specifically designed for this type of call. If this is not available, the EMT should practice using standard statements that cover the required points. As an example: "This 27-yr-old patient is alert and oriented ×3 and refuses to allow further medical care or transport. He verbalizes an understanding of the potential consequences of his refusal to include loss of life or limb. He and his wife signed the RMA form. The patient has been encouraged to seek further medical attention and to call back if he changes his mind."

A written statement such as this at the end of an open-style PCR addresses the necessary questions and requirements for RMA. If a supervisor or physician was contacted regarding the situation, that contact should also be documented.

CONCLUSION

The PCR is the EMT's primary record of patient care. Although the PCR may be used for administrative and legal purposes, its primary purpose is as a medical record. The prehospital PCR is used in the continuity of patient care, quality assurance, education, and research. The EMT must be mindful that other health care professionals will want to read and understand what happened to the patient in the field. An EMT should focus on providing a clear and accurate representation of what occurred during the patient encounter, including assessment, physical examination, and history and how the patient was managed.

The PCR must be legible and accurate, using acceptable abbreviations and objective and subjective information pertinent to the situation. Falsification of any information within the PCR cannot be allowed as it would compromise continued patient management and the EMT's certification.

Documentation of a patient's refusal of care and transport must reflect that the patient fully understood the potential consequences of the decision, including the benefits of allowing treatment and potential risks of refusing.

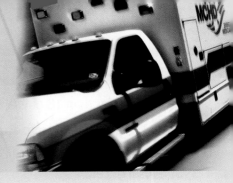

CASE STUDY Continued

After completing the demographic information and recording Mr. Thominnson's vital sign measurements, Casey proceeds to record her subjective and objective observations, assessment findings, and treatment of Mr. Thominnson using the SOAP method. After completing the PCR, Casey has her partner read what she has written, double checking for accuracy in spelling and ensuring her writing is legible and easy to understand. Casey signs her report and leaves a copy with the nurse who has assumed Mr. Thominnson's care.

Key Concepts Revisited

- Complete and accurate documentation of medical care is a fundamental function of the EMT.
- The function of the prehospital PCR is documentation of the patient's condition, treatments, and administrative elements:
  - Quality improvement
  - Research
  - Skills tracking
  - Billing
- The PCR is a legal document.
- State and federal governments have established minimum data sets:
  - Administrative information
  - Patient information
- Documentation can use a variety of formats:
  - Written PCR
    - Open PCR
    - Closed PCR
  - Electronic PCR

- The EMT can use certain principles of documentation to ensure complete, accurate, and timely patient care record keeping.
- Documentation standards include use of standardized abbreviations.
- The EMT must not attempt to omit or alter facts in documentation to cover up an error of omission or treatment.
- A special report form is used for documentation of incidents:
  - Injuries to EMS personnel
  - Infectious disease exposure
  - Equipment failure
  - Crime scene management
- The EMT must document the patient's decision to refuse treatment and transport very carefully.
- The PCR is the EMT's primary record of patient care.

Review Questions

1. Why is it important for an EMT to document care?
2. What essential elements should be included in every PCR?
3. Where does the PCR fit into the patient's medical record?
4. What are the four primary functions of the PCR?
5. What is a minimum data set?
6. What do the letters in SOAP mean?
7. What do the letters in CHEATED mean?
8. What problems may arise by using nonstandardized abbreviations?
9. How is an error corrected on a PCR?
10. Why is a special incident report written?
11. How is documentation handled for multiple-casualty incidents?
12. What are the critical elements of a patient refusal form?

Key Terms

Affidavit
CHEATED
Minimum data set
Objective information
Patient care report (PCR)

Patient refusal form
Sentinel PCR
Special incident report
Subjective information
Triage tag

Further Study

Milewski, R., and R. Lang. *EMS Documentation Field Guide.* Boston: Jones & Bartlett, 2003.

Ornato, J. P., M. L. Doctor, L. F. Harbour, M. A. Peberdy, J. Overton, E. M. Racht, et al. "Synchronization of Timepieces to the Atomic Clock in an Urban Emergency Medical Services System." *Annals of Emergency Medicine* 31, no. 4 (1998): 483–487.

Weaver, J., K. H. Brinsfield, and D. Dalphond. "Prehospital Refusal-of-Transport Policies: Adequate Legal Protection?" *Prehospital Emergency Care* 4, no. 1 (2000): 53–56.

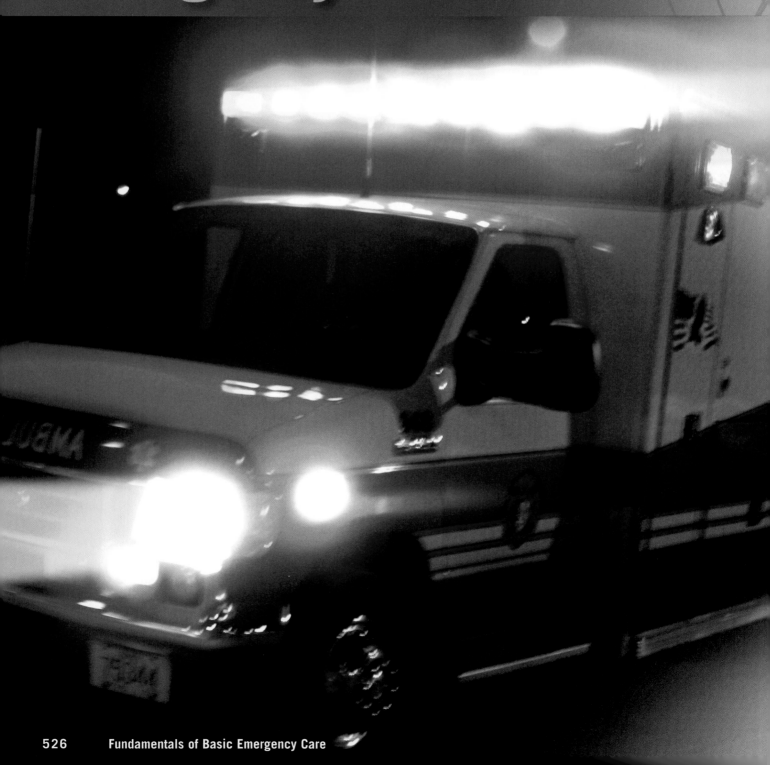

CHAPTER 5

Emergency Medical Care

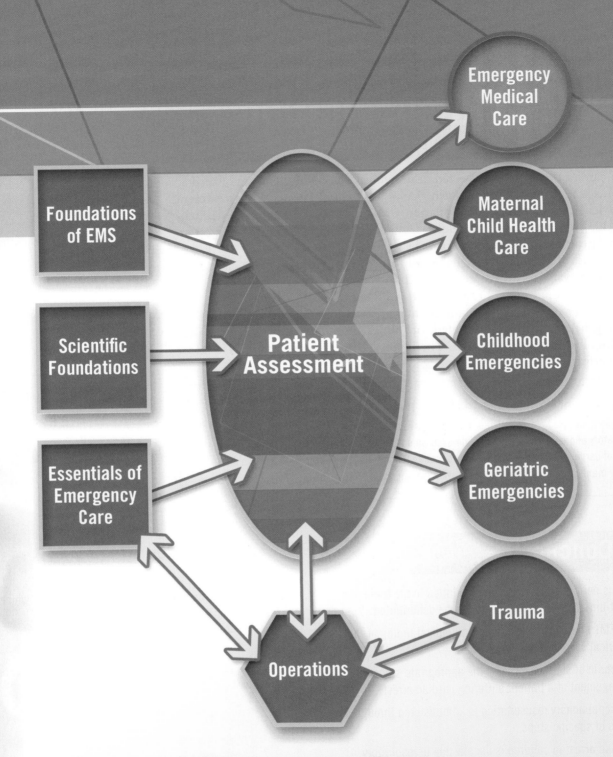

Medical Emergencies

Patients often call EMS because they are suffering from an illness or affliction. It is the EMT's responsibility to determine the nature of the illness, provide immediately necessary interventions, prioritize transport, and offer the patient some symptomatic relief, if possible. The EMT's treatment is therefore based on assessment of the patient's condition.

Many illnesses may affect a person. EMT training focuses on the most common concerns an EMT is likely to encounter. This chapter provides an overview of the medical emergencies an EMT would be expected to assess, treat, and transport to an emergency department.

Sudden cardiac death, an unexpected death within 1 hour of the onset of cardiac symptoms, is typically the result of ventricular fibrillation. The definitive treatment for ventricular fibrillation is defibrillation with an **automated external defibrillator (AED).** *Defibrillation* is an electric shock delivered to the heart to stop an abnormal heartbeat and restore a normal rhythm.

In the case of a cardiac arrest that is not witnessed and in cases in which an AED is not readily available, an Emergency Medical Technician (EMT) will be required to perform cardiopulmonary resuscitation (CPR) until the AED arrives.

CPR is performed to maintain circulation to the brain and heart until the fibrillating heart can be defibrillated, or "shocked," back into a normal pulse-producing, life-sustaining rhythm. Therefore, it is imperative that EMTs know how to perform CPR.

National Education Standards

The Emergency Medical Technician (EMT) will have the fundamental knowledge to recognize respiratory and cardiac arrest based on assessment findings and be able to demonstrate the skills of cardiopulmonary resuscitation to manage respiratory and cardiac arrest, foreign body airway management, and post-resuscitation management.

Key Concepts

- CPR is performed to maintain circulation to the brain and heart until the fibrillating heart can be defibrillated.

- The EMT must have a fundamental understanding of the electrical system of the heart.

- The chain of survival outlines the appropriate steps in management of a patient suffering cardiac arrest.

- Cardiopulmonary resuscitation is administered through a series of specific steps.

- Cardiac arrest in children is usually due to respiratory compromise.

- CPR in infants and children is different only in the case of two-rescuer administration.

- Special situations in administration of CPR present additional challenges for EMTs.

- Defibrillation is the most definitive management for the patient in cardiac arrest whose heart is fibrillating.

- Postarrest care of the patient may require manual ventilations.

- The EMT must be familiar with circumstances in which resuscitation will not be indicated.

Daniel and Mike have just finished cleaning up the ambulance from the last call when the tones go off: "Ambulance 12-57, respond to the airport lobby, man having a heart attack. Time out 12:45."

As Daniel climbs into the driver's seat, he goes over the events of the last cardiac call he had at the airport. It was a full arrest and airport security and a couple of off-duty flight attendants were already on scene performing CPR and using the AED. It was a save, thanks to the good work of those citizens.

Critical Thinking Questions

1. What unique challenges do EMS providers face when confronted with citizens performing CPR or using an AED?

2. How does the EMT interface with citizen CPR?

3. Are there any differences between citizen CPR and rescuer CPR?

INTRODUCTION

Many states require students to obtain certification in CPR before they begin the EMT course. Other states require EMTs to recertify their CPR certification or obtain one during the EMT class. In any case, EMTs are well served if they review and practice the skills of CPR during the EMT course. EMTs need to be experts at CPR and skilled at administration of defibrillation through the use of the automated external defibrillator (AED). This unit reviews the principles of CPR and AED administration for the EMT.

CARDIAC ARREST

A common consequence of acute myocardial infarction (AMI) is cardiac arrest and clinical death. This event, defined as the unexpected cessation of heartbeat within 1 hour of the onset of chest pain, is called *sudden cardiac death (SCD)*.

More than 50% of the cases of sudden cardiac death occur outside of the hospital. Therefore, it is imperative for the EMT to understand why cardiac arrest occurs and how to respond to it.

SIGNS AND SYMPTOMS

When a patient experiences chest pain or any of the other cardiac-related symptoms described in Unit 25, he may be experiencing a threatened AMI or what is known in lay terms as a heart attack. Without prompt treatment, the AMI can lead to complications such as congestive heart failure, cardiogenic shock, or SCD. Why does SCD occur? To understand the cause of SCD, the EMT must first understand the heart's normal electrical activity.

NORMAL SINUS RHYTHM

To review, the heart is a pump. Pumps essentially have two interrelated components: An electrical system triggers the mechanical portion to do its job. The human heart is such a pump. It has an electrical system that triggers the muscle, the mechanical portion, to pump blood.

Street Smart

Normally when a patient's blood pressure drops, for whatever reason, the heart races to compensate for the loss. This reflexive tachycardia is a hallmark of shock.

When an EMT determines that the patient has a low blood pressure, she naturally assumes that the heart will be tachycardic. This is not always the case. If the electrical system of the heart is damaged by an AMI, then an escape pacemaker will take over and the result will be a slow escape rhythm.

When an EMT sees both hypotension and bradycardia in a medical patient, she should be thinking about a possible AMI.

The electrical impulse begins at the sinoatrial node (SA node), a group of specialized cells located high in the right atrium. The impulse then proceeds through the atria to the atrioventricular node (AV node), another specialized group of cells that is situated between the atria and the ventricles. From the AV node, the spark travels through a defined bundle of muscle fibers, called the bundle of His. This bundle of conductive fibers then splits into several branches known as bundle branches. These bundle branches carry the electrical impulse to the ventricular muscle. Within the ventricular muscle are additional specialized conductive fibers called Purkinje fibers, which will then stimulate the remainder of the ventricular muscle. For a review of these structures, see Unit 5.

As the electrical impulse is carried in this organized fashion through the heart, the muscle is stimulated to contract in a coordinated fashion. Because the atria are stimulated by the electrical impulse first, they will contract first, moving blood into the ventricles.

The ventricles will contract after they have been stimulated by the electrical impulses received by the bundle branches and Purkinje fibers. When the ventricles contract in an organized fashion, the effect is for blood to be ejected out through both the aorta and the pulmonary artery. Figure 24.1 depicts the path of the heart's electrical stimulation.

Every heartbeat has an electrical event that precedes the mechanical event. The normal electrical event within the heart is the propagation of electrical impulses from the SA node to the ventricles, as outlined. This electrical activity from the heart can be detected by an ECG machine and graphically displayed on an oscilloscope or printed on paper. This display is called an **electrocardiogram (ECG).**

An ECG normally displays a pattern of grouped waves, called *complexes.* These regularly repeating complexes are seen as a rhythm (a regularly recurring or repeating pattern) on the ECG. The natural source of a normal cardiac complex is the sinus-atrial (SA) node. Therefore, the electrical rhythm that is seen when the heart's electrical system is functioning properly is called a **normal sinus rhythm (NSR).** A normal sinus rhythm is the predominant natural rhythm of the heart.

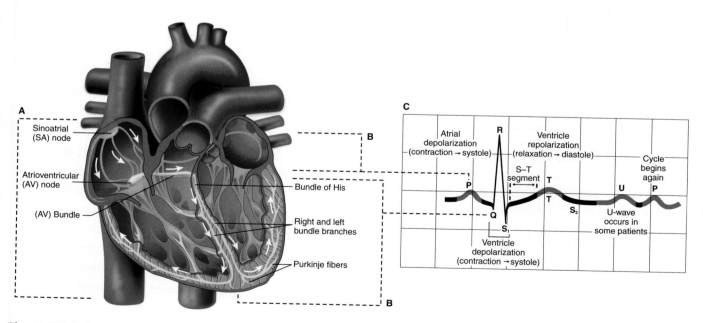

Figure 24.1 An electrical impulse from the SA node travels to the AV node and the ventricle, causing the ventricle to contract and creating a pulse

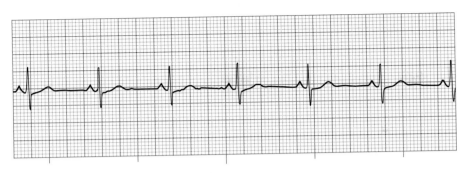

Figure 24.2 Normal sinus rhythm

Although it is not within the scope of practice for an EMT to interpret an ECG, it is helpful in understanding the physiology of cardiac arrest. Figure 24.2 shows an example of a normal sinus rhythm.

ESCAPE PACEMAKERS

The normal source of a heartbeat is the SA node. The SA node is therefore referred to as the heart's pacemaker because it establishes the rate of stimulation and, therefore, contraction.

Heart muscle, or myocardium, has a unique ability to be its own pacemaker. If for some reason the SA node or AV node fails to function properly, the ventricles have the ability to pace themselves, although not as efficiently as the normal conduction system. This ability of the myocardium to self-pace is called **automaticity.**

The special ability of the myocardium to function independently is valuable when the electrical system fails. The resulting rhythm, called an **escape rhythm,** may provide the patient with enough blood flow to stay alive until a physician can insert an artificial pacemaker (a manmade electronic device that will create an electrical impulse signaling the heart to beat). An escape rhythm is slower and less efficient than a normal sinus rhythm. Pacemakers are discussed later in the unit.

DYSRHYTHMIA

When the heart's muscle is injured during an AMI, the muscle becomes irritable, firing chaotically. This irritability can lead to disruptions in the normal sinus rhythm. Any disruption of the normal sinus rhythm is called a *dysrhythmia.*

Occasionally, a small group of irritated cells in the ventricles will start to fire earlier than expected. This unnatural pacemaker creates a **premature ventricular complex (PVC)** (Figure 24.3). A PVC interrupts the regular sinus rhythm and is therefore a dysrhythmia. PVCs can disturb blood flow and are felt as an irregular pulse. PVCs can be an indication of ventricular irritability.

If the signal from this small group of cells in the ventricles is fast enough and strong enough, it can take over the heart's own inherent pacemaker. The ventricles often race at rates from 100 bpm to 250 bpm. The resulting ECG rhythm is called *ventricular tachycardia.* Ventricular tachycardia creates a distinctive ECG, similar to a sine wave pattern (Figure 24.4).

Racing ventricles with a heart rate over 150 bpm do not have enough time to fill with blood and then empty. The result is little or no blood flow to the body, particularly to the coronary arteries. Pulses are quickly lost, and the patient loses consciousness. If a normal heartbeat does not resume quickly, the patient eventually dies. Defibrillation can help to halt this rapid firing of irritable ventricular cells when there is no pulse.

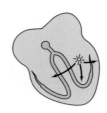

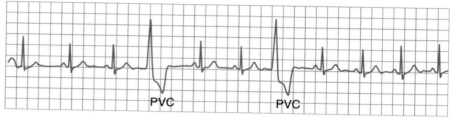

Figure 24.3 Unnatural pacemakers, created by an AMI, interrupt the normal sinus rhythm

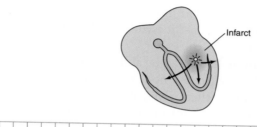

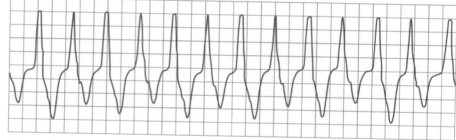

Figure 24.4 Ventricular tachycardia robs the heart's coronary arteries of life-giving blood

If the area of damage from an AMI is extensive, a large group of cells in the ventricle becomes irritable. These irritable cells misfire and can lead to sudden cardiac death. This process can be compared to a nuclear explosion. A pound of uranium is dangerous and potentially lethal. Several pounds of uranium are enough to create a spontaneous nuclear reaction and even a nuclear explosion.

Similarly, if enough irritable ventricular myocardial cells fire prematurely, they can result in **ventricular fibrillation,** or "v-fib," a chaotic firing of multiple ventricular cells resulting in no organized rhythm. During ventricular fibrillation, the heart simply quivers and does not create any forward blood flow. The ECG looks like a chaotic collection of waves that have no discernible rhythm (Figure 24.5).

Without a coordinated rhythmic contraction, blood flow stops and pulses are lost. The patient is in cardiac arrest. Without any blood pressure, the coronary arteries are not filled and the heart muscle goes without oxygen. Defibrillation can halt this chaotic firing of cells.

Eventually, the damage is so extensive, and the cells so damaged, that all cardiac activity stops. The heart, in **cardiac standstill,** will lie flaccid and unable to respond to any stimulus. The inert heart is in a flatline ECG rhythm

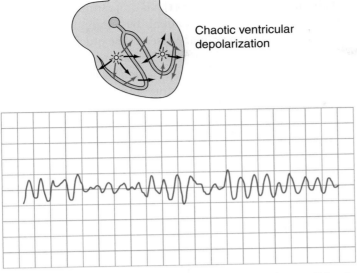

Chaotic ventricular
depolarization

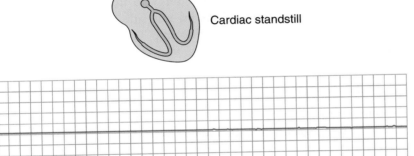

Figure 24.5 Lethal ventricular fibrillation has no discernible rhythm

Cardiac standstill

Figure 24.6 Asystole, a true arrhythmia, occurs in cardiac standstill

called asystole, meaning "without contraction." Because there is no electrical activity, it would not help to defibrillate the patient in asystole. CPR and rapid transport are indicated.

Asystole is a true arrhythmia, meaning "without rhythm." Without any electrical activity in the ventricles, the patient's ECG will be flatline, or asystolic (Figure 24.6).

PULSELESS ELECTRICAL ACTIVITY

Certain conditions, such as severe blood loss, result in no forward blood flow from the heart despite adequate electrical activity. This is called **pulseless electrical activity (PEA)**. It is important for the EMT to realize that despite normal-appearing electrical activity on an ECG, the patient may have cardiac compromise. The best bet is to pay close attention to the patient and not to the monitor. If the patient has no pulse, CPR should be begun, despite the ECG findings.

PEA is not treated with a shock, because there is nothing wrong with the electrical activity. The proper course of action is CPR, 100% oxygen, and rapid transport to the closest appropriate hospital where the cause can be determined and treated.

Street Smart

Doctors, nurses, paramedics, and EMTs often use the terms *arrhythmia* and *dysrhythmia* interchangeably. Although not strictly correct, it is accepted practice.

The assessment of the cardiac arrest victim is done similarly to the assessment of any other unresponsive medical patient. Beginning with a scene size-up, the EMT moves through the primary assessment quickly, providing airway, breathing, and circulatory (ABC) support, in that order. Because cardiac arrest requires significant work before the completion of even the primary assessment, the EMT may never get to a history and secondary assessment. It is, however, important that the EMT gather any known history from the patient's family while care is being provided to the patient. Such historical information will be useful to both advanced providers and hospital personnel.

SCENE SIZE-UP

As discussed in Unit 15, scene safety must always be addressed. Fluids present a hazard to the EMT using an AED. Fluids can transmit the electrical energy to the EMT instead of to the patient, resulting in injury to the EMT. Examples of fluids that can potentially transmit electricity include snow, vomit, rain, urine, and pooled water. If the patient is wet, he should be immediately moved to a dry place. Then the patient should be toweled dry before proceeding. Never defibrillate a patient who is still lying in a puddle of liquid.

The patient's body should also not be in contact with any metal objects. Again, the metal can transmit the energy to the EMT instead of to the patient. Examples of metal objects include sidewalk grates, catwalks, beds of pickup trucks and aluminum flooring. The patient should be moved immediately, in an emergency carry, to a safe location before an AED is used (Figure 24.7).

GENERAL IMPRESSION

The initial dispatch information may have been for a cardiac arrest. CPR may already be in progress when the EMT arrives. In those cases, the EMT enters the scene prepared.

In some cases, the dispatch information does not match the patient's situation. The call may have been received for a "person passed out" or, commonly, for a "person seizing." The EMT walks into those calls unaware of the situation.

Stop and look around the scene first. Get the global picture. Tables or lamps that are knocked over indicate a sudden collapse. If the telephone is off the hook, the patient may have been calling for help. Medications, both over-the-counter and prescription, left out may give a clue to the patient's condition.

Gather a quick impression from the patient's overall appearance. Whether the patient is on the ground, sitting in a chair, or lying in a bed, he will be unconscious if in cardiac arrest. Without blood circulating, the patient will be grossly cyanotic.

Try to obtain a chief concern from any available family member or bystanders. Ask whether anybody witnessed the patient's collapse. If the patient fell, ask whether the head struck anything on the way down. If no one is available, or the answers are questionable, assume spinal trauma.

Position the patient for further assessment. If the patient is unconscious and CPR is likely to be needed, then the patient needs to be on a firm surface. Move the patient out of the bed or chair and onto the floor. If the room is small, such as a bathroom or a cramped bedroom, consider quickly moving the patient to a larger room, such as the hallway or living room (Figure 24.8).

If the patient is unconscious or is in cardiac arrest, the assistance of ALS personnel is required. If ALS is available, then request assistance to the scene right away.

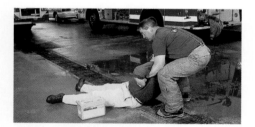

Figure 24.7 Before using the AED, make sure the scene is safe

PRIMARY ASSESSMENT

After completing the scene size-up, the EMT should immediately determine the patient's level of consciousness. If trauma is suspected, an EMT should take manual stabilization of the head and spine first.

If the patient is unconscious and unresponsive to pain, the EMT should immediately open the airway; please refer to Unit 9 for further details on how to open an airway. After the airway has been opened, the EMT should assess for the presence of breathing. If the patient is not breathing, the EMT should deliver two rescue breaths using an appropriate ventilation device. After these breaths have been given, the EMT should check for a carotid pulse.

If the patient is pulseless and the arrest was witnessed by the ambulance crew, the AED must be immediately prepared. If the arrest was not witnessed, then 2 minutes of CPR should be performed. Think of the assessment priorities as changing from ABC to ABCD: airway, breathing, circulation, and defibrillation. A detailed description of CPR will be presented later in this unit.

MANAGEMENT

The first step in management of cardiac arrest depends on whether the arrest was witnessed or not. The American Heart Association recommends 5 complete cycles or 2 minutes of CPR prior to using the AED, based on studies showing CPR first improves the effectiveness of defibrillation.

When cardiac arrest has been witnessed and CPR provided immediately, then the defibrillation should take place as soon as the AED can be gotten to the patient's side and ready to use.

The rest of this unit will explain how to perform CPR and use the AED in the patient experiencing cardiac arrest.

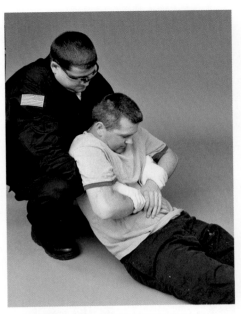

Figure 24.8 Quickly move the patient to a large enough area for CPR

CARDIAC ARREST AND CPR

It is important for the EMT to understand that CPR is only a stopgap measure intended to preserve the brain and heart until the arrival of the AED and a subsequent conversion, by defibrillation, of the deadly rhythm into a normal perfusing rhythm.

While the **return of spontaneous circulation (ROSC)** with CPR alone— that is, pulses returning with just CPR—does occur, these cases are rare, and the patient's survival more likely depends on the well-timed use of an AED.

For every minute of delay getting an AED to the patient, survival from ventricular fibrillation and sudden cardiac death decline by approximately 7–10%; therefore, the priority in emergency care of cardiac arrest is to get an AED to the patient.

CPR is also performed whenever a patient is pulseless and the AED indicates "no shock advised." In those cases, CPR is intended to help convert the nonshockable rhythm into a shockable rhythm, such as ventricular fibrillation, or simply to promote perfusion to the vital organs until a more definitive treatment is successful in restoring spontaneous circulation.

CPR is also performed in cases of near-cardiac arrest; for example, the patient who is in respiratory failure/arrest and the EMT performs rescue breathing, forestalling the inevitable cardiac arrest that would normally follow. This case is especially true in children, who more often die from respiratory failure than from cardiac disease.

CHAIN OF SURVIVAL

Using an AED on the patient in cardiac arrest is only part of the formula for a successful cardiac arrest reversal. Because ventricular fibrillation quickly

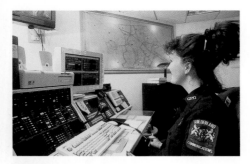

Figure 24.9 Early notification using 9-1-1, the first link in the chain of survival

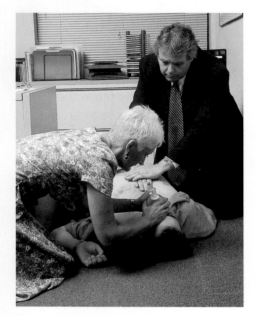

Figure 24.10 Early CPR buys time for the arrival of the AED

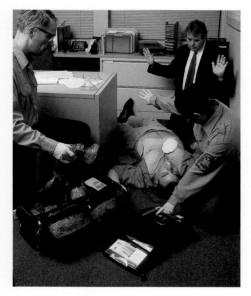

Figure 24.11 Early defibrillation saves lives

degenerates from active, yet chaotic, electrical activity to minimal electrical activity and then no activity at all, time is of the essence when treating the cardiac arrest victim. Every minute of delay calling EMS or getting a defibrillator to the patient decreases the chance that the heart will respond to the shock.

The American Heart Association recognized the importance of speed and started to advance the concept of the **chain of survival.** Simply, the chain of survival links all the elements of a cardiac arrest reversal together. The chain of survival depicts the important steps that must be taken to improve cardiac arrest survival.

EARLY ACCESS

Quick notification of EMS is key to getting EMTs trained in the use of an AED to the patient. Typically, EMS is accessed by calling 9-1-1. Unfortunately, 9-1-1 service is still not universally available in the United States.

One of the attractions of E9-1-1 is that it can provide the communications specialist the location of the call (Figure 24.9). Underlying this ability to locate a call is the assumption that the call is being placed from a stationary landline.

Although cellular telephones have made it easier for people to make calls from the scene of an incident, location identification was often difficult to acertain. Today, the FCC has implemented rules requiring that wireless phones be equipped with software to permit Automatic Location Identification. Current cellular phones have a GPS or similar system installed that can be used for location identification when 911 is initiated from that phone.

EARLY CPR

CPR saves lives. There are some documented instances in which CPR alone reversed a cardiac arrest; however, in most cases CPR is an important but temporary measure. Once EMS has been called, CPR helps preserve the brain until the EMT and AED are at the patient's side. Therefore, citizen CPR remains crucial to patient survival in a prehospital cardiac arrest (Figure 24.10).

EARLY DEFIBRILLATION

The definitive treatment for cardiac arrest due to ventricular fibrillation is defibrillation. The AED is an easy tool to use and allows rapid application of defibrillation to the cardiac arrest victim. EMTs have been targeted to learn AED use because they are the largest group of prehospital care providers (Figure 24.11). Citizens are also being encouraged to use the AED. These devices are commonly placed in work areas, airports, common areas, and any place where a cardiac arrest might occur and bystanders may be able to use an AED to reverse sudden cardiac death. These public access defibrillation programs have become common in industry, business, and community venues that support mass gatherings.

EARLY ADVANCED CARDIAC LIFE SUPPORT

Although an AED can reverse the fibrillation that led to the cardiac arrest, it does not address the cause of the fibrillation and recurrence is likely. Advanced life support (ALS) providers trained in advanced cardiac life support (ACLS) have the skills and knowledge to help protect the patient from further episodes of cardiac arrest. These ALS providers can help to stabilize the patient before and during transportation to the hospital.

SURVIVAL FROM CARDIAC ARREST

Any chain is only as strong as its weakest link. If CPR is provided in less than 4 minutes and defibrillation is provided in less than 8 minutes, the patient potentially has a 49–75% chance of survival, according to the American Heart

Association. For every minute that defibrillation is delayed to the victim of ventricular fibrillation, the chances of survival decrease by at least 10%. In the situation of cardiac arrest, every minute counts.

EMS AND CARDIAC ARREST

"Unknown, man down" or "person collapsed, CPR in progress" can alert the EMT to the possibility of cardiac arrest and the need for CPR. However, many cardiac arrest calls start out less clear. Some callers report a patient having a seizure, the last convulsion of an oxygen-starved brain before death. Other callers report a person with difficulty breathing, as the patient takes his last agonal breath. Because cardiac arrest can be sudden and unexpected, the EMT must always be prepared to perform CPR if needed.

When exiting the emergency vehicle on the scene of a suspected cardiac arrest, the EMT should have a selection of airway devices, including suction, oxygen, and a bag-valve-mask (BVM) as well as an AED.

Despite the excitement and anticipation surrounding a cardiac arrest, the EMT's first consideration must be scene safety when she enters the scene. This is especially true if more than one person has collapsed. Paying no heed to signs of danger leaves the EMT at risk for being the next victim.

OBVIOUS DEATH AND DNR

In some cases, death is obvious and it may not be appropriate to start CPR on the patient. For example, if the patient has **advanced lividity,** pooling of blood in the dependent portions of the body with a clear line of demarcation, or **rigor mortis,** a generalized stiffening of the body following death, then CPR may not be indicated. Other reasons to withhold CPR include decomposition of the body, incineration of the body, decapitation, hemicorporectomy (division of the body in half), and other obviously mortal wounds. The EMT should follow medical protocols regarding when to withhold CPR.

If family or bystanders are present, the EMT should inquire about a do not resuscitate (DNR) order. Some jurisdictions permit an EMT to honor a DNR order in the field. If the DNR can be produced and the EMT, following medical protocols, can honor the DNR, then CPR should not be started. If there is a delay in obtaining the DNR, the EMT might consider starting CPR while trying to contact medical control for more direction.

RESPONSIVENESS

The first step in CPR is determining whether the patient is responsive.

While donning personal protective equipment, minimally a pair of gloves and goggles, the EMT should decide if the situation is a medical circumstance, a trauma circumstance, or perhaps both. This decision affects the EMT's early care of the patient. If the patient is a trauma patient, the EMT must first maintain manual cervical spine stabilization in order to prevent further cervical injury before proceeding. If the patient is a medical patient, then manual cervical spine stabilization is unnecessary.

The EMT must then establish the patient's level of responsiveness. She should determine if the patient is responsive to voice by calling out to the patient, preferably using the patient's name, in a loud, firm voice. If the patient is unresponsive to voice, the EMT should tap the patient on the shoulder to determine unresponsiveness. Patients who appear unresponsive may actually be in deep sleep. The EMT should then proceed to give the patient a painful stimulus, like a sternal chest rub. If there has been no response to loud verbal and painful stimulus, then the patient is determined to be "unresponsive."

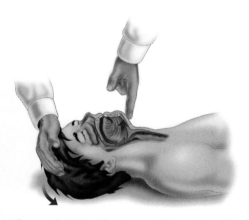

Figure 24.12 The head-tilt, chin-lift airway technique

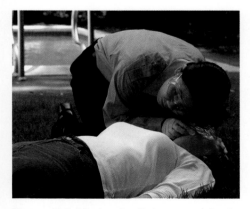

Figure 24.13 Look, listen, and feel for breathing

If the decision is made to start resuscitation, it may be necessary to move the patient from the position in which he was found. The patient should be positioned supine on a firm surface, such as the floor. It may be necessary to drag the patient off a bed and onto the floor before CPR can begin. If the patient has a suspected cervical spine injury, efforts should be made to maintain neutral cervical spine alignment. Often a long axis drag coupled with manual cervical spine stabilization is all that is needed.

A minimum of time should be taken to move the patient to a firm surface. Delays getting a patient to another room, for example, decrease the patient's chances of survival.

AIRWAY

With the patient on the firm surface, and the rescuer typically positioned at his side, the airway must next be opened. The tongue of an unconscious patient can obstruct the airway, so the head must be repositioned to open the airway. The method used for the medical patient, for whom no neck injury is suspected, is the head-tilt, chin-lift, as illustrated in Figure 24.12.

Placing the heel of one hand on the forehead of the patient and using the index finger and thumb to grasp the mandible (chin), the EMT gently tilts the head backward, feeling for resistance. If resistance is felt, it may mean that the patient has a neck injury or another reason for limited neck mobility, requiring the EMT to use the jaw thrust maneuver.

If the patient is a suspected trauma patient or has limited neck mobility, then the EMT should reposition at the head of the patient and, reaching toward the chest, grasp the angle of the patient's lower jaw with both hands, placing the thumb on the patient's zygoma (cheekbones) and lifting the jaw upward. These two airway maneuvers are discussed in Unit 9.

Occasionally, when the EMT opens the airway and inspects the oropharynx, secretions or vomitus may be present. If this is the case, the airway should be aggressively cleared. If large pieces of food are seen, the EMT should use the forefingers like a hook and scoop out the pieces. A bite block, a large airway inserted sideways between the molars, will prevent the EMT's fingers from being inadvertently bitten. The EMT should then proceed to mechanically suction to remove the remaining secretions.

If these secretions are not removed and the patient is ventilated, either by mouth-to-mouth rescue breathing or with a BVM, they will be forced into the lungs and cause an aspiration of foreign liquids or solid material into the lungs. Aspirates block narrow airways, prevent adequate ventilation of the lungs, and can produce hypoxia.

BREATHING

With the airway opened, the EMT should proceed to check for breathing. The mnemonic "look, listen, and feel" summarizes the three-step approach to verify the presence or absence of breathing (Figure 24.13). The EMT should turn her head and place her ear near the patient's mouth. While in this position, the EMT should look to see if there is adequate chest rise, listen for the sound of breathing from the mouth, and feel the breath against the cheek.

If the patient is breathing and just unconscious, the EMT should evaluate the quality of the breathing. Breathing that is shallow and rapid or slow and agonal is not adequate and the patient should be supported by either rescue breathing or BVM.

If the patient is breathing adequately, then the EMT should proceed with the rest of the primary assessment, taking precautions in the case of suspected cervical spine injury.

If the patient is not breathing, then the EMT should proceed to breathe for him by either doing rescue breathing or using a BVM. The procedure for using a BVM is discussed in Unit 10. Figure 24.14 illustrates mouth-to-mouth rescue breathing; it should be noted that the face shield is present.

To perform mouth-to-mouth rescue breathing, the EMT uses a barrier device or pocket mask and provides two breaths that cause the chest to start to rise without overinflating the lungs.

Overinflation of the lungs can cause air to spill over into the esophagus and stomach. Gastric filling can result in decreased lung expansion and regurgitation followed by aspiration. To prevent this problem the EMT could use cricoid pressure, provided sufficient personnel are on hand to assist (see Unit 10 to review this technique).

The process of assessing for breathing should take about 10 seconds. It is important to adequately check for breathing. A short 5-second assessment of breathing may miss the person who is breathing agonally, while a prolonged assessment of breathing, greater than 10 seconds, may delay the time to defibrillation.

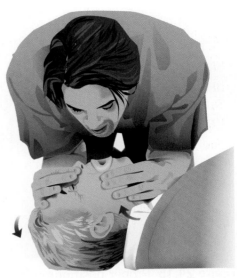

Figure 24.14 An EMT using a face shield and performing mouth-to-mouth rescue breathing

CIRCULATION

After delivering two measured breaths, the EMT should proceed to check the patient for a pulse. In adults, the pulse is verified at the carotid artery in the neck. A pulse here generally indicates that the brain is getting blood flow.

To find a pulse the EMT should place her index and middle finger on the patient's larynx (Adam's apple) at the midline of the anterior portion of the throat and then proceed, on the side closest to the EMT, to run the fingers posteriorly until they fall into a groove, about two or three finger breadths below the larynx. The carotid artery is found in the groove created by the sternocleidomastoid (SCM) muscle, also known as the strap muscle. The EMT should maintain the head-tilt, using one hand on the forehead. This position makes palpating (feeling) the carotid artery easier.

Finding a pulse on a living person is relatively easy; confirming the absence of a pulse on a pulseless patient is more difficult. The EMT should frequently practice finding the carotid pulse so during an emergency she can locate it quickly and easily.

Once the EMT has found the carotid artery pulse point, she should palpate (feel) for a pulse for approximately 10 seconds. If a pulse is present, then the EMT should proceed with the rest of the primary assessment. If the pulse is absent, then the EMT should proceed to chest compressions.

If the EMT suspects that the patient is hypothermic from the cold, a longer pulse check may be necessary. Some experts advocate taking as long as 30 seconds to confirm pulselessness. The EMT should follow the medical protocol for assessing and treating hypothermia in these cases.

CHEST COMPRESSIONS

After confirming pulselessness, the EMT performs external chest compressions, also known as *cardiac massage*. Chest compressions are a series of rhythmic compressions of the anterior chest to compress the heart and great vessels and, in turn, create a blood flow to the vital organs.

It should be noted that even expertly performed manual CPR produces only about 25% of normal blood flow, an inadequate blood flow to sustain life. It is imperative that the heart start pumping on its own, which requires a restart of the heart using the defibrillator.

To perform manual external chest compressions, the EMT must first expose the patient's chest to find landmarks for proper hand placement. The chest needs to be bared to facilitate proper hand placement on the sternum

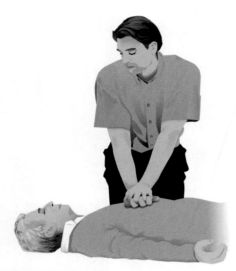

Figure 24.15 Proper positioning for chest compressions

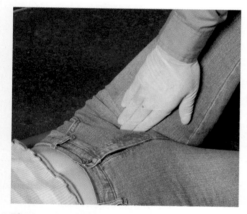

Figure 24.16 Palpation of the femoral pulse to verify compressions

for chest compressions. Using physical landmarks that can be visualized on the bare chest to find proper hand position for compressions, the EMT should lay the heel of one hand on the lower half of the sternum, between the nipples. The EMT should then place the other hand on top of the first hand.

The EMT may choose to either interlace fingers or extend them to keep them off the chest wall. In every case it is important that the fingers of the EMT do not touch the chest wall.

The EMT should take the time to find the proper placement of the hands. Compression of the bottom portion of the sternum may result in injuries to the liver, spleen, and stomach, and compressions of the upper half of the sternum will not be effective.

While kneeling, with legs slightly apart and with both hands positioned perpendicular to the long axis of the sternum, the EMT should make sure her shoulders are squared directly over the patient's chest.

The EMT's elbows should be locked with the arms straight, permitting the EMT to use shoulder and back strength to produce the force of compression. Arm muscles quickly tire after only a few minutes of compressions, but the back and shoulder muscles are more capable of sustaining the compressions for a longer period of time. Figure 24.15 illustrates proper position of the EMT to perform compressions.

The EMT then compresses the sternum downward, toward the ground, approximately 1½–2 inches in depth. Production of a carotid or femoral pulse is evidence of adequate compression. Figure 24.16 illustrates palpation of a femoral pulse.

The EMT should deliver chest compressions using the "push hard and push fast" method. It is vital to allow for complete chest recoil to allow blood to flow back into the heart. Complete chest recoil is achieved when the chest returns to its normal position between every compression. During the recoil phase the EMT should leave her hands on the chest wall, prepared to begin the next chest compression immediately following adequate chest recoil. By keeping her hands lightly on the patient's chest wall—so that a sheet of paper could be slipped under them—the EMT can feel the chest recoil and be ready to begin the next compression.

The EMT should be able to complete 30 compressions at a rate of 100 compressions per minute. The compression should not be abrupt, stabbing, or springy, with the arms recoiling from every compression, but rather a steady rhythmic up-and-down motion. Properly performed CPR can produce systolic blood pressures of 60–80 mmHg.

The chest compression rate for one-rescuer CPR is 30 compressions to two ventilations for five complete cycles. The compressor should be switched every 2 minutes to maintain effective chest compressions with adequate chest recoil. After five complete cycles or 2 minutes, reassess the patient for circulation and breathing. If there is no pulse, resume CPR by completing five cycles of 30 compressions to two ventilations.

If two EMTs are present, one performs chest compressions while the second EMT ventilates the patient with either a BVM or pocket mask. The compression to ventilation rate for two-rescuer CPR is the same as one rescuer CPR, 30 compressions to two ventilations at a rate of 100 compressions per minute.

After two slow breaths of one second each, providing approximately 500 cc of volume delivered to the patient, the first EMT should resume compressions, completing five cycles of 30 compressions to two ventilations. After five cycles the EMT at the head should first attempt to palpate for a carotid pulse during compressions to determine if they are effective, and then call for compressions to stop. Reassessing the patient for a carotid pulse for 5 to 10 seconds, and finding

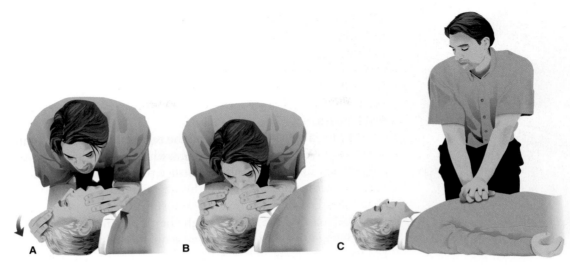

Figure 24.17 The cycle of airway, breathing, and circulation

none, the EMT at the head should deliver two breaths and call for compressions to continue. Figure 24.17 illustrates the cycle of opening the airway, ventilating the patient (barrier device present but not visible), and chest compressions.

If an advanced airway (endotracheal tube, esophageal tracheal combitube, or supraglottic airway) has been placed, there should not be a pause for ventilations. The compressor should deliver continuous chest compressions at a rate of 100 per minute while the EMT providing ventilations should deliver breaths at 8–10 per minute.

AUTOMATED CHEST COMPRESSION DEVICES

Adequate manual chest compressions are also dependent on the fatigue of the provider, the firmness of the surface the patient is lying on while compressions are being delivered, and the accuracy of the compressions being performed—that is, good depth, rate, and sequence and allowing for full chest recoil. Recent studies have shown a higher incidence of return of spontaneous circulation (ROSC) occurs when there is a minimum interruption of chest compressions. In other words, one rescuer will be tasked to perform continuous compressions with little interruption.

Rather than manual compressions, some EMS systems use mechanical compression devices. Several such devices have either been approved for use or are under research.

The mechanical piston device depresses the sternum with a compressed-gas–powered plunger affixed to a backboard. The plunger is centered over the portion of the sternum where manual compressions would be applied and the piston device is positioned above the patient. This device can be configured to deliver a specific rate and depth of compression, allowing for uniform delivery of compressions that do not diminish in quality due to rescuer fatigue.

The load-distributing band CPR or vest CPR is a device that comprises a wide band applied to the chest circumferentially and sometimes attached to a backboard. This device is driven either pneumatically or electronically to provide inward constrictive pressure on the thorax, which causes the heart to be compressed.

Devices such as these can be deployed quickly, performing consistent depth and rate of compressions that can be adjusted to each patient. However, the greatest advantage, as illustrated in Figure 24.18, may be that it helps to free the EMT to attend to other functions, such as helping to maintain the airway.

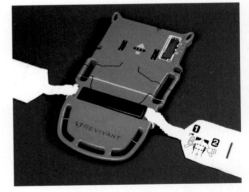

A.

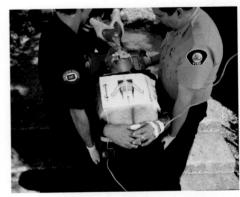

B.

Figure 24.18 A. The Autopulse device B. The Autopulse in position and performing compressions

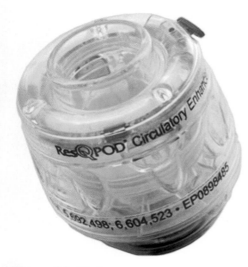

Figure 24.19 Impedance threshold device

IMPEDANCE THRESHOLD DEVICE

The impedance threshold device is another tool that has been shown to improve blood flow through the heart during CPR. The device is placed between the advanced airway device and the ventilatory adjunct, usually a BVM, being used to provide ventilations and is designed with a valve that limits the amount of air allowed to enter the chest and lungs during the chest recoil phase of chest compressions.

The recoil of the chest during the relaxation phase of compressions creates a negative intrathoracic pressure, which normalizes as air moves into the lungs. The impedance threshold device prohibits air from rushing in during the relaxation phase, allowing the negative intrathoracic pressure to draw more blood toward the heart. The result is better cardiac filling before the next chest compression. Although the impedance threshold device is currently being used with advanced airways, it is being considered for use by the EMT in the non-intubated patient where a tight mask seal can be constantly maintained (Figure 24.19).

PEDIATRIC CPR

It is rare for children to go into isolated cardiac arrest, unless they have congenital heart disease. Instead, another event, usually respiratory in nature, precedes the cardiac event. For this reason the EMT should first perform rescue breathing before calling for help. Phone fast for children as opposed to phone first for adults is a useful mnemonic.

Newborns occasionally need stimulation to breathe and even ventilation in a very small percentage of deliveries. This subject is covered in Unit 41 under newborn care.

The process of resuscitation for a child is similar to that of an adult, with the exception that was just noted about phone fast. The differences between pediatric resuscitation and adult resuscitation lie in the unique characteristics of a child's anatomy. For purposes of this discussion, the term *infant* will be used for patients under one year of age and the term *child* for the patient one year of age to adolescence. Adolescence is defined as nipple budding on girls and armpit hair on boys.

The first difference is the airway of the child. A child's head is noticeably larger in proportion to the body than is an adult's head. For this reason it is important to pad the area behind the child's chest to elevate the chest to a neutral position. Although the sizes of children vary, a dependable measure of proper placement is when the opening of the ears is in line, horizontally, with the midline of the shoulder.

With the head in a neutral position, the EMT should gently open the airway. When using the head-tilt, chin-lift technique, the EMT should use caution placing her fingers in position. The soft underside of the chin can easily be displaced upward, pushing the tongue against the hard palate and obstructing the airway. Figure 24.20 illustrates the airway position and ventilation of an infant.

If a child is suspected of having a foreign body obstruction, a common occurrence because of children's smaller airways, the EMT should use the techniques described for pediatric medical emergencies in Unit 42 to relieve the obstruction.

If the airway is clear, the EMT should assess for breathing, using the same look, listen, and feel technique described for adults. If the breathing appears at all distressed—that is, gasping and ineffective—the EMT should ventilate the child.

The EMT should proceed to check the child's pulse. Depending on the size of the child, either the carotid or brachial pulse will be palpated. The

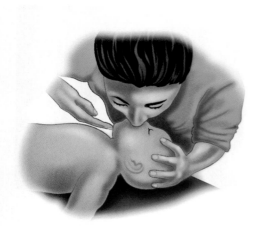

Figure 24.20 Neutral head position for rescue breathing for an infant

brachial pulse is palpated instead of the carotid, typically in children less than 1 year of age, when the EMT is unable to find landmarks on the throat because the child's neck is short and chubby.

The brachial pulse is found on the inner aspect of the upper arm, proximal to the bicep muscle, midline between the elbow and the shoulder.

If no pulse is present the EMT should proceed with chest compressions, depressing the chest approximately one third to one half the depth of the chest, after finding the correct compression site.

The compression site for an infant less than 1 year of age is approximately one finger width below the imaginary line that runs between the nipples, also called the **intermammary line.** Figure 24.21 shows the proper finger position for an infant for compressions.

During two-person CPR on an infant, the EMT should encircle the infant's chest with her hands and perform compressions with the thumbs. This technique is both effective and less tiring for some EMTs.

The compression point for a child is the same as for an adult, except only one hand is used to compress the chest approximately 1–1½ inches. Figure 24.22 shows the proper hand position for chest compressions on a child.

Compression-to-ventilation ratios for children and infants are the same as for adults, 30 compressions to two ventilations. However, the compression-to-ventilation ratio changes when two-person CPR is being administered to infants and children. For infants and children 1 year to adolescent, the compression-to-ventilation ratio in two-rescuer CPR is adjusted to 15:2.

ADULT FOREIGN BODY AIRWAY OBSTRUCTION

Choking, although common, is a rare cause of cardiac arrest, because most people are able to clear their airway without assistance. For this reason, the first step in assisting a person who is experiencing an airway obstruction, typically from meat, is to allow him to attempt clearing his own airway as long as good air exchange occurs. During this time the EMT should remain with the patient and stand by in case his needs should change.

It is when the patient has poor air exchange, as evidenced by cyanosis, a weak or weakening cough, and subsequent loss of consciousness that the EMT must act.

Initially the EMT should ask the patient, "Are you choking? Can you speak?" The patient with an obstructed airway will be unable to speak and may clutch his neck, in a demonstration of the universal choking sign illustrated in Figure 24.23.

With the victim either standing or sitting, the EMT should come around to the back of the patient and place her fist into the area below the xiphoid process, midway and midline between the sternum and the umbilicus.

Grasping the fist with the other hand, the EMT should perform forceful upward abdominal thrusts. This series of forceful upward abdominal thrusts forces air out of the lungs and the trachea. It is often necessary to perform the procedure repeatedly until the obstruction is relieved or the patient becomes unconscious.

Signs that the obstruction has been relieved include seeing the object that has obstructed the airway forced out, the patient taking a gasp of air, or the patient speaking. Figure 24.24 illustrates two positions to relieve obstruction in the conscious patient.

If the patient becomes unconscious, the EMT should help protect him from falling and striking his head by easing him to the floor. Then the EMT

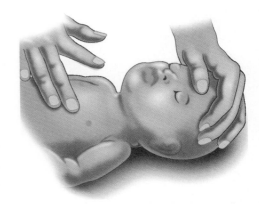

Figure 24.21 Proper finger position for infant CPR

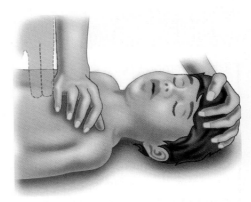

Figure 24.22 Proper hand position for child chest compressions

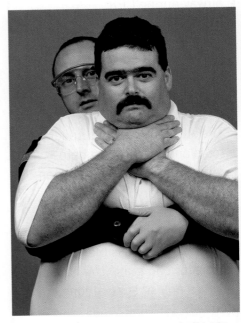

Figure 24.23 The universal choking sign

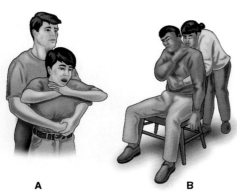

Figure 24.24 Abdominal thrusts performed while standing and seated

should be sure that EMS has been dispatched and that additional help, especially ALS, is on the way before proceeding.

Once the patient is on the floor, the EMT should begin CPR. She should look into the mouth while opening the airway during CPR. If the object is visible, then the EMT should insert a gloved finger formed like a hook into the side of the mouth and scoop the object out. If there is concern about the patient biting, an oral airway may be placed between the molars to act as a bite block.

If the object is not visible, the EMT should continue CPR for 2 minutes, checking to see if the object can be visualized with each pause for ventilations. If the obstruction cannot be visualized and removed, continue CPR until ALS arrives, providing ventilations in the interim.

SPECIAL SITUATIONS IN CPR

The EMT performing CPR is doubly tasked to perform effective CPR while moving the patient toward the ambulance and to the hospital.

For ease of movement of the patient, an EMT may elect to place him on a backboard or similar rigid device, regardless of the presence or absence of spine injury. It is important that the EMT tell emergency department personnel, upon arrival, that the patient is not a trauma patient and that the backboard was used as a convenience for moving the patient.

If the patient lives on an upper story of a building, it will be necessary to move him down to the ground floor and the awaiting ambulance. In some instances an elevator will accommodate the patient lying supine. In many cases the patient will have to be carried down the stairs. In those instances, CPR should be performed for a minimum of 2 minutes and the patient reassessed. If no pulse is found, the patient should be moved quickly to the next landing, or to the foot of the stairs, and CPR should resume for another five cycles of 30 compressions to two ventilations or 2 minutes. If necessary, the process can resume for each flight of stairs.

Once on the ground floor the patient should be placed on the ambulance stretcher, with the stretcher remaining in the low position. The EMT can continue ventilations and compressions while the stretcher is moved to the ambulance.

As space inside an ambulance is often limited, it may be necessary for the EMT to either kneel beside the patient to continue compressions or to straddle the stretcher, placing her back against the ceiling and bracing their legs against the walls of the ambulance. The EMT should attempt to be in a position that will allow for safe and effective chest compressions to be delivered to the patient.

BYSTANDER CPR

An EMT may come across a bystander who is performing CPR, presenting some unique challenges to the EMT when working with these good Samaritans, because there are several differences between layperson CPR and the CPR that an EMT is trained to do.

To begin, the bystander may not have checked a pulse before beginning CPR. Several studies have indicated that laypeople are unfamiliar with, and have trouble finding, the carotid pulse; bystanders correctly assess for a pulse approximately 35% of the time.

For this reason lay rescuers are taught to assess for **signs of circulation,** such as responsiveness, breathing, coughing, and movement, instead of a carotid pulse.

The EMT may also observe that no ventilations are being performed. The bystander is performing hands-only (compression-only) resuscitation. Many bystanders are reluctant to perform mouth-to-mouth rescue breathing, particularly on a stranger, and especially in the absence of a barrier device such as a face shield.

The bystander may have received instruction on CPR from an emergency medical dispatcher. These EMS dispatchers can provide only limited instruction on the telephone and, to conserve time, provide bystanders with only instructions on how to perform compressions.

Finally, the bystander may be physically unable to perform ventilations, perhaps due to advanced lung disease. Some respiratory conditions preclude the well-meaning bystander from performing ventilations.

Although cardiopulmonary resuscitation with both ventilations and compressions is desirable, the usefulness of hands-only resuscitation has been supported by evidence. None of the studies demonstrated there was a negative impact on the survival of the patient when mouth-to-mouth ventilations were not delivered by the lay provider.

BYSTANDER–EMT CPR

Bystanders are not taught two-person CPR, only one-person CPR. If the EMT arrives on scene—assuming that other EMT responders have been notified—and bystander CPR is in progress, the EMT has several options depending on the circumstances.

If the EMT determines that the bystander appears to be comfortable with doing CPR, perhaps by asking if he wants relief and being told no, the EMT should attend to other tasks and permit the bystander to continue one-person CPR. In the interim, while awaiting the arrival of more EMS, the EMT could assess the effectiveness of CPR by checking a carotid pulse or prepare the BVM assembly.

If the bystander appears exhausted and CPR appears ineffective, the EMT should offer to take over compressions from the bystander. In those instances, the EMT should first confirm the absence of a pulse and breathing and then commence CPR as indicated.

The bystander may be willing to continue CPR and provide assistance valuable to the resuscitation. In that case the EMT should ask if the bystander is fatigued (the EMT would replace the bystander and perform one-person CPR) or would like to continue to perform compressions only. If the bystander is willing to perform compressions, then the EMT should call for a halt to CPR and reassess the patient's airway, breathing, and circulation. If no pulse or breathing is present, the EMT should deliver two rescue breaths and instruct the bystander to begin compressions. The rate for one-person CPR and two-person CPR is the same—a compression-to-ventilation ratio of 30:2. The bystander should be replaced when a second EMS provider arrives. Figure 24.25 shows a bystander helping with CPR.

THE AUTOMATED EXTERNAL DEFIBRILLATOR

The obvious problem in a cardiac arrest is that no blood flows from the heart to the body. Although CPR provides some blood flow, this technique cannot sustain the body for a long period. The best CPR provides only about 30% of the normal cardiac output. The preferred option would be to have the heart beat naturally.

If an electrical current is passed through the fibrillating heart muscle, the electrical current will stun, or shock, the heart. In the ideal situation, all uncoordinated contractions of the heart stop immediately and simultaneously.

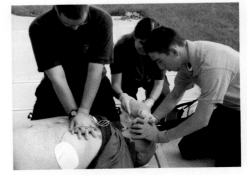

Figure 24.25 Citizen helps to hold the mask seal as the EMT performs CPR after a "no shock advised" by an AED

Street Smart

In many instances the bystander may know the patient. The patient may even be a family member. In these cases, the bystander who has performed CPR has an obvious interest in the outcome. The EMT should consider contacting the bystander later to relay the outcome of the resuscitation or, minimally, to thank him or her for assisting.

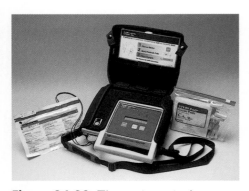

Figure 24.26 The automated external defibrillator, or AED

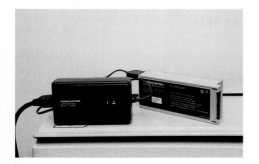

Figure 24.27 The rechargeable battery is the power source for the AED

Then natural sinus pacemakers can assume dominance over the heart and a normal sinus rhythm can begin again.

For defibrillation to work there must be some muscular activity in the heart. Pulseless ventricular tachycardia and ventricular fibrillation are two examples of shockable rhythms.

Asystole is an example of a nonshockable rhythm. Without any muscular activity, the heart will not respond to the defibrillation. In those cases, CPR should be continued until ventricular fibrillation appears.

The purpose of the AED is to assess the rhythm of the heart in a pulseless patient and deliver the appropriate shock when a shockable rhythm is detected.

ELEMENTS OF THE AED

The AED consists of two large electrodes (pads that are placed on the patient's chest) and cables (leads) that connect the patient to the machine. A battery power source is also necessary to generate the electricity used to perform the defibrillation. Figure 24.26 shows the components of the AED.

At the beginning of every shift, the EMT must ensure that the AED is properly prepared for use. An overall inspection should be performed. The case should be intact. Cases may be broken when an AED is accidentally dropped. All electrodes should be sealed within a protective wrapper. Check the expiration date on the electrode package. Electrodes should never be opened until used because they can become dried out and useless. An extra pair of electrodes should be carried just for this reason.

BATTERIES

The AED uses a battery for its power source. Batteries have a tendency to stop working when they are needed most. Every AED should be equipped with a backup battery. The EMT should always ensure that the primary battery and backup battery are adequately charged.

Some types of batteries require regular recharging; others have a charge that lasts for years without a need for a recharge (Figure 24.27). The EMT should familiarize herself with the type of battery her agency uses in its AED.

SUPPLIES

In every routine equipment check, the EMT should ensure that the proper accessory supplies are with the AED. Most AEDs used by EMTs are equipped with a case that has several pockets used to hold additional supplies that may be needed.

It is always advisable to have a spare set of electrode pads as well as a spare battery on hand. Because an AED is used in life-or-death situations, it is important to have redundancy in critical supplies. Families of patients have successfully sued EMS providers that responded with an AED that had dead batteries.

The electrode pads must tightly adhere to the chest wall for optimal delivery of the electrical energy. Moisture prevents proper adhesion. A gauze 4-by-4 pad or a towel should be immediately available to wipe down the chest before applying the electrodes.

Excessive chest hair can also interfere with adhesion of electrodes. A razor may be used to shave hair from the chest for ideal electrode adhesion; however, it is often not necessary and may waste precious time. A safety razor should, however, be available so that if it is necessary to shave a portion of the patient's chest, it can be done quickly.

After completing an AED equipment check, always document the inspection and testing of the AED. Failure to document an inspection leaves the EMT vulnerable should a lawsuit occur owing to equipment failure. Be sure to report malfunctions and take the faulty AED out of service until it can be serviced by a qualified biomedical engineer.

AED INDICATIONS AND CONTRAINDICATIONS

The AED was developed to provide for rapid defibrillation of the fibrillating heart in the adult, non-traumatic cardiac arrest patient. Recent studies have shown the AED can and should be used in children over 1 year of age. By simply placing the pediatric electrodes in the AED, the machine automatically lowers the defibrillation energy to a pediatric dose.

For infants under 1 year of age, begin CPR and DO NOT apply the AED. AED use in infants has not been shown to be beneficial. The primary cause of cardiac arrest in children is respiratory compromise and sudden infant death syndrome, neither of which normally present with ventricular fibrillation.

AED is also not intended for patients suffering cardiac arrest due to traumatic injury. The cause of cardiac arrest in these patients is usually blood loss, and defibrillation will not help. In trauma, cardiac arrest is more commonly caused by the trauma than from a cardiac cause. Trauma patients in cardiac arrest require immediate CPR with bleeding control and spinal immobilization. However, in cases in which it is unclear if trauma caused the cardiac arrest or the cardiac arrest was the cause of the trauma, possibly seen in a motor vehicle crash (MVC), consult medical direction and follow local protocols concerning the use of the AED.

USE OF THE AED

The AED has an internal computer that samples the heart's electrical rhythm through sensors in the electrodes. The computer measures the waves in the heart's electrical activity against a logic formula. If the computer analysis indicates that the rhythm is ventricular fibrillation, or any other rhythm that will potentially respond to defibrillation, then an audible and/or visual warning advises the operator (EMT) that a shock is indicated.

The single largest advantage of an AED is that it does not require the EMT or operator to learn the complex rules of ECG interpretation. The ECG is the record of the heart's electrical activity. There are many different patterns of electrical activity the heart can exhibit, each of which requires a different management strategy. Advanced training is required to learn the technique of ECG interpretation and is not within the scope of practice for the EMT. The EMT should allow the AED to interpret the rhythm and advise if a shock is indicated.

Street Smart

Do not be surprised if an AED has already been used before EMS is on scene. AEDs have so improved in simplicity and dependability that certain segments of the public are being trained in the use of an AED. Airlines routinely train flight attendants in the use of the AED.

Public access defibrillation (PAD), the availability of a defibrillator to the lay public, has become commonplace in the shopping mall, on the factory floor, and in the business office. CPR courses routinely include AED training for rescuers.

Street Smart

Large public gatherings, such as county fairs or sporting events, are often scenes of cardiac arrests. EMTs assigned to stand by at these events should have an AED readily available. The AED left in the ambulance is of no value to the patient who is in the middle of the bleachers in cardiac arrest.

CPR should be performed for five cycles of 30:2 (approximately 2 minutes) prior to AED application in unwitnessed cardiac arrest for patients who are 1–8 years of age. CPR is performed prior to AED application in children to ensure the airway of the child is clear and to provide good ventilations, because the most common reason for a child to go into cardiac arrest is due to an occluded airway or respiratory failure.

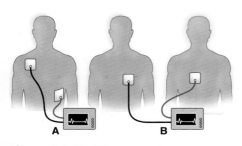

Figure 24.28 There are two acceptable positions for the AED pads: (A) anterior-anterior or (B) anterior-posterior

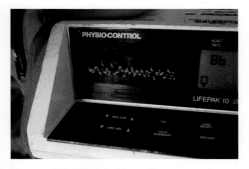

Figure 24.29 Motion, from road vibrations or CPR, creates ECG motion artifact

After completing the primary assessment and determining the patient is pulseless and breathless, CPR should be performed while the AED is prepared for use. For patients over 8 years of age if cardiac arrest was not witnessed or the "down time" is suspected to be greater than 4–5 minutes, five cycles of 30:2 or approximately 2 minutes of CPR should be performed prior to AED application.

If an AED is immediately available and the cardiac arrest was witnessed by the EMT, immediately apply the AED and follow the voice prompts. First, attach the electrode pads to the cables. Then place one pad under the patient's right clavicle and the other pad on the patient's lower left rib cage. Alternatively, one pad may be placed on the anterior chest and one on the posterior chest as indicated in Figure 24.28.

A diagram for electrode pad placement is often found either on the electrodes or on the AED. The cables may also be color coded. The white cable and pad are attached under the clavicle on the right. The red cable and pad are attached to the lower left rib cage (see Figure 24.28).

Once the AED has been attached to the patient, the power should be turned on. Usually the "power on" switch is prominently displayed. Every EMT should take a moment before the call to review the operational features of the AED before using it.

Following the voice prompt, the next step once the AED is operational, is to press the analyze button to activate the AED. The voice prompt will then advise the EMT or operator that the AED is analyzing.

If CPR is in progress, the EMT or operator should instruct everyone to stop. The usual command to the rest of the team is "all clear." **All clear** means that nothing, not even the bag-valve-mask, should touch the patient. Motion from CPR may create **motion artifact** (a false ECG reading created by vibration), causing the AED to mistakenly identify the ECG as ventricular fibrillation (Figure 24.29).

If the patient is already aboard the ambulance when he arrests, and the ambulance is moving, instruct the driver to stop the vehicle. Road vibrations can also create motion artifact that the AED could misinterpret as ventricular fibrillation. Some AEDs are designed to detect road noise and vibration and will direct the EMT to stop.

The AED may take a few seconds, after the analyze button has been pressed, to determine whether the ECG is a shockable rhythm, or a rhythm that will respond to defibrillation. If a shockable rhythm is identified, the AED will start to automatically charge. Most machines create an audible warning or a verbal prompt or both. The audible warning indicates that the AED is energizing. The verbal prompt typically states "shock advised" or a similar statement.

While the AED is charging, call all clear again. Be sure that nothing is touching the patient. Be sure no one is touching the patient while the AED is charging to prevent injury to a member of the resuscitation team should an accidental shock occur.

For the third and final time, the EMT or operator should call all clear. Some EMTs use the mantra "I'm clear, you're clear, we're all clear" while making a visual sweep of the patient before actually defibrillating the patient.

Always perform a head-to-toe visual sweep with every defibrillation. Make a habit of looking at the patient's nose, then looking at his toes, and looking again at his nose, before pressing the button to activate the defibrillator. The EMT should never become complacent about safety when using the AED, even if using the AED has become somewhat commonplace.

Once all team members are physically clear of the patient, the EMT or operator then presses the shock button. The shock button will deliver the defibrillation from the AED to the patient. It is normal for the patient's body to shudder from the defibrillation. This is the result of muscular contraction in the chest. This motion is minor and the patient will remain on the stretcher or backboard.

The EMT or operator should follow the voice prompt immediately following defibrillation. The AED will advise to start CPR immediately following the shock. CPR will be conducted for five cycles of 30:2 or 2 minutes, with the AED counting down the time frame. After 2 minutes of CPR, pause to check the patient's pulse, for no more than 10 seconds. If the patient has a pulse, check for breathing.

If the patient is breathing adequately, place him on oxygen via a non-rebreather mask and transport. If the patient is not breathing or not breathing adequately, continue to ventilate using positive pressure ventilation with supplemental oxygen.

If the patient does not have a pulse, push to reanalyze the rhythm. The AED will again go through the rhythm analysis and determine if a second shock is needed. Follow the voice prompts of the AED, repeating the previous sequence if the shock is advised.

If the patient is still in a shockable rhythm—that is, ventricular fibrillation—the AED automatically recharges the energy used for the next shock, according to a setting entered in its programming. After delivering the second shock, resume CPR for 2 minutes and transport as soon as possible. Some EMS systems will require a third shock prior to transport. Always follow local protocols or guidelines.

Some EMTs may be taught to use a manual defibrillator. In those cases, the first shock should be set at usually 360 joules or equivalent biphasic energy setting. Always follow the manufacturer's recommendations regarding the use of a manual defibrillator.

The EMT should check for pulse and breathing after each sequence of shock and 2 minutes of CPR. If none is present, the CPR should be resumed. The AED can be used again in 2 minutes to analyze the heart's rhythm to see whether a shockable rhythm is present. Remember that several rhythms will result in cardiac arrest yet are not amenable to defibrillation; therefore, the machine will say "no shock advised." If the patient does not have a pulse, however, CPR must be done and the patient should be transported quickly to the closest appropriate hospital. Skill 24-1 at the end of this unit describes the operation of an AED.

Street Smart

If the patient needs to be moved to the floor, consider sliding the seated patient onto a backboard. Place the backboard under the patient's feet and then slide the patient down the ramp. Once the patient is on the backboard, move the backboard to the floor. If the patient is in bed, consider logrolling the patient onto the backboard and then lifting the board onto the floor.

Street Smart

During an emotionally intense event such as a cardiac arrest, some new team members may become so focused on what they are doing that they mentally block out extraneous noise, including the command all clear.

Some EMTs or operators will physically sweep above the body with one hand, in a circular motion. This action will break another team member's concentration and redirect his attention to the EMT or operator. This technique is very useful in noisy environments as well. It is good practice to have all personnel step one step back and raise their hands, indicating they are clear of the body.

Safety Tips

If the patient is on the gurney, be sure that no one's foot is touching the metal carriage. It is common for an EMT to rest her feet on the lower bar of the gurney, out of sight of the EMT or operator handling the AED. Because the hard rubber wheels of the gurney electrically isolate the gurney, the EMT's foot creates a new electrical pathway, and the EMT may get shocked.

SPECIAL SITUATIONS FOR AED USE

Several situations may require slight deviation from the usual protocol in assessing and managing the patient in cardiac arrest. The EMT should be familiar with these few situations.

ARTIFICIAL PACEMAKERS

When the electrical system of the heart fails, causing bradycardia, a cardiologist will place an artificial pacemaker into the patient. The **artificial pacemaker** creates the impulse that signals the heart to beat, ensuring a heart rate that will support a normal blood pressure.

An artificial pacemaker has a pulse generator and a set of wires that lead to the heart. The pulse generator may be placed in a pocket under the skin below the right clavicle, and the pocket is sewn shut.

The AED electrode pad is placed in about the same location as the pacemaker. If a pacemaker is located under the skin, as indicated by a bulge about the size of a silver dollar, then the AED pads should be moved slightly to the left and down several inches toward the feet so that the electrode is not over the pacemaker.

If the AED electrode is placed immediately over the pacemaker, the AED may sense the pacer's impulse, seen as a spike on the ECG, and record that the heart is beating regularly. Even more important, if the AED functions correctly, detects the ventricular fibrillation, and delivers a defibrillation, the pacemaker will absorb some of the defibrillation energy and may not work properly afterward.

AUTOMATIC IMPLANTABLE CARDIOVERTER DEFIBRILLATOR

Using state-of-the-art microelectronics and more powerful microprocessors, physicians and biomedical engineers have created an AED that can be placed within the body. The **automatic implantable cardioverter defibrillator (AICD)** is used for patients who are at risk for developing recurrent ventricular tachycardia or fibrillation.

Often the patient's family will tell the EMT that the patient has an AICD. Many patients also carry an instruction card in their wallet or purse.

Similar to a pacemaker, the AICD has a generator/defibrillator and a set of wires that leads to the heart. When the AICD senses an event, such as ventricular fibrillation, it signals the defibrillator, which in turn shocks the heart.

Because the AICD is internal and the wires are attached directly to the heart, it takes very little energy to defibrillate the heart, 5–15 joules. The energy is so low and the shock so small that if the AICD should function, or fire, while the EMT is doing CPR, he may feel a mild tingling in the arms. This is not dangerous to the EMT but can be diminished by use of gloves, which act as an insulator.

The most common type of AICD looks very similar to an artificial pacemaker and may be located in the same location under the right clavicle (Figure 24.30) or in the left lower abdomen.

When an AICD is detected in the upper right side of the chest, the AED electrode pads should be moved slightly to the left of normal and several inches toward the feet, in the same placement as used for a patient with a pacemaker.

MEDICATION PATCHES

The use of transdermal patches has become increasingly popular. These self-adhesive patches contain medication that is slowly absorbed through the skin. Patches are an easy and convenient way of administering a medication that must have a steady level in the bloodstream. Alternatively, the patient would have to take a pill several times a day.

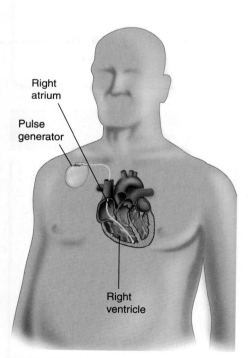

Right atrium

Pulse generator

Right ventricle

Figure 24.30 An automatic implantable cardioverter/defibrillator works like an internal AED

Examples of transdermal patches include nitroglycerin patches, used for cardiac patients; nicotine patches; analgesics used in patients with chronic pain; and hormone replacement patches, used in cancer prevention or treatment.

These transdermal patches often have an aluminum backing, or the drug's paste medium may be reactive to the defibrillation. Consequently, when the patient is shocked, the patch either ignites, making a popping sound, or heats up, burning the patient.

Patches are generally worn on the upper chest, on the upper back, or on the shoulders. Before operating the AED, the EMT must completely expose the patient's chest wall and look for patches.

Gloves should always be worn when removing a patch. Lift the corner of the patch by the tab and pull. The patch should come off easily. If medication is still visible on the patient's skin, use a 4-by-4 pad to wipe it off.

HYPOTHERMIA

Hypothermia is a condition in which the body temperature drops below 95°F (normal body temperature is 98.6°F). When the body temperature drops even further, to 90°F, the heart becomes quite irritable and the patient is at risk for ventricular fibrillation.

Examples of patients who could suffer hypothermia include winter hikers, persons immersed in cold water, homeless persons, and the elderly or very young. Hypothermia is most often associated with persons who have been outdoors for a prolonged period of time; however, it can also occur indoors if the room is insufficiently heated or the patient is inappropriately clothed.

The cold heart is resistant to attempts at defibrillation. Most medical protocols and the American Heart Association's ACLS course advocate delivering one shock after 2 minutes of CPR in an unwitnessed arrest, resuming CPR, and immediately transporting the patient to the most appropriate emergency facility.

TRANSPORT

The patient in cardiac arrest, or having been reversed from cardiac arrest, is a critically ill patient. Transport should be accomplished quickly, and the patient should be brought to the closest appropriate hospital. Local protocols often govern the destination of particular patients on the basis of hospital capability.

ALS should always be requested early in the resuscitation of a cardiac arrest victim. ALS providers can offer additional medications and other procedures to the patient. If no ALS provider has arrived on the scene by the time the patient is packaged and ready to go, an intercept should be attempted while en route to a hospital.

PUBLIC AED USE AND THE EMT

With the increasing use of public AEDs, by flight attendants, casino security, lifeguards, and school teachers, for example, there is an increased likelihood that an EMT will encounter a bystander using one.

Assuming that the EMT is present because the bystander verified that the patient was unresponsive and therefore activated the EMS system, the EMT should allow the bystander to confirm that the patient is breathless and pulseless. CPR should be administered for 2 minutes in an unwitnessed arrest, and then the EMT should proceed normally with use of the AED.

If the bystander has already attached the AED pads, then the EMT should permit the bystander to continue with the sequence. An interruption to reconfirm pulselessness and apnea only delays defibrillation and decreases the chance of defibrillation success. Figure 24.31 shows a citizen using an

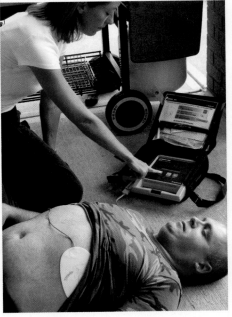

Figure 24.31 Citizen uses AED

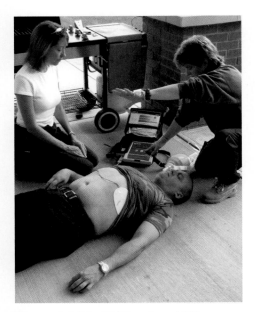

Figure 24.32 EMT using AED following bystander use

AED before the arrival of EMS. Figure 24.32 shows the EMT using the AED after 2 minutes of CPR following the first shock.

POSTARREST CARE

It is common that for several minutes after a successful defibrillation and cardiac arrest reversal that the patient will need manual ventilation, using a bag-valve-mask or similar device.

If the patient is breathing adequately, place him on a high-concentration oxygen mask and proceed to check the patient's level of consciousness.

If the patient remains unconscious and has no evidence of trauma, turn the patient onto his side in the recovery position. The recovery position facilitates drainage of secretions from the mouth and decreases the risk for aspiration. The electrodes should be left in place so that defibrillation may be quickly performed if cardiac arrest should recur.

ONGOING ASSESSMENT

During transport, the patient should be closely monitored. The ongoing assessment should involve continuous monitoring of breathing and pulse.

Recurrence of cardiac arrest is not uncommon. The sooner it is discovered, the more likely the EMT will be successful in reversing it again. Should pulse and breathing be lost, the patient should again be placed on his back; everyone should be clear of the patient; and the AED should be allowed to analyze the rhythm.

FIELD TERMINATION

There are some circumstances in which resuscitative efforts will not be indicated. Circumstances in which death is obviously irreversible are discussed earlier in this unit.

In some areas, ALS personnel may have a protocol to terminate resuscitative efforts once they have become futile. Termination is often done with direct contact with a physician.

When a patient dies, it is important for the EMT to offer support to the family or friends who are present. Family on scene will need support when the decision is made that the patient is dead.

After death has been declared, the EMT must remember to show respect for the deceased. Speak to the family, calling the patient by his or her common name. Use direct language, including the word *dead*. Do not use terms such as "gone to a better place," as these could leave room for misinterpretation.

This is not the time for morbid humor. It is a time for reverence. Though humorous situations do sometimes occur at death, leave the laughter until later.

Be prepared for the family's reactions to death. Any reaction is possible, from denial to anger and rage to bargaining. These normal behaviors represent either some way of fleeing the message or fighting the messenger. Do not take any behaviors personally.

EMTs can provide comfort by contacting clergy to deal with grieving family members, if appropriate. Any death notification is a time for high emotions and can lead to surprising reactions.

POST-RESPONSE

After a cardiac arrest call, the EMT needs to document all actions accurately on the Patient Care Report (PCR). If CPR was not initiated, the rationale for no CPR must be explained. If CPR and the AED were used, then all care surrounding the event must be documented. A readout of the AED's memory or a copy of the tape should be attached to the PCR.

This documentation is generally reviewed by the quality improvement committee. A physician is often a part of this committee when cardiac arrest calls are reviewed (Figure 24.33). The committee will review the call for adherence to protocols as well as for comparison with EMS standards. Nationally, EMS strives to have CPR begin within 4 minutes, and defibrillation within 8 minutes.

All supplies used during cardiac arrest resuscitation should be replenished immediately. Supplies typically used include defibrillation electrode pads (with cables) and the cassette tape or module. The batteries should be rotated out of service for recharging, and replaced with fresh batteries if recommended by the AED manufacturer. Use of a checklist can make this process easier.

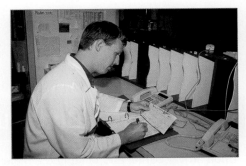

Figure 24.33 Medical control will want to review the Patient Care Report whenever an AED is used by EMTs

COMPETENCY ASSURANCE

Many EMTs do not have an opportunity to use an AED regularly. However, EMTs are expected to be proficient with the use of an AED at all times. Therefore, it is important that EMTs practice AED use regularly. A semiannual refresher course in the use of an AED is a minimum expectation for many EMTs.

Physician oversight is an important component to any defibrillation program. The involvement of a physician in the refresher courses as well as call reviews can help improve the medical care given by the EMT. Physicians are also involved in protocol development regarding the use of AEDs and resuscitation situations. The EMT should be familiar with all relevant protocols in her area.

DEBRIEFING

A cardiac arrest can be one of the most stressful calls to which an EMT will respond. In some cases, the EMT may know the patient or the patient's family. This personal involvement creates some special stress for the EMT.

Whenever a patient dies, an EMT will reflect on the care that was given. It is normal for concerns about errors that may have been made and questions about personal competency to surface. It is important that the EMT explore these questions and resolve them.

A post-response debriefing may help the EMT work through the problems and, more important, improve performance for the next call.

CONCLUSION

Although under the best of conditions survival from cardiac arrest is poor, the knowledge that an EMT's actions have saved even one person's life can sustain morale and reinforce the optimism that EMS can make a difference.

For these reasons alone, the EMT should become expert in CPR, practice CPR in a variety of predictable scenarios, and learn to work together as a team.

The advent of AED technology has improved the chances of survival from prehospital cardiac arrest. An EMT, armed with an AED, can provide definitive care in this critical situation. Combining assessment, AED, and CPR, the EMT can contribute to the successful resuscitation of a victim of cardiac arrest.

CASE STUDY Continued

Upon arrival Daniel and Mike find a male lying on the floor of the airport with CPR in progress. Daniel immediately notices an AED next to the patient's left ear and the patches applied to the patient's chest. There are several people near the patient, and Daniel notices a woman standing above the man who is doing compressions, crying.

They are told CPR was started immediately when the man collapsed, and there has been one shock given by the AED. Mike opens the patient's airway and gives the patient two breaths using a BVM during a pause in the compressions. Ken, the man giving compressions, states he has one last set of 30 compressions in this cycle.

The woman crying says her husband has had two previous heart attacks. As they were getting ready to get on the plane, he suddenly grabbed his chest and complained of severe pain. While she was trying to find his nitroglycerin tablets, he suddenly collapsed and the man doing compressions laid him on the floor and began CPR.

While reassessing the patient at the end of the last set of compressions, Daniel palpates a carotid and radial pulse. Mike states the patient is still not breathing and continues to provide manual ventilations, one every 6 seconds.

The ALS crew arrives and takes over management of the patient after getting a verbal report. As the ALS crew leaves with the patient, Daniel tells Ken what a great job he did providing immediate CPR and the AED. Ken states he has taken a CPR course every couple of years for the past 10 years, but this was the first time he'd used his training on a real person. Daniel knows if the patient survives, it will be because of Ken's quick actions and knowledge of CPR and the AED.

Later that night, Daniel calls the hospital to see how the patient, Mr. Andrews, is doing. Daniel learns the patient is awake and talking after having a procedure to clear another blockage in his coronary artery.

PURPOSE: To perform an external defibrillation, when indicated, on a patient in cardiac arrest.

STANDARD PRECAUTIONS:

☑ Automated external defibrillator

☑ Personal protective clothing

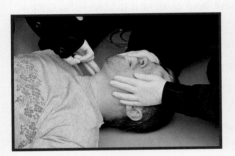

1 The EMT must confirm that the patient is in cardiac arrest.

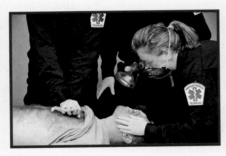

2 Two minutes of CPR is performed in the unwitnessed cardiac arrest or while the AED is being prepared for application.

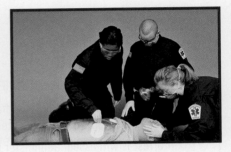

3 The EMT applies the electrode pads to the anterior chest wall, one to the apex of the heart at the lower left rib cage and the other to the right sternal border below the clavicle.

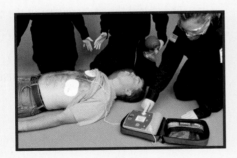

4 The EMT then presses the analyze button and presses the shock button, as advised. Again, the EMT must ensure that no one is touching the patient.

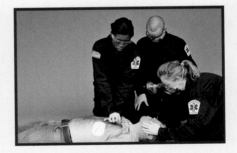

5 After the AED has delivered one shock, CPR must be resumed for five cycles of 30 compressions to two ventilations or 2 minutes. If the patient's pulse returns, then the EMT checks for breathing. The patient will be reassessed for breathing and a pulse after 2 minutes of CPR. If the patient does not have a pulse, the EMT will have the AED analyze and prepare for a second shock to be delivered.

Key Concepts Revisited

- CPR is performed to maintain circulation to the brain and the heart until the fibrillating heart can be defibrillated.

- The EMT needs to be expert at CPR and the use of the AED.

- The EMT must have a fundamental understanding of the electrical system of the heart.
  - Normal sinus rhythm
  - Escape pacemakers
  - Dysrhythmia
    - PVCs
    - Ventricular tachycardia
    - Ventricular fibrillation
    - Asystole
    - Pulseless electrical activity (PEA)

- The first step in management of cardiac arrest is determining the approximate time the arrest occurred.
  - If arrest is witnessed, administer immediate AED if possible.
  - If unwitnessed arrest, perform 2 minutes of CPR prior to AED.

- CPR is intended to preserve the brain and heart until the AED can be applied and the heart defibrillated.

- The chain of survival outlines the appropriate steps in management of a cardiac arrest patient.
  - Early access
  - Early CPR
  - Early defibrillation
  - Early advanced cardiac life support

- CPR should be provided to the cardiac arrest patient within 4 minutes and defibrillation provided in less than 8 minutes.

- In cases in which death is obvious, CPR may not be appropriate.
  - Do not resuscitate orders
  - Lividity
  - Rigor mortis
  - Decomposition
  - Decapitation
  - Incinerations
  - Hemicorporectomy

- Cardiopulmonary resuscitation is administered through a series of specific steps.
  - Check for responsiveness
  - Airway
  - Breathing
    - Manual ventilations
  - Circulation
    - Chest compressions

- Special devices have been developed to provide for more effective CPR:
  - Automated chest compression devices
  - Impedance threshold device

- Cardiac arrest in children is usually due to respiratory compromise.

- CPR in infants and children is different only in the case of two-rescuer administration:
  - Compression to ventilations ratio changes to 15:2.
  - Infant compression is administered with the hands encircling the body, thumbs compressing the sternum.

- Foreign body airway obstruction is managed using CPR in the unresponsive victim.
  - Abdominal thrust maneuver in the conscious patient

- Special situations in administration of CPR present additional challenges for EMTs:
  - Moving the patient prior to administration
  - Obese or pregnant patients
  - Bystander CPR
  - Bystander-EMT CPR

- The automatic external defibrillator (AED) is the most definitive management for the cardiac arrest patient whose heart is fibrillating.

- Defibrillation will only work when there is some muscular activity in the heart.

- The EMT must be familiar with the elements, supplies, and steps in operating the AED.
  - Two electrodes
  - Batteries
  - Case
  - Razor

- The EMT must be familiar with the indications, contraindications, and special situations for use of the AED.
  - Indications
    - Nontraumatic cardiac arrest patient
  - Contraindications
    - Infants under 1 year of age
    - Cardiac arrest due to traumatic injury
  - Special situations
    - Medication patches
    - Hypothermia
    - Wet or metal surfaces
    - Public AEDs

- Postarrest care of the patient may require manual ventilations.
- The patient must be continuously monitored throughout transport.
- The EMT must be familiar with circumstances in which resuscitation may be terminated.
- The EMT must completely document all actions accurately and immediately following a resuscitation attempt.
- Regular practice using the AED ensures competency assurance by the EMT.
- A post-response debriefing may help the EMT deal with related emotions and improve performance through quality assurance following a resuscitation attempt.

Review Questions

1. What is sudden cardiac death?
2. What is the purpose of CPR?
3. When would CPR be withheld from a pulseless patient?
4. What are the two main techniques for opening an airway, and when are they used?
5. What does the phrase "look, listen, and feel" mean?
6. What are some of the differences between citizen CPR and the CPR an EMT performs?
7. What are the anatomic differences between children and adults in relation to CPR?
8. What are the compression–ventilation ratios for infants, children, and adults?
9. What is the method used to clear a foreign body airway obstruction in the unconscious patient?
10. Why is early defibrillation important?
11. What are the indications for the AED?
12. Which ECG rhythms are "shockable" and which are "nonshockable"?
13. What special situations may require a deviation from the usual procedure for using the AED?
14. What is a debriefing useful for?

Key Terms

Advanced lividity
All clear
Artificial pacemaker
Asystole
Automated external defibrillator (AED)
Automatic implantable cardioverter defibrillator (AICD)
Automaticity

Cardiac standstill
Chain of survival
Electrocardiogram (ECG)
Escape rhythm
Hypothermia
Intermammary line
McGill forceps
Motion artifact

Normal sinus rhythm (NSR)
Premature ventricular complex (PVC)
Public access defibrillation (PAD)
Pulseless electrical activity (PEA)

Return of spontaneous circulation (ROSC)
Rigor mortis
Signs of circulation
Ventricular fibrillation

Further Study

American Heart Association. *Fundamentals of BLS for Healthcare Providers*. Dallas, TX: Author, 2005.

American Red Cross and K. A. Handal. *American Red Cross First Aid and Safety Handbook*. Boston: Little, Brown, 1992.

National Safety Council. *CPR and AED*. 4th ed. Itasca, IL: Author, 2002.

Ornato, J., and M. A. Peberdy. (2004). *Cardiopulmonary Resuscitation*. Totowa, NJ: Humana Press.

For additional resources on cardiac arrest and defibrillation, see these Web sites:

- American Heart Association, http://www.americanheart.org
- HeartCenterOnline, http://www.heartcenteronline.com
- National Center for Early Defibrillation, http://www.early-defib.org

UNIT 25 Chest Pain

Chest pain is often a symptom of heart disease. Emergency Medical Technicians (EMTs) are frequently called to the scene of a patient complaining of chest pain. Although only 1 in 12 of these patients is actually experiencing a heart attack, in those cases the patient is at risk for heart failure or even death.

Despite the great strides made in medicine over the past several decades, heart disease remains the number one cause of death among Americans. The prevalence of cigarette smoking and obesity likely contributes to this statistic. Moreover, Americans are at greater risk for a heart attack if they have a family history of diabetes or heart disease. Some risk factors, such as cigarette smoking, are controllable, but others, such as family history, are not. These risk factors, controllable and uncontrollable, leave Americans prone to heart disease. In fact, heart disease strikes one in three Americans.

National Education Standards

The Emergency Medical Technician (EMT) will have a fundamental depth and foundational breadth of understanding of the anatomy, physiology, pathophysiology, assessment, and management of chest pain or discomfort and the associated cardiovascular emergencies.

Key Concepts

- Cardiovascular disease is the number one killer of Americans over the age of 35.

- Acute coronary syndrome (ACS) is a continuum of conditions affecting blood flow to the heart.

- Acute myocardial infarction takes place when myocardial cells die.

- The risk factors of heart disease fall into two categories, modifiable and nonmodifiable.

- The EMT should assess every patient complaining of chest pain or discomfort as if he or she is having a heart attack.

- The time of onset and duration of the pain are of critical importance in getting the patient to definitive treatment.

- It is important to determine if the patient has experienced any medical conditions that have caused the same symptoms of chest pain or discomfort.

- Hypertension is a common sign in patients with chest pain or discomfort.

- Chest pain or discomfort must be treated immediately, with ALS intercept during transport.

- Nitroglycerin should be administered by the EMT only if it has been prescribed to the patient.

- Fibrinolytics are most effective within the first few hours after the onset of symptoms.

- A direct way to open a blocked vessel is to mechanically remove the blockage through angioplasty.

The Morgan family has just finished Thanksgiving dinner. Grandma and Mom are busy washing the dishes in the kitchen when Grandpa comes in and asks Mom if she has anything for indigestion. Sitting down at the kitchen table to rest, Grandpa suddenly clutches his chest, becomes very pale, and starts to sweat. Mom asks if he is in pain, and he says, "Yes, just like that last heart attack I had 5 years ago."

Grandma goes to her purse to find Grandpa's pills and gives him one, saying the doctor said to give him one pill every 5 minutes if he experiences chest pain. She also gives Grandpa an aspirin and tells him to chew it up.

Mom immediately calls 9-1-1 and tells the dispatcher that Grandpa is having chest pain and had suffered a heart attack 5 years ago. She asks the dispatcher to please send an ambulance right away and gives directions so they can find the house more easily.

Critical Thinking Questions

1. What are the priorities in this patient's assessment?
2. What part of the patient's history is critical information?
3. What are the treatment priorities?

INTRODUCTION

Some patients who present with a concern of chest pain or discomfort are not experiencing a heart attack; however, many patients are experiencing some type of cardiovascular event. Cardiac chest pain (*angina*) or discomfort is often a red flag, indicating an occlusion is beginning and a more serious event, such as an acute myocardial infarction, may occur in the near future. All suspected cardiac events have the potential to progress to cardiac arrest, and the EMT must treat all patients experiencing signs and symptoms of a cardiovascular event as emergencies.

The accurate assessment and quick management of the patient with chest pain or discomfort are the keys to survival. This Unit reviews the care of the patient with a concern of chest pain.

ANATOMY AND PHYSIOLOGY REVIEW

Before learning about heart disease, the EMT must have a basic knowledge of cardiac anatomy. The following is a review of cardiac anatomy. The student should review Unit 5 as well.

THE LEFT HEART

The heart can be thought of as a pair of pumps separated by a common wall. This anatomic arrangement allows the two pumps to work in unison. Each half of the heart pumps blood around its own circuit, or circular pathway.

The left ventricle pumps blood around the systemic circuit. The systemic circuit encompasses the entire circulatory system outside of the lungs. Left ventricular failure can lead to cardiogenic shock and, ultimately, to death. This principle was previously defined in Unit 11.

The function of the left ventricle can be grossly estimated by blood pressure. The systolic blood pressure represents the pressure in the arteries during contraction of the heart. If the left ventricle is not pumping adequately, the systolic blood pressure will be low. The diastolic pressure represents the pressure remaining in the circulatory system during the relaxation phase of a heartbeat.

Increased resistance to the blood ejected from the left ventricle, sometimes caused by narrowing of blood vessels, forces the heart to beat harder to overcome the resistance. The result is a higher blood pressure than normal, or *hypertension*. Hypertension can contribute to heart disease.

THE RIGHT HEART

Compared with the left ventricle, the right ventricle has a relatively easy job. The right ventricle pumps the same amount of blood as the left, except exclusively to the lungs. Because the resistance is relatively low in the pulmonary circuit, the right ventricle need not work as hard as the left to circulate blood through the lungs. Figure 25.1 illustrates the pulmonary and systemic circuits.

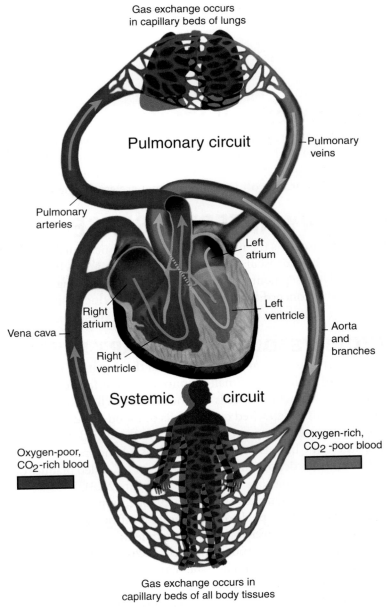

Figure 25.1 The left heart pumps blood to the entire systemic circuit, while the right heart pumps blood through the short pulmonary circuit

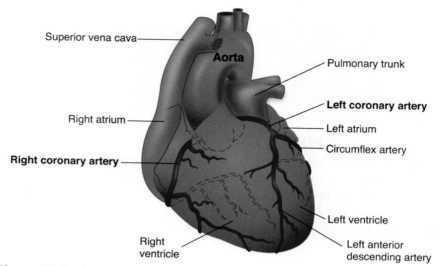

Figure 25.2 The right and left coronary arteries supply oxygenated blood to the heart

CORONARY CIRCULATION

The heart's circulation is derived from the first two arteries that arise from the base of the aorta. These vessels that supply the heart with oxygenated blood are the *coronary arteries*. There are two main coronary arteries (the right and left) that branch off into several smaller vessels (Figure 25.2).

CORONARY ARTERY DISEASE

Cardiovascular disease is the number one killer of Americans over the age of 35. The fact that cardiovascular disease is so common, and is becoming more common as a large segment of the U.S. population is passing 35, makes it a significant health concern in this country. EMTs are increasingly more frequently getting calls to the house of a person having chest pain.

PATHOPHYSIOLOGY OF HEART DISEASE

As blood circulates oxygen and nutrients to all the organs of the body, it also carries foodstuffs called fats. Small amounts of these fats, called lipids, are important for the function of cells and hormones. When too much fat is in the bloodstream, it is deposited on the walls of blood vessels in fatty streaks. These fatty streaks build up over time in a process called *atherosclerosis*. At any place where the bloodstream slows, such as a bend in the vessel, the fat, like sand in a river, is deposited. These deposits of fat, called plaques or **atheromas,** can restrict the passage of blood flow (Figure 25.3).

A blood vessel, when narrowed by a plaque, is prone to blockage, or occlusion. Occasionally a piece of the plaque itself breaks off and can plug the blood vessel. Alternatively, a blood clot, called a **thrombus,** can form in the already narrowed vessel and completely occlude the flow of blood. The result in either situation is that all tissue beyond the occlusion is deprived of oxygen-enriched blood.

When the coronary arteries become narrowed, the heart muscle, or **myocardium,** receives less oxygenated blood. If the amount of oxygen supplied to the heart is insufficient for the needs at that time, the patient may experience

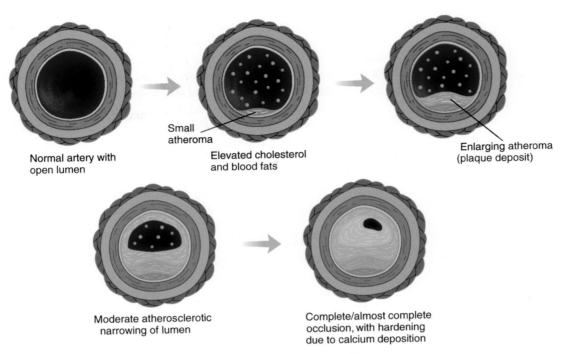

Normal artery with
open lumen

Small
atheroma

Elevated cholesterol
and blood fats

Enlarging atheroma
(plaque deposit)

Moderate atherosclerotic
narrowing of lumen

Complete/almost complete
occlusion, with hardening
due to calcium deposition

Figure 25.3 Atherosclerosis narrows arteries and impedes blood flow

chest pain or other symptoms. This condition is referred to as *angina*. Angina often occurs in patients with narrowed coronary arteries during exertion. This is when the oxygen requirements of the heart are increased.

If the coronary arteries become more narrowed, the person may experience angina with less exertion than previously or even at rest. This is referred to as **unstable angina** and is reflective of more serious disease.

At some point, the coronary arteries may become so narrowed, due to atherosclerosis, spasm of the vessel, or blockage due to thrombus formation, that no oxygenated blood gets through to the myocardium, and death of myocardial cells occurs. This extreme situation is called an *acute myocardial infarction (AMI)* (Figure 25.4).

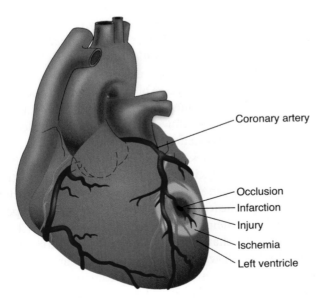

Coronary artery

Occlusion

Infarction

Injury

Ischemia

Left ventricle

Figure 25.4 When a coronary artery is occluded, the heart muscle, the myocardium, dies

An AMI interferes with the heart's ability to effectively pump blood. It causes the injured tissue around the infarction site to become irritable. This irritability may result in inadequate pumping action, leading to cardiogenic shock (Unit 11), or it may cause the heart to beat erratically, resulting in *sudden cardiac death (SCD)*, meaning sudden death related to an arrhythmia as defined in Unit 24.

A term that is often used to describe this continuum of conditions affecting blood flow to the heart is **acute coronary syndrome (ACS).** An EMT will not know the extent of the injury to the heart muscle when caring for a patient with chest pain or other cardiac-related symptoms. As with most other conditions an EMT will treat, the wisest course of action is to provide whatever treatment would be appropriate for the worst possible situation. The treatment an EMT can provide for a patient with an ACS is discussed later in this unit.

RISK FACTORS

Cardiovascular disease has been associated with several risk factors. Identifying these risk factors in ourselves, and in our patients, provides an opportunity to respond appropriately.

Some risk factors for cardiovascular disease are a result of voluntary behaviors that can be eliminated. These *modifiable risk factors* include smoking and drug use (particularly cocaine) and lack of exercise. Other modifiable risk factors include a diet that is high in cholesterol or a diet that leads to obesity.

Other factors are characteristics of the person. These risk factors are *non-modifiable*. Males are more likely to have a heart attack than females, whereas females are more likely to die if they have a heart attack. Family history plays an important role in cardiovascular disease. If the patient's parent or sibling had a heart attack, the patient is at increased risk for having cardiovascular disease.

Nonmodifiable risk factors that may be controlled somewhat include chronic hypertension and diabetes. Medications are available to control both these conditions, although controlling them will not entirely eliminate the increased risk of cardiac disease. Table 25-1 lists both modifiable and non-modifiable risk factors of cardiovascular disease.

SIGNS AND SYMPTOMS

When an acute myocardial infarction affects the heart muscle, impeding its ability to pump, the rest of the heart muscle has to compensate. The result is that the heart tends to beat more rapidly. The normal heart rate is 60 to 100 beats per minute. A rate of over 100 beats per minute means the heart is beating faster than normal, called *tachycardia.* Profound (greater than 150) tachycardia can result in hypotension.

Sometimes AMIs affect the electrical conduction of the heart, causing the heart to beat more slowly than usual, sometimes as slowly as 20 to 30 beats per minute. A heart rate that is slower than 60 bpm is called *bradycardia.* Severe bradycardia may be associated with hypotension.

A feeling of general weakness and nausea may also accompany an AMI. The patient often appears very ill, pale and sweaty, or **diaphoretic.**

Whenever laypeople hear the words *chest pain,* their first thought is the patient is experiencing a heart attack (AMI). Many people experiencing an AMI have chest pain as their initial presenting symptom. Chest pain is a broad, sweeping concern that has a number of descriptors. Some patients say the discomfort is "a dull ache" or "stabbing," whereas others describe it as crushing and oppressive, "like an elephant is sitting on my chest."

All of these concerns may be an accurate description of the chest pain experienced by a person who may be having an AMI. Every patient experiences pain a little differently and, therefore, may describe chest pain differently.

Table 25-1 Risk Factors for Cardiovascular Disease

Modifiable Risk Factors

- Smoking
- Obesity
- Cocaine use
- Lack of exercise
- Diet
- High cholesterol

Non-modifiable Risk Factors

- Sex
- Diabetes
- Age
- Hypertension
- Heredity

Although the concern "I'm having chest pain" is common, particularly among males, it is common for other concerns to represent cardiac disease pain (Figure 25.5). For example, some patients complain of lower jaw pain or neck pain. Other patients may complain of indigestion or shortness of breath. Significant groups of patients complain of left shoulder or arm pain, and there are also patients who do not complain of any kind of pain or discomfort. Some cardiac patients may complain of vague, flu-like symptoms.

An EMT is not expected to diagnose the cause of chest pain in the field. Fortunately, the initial treatment for shortness of breath is very similar to the treatment for an AMI. The assessment and treatment of shortness of breath are discussed in Unit 26. The key to recognition of the possibility of an AMI even without the presence of chest pain is to identify that the patient has risk factors and has any of the classic associated symptoms listed in Table 25-2.

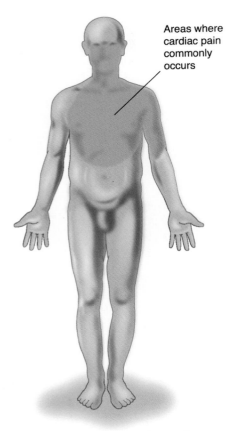

Areas where cardiac pain commonly occurs

Figure 25.5 Any pain from the "nose to the navel" is cardiac until proven otherwise

Table 25-2 Symptoms of an Acute Myocardial Infarction

Common

Symptom	Description
Chest pain	"Pressure" "Elephant sitting on my chest" "Viselike"
Left arm pain	"Dull ache" "Numbness"
Left shoulder pain	"Ache"
Lower jaw pain	"Toothache"
Throat pain	"Burning"
Epigastric discomfort	"Indigestion" "Heartburn"
Fainting (Loss of Consciousness)	"Passed out"
Shortness of breath	"Trouble catching breath" "Not enough air"
Sudden unexplained weakness	"No energy"
Nausea	"Sick to my stomach"
Diaphoresis	"Sweaty"

NONCARDIAC CHEST PAIN

Chest pain may be due to many disorders other than an AMI. Injury or disease of the lungs, or of the muscular chest wall surrounding the lungs, can give rise to a concern of chest pain. Stomach disorders, such as ulcers, can create a similar sort of pain. Because of the proximity of the stomach to the heart, this pain can be mistaken for cardiac pain.

Table 25-3 lists several common disorders that create chest pain. A large number of disorders can mimic a heart attack.

Table 25-3 Noncardiac Chest Pain, by Organ System	
Esophageal spasm	A paroxysmal difficulty in swallowing often associated with a feeling of constriction, or tightness, in the chest.
Pleurisy	An inflammation of the lung's external lining resulting in severe localized chest pain, worsened by deep inspiration.
Pneumonia	Inflammation or infection of the lungs caused by bacteria, viruses, or chemical irritants. Chest pain, chills (shaking from fever), and a cough are symptoms associated with pneumonia.
Pneumothorax	A puncture of the lung that leads to air filling the pleural space. The onset of a sharp chest pain is sudden and associated with marked difficulty breathing.
Rib fractures	A swollen, painful deformity of the rib cage indicating a broken rib. Pain increases with deep inspiration.
Gastric ulcer disease	An open sore, or lesion, of the stomach lining often associated with epigastric pain.

Cultural Considerations

Pain is a personal feeling. Pain means something different for every person. Some people will deny they are having chest pain despite the fact their discomfort is obvious. To admit in public that they are having pain might be seen as a sign of weakness. They may deny pain to avoid frightening loved ones. Whatever the reason, some patients will not admit to having chest pain.

By carefully choosing words, the EMT can often get patients to concede they are having some difficulty and need medical attention. Instead of asking the patient "Are you having chest pain?" it might be more productive to ask "Are you having any chest discomfort?" This wording provides the patient an opportunity to answer the question positively without loss of face.

ASSESSMENT

A broad array of chief concerns may indicate an AMI in progress. The EMT is not expected to differentiate whether the patient's chest pain is cardiac or noncardiac in origin. A common rule of thumb states, "Any pain from the nose to the navel is cardiac until proven otherwise." Failure of the EMT to assess and treat all chest pain as a potential cardiac event may result in an unfortunate outcome for the patient.

The EMT should always err on the side of safety. Assess the patient with chest pain as if she were having a heart attack.

PRIMARY ASSESSMENT

The all-too-common result of an AMI is death. The EMT must act quickly and decisively to protect the patient from further injury and to transport her rapidly to definitive care.

After establishing that the scene is safe, the EMT should form a general impression of the patient's condition and mental status, then assess and manage the airway, breathing, and circulation. Further assessment techniques are determined by the patient's general mental status. Unit 16 addresses the primary assessment in detail.

UNRESPONSIVE CARDIAC PATIENT

A quick check for breathing and circulation should confirm whether the patient is in cardiac arrest. If no pulse or no breathing is found, cardiopulmonary resuscitation (CPR) must begin immediately. Unit 24 reviews the care of the unresponsive cardiac patient.

RESPONSIVE CARDIAC PATIENT

For the responsive patient with potential cardiac concerns, after performing a primary assessment, the EMT should proceed to a history of the present illness and a focused physical examination.

HISTORY

Using the mnemonic SAMPLE (see Table 18-5), the EMT can gather a quick past medical history (Unit 18). The mnemonic OPQRST will provide more details regarding the patient's current symptoms.

ONSET

An EMT should ask the question, "What were you doing when you first noticed the discomfort?" It is important to know what the patient was doing when the symptoms started.

More than half of heart attacks occur while the patient was resting or sleeping. However, a significant number of heart attacks occur during times of high emotional or physical stress. The death of a loved one or the excitement of a surprise party can induce an AMI. The EMT should note and report to the hospital if the chest pain was preceded by some specific stressor.

PROVOCATION

The EMT should determine whether anything makes the discomfort better or worse. For example, does the pain subside when the patient is sitting up or lying down? Does the discomfort change at all with deep inspiration? These types of descriptors can help the physician determine the cause of the chest pain.

Ask the patient whether she has taken any over-the-counter (OTC) medications. Often an AMI is mistaken for indigestion. Many patients will self-treat with antacids (Figure 25.6). Ask the patient whether the medications affected the chest pain.

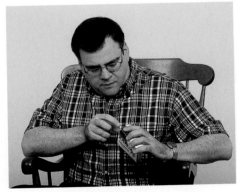

Figure 25.6 Many patients deny that they are having a heart attack, thinking that "it's only indigestion"

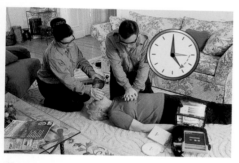

Figure 25.7 Time is crucial. Many AMI patients die within the first 2 hours from the onset of chest pain. Note: Normally the chest is bare in order to expose landmarks for proper hand placement

QUALITY

Patients will have many descriptions of their chest discomfort. Try to have the patient describe the discomfort in her own words. Ask open-ended questions such as, "How would you describe the pain or discomfort?"

If the patient is unable to arrive at an answer, it is acceptable to give the patient a list of descriptive terms. "Is the discomfort sharp, dull, heavy, or tight?" The EMT should be cautious when providing terms so as not to "put words into the patient's mouth."

RADIATION

The same nerves that convey chest pain to the brain are shared by the left shoulder. For this reason, some patients suffering from an AMI may complain of left shoulder or left arm pain, without having any history of injury to that limb. Similarly, neck or jaw pain is also associated with cardiac chest pain.

SEVERITY

Although it is useful for an EMT to ask the patient to gauge her chest pain or discomfort on a scale of 0 to 10, no amount of discomfort should be dismissed. The therapeutic goal for the cardiac patient is zero chest pain or discomfort.

TIME/DURATION

The duration of the pain takes on critical importance when the EMT realizes that most patients will initially deny their chest pain is cardiac in origin. This denial often results in a significant loss of time before medical assistance is sought.

A significant number of heart attack victims die within the first 2 hours from onset of chest pain. Some therapies offered in the hospital are dependent on the length of time the symptoms have been present. Therefore, it is essential that the EMT know the symptoms of a heart attack and the exact time of onset of those symptoms (Figure 25.7).

PREEXISTING MEDICAL CONDITIONS

It is important to determine if the patient has experienced any medical conditions that have caused the same symptoms of chest pain or discomfort. If the patient states she has, the EMT should investigate further by asking specific questions pertaining to that medical history.

If the signs and symptoms are pointing to a possible acute myocardial infarction, ask the patient about any risk factors she may have, including a history of previous angina, AMI, hypertension, diabetes, smoking, and/or elevated cholesterol. The EMT should also inquire if the patient's family has any history of cardiac disease, particularly a close family member such as a parent or sibling.

HYPERTENSION

Hypertension is a common sign in patients with chest pain or discomfort. It is important to not only assess the patient for hypertension, but to also determine if the patient has an underlying history of hypertension, a risk factor for AMI. Hypertension is also a risk factor for an aortic dissection, a life-threatening condition that may also present with chest pain. Blood pressure should be taken in both arms, and a difference of more than 20 mmHg may be found in patients who have an active dissection.

The EMT should also be immediately alert to a patient experiencing chest pain who is hypotensive, or experiencing low blood pressure. Hypotension could be indicative of a right-sided AMI, pulmonary embolism, aortic dissection, cardiac tamponade, or esophageal rupture. These are all life-threatening diagnoses that mandate expeditious transport to a hospital.

BASELINE VITAL SIGNS

It is important to get an accurate baseline set of vital signs. The condition of cardiac patients can change rapidly, and a baseline helps determine the speed at which the patient's condition is changing. If pulse oximetry is available, a reading should also be obtained at this time.

SECONDARY ASSESSMENT

The secondary assessment in the medical patient includes a focused physical examination. The physical changes the patient will demonstrate are the result of hypoperfusion to the heart and the body's efforts to compensate, using endogenous adrenaline (epinephrine).

The pupils are typically dilated as a result of the body's circulating epinephrine. Sluggish pupils may suggest that the patient is hypoxic. Note any distension of the jugular neck veins in a seated patient. Swollen neck veins, jugular venous distention (JVD), often occur when the heart fails as a pump, and blood backs up from the right side of the heart into the visible veins in the neck.

Blood backing up from the left heart also swells blood vessels in the lungs, resulting in **pulmonary edema.** After a time, this excess fluid in the vessels in the lungs will cause narrowing of the airways. Air moving through narrowed airways makes high-pitched, squeaking sounds called wheezes. Eventually fluid leaks into the airways, and the air passing through this fluid crackles with each inspiration. Breath sounds often reveal the degree of failure the heart is experiencing and should be assessed by the EMT on every patient.

MANAGEMENT

The patient should be immediately placed in a position of comfort. If the patient is standing, then assist her to a seated or lying position, whichever is more comfortable. The EMT should bring the stretcher or a chair to the patient to avoid unnecessary exertion in walking. This treatment is more than a mere courtesy. By resting the patient, the EMT is also helping to rest the heart.

Loosen constricting clothing, particularly around the neck. Reassure the patient that everything that can be done is being done. Maintain a calm but deliberate demeanor. High-flow oxygen via non-rebreather face mask should be applied at this time, if it is not already in place.

Street Smart

Some EMS system protocols allow EMTs to administer oxygen via nasal cannula, usually at 2–4 liters per minute. Some patients feel the mask is restrictive and are more comfortable with the "nose prongs."

Although there are a number of advantages to using a nasal cannula, an EMT should carefully weigh the patient's need for oxygen against the patient's desire for comfort. Never deprive a patient of much-needed oxygen when she is hypoxic. Lean toward giving high-flow oxygen via a non-rebreather face mask rather than not giving enough using a nasal cannula.

ASPIRIN

As discussed in Unit 13, aspirin has anti-platelet effects and reduces the incidence of coronary artery reocclusion in AMI. The anti-platelet effect will decrease the ability of platelets to clump together, reducing the formation of a clot within the coronary artery at the site of the occlusion. Aspirin is not being given for pain relief in AMI, but rather to enhance the short- and long-term outcome of the patient with this life-threatening condition. Follow local protocols for administration of aspirin in AMI.

NITROGLYCERIN

If the patient has been prescribed nitroglycerin, and the EMT is trained in assisting the patient with administration, then the patient's nitroglycerin may be given according to local protocols (Figure 25.8). Before assisting with the administration of any patient medications, the EMT must review any precautions that should be taken, as discussed in Unit 13.

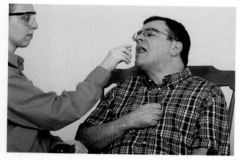

Figure 25.8 Nitroglycerin, a potent vasodilator, is used to relieve some of the work of the heart

REASSESSMENT

The EMT should repeat vital signs as often as the patient's condition requires. Minimally, a set of vital signs is needed before and after the administration of nitroglycerin.

The EMT should review the history, paying close attention to the history of the present illness. Did the pain lessen after the oxygen was given? Did the nitroglycerin help relieve the pain at all? What is the pain, on a scale of 0 to 10, now?

The EMT must be alert to the possibility of sudden cardiac death and the need to do CPR (Figure 25.9).

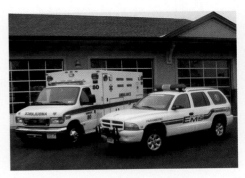

Figure 25.9 The EMT is always prepared for the emergency so that he can react quickly and effectively

TRANSPORT

Never allow the patient to walk to the ambulance or even to the stretcher. The resulting strain to the heart creates more work for an already strained heart. If the cot cannot be brought in to the patient or another method, such as a stair chair, is not available, carry the patient, using any of the techniques discussed in Unit 14.

Ensure that the patient is in a comfortable seated position before beginning transport. Continuously monitor the patient during this time.

The blare of the siren and the flashing red lights may increase the stress the patient is experiencing. It is rarely necessary to use the flashing lights and siren for the cardiac patient. Transport the patient safely, without lights and siren, to the emergency department or appropriate facility in as expeditious a manner as possible.

AEROMEDICAL TRANSPORTATION

The advantages of heart centers with interventional cardiac catheterization labs may not be readily available to the cardiac patient when transportation methods delay their arrival to one of these specialty centers for several hours. This is a serious concern in some rural or remote areas of the United States. Residents of remote or rural areas may be better served if EMS intercepts with an air medical service.

Some urban areas can see substantial delays in transportation owing to traffic tie-ups and gridlock. Air medical services, which have the ability to fly over traffic, may markedly improve transportation times in a large city. The EMT must refer to local protocols when considering use of a helicopter for the cardiac patient.

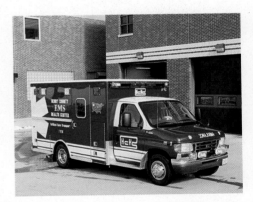

Figure 25.10 Advanced life support personnel bring an added level of care and safety to the patient (Courtesy of Henry County Health Center EMS, Mt. Pleasant, IA)

ALS INTERCEPT

Advanced life support (ALS) personnel can provide additional life-saving care to patients suffering a cardiac event. Using the newest technology, advanced providers may perform many traditional emergency department functions while in the field. These skills and procedures have demonstrated a significant benefit to the cardiac patient. ALS care is an important addition to patient care (Figure 25.10) and should be used whenever feasible.

FIBRINOLYTICS

Fibrinolytics, formerly called *thrombolytics*, is a class of drugs often used in the treatment of AMI. The majority of AMIs, about 70%, are caused by fibrin, a blood clot. ("Fibrinolytic" literally means to divide the fibrin.) With these new fibrinolytics, the emergency physician can attempt to open blocked arteries and reestablish blood flow to damaged heart muscle.

Fibrinolytics are most effective within the first few hours after the onset of symptoms. For this reason, it is important that the EMT quickly transport the AMI patient. The goal of EMS is to decrease the time it takes to get the patient to the treatment. "Time is muscle" accurately describes the challenge EMTs face. The key to appropriate management of the cardiac patient involves getting the patient to definitive care, safely and with a minimum of interruptions.

In some rural areas of the country, ALS personnel are using fibrinolytics to treat heart attack victims in the field under the close direction of a physician.

INTERVENTIONAL CARDIOLOGY

Perhaps a more direct way to open a blocked vessel is to mechanically remove the blockage. Using special catheters, the cardiologist will advance the catheter into the center of the blockage and then expand a balloon on the tip of the catheter. This procedure, called *angioplasty*, has made remarkable progress in reducing the incidence of permanent damage to the heart, by allowing "reperfusion." Sometimes a tiny tubelike stent is left in the lumen of the vessel to hold it open after the balloon and catheter are removed.

Ongoing advances in the field of interventional cardiology use different combinations of tools and medications to aim for the highest success rate for opening the occluded vessel and to prevent reocclusion for the greatest amount of time.

The most recent literature regarding the management of the patient with an AMI supports the use of interventional cardiology techniques when rapidly available rather than fibrinolytic medications to open blocked coronary arteries. Studies are indicating that angioplasty may be more successful with fewer side effects than the fibrinolytic medications alone. The bottom line is that no matter which therapy is chosen, the blocked vessel must be opened as quickly as possible. Sometimes, the technique that is chosen depends on what services are available to the patient in the most rapid fashion. Not infrequently, a combination of both techniques is used if felt to be appropriate for an individual patient.

Some hospitals have designated heart centers, with the capability to perform interventional cardiac procedures. Some EMS systems direct EMTs to transport all cardiac patients to a heart center. Follow your local protocols when making the decision on the transportation destination.

CONCLUSION

The concern of chest pain is one of the most common reasons that EMS is called. The ever-present possibility of sudden cardiac death makes these EMS calls challenging. The EMT's skills and knowledge are put to the ultimate test in caring for these critically ill patients. Thoughtful consideration of the patient's situation and deliberate action on the part of the EMT will improve the patient's overall chance for survival.

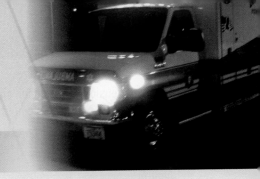

CASE STUDY Continued

Jess and Matt arrive on scene and find an elderly male seated at the kitchen table. As Matt applies oxygen by NRB at 12 lpm, an elderly woman identifies herself as Cleo, the wife of the patient, Henry. Cleo states she has given Henry two nitro tablets, which have not seemed to help, and he has also had one adult aspirin, which he chewed up.

As Jess begins her assessment, she finds Henry is pale, cool, and diaphoretic with clear lung sounds. Henry describes the discomfort as crushing, like an elephant sitting on his chest, and the pain goes down his left arm. Henry rates the pain at an 8 on a 0 to 10 scale and says it started about 25 minutes ago but has gotten worse over the past 5 minutes. Henry denies any shortness of breath, although Jess notices he cannot speak more than two or three words without taking a breath.

As Matt and Jess reassure Henry everything will be done to make him more comfortable, they lift him to the cot. Cleo hands them the nitroglycerin bottle she says the doctor gave them after Henry's heart attack 5 years ago. Jess knows the nitro was too old to be effective and takes note to make sure they tell the ALS crew they will be meeting en route to the hospital.

Jess and Matt meet the ALS crew en route to the hospital. Once on board and after hearing Jess's report, they administer a sublingual nitroglycerin spray to Henry and start an IV. As they arrive at the hospital 5 minutes later, Henry states the pain has gotten much better, rating it at a 4 on the 0 to 10 scale.

Key Concepts Revisited

- Cardiovascular disease is the number one killer of Americans over the age of 35.
- Acute coronary syndrome (ACS) is continuum of conditions affecting blood flow to the heart.
- Acute myocardial infarction takes place when myocardial cells die.
- The risk factors of heart disease fall into two categories:
  - Modifiable
    - Smoking
    - Obesity
    - Cocaine use
    - Lack of exercise
    - Diet
    - High cholesterol
  - Nonmodifiable
    - Sex
    - Diabetes

- Age
- Hypertension
- Heredity
- The EMT should assess every patient complaining of chest pain or discomfort as if he or she is having a heart attack.
  - Primary assessment
  - History taking
    - SAMPLE
  - Baseline vital signs
  - Secondary assessment
- The time of onset and duration of the pain is of critical importance in getting the patient to definitive treatment.
  - OPQRST
- It is important to determine if the patient has experienced any medical conditions that have caused the same symptoms of chest pain or discomfort.
  - Preexisting medical conditions

- Hypertension is a common sign seen in patients with chest pain or discomfort.
- Chest pain or discomfort must be treated immediately.
  - Oxygen
  - Aspirin
- Nitroglycerin should be administered only if it has been prescribed to the patient.
- Transport the patient quickly, without lights and siren, to the emergency department or appropriate facility.
  - Aeromedical transportation
  - ALS intercept
- The ongoing assessment determines the effectiveness of treatment.
- Fibrinolytics are most effective within the first few hours after the onset of symptoms.
- A direct way to open a blocked vessel is to mechanically remove the blockage through angioplasty.
- The concern of chest pain and the ever-present possibility of sudden cardiac death are among the most challenging of EMS responses.

Review Questions

1. Why is early cardiac care important?
2. What are the modifiable risk factors of heart disease?
3. What are the nonmodifiable risk factors of heart disease?
4. What path does a drop of blood take to get from the left ventricle back to the left ventricle?
5. What are the signs and symptoms of a heart attack?
6. What other or preexisting medical conditions may present with chest pain or discomfort?
7. What are the treatments an EMT should give a heart attack victim?
8. What are the side effects of nitroglycerin?
9. How should an AMI patient be transported?
10. What are fibrinolytics, and how have they affected EMS?

Key Terms

Acute coronary syndrome (ACS)
Atheromas
Diaphoretic
Fibrinolytics

Myocardium
Pulmonary edema
Thrombus
Unstable angina

Further Study

Henry, M., and E. Stapleton. "A Voyage to Chest Pain." *Journal of Emergency Medical Services 23*, no. 5 (1998): 74–79.

Kerschenbaum-Cohn, J., and P. F. Cohn. "Modern Treatment for Heart Attacks: Opening Blocked Arteries Quickly." *Circulation* (2006): 114: e578–e580.

Ornato, Joseph P., and Mary M. Hand. "Warning Signs of a Heart Attack." *Circulation* 104 (2001), http://circ.ahajournals.org/cgi/content/full/104/11/1212.

Thygesen, Kristian, Joseph S. Alpert, and Harvey D. White. "Universal Definition of Myocardial Infarction." *Circulation* 116 (2007): 2634–2653.

Wilcox, D. "Angina: Improving the Outcome." *RN* 60, no. 7 (1997): 34–40.

UNIT (26) Shortness of Breath

Difficulty breathing can be caused by many different problems. Each of these problems may arise from a different disease process; however, each causes dysfunction of the respiratory system.

The respiratory system is a vital organ system responsible for providing oxygen to the body and removing the metabolic waste product carbon dioxide. The body has backup systems for times when the respiratory system is not functioning ideally; however, if the problem goes on long enough, these backup systems can also fail.

National Education Standards

The Emergency Medical Technician (EMT) will demonstrate a fundamental depth and foundational breadth of understanding of the anatomy, physiology, assessment, and management of respiratory medical emergencies.

Key Concepts

- The respiratory system provides oxygen to the body and removes carbon dioxide.

- Knowledge of normal breathing patterns enables appropriate assessment and management of breathing problems.

- A person breathing normally appears comfortable during both inhalation and exhalation.

- Respiratory difficulty usually presents easily recognized classic signs and symptoms.

- Clues to respiratory difficulty can be evident during scene size-up.

- Mental status may be the first indicator of respiratory compromise.

- Patient position can indicate the severity of the distress.

- The assessment of the medical patient is guided by the patient's level of responsiveness.

- The primary management of the dyspneic patient is providing high-flow oxygen.

- Position the patient in respiratory distress to support breathing.

- Assist patient with medication administration per local protocols.

- Obtain history from the family or friends prior to transporting unresponsive patients.

- Arrange ALS intercept with severe respiratory distress or arrest.

- Numerous diseases can compromise the respiratory and circulatory systems.

- Appropriate ventilatory assistance and oxygen administration are key to management of respiratory emergencies.

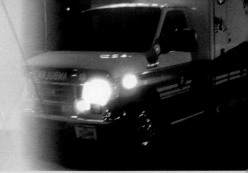

CASE STUDY

Brandon and Christopher are eating lunch at the station when the tones go off for an elderly male having difficulty breathing. Upon arriving on scene they encounter an approximately 70-year-old, thin male sitting hunched over at a small table. His eyes were half open. A half-empty cup of coffee, an ashtray overflowing with cigarette butts, and about a half-dozen prescription medicine bottles as well as two inhalers are visible on the table.

"Good afternoon, Mr. Abernathy. What can we help you with today?" asks Brandon. Mr. Abernathy struggles to say the words, "Trouble. . . breathing." Looking more closely, the EMTs note that Mr. Abernathy's lips are bluish. Brandon notes that he is unable to say more than one word without gasping for breath.

Christopher begins gathering the medicine bottles sitting on the counter and the inhaler to take with them to the hospital. Mr. Abernathy shakes his head no when asked if there is anyone home who can answer questions for him.

As Brandon places high-flow oxygen on, he notices the pulse oximetry is not reading and Mr. Abernathy's nail beds are bluish in appearance.

Brandon and Christopher place Mr. Abernathy on the cot, sitting upright to help him breathe. Christopher contacts dispatch and requests an ALS intercept as they leave the scene.

Critical Thinking Questions

1. What signs of respiratory distress are present?
2. What environmental clues may suggest respiratory disease?
3. What assessment findings will Brandon likely find?
4. What are the treatment priorities?

Pediatric Considerations

The respiratory system of infants and children functions essentially the same as that of adults, but the airway anatomy is somewhat different in relation to size. The pediatric patient has a relatively smaller airway and relatively bigger tongue and epiglottis. This difference allows for much easier obstructions of the pediatric airway because it would take a smaller amount of blockage to completely occlude a small airway.

INTRODUCTION

Emergency Medical Technicians (EMTs) are often called to assist patients whose respiratory system is not functioning normally, causing them to feel as though they cannot breathe. *Dyspnea* is a term that means difficulty breathing. Dyspnea, a Latin word, comes from "dys," difficulty, and "pnea," breathing. It is one of many medical terms that have Latin or Greek origins for their meanings. These roots can also be used in other combinations; for example, *apnea,* which comes from "a," without, and "pnea," breathing, is the medical term for lack of breathing. EMTs encounter many medical terms in their practice.

This unit reviews the normal anatomy of the respiratory system and why it can fail. The common signs and symptoms and the appropriate history and physical examination are outlined. In addition, the appropriate management of the patient who is short of breath is discussed.

ANATOMY REVIEW

The respiratory system is made up of airways, lungs, and blood vessels. Each will be reviewed separately, and their interaction with the muscular diaphragm and the muscles of the chest wall to take in oxygen and get rid of carbon dioxide will also be reviewed. Additional discussions of respiratory anatomy and physiology are found in Unit 5.

UPPER AIRWAY

Air enters the lungs through the nose and mouth, where it is warmed and humidified. The warm, moist air then moves through the pharynx, where it passes the epiglottis and the larynx to enter the trachea.

RESPIRATORY TREE

The trachea is made up of cartilaginous rings and branches into two main bronchi (the left and the right). The bronchi further branch into smaller airways called bronchioles, which eventually empty into small grapelike clusters of tiny air spaces, called alveoli.

The alveoli are surrounded by tiny blood vessels called capillaries. These capillaries carry all of the deoxygenated blood from the body to be reoxygenated at the alveoli. Figure 26.1 reviews the anatomy of the respiratory system, illustrating the branching of the airways and the movement of air into and out of the alveoli.

Street Smart

Some patients who have sustained serious injury to their neck may have damage to the nerves controlling the diaphragm. These patients may have difficulty breathing or may not be able to breathe at all. The EMT should carefully observe the breathing of patients with neck injuries.

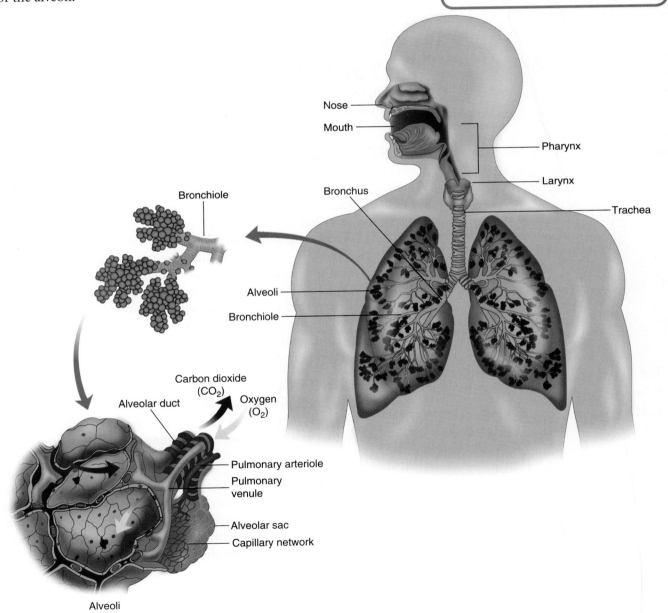

Figure 26.1 The respiratory system is composed of branching airways that get progressively smaller as they get farther away from the trachea

MUSCULATURE

Multiple muscles are actively involved in ventilation. *Ventilation* refers to the movement of air into and out of the lungs. These muscles are generally controlled by the nervous system without conscious effort.

DIAPHRAGM

The diaphragm is a large muscle inside the bottom of the chest. It contracts during inspiration and relaxes to allow exhalation. Nerves from the cervical spinal cord in the neck, the phrenic nerve, control this large muscle.

CHEST WALL MUSCLES

Within the chest wall itself are many other smaller muscles that assist in breathing. These muscles are located between the ribs and in the neck, and other external chest muscles are also used in ventilation, especially when the patient is having difficulty breathing. This muscular system helps to raise the chest during inspiration and is especially important when the diaphragm is unable to work efficiently. These muscles are commonly referred to as the *accessory muscles* of respiration.

PHYSIOLOGY REVIEW

It is important for the EMT to understand how normal breathing occurs to appropriately assess and manage the patient when there is potentially a breathing problem.

RESPIRATORY DRIVE

Among the many elements the brain monitors in the body is the pH, or acid levels, in the blood. The blood level of carbon dioxide directly influences this acid level. When carbon dioxide levels are too high, the acid level rises, causing the body to react in a number of ways.

The first natural response to this abnormality is for the body to try to lower the carbon dioxide level. The initial response is to increase respirations to lower the carbon dioxide because each exhalation should get rid of more of this waste product. As discussed in Unit 6, the healthy individual's respiratory rate is determined by his carbon dioxide levels. A high level of carbon dioxide or acid creates a stronger stimulation to breathe. It is important to realize that, in the healthy individual, it is not the *oxygen* level that normally stimulates a person to breathe.

VENTILATION

Once the brain indicates to the respiratory system that breathing should occur, the message is sent through the nervous system network to the muscles of respiration that work is needed for breathing to be accomplished.

INHALATION

A breath begins when the diaphragm contracts and pulls down toward the abdomen as the ribs rise. This action generates a negative pressure within the chest, similar to a vacuum. Air is pulled into the chest through the mouth and nose and the rest of the airways until the air spaces are full. This concept of negative pressure generating inspiration can be visualized in Figure 26.2.

EXHALATION

After enough time has been allowed for gas exchange between the alveolar sacs and the capillaries, exhalation occurs. The diaphragm relaxes and allows the air to rush back out of the airways and the mouth and nose into the surrounding environment, ending the breath.

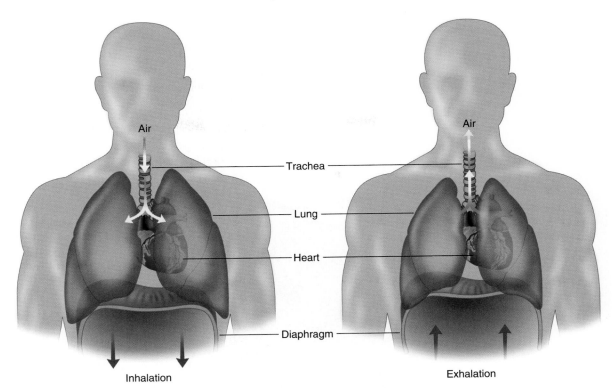

Figure 26.2 Air is drawn into the chest during inhalation by a negative pressure created by diaphragmatic contraction. As the diaphragm relaxes, air is passively released during exhalation

RESPIRATION

The term *respiration* refers to the gas exchange that occurs in the lungs and in the peripheral tissues, not to the act of moving air into and out of the lungs. The mechanical act of breathing is referred to as *ventilation*.

PULMONARY RESPIRATION

As the capillaries pass between the air-filled alveoli, a process called *diffusion* occurs. This means that the oxygen passes from the air space into the blood, where the concentration of oxygen is lower and the carbon dioxide passes from the blood into the air space, where the concentration of carbon dioxide is lower. This **alveolar-capillary gas exchange** occurs passively since the natural preference of these molecules is to be in balance, or in equal amounts on both sides.

The success of this exchange relies on several factors. The air in the air space must be rich in oxygen, the blood must pass closely to the alveoli, and the wall between them must be very thin (one cell layer, in fact!).

CELLULAR RESPIRATION

After oxygenated blood is pumped out of the heart, it must be delivered to the peripheral tissues. It is in the peripheral tissues where carbon dioxide is picked up for delivery back to the lungs to be exhaled.

The process that allows the exchange of gases in the periphery is called *cellular respiration*. This process uses the similar process of diffusion, this time between the oxygen-poor tissue and the oxygen-rich blood in the peripheral capillaries. The process of pulmonary and cellular respiration is illustrated in Figure 26.3.

As discussed in Unit 6, a disruption to ventilations or respiration through injury or a disease process will result in hypoxia, an inadequate supply of oxygen. Discussion of specific illness resulting in respiratory abnormalities is discussed in more detail throughout this unit.

Street Smart

A patient who has been having respiratory difficulty and who begins to look tired may have become physically exhausted from the extra respiratory effort. This patient is in danger of respiratory arrest and will need ventilatory assistance. The EMT should learn to recognize this warning sign and act appropriately.

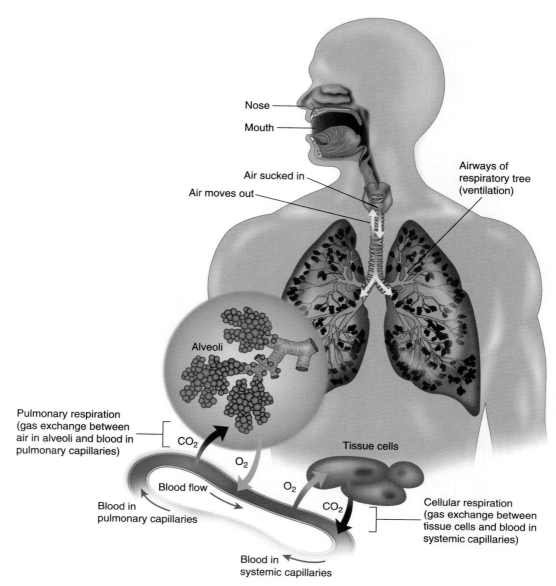

Labels on figure:
- Nose
- Mouth
- Air sucked in
- Air moves out
- Airways of respiratory tree (ventilation)
- Alveoli
- Pulmonary respiration (gas exchange between air in alveoli and blood in pulmonary capillaries)
- CO_2
- O_2
- Blood flow
- Blood in pulmonary capillaries
- Tissue cells
- O_2
- CO_2
- Cellular respiration (gas exchange between tissue cells and blood in systemic capillaries)
- Blood in systemic capillaries

Figure 26.3 Oxygen and carbon dioxide are exchanged between the alveoli and the pulmonary capillaries surrounding them. Oxygen is delivered to the tissues and carbon dioxide is removed in a process called cellular respiration

NORMAL BREATHING

Breathing normally takes minimal effort. The breathing rate is set by the brain as determined by blood levels of carbon dioxide, as previously discussed. Problems affecting the respiratory system will be evident in several ways.

PATIENT APPEARANCE

A person breathing normally appears comfortable during both inhalation and exhalation. The diaphragm and other chest muscles of respiration smoothly contract to pull air into the chest, then easily relax and allow air to exit the airway.

Respiratory difficulty is often obvious when looking at the patient. The patient may appear to be exerting an abnormal amount of effort in breathing, also referred to as *labored breathing*, and may begin to look tired with the effort to breathe.

LUNG SOUNDS

All of this air movement into and out of the lungs creates a characteristic sound that can be heard with a stethoscope held to the chest. Any alteration in this normal pattern of airflow can create abnormal sounds as air rushes into and out of the chest.

A high-pitched, whining sound may be heard as air passes through abnormally narrowed airways. This sound, called *wheezing*, is usually heard during exhalation but may be heard during both phases of ventilation.

If mucus or other foreign material accumulates in the larger airways, the air passing through the airway may cause a coarse sound that can be easily heard on both inspiration and exhalation. This loud coarse crackling sound is called **rhonchi.**

The next common sound heard when auscultating lungs are **rales.** This term is used to describe a bubbly or soft crackling sound, like hair rubbed between the fingers next to the ear, that is created as tiny air spaces that were stuck together by abnormal fluid accumulation pop open. The diseases that cause these common abnormal lung sounds will be reviewed later in this unit.

RATES AND PATTERNS

To maintain normal oxygen and carbon dioxide levels, the body must repeat a full respiratory cycle 12–20 times each minute (the normal respiratory rate).

Respiratory rates lower than normal will be inadequate and result in problems. Abnormally high respiratory rates will also be inadequate and indicate an abnormality affecting the respiratory system.

VITAL SIGNS

As mentioned previously, a smoothly running respiratory system requires minimal conscious effort. The vital signs reflect this relaxation with a normal heart rate and blood pressure. Any extra effort in breathing may be reflected in an abnormally high heart rate and sometimes in a higher-than-normal blood pressure.

COLOR

When adequate gas exchange occurs, the mucous membranes have a pink color. If the blood is poorly oxygenated because of inadequate gas exchange, the mucous membranes may take on a bluish color, especially in the lips. This blue to gray color is called cyanosis and is a sign of serious respiratory disease.

RESPIRATORY DISTRESS

The patient who has a problem within the respiratory system will often present with classic signs and symptoms that the EMT must be able to recognize. The ability to recognize the patient in respiratory distress will enable the EMT to initiate the proper treatment quickly. Without rapid treatment, some patients with respiratory distress will deteriorate and stop breathing. Providing rapid, appropriate assessment and management of the patient in respiratory distress can prevent respiratory arrest.

SIGNS AND SYMPTOMS

Patients who are having respiratory difficulty may describe their symptoms differently. Some patients say they can't breathe or are having trouble breathing. Others may describe an inability to catch their breath or say they are short of breath.

Some very sick patients may not be able to talk or describe their problem at all. The EMT may have been called by friends or family members who noted the patient's distress. In this situation, the EMT must obtain the symptoms from the people who called.

Pediatric Considerations

A child must breathe 15–30 times per minute. Infants have smaller lungs and therefore must breathe 25–50 times each minute.

Cultural Considerations

The pink or bluish color may be difficult to visualize on darker-skinned patients. It is useful to pay careful attention to the lips and oral mucous membranes of these patients and to note any changes in color there.

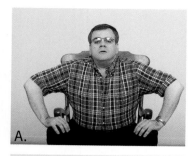

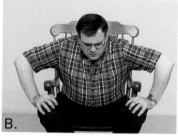

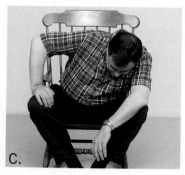

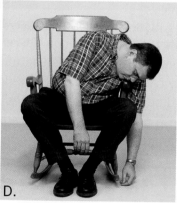

Figure 26.4 A. The patient with respiratory distress will often be found sitting bolt upright in the tripod position, using accessory muscles to assist in breathing B. As hypoxia worsens, the patient will often become anxious C. The dyspneic patient may become tired, as working to breathe has been taxing. This is an ominous sign D. The patient who is cyanotic and not alert is extremely sick and in need of immediate ventilatory support

The dyspneic patient is working hard to breathe and usually presents with a respiratory rate notably higher than normal. The heart rate also may be elevated, as is seen in other circumstances of exertion. As the respiratory system fails and tissues are no longer receiving oxygen, the patient's skin may become cyanotic.

Eventually, if not treated effectively, the patient will no longer be able to compensate for the abnormality in the respiratory system and will become tired. The respiratory rate may drop, and the patient will take on a more slumped, tired position. Finally, if the condition worsens, the patient may stop breathing. Figure 26.4 illustrates the progression of respiratory distress that may be seen without proper treatment.

ASSESSMENT

The EMT must use skills of observation and note the environment the patient is in and how the patient looks upon initial approach. This general impression of the severity of the patient's illness comes within the first 30 seconds and is often quite accurate.

The history and physical exam of the patient with difficulty breathing can be focused on the respiratory system. As always, the airway, breathing, and circulation (ABC) are the crucial initial exam points. This exam should include ensuring that the patient is maintaining his own airway, is breathing spontaneously, and has a pulse.

SCENE SIZE-UP

Clues to whether the patient is experiencing difficulty breathing are often immediately evident. It is important to look for indications of the possible cause of breathing difficulty as part of the scene size-up. Is the patient experiencing respiratory distress because of a traumatic injury, or is a medical condition involved?

Check the scene for a mechanism of injury. There may be a chest wound from a gunshot or knife following a crime, or the patient may have fallen, causing a fracture to the rib area. Are there any objects or indications of a meal present that could indicate a possible airway obstruction?

The presence of oxygen tanks or concentrators, oxygen tubing, or metered dose inhalers indicate a history of chronic respiratory difficulty or disease.

PRIMARY ASSESSMENT

The primary assessment is done very quickly and is meant to briefly assess the patient's mental status, airway, breathing, and circulation.

The conscious patient who is speaking easily may have no immediate life-threatening issues. If life-threatening problems are found during the primary assessment, such as the need for airway maintenance or ventilatory assistance, the EMT should address these problems as soon as she identifies them.

The patient's mental status is the first, best indicator of respiratory compromise. Patients who are confused, restless, and agitated are showing signs of hypoxia, indicating the brain is not getting adequate oxygen. A patient who is becoming lethargic, dropping his head as if he is beginning to go to sleep is on the verge of respiratory arrest and requires immediate intervention with positive pressure ventilations.

GENERAL IMPRESSION

Several common signs and symptoms are associated with respiratory distress. These signs and symptoms help the EMT to form an immediate general impression of the severity of the patient's condition following the scene size-up and primary assessment.

INDICATIONS OF SEVERITY

The patient's position can be an immediate indicator to the severity of the patient's distress. The patient seated in the tripod position, upright and leaning slightly forward, supporting himself on his hands holding onto something in front of him is usually in severe respiratory distress. The patient leaning back or lying back may either be in mild respiratory distress or exhausted with the effort to breathe and may be close to respiratory arrest.

Look at the patient's lips to see if they are pursed while exhaling in an effort to keep the smaller airways from collapsing and making the next breath easier to inhale. Nasal flaring with inhalation is an indication the patient is working hard to breathe and can be an ominous sign in children.

The patient's skin color and quality are also important signs indicating severity of distress. The patient who is pale may be showing early signs of hypoxia, whereas a patient who has advanced to cyanosis (bluish-gray color) is showing clear indications of hypoxia. A patient experiencing respiratory distress is commonly diaphoretic (moist, sweaty skin) because of the increased work of breathing. Pale, cool, clammy skin is an early indicator of hypoxia and may also indicate the patient is in shock.

Patients who can talk in complete sentences, without gasping or obvious difficulty have a clear, open airway. These patients may be in the early stage of difficulty. The patient who can speak only one or two words before gasping for air is in severe respiratory distress. The number of words a patient can speak before gasping for breath is a good indicator of the severity of distress.

Along with the position the patient is in, is the patient using accessory muscles in the neck or are there retractions of the intercostal muscles (between the ribs) to help him breathe? The use of accessory muscles and retractions are clear indicators of significant respiratory difficulty.

HISTORY AND SECONDARY ASSESSMENT

The history and secondary assessment will be completed after the primary assessment and any life threats have been appropriately managed. If the patient is considered to be critically ill or unstable, the focused exam of the secondary assessment will be done in the ambulance while en route to the hospital.

If the patient is stable, the EMT can spend a few moments gathering relevant history and performing a focused physical exam before transport.

RESPONSIVE PATIENT

The patient who is responsive and able to speak well enough to provide the EMT with a history should be asked questions regarding the nature of the illness.

HISTORY

Every patient should be asked the SAMPLE (see Table 18-1) history questions to gather information relating to signs and symptoms, allergies, medications, pertinent past history, last oral intake, and the events leading up to the illness. The OPQRST history is important in determining the history, severity, and progression of the present illness. Also important to note are any interventions the patient may have tried and any other symptoms associated with the original concern. The details of obtaining the history of the medical patient can be reviewed in Unit 18.

SECONDARY ASSESSMENT

Once the history has been obtained in the responsive patient, it is then appropriate to move into the secondary assessment. The EMT can focus on the respiratory assessment by noting lung sounds heard by listening through a

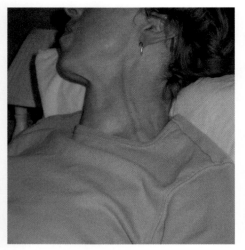

A.

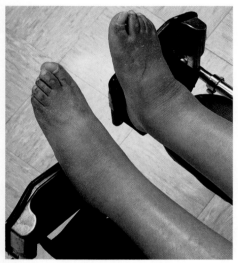

B.

Figure 26.5 A. Jugular venous distention is a sign of excess fluid buildup, often seen in the patient with chronic congestive heart failure B. Edema is often seen in the ankles and legs of patients with chronic congestive heart failure

Street Smart

Pulse oximetry should improve if treatments provided are effective. A falling pulse oximetry may be a sign of deterioration in the patient with a respiratory illness.

stethoscope. Carefully watch the patient's breathing and note any irregular patterns, sounds, or extra work of breathing. Remember that normal breathing is regular, effortless, and quiet.

The presence of jugular venous distention (JVD) and swelling of the legs should be noted as both are associated with the backup of fluids seen in congestive heart failure (CHF), discussed later in this unit. These physical findings can be seen in Figure 26.5. The patient's skin should be briefly examined for a rash or hives, which may indicate an allergic reaction. Abnormal skin colors, such as cyanosis, should also be noted.

VITAL SIGNS

The remainder of the exam of the responsive patient who is short of breath should include a full set of baseline vital signs, including blood pressure, pulse rate and quality, respiratory rate and quality, and pulse oximetry when available.

UNRESPONSIVE PATIENT

The EMT alters her assessment somewhat for the unresponsive patient. The priorities will be to complete a rapid physical examination, obtain vital signs, and obtain relevant history from any family or bystanders.

RAPID PHYSICAL EXAMINATION

After completing the primary assessment, the EMT should perform a rapid physical examination. The point of this quick head-to-toe survey is to find any abnormalities that may help the EMT to understand what has happened to the patient.

For example, the patient who was complaining of shortness of breath who is now unconscious may have a stab wound to the back of the chest. This injury is relevant to the patient's condition and will likely affect the EMT's priorities and management. Without looking for them, the EMT may not find important clues to the patient's illness.

VITAL SIGNS

After the primary assessment and rapid physical exam, the next priority is to obtain a complete set of baseline vital signs. The rate and quality of respirations and pulse should be measured. Blood pressure should be measured. Pulse oximetry is a useful tool in caring for the patient who has a respiratory problem because it can be used to follow the effectiveness of treatment provided.

HISTORY FROM OTHERS

An unresponsive patient is unlikely to provide the EMT with much useful history. It is important that the key parts of the history be obtained from friends, family, or bystanders prior to transport, if possible. These people may be able to provide important information that may be relevant in patient care. The EMT should quickly elicit a SAMPLE history as well as much of the OPQRST history available from these sources.

MANAGEMENT

The management of the patient with difficulty breathing should begin during the primary assessment. No matter the cause of the problem, oxygen is always appropriate as difficulty breathing will result in a lack of oxygen to the body tissues.

Other specific treatments, such as inhaled medications, may be indicated depending on the cause of the problem. It is not important for the EMT to diagnose the underlying cause of the shortness of breath. It *is* important to treat the patient on the basis of their signs and symptoms and pertinent history.

OXYGEN

Because shortness of breath may either be due to or result in low oxygen levels, a crucial part of the management of the dyspneic patient is providing high-flow oxygen in whatever manner is appropriate (Figure 26.6).

SPONTANEOUSLY BREATHING PATIENT

If the patient is moving air well on his own but feeling short of breath, a non-rebreather face mask with 10–15 liters per minute of oxygen is appropriate.

If the patient cannot tolerate the mask, a nasal cannula is a reasonable alternative. Although it delivers less oxygen than a mask, a little is certainly better than none at all.

Children often will not allow either a mask or a cannula to be placed on their face. In this case, a blow-by technique can be used, as shown in Figure 26.7. Newer toy-like devices are available that blow oxygen into children's faces as they play with the toy.

ASSISTING VENTILATIONS

The patient who cannot maintain an airway or whose respiratory effort is inadequate must be assisted by manual ventilation. Adequate respiratory effort can be judged by several factors. A patient whose color is pink, who has a respiratory rate within the normal range for his age and size, and whose chest is moving up and down with each breath is ventilating adequately for the time being.

If the patient becomes cyanotic or the respiratory rate becomes too fast to be efficient or too slow to be adequate, the patient may need ventilatory assistance. Using a bag-valve-mask attached to 100% oxygen to assist respiratory effort is appropriate (Figure 26.8).

POSITIONING

It is important for the EMT to pay attention to the position the patient is placed in. Most patients who are short of breath will prefer to sit upright. In the upright position, breathing may be more effective and easier.

If the EMT finds the patient lying down, it may be worthwhile to sit him up to see if sitting helps ease his breathing. In all cases, the EMT should allow patients to be in whatever position they feel is most comfortable.

PRESCRIBED MEDICATIONS

If a medication such as an inhaler is prescribed to the patient, the EMT may contact a medical control physician and request an order to assist the patient in using the medication. Only medications prescribed specifically for that patient should be used and only if the patient is able to self-administer the drug with only *assistance* from the EMT (Figure 26.9).

BRONCHODILATOR INHALERS

If a patient who is prescribed a bronchodilator inhaler is having trouble breathing and would normally use the medication, the EMT should consider assisting the patient to use this medication according to local protocols.

These medicines are meant to be inhaled directly into the airways. Upon contact with the bronchioles, the medications should help relieve the spasm and allow easier passage of air. An example of such medications is albuterol (common trade names Ventolin and Proventil). The EMT should be familiar with the trade names of albuterol and should refer to local protocol for

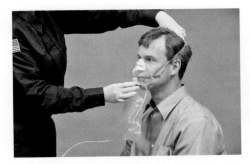

Figure 26.6 No matter the cause of shortness of breath, supplemental oxygen is always indicated

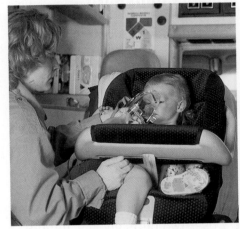

Figure 26.7 Some children will not tolerate having an oxygen mask placed on their face. Oxygen may be administered by a blow-by technique

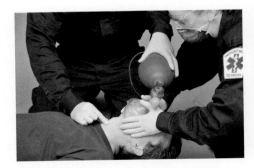

Figure 26.8 The EMT should be prepared to assist a patient's ventilations, if necessary

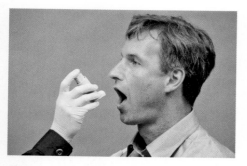

Figure 26.9 The EMT should be familiar with the use of an inhaler so that she may assist a patient with its use

Medication Card

Generic name: Albuterol
Trade name: Ventolin, Proventil
Indications: Signs and symptoms of respiratory distress in a patient who has a physician-prescribed handheld inhaler
Contraindications: The nonalert patient cannot cooperate with administration of an inhaler.
Dose: Two puffs given 1 minute apart
Route: By inhalation
Side Effects: Nervousness, heart racing

regulations on which of these medications may be used. Review Unit 13 on the administration of bronchodilator inhalers.

TRANSPORT

The EMT should initiate transport after determining patient priority. If after completing the primary assessment, the EMT finds that the patient has a potentially life-threatening problem, transport should be initiated immediately.

A quick history should be obtained from the family or friends present while the patient is being prepared for transport. The remainder of the exam should be provided in the ambulance while en route to the hospital.

DESTINATION DECISIONS

The patient should be transported to an appropriate facility, and the EMT must notify that facility as far in advance of arrival as possible. The unstable patient may require transport to the closest facility rather than to a preferred hospital. The EMT should be familiar with local protocols regarding destination determinations for unstable patients.

ADVANCED LIFE SUPPORT

When the patient is considered unstable or is still in distress upon initiation of transport, a basic life support (BLS) agency should make arrangements to intercept with an agency that provides a higher level of care when possible. The EMT, however, should never delay transport to wait for such care. It is sometimes necessary to intercept with the advanced life support (ALS) unit while en route to a hospital.

It may also be appropriate, depending on local protocols, for the EMT to establish on-line medical control to ask the physician for advice. Physicians provide guidance to the EMT in the form of general protocols. If the patient is not improving despite management according to those protocols, a medical control physician may instruct the EMT to provide different or additional therapies.

ONGOING ASSESSMENT

It is important for the EMT to remember that assessment is not static but ongoing. Key elements of assessment must continually be reassessed because a patient may quickly deteriorate.

To provide appropriate emergency care, continue to reassess and recognize significant changes in the patient's condition. The primary assessment should be repeated frequently, as should vital signs. Any significant changes should be relayed to the receiving hospital.

REASSESSMENT

After any treatment has been provided to the patient who is short of breath, the EMT should perform a careful reassessment. The primary assessment, vital signs, and secondary assessment all should be repeated after any therapy. The patient should also be asked how he is feeling in relation to how he felt before the therapy. The EMT should always be prepared for the dyspneic patient to decompensate and need ventilatory assistance.

CAUSES OF SHORTNESS OF BREATH

Problems can arise within any part of the respiratory system, all of which may result in inadequate respiration or poor oxygenation of the blood. This section briefly describes some of the disease processes that may affect each component of the respiratory system. It may be helpful to separate these illnesses into whether they primarily originate from the airway, breathing, or circulation.

AIRWAY

The airways cannot adequately transmit oxygen from the environment into the alveoli for gas exchange if they are obstructed. Airways can be obstructed by many things. Foreign bodies are probably the most common, although it is not unusual for parts of the airway itself to cause partial or even complete obstruction.

FOREIGN BODY OBSTRUCTION

If a foreign body such as a large piece of poorly chewed meat becomes lodged in the trachea or one of the bronchi, air cannot pass beyond it. If air cannot get to the alveoli to deliver oxygen, the body organs cannot function properly and may suffer permanent damage. Figure 26.10 illustrates an airway foreign body obstruction.

The brain and heart suffer permanent damage in as little as 4 minutes when deprived of oxygen. This situation requires rapid attention by the EMT. In the case of a complete obstruction, in which the patient cannot move any air or speak at all, the EMT should perform the abdominal thrust maneuver. The techniques for removal of airway foreign bodies are taught in a cardiopulmonary resuscitation (CPR) class.

The upper airways can also be partially occluded by a foreign body or even by excessive secretions seen in upper respiratory infections.

EPIGLOTTITIS

Another possible source of partial or complete obstruction of the upper airway is the airway structures themselves. The leaf-shaped flap of tissue called the epiglottis sits at the beginning of the larynx, above the opening to the trachea, and flaps open and closed to protect the trachea and lungs from foreign bodies as we swallow. This structure can become inflamed and swollen in a bacterial infection called **epiglottitis.** The enlarged epiglottis can completely occlude the airway quickly in this aggressive disease.

Although this condition can be seen in a patient of any age, the patients at risk for the most severe complications from epiglottitis are those with smaller airways—pediatric patients.

SIGNS AND SYMPTOMS

The child with epiglottitis will appear frightened owing to the difficulty in air movement. The classic history is that of a sudden-onset fever, cough, and now difficulty breathing. The child will most often be seated bolt upright with his head held forward, often drooling. The inability to swallow even saliva indicates severe upper airway narrowing.

MANAGEMENT

The best thing to do for a child who presents in this way is to remain calm while moving the child out to the ambulance and place the child in a position of comfort for a safe ride to the hospital. The parents should be encouraged to remain calm and to comfort the child. If tolerated, humidified oxygen can be administered using the blow-by method. Under no circumstances should the EMT attempt to examine the child's mouth or throat because doing so could cause laryngospasms and precipitate rapid and complete airway obstruction.

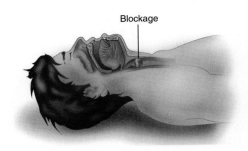

Figure 26.10 A complete airway obstruction will cause death in a matter of minutes if not relieved

Pediatric Considerations

Airway obstruction by secretions or swelling is especially relevant in pediatric patients because their airways are relatively smaller and would require fewer secretions to significantly narrow the air passages.

Early notification of the destination hospital is helpful so the emergency department staff can prepare necessary equipment and call in any needed specialists.

If the child's airway becomes completely occluded with no air movement and he develops cyanosis, the EMT should use a bag-valve-mask to ventilate the child with 100% oxygen. Still, no probing of the airway should be attempted because it may worsen the condition.

CROUP

Croup (laryngotracheobronchitis) is a viral infection usually affecting young children, causing irritation and swelling of the larynx, trachea, and bronchi. This disease is not as aggressive as epiglottitis and tends to cause a partial airway obstruction only. Croup can progress to complete obstruction; however, this is a rare occurrence.

SIGNS AND SYMPTOMS

The child with croup classically presents after several days of upper respiratory congestion and mild fevers. The irritation of the larynx produces a characteristic barking sound when the child coughs. The sound, which has been likened to the barking of a seal, is a significant diagnostic sign of croup.

In addition, if the inflammation is severe, the airway may be narrowed to the point that stridor is heard on inspiration. You will recall that stridor is a low-pitched inspiratory sound as a result of partial upper airway obstructions.

MANAGEMENT

The child with croup should be managed similarly to children with epiglottitis. It is sometimes difficult to tell these two illnesses apart. The priorities are to make the child as comfortable as possible, remain calm, and move quickly to the hospital. Cool, humidified oxygen is often helpful in relieving some of the child's discomfort and should be offered if tolerated.

The EMT has several methods of delivering humidified oxygen to the patient, such as using an in-line humidifier or a **small volume nebulizer (SVN).** The advantage of the SVN is that it can be started in the field and continue while the patient is being transferred to the ambulance. However, an SVN lasts for only about 15 minutes, whereas an in-line humidifier can last for hours.

The EMT may elect to use the SVN, the same one patients use to administer medications such as albuterol, although in this case no medicine is added. Like the in-line humidifier, the nebulizer has several components. The nebulizer has a bowl, sometimes called an acorn, in which approximately 3 milliliters (ml) of sterile saline is added. The sterile saline can come from a larger bottle, or more conveniently, from a small prepackaged ampule of saline flush, referred to as a pearl of saline, that is commercially available. Then the T-piece portion of the nebulizer is screwed into place, oxygen tubing is connected to the portable oxygen regulator, and the regulator is set at 8 liters per minute (Figure 26.11). The other end of the T-piece can either attach to a non-rebreather mask by removing the reservoir and replacing it with the nebulizer or be handheld to blow mist over the patient's face.

BREATHING

As expected, many illnesses that cause a patient to feel short of breath originate from the lungs themselves. A problem with air exchange is evident and results in shortness of breath.

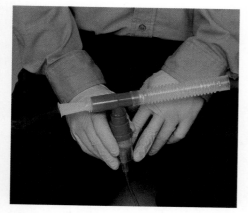

Figure 26.11 Humidified oxygen can be administered via a nebulizer

BRONCHOSPASM

One of the most common causes of shortness of breath is **bronchospasm,** which refers to constriction of the lower airways in the lungs. This can occur as a part of several disease processes, the most common of which will be discussed here.

ASTHMA

The lower airways can be affected by disease processes causing partial obstruction just as diseases such as croup and epiglottitis affect the upper airways. Hyperreactive airways found in some individuals respond to certain irritants (cigarette smoke, pollen, and cold air) by going into spasm and producing secretions. Both spasm and production of secretions can cause narrowing of the air spaces. This narrowing in the bronchioles causes a characteristic musical sound, known as wheezing, when air passes through them.

This disease process characterized by hyperreactive airways is known as reactive airway disease, or *asthma*. Chronic exposure to certain irritants (such as cigarette smoke) and other factors not completely identified can cause previously normal airways to become hyperreactive.

The patient with shortness of breath as a result of asthma will often describe some precipitating factor such as a respiratory infection, exposure to some airway irritant (smoke, animals, cold air), or sometimes just exertion such as exercise. This exposure will lead to a feeling of shortness of breath as bronchospasm occurs and it becomes more difficult to move air into and out of the chest. Figure 26.12 illustrates the basic problem in the airways in an asthma attack.

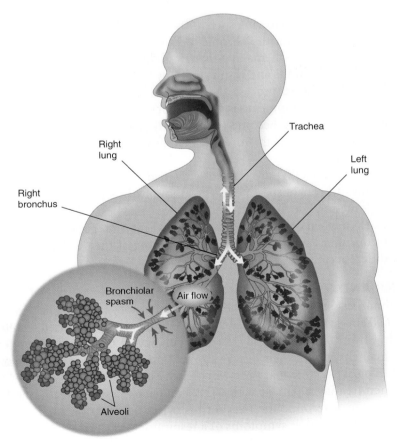

Figure 26.12 Asthma is a disease that involves bronchospasm and excessive airway secretions

SIGNS AND SYMPTOMS

The patient will often look distressed and is usually sitting upright, in the tripod position. He will have an elevated respiratory rate and when the lungs are auscultated, wheezes may be heard. Patients with a history of asthma often do not call for help unless the asthma attack is not responding to their inhalers or home nebulizers. By this time, they are often becoming more significantly distressed and may be anxious and uncooperative, refusing to allow an oxygen mask to be placed over their face.

MANAGEMENT

Patients who suffer from asthma are often prescribed medications that are meant to relieve the bronchospasms causing the breathing difficulty. In certain circumstances, the EMT will assist the patient to use these medications in an attempt to relieve the patient's symptoms.

For all patients who complain of difficulty breathing, the first priority in management is to ensure an adequate airway and to be sure that they are adequately ventilating themselves. Oxygen should be applied immediately, and ventilations should be assisted if the patient is not managing well with their own respiratory effort.

CHRONIC OBSTRUCTIVE PULMONARY DISEASE

Another group of diseases that can lead to bronchospasm is *chronic obstructive pulmonary disease (COPD)*. Emphysema and chronic bronchitis make up a majority of this group.

COPD, as the name suggests, is a chronic disorder involving obstruction of the airways in the lungs. This obstruction is a combination of bronchospasm and inflammation as seen in asthma but also includes other *nonreversible* causes of airway narrowing such as scarring and alveolar destruction.

Over the long term, the chronic airflow obstruction causes degenerative changes in the alveoli, making them less efficient. This chronic disease is often seen in older adults and results in many EMS calls.

COPD is a disease process that remains incompletely understood. It is known that something causes the patient's airways to become hyperresponsive and over time become permanently damaged. Cigarette smoking is highly correlated with this disease. People who suffer from COPD have chronic bronchospasm.

Patients with COPD are treated with medications aimed at decreasing the amount of bronchospasm and the amount of secretions present in the airways. Sometimes doctors will prescribe oxygen to be used at home by these patients. Even when compliant with their medication regimen, patients with COPD can suffer exacerbations (acute worsening of the disease) because of many different causes.

SIGNS AND SYMPTOMS

A common cause for an exacerbation is a respiratory infection. The already tightened airways become even smaller when plugged by increased secretions resulting from these infections. People with severe COPD cannot tolerate even small changes in their airway size without becoming severely short of breath. This is the time that EMS will often be called to assist.

When treating a patient with COPD and shortness of breath, the EMT should try to determine the relevant historical information such as recent fevers, coughs, or other symptoms of a respiratory infection.

Hypoxic Drive Because of their chronic respiratory insufficiency, some patients with COPD may breathe on a hypoxic drive. *Hypoxia* means low oxygen levels. A hypoxic drive means that the stimulus to breathe is low oxygen levels in the blood. The normal stimulus to breathe in healthy individuals is a high carbon dioxide level.

The patient with chronic airway obstruction has an inability to clear much of the carbon dioxide and will therefore have higher levels in the blood all the time. Some of these patients will adapt to that condition and begin to breathe on the basis of the oxygen levels instead, or with a hypoxic drive.

If a patient who breathes with a hypoxic drive is given 100% oxygen, the body may see the additional oxygen as an overabundance and decrease the respiratory efforts, sometimes even allowing breathing to stop altogether. EMTs must therefore pay close attention to the respiration of the patient with COPD who is breathing 100% oxygen and assist the patient's respiration if needed.

However, oxygen should never be withheld from someone who is short of breath. Understanding the importance of providing oxygen to the body organs is essential in treating COPD patients.

MANAGEMENT

If the patient is unable to get enough oxygen into the blood by his own respiratory efforts, the EMT must provide more oxygen via the best available method. It is also appropriate to assist a patient in using prescribed medications when authorized to do so by medical control.

RESPIRATORY INFECTION

Just as a respiratory infection such as pneumonia can cause bronchospasm in the patient with asthma or COPD, it can also cause a patient with previously healthy lungs to become short of breath. Pneumonia, bronchitis, pertussis, and other respiratory infections cause inflammation and excess secretions in the lower airways within the lungs. These may result in lower airway narrowing, even in the patient with healthy lungs.

SIGNS AND SYMPTOMS

Lower airway narrowing along with the buildup of secretions in the lungs can impair oxygen exchange and lead to shortness of breath. Fever and productive cough are common concerns in the presence of a pulmonary infection.

MANAGEMENT

Oxygen administration is indicated for the patient with a respiratory infection causing shortness of breath. Allowing the patient to stay in a position that is most comfortable, usually sitting upright, may also help the patient to feel less short of breath during transport.

OTHER CHRONIC LUNG DISEASES

In addition to those we have discussed so far, there are many other chronic lung diseases, all of which usually create a problem with oxygenation of the blood. If a patient is short of breath and has a chronic lung disease, the EMT should find out exactly what medications are taken and how this problem is related to the disease. Administration of oxygen is always the right treatment in management of the patient with shortness of breath, no matter what the underlying disease is.

CIRCULATION

Because the function of the lungs is so closely related to the function of the heart and blood vessels, a problem with one system will often result in a problem with the other.

Table 26-1 Disease States or Conditions That May Increase the Risk for Developing Blood Clots

Cancers

Prolonged immobility

Casts

Splints

Bedbound

Long car or plane trips

Smoking

Oral contraceptive use (birth control pills)

Prior history of blood clots

Recent surgery

PULMONARY EMBOLUS

If the airways are functioning efficiently and delivering oxygenated air to the alveoli, but there is no blood for the oxygen to diffuse into, the system fails. This condition occurs when blood flow to the alveoli is blocked by a blood clot, or embolus. This is known as a **pulmonary embolus** and is seen in people who are at risk for developing clots in their blood. Table 26-1 lists disease states or conditions that result in an increased risk of developing blood clots.

If the blood is prevented from being oxygenated, the organs do not get this necessary fuel and do not function properly. Figure 26.13 illustrates this sometimes-fatal condition.

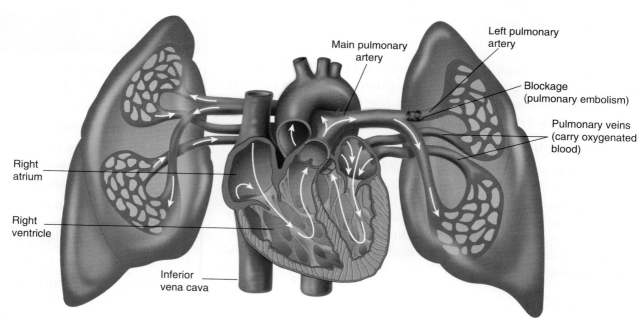

Main pulmonary artery

Left pulmonary artery

Blockage (pulmonary embolism)

Pulmonary veins (carry oxygenated blood)

Right atrium

Right ventricle

Inferior vena cava

Figure 26.13 A blood clot in the pulmonary vessels will block oxygenation of the blood, resulting in hypoxia and shortness of breath

SIGNS AND SYMPTOMS

The patient with a pulmonary embolus will often complain of a sudden onset of shortness of breath. Sometimes these patients will also complain of a sharp chest pain or dry cough. A patient who has had a pulmonary embolus or any type of blood clot before is at high risk for developing this problem again.

Because there is no problem with airflow, the patient's lung sounds will be clear. The respiratory rate will be elevated as the patient tries to increase the amount of oxygen breathed in.

MANAGEMENT

Because the problem is a decrease in oxygen in the blood, the EMT should apply 100% oxygen if she suspects pulmonary embolus to be the source of the patient's symptoms. If the clot is extensive, the oxygen may not significantly improve the patient's symptoms or appearance. Continued cyanosis despite 100% oxygen administration indicates a critical condition and should be reported to the receiving hospital.

PULMONARY EDEMA

We have described diseases that result in difficulty in getting air past narrowed airways and problems with getting blood to the alveoli to pick up the oxygen. A slightly different situation arises when the blood is in the capillaries next to the alveoli but the space between them is thickened. This condition can occur in several situations.

The alveoli can become filled with infectious secretions as when a patient has pneumonia or other respiratory infection, as described earlier. These secretions hinder the exchange of gases that occurs normally. The alveoli can also become filled with fluid that may leak out of the capillaries when the pressure in them is very high, as seen in *congestive heart failure (CHF)*.

This condition occurs when the left side of the heart is not strong enough to pump the blood out of the pulmonary circulation as quickly as it enters. This delay results in a backup of pressure in the small pulmonary vessels and leakage of part of the blood into the alveoli, making gas exchange difficult. Figure 26.14 illustrates this disease process.

SIGNS AND SYMPTOMS

Any condition that results in fluid accumulation results in crackles being heard upon auscultation of the lungs over the fluid-filled area. Whereas pneumonia will result in crackles over the area affected by the infection, CHF will result in diffuse crackles, most often beginning at the bases of the lungs and progressing upward as the condition worsens. Severe CHF is associated with crackles heard throughout the lungs, and the patient may even have pink frothy sputum.

The patient suffering from CHF often has a history of heart trouble, hence the poor function of the left ventricle. These patients will often complain of shortness of breath that has gotten progressively worse over several days.

Their symptoms are often aggravated by lying down because the excess fluid redistributes and spreads throughout the lungs in this position. Any exertion will usually create worsening symptoms as well. Chest pain may be present in some patients.

MANAGEMENT

Because the problem is inadequate oxygen delivery to the blood, the appropriate treatment is to increase the oxygen content in the air in the alveoli. The more oxygen that is there, the more oxygen can diffuse across into the

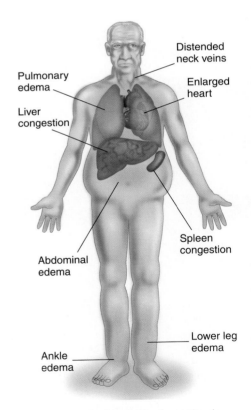

Figure 26.14 A poorly functioning left ventricle will result in a backup of fluid pressure in the pulmonary circulation. Leakage of fluid into the alveoli will result

bloodstream. The EMT should provide the patient with CHF and shortness of breath with 100% oxygen. Allowing the patient to sit completely upright and to loosen tight clothing will also help to minimize the symptoms.

SHOCK

As we discussed in Unit 11, one of the body's reactions to hypoperfusion is to increase the respiratory rate. This increase will bring more oxygen into the body to distribute to its hypoperfused tissues. The elevated respiratory rate may cause the patient to feel short of breath. In this case, the EMT should treat the patient according to the priorities outlined in Unit 11.

CONCLUSION

Many disease processes may cause difficulty breathing as a result of inadequate tissue oxygenation or inadequate blood detoxification of carbon dioxide, or both. The EMT must be proficient in quickly assessing these patients and providing emergency care to them.

An EMT's treatment of a patient with difficulty breathing should always include oxygen and appropriate ventilatory assistance. Specific other medications may be indicated, depending on the most likely diagnosis and the patient's history.

It is always appropriate to call for ALS assistance if the patient continues to have difficulty breathing despite BLS measures. Appropriate decisions regarding transport and constant reassessment are also important in good prehospital management of the patient with difficulty breathing.

CASE STUDY Continued

After completing the primary assessment, Brandon's general impression is that Mr. Abernathy exhibits signs of severe respiratory distress. Mr. Abernathy is cyanotic around his mouth and nail beds. He is using the accessory muscles of his neck and chest to breathe, and wheezes are present throughout all fields in both lungs.

Mr. Abernathy can answer questions only by shaking his head. He indicates when questioned that his inhalers are both empty and he has not taken his numerous medicines. A brief history is obtained by asking yes and no questions.

Baseline vital signs reveal a pulse of 128, respirations of 28, and a blood pressure of 158/90. The pulse oximeter reading is initially 86% at the house but had improved to 91% with the oxygen. Mr. Abernathy hands Brandon a paper that states he has a history of COPD, specifically emphysema.

Upon intercept with the ALS crew, Mr. Abernathy is able to speak 3 or 4 words before gasping for breath and conveys that he had used his inhalers up the night before when he started having problems breathing.

As the ALS crew begins respiratory treatment, using an albuterol nebulizer, Brandon provides a full report of what they saw on scene and hands the bag of medications they had brought along to the paramedic.

As Mr. Abernathy relaxes, appearing to have less difficulty breathing, the paramedic asks Brandon to begin the reassessment while she radios into the hospital. Mr. Abernathy's vitals signs are reassessed, and his pulse is 116, respirations 24, and blood pressure 146/86. Mr. Abernathy's skin is pale and warm, and he is no longer sweating. Lung sounds are still wheezy, but Brandon can actually hear air moving through the lung fields now.

Brandon provides this information to the paramedic for his radio report and begins the documentation that will be left with the patient at the hospital at the time of care transfer.

Key Concepts Revisited

- The respiratory system provides oxygen to the body and removes carbon dioxide.
- Knowledge of normal breathing enables appropriate assessment and management of breathing problems.
  - Respirations are normally driven by carbon dioxide levels.
- A person breathing normally appears comfortable during both inhalation and exhalation.
- Respiratory difficulty usually presents with easily recognized classic signs and symptoms.
- Clues to respiratory difficulty can be evident during scene size-up:
  - Medications
  - Nebulizers
  - MDI
  - Smoking
  - Patient position
- Mental status may be the first indicator of respiratory compromise:
  - Confusion
  - Lethargy
  - Unresponsiveness
- Patient position can indicate the severity of the distress:
  - Tripod
  - Recumbent
- How the medical patient is assessed is based on responsiveness.

- Unresponsive:
  - Primary assessment
  - Rapid physical exam
  - Baseline vital signs
  - History from family
- Responsive patient
  - Primary assessment
  - History
  - Baseline vital signs
  - Secondary assessment with focused physical exam
- The primary management of the dyspneic patient is providing high-flow oxygen.
  - Assisted ventilations with oxygen support
  - Oxygen administration for spontaneous ventilations
- Position the patient with respiratory distress to support breathing.
- Assist patient with medication administration per local protocols.
  - Metered dose inhalers
- Obtain history from the family or friends prior to transporting unresponsive patients.
- Arrange ALS intercept with severe respiratory distress or arrest.

- Numerous diseases can compromise the respiratory and circulatory systems.
  - Obstruction of airways
    - Foreign body airway obstruction
    - Epiglottitis
    - Croup
  - Breathing
    - Asthma
    - COPD
      - Emphysema
      - Chronic bronchitis
  - Infections
    - Pneumonia
    - Pertussis
  - Circulation
    - Pulmonary embolus
    - Pulmonary edema
    - CHF
  - Shock
- Appropriate ventilatory assistance and oxygen administration are key to management of respiratory emergencies.

Review Questions

1. What are the structures and function of the respiratory system?
2. What common signs and symptoms are seen in patients with difficulty breathing?
3. How is the unresponsive medical patient's assessment different than the responsive medical patient?
4. How is the patient with difficulty breathing managed in the prehospital setting?
5. Why is medical direction important to the EMT when caring for the patient with difficulty breathing?
6. What signs or symptoms can be indicators to the severity of the patient's respiratory distress?
7. What are the signs of adequate air exchange?
8. What is hypoxic drive?
9. When is the administration of a prescribed inhaler indicated?
10. What are the key elements in management of patients with epiglottitis, croup, asthma, COPD, and CHF?

Key Terms

Alveolar-capillary gas exchange

Bronchospasm

Croup

Epiglottitis

Pulmonary embolus

Rales

Rhonchi

Small volume nebulizer (SVN)

Further Study

Beebe, R. *Functional Anatomy.* Clifton Park, NY: Thomson Delmar Learning, 2002.

Dalton, A. L., D. Limmer, J. J. Mistovich, and H. A. Werman. *Advanced Medical Life Support.* 3rd ed. Upper Saddle River, NJ: Brady/Prentice Hall, 2006.

Elling, B., and K. M. Elling. *Principles of Patient Assessment in EMS.* Clifton Park, NY: Thomson Delmar Learning, 2002.

Myer, J., M. Neighbors, and R. Tennhille-Jones. *Principles of Pathophysiology and Emergency Medical Care.* Clifton Park, NY: Thomson Delmar Learning, 2002.

Rizzo, D. *Fundamentals of Anatomy & Physiology.* 2nd ed. Clifton Park, NY: Thomson Delmar Learning, 2006.

A patient may act confused or disoriented or may "just not be acting right" for many reasons. Concerned family members or citizens may recognize that the patient is in need of immediate medical attention and call Emergency Medical Services (EMS).

Often people may be frightened by the person or by her actions and call the police. The police, in turn, call EMS when the medical emergency is recognized. In both of these cases, the patient is experiencing a change in behavior that may be due to illness or disease—in other words, an altered mental state.

Several potentially dangerous medical conditions can create altered mental states or unexplained faints (syncopal event). Stroke is an example of a condition that often presents with an altered level of conscious or unexplained loss of consciousness.

As the third leading cause of death and the leading cause of disability in the United States today, stroke is a problem that an Emergency Medical Technician (EMT) is likely to encounter in clinical practice.

It is important for an EMT to understand the conditions that may cause altered mental status or syncope and to be able to assess the patient for those conditions. Early identification of the cause, as in the case of a possible stroke, along with appropriate decision making on the part of the EMT can have a significant impact on the morbidity and mortality associated with these conditions.

National Education Standard

The Emergency Medical Technician (EMT) will apply a fundamental depth and foundational breadth of understanding to provide basic emergency care and transportation, based on assessment findings to an acutely ill medical patient experiencing headache or an altered mental status.

Key Concepts

- Individuals who are confused or disoriented about person, place, or time are considered to have an altered mental state.

- Altered mental status may be due to chronic health conditions or acute changes within the body resulting from disease or trauma.

- A cerebrovascular accident (CVA) or stroke is a disruption of blood flow to part of the brain causing an injury to the brain.

- The causes of stroke can be easily divided into two main categories: ischemic and hemorrhagic.

- The treatment of a stroke in prehospital care is the recognition of the symptoms and expedient transport to a hospital capable of managing the condition.

- Altered mental status may be due to disorders of glucose metabolism associated with diabetes mellitus.

- Seizures are a short circuit of the brain's electrical system resulting in an altered mental status.

- Headaches are classified as primary and secondary and may be the symptom of a more serious disease or condition.

Margeux and John are cleaning the ambulance when they are dispatched to the report of a "man down" on the corner of Cherry and Main streets. They arrive on the scene and note that two police officers have secured the scene. After donning appropriate PPE and gathering the equipment needed, the EMTs perform a scene size-up noting one patient, a male approximately 50 years old.

The patient is sitting on the curb, slightly slumped to one side and leaning on a telephone pole. He is conscious. A police officer informs them he noticed the man sitting there when they drove by approximately 10 minutes ago. The officer indicated that the patient can speak, though with a slight slur, and seems confused, unable to tell them how he got to this place, what happened, or any identifying information.

Critical Thinking Questions

1. What are some possible causes for this man's altered behavior and apparent confusion?

2. How is patient history and information gathered from a patient with an altered level of consciousness?

3. Based on the police officer's report, is the man truly conscious and able to consent to care?

INTRODUCTION

The EMT must quickly assess the patient experiencing an altered level of consciousness, faint (syncope), or stroke. He must also provide the appropriate treatment and transport the patient to the most appropriate facility.

In some of these conditions, the failure of the EMT to quickly assess and intervene may cause the patient to suffer permanent disability or die. This unit addresses the physiology, assessment, and management of patients experiencing a condition causing altered mental status or syncope, including stroke.

MENTAL STATUS

EMTs may encounter many patients who, for some unknown reason, are experiencing an altered mental state. An altered mental state is easiest to define when it is compared with the definition of a normal mental state.

A person who is awake, alert, and appropriately interactive with the environment has a normal mental state. A normal mental state requires that the person have an adequate supply of blood, carrying oxygen and sugar (glucose), circulating in the brain.

The awake, alert patient who is ill or injured will usually cooperate with the care that is being given by answering simple questions. The awake, alert patient will also follow instructions, sometimes described as following commands.

Normally, a person is oriented, meaning the person has the ability to comprehend who she is, where she is, and generally what time or day it is. In other words, the patient is oriented to person (self), place (current location), and time or day.

EMTs determine a patient's mental status at the beginning of the primary assessment, using the AVPU scale (Figure 27.1). Review Unit 16 for further details about AVPU assessment. If the patient is awake and oriented

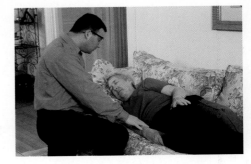

Figure 27.1 The determination of the level of consciousness is made at the beginning of the primary assessment

to person, place, and time or day, then she is alert and considered to be in a normal mental state.

ALTERED MENTAL STATUS

Any time patients are confused or disoriented about person, place, or time, they have an **altered mental state.** The patient who is indifferent, apathetic, and generally detached from her surroundings may also be experiencing an altered mental state.

Examples of statements made by a patient that would lead an EMT to think the patient is disoriented and therefore has an altered mental state include:

- "Where am I?"
- "What just happened?"

A failure to remember what just happened is called *amnesia*. Amnesia can be due to a head injury.

After a motor vehicle collision (MVC), most people are concerned about themselves (Am I hurt?), the other driver (Is he hurt?), and damage to the car (Figure 27.2). A driver who appears to be uninterested in her own injuries should be assumed to have altered mental status.

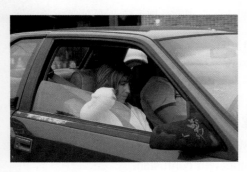

Figure 27.2 A patient's orientation is always relative to her surroundings

CAUSES OF ALTERED MENTAL STATUS

There are many reasons why a patient would have an altered mental state. Some are due to chronic health conditions. For example, elderly patients with Alzheimer's disease are often confused. **Alzheimer's disease** is a progressive, irreversible deterioration of intellectual function.

However, many altered mental states are due to acute changes within the body resulting from disease or trauma. These acute and potentially reversible changes can lead to serious long-term complications or even death, if left untreated. These acute changes usually involve the loss of either sufficient oxygen or sugar in the brain. Table 27-1 lists some potentially reversible causes of an altered mental state. The EMT is trained to identify and treat these causes of altered mental status.

The EMT should never assume that a patient who is not awake, alert, and oriented is normal. Erring on the side of caution, the EMT should always treat every patient as if the patient has a potentially reversible cause for her altered mental status.

A mnemonic to help an EMT remember some of the more common causes of altered mental status is **AEIOU TIPS.** Table 27-2 provides some relatively common conditions an EMT will encounter that could produce an altered mental status. The table explains each letter in the mnemonic, although some providers differ on the meaning of each letter.

Each of the conditions listed in Table 27-2 can lead to potentially life-threatening complications.

STROKE

As stated previously, stroke is the third leading cause of death and the leading cause of disability in the United States today. Early identification of the possibility of stroke as a diagnosis and appropriate decision making on the part of the EMT can have a significant impact on the morbidity and mortality associated with this condition.

Table 27-1 Some Treatable Causes of Altered Mental Status

Problem	Effect
Congestive heart failure	Hypoxia
Diabetes	Hypoglycemia
Gross external hemorrhage	Hypoperfusion
Internal bleeding	Hypoperfusion
Lung disease (e.g., emphysema)	Hypoxia
Oxygen-poor environment (confined space)	Hypoxia
Partial foreign body airway obstruction	Hypoxia
Smoke inhalation	Hypoxia
Stroke	Brain injury

Table 27-2 Conditions That Lead to an Altered Mental Status

Letter	Condition	Contributing Factor
A	Alcohol	Effects of ethanol or any other form of alcohol
E	Epilepsy	Seizures
I	Insulin	Too much insulin results in low glucose levels in the blood
O	Oxygen deprivation or drug overdose	Insufficient oxygen can result in brain hypoxia (Unit 8); overdose on certain types of medications can result in poor brain perfusion
U	Uremia	Kidney failure results in buildup of toxins in the bloodstream (uncommon)
T	Trauma	Injuries to the head
I	Infection	Any overwhelming infection or any infection involving the brain
P	Psychiatric disorder/ Poisoning	Behavioral disorders or poison
S	Stroke	Causes a lack of blood supply to a portion of the brain

PATHOPHYSIOLOGY

A **cerebrovascular accident (CVA),** or **stroke,** is nontraumatic injury to brain tissue that occurs as a result of disruption of blood flow to part of the brain. This disruption can occur in one of two general ways.

A stroke may result in irreversible brain damage, causing the patient to lose a part of her body function, resulting in lifelong disability and necessitating long-term care. Early recognition and diagnosis of stroke is critical, leading to earlier definitive treatment and often better patient outcome.

Despite the profound way that stroke affects so many people, there is general misunderstanding about the condition. It is often thought that once a person has a stroke, nothing can be done in treatment. On the contrary, over the last decade, advances in treatment are resulting in improved recovery of many patients with stroke.

The treatment of stroke is a time-dependent issue. The longer an area of brain is without oxygen, the more damage is done. Many therapies for stroke are only effective when used very early on in the event. This means that public education regarding stroke symptom recognition and how to access emergency services rapidly is paramount if we are to have a chance to treat this disease process.

EMTs must be able to quickly recognize the symptoms and signs of stroke and be knowledgeable regarding the services available in their region to treat this incredibly time-sensitive condition. It is important that patient care protocols address the management of stroke as a true medical emergency.

THE 7 DS

The American Heart Association has identified the 7 Ds in care for a stroke patient. The time factor in stroke care is critical to the reduction of potentially permanent disability and death. Using the 7 Ds—Detection, Dispatch, Delivery, Door, Data, Decision, and Drug—the EMT can address the time factor and improve the patient's outcome.

Early recognition or detection by the patient, bystander, family, and EMT of the signs and symptoms of stroke is the first step in fighting that time "clock." It is equally important for dispatch to recognize the signs and symptoms the caller is describing as a possible stroke and prioritize the call appropriately as an emergency.

Prompt delivery of patient assessment, treatment, and transport is the final step of the 7 Ds in the management of the stroke patient by the EMT in the field. The final four Ds—Door, Data, Decision, and Drug—are management criteria for the patient in the emergency department.

TYPES OF STROKE

Brain cells depend on continuous flow of oxygenated blood to function normally. Anything that interrupts the normal flow of blood will cause malfunction of the cells that depend on it. The causes of stroke can be easily divided into two main categories: ischemic and hemorrhagic.

ISCHEMIC STROKE

Ischemia is the injury of tissue that occurs as a result of blockage of the vessel that normally supplies that tissue with blood. The vast majority of strokes, about 85%, are ischemic in nature. Most **ischemic strokes** occur as a result of chronic narrowing of vessels by atherosclerosis followed by the gradual accumulation of platelets and other blood components, called a *thrombus,* eventually resulting in a complete blockage of the vessel. This process is similar to what is seen in the coronary vessels described in Unit 25. Figure 27.3 illustrates the anatomy of a thrombus.

Street Smart

The lay public sometimes refers to a stroke as a "brain attack" because of its similarity in physiology to a "heart attack," the lay term for a myocardial infarction. Both conditions can involve death of tissue due to lack of adequate blood flow to the area.

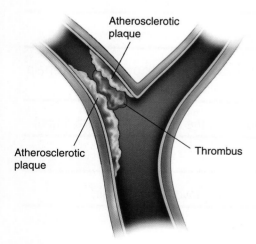

Figure 27.3 Platelets and other blood factors can adhere to the irregular surface of a plaque, resulting in a thrombus

Blood flow may also be interrupted when a blood clot that is formed elsewhere in the body travels through the bloodstream and gets lodged in one of the vessels supplying the brain. This type of traveling debris is called an *embolus* and also interrupts blood flow to the tissue beyond where it is lodged. Figure 27.4 illustrates this concept.

Another less common mechanism whereby the brain is deprived of oxygenated blood is during periods of severe shock when the blood pressure falls so low that flow to the brain is not maintained. In this case, the entire brain is without oxygen and severe brain injury may result.

Regardless of the cause of the interruption in blood flow, the brain cells that are deprived of oxygenated blood die within a very short period of time. A group of cells that has died as a result of prolonged lack of oxygen are referred to as an *infarct*, just as seen in an AMI. When cells die, they release chemicals that may cause injury to the surrounding cells. The area of brain tissue that surrounds an infarct is called the **penumbra.** The penumbra is a group of injured brain cells that has a chance of recovery if appropriate treatment is begun rapidly. Figure 27.5 depicts this concept.

TRANSIENT ISCHEMIC ATTACK

Occasionally, a patient may have decreased blood flow to an area of the brain that is only temporary. When this occurs and the symptoms resolve completely within 24 hours, the term **transient ischemic attack (TIA)** applies. A TIA is usually associated with a thrombus that the body is able to resolve on its own. Patients who have a TIA are at a high risk for having a stroke in the near future. In fact, certain patients have as high as a 25% risk for stroke in the first year after a TIA, the highest incidence being in the first month.

Patients who call EMS for stroke symptoms that resolve spontaneously must still be transported for immediate evaluation. A physician may be able to help the patient modify her risk factors and use medications to try to prevent a more serious event.

Street Smart

Some patients refer to a TIA as a "mini-stroke." Although this usage is not entirely accurate, the EMT needs to be familiar with the common terminology.

HEMORRHAGIC STROKE

The second category of stroke is known as *hemorrhagic stroke*. This category accounts for less than 15% of strokes. In hemorrhagic stroke there is a rupture of one of the cerebral vessels. This may occur as a result of chronic high blood pressure causing a weakening of the vessel or as a result of an abnormality such as an aneurysm in the blood vessel. In either case, rupture of a vessel in the brain will decrease blood flow to the brain tissue supplied by that vessel, resulting in an area of infarct (Figure 27.6).

In addition to the decrease in blood flow to the area supplied by that vessel, the blood that leaks out of the vessel can cause injury to the surrounding brain tissue in several ways. Blood itself is irritating to brain cells and can cause injury when it leaks outside the vessel. Additionally, when a significant amount of blood accumulates, it can compress surrounding brain tissue, also resulting in injury. In this case, intracranial pressure may become elevated, in much the same way it does in a patient with a hemorrhage in the brain caused by trauma. Increased intracranial pressure is discussed in detail in Unit 34.

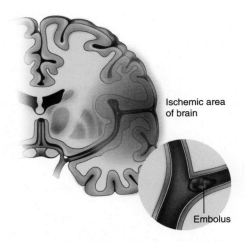

Figure 27.4 An embolus can lodge in a cerebral vessel, resulting in ischemia to the brain tissue supplied by that vessel

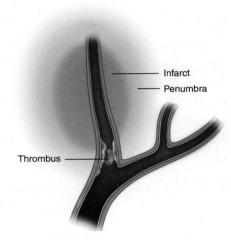

Figure 27.5 The penumbra is a potentially salvageable area of brain tissue

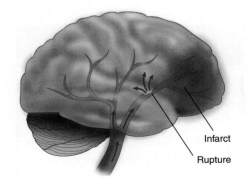

Figure 27.6 In hemorrhagic stroke, the rupture of a blood vessel results in decreased blood flow to an area of brain tissue

RISK FACTORS

Factors that put a person at risk for a stroke include anything that can result in vessel occlusion or vessel weakening and rupture. People with known vascular disease, such as patients with coronary artery disease or hypertension, are at risk. Diabetes over a long period of time can result in vascular abnormalities. Irregular heart rhythms can cause blood clots that can block vessels. Any cause of very high blood pressure, such as amphetamine use (cocaine or methamphetamine) or uncontrolled hypertension, can result in stroke. Anyone who has previously suffered a stroke is at risk of experiencing another.

SIGNS AND SYMPTOMS

The signs and symptoms that are present in a patient experiencing a stroke depend upon the area of the brain affected. The most common cerebral vessel affected by a stroke is the middle cerebral artery. In this case, the patient will present with weakness and/or numbness in the face and arm on one side. Often the leg on the same side is involved to some extent as well. Speech may be difficult to understand, called *dysarthria*, if the muscles in the mouth that normally allow clear speech are affected.

Other symptoms that people suffering from a stroke may complain of are listed in Table 27-3. Many of these symptoms are nonspecific. The EMT must maintain a high index of suspicion when treating patients who may be at risk for stroke.

Although their presentation is sometimes similar to those suffering from an ischemic stroke, patients suffering from a hemorrhagic stroke often present with a headache and signs of increased intracranial pressure.

If the symptoms of stroke are discovered early in the course of the event and the diagnosis is made quickly, therapies may be instituted to reduce the possibility of long-term disability. The symptoms present at the onset of a stroke do not necessarily remain throughout the stroke. Treatment initiated early has shown that some brain tissue may be salvaged and a significant return of function in the affected side is possible. The EMT plays an important role in the long-term outcome for patients suffering a stroke.

ASSESSMENT

During the assessment of a patient with symptoms and signs of stroke, the EMT should assess for immediate life threats, as with any other critically ill patient. Additionally, an accurate history of the events, specifically the time of symptom onset, preceding the call for EMS will be crucial to management decisions made at the hospital. A focused neurologic examination will provide the EMT with information that will allow for decisions to be made regarding management, both by the EMT and by the hospital staff.

PRIMARY ASSESSMENT

Certain patients having a stroke may have problems that present an immediate threat to the patency of the airway, adequacy of breathing, or circulatory status. Immediately after ensuring the safety of the scene, the EMT should perform an initial assessment and immediately address any potential life-threatening issues. Unit 16 details the primary assessment that should be performed on every patient.

HISTORY

If the patient is awake and able to answer questions, the EMT should obtain a history that covers the present illness and questions regarding past medical history, allergies, or medications taken. If the patient is not able to provide the history, the EMT should obtain relevant historical information from family

Table 27-3 Symptoms Associated with Stroke
Generalized or focal weakness
Paralysis on one side of the body
Paresthesias on one side of the body
Difficulty speaking
Headache
Vomiting
Visual changes
Dizziness

Street Smart

Although the incidence of stroke doubles each decade after age 55, the EMT must remember that young patients also have strokes. Signs and symptoms of stroke must not be discounted simply because of the young age of the patient.

or others who are present. Particular attention should be paid to determining the exact time of onset of the current symptoms. The management of stroke is extremely time sensitive. Certain therapies are only employed if they can be initiated within a narrow window of 3 hours from symptom onset. Other therapies have a slightly wider window of opportunity. However, in any case, it is imperative that the time of onset of the symptoms be identified as accurately as possible. Unit 18 discusses the elements of taking a pertinent patient history.

SECONDARY ASSESSMENT

The focused physical examination should include a brief neurologic examination. The neurologic examination should include five pieces of information. The patient's mental status should be described. The level of consciousness on the AVPU scale (see Unit 16) is helpful, as is describing the patient's orientation to person, place, and time or day. If the patient is awake and able to answer questions, the EMT can ask her name, where she is at this time, and what time of day or what day it is. These questions can be repeated as needed by other providers to assess for changes in mental status.

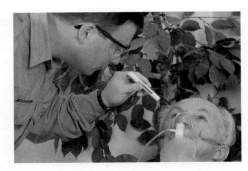

Figure 27.7 Examining the pupils for size and reactivity to light should be a routine part of every assessment

An examination of the patient's pupils is appropriate during the first examination and during each reassessment (Figure 27.7). Their shape and response to light should be assessed. Normally, pupils are round and of equal size and respond by constricting when exposed to a light source. Any irregular shape, size difference from one side to another, or abnormal response to light may be a sign of possible brain injury.

The patient should be asked to perform several tasks as part of the remainder of the neurologic examination. First, the EMT should ask the patient to raise his arms straight out in front of him with palms facing up. Then the patient should be instructed to close his eyes and attempt to keep his arms still for 10 seconds (Figure 27.8). If one arm drifts, it indicates weakness on that side and should be carefully noted. This weakness is called **pronator drift** and is a useful way to test for arm weakness.

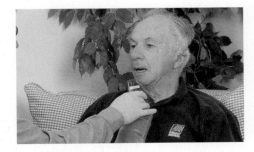

Figure 27.8 The presence of pronator drift indicates arm weakness, sometimes due to a stroke

Next, the patient should be asked to smile and show his teeth (Figure 27.9). Normally, both sides of the face should move equally, and the smile should be equal on both sides. If one side of the face does not move as well, it is called a **facial droop** and indicates facial muscle weakness. This test can be performed easily by the EMT.

Finally, the EMT should note the clarity of the patient's speech (Figure 27.10). If speech seems garbled, slurred, or inappropriate, that should be noted. Garbled speech is called *dysarthria* and can be indicative of a stroke.

Depending upon the area of the brain that is affected, the patient's speech may be affected in a different way. Expressive aphasia is one such condition. If a patient is speaking with inappropriate words, but forming them clearly, she is said to have **expressive aphasia.** This is often frustrating to the patient. In the most extreme case, the patient will be unable to speak at all. **Receptive aphasia** exists when the patient seems to not understand words that are spoken to her. This condition is sometimes difficult to differentiate from uncooperative behavior related to a change in mental status. Each of these speech alterations indicates injury to the area of the brain that controls speech.

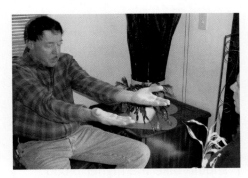

Figure 27.9 Asking the patient to smile can help to demonstrate weakness of the facial muscles on one side of the face

A focused neurologic exam such as this can be rapidly accomplished by the EMT. The combination of assessment of arm drift, facial droop, and speech is known as the **Cincinnati Prehospital Stroke Scale** and has been found to be easily completed by any level of provider, from EMT to physician. Additionally, it is an accurate predictor of the diagnosis of acute stroke and can be used to make decisions regarding the patient's management. Table 27-4 summarizes the Cincinnati Prehospital Stroke Scale.

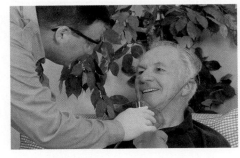

Figure 27.10 Garbled or slurred speech can result from weakness of the muscles in the mouth and throat, sometimes associated with stroke

Table 27-4 The Cincinnati Prehospital Stroke Scale

	Normal	Abnormal
Arm drift	Both arms move equally or not at all.	One arm drifts compared to the other.
Facial droop	Both sides of the face move equally.	One side of the face does not move at all.
Speech	Patient uses correct words without slurring.	Patient uses inappropriate words, slurs, or is mute.

Street Smart

An EMT should consider taking a blood pressure in both arms. Some patients have a difference in blood pressures from the right and left arm. The EMT should take the higher blood pressure as the blood pressure to document.

Other well-known standardized stroke scales are specifically designed to be used in the prehospital environment for the assessment of the patient with an acute stroke. Two such scales are the 3-item Los Angeles Motor Scale and the 15-item shortened National Institutes of Health Stroke Scale. The EMT should become familiar with whatever standardized assessment is recognized in his area of practice.

Some types of strokes affect a part of the brain that does not cause abnormality on any of these tests. Therefore, the EMT should consider stroke not only in patients who have such abnormalities but also in any person who has suspicious symptoms.

BASELINE VITAL SIGNS

As with every patient the EMT encounters, the patient suffering from a stroke will need careful assessment. Baseline vital signs are a part of that assessment. It is not unusual for the blood pressure to be elevated in some types of stroke. The EMT should take careful note of any vital sign abnormalities and report them to hospital staff.

MANAGEMENT

We know that every minute during a stroke, brain cells are being damaged and time is of the essence to try to limit permanent injury of the brain. Although the treatment of a stroke is a true emergency, the prehospital management of stroke is somewhat limited. The job of the EMT is to recognize the symptoms and provide expedient transport to a hospital capable of managing the condition.

HOSPITAL MANAGEMENT

The hospital management of the patient will center on making the diagnosis and ruling out other causes of the symptoms and then in providing definitive therapy to reestablish blood flow to the affected area of the brain when this is possible. In the case of a hemorrhagic stroke, the treatment will focus on controlling the blood pressure and limiting further injury.

In the case of ischemic stroke, intravenous medications may be given to break up the clot and allow blood to flow again to the affected area of the brain. In highly specialized centers, these thrombolytic medications may be administered directly into the affected artery by a specially trained physician. Additionally, similar to what is done in cardiac angioplasty, tiny tools can sometimes be used inside the vessel to assist in the reestablishment of blood flow. These procedures, although available at only certain centers, might offer fewer side effects and a more direct means of reestablishing blood flow to the injured brain.

Hospitals able to offer advanced therapies to stroke victims at all times are referred to as *stroke centers*. Timeliness of transport is of key importance, because these therapies may be used only if the patient presents to the hospital within a short window of time. The EMT should be familiar with the capabilities of hospitals in their region and should follow protocols carefully regarding the appropriate facility to which stroke patients should be transported.

BLS MANAGEMENT

During transport the EMT will continually assess the patient and take steps to prevent worsening injury, if possible. Such steps include appropriate management of the airway, breathing, and circulation (ABCs). If the patient is not able to effectively maintain her own airway, the EMT should take the appropriate action.

Increased intracranial pressure may result in an abnormal breathing pattern. If the patient is not breathing effectively, the EMT must assist ventilations using positive pressure ventilation as described in Unit 10.

Stroke is a condition in which part of the brain is not receiving enough oxygen; therefore, high-flow oxygen should be provided to every patient with a possible stroke.

During a stroke, the brain senses lack of blood flow to the affected area. In compensation, the blood pressure may elevate in an attempt to provide blood flow to the involved area. This may result in very elevated blood pressures. Occasionally, a stroke may result from or cause low blood pressure. If this is the case, the EMT should take steps to support the blood pressure as described in Unit 11.

In the non-hypotensive patient, the head of the bed should be elevated 15 to 30 degrees, which may help to decrease intracranial pressure. This head-elevated position is recommended unless management of the airway and breathing precludes it.

A patient who has severe weakness on one side of her body will likely lean toward that side. If a patient is unable to support herself adequately, the EMT should be sure to provide support for the patient to avoid any falls or injuries during transport (Figure 27.11).

DIFFERENTIAL DIAGNOSES

A focused neurologic examination should be done for any patient suspected of having suffered a stroke. An abnormal finding on any of these tests may indicate a stroke, although other conditions can cause some of them. Table 27-5 lists some of those conditions that should be considered.

The EMT may not be able to differentiate between stroke and many of these other conditions; however, the treatment an EMT can offer is very much the same for each. Management of the ABCs with timely transport to the appropriate facility is indicated in each case.

TRANSPORT

As soon as the possibility of stroke is recognized, the EMT should take steps to initiate transport by the most expedient means to the most appropriate hospital. Advanced life support (ALS) should be requested to intercept if indicated in local protocols. In some areas of the country, stroke patients are specifically triaged to hospitals or facilities that have specialized stroke teams capable of providing advanced therapies very quickly. In some cases, if the most appropriate hospital is a significant distance from the patient, a helicopter might be the most expedient means of transport. EMTs should become familiar with protocols in their area.

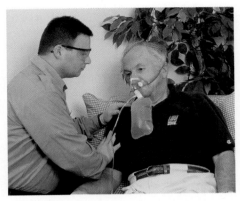

Figure 27.11 The patient suffering from a stroke may be profoundly weak on one side and may need help to keep from falling

Street Smart

If the EMT has the ability to perform blood glucose testing, it is appropriate to do so in the case of a patient with stroke-like symptoms. It is possible for low blood sugar to cause symptoms that mimic a stroke. In that case, glucose administration would be the definitive treatment.

Table 27-5 Other Diagnoses to Consider in the Presence of Stroke-like Symptoms

Hypoglycemia	Low blood sugar
Bell's palsy	An inflammatory condition of the nerve controlling the muscles of one side of the face
Traumatic brain injury	Injury to the brain from trauma
Seizure	Localized paralysis may remain after a seizure for hours to days
Migraine	Complicated migraines may result in neurologic abnormalities that resolve upon resolution of the migraine
Drug toxicity	Toxic levels of some medications (e.g., Lithium, Dilantin, Tegretol) may cause neurologic abnormality

Early notification of the destination hospital is crucial in the case of a stroke patient. Such advanced notification allows the hospital to mobilize necessary resources and prepare to manage this patient in the most expeditious manner.

ONGOING ASSESSMENT

The importance of repeated, ongoing assessments in the stroke patient cannot be overstated. Any changes in the patient's vital signs, mental status, pupils, or focused neurologic examination are of importance to the treating team at the hospital and should be noted carefully.

DIABETES MELLITUS

The brain uses glucose and oxygen to create energy. Without an abundant supply of both, the brain will malfunction. The outward signs of a low glucose level are confusion, combativeness, lethargy, and even coma.

Sugar (glucose) is obtained from the food we eat in a process called *digestion*. However, it is not enough to simply eat large quantities of food. Somehow the glucose has to get to the cells of the brain, where it can be used for fuel.

Glucose is transported to the brain in the blood. Once it is in the brain, it must be carried into the brain's cells, where it can be used for energy. The carrier for glucose into the brain's cells is a hormone called *insulin* (Figure 27.12). Without insulin, the glucose remains in the blood and cannot be used by the cells.

Insulin is produced in a gland called the *pancreas*, which is located under the liver. For reasons yet unknown, the pancreas of some people slows or even stops working, resulting in a disease called **diabetes mellitus.** There are several variations to this disease.

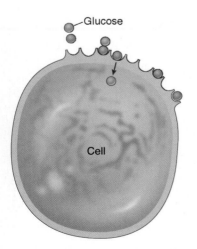

● = Glucose
● = Insulin
⋏⋏ = Insulin receptors

Insulin combines with insulin receptors on cell wall, allowing glucose to enter cell.

Figure 27.12 Insulin is the carrier of sugar from the blood into the cells

INSULIN-DEPENDENT DIABETES

In cases in which the pancreas no longer produces insulin, the patient must take insulin supplements. Insulin is given as an injection. Without these insulin supplements, the glucose the patient eats cannot get to the brain's cells. The result is an increase in the blood glucose levels and a brain that is starved for fuel. Frequently this type of diabetes occurs in children. For this reason, it was once called *juvenile diabetes*. The term *type I* is now more commonly used.

SUPPLEMENTAL INSULIN

Insulin was first obtained from the pancreas of pigs and cows (pork or beef insulin) and was used by physicians to treat diabetic patients. Human insulin used today is artificially created by genetic engineering. This human insulin has fewer side effects than did the pork and beef insulin.

Regular insulin is short-acting insulin. *Longer-acting* insulin, called NPH or Lente, sustains the patient's blood sugar at even levels throughout the day. Many patients with diabetes mix these two types of insulin, depending on the time of day (Figure 27.13).

Insulin is taken in correlation with regular meals. Because glucose levels in the bloodstream rise after a meal, more insulin has to be available at mealtimes to help use this fuel.

NON-INSULIN-DEPENDENT DIABETES

In some other cases, the pancreas does not produce enough insulin for the amount of glucose that is in the bloodstream. The pancreas can be stimulated to produce more insulin by medications called *oral hypoglycemic agents*. Patients with this condition do not require insulin and are referred to as having **non–insulin-dependent diabetes.** Without these oral medications, these patients may also have rising blood glucose levels. Because there is still some insulin production, however, in this case the brain is not completely starved for fuels. The small amount of insulin that is present carries some glucose into the brain's cells. Patients who require supplemental insulin may use intermittent subcutaneous injections throughout the day. Other patients may have a continuous infusion of insulin through an insulin pump.

Table 27-6 lists common diabetic medications, including oral hypoglycemic agents.

OTHER FORMS OF DIABETES

Some diabetic patients do not require any medications to keep their blood glucose under control as long as they carefully regulate their intake of sugars. By controlling their dietary intake of sugars, these patients with type II diabetes, or **diet-controlled diabetes,** can avoid the need to take medications.

When a woman becomes pregnant, her body's need for insulin increases. If her pancreas is unable to supply the insulin her body demands, high blood glucose levels result (Figure 27.14). When her pregnancy is over, her insulin demands drop back to former levels. This type of pregnancy-induced diabetes is called **gestational diabetes.**

SIGNS AND SYMPTOMS

When the pancreas stops creating sufficient insulin, the blood sugar starts to build up. A high blood sugar level, called **hyperglycemia,** has several effects on the patient.

First, the patient's kidneys try to rid the body of the excess sugar. When the kidney starts to excrete sugar, or *spill sugar*, the sweetened urine also removes water as well. The increased volume of urine created is called *polyuria*. This can quickly lead to dehydration.

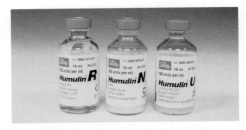

Figure 27.13 Insulin comes in short-acting and long-acting varieties

Table 27-6 Some Common Diabetic Medications	
Injected insulin	Humulin
	Novolin
	Iletin
	Lantus
Oral hypoglycemic agents	Diabinese
	Glucotrol
	Micronase
	DiaBeta
	Glynase
	Orinase

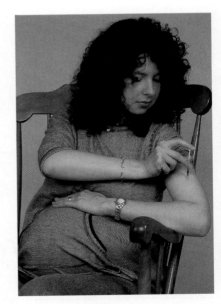

Figure 27.14 A pregnant woman can develop diabetes during her pregnancy

Table 27-7 Signs of Onset of Diabetes Mellitus

Excessive thirst

Frequent urination of large amounts

Excreting sugar into urine

Sudden unexplained weight loss

Constant hunger

With a loss of so much water through urine, the body starts to crave more water and the patient starts to drink water excessively, a condition called *polydipsia*.

In the interim, the cells of the body, including the brain cells, have gone without glucose. These cells continue to send messages for more glucose, and the patient starts to eat larger amounts of food. This condition is called *polyphagia*. Despite the fact that the patient is eating large amounts of food, the sugar is not getting into the cells, and the patient starts to lose weight. Table 27-7 summarizes the signs of the onset of diabetes.

ACUTE DIABETIC PROBLEMS

Even the most attentive diabetic patients will sometimes find themselves having a problem regulating their glucose levels. The EMT will often be called to help manage the diabetic patient when the glucose level has gone to either extreme.

HYPERGLYCEMIA

The development of hyperglycemia, seen in untreated or undertreated diabetes, is a prolonged event, taking from 12 hours to as much as several days to create any significant problem. When glucose cannot be used for fuel, because of an inability to get it into the cells, the body must find a fuel source elsewhere. This alternative fuel source comes in the form of fats. Fats can be broken down to form energy and waste products. This form of energy is much less efficient than the standard glucose breakdown and cannot support normal body functions for long.

When sugar is used, or metabolized, by a cell, the by-products are water and carbon dioxide. Water and carbon dioxide are eliminated by the kidneys or the lungs. When fats are metabolized, an organic acid called a **keto-acid** (or ketone) is created. These keto-acids are the by-products of ineffective metabolism. A diabetic patient who has changed to fat metabolism is at risk for developing a condition called **diabetic ketoacidosis (DKA).**

DKA is a condition characterized by hyperglycemia and a buildup of keto-acids in the blood. Keto-acids are toxic to the body. In addition, the high blood sugar has resulted in excessive urination (polyuria) and loss of significant water and electrolyte stores. DKA occurs only in patients who are dependent upon insulin supplements and only when they have not taken sufficient amounts of the hormone. This condition is potentially life threatening if not recognized and treated immediately.

SIGNS AND SYMPTOMS OF DIABETIC KETOACIDOSIS

Keto-acids, or ketones, are partially eliminated in the urine, like sugar. Ketones are also exhaled on our breath, like carbon dioxide. Ketone-laden breath is sweet-smelling like Juicy Fruit gum. However, this is an ineffective process and not all the ketones are eliminated.

As the ketones build up, and the acid level in the blood increases, the patient starts to breathe faster and deeper, in an effort to *blow off* the excess acid. This deep, almost sighing, breathing is called **Kussmaul's respiration** (Figure 27.15) and is characteristic of diabetic ketoacidosis.

Because of the dramatic fluid level changes that occur in the body, the patient may experience other symptoms. Many patients complain of stomachaches and cramps, followed by vomiting. Most will experience weakness and *malaise,* a sluggishness or lethargy that is associated with sickness.

Unchecked, the combination of dehydration, acidosis, and lack of glucose inside of the brain's cells leads to mental confusion and delirium. Without

Normal breathing

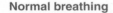

16–20 times/minute

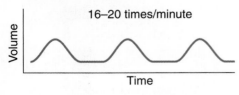

Time

Kussmaul's respiration

Deeper and faster than normal

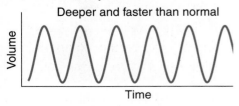

Time

Figure 27.15 Kussmaul's respiration is deep, sighing breaths

any medical intervention, diabetic ketoacidosis can lead to coma and even death. An unconscious diabetic patient who is hyperglycemic is said to be in a **diabetic coma.**

MANAGEMENT OF DKA

Aside from assessing and managing the airway, breathing, and circulation (ABC), there is very little an EMT can do for this high-priority patient in the field. Patients with DKA and any patient with an altered mental status should be given high-flow oxygen. Rapid transport to the emergency department is the best treatment. Whenever possible, an ALS intercept should be arranged while en route.

HYPEROSMOLAR HYPERGLYCEMIC NON-KETONIC COMA

A form of diabetes often seen in obese or elderly patients occurs as the pancreas fails to produce sufficient insulin for the body's needs. Although these patients may supplement their insulin needs with insulin injections, there are times when insulin demands are greater than insulin supply. At those times these patients' blood sugar starts to rise to dangerously high levels. However, unlike patients who are not producing any insulin, these patients do not metabolize fats and therefore do not produce keto-acids, causing a syndrome called **hyperosmolar hyperglycemic non-ketonic coma (HHNK).**

The symptoms of the patient who is hyperglycemic and in diabetic ketoacidosis and the patient who is hyperglycemic and in HHNK are the same, with the notable exception of Kussmaul's respiration and ketones on the breath, that sweet, Juicy Fruit gum smell.

In both cases the patient may experience an altered mental state and may lapse into coma. When faced with these diabetic emergencies the EMT should protect the patient's airway, provide oxygen, and transport the patient immediately.

HYPOGLYCEMIA

DKA or HHNK as a result of high blood sugar is dangerous, but its onset is gradual, generally allowing the patient time to seek medical attention. The opposite condition of a low blood sugar, called *hypoglycemia,* occurs suddenly, usually within an hour, and can quickly lead to brain damage and even death. Hypoglycemia is a true medical emergency.

Insulin allows blood glucose to go into cells, where it is used for fuel. When glucose moves out of the blood and into the cells, the blood glucose level falls. Diabetic patients time their insulin injections around meals. The insulin should "peak" just after the meal.

If the insulin peaks at the wrong time, then the insulin will lower the blood glucose to dangerously low levels. There are numerous reasons why the amount of insulin injected would not match the blood glucose.

If the patient eats a meal later than expected, then the insulin would peak prematurely. If the patient fails to eat a meal, the insulin still works and the blood sugar will drop to dangerously low levels.

SIGNS AND SYMPTOMS OF HYPOGLYCEMIA

When the blood glucose level falls, the body reacts. Adrenaline is excreted into the blood. Adrenaline helps to stimulate the release of stored sugar. Adrenaline also stimulates the heart to beat faster. Adrenaline can make the patient shaky, sweaty, and agitated. Because these body reactions are similar to the reactions that are seen in shock, severe hypoglycemia is sometimes called **insulin shock.**

Street Smart

Despite all the explanations offered about diabetic emergencies, it is sometimes difficult for an EMT to distinguish hypoglycemia from hyperglycemia in the field. It is usually safe to assume that the blood sugar is low if the patient is a confused diabetic. If the patient is unconscious, treat and transport the patient immediately.

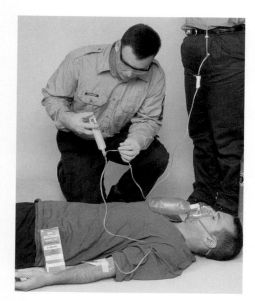

Figure 27.16 Advance life support personnel can rapidly reverse hypoglycemia with sugar (dextrose) via an IV

The lack of glucose to the brain results in its malfunction. Confusion, agitation, and combativeness are commonly seen in hypoglycemia. Without more blood glucose, the patient will progress from confusion to unconsciousness. Often when the blood glucose gets dangerously low, the patient will have a seizure. Without any treatment, the brain starts to suffer damage and the patient may die.

MANAGEMENT OF THE UNCONSCIOUS HYPOGLYCEMIC PATIENT

When a patient with diabetes collapses into unconsciousness, family or bystanders may call EMS. The first-arriving EMT is usually told that the patient is a diabetic. An EMT should also look for a MedicAlert® necklace, bracelet, or wallet card or a patient directive or other similar medical alert identification as part of his assessment. Medical identification or MedicAlert patient directives provide critical information on patient history, especially when the patient is unconscious. Thus, the MedicAlert patient directives speak for the patient when the patient is unable to speak for herself.

If an unconscious patient is thought to be diabetic, the EMT should assume that the patient could be hypoglycemic. The primary assessment should be performed, with time taken to open, assess, suction, and secure the airway. High-concentration oxygen should be given via either a bag-valve-mask or a partial non-rebreather mask, as appropriate.

The EMT should not delay the transportation of the patient and should proceed to package the patient immediately. Minutes count, and the patient should be taken to the closest ALS provider, whether that is the emergency department or interception with an ALS unit. Glucose administered through an intravenous (IV) rapidly reverses the hypoglycemia and can be lifesaving (Figure 27.16).

MANAGEMENT OF THE CONSCIOUS HYPOGLYCEMIC PATIENT

If the patient is conscious, proceed with the initial assessment. If the patient is combative or confused or is altered in mental status and a known diabetic, suspect hypoglycemia. Be sure that the patient can maintain her own airway. That will be critical shortly. Administer high-concentration oxygen via face mask. The patient's body is under stress and will need the supplemental oxygen.

The SAMPLE history (see Unit 18, Table 18-5) will provide the details that confirm that the patient is experiencing a hypoglycemic episode. If the confusion occurred suddenly, consider hypoglycemia. If the change in mental status occurred after missing a meal or after strenuous exercise, consider hypoglycemia.

Check for medications that the patient might be taking. Insulin is usually stored in the refrigerator. The insulin vial is very small, about the same size as a bottle of nitroglycerin. Syringes may be evident as well as sharps containers for used syringes.

The type of diabetes the patient has will help the EMT to look for either insulin or an oral hypoglycemic agent. Many other medications interact with or interfere with the action of these medications. If the patient just started a new medication or recently changed medications or dosages, the change could have affected the patient's blood sugar level. Find and record all medications that the patient is taking.

Safety Tips

Caution is advised when looking for insulin. Insulin is an injected medication, implying that a needle is used. These insulin syringes are small, about the same size as a tuberculin syringe used for tuberculosis (TB) testing.

Sharps containers, the storage space for used needles and syringes, may be too expensive for a patient who is on a fixed income. Some diabetics resort to using empty coffee cans or empty plastic milk jugs in an effort to save money. Although these containers are safe alternatives, they are usually not well marked. Be alert and always keep safety in mind.

The physical examination of the hypoglycemic patient should reveal signs similar to those of a patient in shock. The patient's skin will be cool and moist. The heart rate will be increased, or tachycardiac. However, unlike the lowered blood pressure in hemorrhagic shock, the blood pressure of the hypoglycemic patient will initially be somewhat elevated. (No fluid has been lost to cause the blood pressure to drop.)

Glucose Administration   If the patient is maintaining her own airway, the patient should be placed on high-concentration oxygen. The EMT should then administer oral glucose. Further details regarding this medication and its administration should now be reviewed in Unit 13.

Oral glucose should never be administered to a patient who is unconscious and cannot control her airway. Aspiration of glucose is potentially dangerous. Because the danger of aspiration is always present, if the patient should suddenly become unconscious, the EMT should always have a suction device ready at the patient's side to suction out any remaining material. Table 27-8 summarizes the differences between hypoglycemia and hyperglycemia.

FINGERSTICK GLUCOSE TESTING

Diabetic patients often test their blood glucose at home using special machines. Some EMTs have also started testing the blood glucose of patients with altered mental status while in the field. This quick and simple procedure, outlined here, provides the EMT with a quantitative measure of the patient's blood glucose. However, the EMT should never delay administering oral glucose to a conscious patient who has an altered mental status and a history of diabetes.

There are many commercially available home blood glucose testing machines, called glucometers. All have one common feature: They require a blood sample for analysis. How that sample is obtained and tested varies. Each manufacturer has guidelines for the proper operation of its model of glucometer.

Although glucometers are dependable and rarely need adjustment, it is common practice to test their accuracy regularly, at least once weekly, with a premixed sugar solution of specific strength called a *reagent*.

After the EMT's introduction and assessment, a determination is made to test the patient's blood glucose. Common indications for testing blood glucose include patients with an altered mental status, such as confusion or combativeness, after ingestion of unknown poisons (toxins), after a convulsion, or any diabetic patient with a medical emergency.

Next the EMT should explain to the patient the reason why a blood sample is being taken. This can be done while assembling the necessary equipment such as a lancet (a skin puncture device), alcohol-soaked pads, personal protective equipment (PPE) such as gloves, a sterile gauze pad, and a self-adhesive bandage.

After donning gloves, the EMT should select a site, often a fingertip of the nondominant hand, avoiding areas with burns, rashes, or scars. Next the EMT should prepare the site by cleansing it with the alcohol-soaked pad, allowing time for the alcohol to dry. It is important to allow the alcohol to dry on the skin so that it will not mix with the blood and alter the blood sample. Massaging or warming the selected site will increase blood flow and increase the chances of first-time success.

Table 27-8 Hyperglycemia (Diabetic Coma) versus Hypoglycemia (Insulin Shock)

	Hyperglycemia	Hypoglycemia
Onset	Gradual (12–48 hours)	Sudden (<1 hour)
Level of consciousness	Confused, combative	Confused, combative
Heart rate	Tachycardia	Tachycardia
Skin	Warm and dry	Cool and moist
Pupils	Normal	Dilated
Blood pressure	Normal	Slightly elevated
Respiration	Deep (Kussmaul's)	Rapid and shallow

Medication Card

Generic name: Oral glucose
Trade name: Insta-Glucose, and others
Indications: Suspected low blood glucose
Contraindications: Patients who cannot control their own airway and cannot swallow their own secretions should *not* be given oral medications.
Dose: One tube, or one container
Route: Oral only

The EMT should then grasp the patient's finger with his nondominant hand, place his thumb at the base of the patient's nail bed, and wrap his fingers around the side of the finger. This permits the best leverage for obtaining a blood sample. The EMT should then remove the cover from the lancet, or follow the manufacturer's instructions, and firmly, and with authority, press the lancet against the skin. Any hesitancy may cause the patient unnecessary discomfort. The object of this procedure is to produce a swift, deep puncture.

From the wound, the EMT should squeeze a single large, round droplet of blood and wipe it off on the gauze pad. The EMT should then squeeze a second droplet of blood by milking the patient's finger. The squeezing action (milking) should be gentle; vigorous milking dilutes the sample.

This sample is then placed on the glucometer test strip; some glucometers draw the sample into a sensor using capillary action. The glucometer should then proceed with a countdown to the reading, usually about 10–15 seconds.

While awaiting the results of the blood glucose test, the EMT should apply a sterile gauze pad to the fingertip and ask the patient to apply direct pressure to the site. Once the glucometer provides a reading, it should be recorded and appropriate action should be taken according to the reading.

It is the EMT's responsibility to properly discard the lancet into an approved sharps container and to discard all bloody dressings into an appropriate container. Any blood spilled should be quickly wiped up with an absorbent dressing and the area wiped down with a hypochlorite solution such as 1:10 bleach in water.

After approximately 5 minutes, the EMT should confirm that the bleeding has stopped. If the bleeding continues, then more direct pressure is required. If the bleeding has stopped, a self-adhesive bandage may be applied.

If the patient is a known diabetic and is combative, stand back. The EMT is under no obligation to tackle a combative patient. On the other hand, the EMT cannot sit back and wait for the patient to become unconscious.

Quickly obtain assistance, usually from a law enforcement officer, to restrain the patient. A specific plan should be ready for these types of emergencies. Review Unit 28 for more details on how to handle a combative patient.

When it is safe, quickly proceed with administering the oral glucose. Any delay and the patient may lapse into unconsciousness and lose her ability to protect her airway.

If the opportunity does not present itself, then the EMT should immediately transport the patient to either the emergency department or an ALS unit, whichever is closest.

Time is of the essence. Quick thinking and action on the part of the EMT can prevent a bad situation from getting worse.

SEIZURE DISORDERS

The brain is a group of specialized cells that interact to convey messages to and from every part of the body. The brain controls all activities within the body through these complex interactions. If part of the brain becomes irritated, it can create confusing messages. This event can result in confusion, unconsciousness, or repeated involuntary muscle contractions known as a **seizure.** The events in the brain that result in a seizure can be thought of as a sort of short circuit of the brain's electrical system.

Seizures can indicate a potentially life-threatening problem, which may require prompt medical attention. The EMT should take the necessary steps to stabilize the patient in the field, then transport as soon as possible.

A seizure is not usually life threatening. A patient with a history of seizures may even refuse to be transported to the hospital. When the patient experiences a cluster of seizures, the situation can quickly become life-threatening and warrants immediate definitive advanced management.

The EMT's responsibility is clear in both cases. The EMT should try to protect the patient from further harm and encourage the post-seizure patient to accept transportation for further medical evaluation.

The EMT should remember there are a variety of reasons why a patient might have a seizure, and most cannot be treated in the field. The most appropriate prehospital care for a patient who has had a seizure is transportation to the hospital for further medical evaluation.

CAUSES OF SEIZURES

The most common reason that a person would have a seizure is epilepsy. **Epilepsy** is a condition characterized by recurrent seizures of a similar nature. Although seizures can sometimes be traced to a specific area of the brain, the cause of epilepsy is often unclear.

Isolated seizures, or seizures that have defined causes, are not due to epilepsy. Certain toxins, or poisons, can build up in the blood and cause the patient to have a seizure. Hypoxia and hypoglycemia can cause a patient to have a seizure. Patients with a head injury or experiencing a stroke may experience seizures. Table 27-9 lists some of the more common causes of seizures.

Table 27-9 Causes of Seizures

Alcohol withdrawal

Brain tumor

Eclampsia (toxemia of pregnancy)

Fever (common in children)

Hypoglycemia

Hypoxia

Infectious disease (e.g., food poisoning)

Metabolic disorders (e.g., endocrine disease)

Poisons (e.g., camphor, cyanide, strychnine)

Stroke

Traumatic brain injury

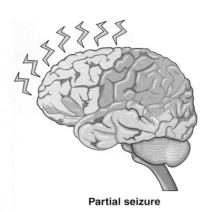

Partial seizure

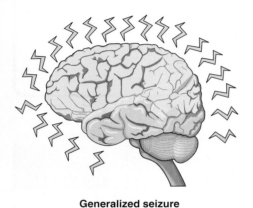

Generalized seizure

Figure 27.17 Chaotic firing all over the brain results in a generalized seizure

TYPES OF SEIZURES

Seizures affect the brain's ability to function. Think of the brain as a large circuit board, with electrical pathways that operate a machine called the body. If a bucket of water is poured over a circuit board, as the water advances, the circuit board starts to short-circuit, and eventually the entire circuit stops working.

When the brain's "electrical circuits" malfunction, owing to a short circuit in the brain, the patient experiences a seizure. If the malfunction is isolated to a small portion of the brain, a **partial seizure** results. This type of seizure may affect the speech or the motor function of a portion of the body.

If the seizure affects the entire brain, the patient will experience a dramatic set of events involving the whole body. These total body seizures are called **generalized seizures** (Figure 27.17).

GENERALIZED SEIZURE

Generalized tonic-clonic seizures are the most common type of epileptic seizure. They were once referred to as **grand mal seizures,** and many laypeople still use that term to describe a generalized seizure.

The source of a seizure is called the *origin.* If the origin is in the visual center, the patient may see a flash of color. If the origin is in the olfactory area, the patient may sense a strange smell. These sensations serve as a warning sign at the onset of a seizure. This phenomenon is referred to as an **aura.** Auras are usually very brief. The patient typically does not have time to react, to sit down, for example, before the next phase.

After the aura passes, the patient loses consciousness. As the irregular electrical activity moves throughout the entire brain, the patient collapses to the ground.

TONIC-CLONIC PHASE

In the beginning of the **tonic phase,** the patient's entire body first stiffens with muscle contractions, followed by the hypertonic phase exhibited by extreme muscular rigidity and arching of the back. The forceful contraction of all the muscles of the body, in the tonic phase, lasts for about 30 seconds.

The sudden contraction of the diaphragm may cause air to be forcefully exhaled against a partially closed voice box. A high-pitched sound can be produced that sounds like a scream and has been referred to as the "epileptic cry." Any sputum in the airway may be forcefully expelled as well. This expulsion results in "foamy" sputum erupting from the mouth.

During the tonic phase, the diaphragm and the chest wall muscles remain contracted and the patient stops breathing. If the tonic phase is prolonged, the patient may become hypoxic and cyanotic.

As the muscles become exhausted, the body relaxes momentarily, only to contract again. This intermittent contraction and relaxation of the muscles is called the **clonic phase.** During this phase, the patient may unintentionally empty her bladder. Additionally, the patient's tongue, lips, or mouth may show signs of being bitten or rubbed raw against the teeth during clonic movements.

The intermittent contraction and relaxation of muscles results in the patient's body thrashing around, striking any nearby objects, and can result in serious injury.

The clonic phase normally lasts approximately 1–3 minutes. Seizure lasting longer than 1–3 minutes without entering the postictal phase may indicate the patient is in status epilepticus, discussed later in this unit.

POSTICTAL PHASE

Most seizures last for only about 3–5 minutes. During that time, the muscles have been working extremely hard; as a result, the patient feels completely exhausted once the seizure ends (Figure 27.18). This phase is called the **pos-tictal phase.** (Postictal translates as "after the blow.") This phase will usually gradually resolve, and the patient will become more awake and oriented but will likely be tired from the event.

PARTIAL SEIZURE

Partial seizures are divided into simple partial and complex partial seizures. A simple partial seizure is also known as a focal motor seizure and sometimes referred to as a *Jacksonian motor seizure*. A **simple partial seizure** produces jerky movements, usually in only one area of the body, such as an arm or leg or the face, which the patient cannot control. The term *simple* is used to describe the "awake" state of the patient. In other words, the patient does not lose consciousness or awareness during the seizure.

The uncontrolled muscle activity may move from one area of the body to another (*Jacksonian March*) and may progress into a generalized tonic-clonic seizure. The EMT should document and report, if possible, in which part of the body the seizure activity originated.

Complex partial seizures, also known as *psychomotor* or *temporal lobe seizures*, usually begins with a vacant or blank stare, followed by a repetitive, random activity such as lip smacking or chewing. The patient does not respond to commands, appearing dazed or unaware of anything around her. The patient may show erratic behavior, abrupt personality changes, and exhibit some violent behaviors.

Complex partial seizures usually last only a few minutes; however, the patient's confusion may last longer. The patient will not remember what has happened or how she behaved.

OTHER TYPES OF SEIZURES

Absence seizures, or **petit mal seizures** as they are more commonly known, are seen mostly in children if recognized as a seizure at all. Absence seizures are characterized by a blank or "absent" stare, usually lasting only seconds, and may begin and end abruptly. The individual may also show signs similar to simple partial seizures, such as rapid blinking or chewing; however, unlike a simple partial seizure, she is unaware of what is happening.

No emergency care is needed for an absence seizure and in fact often times no one is aware one has taken place. If signs of an absence seizure are witnessed, especially if it is believed to be a first-time seizure, the patient should be encouraged to have a complete medical evaluation.

Febrile seizure is caused by a rapid rise in temperature, most commonly seen in children between 6 months and 6 years of age. Febrile seizures are usually generalized seizures, short in duration. Febrile seizures will be discussed in more detail in Unit 42.

MANAGEMENT OF THE PATIENT WITH A SEIZURE

Field treatment of a patient with a seizure disorder is dependent on which phase of the seizure the patient is experiencing. Typically, an EMT arrives to find the patient postictal, after the tonic-clonic phase, and can assist the patient with recovery.

Repeated seizures do occur. The EMT must always be prepared to protect the patient in case of another seizure.

THE ACTIVELY SEIZING PATIENT

Witnessing a generalized tonic-clonic seizure can be frightening. The EMT should calmly proceed with protecting the patient during the seizure. Do not attempt to restrain the patient. Instead, remove any objects the patient

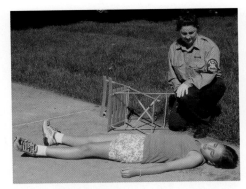

Figure 27.18 The period of time immediately after the tonic-clonic phase is called the postictal phase

Cultural Considerations

Many patients with epilepsy are referred to as "epileptics." The use of a diagnosis to describe a person is demeaning and reduces that person to being thought of only as a "disease." These people are patients with epilepsy and should be referred to, correctly, by their name and not by a label.

Street Smart

Another myth that accounted for epilepsy was the disease theory. It was theorized that the patient with epilepsy was diseased with *rabies*. Epilepsy is not caused by rabies However, a patient with a serious infection of the brain, called *meningitis*, can experience a seizure. The EMT should observe standard precautions when caring for a patient during a seizure. If the patient is feverish, the EMT should wear a mask as well as gloves.

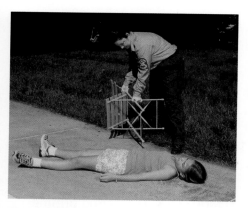

Figure 27.19 Protect the seizing patient from injury

may inadvertently strike during the clonic phase (Figure 27.19). If possible, remove or loosen any tight clothing that may create a strangulation hazard.

When possible, turn the patient's head to the side to allow drainage of saliva, but do not restrain the patient's head. Restraining the patient's head may create whiplash-like muscle injury. Always have suction ready to manage secretions, blood, or vomitus.

Do *not* force anything into the mouth of the seizing patient. If the patient *had* an oral airway in place, leave it. Never force an oral airway, a bite block, or other device between the teeth of a seizing patient. To do so may result in broken teeth, which may then obstruct the airway.

High-flow oxygen should be administered via a non-rebreather mask. If the patient is not breathing adequately, the EMT may need to assist ventilations with a bag-valve-mask device. Constant attention should be paid to the airway and breathing status of the seizure patient until she is able to manage on her own.

Carefully observe the patient during the seizure. Note the time of onset and the duration of the seizure. Note which body parts were involved as well as the presence of any cyanosis. Be prepared to support the patient immediately after all muscle activity stops.

STATUS EPILEPTICUS

If the patient continues to convulse, without interruption, for more than 5 minutes or if the patient has a series of seizures without regaining consciousness, the patient is in a condition called **status epilepticus.**

Status epilepticus is a medical emergency. This condition requires airway management, with positive pressure ventilations and supplemental oxygen. Rapid intervention by advanced-level providers, such as paramedics, is needed to prevent brain damage or even death. Status epilepticus is therefore a high-priority situation.

Street Smart

There are many advantages to using a nasopharyngeal airway for a postictal patient. If the patient should seize again, an airway is in place and the patient can be ventilated if needed. Second, as the patient becomes more conscious, she will not be stimulated to vomit. Finally, as the patient becomes more responsive, she will attempt to remove the nasopharyngeal airway from her nose. This attempt signals the EMT that the patient is improving.

Cultural Considerations

Be sensitive to the patient's right to privacy. Some patients, after having had a seizure, are embarrassed because the seizure occurred in public. In simple-to-understand terms, tell the patient who you are and that she may have just seized. Then tell the patient what you are going to do.

The EMT should cover the patient, if possible. Consider moving the patient to a more private location or the back of the ambulance before proceeding with detailed assessments.

Safety Tips

The EMT should take standard precautions to prevent possible contamination by body fluids. Minimally, gloves should be worn.

THE POSTICTAL PATIENT

When the patient is postictal, the EMT should be sure that the patient has an adequate airway. If the patient has bitten her tongue while seizing, there may be blood in the airway. The blood should be suctioned out using a Yankauer suction tip.

If the airway is clear, consider rolling the patient onto her left side, in the recovery position. This position allows the patient's secretions to naturally drain from the mouth and nose.

If the patient is responsive only to painful stimuli, consider an oral airway. Many EMTs avoid the use of an oropharyngeal airway, concerned that it will stimulate vomiting. In those cases, a nasopharyngeal airway may be used.

The patient should be given high-concentration oxygen. Although the patient's color may have returned, the body just endured an exhausting physical exercise. Oxygen helps the patient to recover.

If the patient's breathing is shallow or inadequate, it is appropriate to assist the patient's breathing with a BVM device. Remember, although epilepsy is the most common cause of seizures, there are other causes. These other causes can produce respiratory depression or arrest.

Usually, there is no serious bleeding unless injury occurred during the seizure. Proceed with obtaining a set of vital signs. Remember that the vital signs obtained are going to be more consistent with those of an athlete who just ran a 100-yard dash than with those of a sleeping patient.

Once the ABCs have been addressed, the EMT should perform a rapid head-to-toe assessment using DCAP-BTLS (Unit 19, Table 19-3) to assess for the possibility of any injuries that may have occurred during the seizure. Note whether the patient has been incontinent of urine (involuntary bladder emptying).

ANTICONVULSANTS

After being diagnosed with recurrent seizures, the patient may be placed on medication. The frequency and severity of seizures can be controlled by medications called **anticonvulsants**. These medications, if taken as directed, are sometimes effective in preventing further seizures. More than half of patients on anticonvulsants remain seizure free. Table 27-10 lists some common anticonvulsants.

Table 27-10 Commonly Prescribed Anticonvulsants	
Generic Name	**Trade Name**
carbamazepine	Tegretol
clonazepam	Klonopin
ethosuximide	Zarontin
phenobarbital	Luminal
phenytoin	Dilantin
valproic acid	Depakote

HEADACHE

A headache is one of the most common concerns people have throughout their lives. Because headaches are so common, people do not typically seek medical attention unless they have chronic headaches and need additional help for pain control. Most people do not associate a headache with a serious medical condition and therefore may ignore the signals being sent of a more serious condition.

The signs and symptoms of a headache can be very subjective, especially when assessing the quality and intensity of the pain, and can develop over a period of time ranging from minutes to hours. Because of the subjectivity, the intensity of the headache may not be a good indicator of the seriousness of the condition or underlying cause. Every patient who calls EMS for a headache should be assessed for changes in mental status and neurological deficits and should be watched closely to see if the headache progresses, indicating a more serious condition.

Headaches can result from a number of mechanisms that include contraction of the muscles of the neck and scalp, dilation of the cranial vessels, inflammation of the vessels of the head and neck, irritation or inflammation of the meninges, and increased intracranial pressure (ICP).

TYPES OF HEADACHES

According to the International Headache Society (IHS), headaches can be classified as primary or secondary. Primary headaches are the most common type seen in patients who seek medical care from their physicians or EMS. A secondary headache is caused by an underlying disease or condition and is actually one of the symptoms of the condition. It is important for the EMT to know that secondary headaches are usually an indicator of a more serious underlying condition.

Headaches can be further categorized based on their etiology or cause. This can include an individual etiology or a combination of etiologies

Table 27-11 Headaches Associated with Serious Etiology

Neurologic dysfunction	New and abrupt onset of head-ache not previously experienced
Altered mental status	Worsening when coughing, sneezing, or bending over
Behavior change	Fever or stiff neck
Seizure	Change in quality of a chronic headache
Stroke (ischemic or hemorrhagic)	Marked elevation of blood pressure

resulting in three main types of headaches: tension-type headaches, vascular headaches/migraines, and cluster headaches.

New-onset headaches, which occur abruptly and can be associated with behavioral or neurological changes, seizure, or altered mental status, require a thorough assessment and complete history.

Table 27-11 lists headaches potentially caused by serious etiology.

HEADACHE MANAGEMENT

Management priorities begin with ruling out or reversing any immediately life-threatening conditions. Management of headaches in the prehospital set-ting will be minimal, focusing primarily on assessment of the potential cause for the headache and the relief of the pain.

Place the patient in a position of comfort and administer high-flow oxy-gen after determining adequate respiratory status. ALS intercept should be considered for any patient showing signs of neurologic dysfunction, altered mental status, behavioral changes, or marked elevation of blood pressure.

CONCLUSION

There are many causes for alterations in mental status. Stroke affects more than 700,000 people in the United States each year. The EMT must be very familiar with stroke, which is a true medical emergency. Protection of the patient from further injury during expedient transport to an appropriate facility will be the cornerstone of the prehospital management of this condition.

Because diabetic emergencies and seizures are commonly seen by the EMT, having a basic understanding of these conditions will help to man-age the situation more effectively. No matter the cause of an altered mental status, the EMT's initial priorities are to assess and manage the ABCs.

In general, quick, effective, and professional behavior on the part of the EMT can prevent a change in the patient's mental status from becoming deadly. Accurate assessment of the situation, coupled with good decision making about treatment and transportation priorities, results in better patient outcomes.

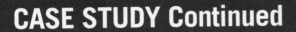

CASE STUDY Continued

John approaches the patient and introduces himself. The patient verbally responds, evidence that his airway is open. His breathing appears adequate. John quickly listens to the patient's chest. Breath sounds are clear, equal, and present bilaterally. Margeux places the patient on oxygen via non-rebreather at 15 lpm. John notes a rapid radial pulse and pale, cool, and damp skin. John notes there are no signs of trauma.

Because the man is unable to provide them with any information, Margeux asks the bystanders if anyone knows the man or saw anything before the police and EMS arrived. A woman informs them that she saw him walking down the street, stumbling, and then sitting down in that spot about 5 minutes before the police arrived. She states that she thought he was drunk. He did not fall down or strike his head, nor did she notice any seizure activity.

While Margeux is interviewing people, John begins his physical exam of the man. He finds a Medical Alert necklace, which notes that the man has an allergy to penicillin and a history of diabetes. Upon physical exam, John finds no signs of trauma. His pupils are equal and reactive, but dilated. His lungs are clear. His abdomen is soft, non-tender, and not distended. Circulation, sensation, and motor function are present in all four extremities. His vital signs show a pulse of 130 and regular, blood pressure 94/66, and respirations 14 and regular. Pulse oximetry on room air is 97%, and 99% with the oxygen.

After loading the patient into the ambulance, the EMTs call for an ALS intercept en route to hospital. Given his history of diabetes and the patient's ability to swallow, John administers a tube of oral glucose to the patient. By the time they meet with the ALS intercept, the patient is alert and oriented to person, place, time, and date but is unable to state the events over the past hour.

John turns patient care over to the ALS crew and begins his documentation after giving the paramedic his verbal report.

Key Concepts Revisited

- Individuals who are confused or disoriented about person, place, or time are considered to have an altered mental state.

- Altered mental status may be due to chronic health conditions or acute changes within the body resulting from disease or trauma.

  - The AEIOU TIPS mnemonic helps the EMT to remember some of the common causes of altered mental status:

    - Alcohol

    - Epilepsy

    - Insulin

    - Oxygen deprivation or drug overdose

    - Uremia

    - Trauma

    - Infection

    - Psychiatric disorder/poisoning

    - Stroke

- A cerebrovascular accident (CVA) or stroke is a disruption of blood flow to part of the brain causing an injury to the brain.

- The causes of stroke can be easily divided into two main categories: ischemic and hemorrhagic.

  - Ischemic stroke results from a blockage of the vessel that normally supplies that tissue with blood.

    - Transient ischemic attack (TIA) is the temporary decrease of blood flow to an area of the brain that resolves completely within 24 hours.

  - Hemorrhagic stroke is a rupture of one of the cerebral vessels.

- The treatment of a stroke in the prehospital management of stroke is the recognition of the symptoms and expedient transport to a hospital capable of managing the condition.

- Altered mental status related to diabetes mellitus is due to inadequate insulin causing glucose to remain in the blood, not reaching the cells of the brain.
  - Insulin-dependant diabetes requires insulin supplements as the pancreas has quit making insulin, resulting in glucose not getting to the body's cells.
  - Non–insulin-dependant diabetes occurs when the pancreas is making a small amount of insulin, resulting in abnormal blood glucose levels.
    - Hyperglycemia results when the lack of insulin prevents glucose from entering the cells, remaining in the blood.
      - Diabetic ketoacidosis (DKA) occurs when insulin-dependant diabetics do not take enough insulin and the body begins to metabolize fat, resulting in a buildup of ketones.
    - Hyperosmolar hyperglycemic non-ketonic diabetes does not produce ketones.
      - It is seen in obese elderly patients whose blood sugar rises to dangerous levels.
    - Hypoglycemia, low blood sugar, occurs very suddenly and can be life threatening if not immediately treated.
- Seizures are a short circuit of the brain's electrical system resulting in an altered mental status.
  - Epilepsy is a condition of seizures that occur recurrently.
  - Generalized seizures involving the phases of tonic (muscle contracture), clonic (muscle relaxation followed by contraction), and postictal (unresponsiveness) phase.
  - Partial seizures can be simple or complex.
    - Simple partial seizures are characterized by jerky movements on one side of the body the patient cannot control, with the patient remaining awake.
    - Complex partial seizures are characterized by a vacant or blank stare followed by a repetitive movement such as lip smacking, with the patient unaware and not able to follow commands.
  - Febrile and absence seizures are seen mostly in children.
  - Status epilepticus is a life-threatening condition that occurs when seizures are sustained for more than 5 minutes with the patient not regaining consciousness between seizures.
- Headaches are classified as primary and secondary, which can be the symptom of a more serious disease or condition.
  - Primary headaches are the most common type of headache seen by health care professionals, including migraines and cluster headaches.
  - Secondary headaches are a symptom of a more serious condition such as a stroke or hemorrhage in the brain.
- Any concern of headache that also shows signs of neurologic dysfunction, altered mental status, behavioral changes, or marked elevation of blood pressure requires further evaluation, and an ALS intercept should be considered.

Review Questions

1. How is an altered mental state determined?
2. What are some general causes of an altered mental state?
3. What is an ischemic stroke?
4. What is a hemorrhagic stroke?
5. What are the appropriate assessment techniques for a patient with signs and symptoms of stroke?
6. What is the most important part of the OPQRST assessment of stroke?
7. What is insulin, and how does it affect metabolism?
8. What is the treatment for diabetes?
9. What occurs if diabetes is left untreated?
10. What is the difference between a generalized and a partial seizure?
11. How does an EMT care for an actively seizing patient?
12. What are some of the common causes of seizures?
13. What are the two types of headaches?
14. What is the primary focus when caring for a patient experiencing a headache?

Key Terms

AEIOU TIPS
Altered mental state
Alzheimer's disease
Anticonvulsant
Aura
Cerebrovascular accident (CVA)
  or stroke
Cincinnati Prehospital Stroke Scale
Clonic phase
Complex partial seizure
Diabetes mellitus
Diabetic coma
Diabetic ketoacidosis (DKA)
Diet-controlled diabetes
Epilepsy
Expressive aphasia
Facial droop
Generalized seizure
Gestational diabetes
Grand mal seizure

Hyperglycemia
Hyperosmolar hyperglycemic non-ketonic
  coma (HHNK)
Insulin shock
Ischemia
Ischemic stroke
Keto-acid (ketone)
Kussmaul's respiration
Non—insulin-dependent diabetes
Partial seizure
Penumbra
Petit mal seizure (absence seizure)
Postictal phase
Pronator drift
Receptive aphasia
Seizure
Simple partial seizure
Status epilepticus
Tonic phase
Transient ischemic attack (TIA)

Further Study

Nicholl, J. "Prehospital Management of the Seizure Patient." *Emergency Medical Services*, 28, no. 5 (1999): 71–79.

Dalton, A. L., D. Limmer, J. J. Mistovich, and H.A. Werman. *Advanced Medical Life Support*. 3rd ed. Upper Saddle River, NJ: Brady/Prentice Hall, 2006.

UNIT (28) Abnormal Behavior

Mental illness is any disorder that affects the mind and is exhibited in a person's behavior. Although mental illness—and **psychiatry,** which is the study of mental illness—is a complex topic, Emergency Medical Technicians (EMTs) need to develop a basic understanding of these disorders related to the patient care they provide.

National Education Standards

The Emergency Medical Technician (EMT) will be able to recognize behaviors that pose a risk to EMS personnel, patients, and others and demonstrate a fundamental depth and foundational breadth of understanding in the assessment and management of behavioral emergencies.

Key Concepts

- A behavioral emergency is any situation in which the patient exhibits a behavior that is unacceptable, dangerous, or intolerable to the person, the family, or the community.

- Behavioral emergencies can be attributed to organic disorders and/or mental disorders.

- Long-term mental illnesses may result in acute behavioral emergencies that pose risks to EMTs.

- The EMT should always be alert and prepared for violence on the scene of behavioral emergencies.

- Management of behavioral emergencies includes verbal persuasion and physical restraint.

- Physical restraint is performed when it becomes medically necessary to ensure the protection of the patient and EMS providers.

- Psychiatric patients may suffer from some impairment of the ability to conduct activities of daily living (ADL).

- Management of suicide focuses on protection from further injury to patients and EMS personnel and treatment of injuries.

- Substance abuse leads to abnormal and sometimes bizarre and violent behavior, especially when the patient has overdosed or is withdrawing from the substance.

- The EMT must focus on personal safety, patient care, and documentation of abnormal behavioral emergencies.

CASE STUDY

Kaleena lives next door to Katharine, an elderly woman who sometimes acts strangely. Kaleena tries to check on Katharine every day because she has no children or family in the area. She knows that Katharine sometimes does not get out of bed or eat properly, so Kaleena tries to take her some food on the days when she isn't working. She doesn't really know much about Katharine's health, except that she sometimes seems anxious and worried that she might be put in the hospital again.

Kaleena approaches Katharine's door and suddenly has a feeling something isn't right. The front door was open and she can hear Katharine speaking as if she is talking to someone in the apartment. Knocking and calling out before carefully entering the apartment, Kaleena can see Katharine standing before her hall mirror talking to her reflection. Katharine has a wild look in her eyes and begins screaming, "You leave me alone; I don't have to listen to you." Calling out, Kaleena asks, "Katharine, are you all right?"

When Katharine spins away from the mirror to look at Kaleena, she sees the rolling pin in Katharine's hand and begins slowly backing out of the apartment as Katharine screams at her, "No! I told you I won't go!"

As Kaleena closes the door of the apartment to keep Katharine from leaving before help arrives, she calls 9-1-1 and says, "My next door neighbor is talking out of her head and not acting right. She is an older lady and usually very nice. Can you send some help?"

Critical Thinking Questions

1. What signs and symptoms of a potential behavioral emergency are present in this case?

2. What are some of the potential causes of this abnormal behavior?

3. What are the EMT's first priorities?

INTRODUCTION

Typically, EMS is called whenever the patient's behavior is seen as dangerous to himself or others or when the patient's behavior is socially unacceptable. Therefore, EMTs are less interested in the specific diagnosis of mental illness than in understanding the types of behaviors that would generate a call for EMS.

This unit discusses mental illness within the context of the accompanying abnormal behavior, with a focus on how an EMT should respond to those behaviors.

BEHAVIORAL EMERGENCY

A **behavioral emergency** can be defined as any situation in which the patient exhibits a behavior that is unacceptable, dangerous, or intolerable to the person, the family, or the community. Attempted suicide is an extreme example of a behavioral emergency. A subtle example of a behavioral emergency is the clinical depression that may have led up to the suicide attempt.

Often, a behavioral emergency is brought to the attention of authorities, such as police, because of the violent nature of the behavior. This is not always the case. Concerned persons who call on the public, such as postal carriers or drivers for Meals on Wheels, may call EMS if they find a person acting in a manner that is not typical for the person and is potentially unsafe (Figure 28.1). Family members, close friends, and interested bystanders often call 9-1-1 when a person is "not acting right."

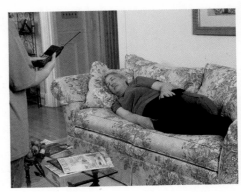

Figure 28.1 Concerned citizens and family members call EMS to report a behavioral emergency

Table 28-1 Some Organic Disorders That Cause Abnormal Behavior

Hypoxia

Hypoglycemia

Hypoperfusion

Head injury

Drug overdose

Excessive cold

Excessive heat

ORGANIC DISORDERS

Abnormal behaviors have been attributed to people who are "not thinking right." This is a simplistic definition, but it points to the core of the matter. Abnormal behavior is the result of a malfunction in the brain.

The brain can malfunction for a variety of reasons. For example, the brain fails without adequate oxygen and glucose. Any disease or physical condition that causes the brain to malfunction is an organic disorder. Table 28-1 is a list of **organic disorders.** It is important for an EMT to understand, evaluate, and treat any organic disorder.

Hypoxia-induced abnormal behavior is a common organic disorder an EMT can treat readily through oxygen administration. Hypoglycemia, as discussed in Unit 27, is another organic disorder an EMT can treat quickly, using oral glucose.

The key is that the EMT must have a suspicion that the patient's abnormal behavior may be due to a medical, or organic, cause, not to a psychiatric cause. If the EMT is wrong, then no harm has come to the patient. If she is right, the EMT may have prevented brain injury and possibly even death.

DANGEROUS ASSUMPTIONS

Some people, when witnessing abnormal behavior, dismiss the patient's illness as "just plain crazy." If an EMT dismisses a patient in this manner, she may be overlooking a life-threatening condition.

As a medical professional, the EMT must safeguard the patient's life. With this responsibility in mind, an EMT must evaluate and treat any serious medical conditions that could create abnormal behavior.

The mnemonic AEIOU TIPS, discussed in Unit 27, is helpful for understanding possible organic causes of altered mental states.

MENTAL DISORDERS

Any disorder that impairs the brain's function, or the way the brain thinks, without a firm physical (organic) cause is considered a mental illness. The outward evidence of mental illness is usually bizarre or irrational behavior.

Substance abuse, depression, and psychosis are examples of common mental illnesses; they are discussed in detail later in this unit. An EMT might encounter a patient suffering from any one of these disorders. The EMT's focus is not to diagnosis the illness, but rather to deal effectively with the potentially dangerous behavior the patient is exhibiting.

THE THREE Ds

Patients, especially those over the age of 65, are at risk for the "three Ds": depression, dementia, and delirium. The EMT should attempt to differentiate between dementia and delirium. Depression is discussed later in the unit.

Dementia is a gradual loss of cognitive (thinking) function. A common cause of dementia in the elderly is Alzheimer's disease. Alzheimer's disease is a progressive neurologic disease that is associated with a gradual loss of intellectual function.

Delirium, on the other hand, is a sudden erratic change in behavior and is seen in younger patients as well. A delirious patient may be frightened, disoriented, incoherent, and combative. Delirium may be the result of a stroke, infection, fever, or accidental overdose of medications (review AEIOU TIPS). A sudden change in mental state, such as confusion and bizarre behavior, requires immediate medical assessment in the emergency department.

SIGNS AND SYMPTOMS

Although each behavioral disorder is characterized by its own specific signs and symptoms, those that will most often result in an emergency call for the EMT are listed in Table 28-2.

SCENE SIZE-UP

The initial dispatch information should alert the EMT to the potential for violence on scene. Radio reports of "shots fired," "suicide attempted," and the like should warn the EMT of the potential for personal injury and an unsafe scene.

Occasionally, the street address is known to EMS. There may have been previous EMS calls at the same location for injuries secondary to fighting, for example. Many communications centers have a location's call history on the computer system.

Never enter an unsafe scene. If the scene involves weapons, the EMT should place, or stage, the ambulance far enough back to be out of sight and out of the line of fire. Turn off any warning lights that might alert those on scene of your presence. Stay in the vehicle until the scene is declared safe by police.

As the EMT approaches the scene, she should perform a visual sweep of the scene, looking for telltale signs of violence, such as broken glass, blood on the ground, empty alcohol containers, and spent gun shell casings.

Table 28-2 Signs and Symptoms of a Behavioral Emergency
Mental confusion
Extreme agitation
Inappropriate anger
Weeping and crying
Violence

Street Smart

EMS is sometimes called to what turns out to be a crime scene. Attention should be paid to the details on scene. Take extreme care to avoid destroying footprints, tire tracks, or broken glass.

Do not touch or move suspected weapons. Call police immediately for assistance, and consider retreating from the scene until they arrive. Always wear gloves whenever handling any object on scene.

SCENE SAFETY

An EMT should take several important safety measures whenever entering a scene. Never enter a potentially violent scene alone. Always have a police officer clear the scene first. Then proceed into the scene with a partner or a police officer. Using the "buddy system" improves the EMT's chances of remaining safe.

Whenever an EMT is approaching a potentially violent scene, she should be thinking and determining routes of escape. The EMT should look for nearby objects that could provide cover (protection from bullets) and concealment.

Carry all portable gear over one shoulder only or in one hand by the straps (Figure 28.2). Never sling portable gear over both shoulders. A violent patient could grab the portable gear bag and use it to drag the EMT off her feet.

If it is necessary to make a hasty retreat, slip the bag off the shoulder and onto the ground in the path of any pursuers.

Have a portable radio immediately available for emergency use. Observe radio silence when approaching the patient. Extraneous radio chatter may be both distracting and alarming to the patient.

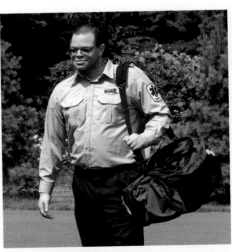

Figure 28.2 Equipment should be carried in a manner that will allow the EMT to make a quick getaway if a patient becomes violent

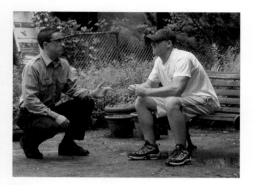

Figure 28.3 Never kneel or sit directly in front of a patient. Instead, crouch in front of the patient at least an arm's length away

At night, only the first EMT should have a flashlight. All personnel should walk in a single file to decrease their target profile. The first EMT should hold the flashlight out to the side of the body, which is another way to decrease the target profile.

If it is a street call and a crowd has assembled, study the crowd carefully. The mood of the crowd, heard in the tone and words of the bystanders, should key the EMT to the potential for further violence.

If it is a house call, stand to the side of the door and knock loudly. Do not depend on doorbells. Call out loudly. Use terms like "ambulance" or "rescue squad." Pick terms that any patient will understand. If possible, leave doors open to provide a ready escape route.

The EMT, or her partner, should always make sure that the path to the exit or doorway is open and clear of obstacles. If a hasty retreat is necessary, the EMT should carefully back out of the situation. The EMT should never turn her back on the potential assailant until clear of the doorway or a considerable distance away.

Finally, the EMT should stand a safe distance from the patient; over an arm's length away is usually sufficient. Never stand too close to the patient. The patient may feel threatened and respond violently.

An EMT should never sit or kneel in front of a seated patient, especially one who is acting abnormally. Instead, the EMT should crouch down while still on the balls of the feet. From this crouched position, the EMT will be able to quickly respond to threats by springing up and retreating to safety (Figure 28.3).

Objects around the patient that could be used as weapons should be removed if possible. Alternatively, the patient can be lured away from them. The EMT should always be alert and prepared for potential violence.

ASSESSMENT

The general approach to assessing a potentially violent patient is to "stop, look, and listen." Observe the patient carefully. Angry patients often stand bolt upright, legs spread slightly apart, ready for a fight. Other signs of potential violence include clenched fists, hands stiffly forced into pockets, or arms folded tightly across the chest.

Look into the patient's eyes. The saying goes that "the eyes are the windows to the soul." Many times the EMT can tell whether the patient is angry, frightened, or confused just by looking into his eyes.

The eyes also often signal when a patient is going to make a sudden move, for example, when reaching for a weapon. Maintain good eye contact. Good eye contact communicates the EMT's confidence to the patient.

The primary assessment can be done at a safe distance. The patient who is awake, on his feet, and exhibiting potentially violent behavior likely has a patent airway, adequate respirations, and no gross circulatory problem. The EMT should not attempt close physical assessment if she feels that might be dangerous.

HISTORY AND FOCUSED PHYSICAL EXAMINATION

As the EMT gathers the history, listen closely to the patient's voice. An angry patient will use angry words and profanity. The patient's speech may be pressured, trying to get a complete thought out in just one breath.

Signs of agitation include rapid pacing, rigid posture (Figure 28.4), and quick irregular movements. Rapid darting eye movements, like those of a trapped animal looking for an escape, may indicate the patient's panic.

If it is safe to do so, a history of the present illness and SAMPLE history can be obtained from family members if the patient is unable or unwilling to

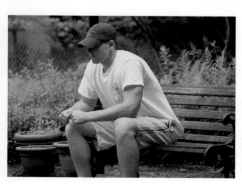

Figure 28.4 Body language often says what the patient is feeling

provide this information. The focused physical examination may be limited for safety reasons, but if able, the EMT should assess the patient from head to toe for signs of obvious injury. Vital signs should be measured when it is safe to do so, and should be repeated as often as necessary.

MANAGEMENT

Regardless of the situation, the EMT must maintain a calm and professional manner. As a matter of practice, only one EMT should talk to the patient, if possible. This approach allows the EMT–patient relationship to be developed. Hopefully, the patient will begin to trust the EMT and then agree to care and transport. The EMTs should identify themselves clearly and tell the patient what their intentions are. The EMT should speak calmly, in a reassuring manner, and maintaining good eye contact with the patient, which helps improve patient rapport, in most cases.

VERBAL PERSUASION

One of the EMT's goals is to defuse the angry situation and convince the patient to cooperate with care. The key to achieving that goal is effective communication. Effective communication with an angry, agitated, or confused patient first requires that the EMT speak slowly and clearly. The EMT should state her name and purpose plainly to the patient. If the patient does not understand what is being said, repeat the message until he does understand.

The EMT should ask the patient about his concerns. If the patient asks a question, answer honestly. Patients will sense when an EMT is lying.

If the patient wants to talk about hallucinations, reassure the patient that the hallucinations are temporary. Hallucinations can be frightening to the patient. Remind the patient that you are there to help and protect him.

Seek the patient's cooperation. Encourage the patient to "speak up." Talking about emotions and feelings starts the therapeutic process. For an EMT to be effective with this aspect of patient care, she need only be a good listener.

If the patient is refusing transportation and needs medical attention, be firm and explain to the patient, in simple terms, that his refusal is unacceptable and that he must go to the hospital.

If the patient remains uncooperative, the EMT should clearly explain the consequences of failing to go to the hospital. Some patients may feel threatened and lash out unexpectedly. The EMT should be prepared to withdraw in case of a physical attack.

Even when the patient is visibly shaken, the EMT must stay calm. The patient may direct hurtful comments toward the EMT. Remember that the patient is ill, and the comments are made under duress. An EMT always maintains a professional attitude, never taking comments personally and remembering that the patient is suffering from an illness that alters his thought processes.

PHYSICAL RESTRAINT

Sometimes in a behavioral emergency, it becomes clear that verbal persuasion is not going to be effective. The patient will display signs of **excited delirium.**

The patient in an excited delirium will demonstrate hyperactive irrational behavior. Often, excited delirium is the result of drug intoxication or mental illness, such as schizophrenia. The patient is frequently described as being *out of control.*

Unchecked, the patient will become increasingly agitated and may become violent. Therefore, the patient who is experiencing excited delirium is clearly in danger of harming others or himself.

Cultural Considerations

Some patients may consider direct eye contact as a challenge or an affront. Staring contests, as these behaviors are called, are counterproductive to the task at hand. The intent is to calm the patient and to get the patient to trust the EMT. If the patient appears to be offended by direct eye contact, then the EMT should avoid it.

When a patient is out of control and is a clear danger to himself or others, then a decision has to be made to restrain the patient for his own protection. The decision to restrain a patient should be made only after all other means of persuasion have been exhausted. Family members may be helpful in convincing the patient to cooperate.

MEDICAL NECESSITY

A patient may be restrained against his will for a legitimate medical necessity. The government provides physicians limited authority, usually under the mental health law, to restrain a person when the patient is a danger to himself or others.

When a restraint is performed for this reason, it is called a **medically necessary restraint.** A medically necessary restraint is ordered by a doctor and done only for the safety of the patient or others.

A medically necessary restraint is a treatment, but it is different from most treatments in that the patient is not permitted to refuse it. To refuse a treatment, the patient must be competent. It is assumed that any person who is thinking of harming himself or others is irrational and therefore incompetent. If the patient is incompetent, then the patient cannot refuse treatment.

Medically necessary restraint differs from police custody. Police officers are afforded wider authority to stop, detain, and, if necessary, restrain citizens—in other words, place them in custody—for the purposes of law enforcement. Medically necessary restraint is a treatment ordered for a patient who is incompetent to make his own decision.

In some jurisdictions, the law allows police to take protective custody of certain incompetent individuals. Review Unit 3 for the medical application of the terms *competency* and *consent.* The idea of protective custody follows logically. If the patient is incompetent, then he cannot refuse treatment. In this case, the patient is restrained by police until EMS arrives.

An EMT is permitted to use only reasonable force to restrain a patient. Reasonable force might be defined as the strength it would take to overpower the patient and no more. In other words, it is the minimum force needed to confine a patient without undue risk of injury to either the patient or the EMT.

The objective of the restraint is to protect the patient from himself, not to harm him. Use of more force than is necessary to restrain the patient might be considered *excessive force.*

If excessive force is used, or if the patient should not have been restrained in the first place, then the patient has been denied his civil rights. In those cases, the patient or patient's family may elect to start legal action against the EMT. Criminal charges for assault could also be filed against the EMT for use of excessive force.

The EMT's best protection when determining when to use restraint is to follow local protocols and carefully document the need for such restraint.

RESTRAINT PROCEDURE

At some point in the patient assessment, it may become apparent that the patient will not cooperate with the plan of care. The patient may be clearly demonstrating that he intends to harm himself or others. A physician (through protocols) or, more commonly, a law enforcement officer makes the decision to restrain the patient and have him brought to the emergency department. When these conditions have been met, then the patient must be restrained using a **takedown procedure.**

A takedown is the planned orderly restraint of a patient for a medical purpose. Before the takedown is actually performed, there must be a strategy on how to proceed. This preplanning helps ensure the safety of all providers involved and, more importantly, the safety of the patient.

To control the patient's extremities is to control the patient. Most takedown procedures involve obtaining and maintaining control of the extremities.

While the first EMT is attempting to verbally persuade the patient to cooperate with the treatment plan—sometimes referred to as "talking the patient down"—another EMT should be establishing a safe strategy for the takedown.

First, always ensure that there are enough crew members, usually a minimum of four people, for a safe restraint. If there are not enough for a safe takedown, the group should withdraw until reinforcements arrive.

Each crew member must be assigned a role for the takedown. Typically, one person is assigned the role of team leader. Each member of the team will be assigned a specific job, often maintaining control of a body part. The team leader will signal the team when to move, quickly, to restrain the patient. The signal, usually a verbal cue such as "OK" or a hand gesture, tells all team members to proceed to restrain the patient's limbs.

With a strategy in place, the team moves into position. The EMT negotiating with the patient should signal the team to move forward at the right moment (Figure 28.5). When the team leader moves the team forward, what they have effectively done is to say that the discussion has failed.

At this time, the EMT talking with the patient should make one last effort to convince the patient to agree to care by pointing out the large number of people behind him. The patient, seeing a large number of determined individuals, called a **show of force,** may see the intelligence in cooperating and quietly comply with the first EMT's request. If the show of force fails, then, on cue, the team should move forward quickly to surround and take the patient down.

Having the stretcher near is convenient. Then the patient can be positioned on the stretcher. At other times, flexible stretchers are used. The next section discusses alternative restraint techniques.

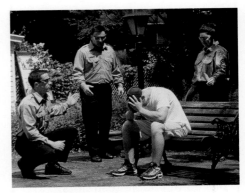

Figure 28.5 A show of force is sometimes all that is necessary to obtain a patient's cooperation

TOTAL BODY RESTRAINT

The most effective restraint would totally encapsulate the patient, preventing the patient from moving while still allowing him to be carried. A blanket, flexible stretcher, or similar apparatus is an effective total body restraint device.

If a flexible stretcher is used, the patient must first be placed on the stretcher. Once the patient is on the stretcher, the bedroll is opened and wrapped around the patient. The sheet is snugly wrapped around the patient, while the patient's arms are down along his sides. Next the blankets are crossed over the patient, opposite the direction of the sheet.

The EMT should layer the linen over the patient while folding the linen in opposite directions, called the *papoose* technique (Figure 28.6). Papoose is effective for children or for weak or elderly patients.

Finally, the stretcher straps are secured at the shoulders, hips, and thighs. Additional 9-foot straps placed around the entire apparatus can help secure the patient.

The EMT should take care to continually monitor the respiratory status of the restrained patient, because overly tight restraints can restrict breathing.

EXTREMITY RESTRAINT

After the team has completed the takedown and the patient's limbs are being physically restrained, the patient must be moved to a transportation device, such as the stretcher.

If the patient is found "hobbled," immediately roll the patient onto his side to allow him the chance to breathe deeply.

When an exhausted patient is placed facedown, after a vigorous physical confrontation, he may not have the strength to lift his chest and breathe deeply. There are reports of people having died because they were placed in hobble restraints.

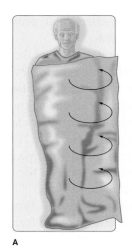
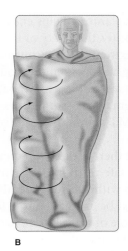
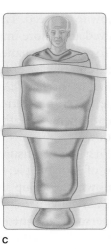

Figure 28.6 The papoose is an effective restraint technique for small or elderly patients

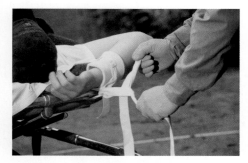

Figure 28.7 Secure one arm over the patient's head

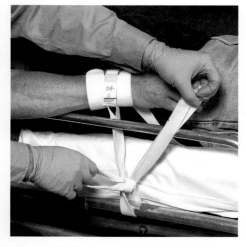

Figure 28.8 A restraint looped over the patient's wrist with a half-hitch is an effective restraint device

If the gurney wheels are lockable, then lock them. If they are not, the EMT must remember to place a foot under a wheel to act as a chock. Nothing is more difficult than trying to restrain a squirming patient on a moving gurney.

The patient is lifted by all four extremities and placed, faceup, onto the stretcher. Placing the patient faceup is important to prevent respiratory compromise in the prone position. It also allows the EMT to monitor the patient's airway, breathing, and circulation (ABCs).

Restraining a patient facedown can result in the patient slowly suffocating and could lead to respiratory arrest. Death from being restrained facedown is called **positional asphyxia.** The use of **hobble restraints,** also known as "hog-tying," which places the patient on his stomach with his wrists and ankles tied together behind him, is not an acceptable restraint method used in EMS. Most police departments now also ban the use of hobble restraints.

Secure one arm above the patient's head, at the crossbar at the head of the gurney. Place the other hand, preferably the nondominant hand, down at the patient's side. By having his arms placed in opposing directions, the patient cannot get leverage and use the large abdominal muscles to sit up (Figure 28.7).

Place the gurney's strap under the patient's armpits. Keep the strap high and tight. Another strap should be placed immediately above the patient's knees. Again, with the knees held down, the patient is prevented from using the large thigh muscles for force. If the legs are strapped at or below the knees, then the patient can squirm out from under the strap.

Finally, if necessary, restrain the ankles. First, secure the two ankles, one to the other. Then secure the ankles to the gurney. Often this last step, securing the ankles to the gurney, is unnecessary and makes the move to the hospital gurney more difficult.

RESTRAINT DEVICES

There are several devices an EMT can use to restrain a patient. A common choice is triangular bandages. Cravats, triangular bandages folded lengthwise, are strong and versatile. EMTs often use cravats for restraint. Cravats fold into small packets about the size of the palm of the hand and fit easily into a uniform pocket, out of sight.

Cravats also apply the force of the restraint across a broad swath, preventing the restraint from cutting into the patient's flesh. When applied to a wrist or an ankle, the cravat is looped *twice* over the limb and then secured with a half-hitch. The *tails* of the cravat are then secured to the stretcher railing (Figure 28.8).

Strong roller gauze (Kling or Kerlix) can be used as well. Caution must be exercised because a roller bandage can cut into the patient's wrists, creating a soft tissue injury.

Psychiatric hospitals use a leather restraint device, a commercially manufactured restraint device that consists of a loop of leather with a locking device on a strap applied to each wrist. The top wrist loops are then secured to a waist belt or to the rails of the stretcher. Like the wrist restraints, in an ankle restraint a leather loop goes around the ankle. Ankle restraints are usually secured to the stretcher by a belt wrapped around the foot of the stretcher.

Although leather restraints are more expensive than other devices, they can be fixed on the patient quickly. Leather restraints have the added advantage of being padded. Padding prevents friction burns to the wrist and ankles as the patient struggles.

In nursing homes, elderly patients who are prone to falling or wandering off are restrained with a chest harness. A chest harness is vestlike and goes over the patient's head in a T-shirt fashion. Some chest harnesses have panels made of cotton; others have panels made of nylon mesh. Both varieties of chest harnesses are strong and durable.

The chest harness has fabric belts sewn into the vest. These belts can be fastened behind the patient's back, out of reach, to keep the patient in the chair.

A chest harness is an effective means of restraining a patient while still allowing him to sit upright (Figure 28.9). Certain elderly patients—those with heart failure, for example—cannot tolerate lying flat for extended periods without feeling short of breath. Furthermore, the chest harness allows the EMT access to the patient's arms for purposes of taking blood pressures.

SAFETY

If a situation deteriorates and safety is compromised, the team should withdraw. Police are trained in effective restraint techniques. In those cases, the police should be encouraged to restrain the patient.

Once the patient has been restrained, the EMT, at her earliest convenience, should replace the police restraints (handcuffs, ties) with medical restraints. Often patients become exhausted after a vigorous restraint and are easier to manage.

If the patient must remain in handcuffs, then the police officer should accompany the patient to the hospital.

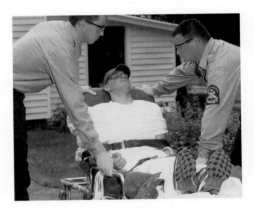

Figure 28.9 A chest restraint allows the patient to remain seated

TRANSPORT

Once the patient has been safely secured to the stretcher and is in the back of the ambulance, the EMT should transport the patient to the closest appropriate

---

Street Smart

When securing a patient to a stretcher, be sure to secure the limbs to a nonmovable rail. If the limbs are secured to lower bars in the carriage and the stretcher is quickly raised to the high position, then the patient's pinned arms will be injured, possibly even broken.

As a matter of practice, all restrained patients should be transported on a stretcher in the low position. This practice prevents a squirming patient from overturning the stretcher.

Safety Tips

If the patient is spitting at people, the EMT should be sure to wear eye protection as well as a mask. Placing a mask on the patient may be effective, but a determined patient will manage to get the mask off and spit at the EMT. Be proactive, and protect yourself by shielding your eyes.

hospital. Every EMT should be familiar with the capabilities of each nearby institution. Some emergency departments have a separate psychiatric facility, which may be appropriate for a patient with an acute mental illness. The EMT should always follow local protocols regarding transport of the psychiatric patient.

ONGOING ASSESSMENT

Whenever a patient is restrained, it is imperative that the EMT maintain a constant vigil. The EMT has eliminated the patient's ability to care for himself. The patient is completely dependent on the EMT for safety. This is no small matter. It is frightening to the patient and places the burden of the patient's safety entirely on the EMT.

The EMT should check pulses, movement, and sensation in the extremities at least every 10 minutes (Figure 28.10). The patient's ABCs should be reassessed at least every 5 minutes.

DOCUMENTATION

A restraint call involves a great deal of documentation. The EMT must document the patient's condition. It is important to document the efforts that were made to avoid using the restraint before it was decided that the restraint had to be used. If medical control was contacted for orders to restrain, that contact must be documented. If a police officer ordered restraint, in some jurisdictions, then the officer's name, badge number, and agency should be noted.

The method of restraint must be noted. The ongoing assessment of the patient must clearly indicate the EMT's attention to the ABCs as well as to the extremities.

PSYCHIATRIC DISORDERS

Although there are a number of psychiatric disorders, they all have some common features. First, the patient may completely lose touch with reality or at least have distorted perceptions of reality. The patient may no longer be able to interact appropriately with the environment and does not see the world as others do. The difficulty lies in the fact that the patient's distorted perceptions of reality can eventually result in a complete loss of touch with reality.

Overall, many psychotic patients suffer from some impairment of their ability to conduct activities of daily living (ADLs). ADLs are the human routines that sustain a person, including eating, sleeping, working, and having hobbies. When ADLs are neglected, patients may either become unhealthy or a danger to themselves.

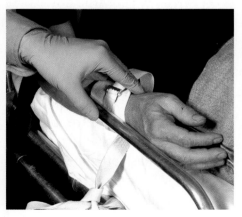

Figure 28.10 Distal pulses should be checked every 5–10 minutes

These patients are truly in need of prompt medical attention. Medications and psychiatric intervention can help these patients regain a grasp on reality and a chance to return to normalcy.

DEPRESSION

Depression is a condition in which sadness and despair dominate the person's mood. These feelings become overwhelming and can lead to neglect of family, friends, and self. Depression is seen in many people, to some extent, under certain almost-predictable circumstances. For example, after a severe life disappointment, a person usually goes through a period of depression. This situational depression resolves itself, usually with support from friends and family, and the person returns to normalcy.

Clinical depression occurs in about one third of the U.S. population, at least once in their lives. Extreme emotional trauma, such as the death of a spouse, can lead to clinical depression. Table 28-3 lists some common causes of depression.

SIGNS AND SYMPTOMS

If the depression is severe or the patient does not have sufficient support mechanisms, the depression can lead to abnormal behavior. The patient will experience mental apathy, or melancholy. As the patient becomes increasingly depressed and despondent and starts to neglect ADLs, *clinical depression* may ensue. This condition is present when the mental condition results in physical problems such as changes in appetite, weight gain or loss, sleeping difficulties, and illness. Table 28-4 lists signs and symptoms of clinical depression.

ASSESSMENT

When called to the scene of a depressed patient, the EMT should take careful note of her surroundings. Any description of the living conditions and any evidence of an overdose, drug use, or other means of self-harm are important to pass on to hospital personnel.

Table 28-3 Causes of Depression

Death of child

Loss of job

Death of spouse

Divorce

Financial catastrophe

Terminal illness

Safety Tips

Note that all of the causes of depression listed in Table 28-3 are common life stresses. During the course of a lifetime, most individuals develop coping mechanisms to deal with these stresses. If the individual becomes overwhelmed by these stresses or has insufficient coping mechanisms to deal with them, the individual may become victim to depression.

EMTs encounter these stresses frequently. Both sympathy and empathy for these patients add to the stress that the EMT feels, possibly leading the EMT into depression. It is important that EMTs know how to cope with stress successfully. Unit 4 provides some insight into commonly encountered stress in EMS and how to cope with it.

Table 28-4 Signs and Symptoms of Clinical Depression

Loss of appetite

Loss of weight

Overeating

Insomnia (sleeplessness)

Hypersomnia (sleeps all day)

Decreased libido (loss of sex drive)

Feelings of worthlessness, helplessness, or hopelessness

Excessive guilt

Recurrent thoughts of death

Suicidal ideation

Frequent crying

Emotional lability (mood swings)

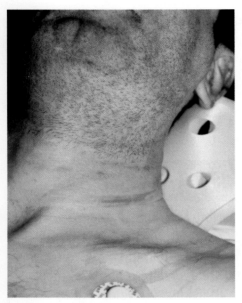

Figure 28.11 Suicide is the final result of depression in many cases. Note the rope marks on the neck of this man who attempted suicide (Courtesy of Wayne Triner, DO, Albany Medical Center, Albany, NY)

Table 28-5 Methods of Suicide
Gunshot
Hanging
Drowning
Poisoning
Lacerating arteries (slashing)
Burning
Jumping from a height
Intentional overdose
Inhalation of toxic gases
Intentional motor vehicle collision

MANAGEMENT

In the care of the depressed patient, it is important for the EMT to be supportive. Regardless of the reason for the depression, the EMT cannot begin to understand exactly what the patient is experiencing. Simply to be there and to offer medical help and a hand to hold will be appreciated.

The person with severe depression is often unable to make decisions easily or quickly. Any decisions made, such as which hospital to go to or which shoes to put on before transport, may need significant coaxing by the EMT. A supportive, yet decisive, manner is most useful.

SUICIDE

When a patient voluntarily takes his own life, he has committed **suicide.** Suicide is a national health problem. Every year, about 25,000 Americans attempt suicide. That is one suicide attempt every 90 seconds.

Although EMTs do not perform suicide risk assessments, it is valuable to know the risk factors for suicide so that they can have a "heads-up" attitude about suicide.

Depression is the leading risk factor for suicide. Depressed elderly males who are either divorced or widowed are at greatest risk for committing suicide. There is also an increased incidence of suicide around the holidays, when families traditionally gather. The patient remembers and misses loved ones. These feelings can lead to worsening depression and suicide. Similarly, there is an increased incidence of suicide around anniversaries and birthdays.

More females attempt suicide, but more males actually kill themselves. Any attempt at suicide is a cry for help and should be taken seriously (Figure 28.11). Eighty percent of people who attempt suicide do so repeatedly; eventually, those attempts turn fatal if appropriate help is not obtained. Table 28-5 lists some common mechanisms encountered during an attempted suicide.

SIGNS AND SYMPTOMS

When assessing the potential suicidal patient, the EMT should look carefully for signs of self-inflicted injury or of illness secondary to poisoning or overdose. The specific signs and symptoms present will be related to the method of suicide that the patient attempted.

MANAGEMENT

In caring for the person who is suspected of being suicidal, the EMT should be direct in her questioning. It is important to be clear about whether the patient intended to harm himself. If there is physical evidence of attempted self-harm or if a bystander claims that the patient threatened to harm himself, the EMT should assume that the patient is a potential danger to himself. This patient must be transported to an emergency department for evaluation by a physician regardless of his desires. The EMT should treat whatever injuries are found in a focused physical exam.

BIPOLAR DISORDER

Manic-depressive disorder, or **bipolar disorder,** is a type of mental illness characterized by extremes of emotion ranging from total elation to deep depression.

SIGNS AND SYMPTOMS

One day the patient may feel all-powerful, euphoric, and full of energy. The patient can also become extremely agitated and irritable. On other days, the

Many questions are raised when a dead body is discovered. The police have an interest in determining whether the person died because of suicide or murder. EMS has an interest in determining whether the patient is dead or is in need of medical treatment.

EMS and police, working together, can accomplish both missions without compromising either. Only one EMT need enter a scene to confirm the patient's condition. Carefully noting what she touches and where she steps, and trying to preserve evidence, the EMT should approach the patient.

Once the EMT is at the patient's side, she should determine whether resuscitation is possible. If it is not, then the EMT should carefully withdraw. If the patient is in cardiac arrest and cardiopulmonary resuscitation (CPR) is needed, the EMT should consider dragging the patient, using an emergency move, to another area.

In the meantime, other EMS personnel should stand by, or stage, in an adjacent area. When the patient is brought out, CPR may be started.

The nature of a suicide attempt implies that a dangerous instrument may have been used by the patient. An EMT must cautiously proceed into every scene of an attempted suicide. Obvious dangers, such as a loaded handgun, may be evident.

Hidden dangers, such as carbon monoxide, can make the EMT an unwitting victim. The EMT approaching the scene must be aware of these potential dangers. The EMT must predict these dangers, on the basis of all available information, and proceed prepared to protect herself and her crew. In other words, the EMT must have a heads-up attitude about the scene before proceeding.

Some patients choose a weapon, such as a shotgun, as their instrument of death. If EMS interrupts the patient during his suicide attempt, the patient may become angry and turn on the responders. The police should always be asked to secure any weapon before EMS enters the scene.

patient is depressed and withdrawn and feels worthless. The patient has all the signs and symptoms of clinical depression.

MANAGEMENT

The drug lithium is often prescribed to control the manic phase of the disorder. Along with lithium, an antidepressant medication may also be prescribed. Although certain medications can control the extreme emotional swings, the patient must be compliant with his medications to get the desired effect. Table 28-6 lists common antidepressants.

The patient with bipolar disorder who seems to be out of touch with reality or in any danger of causing harm to himself or others must be transported safely to the emergency department.

SCHIZOPHRENIA

Schizophrenia is a poorly understood mental disease that may be due to a neurochemical imbalance. Schizophrenia is defined by its several distinguishing elements or psychotic features.

Whenever a patient attempts suicide by hanging, the assumption is that a neck injury has occurred. Quickly have one EMT support the body, lifting the patient's weight off the rope. Another EMT should quickly stabilize the head, while cutting the rope. Do not cut through, or try to untie, the knot. Cut the rope far enough away from the knot so that it can be loosened. Proceed treating the patient as a trauma patient.

Table 28-6 Common Antidepressants

Generic Name	Trade Name
Amitriptyline	Elavil
Amoxapine	Asendin
Bupropion	Wellbutrin
Doxepin	Sinequan
Fluoxetine	Prozac
Imipramine	Tofranil
Nortriptyline	Pamelor
Sertraline	Zoloft

SIGNS AND SYMPTOMS

In general, the schizophrenic patient is out of touch with reality. The patient imagines a fantasy world and lives out his life in that fantasy. Part of that fantasy may involve **hallucinations.** Hallucinations are sensations or perceptions that have no basis in reality.

For example, some patients with hallucinations may feel as if bugs are crawling on their skin when that is not the case. These hallucinations are called **tactile hallucinations.**

Other hallucinations may be **visual hallucinations.** Seeing snakes all around is an example of a visual hallucination. Finally, the patient may have an **auditory hallucination** in which he hears voices or other non-existent sounds.

MANAGEMENT

The EMT should ask the psychotic patient, "Are you hearing voices?" Certain auditory hallucinations are called **command hallucinations.** The voices in a command hallucination are telling the patient what to do.

If the patient answers yes, continue to probe. Ask the patient what the voices are saying. Do not act surprised if the patient answers something to the effect that "The voices say you are the devil and I should kill you." Remember that the patient is out of touch with reality. The patient does not see the EMT as someone who will help him, but rather as someone who may harm him.

Command hallucinations can be compelling and powerful to the patient. The patient may act violently toward the EMT. The EMT should always be prepared for a tactical retreat. Continually reassure the patient that he has control and the hallucination will pass. Encourage the patient to keep you informed of what the voices are saying. Table 28-7 lists other common psychotic features.

Patients with schizophrenia are often prescribed medications to try to calm their symptoms and help them live normal lives. These medications are called *antipsychotics,* some of which are listed in Table 28-8.

Table 28-7 Psychotic Features

Feature	Definition
Delusions of grandeur	False belief that the person is something he is not
Hallucinations	False perceptions having no basis in reality
Muted catatonia	Inability to speak or respond
Paranoia	Persistent persecutory delusions
Persecution complex	Belief that everyone is intent on harming the patient
Somatic illness	Concern of illness with no physical evidence

Table 28-8 Common Antipsychotic Medications

Generic Name	Trade Name
Chlorpromazine	Thorazine
Clozapine	Clozaril
Fluphenazine	Prolixin
Haloperidol	Haldol
Mesoridazine	Serentil
Perphenazine	Trilafon
Thioridazine	Mellaril
Thiothixene	Navane

Table 28-9 Anxiety Disorders

Feature	Definition
Obsessive-compulsive disorder (OCD)	Irresistible urge to do an act repeatedly (ritualistic behavior)
Panic disorder	State of extreme uncontrollable fear; also called panic attack
Phobia	Intense and irrational fear of something (there are 700 described phobias)
Post-traumatic stress disorder (PTSD)	Maladaptive response seen after a psychologically distressing event

ANXIETY DISORDER

Anxiety is a normal response to stress. Anxiety becomes abnormal when the response is exaggerated or inappropriate to the situation. Abnormal anxieties, or **anxiety disorders,** collectively represent the largest group of mental illnesses in the United States.

The causes of anxiety disorders are varied. Table 28-9 provides a partial listing of causes of anxiety disorders. Regardless of the cause, the results are the same—exaggerated or inappropriate anxiety.

SIGNS AND SYMPTOMS

The patient suffering from an anxiety disorder becomes anxious when exposed to a stimulus that frightens him. Sometimes the stimulus is a tangible thing, such as a bee; other times, it is not as readily found, as in the case

Table 28-10 Signs and Symptoms of an Anxiety Disorder

Anxiety

Diaphoresis

Dilated pupils

Fear

Hyperventilation

Palpitations

Pins and needles sensation

Shortness of breath

Sweatiness

Tachycardia

Tremulousness

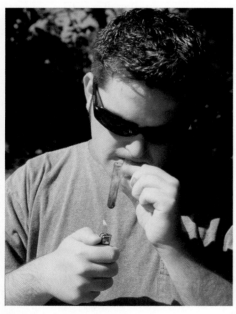

Figure 28.12 Substance abuse, including drug abuse, can lead to behavioral emergencies

of panic attacks. Table 28-10 lists some of the more common signs and symptoms found in the patient suffering from an anxiety disorder.

MANAGEMENT

Patients who are experiencing panic attacks or extreme anxiety often hyperventilate (breathe too deeply), causing physical symptoms such as dizziness, tingling in their hands and around their mouths, and heart palpitations; they also may experience spasms of the hands and feet, called *carpal-pedal spasms*. When caring for an anxious patient, the EMT should speak in a calm, reassuring voice. She should allow the patient to talk about the cause of his increased anxiety if he desires and lend a sympathetic ear. The crew should transport the patient in a position of comfort and consider ALS intercept for a patient who is experiencing extreme symptoms and not responding to emotional support.

SUBSTANCE ABUSE

The misuse of a drug or other substance to alter the person's perception or mood is called **substance abuse.** Substance abuse, including alcoholism, is a significant health problem in this country. Substance abuse can lead to a number of chronic debilitating diseases that cost Americans almost $1 trillion a year in health care and related costs.

Substance abuse often leads to abnormal behavior. The EMT is expected to be able to deal with the patient who is under the influence of a mind-altering substance (Figure 28.12).

Often people use illicit (illegal) drugs to alter their mood or mental state. Most illicit drugs create a heightened sense of well-being, or euphoria, called *getting high*. Often these drugs are impure. Numerous materials—including baking soda, talcum powder, and rat poison—are used to dilute, or *cut,* these drugs, in order to sell more drugs. Many of these substances are toxic. For this and other reasons, any patient who is suspected of substance abuse should be seen in the emergency department. Table 28-11 lists some commonly abused street drugs.

As a patient repeatedly consumes certain drugs, his body will start to need that drug. This physical need for a drug is called an **addiction.** Not all drugs are physically addicting. Over time, patients may develop a craving for a drug. Called **dependency,** this craving is largely psychological. The combination of dependency and addiction, often terms used interchangeably, helps explain why drugs are so widely abused.

OVERDOSE

When too much of a substance is ingested, inhaled, or injected into the body, the substance becomes toxic to the body. A toxin, or poison, interferes with the body's metabolism. Too much of a toxin can be fatal. Any intoxication is, by definition, an overdose of the drug.

DRUG WITHDRAWAL

Withholding a drug from an addicted patient can have many unpleasant physical and psychological effects, called **withdrawal symptoms.** Withdrawal symptoms vary widely according to the type of drug, the patient's length of addiction, and the drug's effect on the body.

A program of gradual drug withdrawal, under medical supervision, is called *detoxification.* A detoxification program minimizes the impact of withdrawal symptoms while ridding the body of the unwanted drug.

Withdrawal from any drug without medical supervision can be dangerous. Sudden withdrawal from heroin, for example, can lead to sweating, tremors, diarrhea, vomiting, and cramps in the stomach and legs. Unexpected withdrawal from other drugs can lead to sudden cardiac death.

Table 28-11 Commonly Abused Drugs

Name	Street Names	Source	Effect
Amphetamines	Uppers, speed	Manufactured	Stimulant
Caffeine	N/A	Coffee, chocolate	Stimulant
Cocaine	Coke, crack	Coca plant	Stimulant/Euphoria
Ecstacy	E, Adam, E-bomb	Manufactured	Hallucinogen/Stimulant
Hashish	Tar	Resin of cannabis	Euphoria
Heroin	H, smack, horse	Opium plant	Depressant/Euphoria
Inhalants	Huffing, bagging	Lighter fluid, gas	Depressant/Euphoria
Lysergic acid diethylamide (LSD)	Acid	Chemistry lab	Euphoria
Marijuana	Pot, grass, weed	Cannabis plant	Euphoria
Methamphetamine	Crank, ice, stove top	Manufactured	Stimulant/Euphoria
Nicotine	N/A	Cigarettes, tobacco	Stimulant
Sedatives	Downers, barbs	Manufactured	Sedative

ALCOHOL WITHDRAWAL

Alcoholic patients are both psychologically dependent on and physically addicted to alcohol. Chronic alcoholism causes damage to every organ system, especially the liver and heart. Common physical problems associated with alcoholism are heart disease, hypertension, cirrhosis of the liver, pancreatitis (inflammation of the pancreas), and gastrointestinal problems. Alcoholic patients also suffer from depression (alcohol depresses the functions of the central nervous system), insomnia, impotence, and amnesia (blackouts).

SIGNS AND SYMPTOMS

For all these reasons, alcoholic patients may try to stop drinking. Within 24 hours, the patient may start to experience acute alcohol withdrawal symptoms. The symptoms of alcohol withdrawal include marked tremors (shaking), sweating, weakness, nausea, vomiting, and diarrhea. In addition, the EMT may find that the patient is tachycardiac and hypertensive.

Sudden alcohol withdrawal can lead to **delirium tremens (DTs).** DTs is a state of mental confusion, anxiety attacks, and hyperexcitability, frequently with visual hallucinations.

Some patients may be quiet and paranoid, possibly fearful of snakes or monsters that are frequently hallucinated. Others may be excited, trembling, or talking or yelling incoherently.

EMTs caring for a substance abuser must also consider the possibility of other disorders such as a head injury or ingestion of other poisons. Confusion, nausea, and vomiting are all common signs seen in many disorders.

The EMT should inquire whether the patient fell and struck his head. If the patient did fall, then the EMT should take appropriate spinal precautions.

The EMT should ask the patient whether he drank or ingested anything else. Alcoholics will sometimes find sources of alcohol other than the local bar. Automobile antifreeze, isopropyl (rubbing) alcohol, and mouthwash contain alcohols that may satisfy the alcoholic's craving for alcohol, despite their toxic nature. The EMT should bring any containers found on scene to the emergency department.

MANAGEMENT

Without immediate medical treatment, the patient experiencing DTs may suffer seizures, status epilepticus, and possible cardiac arrest. The EMT should provide supportive care, including oxygen administration; close observation of the airway, breathing, and circulation; a darkened room; and quiet transportation. Any patient who is going through DTs must be evaluated in the emergency department immediately.

AGITATED DELIRIUM

Agitated delirium (AD), or **excited delirium** as it is sometimes called, is a behavioral emergency involving patients exhibiting bizarre and violent behavior. AD may result from psychiatric disorders such as manic-depressive psychosis and chronic schizophrenia, alcohol withdrawal, or head trauma. Agitated delirium is also associated with substance abuse such as cocaine or methamphetamine. Medical history and the history of events leading up to AD may be difficult to obtain.

EMS is often the first to encounter individuals in agitated delirium. Establishing scene safety and ensuring the safety of EMS personnel must be the primary focus. Law enforcement should be present before approaching the patient and attempting to provide patient care.

SIGNS AND SYMPTOMS

Patients experiencing agitated delirium often have a history of drug or alcohol abuse, schizophrenia, or bipolar disorders; however, head trauma should also be considered until ruled out. These patients may exhibit bizarre behaviors such as partially or completely undressing. They are usually violent, aggressive, combative, loud, obnoxious, agitated, and uncooperative, with bizarre thoughts and actions, paranoia, delusions, or confusion.

Physical signs of AD include rapid, heavy or labored breathing, tachycardia, and increased blood pressure. Skin may be cool, moist, and pale or dry, warm, and flushed.

MANAGEMENT

Management will include restraint (physical or chemical) of the patient to reduce threats to self and others. Blood glucose should be checked to rule out hypoglycemia. Monitor vitals signs and assess for head injury or other traumatic injuries. Consider ALS intercept for administration of **chemical restraint,** the use of medications to keep the patient calm or sedated.

Patients with agitated delirium, especially involving a history of cocaine or methamphetamine use, are at risk for sudden death. Respiratory and cardiac function should be monitored closely, especially in patients who have been physically restrained.

CONCLUSION

Behavioral emergencies present a unique challenge to the EMT. The EMT must maintain professional dignity, often in the face of personal attack. The EMT must attempt to assess and treat any medical conditions that may be causing the abnormal behavior. Finally, the EMT must maintain safety for herself, the crew, and the patient.

The single most important principle an EMT must keep in mind is that this is a patient, a person in need of medical attention. This patient needs help and compassion, despite appearances to the contrary.

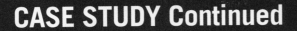

CASE STUDY Continued

Lataesha, Monica, and a local police officer meet outside the door of an apartment to which they were dispatched, for a woman acting strangely, by a neighbor who had called for help. Lataesha learns Mrs. Wilson is normally a kind, elderly female who keeps to herself. Today she is agitated and may be violent.

The law enforcement officer knocks on the door, calling out to Mrs. Wilson as he enters the apartment. After he indicates it is safe, Lataesha and Monica enter to find Mrs. Wilson standing in her bedroom talking as though someone else is in the room. She is muttering quietly and seems not to be aware she is alone in the room.

Lataesha slowly approaches and introduces herself. Mrs. Wilson looks at her and says, "They told me you were evil, but I told them to leave me alone." She appears confused, quietly repeating, "Be quiet. I'm not listening to you" to no one specifically. Lataesha asks her who she is talking to and she says, "The voices say evil is all around me."

Monica finds a folder with Mrs. Wilson's medical history on the kitchen counter next to empty medication bottles for clozapine and Seroquel. Mrs. Wilson has a history of schizophrenia and has been out of medicine for a couple weeks.

Lataesha reassures Mrs. Wilson that she is doing a great job with the voices and that they will give her a ride to the hospital to get more medicine. Mrs. Wilson is cooperative and goes to the ambulance without resistance, repeatedly telling the voices to be quiet.

Mrs. Wilson has occasional outbursts on the way to the hospital, telling the voices to "Leave me alone." Lataesha provides a report to the hospital of Mrs. Wilson's history and how she had been potentially violent prior to their arrival but has remained cooperative throughout transport.

Key Concepts Revisited

- A behavioral emergency is any situation in which the patient exhibits a behavior that is unacceptable, dangerous, or intolerable to the person, the family, or the community.

- Behavioral emergencies can be attributed to organic disorders and/or mental disorders.

  - Organic disorders are any disease or physical condition causing the brain to dysfunction.

  - Mental illness is any brain disorder not related to a physical condition or disease.

- Long-term mental illnesses may result in acute behavioral emergencies that pose risks to EMTs.

- The EMT should always be alert and prepared for violence on the scene of behavior emergencies.

- Management of behavior emergencies includes verbal persuasion and physical restraint.

  - Verbal persuasion requires calm, clear, slow communication that reassures the patient.

  - Physical restraint is performed when it becomes medically necessary to ensure the protection of the patient and EMS providers.

    - Total body restraint using a "papoose" method

    - Extremity restraint of hands and legs/ankles

- Psychiatric patients often suffer from some impairment of the ability to conduct activities of daily living (ADL).

- Depression causes feelings of sadness and despair that can lead to suicide.

- Management of suicide focuses on protection from further injury and treatment of injuries.

- Bipolar disorders are a mental illness characterized by extremes of emotions.

- Schizophrenia is characterized by tactile, visual, and/or auditory hallucinations.
  - Tactile hallucinations may be a feeling of something crawling on the skin.
  - Seeing snakes where there are none is an example of visual hallucinations.
  - Auditory hallucinations involve hearing nonexistent voices and other sounds.
- Anxiety is a normal response to stress that becomes abnormal when it is exaggerated or inappropriate to the situation.

- Substance abuse leads to abnormal and sometimes bizarre and violent behavior, especially when the patient has overdosed or is withdrawing from the substance.
  - Alcohol withdrawal involves physical signs and symptoms that may include marked tremors (shaking), sweating, weakness, nausea, vomiting, diarrhea, tachycardia, and hypertension.
  - Agitated delirium is an extreme condition characterized by bizarre and violent behavior.
- The EMT must focus on personal safety, patient care, and documentation of abnormal behavior emergencies.

Review Questions

1. What is a behavioral emergency?
2. What are several reasons that a patient might have a behavioral emergency?
3. What mental illnesses could cause the patient to have a behavioral emergency?
4. What are the signs and symptoms of severe depression?
5. What is a psychotic feature?
6. What are several drugs of abuse that can lead to behavioral emergencies?
7. What are some of the methods EMTs can use to protect themselves on scene?
8. What does it mean when it is said that the patient was restrained out of a medical necessity?
9. What is a show of force?
10. How would a patient be restrained to a stretcher?
11. How often does an EMT check a restrained patient?
12. What is agitated delirium?

Key Terms

Addiction
Agitated delirium (AD)
Anxiety disorder
Auditory hallucination
Behavioral emergency
Bipolar disorder
Chemical restraint
Command hallucination
Delirium
Delirium tremens (DTs)

Dependency
Depression
Excited delirium
Hallucination
Hobble restraint
Medically necessary restraint
Mental illness
Organic disorder
Positional asphyxia
Psychiatry

Show of force
Substance abuse
Suicide
Tactile hallucination

Takedown procedure
Visual hallucination
Withdrawal symptoms

Further Study

Abdon-Beckman, D. "An Awkward Position: Restraints and Sudden Death." *Journal of Emergency Medical Services* 22, no. 3 (1997): 88.

Ball, R. "Waiting to Exhale: Treatment of Hyperventilation." *Journal of Emergency Medical Services* 23, no. 1 (1998): 62–69.

Doyle, T., and R. Vissers. "An EMS Approach to Psychiatric Emergencies." *Emergency Medical Services* 28, no. 6 (1999): 87–88.

Park, K. S., C. S. Korn, and S. O. Henderson. "Agitated Delirium and Sudden Death: Two Case Reports." *Prehospital Emergency Care* 5, no. 2 (2001): 214–216.

UNIT (29) Abdominal Pain

Abdominal pain is one of the most common concerns for patients visiting emergency departments, accounting for 5% to 10% of adult emergency department visits in the United States. Accordingly, abdominal pain is a common reason for a call to Emergency Medical Services (EMS). Although the etiology of the pain does not usually have an impact on the emergency management provided by an Emergency Medical Technician (EMT), it is useful for prehospital providers to understand the potential for serious illness when a patient complains of abdominal pain.

National Education Standards

The Emergency Medical Technician (EMT) shall demonstrate a fundamental depth and foundational breadth of understanding in the anatomy, physiology, pathophysiology, assessment, and management of acute and chronic abdominal pain.

Key Concepts

- The EMT must have knowledge of the organ systems contained within the abdomen.

- The three types of abdominal pain are visceral pain, parietal pain, and referred pain.

- Common diseases that may cause abdominal pain affect the gastrointestinal, genitourinary, vascular, and extra-abdominal systems.

- Peptic ulcer disease involving a blood vessel can produce serious gastrointestinal bleeding that may lead to shock.

- Pyelonephritis is a severe infection of the kidneys that can result in significant morbidity and mortality if left untreated.

- An abdominal aortic aneurysm (AAA) leads to massive internal bleeding and death if a rupture or leak is not rapidly identified and surgically repaired.

- Acute coronary syndrome and pneumonia are two extra-abdominal conditions that can cause abdominal pain.

- Abdominal pain may be a symptom of a variety of disease states that can lead to shock and hypoperfusion.

- The EMT should always treat concerns of abdominal pain as potentially life threatening and high priority.

- The management priorities for a patient with abdominal pain include a thorough assessment of the ABCs and transport to the appropriate hospital.

CASE STUDY

Jamal and Daisy are called to a local residence for a 17-year-old female with severe abdominal pain. Upon arrival they are met at the door by a woman who states, "Please help my daughter, she is in the bathroom with severe stomach pains. She has been vomiting for the past hour, but nothing is coming up. I thought she just had the flu, but she feels hot, like she is running a fever and can't stand up without doubling over."

As Jamal and Daisy enter the bathroom they find a thin, young woman lying on the floor next to the toilet. She has her knees drawn up to her chest and her arms wrapped around her legs. She is shivering, but Jamal notices she looks flushed and her skin is very warm.

Daisy approaches the young woman, who is lying very still, as if she is afraid to move. Daisy introduces herself, reaching for the patient's wrist and asking her name. The young woman whispers, "My name is Ashley, and please don't make me move."

Because Ashley is able to answer questions, Daisy knows her airway is clear, she is breathing, and her pulse is rapid and bounding. She feels very warm to touch, with flushed, moist skin. When asked to point to her pain, using one finger, Ashley states she cannot, her whole stomach hurts but mostly on her right side.

Critical Thinking Questions

1. What are the priorities of assessment for a patient with abdominal pain?
2. Is this patient a high-priority or low-priority patient?
3. What are the priorities of care for patients with abdominal pain?

INTRODUCTION

Abdominal pain can have a variety of causes and may be the symptoms of a serious medical illness. Abdominal pain must be thoroughly assessed for any potentially life-threatening conditions. Management includes making the patient as comfortable as possible during transport to the hospital. This unit describes the more common nontraumatic conditions that cause abdominal pain and outlines the appropriate management techniques to be used by the EMT.

ANATOMY REVIEW

Prior to a detailed discussion of the management of patients with abdominal pain, it is wise to briefly review the relevant anatomy that was introduced in Unit 5. The abdomen is defined as the space bordered superiorly by the muscular diaphragm, posteriorly by the retroperitoneum, anteriorly and laterally by the abdominal wall musculature, and inferiorly by the bony pelvis. This is illustrated in Figure 29.1.

The four quadrants of the abdomen are the right upper quadrant, right lower quadrant, left upper quadrant, and left lower quadrant. Several organ systems are contained within the four quadrants of the abdomen. The digestive organs of the gastrointestinal tract include the hollow organs—stomach, gallbladder, and small and large intestines—and the solid organs—the liver and pancreas. These organs are responsible for a number of functions, most notably digestion of nutrients that are ingested.

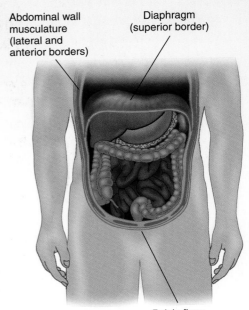

Abdominal wall musculature (lateral and anterior borders)

Diaphragm (superior border)

Pelvic floor (inferior border)

Figure 29.1 The abdomen has defined borders

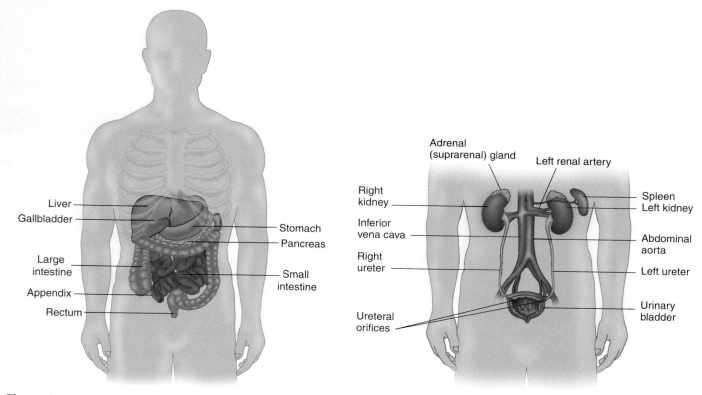

Figure 29.2 Several organ systems are found within the abdomen

The genitourinary system, comprised of the kidneys (solid organs), ureters, and bladder (hollow organ), excretes bodily wastes, and maintains a fluid and electrolyte balance within the body. Additionally, while the male genitals are largely located outside the borders of the abdomen, both male and female genital organs serve important functions in hormone regulation and can lead to abdominal pain when disease occurs.

The spleen (solid organ) and blood vessels that are located in the abdomen are part of the hematologic system and are involved in the flow of blood through the body. Figure 29.2 illustrates the location of each of these organs within the abdomen.

When discussing abdominal anatomy, it is useful to use the commonly known topographic descriptions noted in Figure 29.3. Although this is not the only means of describing abdominal anatomy, it is likely the most commonly used in the prehospital setting.

TYPES OF ABDOMINAL PAIN

The three types of abdominal pain are visceral pain, parietal pain, and referred pain, which can be linked to the organ involved. Referred pain can be experienced in an area of the body not connected to a specific organ. The types of abdominal pain are discussed in more detail in this section.

VISCERAL PAIN

Visceral pain is a poorly localized pain, more general in nature, and is a result of an illness directly involving an organ. When asked to point to the pain, the patient will have a hard time pinpointing an exact location. It is usually a less severe pain, dull or aching in nature, that may be constant or intermittent. Although visceral pain may not seem severe, because the underlying

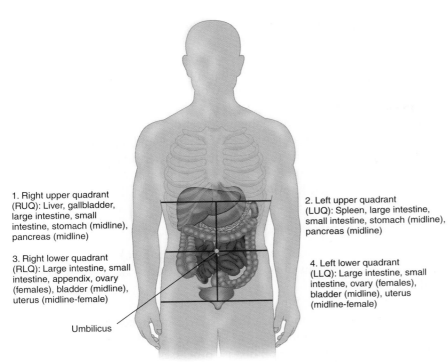

1. Right upper quadrant (RUQ): Liver, gallbladder, large intestine, small intestine, stomach (midline), pancreas (midline)

2. Left upper quadrant (LUQ): Spleen, large intestine, small intestine, stomach (midline), pancreas (midline)

3. Right lower quadrant (RLQ): Large intestine, small intestine, appendix, ovary (females), bladder (midline), uterus (midline-female)

4. Left lower quadrant (LLQ): Large intestine, small intestine, ovary (females), bladder (midline), uterus (midline-female)

Umbilicus

Figure 29.3 Abdominal topography can be described in four quadrants

cause is directly related to an organ, a serious illness may be involved. Additional signs and symptoms often seen with visceral pain include nausea and vomiting.

PARIETAL PAIN

Parietal pain, also called *somatic* pain, is seen when there is an irritation of the outer lining of the abdominal cavity or peritoneum. The peritoneal lining contains highly sensitized nerve endings; therefore, parietal pain is usually more severe and the patient will be able to point to the area of pain. Parietal pain is intense, localized pain, usually found on one side or the other, and is usually described as sharp and constant. The patient experiencing parietal pain will generally want to lie supine with her knees flexed toward her chest to keep the abdominal muscles from stretching. Further, the patient may be breathing shallowly and not moving in an attempt to lessen the pain. Peritonitis discussed later in the unit is an example of an illness often presenting with parietal pain.

REFERRED PAIN

Referred pain is often similar to visceral pain located in an area of the body away from the point of origin. Referred pain occurs when an organ shares a nerve pathway with a skin sensory nerve. As with all visceral-type pain, it is dull and achy in nature and poorly localized, though usually constant in the area to which it has referred. An example of referred pain is a patient with an inflamed gallbladder (discussed in more detail later in the unit) experiencing visceral pain in the right shoulder or shoulder blade area.

CAUSES OF ABDOMINAL PAIN

Although many disease processes can cause abdominal pain, the specific etiology may not be obvious to the EMT. The focused history and physical exam may lend clues to the underlying problem, but the EMT will often not have sufficient information to exclude the presence of a serious illness. For this reason, the EMT should provide aggressive treatment for the patient with abdominal pain and assume the presence of a significant disease process. Because of this potential, advanced life support (ALS) involvement is often indicated in the prehospital management of the patient with abdominal pain. Local protocols govern this practice.

The EMT should treat the patient with abdominal pain for the potential of serious illness and appropriately manage shock and other obvious threats to life found during the initial assessment. The determination of a diagnosis is not necessary to provide these basic treatments; however, it is useful for the EMT to have a basic knowledge of the specific conditions that can cause abdominal pain.

GASTROINTESTINAL

The gastrointestinal system comprises the organs involved in digestion of foods. This system begins at the mouth and includes all of the organs pictured in Figure 29.4.

Disease in any part of the gastrointestinal system can cause abdominal pain. Alteration of the function of this system can result in serious imbalances in the body's fluid and electrolyte balance as well as in the stores of glucose. Some of the more common disease processes originating in this system are described next.

PEPTIC ULCER DISEASE

The stomach is normally responsible for producing acid that is effective in breaking down foods for digestion. These acids are powerful and have the potential to cause injury to the lining of the stomach as well, if protective

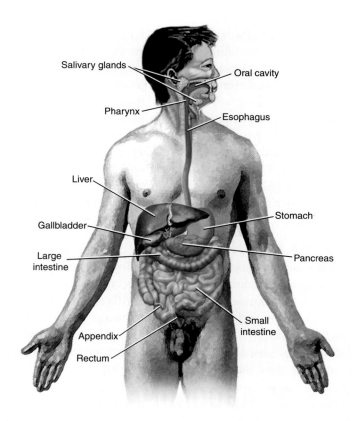

Figure 29.4 The gastrointestinal system includes all organs involved in the digestion of food

mechanisms are not in place. When these protective mechanisms are not functional, the result can be irritation of the stomach lining or even erosion through the entire wall of the stomach (Figure 29.5). Such erosion is referred to as a gastric **ulcer.** Ulcers occur commonly in the first part of the duodenum as well. If an ulcer involves a blood vessel, serious bleeding can occur. The patient with an ulcer may have abdominal pain located in the middle of the upper abdomen, often referred to as the *epigastrium*. If the ulcer involves a blood vessel, the patient may vomit blood, called **hemetemesis.**

Additionally, blood that passes through the gastrointestinal tract will undergo some digestion, resulting in black-colored, tarry stools. This type of stool is characteristic of bleeding in the upper gastrointestinal tract and is called **melena.** Significant blood loss can occur as a result of a bleeding ulcer. The EMT should be aware of the potential for hemorrhagic shock. Definitive treatment involves reduction of acids and enhancement of protective mechanisms within the stomach. In severe cases, surgery may be required to repair perforations of the stomach.

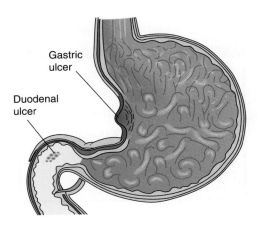

Figure 29.5 Peptic ulcer disease can cause gastric or duodenal ulcers

ESOPHAGEAL VARICES

The veins that run through the distal esophagus can, in certain disease states, become distended and rupture, resulting in ¨massive uncontrolled bleeding. These distended veins are called **esophageal varices** and are most commonly seen in patients with severe liver disease. A patient with ruptured esophageal varices will present with repeated episodes of hemetemesis and likely signs of shock. This patient may or may not complain of pain. The mortality associated with such an event is 50% even with treatment. Hospital treatment involves halting the bleeding and replacing the lost blood.

GASTROENTERITIS

Usually a viral irritation of the stomach and intestines, **gastroenteritis** is a condition that results in vomiting, diarrhea, and, often, abdominal pain and fever. If vomiting and diarrhea are profuse, gastroenteritis can lead to significant dehydration and hypovolemic shock. Definitive goals in management involve slowing the fluid losses and ensuring adequate hydration. Although the condition is most often self-limiting, in its most severe form, gastroenteritis can result in significant morbidity and mortality.

BOWEL OBSTRUCTION

Normal functioning of the gastrointestinal tract involves the passage of solids, liquids, and gases from one end through the other. This movement is dependent on a clear passageway. If there is a narrowing or complete blockage at any point, these materials will not be able to pass and will back up. This backup causes distention of the bowel and sometimes the stomach, resulting in pain and often vomiting. Such a **bowel obstruction** can have multiple etiologies, and curative treatment will depend on the specific cause. Radiologic testing will often be required for diagnosis.

GALLBLADDER DISEASE

The gallbladder stores bile that is secreted into the duodenum when needed to assist in absorption of fatty foods. Occasionally, solid material can accumulate in the gallbladder, forming gallstones. These gallstones can cause a blockage of bile flow (Figure 29.6), resulting in distention of the gallbladder and pain. This distention can lead to inflammation and infection of the wall of the gallbladder. This condition is called **cholecystitis** and results in fever, right upper abdominal pain, and often vomiting. Backup of bile can result in excess accumulation of its

> ### Street Smart
>
> The patient with bleeding from esophageal varices may have such massive hemetemesis that her ability to maintain her own airway may be in jeopardy. The EMT should be prepared to intervene if needed.

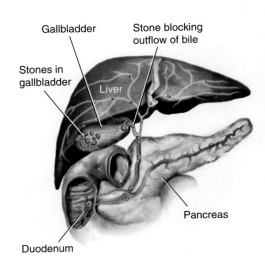

Figure 29.6 Gallstones can block the outflow of bile from the gallbladder

components in the bloodstream, resulting in a yellow color to the skin, called *jaundice*. Jaundice is commonly seen in gallbladder disease. Decompression or surgical removal of the gallbladder is sometimes indicated.

APPENDICITIS

The appendix is a narrow appendage at the junction of the small and large intestines, often located in the right lower quadrant of the abdomen. In 6% of the American population, the appendix becomes obstructed with some solid material, distends, and may rupture (Figure 29.7). This condition is called **appendicitis** and presents most often with right lower abdominal pain. Other associated symptoms may include poor appetite, nausea, and fever. Surgical removal of the appendix is necessary.

DIVERTICULITIS

Many people have small outpouchings of the large bowel called diverticuli. They are most commonly found in the descending colon located in the left side of the abdomen, although they can be found throughout the large intestine. If one of these diverticuli becomes obstructed, it can distend, become inflamed, and perforate similar to the process described in appendicitis (Figure 29.8). When diverticuli become diseased, the resulting condition is called **diverticulitis.** Patients with diverticulitis complain of abdominal pain and may notice red blood in their stool. Passage of bright red blood from the rectum is known as **hematochezia** and is usually indicative of a disease process in the lower gastrointestinal tract. Diverticulitis may require surgery in severe cases.

PANCREATITIS

One of the jobs of the pancreas is to secrete enzymes into the duodenum to aid in digestion. If the ducts that contain these digestive enzymes become blocked, they can become distended and result in inflammation of the organ. Inflammation of the pancreas is called **pancreatitis** and often results in severe upper abdominal pain and vomiting. Patients with pancreatitis can become quite ill and may require prolonged hospitalization.

GENITOURINARY

Although many disease processes involve the genitourinary tract, we discuss the more common acute conditions that might result in a call for EMS assistance.

KIDNEY STONES

As blood flows through the kidneys, salts and water are filtered out into the ureters as urine. Occasionally, particulate material crystallizes in the urine, resulting in a formed piece of solid material referred to as a *stone*. These **kidney stones** can become lodged in the ureter during attempted passage to the bladder. Severe flank pain is often experienced by the patient who has a renal stone that has become lodged in a ureter. Classically, the pain radiates along the anatomy of the genitourinary system—that is, from the flank to the groin. Vomiting is also common, and pain medications are crucial to the management of this condition. Although renal stones are not immediately life threatening, the pain can often be quite severe, and rapid transport is most appreciated by affected patients.

PYELONEPHRITIS

Infection of the urinary tract can involve the bladder alone or may ascend through the ureters into the kidneys, resulting in **pyelonephritis.** The kidneys are extremely well vascularized, and when bacteria infiltrate these organs, the risk for the infection spreading into the bloodstream is high.

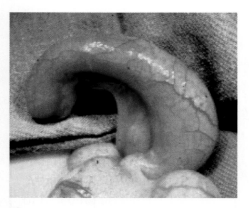

Figure 29.7 Definitive treatment for appendicitis is surgical removal of the inflamed appendix (Courtesy of the Division of Pediatric Surgery, Brown Medical School, Providence, RI)

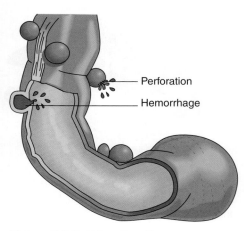

— Perforation

— Hemorrhage

Figure 29.8 Diverticuli can perforate or cause internal bleeding

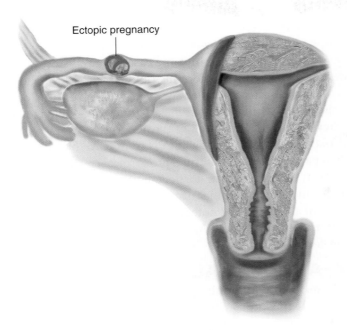

Figure 29.9 An ectopic pregnancy will rapidly outgrow the confines of the fallopian tube

Patients who have infections involving the kidneys may have pain over one or both flanks, vomiting, and high fever. This type of severe infection can result in significant morbidity and mortality if not rapidly treated with appropriate antibiotics. Patients with pyelonephritis may require hospitalization for intravenous antibiotic therapy.

ECTOPIC PREGNANCY

In a small percentage of pregnancies, implantation occurs outside the uterus. This is called an **ectopic pregnancy**; *ectopic* means "misplaced." The most common place for an ectopic pregnancy to occur is in a fallopian tube (Figure 29.9). As the pregnancy advances, the fallopian tube is not large enough to accommodate its occupant. Sometime between 6 and 12 weeks (often before some women realize they are pregnant) the fallopian tube becomes quite distended and is in danger of rupturing. If this should happen, the results would be catastrophic bleeding. For this reason, ectopic pregnancy is the second leading cause of maternal mortality in the United States. Early symptoms of this condition might be lower abdominal pain with or without vaginal bleeding in a woman of childbearing age. The woman may or may not realize she is pregnant so it is important for the EMT to consider the possibility of this life-threatening condition in any woman of childbearing age who complains of lower abdominal pain. Careful evaluation by a physician and sometimes surgical intervention is required. Ectopic pregnancy is further discussed in Unit 40.

VASCULAR

Several large blood vessels pass through the abdominal cavity. Disease within these vessels can result in abdominal pain or, in some cases, what patients perceive as back pain because the aorta and vena cava lie rather posteriorly in the retroperitoneal space.

ABDOMINAL AORTIC ANEURYSM

The abdominal aorta carries blood at arterial pressures out of the chest and to the abdominal organs and lower extremities. As a person ages, the structure of the arteries may change. In some cases, the walls of the vessels may become weakened, allowing a ballooning out to occur. This balloonlike widening of a weakened artery is called an *aneurysm*. When this occurs in the section of the aorta passing through the abdomen, it is called an **abdominal aortic aneurysm (AAA).** If the wall of the aneurysm becomes stretched thin enough, it may leak or rupture. This leads to massive bleeding and death if not rapidly repaired. Even with immediate surgical treatment, many patients who suffer from a rupture of an aortic aneurysm die. Typical symptoms of an AAA might include abdominal or back pain. If there has been any blood loss, evidence of shock may be noted. Syncope is not uncommon as the presenting concern with a ruptured AAA because of the rapid loss of blood and resultant profound shock.

EXTRA-ABDOMINAL

Some conditions can commonly cause the patient to feel abdominal pain when the pathology is not in the abdomen at all. These are referred to as *extra-abdominal sources* of abdominal pain, which result from shared sensory nerves between the diseased organ and the abdomen. The more common serious conditions that mimic an abdominal emergency are discussed next.

ACUTE CORONARY SYNDROME

Women and patients who suffer from diabetes are at higher risk than other populations to have atypical symptoms of an *acute coronary syndrome (ACS)*. These patients may not describe the chest pain and shortness of breath that are commonly associated with a heart problem. In fact, abdominal concerns are not uncommon as symptoms of ACS in these and other patients. The EMT must consider this potentially life-threatening diagnosis presenting with abdominal pain when a patient has risk factors for ACS. Appropriate management for this potential is crucial to decrease morbidity and mortality associated with this condition, discussed in detail in Unit 25.

PNEUMONIA

Fairly common in children and occasionally in adults, pneumonia can cause abdominal pain. Typically, the patient with pneumonia has some symptoms consistent with this respiratory infection, such as cough, fever, or difficulty breathing. Whereas the EMT may have been called for a patient with abdominal pain, if upon assessment the patient appears to be short of breath, appropriate action must be taken as outlined in Unit 26.

ASSESSMENT

The assessment of the patient complaining of abdominal pain will follow the principles of those for all patients with a focus on the history of the present illness and the patient's pertinent past medical history. As always, the first task is to perform a scene size-up and ensure the safety of the situation for the EMT and his team.

PRIMARY ASSESSMENT

The primary assessment is always completed following the scene size-up and must include the EMT's general impression following his initial view of the patient. It is important to take note of the environment as well as the appearance of the patient as the EMT approaches. The findings of the primary assessment will guide the remainder of the assessment. If the patient is responsive, the airway, breathing, and circulation are assessed and any immediate life threats are addressed appropriately.

Because many of the disease states that can cause abdominal pain can be life threatening, the EMT must assume that possibility and manage the patient as a high priority. The airway should be addressed as needed, and any necessary breathing assistance should be provided. Even when the patient is not having trouble breathing, supplemental oxygen should be applied in patients with abdominal pain, given the potential for shock. The patient's circulatory status should be assessed and managed as appropriate, with a focus on treating for any signs of hypoperfusion.

HISTORY

When the patient is able to provide the history of the present illness, the EMT should listen carefully to the events leading up to the call for EMS. Using the OPQRST acronym is helpful in gathering the history of the present illness.

Additionally, questions about the patient's past medical history following the SAMPLE format should be asked. If the patient is unable to provide this information, friends, family members, or bystanders should be briefly questioned.

In the unresponsive patient, most of this historical information will be obtained only after the EMT performs a rapid, focused physical assessment as detailed in Unit 19. If staffing permits, while the EMT performs this assessment, another member of the team can attempt to obtain historical details of the present illness from people nearby the patient.

SECONDARY ASSESSMENT

In the responsive patient, a focused physical exam should be completed after the primary assessment and history have been taken. In a patient with a concern of abdominal pain, the EMT should pay careful attention to the assessment of the abdomen. This assessment should include visual inspection and palpation.

Palpation of the abdomen should be done gently, beginning in an area farthest from the noted site of pain. The EMT should press down in each of the four quadrants of the abdomen. He should note the patient's response to pressure in each area. Tensing of muscles over an area of pain, called *guarding*, is worthy of note. Sometimes, the entire abdomen will feel tense, or rigid, when the intra-abdominal process is generalized. This finding of abdominal rigidity is also important to note. Any obvious masses felt during this examination should be documented carefully. It is important that one person only perform the abdominal palpation when possible. Repeated palpation of the abdomen in a patient complaining of abdominal pain is unnecessary and uncomfortable for the patient.

In the unresponsive patient, the EMT should perform a head-to-toe assessment as detailed in Unit 19, looking for any signs that might point to the reason for unresponsiveness. If it is known that the patient complained of abdominal pain prior to losing consciousness, careful attention should be paid to the abdominal exam during this rapid medical assessment.

VITAL SIGNS

The baseline and repeated measurement of respirations, pulse, and blood pressure can provide important information regarding the state of a patient's health. This should be done immediately after the rapid physical assessment

Street Smart

When a patient complains of abdominal pain, it is important to have her indicate with her own hand exactly where the pain is noted. This allows the examiner to avoid the painful area early on in the assessment. Immediately pressing on a painful area during an assessment may cause the patient such upset that the remainder of the assessment may be unreliable or difficult to complete.

in the unresponsive patient and may be accomplished after the focused physical exam in the responsive patient.

Because abdominal pain can be a symptom of several conditions that can lead to shock and hypoperfusion, careful attention to the vital signs will be paramount as the EMT assesses the patient for signs of shock. The measurement of orthostatic vital signs in the awake patient may be appropriate to assess for signs of hypovolemia. This measurement of blood pressure and heart rate in a supine and standing position is discussed in Unit 12.

MANAGEMENT

It is important to remember that there are many potential causes of abdominal pain and as many as 50% may go undiagnosed. Regardless of the cause, the principles of early management are the same in all cases. Some patients with abdominal pain may be profoundly ill upon presentation to EMS, others may be early in the course of their illness, and yet others may have a condition that is not life threatening. In any case, the EMT is responsible to thoroughly assess the patient and assume the potential for serious disease. Management of the airway, breathing, and circulation will be appropriate for any patient with abdominal pain during transport to definitive care.

TRANSPORT

Transport should be initiated as soon as it is possible during the previously described phases of assessment. It is important to maintain patients in whatever position they find most comfortable during movement and ambulance transport. Often in patients with abdominal pain, drawing the knees up toward the abdomen can be of comfort and should be allowed. The mode of transport and destination facility will be determined based on the patient presentation and local protocols.

In most patients with abdominal pain, ALS assistance would be of potential benefit, although transport should not be delayed. An intercept during transport would be appropriate, although the EMT should take note of local protocols regarding this issue. Additionally, early notification of the receiving facility will ensure that it is adequately prepared for the arrival of a potentially ill patient.

REASSESSMENT

As with any patient, it is important to continually observe for changes in assessment findings. As described in Unit 20, the key parts of the assessment should be repeated during the transport and any changes noted carefully and passed on to the receiving staff at the hospital.

CONCLUSION

The EMT will have multiple occasions to care for patients with the concern of abdominal pain. Some patients will be overtly ill with clear evidence of shock upon presentation. Others may not show physical evidence of hypoperfusion or have abnormal physical findings upon the initial examination. All patients with abdominal pain, no matter their initial presentation, have the potential for serious morbidity and mortality. The EMT must realize this and structure his management priorities around it.

CASE STUDY Continued

Jamal places Ashley on oxygen via NRB at 12 lpm as Daisy begins conducting her OPQRST and SAMPLE history. Ashley states she has been having a stomachache for a couple of days with some diarrhea, but today the pain got really bad and she began vomiting. She states it feels better to keep her knees bent and to lie still. Ashley says the pain became very sharp today and rates it a 9 on the 1/10 pain scale. The severe pain with nausea and vomiting has been going on for over an hour at this time.

As they place Ashley on the cot in a position of comfort, Ashley provides the rest of her SAMPLE history. Daisy documents that Ashley is on birth control pills, with her last menstrual period ending 1 week ago. She has an allergy to penicillin, has never experienced anything like this before, has had nothing to eat since the night before, and was sleeping when the pain started getting bad and woke her up.

Daisy determines Ashley may have appendicitis and needs to go to the hospital immediately. She calls for an ALS intercept based on local protocol and conducts a focused physical examination, noting tenderness of the right lower quadrant, radiating into the left side. Baseline vital signs are blood pressure of 118/70, pulse of 120, and respirations shallow at 22.

Upon arrival with the ALS service, Daisy provides a verbal report, turning patient care over to the ALS provider. As the medic establishes an IV, Daisy begins a reassessment, noting no significant change in Ashley's vital signs or pain.

Later that night as Daisy is leaving the hospital following another run, the ED nurse tells her that Ashley was immediately taken into surgery for a ruptured appendix and is recovering well at this time.

Key Concepts Revisited

- The EMT must have knowledge of the organ systems contained within the abdomen.
  - Gastrointestinal tract
    - Stomach
    - Small and large intestines
    - Liver
    - Gallbladder
    - Pancreas
  - Genitourinary system
    - Kidneys
    - Ureters
    - Bladder
  - Hematologic system
    - Spleen
    - Blood vessels
  - Male and female gonads lie outside the abdominal border but can lead to abdominal pain when disease occurs.

- The three types of abdominal pain are visceral pain, parietal pain, and referred pain.
  - Visceral pain is dull, achy, intermittent, and poorly localized pain directly related to an organ.
  - Parietal pain is sharp, intense, constant, localized pain related to irritation of the peritoneum.
  - Referred pain is visceral in nature, occurring in a part of the body away from the point of origin.

- Common diseases that may cause abdominal pain affect the gastrointestinal, genitourinary, vascular, and extra-abdominal systems:
  - Gastrointestinal
    - Peptic ulcer can produce severe bleeding and shock.
    - Esophageal varices can produce life-threatening hemorrhage when ruptured.
    - Gastroenteritis is a viral irritation of the stomach and intestines.

- Bowel obstruction can result in pain, vomiting, and distention.
- Gallbladder disease causes a blockage of bile flow that may result in inflammation and infection of the walls of the gallbladder.
- Appendicitis is the obstruction of the appendix that may rupture, causing a serious infection.
- Diverticulitis is inflammation of the diverticuli that may cause bleeding from the lower gastrointestinal tract.
- Pancreatitis is inflammation of the pancreas resulting in upper abdominal pain and vomiting.

  o   Genitourinary
- Renal stones are formed pieces of solid material causing flank pain when lodged in the ureter.
- Pyelonephritis is a severe infection of the kidneys that can result in significant morbidity and mortality if left untreated.
- Ectopic pregnancy occurs when the egg implants, usually in the fallopian tube, and can be life threatening if rupture occurs.

  o   Vascular
- An abdominal aortic aneurysm (AAA) leads to massive internal bleeding and death if a rupture or leak is not rapidly identified and surgically repaired.

  o   Extra-Abdominal
- Acute coronary syndrome and pneumonia are two extra-abdominal conditions that can cause abdominal pain.

- Abdominal pain may be a symptom of a variety of disease states that can lead to shock and hypoperfusion.
- The EMT should always treat concerns of abdominal pain as potentially life threatening and high priority.
- The management priorities for a patient with abdominal pain include a thorough assessment of the ABCs and transport to the appropriate hospital.

  o   An ALS intercept is necessary for life-threatening hypoperfusion as a result of internal bleeding and pain management.

  o   Reassessment should continue throughout transport, noting changes in condition to report to receiving facility.

Review Questions

1. What organs lie within each of the following abdominal quadrants?
   a. Right upper quadrant
   b. Left upper quadrant
   c. Right lower quadrant
   d. Left lower quadrant
2. What is the difference between visceral pain and parietal pain?
3. What is meant by referred pain?
4. What are some of the more common diseases affecting abdominal organs that may cause abdominal pain?
5. What is the definitive treatment for appendicitis?
6. What is the cause of renal stones?
7. Why is an abdominal aortic aneurysm potentially life-threatening?
8. What type of pain can be associated with an AAA?
9. Name two extra-abdominal conditions that can cause a concern of abdominal pain.
10. What type of assessment would be appropriate for the conscious patient experiencing abdominal pain?
11. What is the assessment technique used for the unconscious patient experiencing abdominal pain?
12. What are the management priorities for a patient with abdominal pain?

Key Terms

Abdominal aortic aneurysm (AAA)
Appendicitis
Bowel obstruction
Cholecystitis
Diverticulitis
Ectopic pregnancy
Esophageal varices
Gastroenteritis
Hematochezia

Hemetemesis
Kidney stone
Melena
Pancreatitis
Parietal pain
Pyelonephritis
Referred pain
Ulcer
Visceral pain

Further Study

Beebe, R., A. Scott, and E. Fong. *Functional Anatomy for Emergency Medical Services.* Clifton Park, NY: Thomson Delmar Learning, 2002.

UNIT (30) Bariatrics

Over half of Americans are either overweight or obese. It is likely that the Emergency Medical Technician (EMT) will care for an obese patient. With a little preplanning and preparation, the challenges that often arise during these patient encounters can be minimized.

National Education Standard

The Emergency Medical Technician (EMT) shall have a fundamental depth and foundational breadth of wellness principles, scene size-up, patient assessment, and lifting and moving patients as it applies to obese patients.

Key Concepts

- Obesity is an epidemic in the United States.

- Obesity has several definitions that are linked to health risk.

- The EMT will encounter patients with health risks associated with obesity.

- Treating a patient with obesity presents some challenges.

- Transfer and transportation of the patient with obesity requires care and special planning.

CASE STUDY

101 Magnolia Terrace. The address is familiar to Heather, a new EMT. A very large patient lives there, and the last time she called EMS, the fire department, the police department, and even the press showed up. The fire department had to take out the front window of the house to get the patient out. She simply couldn't fit through the doorway. It took time to reinforce load-bearing walls and move the pickup truck that eventually would transport her to the hospital, because she didn't fit into the back of the ambulance. An additional complication was that the patient had waited to call EMS until her symptoms were quite severe.

The police were on scene that day because the large crowd and presence of the television camera crews gave the scene a circus-like atmosphere. Who would want all that attention? Then Heather remembers how the patient cried on the way to the hospital, humiliated by the insensitive comments and embarrassed by the unwanted attention. She only wanted to get to the hospital so that

the doctor could treat the open sore on her ankle that wasn't healing with standard antibiotics. The wound had become grossly infected, and she was starting to go into septic shock.

Heather begins to think about what she might do differently for this patient. She knows the patient must be really sick to call EMS again, and Heather is determined to make this experience more pleasant for the patient.

Critical Thinking Questions

1. What are the special health risks associated with obesity?
2. What are the special transportation concerns associated with obesity?
3. What could be done differently to care for this patient?

INTRODUCTION

Obesity is second only to tobacco smoking as the leading cause of preventable death in the United States, and projections suggest that obesity among Americans is growing at an alarming rate. As these trends continue, EMS will be called to the scene of patients with obesity who are experiencing medical problems. Caring for and transporting these patients can be a problem for some EMS systems.

OBESITY DEFINED

Whenever a patent is 10% greater than his ideal weight, they are considered obese. Health problems typically do not arise from being a little overweight; in fact, a few extra pounds might even be healthy for some people. The problem is when a person's weight starts to have a negative impact on their health and on their activities of daily living. This is the best definition of obesity. Patients with potentially life-threatening weight-related health problems, or **morbidly obese** patients, have a specific set of health issues and will require the assistance of EMS with these health issues.

The branch of medicine that deals with the diagnosis and treatment of problems of obesity is called **bariatric medicine.** To help clinically define obesity, bariatric physicians have developed a classification system based on the body mass index (BMI). The **body mass index** is a system that takes into

Table 30-1 Obesity Scale Using Body Mass Index

- Underweight = <18.5
- Normal weight = 18.5–24.9
- Overweight = 25–29.9
- Obesity
  - Class I = BMI 30–35
  - Class II = BMI 35–40 (Malignant Obesity)
  - Class III = BMI 40–45 (Morbidly Obesity)
  - Class IV = BMI >40 (Super Morbidly Obese)

account not only patients' weight but their height as well. By simply plugging the patient's height and weight into a formula, the physician derives the BMI. Many Web sites have BMI calculators, in both metric and standard measurements, which an EMT can use to calculate BMI.

The normal BMI is between 20 and 25 and generally correlates with good health (see Table 30-1). Anyone with a BMI over 25 is considered overweight, and a BMI over 30 indicates obesity. Serious potentially life-threatening health problems occur when a patient has a BMI of more than 30. Depending on the patient's BMI, the obesity may be labeled morbid—that is, disease producing. Patients with a BMI between 40 and 45 are probably 100% over their ideal body weight and prone to specific ailments that will be discussed shortly.

Although the BMI tables can be helpful in determining risks associated with obesity, the tables tend to not represent patients who are muscular; these patients are over-lean, not overweight. Over-lean athletes may have lower blood pressures and better health than another individual who is merely overweight.

HEALTH RISKS AND OBESITY

Several diseases have been directly linked to obesity, including heart failure, a respiratory failure condition called Pickwickian syndrome, and hypertension. The risk for cancer increases by as much as one third in obese patients, with an increased risk for breast cancer among women and prostate cancer among men. The largest risks are probably cardiovascular complications leading to heart failure and type II diabetes.

The obese patient is at a threefold risk for becoming diabetic. An estimated two thirds of type II diabetes cases result from obesity. As the number of Americans who are obese increases, so does the number of patients with type II diabetes. Diabetes has several severe complications, including hypertension and blood vessel disease. The latter can progress to stroke or a silent heart attack; patients with diabetes often do not feel chest pain when having a heart attack, leading to the term *silent heart attack*. Patients with diabetes can also have eye problems, which can lead to blindness, and distal neuropathy of the feet that makes walking difficult. A neuropathy is loss of function of the nerves of the feet. Blindness and neuropathy, in turn, can lead to falls and injury.

Respiratory difficulties and respiratory failure are common complications of obesity. As a result of the increased body weight, the body demands more oxygen for the tissues. This demand results in both a faster respiratory rate and an increased heart rate. However, the lungs, trying to meet the demand, are impeded by the large mass of adipose tissue and are prevented from expanding. The large abdomen thus causes a functional restriction of the lungs, and the patient cannot adequately exhale. The trapped gases, containing carbon dioxide, remain in the lungs and blood.

The effect of increased levels of carbon dioxide on the brain is to cause drowsiness. This drowsiness can be seen in the excessive daytime somnolence, or sleeping, observed in obese patients. This phenomenon is described in Charles Dickens's novel *The Pickwick Papers*, which inspired the name for hypoventilation–obesity syndrome, or *Pickwickian syndrome*.

Finally, obesity puts a tremendous strain on the heart and cardiovascular system. It has been estimated that for every kilogram (2.2 pounds) of additional weight, the body must create approximately 25 miles of arterioles, venules, and capillaries, if laid end to end. The heart must create the extra pressure to create blood flowing through these blood vessels to maintain perfusion of the adipose tissue. This puts a tremendous strain on the heart to produce an adequate blood pressure. Initially the patient loses endurance and has trouble walking up even one flight of stairs without becoming short of breath. Eventually, the heart fails and the blood starts to back into the lungs and then the body in a syndrome called *heart failure*.

HISTORY AND PHYSICAL EXAMINATION

The obese patient may call EMS for a variety of reasons, but a common cause is a concern of shortness of breath. This shortness of breath may be due to heart failure. The EMT should take the normal history as she would for any patient with shortness of breath, paying special attention to gather the list of medications. Especially if the patient is on multiple medications, that list may offer a great deal of information about the patient's past medical history even if the patient cannot speak.

The EMT should also perform a standard medical examination. It may be difficult to examine the patient for signs of heart failure. The **body habitus,** the unique physical appearance that a patient possesses as a result of his disease, of the obese patient makes assessment difficult. For example, large folds of skin and pendulous breasts make listening for the crackles of pulmonary edema difficult. Similarly a short neck makes it difficult to see jugular venous distention, as shown in Figure 30.1. Even the telltale sign of heart failure, pedal edema, may result from peripheral vascular insufficiency and may be chronic.

VITAL SIGNS

Obtaining vital signs from a morbidly obese patient can be challenging. Pulses at the antecubital space at the elbow or even the carotid pulses are buried deep in the subcutaneous tissue and may be difficult to detect. In those cases the EMT will have to depend on the radial pulse. Even the radial pulse may have an overlying fold of skin.

Typically the patient's pulse will be fast. To maintain perfusion, the heart must beat faster and stronger. To make the heart beat faster and stronger, the body secretes epinephrine. The result is a persistent tachycardia.

Unfortunately, tachycardia is one of the earliest signs of hypoperfusion (shock). An EMT will not know if the patient's tachycardia is compensation for hypovolemia, or if it is normal for the patient, until the blood pressure drops as the patient decompensates and goes into shock. Therefore, the EMT must depend on the blood pressure.

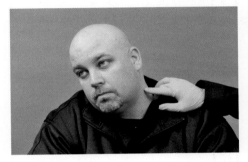

Figure 30.1 The short neck of an obese patient makes it difficult to assess jugular venous distention (JVD)

Cultural Considerations

An EMT may have a feeling of contempt for the obese patient, believing that the patient chooses to be obese. This weight bias is a form of prejudice that interferes with the patient–EMT relationship. The patient can do nothing about his or her weight at this time, and the EMT must focus on the patient's current problem.

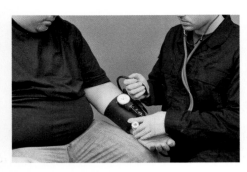

Figure 30.2 An alternative method of obtaining a blood pressure on the forearm

Standard blood pressure cuffs, even large adult sizes, may not fit around the patient's arm. The EMT may have to resort to using a thigh cuff on the arm. Alternatively, the EMT may elect to place a large adult blood pressure cuff on the forearm and place the stethoscope at the radial pulse, as shown in Figure 30.2. Too small a blood pressure cuff may give a falsely high blood pressure and the EMT should compare the blood pressure to the patient's condition. If the blood pressure is normal, but the patient appears lethargic, the blood pressure may be falsely high.

TREATMENT

The first priority in the treatment of the patient with obesity is to keep him sitting upright. These patients do not do well when lying flat. When supine obese patients become extremely short of breath, they may go into respiratory, then cardiac arrest.

If the patient is lethargic or drowsy, due to increased carbon dioxide levels, the EMT could consider inserting a nasopharyngeal airway (NPA). An NPA will slide behind the extra folds in flesh in the airway and help maintain a passage for ventilation. Without a patent airway the patient may experience periods of sleep apnea.

High-flow oxygen should be given to any patient who is lethargic or who has shortness of breath, regardless of the pulse oximeter reading. Some patients may be on home oxygen. The EMT needs to switch the patient over to high flow oxygen before beginning transportation. If the patient's mental status does not improve, or the patient is experiencing respiratory failure, the EMT needs to ventilate the patient with a bag-valve-mask assembly.

If the patient should go into cardiac arrest, the EMT should start cardiopulmonary resuscitation (CPR) while preparing the automated external defibrillator. External cardiac compressions may be more difficult than normal because of the thickness of the chest. Fortunately external landmarks are still easy to identify on the chest of the obese patient.

Defibrillation of an obese patient can also be a challenge. Defibrillation pads should be placed in the standard position. Large pendulous breasts may make placement of the lateral/apex/positive difficult. Alternatively, the patient can be logrolled and the defibrillation pad can be placed on the back just below the left scapula.

The exact energy required to defibrillate an obese patient is unknown. Therefore, the EMT should use the standard defibrillation energy until research indicates otherwise.

OBESITY AND TRAUMA

Although at first it might appear that obese patients would have more protection from blunt trauma, studies have shown that critically injured obese patients tend to experience more injury and death from trauma than patients of normal weight. Obese patients also have the same patterns of injury as other patients. Therefore, the standard of care for obese patients is no different than for other patients. These patients need to be assessed and treated according to their clinical presentation, keeping the mechanism of injury in mind.

When the EMT is assessing the scene of a motor vehicle collision (MVC) that involves an obese patient, the EMT should inspect the seatbelt. Many obese patients do not wear seatbelts because they are either uncomfortable or cannot securely fasten them. Those obese patients who do wear seatbelts may wear the seatbelt high across the abdomen instead of across the hips, where it is supposed to be worn. When a patient wearing the seatbelt high across the abdomen is involved in an MVC, the seatbelt tends to "catch" at the lower floating ribs and injure the liver and/or the spleen. This phenomenon, first seen during the 1960s, was called **lap belt syndrome.**

Treatment of the obese patient can be a problem. In the past an EMT would try to modify an adult device, such as a short board to fit small children. Now there is special pediatric equipment. Presently the EMT may have to adjust or adapt adult devices to fit the obese patient until special bariatric equipment is available. In some cases this is not always possible.

For example, the standard vest-style immobilization device may not have straps long enough to reach around the patient. In those cases the EMT may need to resort to a short board and attach 12-foot straps.

Transferring the patient from the short board to the long board may also be a problem. Standard backboards will support only approximately 300 pounds. Special heavy-duty backboards are available, but not every ambulance carries them. Furthermore, although a bariatric ambulance that carries the right equipment may be called to the scene, the standard of care for critically injured trauma patients is rapid transportation to definitive care within 10 minutes, not enough time for another ambulance to respond.

TRANSPORTATION

The greatest challenge to the EMT caring for a morbidly obese patient may be transportation. First the EMT must move the patient from the bed, or chair, or floor, to the stretcher. Lifting a 500-pound patient takes a minimum of six people working in unison. A misstep can result in a back injury for the EMT and trauma for the patient.

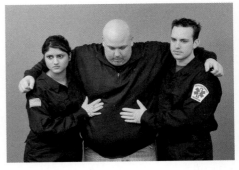

Figure 30.3 These EMTs are using the rescuer assist to help this obese patient walk

If possible, and medically advisable, the patient should be encouraged to self-lift with assistance. Using a "rescuer assist," the patient should sling one arm over two EMTs, one standing on either side of the patient, as shown in Figure 30.3. The EMTs then grasp the patient's wrist and simultaneously stand with the patient, remembering to lift with their legs and not with their back.

Another new lifting device called the *standing and raising aid* (SARA) device is being used to help lift patients up to 420 pounds so they may stand and pivot onto the stretcher.

If available, a mechanical lift that uses a sling device, such as the Hoyer lift, should be used. Although newer generations of these devices have greater weight limits, the device should never be used if the patient exceeds the weight limit or if the EMT is unfamiliar with its use.

Various devices are available to help move the patient from one level surface, such as a bed, to another level surface, such as the stretcher. One such device to help move a patient from a bed to the stretcher is the slide board. The slide board, shown in Figure 30.4, is a plastic or polyurethane flat panel. And although a slide board may look like a backboard, a slide board is not a backboard and is not capable of holding any amount of weight suspended in the air. Therefore, the two surfaces must be held closely together and no gap can exist between the bed and the stretcher. Another patient transfer device is the use of specially coated "slippery" sheets that reduce friction between the patient and the surface and allow EMTs to move the patient more easily.

Some companies have created special heavy-duty vinyl **transfer sheets,** reinforced with webbing, that are capable of holding a maximum weight of 1,600 pounds. These transfer sheets have multiple handles, 10 to 12, for many rescuers. However, the patient must lie flat on these transfer sheets. For this reason the transfer sheet should only be used as an interim device to get the patient to the stretcher, and the patient should be immediately be placed in high-Fowler's position.

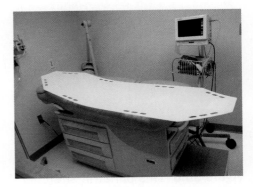

Figure 30.4 A slide board can make the transfer easier from bed to stretcher and stretcher to bed

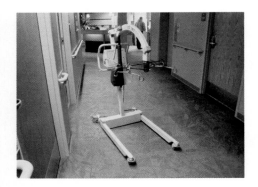

Figure 30.5 Pneumatic lift pads help elevate the patient to a height that allows a slide transfer onto the stretcher

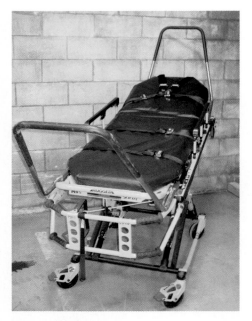

Figure 30.6 This bariatric stretcher has additional handholds for carrying a patient of 700 pounds or more

Other lifting devices in development or commercially available include airbag lift devices or **pneumatic lift pads.** These devices use inflatable air pillows or pads to lift the patient to an acceptable height for a flat transfer, as shown in Figure 30.5. The patient is logrolled onto the device and then the device's pads are inflated.

Moving a large patient can be dangerous, especially to the unorganized team of responders. Some EMS systems have developed special **lift teams,** modeled after hospital lift teams. These teams are specially trained in proper lifting techniques and practice lifting safely. Often members of these teams have special lumbar braces to help to protect their backs. These teams are called to respond to the scene whenever lifting assistance is requested.

Another challenge is the transport of patients living up a flight(s) of stairs, without elevator access. Although stairs may support 300, 400, or even 500 pounds, most stairs will not support the combination of the patient's weight and the weight of the rescuers. Creative alternatives must be considered.

Some EMS systems resort to using technical high rescue equipment, such as Stokes baskets and rope with pulley systems to lower the patient. The difficulty with this approach is that the patient must lie flat to be transported. Many patients who are morbidly obese cannot tolerate lying flat. A suddenly panicked patient, gasping for breath, who sits up in a Stokes basket while it is being lowered can destabilize the entire rigging and cause the patient to fall.

Another common obstacle is the doorway. Most doorways are not designed to be wide enough to accommodate the patient and rescuers. It may be necessary to remove walls and create new passageways. This type of rescue requires special knowledge of building construction and the participation and assistance of experts from an urban search and rescue team (USAR).

With the patient out of the house, the patient should be transferred to an ambulance. However, some ambulances may not have the size or capacity to accommodate the morbidly obese patient. The average floor space of the modular ambulance is 40 to 44 inches; a van ambulance is 4 to 8 inches narrower. A 700-pound patient may be 50 to 55 inches across and would not fit into that narrow space.

The next challenge is the ambulance stretcher itself. Standard ambulance stretchers are rated to carry only 450 pounds. Newer model stretchers, called **bariatric stretchers,** as shown in Figure 30.6, may carry up to 700 pounds in the elevated position and up to 1,100 pounds in the lowest position. However, a morbidly obese patient, with equipment including oxygen tanks may by greater than 700 pounds.

Another advantage of bariatric stretchers are extra handholds for additional rescuers. If these additional handholds are used, the EMT should remember to use the power grip when lifting. In some cases the standard stretcher strap will not be long enough to go around the patient's torso. The use of 12-foot straps, or additional extension straps, may be necessary to secure the patient to the stretcher. It is important to secure the patient to the stretcher to prevent shifting of the patient off the stretcher during routine traffic.

Next the patient must be transferred into the ambulance. There are three systems to move the patient into the ambulance. The first is the ramp system. Some EMS services use folding ramps, the same type used to transfer motorcycles onto a flat bed truck or trailer, which can be placed in the backboard compartment. Other services have gone to a ramp and winch system. These systems depend on a strap and ring apparatus attached to the stretcher's frame that is attached to a cable. The cable is part of an electronic winch system, such as might be found on the front of an off-road rescue truck. The final system is a tail-lift system similar to the type of tail-lift used by delivery trucks. Each of these systems has its advantages and disadvantages, but all help the EMT move the patient with minimal effort.

Ambulances also have limitations on their payload. The average payload allowance is 1,500 to 1,750 pounds, without equipment. With a 700-pound patient and two EMTs, each weighing 200 pounds, plus all of the equipment stored and carried into the ambulance, it is possible that the ambulance could be overloaded. An overloaded ambulance can be dangerous, especially if being driven at high speeds around bends or coming to a sudden stop.

Many EMS services have developed a special bariatric response unit, like the one shown in Figure 30.7, accompanied by a special lift team, to calls involving a morbidly obese patient. Because these special ambulances, stretchers, and personnel are expensive, many EMS services that support these special operations offer their service to other systems as mutual aid.

As with EMS, hospitals are mandated to meet the challenges of treating the morbidly obese patient. Hospitals have obtained special bariatric equipment and prepared special rooms. It is important that the EMT alert the hospital at the earliest convenience so that the hospital can prepare for the arrival of the patient.

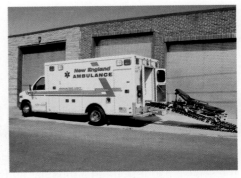

Figure 30.7 This bariatric ambulance, with a ramp and winch system, is specially designed to convey the morbidly obese patient to the hospital (Courtesy of New England Ambulance Service)

CONCLUSION

The morbidly obese patient presents special challenges to the EMT. In many cases EMS is not ready to care for these special patients. While EMS retools to meet this new demand, the EMT will need to rethink answers to problems on scene. With proper preparation and persistence, the EMT can provide high-quality patient care to this particularly vulnerable patient population.

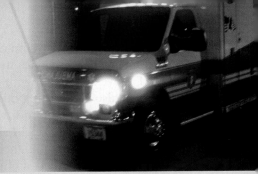

CASE STUDY Continued

Since the last time EMS had been at 101 Magnolia Terrace the service had retrofitted a modular ambulance with a bariatric stretcher that is hoisted into the ambulance with a winch and ramp system. The crew bench has been removed and the captain's chair moved toward the center.

The house has also been remodeled, thanks to some money from the health insurance provider, and a wide ramp has been placed in front of the house that leads to a widened doorway.

Stepping out of the ambulance with the special "barry bag," Heather feels strongly that she can treat and transport this patient with compassion while maintaining the patient's dignity.

Key Concepts Revisited

- Obesity is an epidemic in United States and the second leading cause of preventable death.
- Obesity is defined by body mass index and divided into classes.
- Common health risks associated with obesity include respiratory failure, heart failure, and diabetes.
- Obese patients present unique challenges to assessment.
- Standard equipment may not work in assessing and treating obese patients.
- EMS may need to retool to safely care for obese patients.

Review Questions

1. What is the definition of obesity?
2. What are the major health risks for obesity?
3. What is the difficulty with tachycardia in obese patients?
4. What alternative method can an EMT use to obtain a blood pressure on an obese patient?
5. What happens when the obese patient retains carbon dioxide?
6. Do obese patients experience less death and disability from motor vehicle collisions?
7. What are some of the challenges of transferring a morbidly obese patient to an ambulance?
8. What are some devices that help the EMT transfer the patient to the ambulance?
9. What are some ambulance-specific problems of transporting a morbidly obese patient?
10. What are three approaches to loading the obese patient into the ambulance?

Key Terms

Bariatric medicine

Bariatric stretchers

Body habitus

Body mass index

Lap belt syndrome

Lift teams

Morbidly obese

Pneumatic lift pads

Transfer sheets

Further Study

Beebe, R., and A. J. Heightman. "Handle with Care: Specialized Methods and Devices for Moving Morbidly Obese Patients." *Journal of Emergency Medical Services (JEMS)* 27, no. 1 (January 2002): 31–34, 48, 98–99.

Brunette D. D. "Resuscitation of the Morbidly Obese Patient." *American Journal of Emergency Medicine* 22, no. 1 (2004): 40–47.

Grant, P., and M. Newcombe. "Emergency Management of the Morbidly Obese." *Emergency Medicine Australasia* 16, no. 4 (2004) 309–317.

Zezima, Katie. "Increasing Obesity Requires New Ambulance Equipment." *New York Times*, April 8, 2008.

UNIT (31) Rashes and Fevers

The increasing prevalence of diseases such as SARS and MRSA and the looming specter of a flu pandemic make it more important than ever that Emergency Medical Technicians (EMTs) know how to respond to potentially infectious patients and be able to interface with public health to respond quickly and effectively to an outbreak.

National Education Standard
The Emergency Medical Technician (EMT) will have a simple understanding of the principles of illness prevention to emergency care and a simple depth and simple breadth of understanding of the assessment and management of the patient who may have contracted an infectious disease.

Key Concepts

- Diseases caused by common microorganisms occur through the chain of infection.

- The prodrome for infection can include a fever and rash.

- Infection control is a process that decreases infections for the EMT and the patient.

- EMS and the EMT play a key role the public health response to infectious disease.

CASE STUDY

"A – 3 – 0 – 4, respond to the King's Arms adult community residence for a report of a person with a fever, time out 13:10 hours," crackles the radio. Myra turns to her partner Malinda and asks if she remembers the last time they responded to a report of a person with a fever. The doctors had trouble finding the source of the infection and diagnosed the patient with a "fever of unknown origin." Later, when Myra and Malinda returned to the same hospital with another case of "fever of unknown origin," they learned the patient was also diagnosed with methicillin resistant staphylococcus (MRSA).

Malinda was concerned about what MRSA was and the associated dangers. She has a newborn at home and doesn't want her baby to become sick from something she contracts at work. She understands the risks for infection working in EMS and always diligently uses standard precautions. She also always washes her hands with waterless antiseptic after removing her gloves and washes her hands with soap and water after every patient contact.

Malinda becomes more concerned when she hears that if she has contracted MRSA, she could infect other patients, particularly the elderly. Malinda prides herself on her compassionate care of the elderly and the idea that one of her patients could become sick, even die, because she took care of them makes her sick to her stomach.

Myra, on the other hand, is starting to put one plus one together. This is the fourth case of fever that they have transported from King's Arms adult community residence. Is this a coincidence, or do they have an outbreak on their hands? Myra knows that early reporting of an outbreak to the county's public health department may help limit the number of cases of infection and may even save a life. Myra understands how vulnerable the elderly are to infection and the need for all health care providers to maintain a high index of suspicion about the potential for communicable disease in a communal living arrangement such as King's Arms adult community residence.

Myra understands that early intervention during an outbreak of a communicable disease can prevent needless suffering. As the saying goes, "An ounce of prevention is better than a pound of cure."

Arriving on scene Myra and Malinda enter the building and are escorted by a community aide to the patient's room. While walking with the stretcher, Malinda, who is going to be the "contact" EMT—that is, the EMT speaking to and caring for the patient—dons her gloves. The aide explains that the patient is covered in a strange rash. Both Malinda and Myra stop in their tracks.

Critical Thinking Questions

1. Why is a rash of concern?
2. What are the potentially dangerous causes of rash?
3. What diseases could EMTs bring home to their family?

INTRODUCTION

An EMT may be called to the scene of a patient with a concern of either a rash or a fever of unknown origin (FUO). A rash or a fever can be harmless, but they can also be an indication of a much more serious condition such as a potentially life-threatening infection. The key is differentiating between a relatively minor health problem and a condition that puts the patient and others at grave risk. This unit is an overview of conditions that can cause rashes and fevers and those dangerous conditions that are of concern to an EMT.

Floods and earthquakes disrupt the operations of essential public health services, such water treatment and sanitary sewers. During these disasters the incidence of infection from protozoa, for example, can increase unless preventive, or prophylactic, infection control measures are taken.

MICROBES

Infections are caused by life forms that are not visible to the naked eye. These microscopic life forms are called microbes. The world is teeming with these microbes, and many live within the human body without causing harm; there are literally trillions of these microorganisms within the human body. But occasionally a microbe will enter the body and then work against the body. These microbes are *pathogens,* or disease-causing microbes.

Because of the large number of microbes in the world, scientists divide them into classifications according to some simple criteria so that they can study them. Microbes are classified as worm, fungi, protozoa, bacteria, virus, or prion. Worms are the largest of the microbes. In some cases worms can become large enough to be seen by the naked eye, but most are microscopic. In the next class of microbes, fungi are multicelled microorganisms. Athlete's foot is an example of a fungus. Fungi can survive unfavorable conditions by creating hard encapsulated spores that can be difficult to destroy. This makes treating athlete's foot somewhat of a challenge.

The next classification of microbes is protozoa. These single-cell micro-organisms are mobile and can migrate within the body. These cells form cysts to protect themselves. The body has effective defense mechanisms against worms, fungi, and protozoa, but occasionally the body's defenses become overwhelmed and an infection occurs.

Worms, fungus, and protozoa can all cause infections. However, modern sanitary practices, including water treatment and sanitary sewers, have markedly decreased the number of infections caused by these three classes of microbes. The final three classifications are more traditionally considered the disease-causing microbes: bacteria, viruses, and prions.

Bacteria are single-cell microorganisms that live in a **symbiotic** or interdependent relationship with the body. Most of the time this relationship is mutually beneficial to both the host, in this case the person, and the parasite, or bacteria. In fact, humans depend on certain bacteria to produce by-products for survival. Both helpful and harmful bacteria can exist in the body at the same time. These two groups of bacteria compete for the same food sources and therefore keep each other in check, a phenomenon called *competitive inhibition.* But that balance can be upset, by a new strain of bacteria, for example, or the use in antibiotics that kill off "friendly" bacteria. An overgrowth of pathogenic bacteria may result, and infection occurs. The body's immune system responds to these infections and tries to limit the infection.

Several potentially life-threatening problems can occur if the body is overwhelmed with these bacteria. The infection can attack the blood vessels, and the blood vessels can become damaged and "leaky." As a result, fluid seeps out of the blood into the tissues; this phenomena is called **edema.** An example of edema due to an infection is shown in Figure 31.1. As the edema accumulates, and the patient's blood volume is lost, blood pressure decreases, hypoperfusion occurs, and the patient goes into septic shock.

Viruses are smaller than bacteria and are true parasites. Given the right food, bacteria can survive outside of the body; a virus cannot. A virus is not capable of supporting itself without a host. To survive, a virus enters into a cell within the host's body and reprograms the cell's DNA to produce more of the virus. Thus, the virus multiplies. For example, if the cell is a heart muscle cell, or a myocardial cell, as more and more myocardial cells become infected and dysfunctional, they cannot perform their function of pumping blood. This type of viral infection would be called myocarditis and can be life threatening. In some cases of myocarditis, the patient's only hope for survival is a heart transplant.

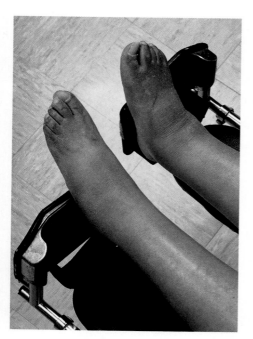

Figure 31.1 Peripheral edema as a sign of infection and/or inflammation

The final class of microbes are the prions. A prion is a protein that can alter its shape and cause a variety of diseases. This is a newly discovered microorganism and is thought to be the cause of mad cow disease and other neurologic diseases. Relatively little is known about prions at this time.

CHAIN OF INFECTION

For an infection to occur, certain essential conditions must exist. These conditions are called the **chain of infection** (Figure 31.2). The chain of infection consists of three parts: reservoir, transmission, and host.

For infection to begin, there must be a source, called the **reservoir,** within which the microbe resides. Common reservoirs for infection can be water, food, and animals. Many animals have the same or similar diseases as humans. These diseases that humans have in common with animals are called **zoonoses**. Table 31-1 lists just a few of the common zoonoses.

For a disease to spread, it must be *contagious,* or able to be spread from animal to person or person to person. Some diseases are spread by contact with a contaminated surface, called a **fomite.** The surface may be contaminated with stool, from unwashed and soiled hands, or from droplets raining on the surface after a sneeze. Sometimes a go-between helps transmit the disease, such as a mosquito. These disease-laden animals that infect other animals are called *vectors*. Other examples of vectors include fleas, which transmit the plague, and ticks, which transmit Lyme disease or Rocky Mountain Spotted Fever. A vector is not infected by the disease; it simply acts as a carrier.

The patient who comes in contact with a vector may be contaminated by a contagious disease (Figure 31.2). Whether the target of an infection, called the **host,** becomes infected is a function of the host's resistance to disease. The host's resistance is the ability of nonspecific defenses, such as the skin and mucous membranes, to keep the disease out for the body. Certain patient populations are at greater risk for infection than others. For example, infants enjoy the immunity passed from their mother through the first breast milk, called *colostrum,* but that immunity is only temporary until the infant's own immune system develops. Another population at risk is the elderly, whose immune system has weakened after years of fighting infections. Adults can be at risk, too. Adults with leukemia or human immunodeficiency virus (HIV) and alcoholic patients can be at greater risk of contracting a contagious disease. An EMT is at greater risk because he may encounter infected patients with a communicable disease on a daily basis. The EMT can protect

Table 31-1 Zoonoses	
Zoonosis and Vector	
1. Anthrax	sheep
2. Bovine tuberculosis	cows
3. Ebola fever	monkeys
4. Distemper	dogs
5. Influenza	pigs
6. Rabies	bats
7. Toxoplasmosis	cats

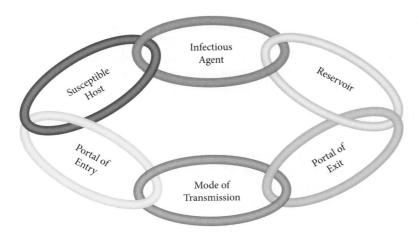

Figure 31.2 The chain of infection from reservoir to host

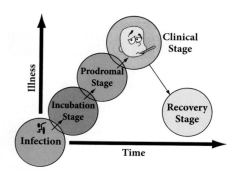

Figure 31.3 The stages of an infection

himself from disease through hand washing and barrier devices, as discussed in Unit 8.

STAGES OF INFECTION

As a microbe enters the body and overwhelms its defenses, it becomes an infectious disease. The life cycle of an infection has four phases: incubation, prodrome, infirmity, and convalescence. These stages can overlap, as shown in Figure 31.3. At the end of an infection the patient is either cured, becomes a carrier, or is overwhelmed by the infection and dies.

The incubation period is that period of time from when the microbe enters the body to when the first symptoms appear. Therefore, a patient can be infected—that is, have the microbe in her body—and be asymptomatic, or without symptoms. These patients are considered to be **subclinical,** or without symptoms that can be detected in a physical exam.

The next period is called the **prodrome.** The prodrome starts when the patient suspects that she is sick. The initial symptoms are often nonspecific; that is, they do not indicate any specific disease. Examples of nonspecific signs are fever, headache, **anorexia** (absence of appetite), and general weakness.

The next phase is infirmity. **Infirmity** is that stage when the patient becomes grossly symptomatic with all of the signs and symptoms specific for that disease. In this stage, the patient may be incapacitated by the disease. It is during this period of time that the infection reaches its peak, called its **acme,** and the patient is either overwhelmed by the infection and dies or survives the infection.

If the patient survives the infection, the body starts to recover and repair itself. This period of time is called **convalescence.** During this recovery period, the patient can either recover completely or be left with complications resulting from the infection. For example, the patient may survive polio but be left crippled and unable to walk for the rest of her life.

Sometime between the incubation and convalescent period, the patient is able to spread the infection to others. This period of time is called the *communicable* period. Some diseases, such as diphtheria, can be transmitted immediately. Other times the disease remains in the patient's body, even after recovery. Patient who are still infected but are asymptomatic for a disease are called *carriers.* Carriers can still infect others.

DISEASES ASSOCIATED WITH RASH AND FEVER

Although an EMT is not expected to remember all of the different infectious diseases, these conditions generally can be grouped into three general categories: diseases that cause upper respiratory infections, infectious diseases that cause urinary tract infections, and infectious diseases that cause skin infections. A simple mnemonic to remember these is PUS, for pulmonary, urinary, and skin. An infection in any of these three areas can cause a rash and/or a fever.

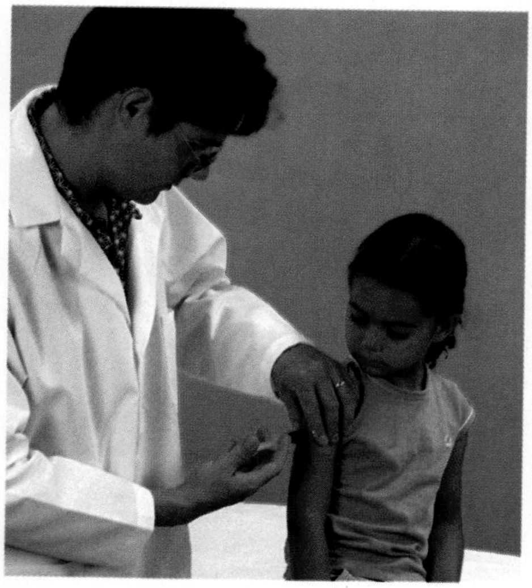

RASHES

Initially, many patients experience nonspecific signs of an impending illness during the prodrome phase. The appearance of a rash confirms that the patient has an infectious disease. Many of these infections can be prevented by immunizations. For example, an MMR immunization prevents mumps, measles, and rubella. Figure 31.4 shows a child receiving a preschool immunization to prevent infection.

Many of these so-called childhood infections are self-limiting, meaning that the disease runs its natural course without any long-term ill effects

Figure 31.4 A child receiving a preschool immunization

on the patient, and the patient recovers without medical intervention. It is unusual for a family to call EMS for these infections. One exception is an infection resulting in excessive itching.

An accompanying symptom of many of these infectious diseases is an intense itching sensation called **pruritus.** To help relieve this symptom, some patients may take medications such as diphenhydramine (trade name Benadryl) or use ameliorants such as calamine lotion. Many patients simply scratch the itch—despite warnings to avoid scratching the skin. As a result secondary bacterial infections can occur. This interruption in the skin, the first defense against disease, can lead to systemic infection, and the patient can become very ill.

Although a rash can be a sign of an infectious disease and the EMT should take precautions to prevent getting infected, some rashes are not due to an infection. For example, a simple allergy to laundry soap can cause a rash but is not infectious. The difference between an infectious rash and an allergic rash is the existence of other signs of infection, such as a fever, cough, or runny nose. It is possible for a child to have an allergic reaction and a cold at the same time. When in doubt, the EMT should wear personal protective equipment (PPE).

One rash-like symptom, called *hives*, is not a sign of infection, but of a severe allergic reaction. Figure 31.5 shows an illustration of hives. One way to distinguish hives from a rash is the speed of onset: Whereas rash may appear gradually, hives appear quickly and are generally not associated with a fever.

The appearance of hives is a warning to watch out for more serious symptoms of a severe allergic reaction, or anaphylaxis. The EMT should listen to the patient's throat for signs of constriction, called *stridor* (the patient may complain that her throat feels tight), and the lungs for signs of bronchoconstriction, or wheezing. The combination of hives and either stridor or wheezes indicates a medical emergency. Anaphylaxis is discussed further in Unit 39.

MENINGITIS

Some childhood infections, such as mumps, can infect the covering that overlies the brain, called the *meninges*. An infection of the meninges, called **meningitis,** can be life threatening. Meningitis can lead to swelling of the brain and increased intracranial pressure (ICP). Increased ICP in a head injury can lead to traumatic brain injury and long-term disability and death. Increased ICP resulting from meningitis is equally dangerous.

The three signs characteristic of a disease, called a **triad,** for meningitis are a severe headache; **photophobia,** or an abnormal sensitivity to light; and and a stiff and painful neck called **nuchal rigidity.** This triad of symptoms accompanied by a high fever is referred to as meningeal signs. When meningeal signs are discovered, the EMT should take immediate steps to protect himself. Whereas most cases of meningitis are viral in origin and typically run their course without long-term harm to the patient, a bacterial infection can cause meningitis. Bacterial meningitis can be lethal in less than 24 hours.

Therefore, whenever meningitis is suspected, the EMT should use appropriate PPE such as gloves and a mask that will protect against inhalation of airborne particles. As meningitis is passed by droplet, an oxygen mask on the patient will suffice to decrease the particles exhaled into the environment. If the patient cannot tolerate an oxygen mask, or oxygen is not needed, then a simple paper surgical mask is sufficient.

It is important that the EMT report his suspicions of meningitis or other infectious disease when he arrives at the hospital or, even better, radio the report ahead to the intended facility. The hospital may want to isolate the patient in a special room to prevent further infection and clear the halls of small children and pregnant women.

A rash without an accompanying fever and other signs of infection may be due to scabies. As the mite burrows under the skin, it lays eggs, which cause an allergic reaction leading to intense pruritus. Scabies are often found along the beltline, on the genitals, and at joints such as arm pits, elbows, and the webs of the fingers.

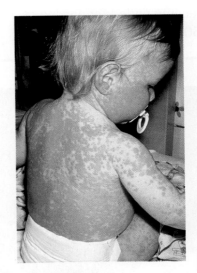

Figure 31.5 Hives

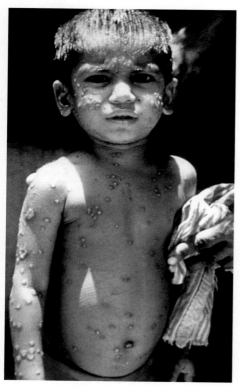

Figure 31.6 Smallpox

After transporting a patient with a possible infection, the EMT should ensure that the hospital has his name and a means to contact him. The EMT should also notify the EMS infection control officer (ICO) or other designated officer of his suspicions. Many EMS services require a special report for suspected contact with an infectious patient. In every case the EMT should follow the agency policy on possible exposure to infection.

SPECIAL CASE OF SMALLPOX

Smallpox is a deadly disease that was thought to be eradicated by a worldwide immunization program in the latter half of the last century. The concern is that there may be a reservoir of smallpox someplace in the world and that terrorists could seize on the opportunity to infect a whole new generation of people who are not immunized against smallpox. There is more discussion of the use of infectious disease as weapons of mass destruction in Unit 51, *The Emergency Response to Terrorism.*

Smallpox looks very similar to its cousin chickenpox, and the unsuspecting EMT may be the first person to encounter a smallpox infection. One key difference between smallpox and chickenpox is the distribution of the blisters. Tiny blisters, called the **pox,** contain fluid loaded with virus and form on the surface of the skin. In the case of chickenpox the pox are primarily found on the chest and face, whereas in the case of smallpox, these blisters are most frequent on the hands and feet. Figure 31.6 shows a picture of smallpox.

INFLUENZA

In the United States between 5% and 20% of the population will contract the flu each year and almost everyone has the flu at one time or another. Flu symptoms include fever, chills, sore throat, and muscle aches. Patients with the flu generally feel weak, experience general malaise, and feel quite ill. As many as 200,000 patients are hospitalized annually with complications from the flu, and approximately 36,000 people die, primarily the elderly.

In recent years, government and public health agencies have been preparing for a widespread flu outbreak, like the flu that caused the pandemic of 1918. Killing between 20 million and 40 million people worldwide, the "Spanish flu of 1918" quickly spread from its suspected American origin in Kansas around the world as a result of World War I. A new flu, called the avian flu, is found primarily in birds but has the potential of crossing the "species barrier" and infecting humans. Avian flu would then be an example of zoonoses.

Both wild birds and domestic chickens and turkeys can shed the virus in their saliva and pass it along from bird to bird, but there are very few cases of bird-to-human infection. Currently the avian virus has not mutated into a highly contagious form of influenza. In the event that such a change in the flu virus occurs, many people would become sick and EMS systems could be overwhelmed.

In April 2009, a new flu virus of swine origin was first detected, with a serious outbreak occurring in Mexico that included several deaths. The Novel influenza A (H1N1) virus was spread from person-to-person, with a growing outbreak occurring throughout the United States and a number of cases also reported internationally. H1N1 spread in the same manner that regular seasonal influenza viruses spread: through the sneezes and coughs of the infected individuals. Because it is a new virus, most people had no immunity to it, possibly making the illness more serious and widespread. Many schools were closed in areas where cases were confirmed in an attempt to keep the virus from spreading. The H1N1 virus prompted many communities, hospitals, and EMS services to review and in some areas activate their pandemic flu action plan.

EMS OUTBREAK RESPONSE

In the event of an outbreak of contagious avian flu or smallpox, EMS systems would be called to respond. To ensure an organized response, many public health departments and emergency services have developed response plans. Part of preparedness planning is stockpiling emergency provisions such as food reserves in the form of meals ready to eat (MRE), water purification systems, and medical supply stockpiles. Medical supplies in the stockpile would include N95 masks, for example.

The first step of an emergency response plan is early detection. An early response permits public health authorities to limit the spread of the contagious disease. Public health authorities have established surveillance systems that monitor for reports of infected patients. Many of these reports consist of concerns of flu-like symptoms; when a cluster of reports occur, health authorities suspect an outbreak and investigate.

EMS is part of that surveillance system. Sometimes an outbreak is discovered by emergency medical dispatchers. In the course of their interrogation, the dispatchers may note that there are numerous reports of fever and flu-like symptoms. Likewise an EMT might note that he has transported several family members or neighbors from the same location with the same or similar symptoms.

The first responsibility of an EMT at the onset of any suspected outbreak is self-protection. The first step of self-protection is obtaining and maintaining up-to-date immunizations. This may include vaccines against the flu, such as Flumist® or other prepared flu vaccines.

Next, on scene, the EMT should use appropriate body substance isolation, including gloves, masks, goggles, and even a gown in appropriate circumstances. The use of these barrier devices and hand washing are explained in Unit 7. The importance of hand washing cannot be overemphasized. Many diseases are spread by contact. Contamination on the EMT's hands may result in self-infection if he inadvertently rubs his eyes or handles food with his bare hands before eating. These are common potential routes of infection. For this reason most EMS systems prohibit eating food, drinking beverages, and applying cosmetics in the ambulance. The EMT should also avoid handling contact lenses without first washing his hands.

In the case of a flu epidemic, extraordinary measures may be needed to prevent further spread of the disease. For example, many ambulances have a team of EMTs who switch roles as attendant and as driver. In the case of a flu epidemic it would be wise to choose only one of the two EMTs to be the attendant. This would reduce the risk of exposure by 50%. Further contamination can be prevented by closing the intercompartment door.

The EMT should use the exhaust fans to keep the patient compartment air moving and wear an appropriate mask. It is also advisable to place a mask on an infected patient. If the patient cannot tolerate an oxygen mask, then a paper surgical mask can be used as an alternative.

Some experts recommend that EMTs should "double glove" to decrease the chance of exposure and immediately use waterless sanitizers after removing the gloves. EMTs are also advised to wear eye protection, such as goggles; corrective eye glasses alone do not provide sufficient protection from infection. If possible, they should avoid cough-producing treatments, such as suctioning and small volume nebulizers, unless absolutely necessary. When the driver assists with patient care, the driver should use the same barrier devices, including double gloves and mask and eye protection.

PUBLIC HEALTH RESPONSE

The key strategy in an epidemic is containment of the disease to a small population of patients. It would be difficult to confine these patients to hospitals, as most hospitals normally operate at or near capacity with limited ability to accept more patients. In other words, hospitals have a small **surge capacity,** which refers to the ability of a health care system, including EMS, to care for a sudden increase in the number of patients.

Public health authorities and EMS systems might have to resort to commandeering hotels and other such facilities to house and confine patients. Or they might elect to take a protect-in-place philosophy. Quarantine is an example of a protect-in-place approach to preventing the spread of a contagious disease.

Strict quarantine that does not permit the patient to leave the residence is difficult to enforce. More likely, especially in the early phases of an epidemic, will be movement restrictions. Movement restrictions prevent potentially contagious persons from traveling outside of the area. Public authorities may also close down mass transportation and institute **social distancing** by closing schools and banning mass public gatherings such as church services. Social distancing serves to limit the number of people coming in contact with an infected person.

The next step in the public health response will be to identify a vaccine for the disease. As vaccine becomes available, the first step is to inoculate the citizens immediately surrounding the area where infection is prevalent, called *ring vaccination,* followed by a mass vaccination of the remaining public. It is anticipated that EMS systems will be involved with supporting public health officials with this vaccination process.

CONCLUSION

Although most patients with a fever and rash have simple viral illnesses, these concerns could indicate a potentially deadly infection. Whenever an EMT encounters a patient with either a fever or a rash, he should take precautions to protect himself. The time to find out that the EMT may have been exposed to a potentially deadly disease and should have protected himself is not after the call.

CASE STUDY Continued

Myra and Malinda elect to take extra precautions after hearing about the rash. They double glove and put on masks as well. Entering the dark apartment, they look at each other with a knowing glance. This may be meningitis. Myra turns to the community aide and asks if she could please get a list of everyone who has been in contact with the patient and make a list, being sure to add herself.

Key Concepts Revisited

- Microbes, such as bacteria and viruses, can cause serious and deadly disease.
  - Worm
  - Fungi
  - Protozoa
  - Bacteria
  - Viruses
  - Prion
- A chain of infection between the reservoir containing the microbe and the human host must exist for an infection to occur.
- An infection within the patient enters into various stages, some clinically apparent while others are not.

  - Incubation
  - Prodrome
  - Infirmity
  - Convalenscence
- A rash can indicate the presence of a potentially infectious disease, and the EMT should take precautions.
- An EMT must take special actions during an outbreak to prevent the further spread of the disease.
- EMS and the EMT will be part of the public health response to any outbreak as part of identification and preventing the spread of the disease.

Review Questions

1. What are the six classifications of infectious microbes?
2. How can a person die from an infection?
3. What are the elements of the chain of infection?
4. How are diseases passed along from one person to another?
5. What are the stages of a disease?
6. What are some infectious and noninfectious causes of a rash?
7. What is the triad of symptoms of meningitis?
8. What are the differences and similarities between chickenpox and smallpox?
9. What are some extraordinary measures that an EMT might take at the first sign of an outbreak of influenza, for example?
10. What are some public health techniques used to reduce the spread of infection?

Key Terms

Acme

Anoxeria

Chain of infection

Convalescence

Edema

Fomite

Host

Infirmity

Meningitis

Nuchal rigidity

Photophobia

Pox

Prodrome

Pruritus

Reservoir

Shingles

Social distancing

Subclinical

Surge capacity

Symbiotic

Triad

Zoonoses

Further Study

For more information, visit these Web sites:
Centers for Disease Control and Prevention,
http://www.cdc.gov

World Health Organization, charged with controlling the spread of infectious diseases,
http://www.who.int

UNIT (32) Poisoning

The term **poison** has been used for hundreds of years to describe a deadly substance, solid, liquid, or gas, that is detrimental to an individual's health or causes death. Exposure to such substances can cause predictable or unpredictable chemical reactions. When a person is exposed to a substance and becomes ill as a result, it is referred to as **poisoning.** Poisoning can be a deliberate exposure, sometimes called an *overdose*. If a generally harmless substance causes an unexpected activation of the person's immune system, it is called an *allergic reaction*. Such reactions can become life threatening when severe.

It is important that the Emergency Medical Technician (EMT) be familiar with the concepts of poisoning and understand the priorities in the management of poisoned patients and patients suffering from allergic reactions.

National Education Standards

The Emergency Medical Technician (EMT) will demonstrate a fundamental depth and foundational breadth of understanding of the anatomy, physiology, pathophysiology, assessment, and management of poisoning emergencies.

Key Concepts

- The EMT must be familiar with the types of poisoning and management priorities.

- Poisons can enter the body through four basic routes of exposure.

- Scene safety has a high priority when poisons are suspected.

- The signs and symptoms can vary based on the type of poison.

- Recognition of airway issues in the poisoned patient is a priority during the primary assessment.

- Medical control and advanced life support should always be considered in the poisoned patient.

- The EMT must be able to quickly recognize an allergic reaction.

- The EMT must be able to recognize the differences between a simple allergic reaction and anaphylaxis.

- Airway management is the highest priority in the patient suffering from an anaphylactic reaction.

- ALS providers carry medications useful in the management of anaphylactic reactions, and an ALS intercept should always be considered in anaphylaxis.

Jackie and Devon have just finished dinner when they are paged for a woman having difficulty breathing. While en route, they are advised by dispatch that the patient's neighbors state the patient is sitting on the steps in front of her home with a strong order of something coming from the windows of the house. The fire department and hazardous materials team have also been dispatched.

Upon arrival, they notice a strong smell of chlorine in the air, and Jackie stages the ambulance upwind of the residence. Fire department personnel approach the residence wearing air packs. After determining that the patient is not in need of decontamination and is able to walk without difficulty, the firefighters assist her to the ambulance.

Once in the ambulance, Devon begins his primary assessment, noting that Mrs. Smythe can speak her name but is coughing harshly and her voice is hoarse. Devon provides oxygen at 12 lpm via non-rebreather mask, and after a few minutes, Mrs. Smythe is able to speak more clearly and easily.

Mrs. Smythe explains that earlier that day, her husband had unplugged the kitchen drain using a drain opener. A few minutes ago, she poured bleach down the drain to get rid of a lingering odor. Immediately after pouring the bleach, the room filled with the strong odor and she felt her throat begin to burn. She realized something must be wrong and tried to open the windows in the house; however, she started coughing and her chest started hurting, so she went outside and called 9-1-1 from her portable phone.

Critical Thinking Questions

1. What are the immediate priorities when responding to this type of emergency call?
2. What are the priorities of emergency medical care for this patient?
3. What type of poisonous exposure has this patient experienced?

INTRODUCTION

A **toxin** is any drug or substance that is poisonous to the human body, causing a decline in health and the potential for a fatal reaction. **Toxicology** is the study of toxins, antidotes, and the effects of toxins on the body. This unit will discuss types and routes of exposure of poisons as well as the effects, assessment, and management of poison emergencies. In addition, although an allergic reaction is not truly a toxicologic emergency, the body reacts to a foreign substance in a similar manner as to a toxin. Assessment and management of patients with allergic reactions will also be reviewed in this unit.

POISONING

Thousands of children are poisoned each year as they explore their environments. Many adults become ill each year as a result of poisoning as well. Some poisonings are unintentional; others are deliberate.

People can become ill after exposure to harmful substances via several routes. Although the general concepts are similar, each mechanism has unique differences in management.

ROUTES OF EXPOSURE

There are four main routes a poison can enter the body. These routes of exposure are important information because how the poison enters the body may also determine how quickly the body reacts to it. As an example, an individual has taken more sleeping pills than he needed in an attempted suicide, but changes his mind and calls 911. This route of exposure, through ingestion of pills, takes several hours for the poison to be broken down by the stomach and absorbed into the stomach. Therefore, type of poison, route of exposure, and OPQRST history become important information in the management of this poisoning. The routes of exposure include ingestion, inhalation, injection, and absorption.

INGESTION

When a substance is swallowed and absorbed through the stomach and intestines (gastrointestinal tract), the route of exposure is called *ingestion*. Ingestion is the most common route of exposure in poisoning. Ingested poisons tend to be delayed in their absorption by the body, and signs and symptoms of poisoning may not appear for hours following ingestion. Examples of ingested substances that could be poisonous are drugs and medications in pill or liquid form, household cleaners, and alcohol.

INHALATION

Poisons in the form of gases, vapor, fumes, or aerosols are breathed or inhaled into the body and into the lungs. Inhaled poisons are rapidly absorbed into the body through the lungs and transported throughout the body. The inhalation route produces signs and symptoms of poisoning that appear more rapidly and throughout the body (systemic) than ingested poisons. Additionally, inhaled poisons can have a direct effect on the pulmonary system, destroying the tissues along the respiratory tract and the lungs. Examples of inhaled poisons include carbon monoxide, carbon dioxide, chlorine gases as seen around swimming pools, and solvents often found in household cleaners.

INJECTION

Poison can be injected into the bloodstream through a puncture of the skin, entering the subcutaneous layer of skin or muscle. Often injected poisons will cause an immediate reaction at the site of the injection, seen as swelling, redness, irritation, and pain. Injected poisons can have an immediate systemic reaction, or they can have a delayed reaction depending on the type of poison, speed of absorption, and speed of distribution throughout the body. Injected poisons include both drugs or other substances an individual may intentionally inject and poisons injected through insect bites or stings of bees or wasps. Some individuals are allergic to the venom injected by these insects and experience an anaphylactic reaction, discussed later in this unit.

ABSORPTION

When a poisonous substance comes in contact with the skin or mucous membranes, it can enter that body through absorption. The substance can be a dry powder or liquid and may cause a local reaction of the skin or mucous membrane or may lead to a more systemic reaction to the poison. An example of a localized reaction to a poison is poison ivy initially causing irritation of the area that came in contact with the plant. An example of a more serious absorption poisoning is organophosphates, commonly found in pesticides and fertilizers. Organophosphates can be absorbed through the skin and may result in a severe systemic reaction that can lead to death if not reversed.

GENERAL ASSESSMENT

As with all emergency situations, it is important that the EMT evaluate the scene for safety before approaching the patient. Some poisons, if still present on the scene, can be harmful to emergency providers. Appropriately trained hazardous materials technicians should be called to assist if it is thought that the substance involved makes the scene unsafe. Hazardous material scene safety is discussed further in Unit 50.

Once safely removed from any danger, poisoned patients all require a thorough assessment and history by the EMT. If the patient does not have any acutely life-threatening issues, the EMT should carefully look for specific evidence of illness related to the poisoning.

The history obtained should include specific information regarding the poisoning using the OPQRST history as well as the SAMPLE history and relevant medical history.

SPECIFIC HISTORY

If the exact name of the substance to which the patient was exposed is available, the EMT should carefully record it and relay it to hospital personnel. If the container or a sample of the substance is available and can safely be collected, the EMT should consider bringing it to the hospital for identification.

The exact time and route of exposure to the poison should be determined. Some remedies are useful only during a certain time frame. If the exposure was more than a single event, the EMT should determine over how long a period of time the patient was exposed to the substance. If the amount of the substance that was involved is measurable, the EMT should record the amount as well.

The EMT should determine and document whether anyone provided any type of treatment for the patient before the EMT's arrival. There are **Poison Control Centers** all over the United States with a nationally recognized phone number that will route the caller to the Poison Control Center nearest the caller. The telephone number (1-800-222-1222) is a useful resource for laypersons and medical personnel as well. Some EMS systems recommend that EMTs call Poison Control from the scene for advice in managing a poisoned patient. The EMT should follow local protocols regarding whom to contact.

Many decisions regarding treatment of the poisoned patient involve calculations based on the patient's weight. If possible, the EMT should determine what the patient weighs. Parents often know what their child weighs and can relate that information if asked.

GENERAL MANAGEMENT

Although every situation is unique and each toxic substance creates its own problems that need individualized care, the EMT can use some general management principles when caring for all poisoned patients.

LIFE-THREATENING PROBLEMS

The EMT should use her general impression and primary assessment to identify and treat any immediately life-threatening problems. It is not uncommon for a poisoned patient to develop airway, breathing, or circulatory compromise. The EMT should follow the principles of supporting these systems.

Specific management techniques should be used as appropriate for the situation and as directed by medical control.

MEDICAL DIRECTION

After addressing any immediate life threats, the EMT should consult with medical control regarding further management. Some systems have set up protocols to be used as off-line medical control in this circumstance. The EMT should be familiar with local protocols and follow them carefully.

Other systems require on-line consultation with a physician or the physician's designee. That designee may be the Poison Control Center in the case of the poisoned patient. Again, the EMT should follow local protocol.

TRANSPORT

After addressing any immediate life threats, the EMT should collect any remaining pills, containers, or labels that can identify the potential poison and transport the patient to the most appropriate medical facility or meet up with an advanced life support (ALS) provider, whichever is quicker. In some cases, identification of the substance will be crucial in providing appropriate in-hospital care (Figure 32.1).

ONGOING ASSESSMENT

The EMT should realize that the poisoned patient has the potential to decompensate quickly. Even if the patient appears well upon first assessment, the poison may not yet have absorbed fully into the bloodstream. Once this has absorbed, the patient may rapidly decompensate. Consequently, the EMT must continually reassess the poisoned patient for hints of such decompensation. Table 32-1 lists some signs of decompensation in the poisoned patient.

Certain poisons cause characteristic changes in the patient's vital signs. The EMT should carefully monitor the patient's heart and respiratory rates, blood pressure, skin color and temperature, and pulse oximetry.

ANTIDOTES

An **antidote** is a substance that will counteract or neutralize the effects of a poison or toxic substance. Family and patients often believe there is an antidote for many poisons or toxic substances when in fact a limited number of antidotes is available for only a small number of specific poisons. The general management of poison exposures is to limit or prevent further absorption of the poison and to manage the patient's airway, breathing, circulation, and other signs and symptoms as absorption progresses.

ALS INTERCEPT

If the patient's condition exceeds the EMT's abilities, an ALS intercept should be considered. ALS units may be able to administer medications that can reverse the effects of specific drugs or poisons. An example would be the drug naloxone (**Narcan**), which can reduce the effects of a narcotic, as seen with heroin overdose. Medical control may be helpful in deciding when the use of ALS intercept is beneficial.

Transport should be accomplished in a timely fashion, and the EMT should continually reassess the patient and be prepared for possible decompensation.

If any further decontamination is needed, notification of the destination facility is critically important so that it may make appropriate arrangements.

INGESTED POISONS

As previously stated, the most common route of poisoning is by oral ingestion. Young children will put just about anything into their mouths. If he has access to a potentially harmful substance, a child may unintentionally poison himself.

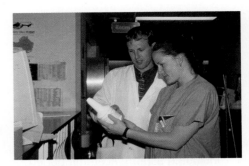

Figure 32.1 Some therapies for poisoned patients are dependent on accurate identification of the substance involved

Table 32-1 Signs of Decompensation— Poisoning

Decreasing mental status

Increasing heart rate

Seizure

Decreasing respiratory rate

Respiratory arrest

Hypotension

Cardiac arrest

Table 32-2 Commonly Ingested Poisonous Substances

Prescription Medications

Over-the-counter medications, including aspirin, acetaminophen (Tylenol), cough and cold medications

Illegal drugs (heroin, methamphetamine, cocaine, ecstasy)

Household products, including cleaning agents (detergents, bleaches, pine oil)

Foods

Insecticides

Petroleum products (kerosene, gasoline)

Plants

A different situation may exist in adults. Certainly the possibility of unintentional poisoning exists, but the rates of deliberate poisoning increase in adulthood. Care of these patients involves some different considerations. Table 32-2 lists commonly ingested poisons.

INTENTIONAL INGESTIONS

When a person deliberately ingests a substance that is believed to be harmful, it is referred to as an *overdose*. Often the patient is suffering from severe depression and is attempting to harm or even kill himself.

In this situation, it is the duty of the EMT to treat the patient and prevent any further harm. A patient who has attempted or threatened to harm himself should be transported to an appropriate hospital for medical and psychiatric treatment. This person should not be given the option to refuse further treatment, even if he does not appear to need acute medical care. The care of patients who may be a danger to themselves is covered in detail in Unit 28.

SIGNS AND SYMPTOMS

Ingested poisons can cause myriad physical findings and symptoms (Figure 32.2). The earliest are often related to the gastrointestinal tract, as this is the part of the body first contacted by the substance. The airway can also be affected if the poison injures the mouth and throat. The EMT should look for these specific signs and symptoms when evaluating the patient who has ingested a poison. Table 32-3 lists these signs and symptoms.

Table 32-3 Signs and Symptoms of Ingestion Poisoning

Nausea

Vomiting

Diarrhea

Altered mental status

Abdominal pain

Chemical burns around the mouth

Breath odor of chemical

Difficulty breathing

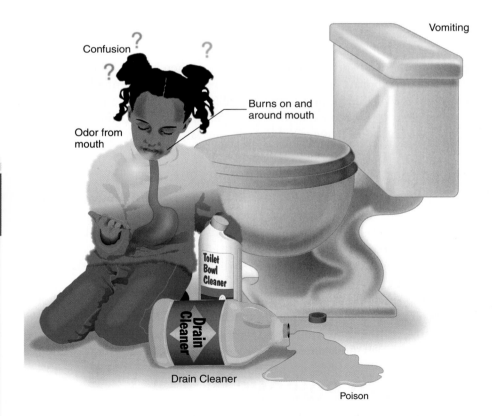

Figure 32.2 Ingested poisons can cause injury to the mouth and throat and will absorb into the stomach vessels and be distributed throughout the body

MANAGEMENT

A general impression and primary assessment will identify any potential airway, breathing, or circulatory problems. These issues must be addressed immediately upon their recognition.

Potential life-threatening problems in the patient who ingested a poison may include loss of airway patency because of mouth and throat burns if the substance ingested was a caustic substance. The patency of the airway may also be in jeopardy if the patient is unconscious as a result of the effects of the ingested poison.

Any pills or harmful materials that remain in the patient's mouth should be removed. If the patient is conscious, he should be asked to spit into a basin. Often a suction catheter can be used to remove any material from the unconscious person's mouth. Certain ingested substances can rapidly cause heart or brain malfunction, resulting in shock, seizures, or decreased level of consciousness. If faced with a patient with evidence of hypoperfusion, the EMT should treat him as outlined in Unit 11. Seizures and altered mental status can be managed according to the priorities discussed in Unit 27.

ACTIVATED CHARCOAL

The ideal way to manage a potentially harmful oral ingestion is to prevent some or all absorption of the poison. Activated charcoal can prevent absorption of certain ingested substances if administered within 1–2 hours of ingestion.

This suspension of charcoal in a liquid binds to some poisons, preventing them from being absorbed. It should be given only to patients who have ingested a noncaustic substance and who are awake and able to drink the liquid without potential for airway compromise. Charcoal does not appear appealing to the eye. For this reason a cover is put over the cup. To make it more palatable, activated charcoal is often flavored with grape or cherry flavoring.

Activated charcoal should never be administered to a patient with an altered mental status or who has ingested a caustic substance. Caustic substances found in drain cleaners, toilet bowl cleaners, and even some dishwasher detergents, when accidentally ingested will cause serious burns and tissue damage to the lips, mouth, esophagus, and stomach. If the patient vomits, as often occurs with activated charcoal, additional damage may occur from the caustic substance returning up the esophagus as it did when it was originally ingested. Therefore, activated charcoal or any substance that may induce vomiting must be avoided in poisonings involving caustic substances. The EMT should follow local protocol for specific recommendations.

INHALED POISONS

The priority of emergency personnel responding to the scene of a potential poisoning by inhalation must be their own safety. If the dispatch information is suspicious for an airborne poison, personnel trained to operate in such an environment should immediately be called to assist. The EMT should take the time to survey the scene for any potential airborne poison and should not enter a scene that is considered to be potentially dangerous. Table 32-4 lists commonly inhaled poisons.

SIGNS AND SYMPTOMS

After inhaling a poison, a patient will likely experience respiratory problems (Figure 32.3). Depending on the nature of the substance, however, the signs and symptoms may be quite extensive. Table 32-5 lists common signs and symptoms seen in the patient who has inhaled poison.

Street Smart

Certain poisons can create a characteristic odor to the breath. During the assessment of the airway, the EMT should note any odors on the patient's breath.

Medication Card

Generic name: Activated charcoal

Trade name: Actidose, Super-Char, and more

Indications: Recent ingestion of poison

Contraindications: Patients who cannot control their own airway and swallow their own secretions or who have been given ipecac should not be given oral medications or who have ingested a caustic substance.

Dose: 1 g/kg body weight (50–100 g for typical adult)

Route: Oral

Table 32-4 Commonly Inhaled Poisons

Carbon monoxide

Carbon dioxide

Chlorine gas

Liquid chemicals and sprays

Ammonia

Aesthetic gases (ether, nitrous oxide)

Solvents (dry cleaning, degreasing agents, fire extinguishers)

Natural gas

Table 32-5 Common Signs and Symptoms of Inhalation Poisoning
Difficulty breathing
Chest pain
Cough
Hoarseness
Dizziness
Headache
Confusion
Seizures
Altered mental status
Residue on hands and/or face

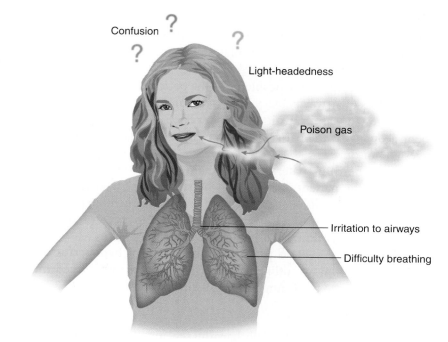

Figure 32.3 Inhaled poisons can cause irritation and injury to the upper and lower airways and may impede effective oxygenation

MANAGEMENT

Once properly trained providers have removed the patient from the potentially harmful area, the EMT can safely assess and treat the patient.

The general impression and primary assessment will allow the EMT to identify and treat any potentially life-threatening conditions immediately. Oxygen should always be administered to the patient who appears to have inhaled a potentially harmful substance, and the EMT should be prepared to ventilate the patient with a bag-valve-mask assembly if necessary.

INJECTED POISONS

Another type of poisoning involves the injection of a harmful substance. Intentional injection of a substance known to be harmful falls under the category of overdose.

Sometimes a patient will not know of the toxic nature of the substance; in those cases, the poisoning is unintentional. Another unintentional source of toxic injection is from creatures such as snakes, spiders, scorpions, wasps, bees, ticks, and marine animals such as jellyfish, coral, and stingrays. The management of venomous injections is discussed in Unit 39.

SIGNS AND SYMPTOMS

The signs and symptoms associated with an injected poison depend significantly on the specific poison (Figure 32.4). Some commonly seen signs and symptoms that the EMT should look for are listed in Table 32-6.

MANAGEMENT

In keeping with the high priority of safety in the management of any patient, the EMT should be aware of the sharp nature of the injecting device and should take care to ensure proper disposal of any contaminated sharps.

The patient should be removed from any potential danger. If any systemic signs and symptoms are present, the EMT should encourage the patient to lie

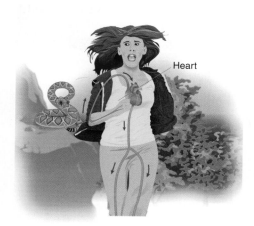

Figure 32.4 An injected poison will directly enter the bloodstream and be distributed around the body. Local blood vessel irritation is often seen

quietly, with the affected part (the body part that suffered the bite, sting, or injection) lower than the heart. This position will decrease the flow of toxin toward the heart. Oxygen should be administered, and the patient should be transported as appropriate.

ABSORBED POISONS

Certain types of substances have the ability to be absorbed through intact skin. Others can cause injury to the skin on contact. Absorbed poisons can be dry powder or liquid substances used in common cleaning supplies and farming. Examples of absorbed poisons are insecticides and dry lime or organophosphates used in farming as a fertilizer. Biological agents used in warfare may also be absorbed through the skin or mucous membranes.

SIGNS AND SYMPTOMS

The patient who is exposed to an absorbable poison will have symptoms that are specific to that agent but will often exhibit signs and symptoms such as those listed in Table 32-7 and shown in Figure 32.5.

MANAGEMENT

The principles of scene safety are crucial in the case of absorbed poisons. Often, the offending agent is still in contact with the patient, presenting a significant danger to the unprepared EMT. Only emergency providers with training specific to this situation should attempt to enter the scene. These providers will appropriately decontaminate the patient and bring her to a safe area where the EMT can then provide the appropriate medical treatment.

If the exposure is limited and the substance easily recognized and dealt with, the EMT may choose to initiate decontamination according to local protocols. The appropriate initial care for any potentially harmful substance on the skin is to remove the substance by first brushing away any solid material. This step should be followed by extensive flushing with copious amounts of clean water. All clothing around the site should be removed before flushing. This decontamination should be done on scene.

If the patient's eyes were exposed to the substance, they should be irrigated thoroughly with clean water or saline solution for at least 20 minutes. Contact lenses should be removed promptly. Care should be taken not to contaminate the unaffected eye by directing the irrigation from the middle of the face toward the affected eye as illustrated in Figure 32.6.

Care should be taken to properly collect and dispose of any contaminated runoff from the irrigation or flushing of a contaminated patient.

Street Smart

Large-scale flushing may be impractical in the back of a moving ambulance; therefore, any flushing should be accomplished on scene. The only exception would be if the patient's condition warrants immediate transport or if only eyes are involved. The irrigation of eyes involves a more controlled flow of water and can be more easily accomplished in the rear of an ambulance.

Table 32-6 Signs and Symptoms of Injection Poisoning
Pain at injection site
Weakness
Dizziness
Chills
Fever
Nausea
Vomiting

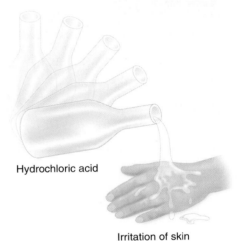

Hydrochloric acid

Irritation of skin

Figure 32.5 Some substances can be absorbed directly through the skin into surface blood vessels; others cause injury to the skin itself

Table 32-7 Signs and Symptoms of Absorption Poisoning
Liquid or powder on skin
Burns
Itching
Irritation to skin
Redness to area of exposure
Difficulty breathing

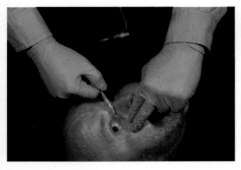

Figure 32.6 When the EMT is irrigating a contaminated eye, it is important to avoid cross-contaminating the uninvolved eye

Street Smart

There are many different ways to effectively provide eye irrigation. If one eye is involved, intravenous (IV) tubing can be hooked up to normal saline and used to irrigate the eye. Alternatively, if these supplies are not available, oxygen tubing can be pushed through the punctured cap of a plastic bottle of normal saline with the same effect.

If both eyes are involved, a nasal cannula attached to IV saline may be placed over the bridge of the nose, allowing even flow to both eyes simultaneously.

Table 32-8 Common Allergens
Insect stings (bees, wasps, etc.)
Foods (nuts, seafood, peanuts, etc.)
Plants
Medications

ALLERGIC REACTIONS

An **allergic reaction** occurs when the body is exposed to a particular substance to which the immune system is particularly sensitive. The immune system is the part of the body that responds to foreign materials such as viruses and bacteria and fights them to prevent illness.

Occasionally a person's immune system may be particularly sensitive to a material that may otherwise be considered harmless. Every person's immune system responds to substances differently. A substance that causes an exaggerated immune system response resulting in an allergic reaction is called an **allergen**. Some common allergens are listed in Table 32-8.

ANAPHYLAXIS

The actual effects on the body of an activation of the immune system can range from a local irritation at the site of the exposure to a life-threatening reaction called *anaphylaxis* (see Unit 11). Anaphylaxis is a serious form of allergic reaction that may result in shock and even death.

PATHOPHYSIOLOGY

The body's reaction to an extreme immune response involves several body systems, and substances are released from different cells throughout the body. These substances cause the signs and symptoms that are classically seen with an allergic reaction. Figure 32.7 illustrates the physical findings seen in an allergic reaction.

SKIN

One of the most common signs of an allergic reaction is a rash. The rash associated with an acute allergic reaction is a characteristic pattern of raised reddened areas of skin called hives, or urticaria. The hives are actually created by tiny patches of dilated blood vessels with localized swelling caused by the chemicals released when triggered by the immune system. Figure 32.8 illustrates the pathophysiology behind hives.

Hives can be localized to just the area of exposure, as is seen in a bee sting. If the allergy is from ingestion, such as peanuts, the hives may be more generalized. Hives tend to be very itchy, and the patient will want to scratch all over.

A mild allergic reaction may be limited to hives. Although this condition is uncomfortable, isolated urticaria is not life threatening. The patient with

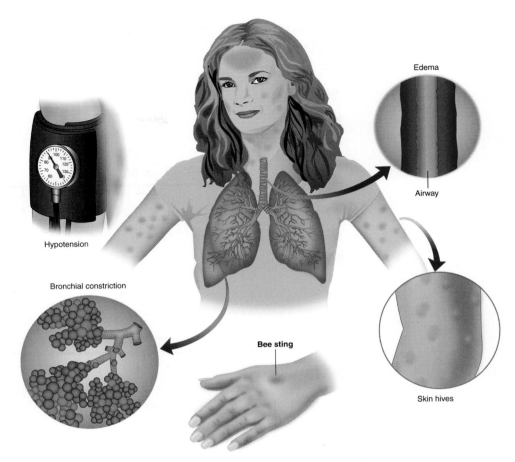

Edema

Airway

Hypotension

Bronchial constriction

Bee sting

Skin hives

Figure 32.7 A severe allergic reaction involves several body systems

hives, however, should be assessed for the presence of other signs of a severe allergic reaction.

RESPIRATORY

In addition to causing localized inflammation of the skin, the immune response can cause inflammation and edema in the upper airway and lungs.

Swelling of the face, lips, and tongue is an ominous sign of a severe allergic reaction. The swelling can continue and completely occlude the patient's airway, making breathing impossible, if allowed to progress.

Signs of significant swelling in the airway are a hoarse voice, indicating swelling of the vocal cords, or an inspiratory upper airway sound called *stridor*. These signs indicate a dangerously narrowed upper airway.

Inflammation in the lower airways and lungs will result in constriction of the bronchioles. As the space for airflow is narrowed, the patient will begin to feel short of breath. The sound of the air rushing through the narrowed airways is called *wheezing* and can be heard on auscultation of the chest.

These signs of airway and respiratory compromise may become increasingly obvious but may initially be quite subtle. The EMT must specifically look for these signs of a severe allergic reaction to begin treatment immediately.

CARDIOVASCULAR

The generalized effects on the cardiovascular system are usually seen only with a severe reaction. This exaggerated immune system response results in dilation of blood vessels throughout the body. Such generalized dilation of

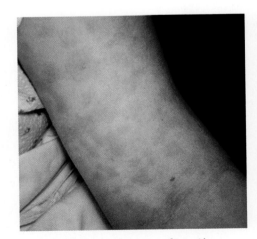

Figure 32.8 Hives are often the result of allergic reactions such as this reaction to penicillin (Courtesy of the Centers for Disease Control Public Health Image Library)

Table 32-9 Signs and Symptoms of an Allergic Reaction*

Severe

Mild Allergic Reaction	Allergic Reaction (Anaphylaxis)

Skin

Warmth	Warmth
Redness	Redness
Hives	Hives
Itching	Itching
Localized swelling	Swelling

Respiratory

No signs or symptoms	Throat tightness
	Shortness of breath
	Cough
	Wheezing
	Stridor
	Hoarseness
	Tachypnea

Cardiovascular

No signs or symptoms	Tachycardia
	Hypotension
	Dizziness
	Other signs and symptoms of a hypoperfused state

Other

Itchy, watery eyes	Itchy, watery eyes
Headache	Headache
Runny nose	Sense of impending doom
	Runny nose

blood vessels causes a fall in blood pressure and a sharp rise in heart rate. These will result in hypoperfusion if not quickly treated.

SIGNS AND SYMPTOMS

It is important to realize that the patient suffering from an allergic reaction may initially have signs of only a mild reaction but can progress to severe anaphylaxis in a matter of minutes. The typical allergic reaction begins within 30 minutes of exposure to the allergen. Table 32-9 lists the most common signs and symptoms of an allergic reaction.

ASSESSMENT

The key in management of the patient with an allergic reaction is for the EMT to recognize the signs and symptoms of anaphylaxis. A mild allergic reaction requires little treatment by the EMT. Anaphylaxis will result in death if not quickly and properly treated.

PRIMARY ASSESSMENT

During the primary assessment, the EMT should look specifically for any evidence of airway swelling and respiratory or cardiovascular compromise.

High-flow oxygen should be administered and, if signs of hypoperfusion are evident, the patient should be kept warm and immediately transported to the closest hospital, with an ALS unit called to intercept if available.

If the patient's breathing is inadequate, ventilations should be assisted with 100% oxygen. If the patient suffers a cardiac arrest, the EMT should institute appropriate supportive measures and rapidly transport.

The ongoing assessment should be repeated frequently because patients suffering from an allergic reaction can quickly worsen and require additional treatments.

HISTORY AND SECONDARY ASSESSMENT

A history and focused physical exam of the secondary assessment can provide crucial information to the EMT. Table 32-10 lists some important historical questions the EMT should ask of the patient with evidence of an allergic reaction.

MANAGEMENT

The patient with a severe allergic reaction will decompensate quickly without rapid treatment. The EMT should initiate treatment as appropriate through the primary assessment, including oxygen and ventilatory assistance, if needed.

Street Smart

Some states allow EMS services to carry and administer epinephrine in the case of a severe allergic reaction. The EMT should be familiar with local regulations and obtain the relevant training if she is expected to administer this medication without a physician's prescription.

Table 32-10 Questions Related to Allergic Reactions

Is there a previous history of allergic reaction?

How severe was the previous reaction?

To what was the patient exposed?

What were the nature and timing of the exposure?

What symptoms are evident?

Has there been any progression of the symptoms?

Has your doctor prescribed medication for you to use in this situation?

What interventions have been attempted?

Medication Card

Generic name: Epinephrine
Trade name: EpiPen
Indications: Life-threatening allergic reaction
Contraindications: None in the presence of an indication
Dose: 0.3–0.5 mg for adults 0.15–0.3 mg for children
Route: Intramuscular

Table 32-11 Indications for Use of Epinephrine

Airway	Throat tightness
	Hoarseness
	Stridor
Breathing	Shortness of breath
	Wheezing
	Dyspnea
Circulation	Hypotension

Table 32-12 Signs of Decompensation— Allergic Reaction

Decreasing mental status

Increased difficulty breathing

Decreasing blood pressure

Some patients who have experienced previous anaphylactic reactions are prescribed a lifesaving medicine, epinephrine, by their physician. The EMT may assist the patient to use this medication with approval from medical control.

EPINEPHRINE

Epinephrine is an injectable medication that dilates the bronchioles and constricts the blood vessels. These effects are useful in the patient suffering from an anaphylactic reaction.

Along with these useful effects, epinephrine has many unwanted and potentially harmful side effects. Therefore, the EMT must be thoroughly familiar with its indications and should consider its use only for a patient who has been prescribed it by a physician, unless local protocols allow differently.

Clear indications for use of epinephrine include those signs and symptoms listed in Table 32-11. Epinephrine is not indicated for use in a mild allergic reaction without evidence of airway, breathing, or circulatory compromise. Further details regarding the assisted administration of this medication can be found in Unit 13.

TRANSPORT

The patient suffering from an allergic reaction should be transported to the closest appropriate hospital. If any evidence of a severe reaction is present, an ALS intercept should be requested, if available. ALS providers carry additional medications that may be useful in the management of the anaphylactic reaction.

Frequent reassessments during transport are critical so that any decompensation can be recognized quickly and dealt with appropriately. Table 32-12 lists signs of patient decompensation.

If these signs of deterioration become evident, the EMT should contact medical control for advice on further management. High-flow oxygen with ventilatory support if necessary are indicated for the patient with evidence of hypoperfusion.

If the patient continues to decompensate, the EMT should be prepared to initiate basic cardiac life support measures to include cardiopulmonary resuscitation (CPR) and automated external defibrillator (AED).

In most cases, with appropriate therapy, the patient with an allergic reaction will improve quickly. If the patient does not improve, the EMT should continue to administer high-flow oxygen and monitor the patient for deterioration.

All patients suffering from an allergic reaction should be transported to the hospital for further treatment and observation.

CONCLUSION

The body reacts to different substances in different ways. Some reactions can be predicted on the basis of the type of exposure, but some are quite unpredictable.

Exposures can be to substances known to be harmful or to harmful amounts of otherwise harmless substances. These poisonings can result in severe illness. Exposure to a substance that causes an allergic reaction can also cause severe illness.

No matter the nature of the exposure, the EMT must be familiar with the concepts of assessment and management of these patients.

CASE STUDY Continued

Mrs. Smythe can speak with less difficulty following oxygen administration. Her airway is open, she is breathing adequately with respirations at 22, and her pulse is regular and strong at 98. Breath sounds indicates some wheezes on inspiration and a SpO$_2$ of 98% on oxygen.

Devon advises Mrs. Smythe that she most likely inhaled a toxic or poisonous substance, due to a chemical reaction caused through the combination of bleach and the drain opener her husband used earlier in the day. Devon explains she needs to be evaluated at the hospital to ensure she has no further breathing difficulties or other adverse reactions to the toxic fumes she has inhaled.

Mrs. Smythe is advised by the fire department that her home will be ventilated while she is at the hospital and that her husband has been contacted and will meet her in the emergency department.

During transport to the hospital, Mrs. Smythe's breathing continues to improve with oxygen. She continues to complain of a sore throat but states the tightness in her chest has gone away. Devon provides the hospital with a report of the incident during transport and follows up with an additional report upon transfer of Mrs. Smythe's care.

Later that night Devon and Jackie receive a phone call from Mr. and Mrs. Smythe thanking them for their professionalism and good care of Mrs. Smythe.

Key Concepts Revisited

- The EMT must be familiar with the types of poisoning and management priorities.
- Poisons can enter the body through four basic routes of exposure:
  - Ingestion
  - Inhalation
  - Injection
  - Absorption
- Scene safety has a high priority when poisons are suspected.
- The signs and symptoms associated can vary based on the type of poison.
  - Signs and symptoms of ingested poisons include nausea, vomiting, diarrhea, altered mental status, abdominal pain, chemical burns around the mouth, breath odor of chemical, and difficulty breathing.
  - Signs and symptoms of inhaled poisons include difficulty breathing, chest pain, cough, hoarseness, dizziness, headache, confusion, seizures, and altered mental status.
  - Signs and symptoms of injected poisons include pain at the injection site, weakness, dizziness, chills, fever, nausea, and vomiting.
  - Signs and symptoms of absorbed poisons include liquid or dry powder on the skin, burns, itching, irritation to skin, redness to area of exposure, and difficulty breathing.
- Recognition of airway issues in the poisoned patient is a priority during the primary assessment.
- Medical control, poison control centers, and advanced life support should always be considered in the poisoned patient:
  - Management of life threats
  - Poison control—management options
  - ALS—medications to reverse the effects of some drug overdoses
- The EMT must be able to quickly recognize an allergic reaction.
- The EMT must be able to recognize the differences between a simple allergic reaction and anaphylaxis.
  - Simple allergic reaction
    - Skin signs and symptoms include warmth, redness, hives, itching, and localized swelling.
    - Other signs and symptoms include itchy, watery eyes, headache, and runny nose.

- No signs or symptoms of compromise to the respiratory or cardiovascular symptoms are evident.
  - ○ Anaphylaxis
    - Skin signs and symptoms include warmth, redness, hives, itching, and swelling.
    - Respiratory signs and symptoms include throat tightness, shortness of breath, cough, wheezing, stridor, hoarseness, and tachypnea.
    - Cardiovascular signs and symptoms include tachycardia, hypotension, dizziness, and other signs and symptoms of a hypoperfused state.
    - Other signs and symptoms include itchy, watery eyes, headache, sense of impending doom, and runny nose.
- Airway management is the highest priority in the patient suffering from an anaphylactic reaction.
- ALS providers carry medications useful in the management of anaphylactic reactions and should always be considered in anaphylaxis.

Review Questions

1. What are the four routes poisons can enter the body?
2. What are the signs and symptoms associated with different types of poisonings?
3. What is the emergency medical care for the patient who has been poisoned?
4. What are the special considerations required in the emergency medical care of the patient with an intentional overdose?
5. What are the indications and contraindications for activated charcoal in the poisoned patient?
6. What is the role of medical control and advanced life support in the poisoned patient?
7. What are the typical signs and symptoms of an allergic reaction?
8. What is the emergency medical care for the patient with an allergic reaction?
9. What is the difference between a simple allergic reaction and anaphylaxis?
10. What are the implications of anaphylaxis in regard to airway management?
11. What are the indications and contraindications for the epinephrine auto-injector?

Key Terms

Allergen
Allergic reaction
Antidote
Narcan
Poison

Poison Control Center
Poisoning
Toxicology
Toxin

Further Study

Haynes, B. E., & J. Pritting. "A Rural Emergency Medical Technician with Selected Advanced Skills." *Prehospital Emergency Care* 3, no. 4 (1999): 343–346.

Hunt, D. "Curse of the black scorpion." *Emergency Medical Services 26,* no. 10 (1997): 37–44.

Marciano, S. (1997). "Mammalian Animal Bites." *Emergency Medical Services* 26, no. 10 (1997): 50–55.

Myer, J., M. Neighbors, and R. Tannehille-Jones. *Principles of Pathophysiology and Emergency Medical Care.* Clifton Park, NY: Delmar-Thomson Learning, 2002.

Phillips, K. "Nicotine Poisoning." *Emergency Medical Services* 26, no. 9 (1997): 38–40.

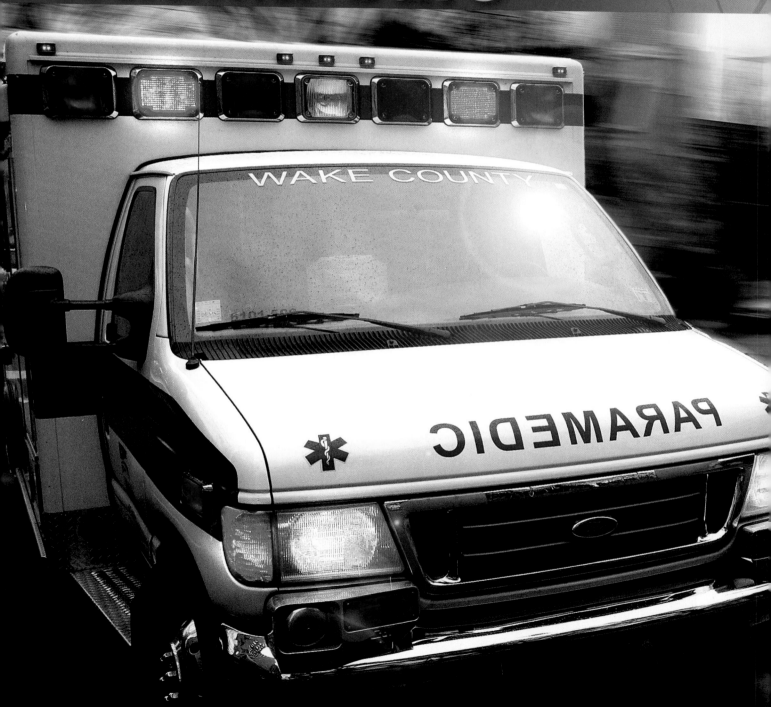

CHAPTER 6

Trauma Care

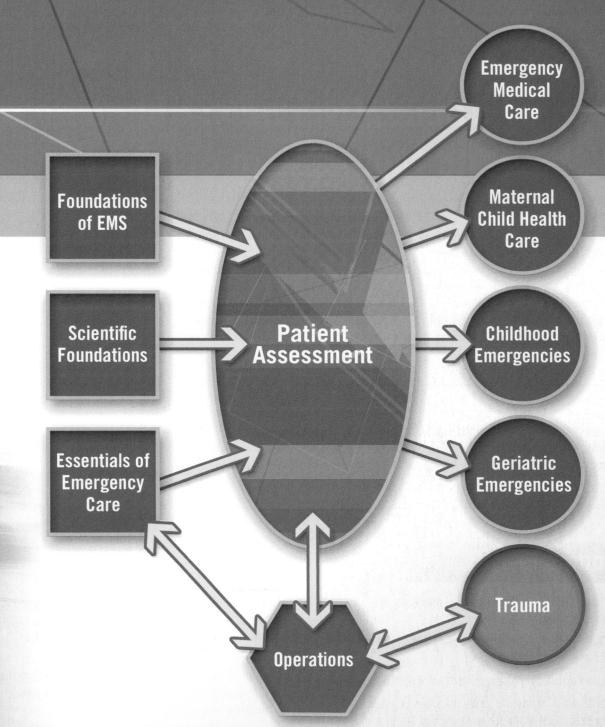

Trauma Emergencies

Emergency Medical Services (EMS) was formed to provide trauma care, and even today, despite the incredible growth of EMS and trauma systems, trauma remains the number one killer of young people.

The challenge to the Emergency Medical Technician (EMT) is to be able to accomplish all the tasks necessary for assessment and management of the injured patient as quickly as possible. The EMT must quickly identify and manage traumatic injuries in minimum time and initiate rapid, safe transportation to a trauma center. In many cases, the survival of the patient is dependent on the EMT's ability to provide basic stabilization and get the patient to the trauma surgeon center quickly.

This section reviews the fundamentals of trauma care and the role of the EMT in the trauma care system.

Trauma is a physical injury or wound caused by external force or violence. Trauma is the leading cause of death for persons 1 to 44 years of age. The goal of trauma care is to get the patient to the appropriate facility, using the right mode of transportation, within the shortest amount of time, while providing the appropriate management while en route to definitive care. To accomplish this, the Emergency Medical Technician (EMT) must be able to determine the mechanism of injury and use his understanding of the kinematics of trauma to determine the extent of injury and priority decisions.

National Education Standards

The Emergency Medical Technician (EMT) will demonstrate a fundamental depth and foundational breadth of understanding of the pathophysiology, assessment, and management of the trauma patient, including trauma scoring, rapid transport, and destination issues and mode of transportation.

Key Concepts

- Kinematics of trauma is the science of analyzing the mechanism of injury.

- The amount of kinetic energy of a moving object depends on the mass and velocity of the object.

- The mechanism of injury refers to how the patient was injured.

- The mechanism of injury will guide the steps of assessment following evaluation of the patient's mental status and primary assessment.

- The secondary assessment of the trauma patient is divided into the rapid method and modified method.

- The secondary assessment of a trauma patient with a significant mechanism of injury uses the rapid method, brief head-to-toe assessment prior to gathering the history.

- The secondary assessment of a trauma patient with a nonsignificant MOI is modified to focus on the injured body part.

- The components of DCAP-BTLS guide the types of injuries being looked for in the secondary assessment.

- The trauma score, which includes the GCS, is a numerical method of communication between EMS and hospital staff to signify the severity of the trauma patient's condition.

- An organized trauma system provides the EMT with guidelines for making transport decisions, including the best mode of transport and most appropriate trauma center destination for a given area.

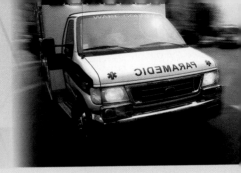

CASE STUDY

"Dispatch to Medic 12, respond to a high-speed crash, possible rollover on Berwick Hill."

Jason and Michele acknowledge the call and go en route, preparing for a trauma call and donning the appropriate PPE prior to arrival to the scene of the motor vehicle crash.

Upon arrival, the ambulance pulls ahead of the crash scene. A teenager can be seen lying on the side of the road, covered with a blanket. Michele, the EMT in charge, prepares to care for the patient, while Jason carefully proceeds down the hill to check out the car in the ravine.

As Jason walks completely around the car, he observes the driver's-side front fender damage. He also notices that, although the car is now on four wheels, the roof is caved in.

Jason peers into the driver's-side window, taking note of the broken windshield and the deflated air bag

hanging from the steering wheel. He lifts the air bag off the steering wheel and observes that the steering wheel is bent. Jason tugs on the seat belt and notes that it unrolls easily.

Returning to the ambulance, Jason finds that Michele has completed her primary assessment. The patient's only concern is sore wrists.

Critical Thinking Questions

1. What potential does this mechanism of injury have?
2. What observations should make an EMT have a high index of suspicion that there may be serious hidden injury?
3. How does the possibility of hidden injury affect the patient's priority?

INTRODUCTION

The EMT must learn how to quickly recognize serious trauma through an understanding of the kinematics of trauma and identification of the mechanism of injury. The mechanism of injury provides significant information concerning the seriousness and type of injury. The patient must further be assessed for injury secondary to that mechanism, and immediate lifesaving measures must be instituted on scene. This unit discusses the process of identifying the mechanism of injury through understanding of the kinematics of trauma.

KINEMATICS OF TRAUMA

Kinematics of trauma is defined as the science of analyzing the mechanism of injury. The *mechanism of injury* is how the patient was injured. **Kinetics** is the mechanics dealing with the motions of material objects and the *kinetic energy* contained in those objects. Mechanism of injury may be a motor vehicle crash (MVC), a fall, a gunshot, or being hit with an object such as a bat. Analyzing the mechanism of injury through the kinematics of trauma, the EMT will be able to make priority decisions regarding the assessment, management, and transport of the trauma patient.

Trauma almost always involves the collision of a body part or parts with another object, with the exception of blast injuries, which are caused by waves of pressure sometimes referred to as *shock waves*. The severity of a patient's injury depends on the force of the impact between the body and with which it collides.

VELOCITY AND MASS

The body's **mass,** the weight of an object, and **velocity,** or speed, determine the amount of kinetic energy of a moving body. The formula for the kinetic energy in a moving body is the mass or weight of the body in pounds, multiplied by the velocity (speed in feet per second) squared, and divided by 2. The formula can be written as:

$$\text{Kinetic energy} = \frac{\text{Mass} \times \text{velocity}^2}{2}$$

The formula demonstrates that when the mass of a moving object is doubled, its kinetic energy doubles. In other words, the injury sustained when struck by a 4-pound ball is 2 times more severe than if injury was caused by a 2-pound ball.

Although the weight or mass of the object is significant for the severity of the injury, the velocity at which the object is moving at the time of impact is more significant. In other words, if a ball was thrown at 1 foot per second and a second ball was thrown at a speed of 2 feet per second, the injury incurred by the ball thrown at 2 feet per second would be four times more serious rather than twice as serious.

The velocity each vehicle was traveling is important in evaluating the mechanism of injury in MVCs. The EMT should attempt to obtain or estimate the rate of speed of each vehicle at the time of the collision. A high-velocity collision will cause greater injury than low-velocity collisions. It is also important to remember that when two vehicles collide, the kinetic energy is a combination of the velocity of both vehicles. If each vehicle involved in the collision is traveling at 55 mph at the time of a head-on collision, the kinetic energy is the same as if one vehicle were traveling at 110 mph when it struck a stationary object.

Velocity also plays a role in penetrating injuries, such as gunshot wounds or knife wounds. Bullets generally have a small mass; however, the speed at which they leave the barrel of the gun causes the bullet to impact the body at a high velocity. A knife wound is a lower-velocity injury because the speed at which it is thrust into the body by a human hand has considerably less velocity.

BLUNT TRAUMA

Any force that impacts the body without penetration and causes an injury is blunt trauma. MVCs, falls, fights where blows to the body occur, or crushing injuries from an extremity being caught in a machine are examples of blunt trauma. Clues to blunt trauma are usually evident from the scene. As an example, the EMT should have a high index of suspicion that a bent or broken steering wheel may be indicating a mechanism of injury suggestive of chest injuries resulting from blunt trauma. Blunt trauma should be suspected when an individual is showing signs of an altered mental status or signs of shock following a traumatic event where no external bleeding is obvious.

Blunt force trauma is often multisystem, involving multiple impacts within the body. As an example, during an MVC, when the vehicle strikes another object, the first or initial impact occurs. The individual inside the vehicle continues to travel forward, moving at the same speed the vehicle was traveling prior to impact. The individual will continue to move forward until stopped by another object.

As the individual's chest encounters the steering wheel, the second impact occurs. If the individual is unrestrained, her head may encounter the windshield and a third impact occurs. Finally, the body's organs, held in place by a single ligament, vessel, or container, such as the skull, continue to move forward until they are stopped by another structure in the body. Based on the number of impacts, the index of suspicion is high that the patient has suffered multisystem blunt trauma.

PENETRATING TRAUMA

Any injury caused by the penetration of an object into the body is considered penetrating trauma. Examples of objects that penetrate are bullets, nails, and knives. The severity of penetrating trauma is related to the velocity or kinetic injury and the area of the body the object penetrates.

A knife impaled into the body damages the tissue surrounding the entry side of the impact and the structures immediately around that site. The amount of damage also depends on the size of the blade, with a longer blade reaching farther into the body. However, the force behind the impalement of the knife is low-velocity; therefore, the damage is predictable and limited to the path that the knife traveled.

Objects that are propelled as projectiles causing injury are considered medium- and high-velocity injuries. Shotguns and handguns are generally fired at medium velocity, whereas high-powered weapons such as high-speed rifles, are considered high-velocity weapons. The damage to the body caused by medium- and high-velocity weapons is dependent on two factors: (1) the path or motion of the projectile during travel, called the *trajectory,* and (2) the way the energy is transferred to the body when the projectile enters the body, called *dissipation of energy.*

A shotgun is a medium-velocity weapon resulting in a wound that is characterized by a "spray" or multiple sites where the pellets contained within the shell have struck the body. The area of damage is usually larger than a rifle or handgun wound, which impacts at a higher velocity, causing more extensive damage deeper into the body.

MECHANISM OF INJURY

As stated previously, the mechanism of injury is the cause of the injury. When the EMT arrives on the scene of an MVC and performs a scene size-up, he should look at the damage to the vehicles involved. Understanding the mechanism of injury allows the EMT to determine the possible injuries based on his observation of that damage. The variety of mechanisms of injury will be discussed later in this unit.

MVCs, falls, penetrating gunshot wounds or knife wounds, and explosions are all examples of mechanisms of injury. A common mechanism of injury the EMT may see are falls, especially in the elderly. Table 33-1 lists mechanisms indicating potentially serious trauma.

ASSESSMENT

Assessment of the trauma patient follows the same steps as assessment of the medical patient. General assessment of the trauma patient begins with the initial scene size-up, which includes a consideration of the mechanism of injury. The primary assessment of airway, breathing, and circulation and identification and management of life-threatening injuries is immediately followed by the EMT determining if the patient is high priority or low priority. This decision is important to determining the next step.

If the patient is high priority, then efforts should be made to immediately package and transport the patient before proceeding with the physical examination and history. In some cases, with sufficient personnel, the EMT may continue with physical examination while the patient is being prepared for transport.

Alternatively, if the patient is low priority, then the EMT may elect to obtain baseline vital signs and conduct the secondary assessment, including a thorough physical examination, followed by a history of the patient on scene.

Table 33-1 Serious Trauma by Mechanism

Falls
- Adults—> 20 (two stories)
- Pediatrics >10 feet (one story or 2 to 3 times child height)

High Risk Auto Crash
- Intrusion: 12 inches from occupant or 18 inches any side
- Ejection (partial or complete)
- Death of another occupant
- Vehicle telemetry data consistent with high risk injury

Auto vs Pedestrian/Bicyclist Thrown/Run Over or Significant Speed (>20 mph)

Motorcycle Crash > 20 mph

Source: CDC

PRIMARY ASSESSMENT

The primary assessment of the trauma patient begins by assessing for a clear, patent airway. Cervical spinal immobilization should be immediately applied and the jaw-thrust used to open the airway for unconscious trauma patient. The EMT must be prepared to keep the airway clear by suctioning and protect the airway, especially when head and facial trauma is present.

Breathing and circulation should then be assessed, with any life-threatening injuries immediately managed. High-concentration oxygen via non-rebreather mask at 12–15 lpm is appropriate at this point in the significantly injured patient.

HISTORY AND SECONDARY ASSESSMENT

The secondary assessment of the trauma patient is geared toward finding the patient's specific injuries. The mechanism of the accident often allows prediction of the type and severity of injury. The more significant the mechanism, the more serious the injuries may be. Whenever a major mechanism of injury is encountered, the EMT should perform a complete rapid trauma assessment. By performing an organized examination of the patient from head to toe, the EMT can quickly discover hidden or suspected injuries.

The secondary assessment of the trauma patient is divided into two methods, depending on the significance of the potential injuries. The rapid method consists of a brief head-to-toe assessment performed on the patient who has suffered a significant mechanism of injury and is considered a serious or critical high-priority patient. Because early identification of injuries will guide the management of the serious trauma patient, the physical assessment is performed before the medical history.

However, most traumas involve an isolated minor injury. It is unnecessary for an EMT to perform a complete head-to-toe assessment on a patient with an isolated minor injury. For example, a patient who cut his finger with a knife while slicing bread has an injury that is obviously isolated to the finger. The chances of hidden injury as a result of this mechanism are fairly low. A rapid head-to-toe trauma assessment is unnecessary and would be an unwarranted intrusion into the patient's privacy. In cases in which there is minor isolated trauma, the EMT should perform a modified secondary assessment based on the patient's specific injury.

The modified secondary assessment is performed on patients who have suffered a nonsignificant mechanism of injury. The modified assessment focuses on the chief concern or primary injury. After the modified secondary assessment is complete, the EMT should obtain a baseline set of vital signs as well as a SAMPLE history, as described in Unit 18. In some cases, the injury is treated at the same time as, or immediately after, the vital signs are taken.

RECONSIDER THE MECHANISM OF INJURY

Although obvious injuries are usually easily discovered and managed during the primary assessment, it is important to reconsider the mechanism of injury while performing the secondary assessment on the trauma patient. Often a significant internal injury will not be obvious until the secondary assessment. Reconsidering the mechanism of injury while performing the physical assessment can help identify serious injuries not previously identified.

As discussed in Unit 19, the mechanism of injury for a trauma patient is similar to the history of the present illness (HPI) in the medical patient. The EMT should always reconsider the mechanism of injury and be prepared for signs and symptoms of additional injuries to appear at any time as the call progresses.

ALS INTERCEPT

Trauma can produce injuries that will have serious consequences that may require treatment only available through an ALS intercept. If the patient's airway is compromised, the EMT may not have the tools and skills required to maintain a patent airway. ALS personnel are trained in the insertion of advanced airway adjuncts, such as the endotracheal tube that will ensure a patent airway. If ALS personnel (i.e., EMT–Intermediates or paramedics) are not on scene, then an ALS unit should be called to the scene or to intercept the ambulance while it is en route to the closest appropriate hospital (Figure 33.1).

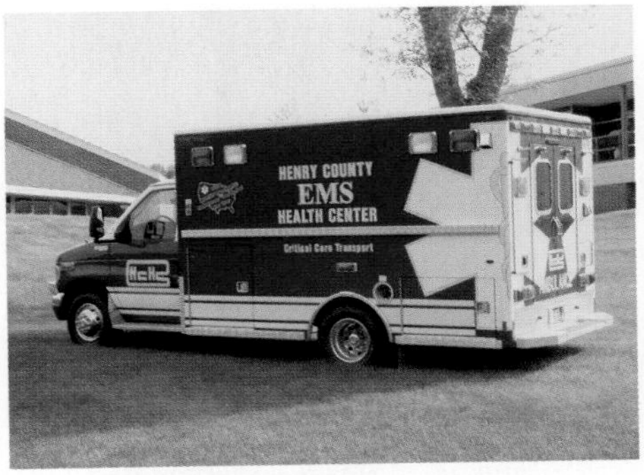

ALS backup should be called following the scene size-up and based on the mechanism of injury and initial general impression of the patient's condition. ALS intercept can be called at any time as the call progresses, for patients who initially appear stable with minor injuries but whose vital signs become unstable or for whom new signs and symptoms indicate a more serious injury than first indentified. The EMT should remember that three factors—unstable vital signs, significant physical injuries, or a significant past medical history—are reasons to call for ALS backup at any point in the patient's care. Review Table 19-2 in Unit 19 on when to call for ALS intercept.

Figure 33.1 Consider advanced life support (ALS) backup for a seriously injured patient (Courtesy of Henry County Health Center, Mt. Pleasant, IA)

RAPID TRAUMA ASSESSMENT

Any trauma patient who has been exposed to a significant mechanism of injury should undergo a primary assessment followed by a **rapid trauma assessment.** As discussed previously, this rapid head-to-toe assessment is geared toward identifying injuries that may be quite serious although they are not initially obvious. The rapid trauma assessment, as the name suggests, is quick. It should take an EMT about 1–2 minutes to complete a rapid trauma assessment. Taking longer than 2 minutes is wasteful and unnecessary and could compromise the patient by further worsening a serious injury or condition.

While the EMT is performing the rapid trauma assessment, he must also be continually monitoring the patient's condition. Is the patient still awake? Is the patient maintaining her airway? Is the patient breathing adequately? If at any point the patient's condition changes, the EMT must immediately stop the rapid trauma assessment and resolve the life-threatening problem.

During the rapid trauma assessment, the EMT is looking for indications of obvious or hidden trauma. Although accuracy is important, time should not be wasted on details that are not significant at this point. The rapid trauma assessment is short and to the point. A more detailed physical exam of areas of injury will be performed later.

PHYSICAL SIGNS OF INJURY

The signs an EMT looks for that may indicate serious underlying injuries are abbreviated by the initials DCAP-BTLS. Table 33-2 lists the initials and their meanings. The EMT should memorize this abbreviation and use it every time a rapid trauma assessment is performed.

DEFORMITY

Any irregularity outside of the normal body shape should be considered a **deformity** and possibly the result of trauma. For example, a deformity is often the first indication of a broken or fractured bone under the skin. The forearm of the patient in Figure 33.2 is deformed.

CONTUSION

A bruise is a layperson's term for a **contusion.** Bruises are the result of blood pooling under the skin. Therefore, any contusion should be considered a sign of potentially serious bleeding under the skin. Contusions usually take around 15–20 minutes to form and therefore may not be immediately apparent to the EMT. The presence of a contusion, as seen in Figure 33.3, may indicate that the trauma occurred some time ago. The exact location and size of any contusion should be noted in the report.

ABRASION

Abrasions occur whenever the skin is scraped and underlying tissue is exposed. A skinned knee from a fall off a bike is an example of an abrasion. An abrasion in and of itself is not serious, but it delineates the area where a force was applied, as in a fall. Most of the bleeding, as seen in Figure 33.4, is self-controlled.

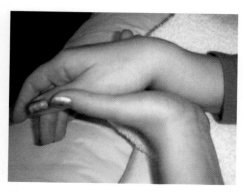

Figure 33.2 A fractured bone can result in a painful, swollen, deformed extremity (Courtesy of Deborah Funk, MD, Albany Medical Center, Albany, NY)

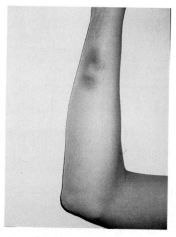

Figure 33.3 A large bruise, or contusion, can represent serious bleeding

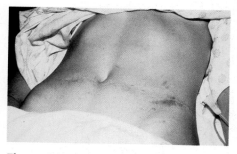

Figure 33.4 Abrasions indicate that force was applied to the body (Courtesy of Deborah Funk, MD, Albany Medical Center, Albany, NY)

Table 33-2 DCAP-BTLS

Term	Meaning	Lay Term
Deformity	Distorted, unnatural	Looks funny
Contusion	Injury where the skin is not broken	Bruise
Abrasion	Scraping away the top layer of skin	Skinned knee
Puncture	A wound that pierces the skin	Knife wound
Burns	Tissue injury due to heat or chemicals	Burn
Tenderness	Pain when pressure is applied	Tender, sore
Laceration	Torn skin	Cut
Swelling	Abnormal enlargement	Swollen

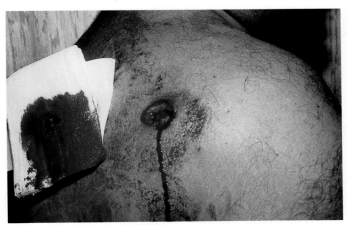

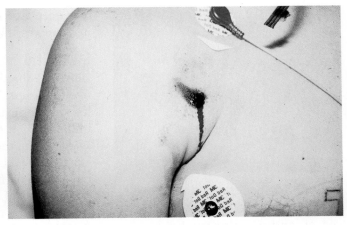

Figure 33.5 Puncture wounds can result in serious underlying injury (Courtesy of Deborah Funk, MD, Albany Medical Center, Albany, NY)

PUNCTURE

A **puncture** wound is an injury caused by an object penetrating the skin and soft tissues. Puncture wounds can be quite deep despite a relatively small skin wound. Any penetrating wound to the head, neck, chest, abdomen, or pelvis should be considered serious. The EMT cannot know how deep the puncture could have gone or what organs may have been damaged along the way. The gunshot wound in Figure 33.5 may have damaged organs that are 6 inches, or farther, away from the entrance wound. All wounds need to be reported to the hospital staff immediately so that further assessment of underlying organs may be immediately initiated.

BURN

Burns are created whenever a significant source of heat damages the outer layers of the skin. Although a superficial burn, such as sunburn, may not be serious, other deeper burns are considered more serious. Any burn involving the hands, face, feet, or genitals, such as the burn seen in Figure 33.6, is considered a serious burn regardless of the depth of the burned skin.

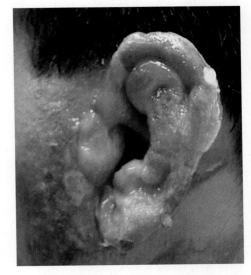

Figure 33.6 Burns can range from minor in severity to life threatening (Courtesy of Deborah Funk, MD, Albany Medical Center, Albany, NY)

TENDERNESS

While assessing the patient, the EMT should be gently pressing his fingertips against the skin. Any area that is sensitive or even painful to the touch is said to be **tender.** Such areas, or points, of tenderness usually indicate tissue damage under the skin. Signs of tenderness include a facial grimace or guarding of the injured area (Figure 33.7). The patient may even push the EMT's hand away from her body. If the area is tender, the patient will usually complain of pain, a symptom.

LACERATION

Any deep cuts in the skin, called **lacerations,** should be noted and reported. Lacerations often need to be *sutured*, or sewn closed. More important, lacerations can indicate where a significant external force was applied to the body.

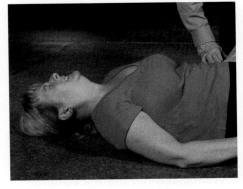

Figure 33.7 Facial expressions often reveal areas of tenderness

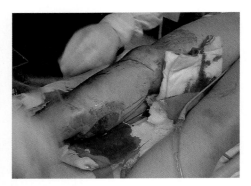

Figure 33.8 Lacerations can result in injury to underlying nerve, vessel, and muscle structures (Courtesy of Deborah Funk, MD, Albany Medical Center, Albany, NY)

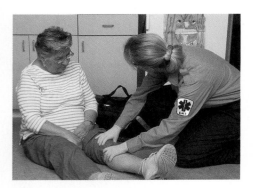

Figure 33.9 Swelling is often felt and not seen

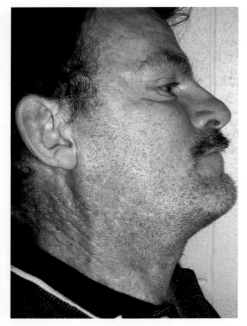

Figure 33.10 Jugular venous distention in the trauma patient can indicate serious internal chest injuries

The deep laceration seen on the patient's leg in Figure 33.8 may have damaged nerves and tendons as well as ¨muscle.

SWELLING

The EMT should note any **swelling** under the skin. This final sign can be difficult to assess. The best method of determining whether something is swollen is to compare the suspect area with the other side of the body, as shown in Figure 33.9. Often, an EMT can feel, rather than see, that one leg is more swollen than the other leg.

DCAP-BTLS represents an excellent foundation for a descriptive assessment of injury findings. EMTs may always add to this list of descriptive terms, but DCAP-BTLS should remain the main staple of any assessment.

STEPS OF THE RAPID TRAUMA ASSESSMENT

Starting at the head, the EMT uses his senses of hearing, touch, and sight to rapidly assess the patient for injuries. The mnemonic DCAP-BTLS serves as a reminder of all the points of the assessment. Starting at the head, methodically work down the patient's body.

HEAD AND NECK

Injuries to the head and neck are often very serious. Bleeding can cause problems with the airway. Blows to the head can injure delicate brain tissue, causing the patient to lose consciousness. Neck injuries can lead to permanent paralysis. Therefore, the EMT should take a moment to carefully assess the head and neck. The abbreviation DCAP-BTLS should be recalled as the EMT looks for signs of injury to the head and neck.

Starting at the top of the head, the EMT should run fingers through the patient's hair, somewhat like kneading bread dough, looking for deformities and checking often for blood on his gloves.

Attention should then be given to the bony structures that surround and support the airway. Grasping the angle of the jaw, the EMT should feel over the length of the jawbone, ending by pressing gently on the teeth. Next, check inside the mouth and nose for any signs of bleeding or foreign objects.

The EMT moves down to assess the neck, beginning by checking the anterior neck for DCAP-BTLS. Is the trachea damaged? Is the trachea midline? Is there any swelling that could threaten the airway?

An important sign to assess for is **jugular venous distention (JVD).** Veins on the side of the neck, running from the angle of the jaw to the shoulders, are normally visible but not bulging. Bulging jugular veins in the neck can be a sign of fluid overload in the medical patient or serious internal chest injuries in the trauma patient. Significant JVD, as seen in Figure 33.10, should be reported.

Sliding his hands downward to the posterior neck, the EMT should palpate for point tenderness along the midline, starting at the base of the skull and ending at the shoulders. Any pain or tenderness should be reported. All seriously injured patients are assumed to have spinal injury until proven otherwise. Therefore, if a rigid cervical immobilization device (CID) has not already been applied, then one should be applied now.

CHEST

The chest cavity contains the heart and the lungs. Injuries to the chest are potentially life threatening. An EMT's skill in quickly, but accurately, assessing the chest wall for signs of chest injury can mean the difference between life and death.

"You can't treat what you don't see." This statement is especially true when it comes to chest injuries. It is important for the EMT to balance the patient's right to privacy with her need for effective medical attention. The two can be accomplished simultaneously. Unbutton or pull down the shirt, one section at a time. Perform all aspects of the assessment at one time, and then re-cover that section of the patient. If serious injury, such as a gunshot wound, is discovered, then the need for immediate lifesaving treatment should supersede any concerns about privacy.

The EMT should begin assessment of the chest by looking carefully at the entire chest wall. What is the quality of breathing? Does the patient appear to be straining or working hard at breathing? Problems with breathing should be addressed immediately.

Then the EMT should proceed to assess each section of the chest—upper, lower, and sides—for DCAP-BTLS. Starting at the top of the anterior chest wall, the EMT should first look and listen, then feel, that section.

Look, or inspect, for signs of chest injury: DCAP-BTLS. Are there abrasions from seat belts, or punctures from gunshot wounds? A quick visual inspection of the chest wall usually reveals any injuries. Paradoxical motion from a flail chest or air escaping from a sucking chest wound should be noted now if they were not picked up in the primary assessment. These findings are discussed in Unit 16.

Using a stethoscope, the EMT should listen to, or auscultate, the lungs. Place the stethoscope against the bare skin; clothing can muffle the breath sounds. The head of the stethoscope rubbing against clothing can also create false impressions of the lung sounds. A more thorough assessment of lung sounds is done in the rapid trauma assessment than was done in the primary assessment.

At this time, the EMT should listen minimally in four places. The most useful areas to hear breath sounds are in the apices at the midclavicular lines and at the bases, in the midaxillary lines, high in the axillae. The EMT should determine whether breath sounds are present in each of these places, and, if they are present, whether they sound equal from one side to another.

Next, the EMT should feel, or palpate, the entire chest wall, looking for any injuries. In addition to the usual DCAP-BTLS, when assessing the chest, the EMT should note the presence of crepitus. Crepitus is a crunching sensation felt during palpation of an injury. Crepitus can be caused by air accumulation under the skin from a lung injury, creating the sensation of Rice Krispies when palpated, or by broken bone ends rubbing together. These physical findings indicate serious chest injury and should be reported to the hospital staff immediately upon arrival.

ABDOMEN AND PELVIS

The abdominal cavity is home to a large number of solid and hollow organs. These organs all lie within a large bowl-like cavity formed by the pelvis and the diaphragm. This abdominal bowl can hold a great deal of blood without demonstrating significant outward signs. The rapid trauma assessment will not only discover some of the more subtle signs of intra-abdominal injury but also, and perhaps more important, can establish a baseline abdominal exam for comparison later.

The abdomen lacks any distinct landmarks. For this reason, the belly button, or umbilicus, serves as the midpoint of the abdomen, and the abdomen is divided into four quadrants. Each quadrant is labeled left or right, upper or lower, as the case may be. Review Unit 5 for a discussion of abdominal anatomy.

The EMT should assess the abdomen using the "look first, then feel" concept that was described in the chest assessment section. The abdomen should be exposed for assessment, and the EMT should first look for DCAP-BTLS.

Street Smart

To avoid worsening any injuries, as well as to maintain the patient's trust, most EMTs assess obviously injured areas only after they have looked for less obvious injuries.

Although seat belts are very helpful in reducing injuries sustained in MVCs, they can also cause some injury. A seat belt applies pressure across the abdomen and torso; this pressure can be significant in the event of a high-speed crash. The pressure from the seat belt can cause contusions and abrasions to the abdominal wall, which can be seen by the EMT during assessment, and may result in internal abdominal organ injury. These internal injuries are most often seen when the seat belt is worn incorrectly and are invariably not as severe as the injuries sustained by unbelted occupants of a vehicle involved in a high-speed crash.

After a complete visual inspection, the EMT should gently palpate each quadrant. The abdomen should be soft and not distended. Any distension should be noted as well as any attempt by the patient to guard the abdomen. **Guarding,** a tightening of the abdominal muscles, is a protective reflex when abdominal injury exists and is evidenced by a localized firm feeling upon palpation of the abdomen. A patient's grimace or loud protest may indicate that an area is very painful. The exact location of any tenderness should be carefully noted and reported.

The pelvis is a strong ring of bone that protects many important organs and large blood vessels. Damage to these organs and vessels can lead to a substantial amount of blood loss. It takes a great deal of force to break this bony ring. However, if the pelvis is fractured, then it is likely that the underlying structures are also damaged.

To assess the bony pelvis, the EMT should gently press downward, then inward on the pelvic wings. A fractured pelvis is painful, and the conscious patient will likely make this discomfort known. If bony fractures are present when this compression is done, the EMT may feel crepitus as bone ends grate against one another. If tenderness or crepitus is elicited during the exam, that maneuver should not be repeated.

Finally, the EMT should press downward on the pubic bone to assess for fractures of the anterior pelvis. Some EMTs find it more acceptable to take the patient's hand, provided it is not injured, and place it over the pubis. Then the EMT lays his hand on top of the patient's hand and gently presses down. Again, patient modesty or EMT inhibition should not prevent the patient from receiving a complete medical assessment.

EXTREMITIES

Although a broken bone itself is usually not life threatening, the bleeding that can come with a broken bone can be significant. Therefore, one of the objectives of an extremity check is to determine whether there is severe bleeding within the tissues.

As usual, the EMT should assess each extremity using DCAP-BTLS. Any deformity noted may be an indication of a broken bone. Contusions and abrasions indicate where a force has been applied. The EMT should carefully assess for deformity and tenderness in those areas particularly. Often the only sign of bleeding into the soft tissues, such as the thigh, is swelling. Again, this swelling may not be readily apparent to the naked eye, but careful comparison of one leg with the other will reveal the swelling occurring inside.

Any lacerations that are accompanied by deformity may indicate that an open fracture of the bone has occurred. An open fracture carries with it serious risk for bleeding and infection and will be discussed further in Unit 38.

Major arteries, veins, and nerves run parallel to the large bones of the body. Therefore, if a large bone breaks, there is a great likelihood that the sharp, broken ends will puncture these vessels or damage the nerves. The result is severe bleeding or loss of function. To assess whether a blood vessel has been damaged, the EMT should check for peripheral pulses.

The most accessible peripheral pulse in the arm is the radial pulse at the wrist. The radial pulse can be found on the palmar surface of the wrist proximal to the thumb. The most accessible peripheral pulse in the leg is the pedal pulse. The pedal pulse can be found along the midline of the top of the foot, about halfway between the ankle and the great toe.

Whenever an EMT is checking for the pulse in an extremity that has been injured, he should also check for nerve function. Nerves have both fibers that create movement, or motor nerves, and fibers that create feeling, or sensory nerves. Therefore, a check of motion and sensation is part of the assessment.

A complete assessment of peripheral pulses and motor and sensory nerve functions (PMS, for pulses, movement, and sensation) should be completed on all four extremities. Typically, an EMT will report "PMSx4 intact." Any loss of these functions should be reported.

BACK AND BUTTOCKS

When the patient is being logrolled onto a backboard, a moment should be taken to assess the back and buttocks. The EMT should quickly perform a check for DCAP-BTLS. After a visual inspection for signs of injury, a hand should be run down the length of the spine from the top of the shoulders to the top of the buttocks. Any wounds or tenderness should be noted and reported.

Careful control of the spine, using a rigid cervical immobilization device as well as continuous manual in-line stabilization, is required. It takes a minimum of three providers to properly logroll the patient to assess the back and buttocks. The concepts involved in spinal immobilization are discussed further in Unit 35. Skill 33-1 at the end of this unit describes the procedure for a rapid trauma assessment.

BASELINE VITAL SIGNS AND HISTORY

A baseline set of vital signs is a part of every physical assessment. Some EMTs will clear an arm so that another EMT can start vital signs while the rapid trauma assessment is being performed.

A SAMPLE history is then performed. An abbreviated history of the present illness is often obtained on scene. Once the rapid assessment is complete, the EMT must take the time to obtain as complete a SAMPLE history as possible. Frequently, this history is taken while en route to the hospital. Skill 33-1 at the end of this unit describes the procedure taking a history as part of a rapid trauma assessment.

THE MODIFIED SECONDARY ASSESSMENT

Not every trauma call is a life-or-death emergency. In fact, most are not. That is not meant to imply that these patients do not need prompt medical attention but simply that the nature of the injury permits the EMT to assess and stabilize the injury on scene. This modified secondary assessment and stabilization before transport prevents further injury from occurring.

If the injury is obviously isolated and the mechanism does not suggest further injury potential, it is unnecessary to perform a head-to-toe rapid trauma assessment. If the mechanism of injury is minor or the injury is isolated, it is more appropriate to focus on the injured part.

A physical assessment that is limited to the area of injury is called a **focused trauma assessment.** Except for the fact that it is limited to one body part or region, it is otherwise performed in the same manner as the rapid trauma assessment.

After an appropriate scene size-up and primary assessment reveal that the patient has no significant mechanism or obvious signs of serious injury, the EMT should begin a focused trauma assessment based on the patient's specific injury. Focusing on the affected area, the EMT should assess for DCAP-BTLS.

Naturally, treatments will follow in accordance with the type and severity of the injury. It is a safe practice to assume the worst injury and hope for the best.

Every patient, regardless of the severity of the injuries, needs a baseline set of vital signs and a SAMPLE history. Appropriate preparation for transport should be accomplished, and the patient should be brought to the most appropriate hospital for further evaluation of the injury. Skill 33-2 at the end of this chapter demonstrates the modified secondary assessment focused physical examination.

TRAUMA SCORING

Many EMS systems and hospitals use a trauma score as the means of communication to identify the severity of the trauma patient. A trauma score is a numerical way to identify that severity. The EMT should be familiar with the scoring methods used in their region.

REVISED TRAUMA SCORE

The **Revised Trauma Score** is a standard method of trauma scoring that uses results of the Glasgow Coma Scale, and the patient's respiratory rate and systolic blood pressure, assigning a number to each element that sets the level of severity. The lower the number of the Revised Trauma Score, the more severe the patient's condition and percentage of survival. Table 33-3 shows the scoring parameters of the Revised Trauma Score.

Table 33-3 Revised Trauma Score		
Respiratory Rate	10 to 29/min	4
	>29/min	3
	6 to 9/min	2
	1 to 5/min	1
	None	0
Systolic Blood Pressure	>89 mmHg	4
	76 to 89 mmHg	3
	50 to 75 mmHg	2
	1 to 49 mmHg	1
	No Pulse or 0 SBP (systolic blood pressure)	0
Total Glasgow Coma Scale Points	13 to 15	4
	9 to 12	3
	6 to 8	2
	4 to 5	1
	<3	0
Total Trauma Score (Trauma Scale + GCS)		1 to 12

THE GLASGOW COMA SCALE

The patient's mental status is first established during the primary assessment, using the AVPU scale. The **Glasgow Coma Scale** is a means to rank the level of an individual's neurologic status. The Glasgow Coma Scale should be rescored during the rapid secondary assessment and reassessment of mental status. Changes in the score can indicate the deterioration or improvement of the patient's condition and is extremely important information in tracking the effectiveness of trauma management.

The Glasgow Coma Scale rates the level of responsiveness based on eye opening, verbal response, and motor response (Table 33-4). The Glasgow Coma Scale is also used on pediatric trauma patients, discussed further in Unit 43.

EYE OPENING

As the EMT approaches the patient and begins the primary assessment, the patient's mental status can be initially assessed based on whether her eyes are open or closed. If the patient's eyes are open as the EMT approaches, the patient is said to have spontaneous eye opening, a score of 4 on the Glasgow Coma

Table 33-4 Glasgow Coma Scale

Eye Opening	
Spontaneous	4
To verbal command	3
To pain	2
No response	1

Verbal Response	
Oriented	5
Disoriented/Confused	4
Inappropriate words	3
Incomprehensible sounds/words	2
No response	0

Motor Response	
Obeys verbal commands	6
Localizes pain	5
Withdraws from pain	4
Abnormal flexion (decorticate posturing)	3
Abnormal extension (decerebrate posturing)	2
No response	1

Scale. If the patient's eyes are closed, what will cause the patient to open her eyes? The next three scoring elements of eye opening are based on the patient opening her eyes to a verbal command, painful stimulation, or no response.

VERBAL RESPONSE

A verbal response by the patient should not be confused with the eye opening response to a verbal command to "open your eyes." The patient's verbal response is how she answers the EMT when asked questions. There are five possible responses the patient can make with the score decreasing based on the way she responds to verbal stimulus.

The patient may respond to verbal stimulus with appropriate orientation, conversing easily with the EMT. If the patient converses but is disoriented or confused, she is showing some abnormality in neurologic function. Patients who respond with incomprehensible sounds such as mumbling or who do not respond at all to verbal stimuli are showing serious deterioration of their neurologic function.

MOTOR RESPONSE

The motor response of the Glasgow Coma Scale measures the patient's response to painful stimulus. Patients may have purposeful movements, attempting to remove the painful stimulus, such as attempting to push away or grabbing at the hand or object causing the pain.

Patients may also respond with nonpurposeful movements in response to painful stimulation. Nonpurposeful movements include flexion or extension posturing that is not an attempt to remove the stimulus. Flexion posturing, also called decorticate (to the core) posturing, involves a strong movement of the arm pulled upward toward the chest. Extension posturing, also called decerebrate posturing, involves extending the arms parallel to the body. Patients may also have no response to painful stimulus.

MANAGEMENT

Management of the trauma patient focuses on packaging, including spinal immobilization, and rapid, timely transport to the appropriate facility. Critical trauma patients should be rapidly packaged and transported immediately following the primary assessment and management of life threats. Additional treatments should completed in the back of the ambulance while en route to the hospital. ALS should be requested; however, the EMT should not remain on scene but rather arrange an intercept on the way to the hospital. Scene time should be limited to 10 minutes when possible for the critical trauma patient.

TRANSPORT

Transporting trauma patients requires the EMT to make important decisions quickly. Where is the best place for the patient to receive definitive trauma care? What is the quickest, most beneficial mode of transport to that facility?

MODE OF TRANSPORT

Transportation of the trauma patient depends on several factors, including the type of traumatic injury, the anatomy most likely to need urgent surgery, mechanism of injury (life or limb), and preexisting conditions. Appropriate triage of trauma patients along with the distance from the appropriate facility will determine the mode of transport: air medical transport or ground ambulance transport.

Many remote or rural areas rely on air medical transport, either helicopter or fixed-wing, because the distance to the closest trauma center exceeds a recommended transport time. However, recent studies covering response times for air transports over-ground transports of the trauma patients have proven inconclusive. The EMT should be familiar with territorial, state, regional, or local trauma protocols in determining the most appropriate mode of transport for the critical trauma patient.

DESTINATION DETERMINATION

Trauma systems developed over the years in each state are providing an organized approach to treating trauma patients. The trauma care systems provide around-the-clock care and equipment at facilities developed specifically for the definitive treatment of traumatic injuries.

TRAUMA CENTER

Trauma centers are hospitals that provide definitive emergency care to trauma patients. In order for a hospital to qualify as a trauma center, specific criteria must be met. Additionally, the hospital will be designated by a level, depending on the level of trauma services it offers. In most areas, there are four levels of designation with a Level I being the highest level of service. Trauma centers are ranked by the American College of Surgeons (ACS) in the United States, by category from Level I (comprehensive trauma service) to Level III (limited-care). Some states rank their own trauma centers, separate from ACS, ranging from Level I to Level IV (Table 33-5).

The EMT should be familiar with local out-of-hospital trauma triage protocols. All transport decisions are based on the type and severity of injury, mental status, primary assessment findings, and distance to the facility best capable of providing definitive trauma care. The EMT should be familiar with local protocols that usually provide an algorhythm to aid the EMT in determining the most appropriate destination and mode of transport for the critical trauma patient.

Table 33-5 Trauma Center Levels and Criteria

Level I—24/7 definitive trauma services including Resuscitation Unit, Operating Room, and Intensive Care Unit (ICU). Physician requirements include in-house trauma surgeon, anesthesiologist, orthopedic surgeon, neurosurgeon, critical care physician in ICU, and surgical director of ICU; also includes a comprehensive trauma research program, surgery residency program, and outreach professional trauma educational program.

Level II—24/7 trauma services including a Resuscitation Unit, Operating Room, and Intensive Care Unit. Physician requirements include in-house trauma surgeon, anesthesiologist, and critical care ICU physician, and on-call orthopedic and neurosurgeons available within 30 minutes. Additional requirement include an outreach trauma education program.

Level III—24/7 trauma services including a Resuscitation Unit, Operating Room, and Intensive Care Unit. Physician requirements include on-call trauma surgeon, anesthesiologist, and orthopedic and neurosurgeons available within 30 minutes.

Level IV—state-specific level; common criteria is the ability to provide initial evaluation, stabilization, diagnostic capabilities with ability to transfer to a higher level trauma center. Level IV may be able to provide surgery and critical care services, with nurse trained in trauma management on site and emergency physicians able to be available at the time of patient's arrival to the Emergency Department. Level IV trauma centers usually have transfer agreements with other trauma centers with higher levels.

CONCLUSION

The decision whether to perform a rapid physical examination or a modified focused physical examination is determined based on the mechanism of injury as well as the potential severity of the injury. Whenever an EMT is in doubt about which type to perform, the the EMT should perform a rapid trauma assessment.

The usefulness of a rapid trauma assessment is in discovering potentially life-threatening injuries. To find an injury, one has to suspect an injury might exist in the first place. A basic understanding of the kinematics of trauma and consideration of the mechanism of injury can help the EMT obtain a high index of suspicion that a serious underlying injury may exist.

Most injuries are minor and a modified secondary assessment, focused physical examination is sufficient to determine the right course of treatment. However, keep an open mind and always suspect that other injuries may have occurred.

The mode of transport of the trauma patient is based on the available resources, severity of injuries, and distance from the appropriate level trauma center. Transport of critical trauma patients should be to the facility best able to provide definitive care.

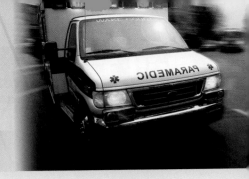

CASE STUDY Continued

Jason discusses his finding with Michele, including the caved-in roof on the car indicating the vehicle had rolled over at least once, the broken windshield, bent steering wheel, and loose seatbelt. Michele determines a rapid trauma assessment is warranted based on the mechanism of injury.

Although the patient denies any concerns other than her wrist, Michele notices she is not keeping her eyes open without being told to open them; she is withdrawing from pain and not following commands. The first responder is holding cervical spinal immobilization while Michele begins her rapid trauma assessment. Jason obtains a quick set of baseline vital signs; blood pressure 118/64, pulse 110, and respirations of 22 with good air exchange. The patient has a Glasgow Coma Score of 12 at this time.

During the brief head-to-toe, Michele notes additional injuries to the patient including a bruise to the patient's chest, tenderness in the lower left quadrant of the abdomen and abrasions on her left arm and leg. There is a deformity to the left wrist with bruising and swelling becoming evident.

Michele determines this is a priority transport and requests an ALS intercept on the way to the closest

trauma center 20 minutes away. En route Michele obtains a patient history, noting that the patient appears to be having increasing difficulty responding. Baseline vitals following the primary assessment are repeated with the blood pressure now 92/56, pulse 132, and respirations of 24 and shallow with diminished breath sounds on the left side. Oxygen at 15 lpm via non-rebreather mask is maintained, and Michele prepares to ventilate if needed.

ALS intercept is met approximately 10 minutes from the scene, and Michele gives a report, including the results of the brief head-to-toe, vitals, and history. Michele provides the ALS crew with an updated GCS of 8 as the patient is now only opening her eyes to painful stimuli, making incomprehensible sounds, and withdrawing from pain. She also gives a Revised Trauma Score of 10 out of 12.

Michele continues to assist the ALS crew throughout transport to the Level I trauma center, where the patient is taken immediately into surgery to relieve pressure that had begun to build on her brain from a closed traumatic brain injury. Michele knows the rapid assessment, packaging, and quick transport of the patient to a facility that could immediately treat her life-threatening brain injury will be vital to the patient's complete recovery.

PURPOSE: To assess the major trauma patient for injuries that are not life threatening.

STANDARD PRECAUTIONS:

☑ Gloves
☑ Goggles

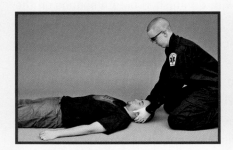

1 After completing an appropriate scene size-up and primary assessment, the EMT considers a request for ALS backup and transport priority. The EMT then performs a rapid trauma assessment on the trauma patient with a significant mechanism of injury. Manual head stabilization should be maintained for the duration of the rapid trauma assessment.

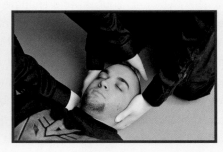

2 The EMT next assesses the head by careful inspection and palpation for any signs of injury. Deformities, contusions, abrasions, punctures or penetrations, burns, tenderness, lacerations, or swelling should be noted. Moving in a methodical fashion, the EMT then inspects and palpates the neck.

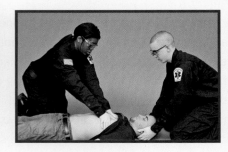

3 The EMT next looks and feels the chest to assess for the presence of any signs of injury. The EMT should also listen to breath sounds carefully assessed at the apices and the bases. Presence and equality of air movement should be noted.

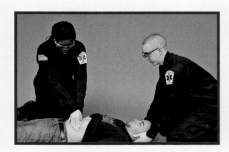

4 The abdominal assessment includes looking and feeling for any signs of injury. The pelvis is visually inspected, then gently compressed downward and inward in order to find any signs of injury.

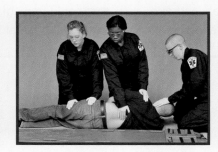

5 After rolling the patient to the side, using a logroll technique and maintaining spinal immobilization, the EMT inspects and palpates the back and buttocks to find any signs of injury.

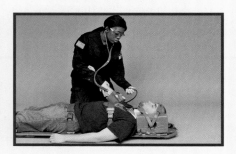

6 After the rapid trauma assessment has been completed, a complete baseline set of vital signs must be taken.

PURPOSE: To obtain a baseline physical examination for assessment and comparison of the minor trauma patient.

STANDARD PRECAUTIONS:

☑ Stethoscope
☑ Blood pressure cuff
☑ Penlight
☑ Gloves
☑ Goggles

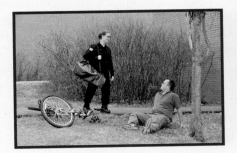

1 The EMT considers the mechanism of injury. Depending on the mechanism of injury, the EMT decides whether to perform a rapid trauma assessment or a focused physical examination.

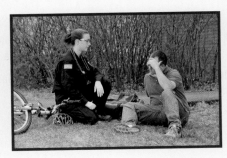

2 The EMT next determines the chief concern.

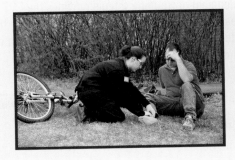

3 The EMT performs a focused examination specific to the injury.

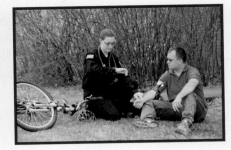

4 The EMT then obtains baseline vital signs.

Key Concepts

- Kinematics of trauma is the science of analyzing the mechanism of injury.

- The amount of kinetic energy of a moving object depends on the mass and velocity of the object.

  - Mass = weight

  - Velocity = speed of travel

    - Blunt force trauma

    - Penetrating trauma

- The mechanism of injury refers to how the patient was injured.

- The mechanism of injury will guide the steps of assessment following evaluation of the patient's mental status and primary assessment.

  - Serious mechanism

    - Refer to Table 33-1

- The secondary assessment of the trauma patient is divided into the rapid method and modified method.

- The secondary assessment of a trauma patient with a significant mechanism of injury uses the rapid method, brief head-to-toe prior to gathering the history.

  - Immediately follows the primary assessment

  - Includes baseline vital signs

- The secondary assessment of a trauma patient with a nonsignificant MOI is modified to focus on the body part that has been injured.

  - Done after history and baseline vital signs

  - Focuses on injury of chief concern

- The components of DCAP-BTLS are the types of injuries being looked for in the secondary assessment physical examination:

  - Deformity

  - Contusion

  - Abrasion

  - Puncture

  - Burn

  - Tenderness

  - Laceration

  - Swelling

- The Revised Trauma Score, which includes the Glasgow Coma Scale, is a numerical method of communication between EMS and hospitals to signify the severity of the trauma patient's condition:

  - Glasgow Coma Scale

    - Eye opening

    - Verbal response

    - Motor response

  - Trauma score elements

    - Respiratory rate

    - Systolic blood pressure

    - Glasgow Coma Scale

- The development of trauma systems provides the EMT with guidelines for making transport decisions, including the best mode of transport and most appropriate trauma center destination

  - Mode of transport

    - Air medical, including helicopter and fixed wing

    - Ground ambulance

  - Trauma Centers

    - Level I—highest level with greatest trauma services

    - Level II—second highest level

    - Level III—lowest level by ACS criteria

    - Level IV—lowest level by specific state criteria

Review Questions

1. What is meant by the kinematics of trauma?
2. How do mass and velocity affect the mechanism of injury?
3. What is the main objective of the rapid trauma assessment?
4. Give several examples of trauma patients who would receive a rapid trauma assessment.
5. Give examples of mechanisms of injury that have a high potential for serious bodily harm.
6. List each step in the assessment of a seriously injured trauma patient, starting at the scene size-up.
7. What does each of the initials in DCAP-BTLS mean?
8. In addition to DCAP-BTLS, list one extra assessment finding for each of the following body regions: head, neck, chest, abdomen, pelvis, extremities, and back.
9. What is the importance of a trauma score?
10. What are the elements of the Glasgow Coma Scale?
11. Which level trauma center provides the best resources caring for trauma patients?
12. What elements should the EMT consider to determine the mode of transport and destination for the critical trauma patient?

Key Terms

Abrasion
Burns
Contusion
Deformity
Focused trauma assessment
Glasgow Coma Scale
Guarding
Jugular venous distention (JVD)
Kinematics of trauma
Kinetics

Kinetic energy
Laceration
Mass
Puncture
Rapid trauma assessment
Revised Trauma Score
Swelling
Tender
Velocity

Further Study

Elling, B., and K. M. Elling. *Principles of Patient Assessment in EMS*. Clifton Park, NY: Thomson Delmar Learning, 2002.

National Association of Emergency Medical Technicians. *PHTLS: Basic and Advanced PrehospitalTrauma Life Support*. 6th ed. Clinton, MS: Mosby, 2006.

UNIT (34) Head, Face, and Traumatic Brain Injury

Approximately half of the trauma-related deaths in the United States are due to head injuries. The mortality rate after a severe head injury is approximately 35%. More than half of those who do survive are left with serious disability as a result of injury to the brain.

Head injuries can appear minor, initially occurring days or weeks before the onset of symptoms and quickly become life threatening. It is important to remember the skull holds the structure that controls the body's functions—the brain. Injury to the brain can be catastrophic, causing a lifelong disability or death.

National Education Standards

The Emergency Medical Technician (EMT) will demonstrate a fundamental depth and foundational breadth of understanding of the pathophysiology, assessment, and management of traumatic brain injury, with a simple depth and breadth of understanding in the assessment and management of facial fracture, skull fractures, foreign bodies in the eyes, and dental trauma.

Key Concepts

- The brain controls all vital functions of life and is housed and protected within the skull.

- Injury to the skull and brain can be catastrophic, causing lifelong disability or death.

- Traumatic injuries to the face, including the eyes, nose, ears, and mouth, may include significant injury to the skull, brain, and cervical spine.

- The mechanism of injury is the indicator for significant injuries to the head and affecting the face, cervical spine, and brain.

- Traumatic injury to the skull is either an open head injury where the brain is exposed or a closed head injury.

- Brain injuries can be divided into two categories: primary and secondary.

- Skull fractures can cause bleeding between the meninges of the brain, increasing pressure within the brain and altering brain function.

- Elevated intracranial pressure causes compression of the brain and neurologic damage.

- Many head injuries have similar signs and symptoms, but one sign or symptom may be specific to one particular type of head injury.

- Management of the patient with injuries to the head, face, and brain focuses on airway management, adequate oxygenation, and control of bleeding.

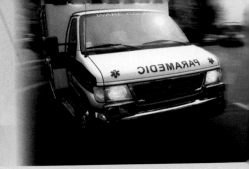

CASE STUDY

"Dispatch to Medic 16—respond to Murphy's Bar for a possible head injury. Law enforcement is on scene. Time out 00:45."

Upon arrival to the scene, Jose and Roberto are directed into the bar. The scene has been secured by law enforcement officers who report there had been a fight between two adult males. One male is in custody at this time after admitting he struck the second male in the head with a beer bottle. Jose notes a broken beer bottle on the floor next to a male in his 20s who is unconscious on the floor. A bar stool is lying on its side next to the patient, and there is considerable blood pooled on the floor beneath the patient's head. The back of the patient's blond hair is red with blood.

Roberto immediately takes spine stabilization, with gloves on, while Jose begins the primary assessment, noting the patient is breathing adequately, with equal chest rise. The patient moans to painful stimuli, attempting to push Jose's hand away when he applies pressure to the fingernail. Bleeding from a large laceration on the top of his head has slowed, with matted hair covering the laceration.

Critical Thinking Questions

1. What are the assessment priorities for this patient?
2. What is the significance of the patient's symptoms?
3. What are the treatment priorities for the patient?

INTRODUCTION

Recognition of the signs and symptoms of a traumatic brain injury is a necessary skill for an Emergency Medical Technician (EMT). Traumatic injuries to the face can mask an underlying traumatic brain injury and should always be considered a sign of a potentially more serious head injury. Appropriate prehospital treatment of these patients is necessary to minimize further injury to the brain. It is crucial that the EMT be familiar with the concepts of managing the patient with a head injury.

ANATOMY REVIEW

To understand the presentation of injuries to the face, head, and brain and the concepts behind their management, the EMT must first have an understanding of the anatomy of the head.

Unit 5 should be reviewed at this time, with special attention paid to discussions of the structures of the head and face, including the scalp, skull, meninges, and brain. Figure 34.1 illustrates this anatomy for review.

TYPES OF INJURIES

Trauma to the head can result in many different types of injuries. Some types of head injuries may be instantly fatal; others are not at all life threatening. It is not crucial for the EMT to identify the exact injury that exists, although understanding the mechanisms for these injuries will help in the assessment and management of the patient with a head injury.

The mechanisms of injury that commonly cause trauma to the head and face include motor vehicle crashes, sports injuries, falls, penetrating trauma,

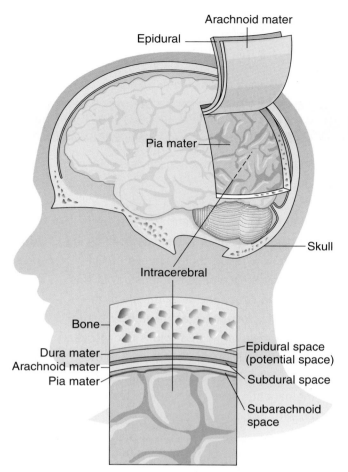

Figure 34.1 The scalp, skull, meninges, and brain are important anatomic structures with which the EMT must be familiar

and blunt trauma to the soft tissue as well as to the bones of the face and skull. Whenever there is a traumatic injury to the head or face, airway compromise and cervical spinal injury should also be considered and quickly managed.

SCALP

Because of the large number of blood vessels present in the scalp, any injury will result in bleeding. If the injury is from a blunt object, such as a baseball bat, there may be no tear in the skin. If sufficient force was applied, vessels may break and cause bleeding under the skin. This resulting collection of blood underneath the skin is known as a **hematoma.** A scalp hematoma can become very large if not treated quickly. Figure 34.2 shows a patient with a scalp hematoma.

If the mechanism of injury involved a sharp edge or sufficient force from a blunt object to break the skin, then the bleeding will be outward. Scalp lacerations often bleed extensively. It is not uncommon for blood loss from an isolated scalp wound to result in hypovolemic shock if the patient is not appropriately treated.

FACE

Traumatic injuries to the face can involve many structures. The nasal bones, orbits of the eyes, maxilla and mandible (jaws), and zygoma/zygomatic arch (cheek bones) all come together to form the face. The structures of the face are covered by a layer of skin containing numerous arteries, veins, nerves, and some muscle. There is usually a minimum amount of subcutaneous fat

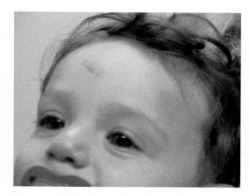

Figure 34.2 A collection of blood between the skull and the scalp is called a scalp hematoma (Courtesy of Deborah Funk, MD, Albany Medical Center, Albany, NY)

tissue; therefore, there is not as much "cushion" available to protect those structures from blunt or penetrating trauma.

The facial bones contain numerous blood vessels, and even minor injuries can bleed heavily. Broken bones, teeth, and soft tissue can easily become an airway obstruction when facial injuries occur. Additionally, the bones of the face are the attachment points for the muscles that control expression and are used in chewing food. Injury to the bones, muscles, and soft tissue can affect an individual's ability to chew and swallow adequately. Airway obstruction must always be considered with injuries to the face. Specific injuries to the structures of the face will be discussed later in this unit.

GENERAL ASSESSMENT

During the scene size-up, it is important to consider the mechanism of injury in relation to potential facial injuries. For example, the broken windshield in a motor vehicle crash can be a significant indicator of trauma to the patient's face, mouth, and cervical spine. Physical assessment must include looking for fractures of the jaw, damaged or broken teeth, fracture of the nasal bones, and serious injury to the brain. Any fracture or soft tissue injury to the face, mouth, or nose creates a potential for airway compromise due to bleeding and foreign bodies (teeth) that can occlude the airway.

Assessment of the face and mouth include conducting a rapid trauma assessment with inspection and palpation for injuries using DCAP-BTLS. Some injuries of the face typically produce signs such as bruising and swelling of soft tissues, away from the actual site of injury. For example, a fracture to the nose often produces black eyes, as does a fracture to the upper jaw (maxilla). Fractures of the lower jaw (mandible) can produce loose or missing teeth and the patient's bite may not align. Assessment of suspected jaw fracture must also include inspection for loose, missing teeth, which pose a significant potential for airway compromise.

TYPES OF FACIAL INJURIES

Soft tissue injuries to the face include burns, lacerations, abrasions, and contusions. It is important to remember that forces that cause injury to the face are often also transmitted to surrounding structures as well. Therefore, injury to the cervical spine, skull, and brain should always be considered when there are significant injuries to the structures of the face.

MOUTH AND JAW

Blunt trauma to the upper and lower jaw and mouth can result from motor vehicle crashes, a gunshot, or a blow from a blunt object or a person's fist. Lacerations and nerve damage can also occur to the soft tissues of the upper and lower jaw and the tongue, lips, and gums of the mouth (Figure 34.3).

Signs and symptoms of injuries to the jaws and mouth include numbness or pain, distortion of facial features due to nerve damage or fractures; bruising and swelling; limited jaw movement or palpable movement of the upper jaw; teeth that do not meet normally; blood collection (hematoma) under the tongue; blood coming from the mouth; drooling due to painful swallowing; missing, loose, or uneven teeth (bite); and pain in or around the ears.

The mechanism of injury combined with any of these signs and symptoms should prompt the EMT to suspect a fracture and treat accordingly. Remember to assess for associated injuries to the eyes, cervical spine, and skull and brain.

Management for trauma to the upper and lower jaw and mouth focuses on establishing and maintaining cervical spinal immobilization, a patent airway,

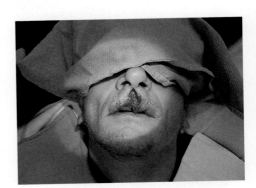

Figure 34.3 Laceration to the mouth/jaw (Courtesy of Larry Torrey, RN, Portland, ME)

breathing, and controlling life-threatening bleeding. Use the jaw-thrust to open the airway as needed and be prepared to suction. Provide supplemental oxygen via non-rebreather mask. ALS intercept should be requested for patients with significant facial trauma, because ventilation may be difficult and an advance airway adjunct may be required.

Teeth Blunt trauma can cause teeth to become loose, break off, or become avulsed. Loose or missing teeth are common when trauma has caused a fracture to either the upper or lower jaw. Assessment of trauma to the mid-face and jaw must always include inspection for fragments of teeth, broken dentures, pieces of bone, or other foreign objects that may cause an airway obstruction.

If dentures are secure and unbroken in the mouth, leave them in place; however, if they are no longer fitting securely, as seen with jaw fractures, or broken, they must be removed. If removal is necessary, transport the dentures and any broken pieces with the patient.

Teeth that have been avulsed can possibly be reimplanted if found and gotten to the hospital with the patient. If time permits, always try to find a missing tooth; however, transport of potentially unstable trauma patients should never be delayed to look for a missing tooth. If the missing tooth is not found, consider the possibility the patient has swallowed or aspirated the tooth. Control bleeding by placing a gauze pad on the tooth socket and gently holding it in place or having the patient gently bite down on it.

Once the missing tooth has been located, rinse it with saline to remove any debris. Never scrub the tooth. Place the tooth in a cup of saline or wrap in moistened gauze and transport with the patient. Never wrap the tooth in dry gauze or allow the tooth to dry out. Do not handle the tooth by the root because the structures of the tooth (ligament fibers) are needed for successful reimplantment.

IMPALED OBJECT IN CHEEK

Objects impaled in the cheek should be stabilized using a bulky dressing unless they are felt to pose an airway risk. If the impaled object needs to be removed, the following steps should be considered:

1. Pull or push the object out of the check in the direction that causes the least amount of injury or compromise to the airway.
2. Using sterile or clean dressing, pack the material between the teeth and the wound, taping some of the dressing outside the mouth to prevent the patient from swallowing the dressing. The dressing must be monitored closely to ensure it does not become loose and become an airway obstruction.
3. Control bleeding by applying a dressing and bandage to the outside of the wound.
4. Consider ALS intercept if an advanced airway adjunct may be needed and suction the throat and mouth frequently during transport.

THE NOSE

A broken nose is a common traumatic injury to the face because the structures of the nose are fairly delicate. Blunt force to the nose, such as being hit with a batted baseball or a fist, can cause nasal fractures. Assessment findings typically include pain, swelling, bleeding, and deformity. Significant bleeding (epistaxis) may occur with nasal trauma, and the potential for airway obstruction exists (Figure 34.4).

Do not pack the nares because clear or bloody fluid from the nose could be indicative of a skull fracture (discussed later in this unit) and packing the

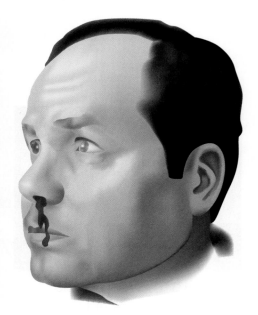

Figure 34.4 Bloody nose

nose could increase in pressure and cause more damage. Place a loose dressing below the nares and control bleeding from the nose as follows:

1. Have the patient sit and lean forward (unless there is a concern for a cervical spinal injury. Cervical spinal immobilization should be maintained with suction available while following the steps to control bleeding.
2. Pinch the fleshy part of the nostrils together.
3. Keep the patient calm and as still as possible.
4. Apply a cold pack over the bridge of the nose if possible.

Patients may present seated with their head thrown back to stop the bleeding. Adjust the patient position by having them lean forward. The patient who has been sitting with the head back may have swallowed a considerable amount of blood. Because blood is an irritant to the lining of the stomach, the patient may vomit. The EMT should be prepared for vomiting and have suction handy.

THE EAR

The most common injuries to the ear are cuts and lacerations. The outer portion of the ear (pinna) is often involved when there is trauma to the head. There is a limited amount of blood flow to the outer structure of the ear, which is made up of cartilage; therefore, injury usually produces minimal bleeding.

Assess and treat ear injuries the same as for soft tissue injuries (Unit 37), using loose dressing to cover the injury and avoid pressure. Remember that clear or bloody fluid can indicate a more serious skull fracture. Never probe into the ear or pack the ear to stop bleeding from the ear canal.

Save any avulsed parts; wrapped in moist gauze, and transport with the patient. If there is a foreign object in the ear, as seen often with children, do not attempt to remove the object. Reassure the patient (and parent if the patient is a child) and transport so the object can be removed at the hospital.

THE EYE

The eye is a globe, made up of many intricate structures confined inside an orbit of the face. The readily visible structures of the eye include the cornea (clear front portion of the eye), the pupils (dark center of the eye), and the iris (colored portion of the eye). The globe itself is covered by a thick membrane or outer layer called the *sclera*. The eyelids and exposed portion of the sclera are covered with a very thin covering called the *conjunctiva*.

Light enters the eye through the cornea, with the pupil opening and expanding or contracting to control the amount of light allowed into the eye through the lens. The light that is allowed through is focused on the retina (back of the eye) by the lens.

The interior of the eye is made up of the front chamber filled with the aqueous humor (watery fluid), and behind the lens is the large vitreous body containing a clear, jelly-like fluid called the *vitreous humor*.

Finally, there are muscles holding the eyes in position and the bones of the orbits, all of which are extremely susceptible to traumatic injuries.

GENERAL ASSESSMENT

Physical assessment of eye injuries should include assessing the eyes separately and together using a light, such as a small penlight. Evaluate the eyes for bruising, swelling, lacerations, and tenderness of the orbits (eye sockets) and eye lids. Look for redness or abnormal coloring, pus, and foreign bodies of the conjunctiva and globe (eyeball). Check the pupils for size, shape, equality, and reaction to light. Ask the patient to follow an object or finger to assess for movement in directions (up/down and right/left), looking for a paralysis of eye movement or pain with movement.

Impaled objects in the eye are often immediately evident; however, small objects that can become lodged, or impaled, in the eyeball may not be immediately evident. Additionally, burns to the eye may initially appear as a simple redness; however, severe pain and loss of vision may appear over a short period of time. Suspect a significant injury to the eye whenever the patient complains of severe pain, partial or complete loss of vision that does not improve with blinking, double vision, or an unusual sensitivity to light.

Time is of the essence when determining the mechanism of injury and management of eye injuries, particularly when chemical burns or impaled objects are suspected.

TYPES OF EYE INJURIES

Injuries to the eye, although usually not life threatening, can create lifelong challenges for the patient. Injuries that occur to the structures of the eyes may cause profuse bleeding, pain, discomfort, disfigurement, and possibly loss of sight.

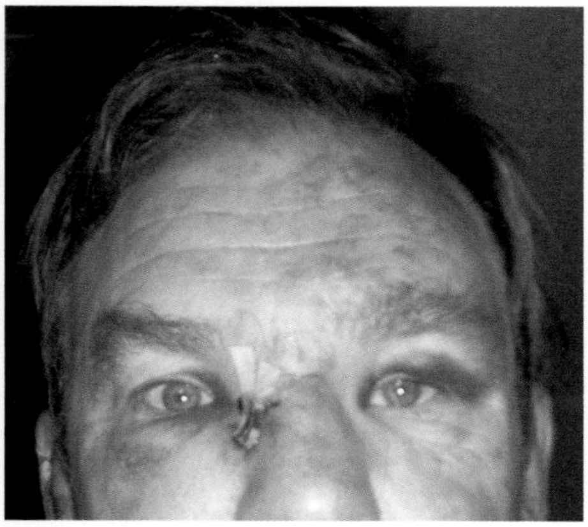

INJURY TO THE EYE ORBITS

Blunt trauma to the face often results in fractures to one or several of the bones that form the orbits containing the eye. Orbital fractures require significant force; therefore, cervical spinal injuries should also be suspected and spinal stabilization applied and maintained when eye orbit fractures are suspected (Figure 34.5).

When assessing the eye for signs of injury to the orbits, look and feel for signs of injuries using DCAP-BTLS. Signs and symptoms of orbital fractures may include deformity of the orbital bones; double vision (diplopia); loss of vision; loss of sensation over the cheek, above the eyebrow, or in the upper lip; tenderness with palpation; nasal discharge; or the inability of the eye to follow an object, such as a finger, upward (paralysis of upward gaze).

Orbital fracture may require surgery and hospitalization. If the eyeball has not been injured, place cold packs over the eye with a suspected orbital fracture to reduce swelling and provide some pain relief. Transport in a seated position. If an injury to the eyeball is suspected, do not place any pressure on the injured eye and transport with the patient lying supine.

FOREIGN OBJECTS

Objects such as dirt, dust, sand, cinders, and fine metal particles can be blown into the eye and get lodged. Foreign objects cause the eye to tear as a preventive mechanism to wash the particles away before any serious damage is done; however, abrasions to the cornea may occur. Patients will complain of "something in my eye," and the eyeball may appear red. It is important to determine if the patient or anyone else has attempted to remove the object, causing abrasions to the cornea.

In most cases, the patient should be transported for further medical treatment without removing the object in the field. If it is necessary to remove the object from the conjunctiva, flushing the eye with clean water while holding the eyelid open is the recommended method of removal (Figure 34.6).

If the object is lodged in the eyeball, do not attempt to remove it, and keep the patient from rubbing his eye by placing a bandage over both eyes and transporting the patient to the hospital for removal.

INJURY TO THE EYELIDS

Black eyes (bruising), lacerations, and burns are injuries that can occur to the eyelid. The eyelids are very vascular, meaning they have a rich supply

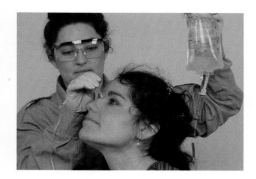

Figure 34.5 Orbital fracture of the eye

Figure 34.6 Flushing the eye

of blood vessels and can bleed profusely when lacerated. It is important to remember that any laceration to the eyelid may also indicate a laceration to the eyeball. The entire eye including the area around the eyelid should be carefully inspected for injury.

Treatment of eyelid injuries begins with control of any bleeding present, using light pressure and a clean dressing. If the eyeball is suspected to be injured, do not use pressure. Carefully cover the lid with sterile gauze, moistened with saline. Save any avulsed skin, transporting it with the patient, as it may be possible to graft the avulsed skin back into place. Place a cold pack over the injured eyelid if no injury to the eyeball is suspected. As with all eye injuries, cover the uninjured eye as well to reduce movement (both eyes will move in response to what one eye sees) and transport.

INJURY TO THE EYEBALL

Foreign objects, abrasions, lacerations, and bruising are some of the injuries that can occur to the eyeball or globe. Contact lenses not made for long-term wear can cause abrasions to the cornea, inflammation of the conjunctiva, and infections. The contents of the eyeball (aqueous and vitreous humor) can spill or leak out because of deep lacerations or penetrating injuries that cut the cornea.

Lacerations, penetrations, and impalements to the eyeball are usually apparent when first encountering the patient. Injuries to the globe causing a pear- or irregular-shape, or blood buildup in the anterior of the eye (*hyphema*) may also be noted upon further examination.

Great care must be taken when treating injuries to the eyeball and are usually best managed at the hospital. Application of lightweight patches to both eyes, avoiding any pressure to the eyeball is the primary field management for injuries to the eyeball. A potentially ruptured eyeball must be treated with extreme caution to avoid the loss of eye fluids. Avoid any pressure or use of ice packs, keep the patient calm, and transport in the supine position.

IMPALED OBJECTS

Emergency care in the field for objects that are embedded or impaled in the eye focuses on stabilization of the object and transport to the hospital for removal. The EMT should not attempt to remove an embedded or impaled object and should prevent accidental movement of the object. Additionally, if the eyeball has been forced out of the eye socket or extruding, never attempt to push the eyeball back in. Impaled or embedded objects in the eye or an eye that is extruding from the socket are true emergencies.

Treatment of both an impaled object and extruded eyeball is the same. Ensuring there is no manipulation of the eyeball during treatment, place the patient in the supine position and immobilize the head and spine. Immobilization of the head and spine will help to prevent further movement of the eyeball or object. Additionally, a force strong enough to cause the eyeball to extrude from the socket may also cause injury to the cervical spine.

Using gauze dressing or soft sterile cloth, encircle the object or extruded eyeball, avoiding placing any pressure on the eye. A hole may be cut in the bulky dressing for an impaled object. Use a metal shield, cone, or paper cup and place it over the impaled object. Make sure the impaled object or eyeball is not touching the top or sides of the cup or cone.

Once the cup or shield and dressing is in place over the eyeball, use a roller bandage or self-adhesive bandage to hold the cup or shield in place. Do not bandage over the cup, which may apply pressure and push the cup down onto the impaled object or extruded eyeball. Again, as with all eye injuries, make sure to bandage both eyes to avoid movement, making sure to close the uninjured eye of the unresponsive patient to prevent drying.

Remember the conscious patient with an impaled object or extruded eyeball will be understandably anxious. Once both eyes have been bandaged, the patient's anxiety will increase because they are now completely blind and must rely on individuals they may not know. Never leave these patients alone and always provide constant verbal assurances, explaining to them what is happening and any additional procedures that may be required. Transport immediately and never give or allow the patient to have anything to eat or drink by mouth.

CHEMICAL BURNS

Chemical burns to the eye can cause permanent damage within seconds. Immediate intervention (within 10 minutes) after the injury occurs can have a profound effect on the long-term outcome for the patient. As with all substances that cause burns, the burning and tissue damage will continue to occur as long as the substance causing the burn—in this case, the chemical—is in the eye. When the mechanism of injury, following scene size-up and primary assessment, indicates a chemical to the eye, treatment must begin immediately.

Signs and symptoms for chemical burns to the eye begin with a history of exposure to a chemical. The patient will complain of severe pain and burning in the eye and blurred or diminished vision. The eye will be irritated, with redness or red streaks over the surface of the eye. The eyelid may be irritated and swollen, and there may be burns to the skin around the eyes.

Treatment for chemical burns to the eyes is focused on removing the chemical as much as possible through continuous irrigation with clear water or saline. The eyelids will have to be held open allowing for any chemical under the lids to be flushed out. The patient may not be able to hold his eyelids open himself due to pain; therefore the EMT may have to force the lids open. Irrigation must be continuous for a minimum of 20 minutes. If the chemical is an alkali, irrigation must be continuous for at least 1 hour or until arrival to the hospital.

The EMT must make sure the patient is positioned so the water will run from the inside corner, across the eyeball to the outer edge of the eye, without contaminating the uninjured eye.

Contact lenses must be removed as soon as possible or flushed out. Chemicals can be trapped between the lens and the eye (cornea) and the eye tissue will continue to be damaged if the contact is not removed.

CONTACT LENSES

Contact lenses can complicate eye injuries and removing them in the field may be necessary, as with chemical burns to the eye. The EMT must first determine if the contact is in the eye. Soft contacts show up as a shadow over the outside of the eye and hard lenses looked like a shadow over the iris when a light is shined in the eyes.

EMTs should follow local protocols and seek advice from medical direction when determining whether to remove contacts. Table 34-1 presents common guidelines for when contacts should be removed and when they should not be removed.

REMOVAL OF HARD CONTACT LENSES

Hard contact lenses are still being worn by many people, although soft lenses are more popular. Hard lenses are small, approximately the size of a button on a shirt made to fit directly over the cornea. In some cases, patients will have already removed their own contacts or request to be allowed to remove

Table 34-1 General Guideline for Removal of Contact Lenses

- Chemical burns to the eyes
- Extended transport time for unresponsive patients wearing hard contact lenses

General guidelines for when contact lenses should NOT be removed.
- The eyeball itself is injured, unless there are chemical burns.
- Transport time is short enough that the lenses can be removed in the emergency department.

them themselves. If the patient can do so without difficulty or causing further injury to the eye, they should be allowed to do so.

Before removing any contact, you must obtain permission from the conscious patient and ensure your gloved hands are clean. The steps for removing hard contact lenses are:

1. Separate the eyelids.
2. After visualizing the lens, use the eyelid to move the lens over the cornea.
3. Gently place your thumbs on the top and the bottom of the eyelids and open the eye wide.
4. Then gently press the eyelids down and forward, to the edge of the lens.
5. Pressing the lower lid slightly harder, move it under the bottom edge of the lens.
6. Finally, moving the eyelids toward each other, slide the lens out, between the upper and lower eyelids.

After removing the contact lenses, place them in a container with saline solution, if possible. Many ambulances carry a contact case for this purpose. If possible, place the appropriate contact in the correct side of the case as indicated by the L or R for right or left eye.

REMOVAL OF SOFT CONTACT LENSES

Soft contact lenses are the most commonly used contacts because they are designed for extended wear. Soft contact lenses that are left in too long can cause damage and injury to the eye by adhering to the cornea. When they are left in too long, they gradually dry out and shrink, making removal difficult.

Soft lenses are a little bigger than a dime, with the edges extending past the iris; covering the entire cornea and some of the sclera. Again, if the patient is requesting to remove his own contacts and can do so without further contamination or injury to the eye, he should be allowed to do so.

One method of soft contact removal is to place several drops of saline into the eye, moistening the contact. The lens can then be gently lifted off the eye by pinching the contact between the thumb and forefinger.

The following steps demonstrate another method of soft contact removal. The EMT should ensure she has on clean gloves and has gotten permission from the conscious patient to remove his contacts and then use the following method:

1. Pull the lower lid down using the middle finger.
2. Place your forefinger on the lower edge of the lens, sliding the lens down onto the sclera (white of the eye).

Children have fusion points in their skulls that do not close until around age 2. These soft spots, or fontanels, leave the underlying brain vulnerable to injury.

When examining a child, the EMT can note the presence of these soft spots on the top and back of the skull. The EMT should note the shape of the scalp over the fontanel.

A bulging fontanel can mean elevated pressures within the skull, whereas a sunken fontanel can mean dehydration. Examination of the fontanels can be a useful tool in the pediatric physical exam.

3. Compress the lens gently between the thumb and forefinger, allowing air to get under the lens, and remove it from the eye.
4. If the lens is sticking to the eye, it may be dehydrated. Run sterile saline across the surface of the eye while sliding the lens off the cornea, and pinching it up to remove it.

Make sure to store the lenses in a container that has saline or water to keep them moist. If possible, label each container with an L or R to indicate from which eye the contact was removed, or place in the corresponding sides of a commercial contact case.

THE SKULL

Significant blunt or penetrating trauma to the skull can result in a break in this bony protective covering, leaving the brain exposed to injury.

There are many specific types of skull fractures. Differentiating among them is unimportant to the EMT, with two exceptions. The ability to differentiate between these two types of skull fractures may affect the care provided by the EMT.

BASILAR SKULL FRACTURE

Blunt trauma to the skull may result in a fracture in any area. When a fracture is at the base of the skull, the area just behind the face, there may be characteristic physical findings. This type of fracture is called a **basilar skull fracture** and will have implications for emergency care of the patient. Figure 34.7 illustrates this fracture.

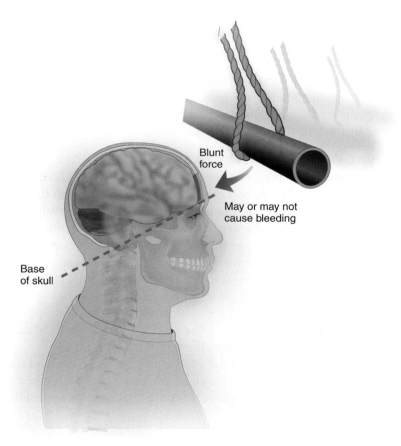

Figure 34.7 A basilar skull fracture may have implications for airway management techniques because it is so close to airway structures

Bleeding associated with this type of fracture will spread from the fracture site and settle into a few characteristic places. Bruising behind the ears over the bony prominence called the **mastoid process** is known as Battle's sign and can develop within a few hours of a basilar skull fracture. Another characteristic physical finding with this type of injury is bruising around both eyes, commonly called raccoon's eyes (Figure 34.8). Although characteristic for basilar skull fracture, these useful physical findings often will not be present until several hours after the injury.

Injury to the base of the skull may disrupt delicate structures within the ear. If it does, cerebrospinal fluid (CSF) may leak out through the fracture into the ear canal. The EMT will see a clear or blood-tinged liquid draining from the patient's ear. This condition is called **CSF otorrhea.**

Similarly, if the fracture is at the base of the skull close to the posterior of the nose, CSF may be seen leaking from the nose. This condition, called **CSF rhinorrhea,** is identified as a clear or thin bloody liquid coming from an otherwise uninjured nose.

The EMT should never attempt to halt the flow of any fluid that may be CSF coming from the ear or nose. A sterile dressing may be used to collect the fluids as they leak out.

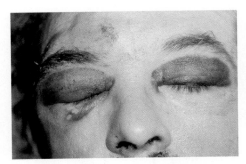

Figure 34.8 Raccoon's eyes (Courtesy of Wayne Triner, DO, Albany Medical Center, Albany, NY)

OPEN SKULL FRACTURE

An open skull fracture is an obvious opening in the skull, sometimes exposing underlying brain. If an open skull fracture exists, the EMT should take care not to touch the underlying brain tissue. The opening should be carefully covered with a dry sterile dressing. Care should be taken not to apply pressure to the brain itself while attempting to control bleeding from the scalp.

Although open skull injuries are frightening to view, they are not necessarily correlated with a poor prognosis. The amount of underlying brain injury is the determinant of the final outcome. Figure 34.9 shows an illustration of an open skull fracture.

PENETRATING INJURY

If an open skull fracture is associated with a penetrating injury, such as a knife or gunshot wound, it should be understood that underlying damage is variable. The extent of intracranial damage is often difficult to determine by looking at the outside of the skull.

Seemingly minor exterior wounds from a gunshot may result in severe intracranial injury. On the other hand, extensive scalp wounds associated with a penetrating injury may not result in serious brain injury.

The EMT should stabilize any remaining foreign body and treat the patient according to the guidelines that will be outlined later in this chapter.

TRAUMATIC BRAIN INJURY

The most significant component of a head injury is the injury the brain sustains. A **traumatic brain injury (TBI)** can be due to a direct cause (penetrating trauma), indirect cause (blow to the skull), or secondary (hypoxia) cause. To understand how trauma affects the brain, the EMT needs to be familiar with the anatomy of the brain and pathophysiology of traumatic brain injury.

The brain, brain stem, and spinal cord are covered by three separated membranes called the *meninges.* The *dura mater* (literally meaning "tough mother") is the outermost layer lining the cranial vault (cranium) and is made up of tough fibrous tissue. The dura mater adheres to the inner surface of the cranial vault with the middle meningeal arteries located in the epidural space (between the temporal bones and the dura mater). Blunt trauma to this

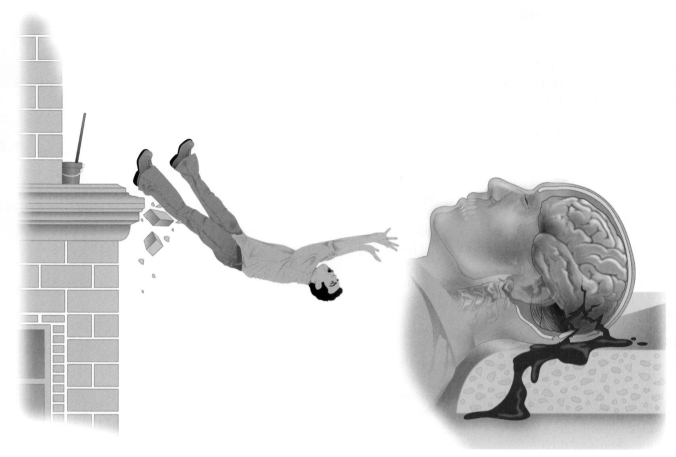

Figure 34.9 Open skull fractures leave the brain susceptible to direct injury. Injuries such as this may also contribute to spinal injury

area producing a skull fracture can damage the artery, causing blood to collect in this space. This is called an *epidural hematoma*, discussed later in this unit.

The next two meningeal layers are the *arachnoid*, which has a spider web appearance and the **pia mater** (literally translated "soft mother"). Between the arachnoid and pia mater is a space called the **subarachnoid space,** which is filled with cerebrospinal fluid. Cerebrospinal fluid is produced in the ventricles of the brain, surrounds the brain and spinal cord, and is thought to cushion the brain. Blunt force trauma can cause blood to collect beneath the dura mater and form a subdural hematoma. An injury that results in bleeding in the subarachnoid space is known as a *subarachnoid hemorrhage*.

The pathophysiology of a brain injury can be divided into two categories: primary brain injury and secondary brain injury. **Primary brain injury** is defined as a direct trauma to the brain and associated vascular structures. The nerve cells (neurons) sustain damage due to the initial assault. Because neurons do not regenerate, permanent neurologic damage may result, depending on the location and number of neurons affected.

Secondary brain injury is an extension of the primary brain injury and is a result of things that occur within the brain after the original insult. Secondary injuries can produce larger, more permanent neurologic deficits and can be separated into systemic factors and intracranial causes. Systemic causes of secondary brain injury include hypoxia, hypercapnia (high carbon dioxide levels), anemia, hypotension, hyperglycemia, and hypoglycemia. Intracranial causes of secondary brain injury are cerebral edema and intracranial hematoma, both causing increased intracranial pressure and compression of brain structures.

Early recognition of brain injury and prevention of secondary injury is the goal of emergency care. The EMT plays a crucial role in minimizing secondary brain injury. This can be done by accurate assessment, good management of the airway, breathing, and circulation, and expeditious transport to the closest appropriate hospital.

An EMT will have no way to tell what type of brain injury exists; however, there are several classic presentations of different types of injuries. It is helpful for the EMT to recognize these injury patterns.

OPEN HEAD INJURY

Open skull injuries will usually result in direct trauma to the brain because there no longer is a protective covering. The EMT should take care to protect the exposed brain from further injury.

CLOSED HEAD INJURY

Closed head injuries are less impressive to see, but they are much more common and often much more severe. Remember, the skull is rigid and can be thought of as a closed container that cannot expand. Bleeding and swelling within the skull will eventually result in pressure on the adjacent brain tissue. Brain tissue does not respond well to compression.

Compression of blood vessels supplying a section of brain with blood will result in hypoperfusion of the tissue. Brain tissue can survive only a few minutes without oxygenated blood before it is irreversibly damaged.

The EMT must recognize early signs of closed head injury and treat the patient appropriately in an attempt to prevent irreversible brain damage.

CONCUSSIONS

A **concussion** is a mild closed head injury that can occur with blunt force trauma. A mild stretching, tearing, and shearing of brain tissue occurs, and there is normally a disturbance in brain function. However, no readily apparent damage is seen to the brain on the CT scan. The CT scan is the most common radiographic imaging used in the emergency department to evaluate for an acute brain injury. These disturbances can range from temporary confusion to loss of responsiveness. If a complete loss of consciousness occurs, it is usually temporary, lasting only a few minutes, and it typically does not recur. Table 34-2 lists the signs and symptoms of a concussion.

Table 34-2 Signs and Symptoms of a Concussion

- Confusion that lasts for several minutes
- Inability to recall the incident, the period of time just before the incident (retrograde amnesia), and after the incident occurred (anterograde amnesia)
- Repeated questions about what happened
- Mild to moderate irritability or resistance to treatment
- Restlessness or combativeness
- Inability to answer questions or appropriately obey commands
- Nausea and vomiting

Concussions are specifically characterized by the appearance of the symptoms immediately or soon after impact, with gradual resolution. If symptoms do not improve over time or the patient experiences a second or prolonged loss of consciousness, it is likely not a concussion but a more serious TBI. It is impossible to differentiate concussion from more serious brain injury in the prehospital environment. Emergency department evaluation and often advanced radiographic imaging such as CT scans are required to make this differentiation.

BRAIN CONTUSION

A **brain contusion** is bruising and swelling of the brain tissue. It may or may not cause an increase in intracranial pressure (ICP) and is usually caused by blunt trauma to the head.

Coup-contrecoup injuries are characterized by damage to the brain tissue at the point of the initial impact to the head and also damage on the side opposite the point of the initial impact, where the brain impacts the skull. In car crashes, **acceleration/deceleration** injuries are common as the brain continues to move back and forth inside the skull after the head has come to a sudden stop. This continued movement of the brain causes potentially severe bruising to the brain. Signs and symptoms of contusions include the same initial signs and symptoms of a concussion plus one or more of the signs and symptoms listed in Table 34-3.

Contusions can lead to permanent disability or death as a result of severe swelling of brain tissue. As with all brain injuries, outcome can be potentially improved through appropriate and immediate airway management and high-flow oxygen with assisted ventilations as needed. Immobilization of the cervical spine should always be established and maintained in a person showing the signs and symptoms of a brain contusion.

SUBDURAL HEMATOMA

One of the more common causes of severe brain injury is a collection of blood between the brain and the dura mater. This type of blood collection is known as a **subdural hematoma.**

A subdural hematoma is caused by tearing of multiple small veins that run between the brain's surface and the dura mater. This is often the result of blunt head trauma. Figure 34.10 illustrates this type of injury.

A subdural hematoma can expand, compressing the adjacent brain tissue significantly. When important brain structures are compressed, the brain will malfunction and may cause the death of the patient. It is the responsibility of the EMT to recognize the early signs of this brain compression and to treat the patient aggressively to attempt to reduce the likelihood of complications.

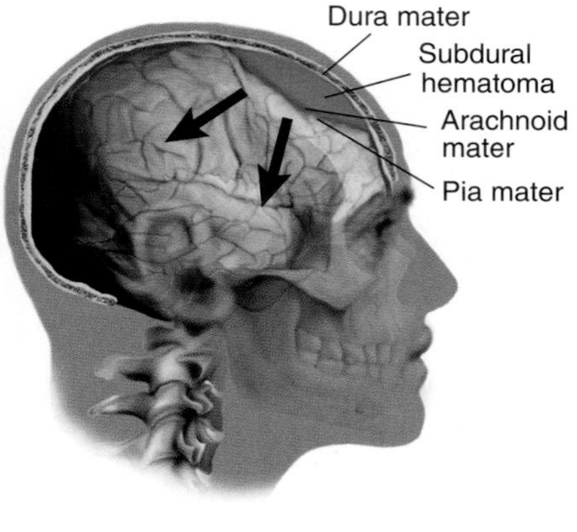

Street Smart

Because a subdural hematoma is the result of venous bleeding, it can sometimes take time to develop. Depending on the size and number of veins that have torn, it may be hours to days before the expanding hematoma causes significant symptoms. The EMT should take a careful history and inquire about any possible head injury over the previous several days and weeks.

Dura mater
Subdural hematoma
Arachnoid mater
Pia mater

Figure 34.10 A subdural hematoma is usually the result of the tearing of small veins under the dura mater

---

Table 34-3 Additional Signs and Symptoms Indicating a Contusion

- Decreasing mental status or unresponsiveness
- Paralysis
- Unequal pupils
- Vomiting
- Changes in vital signs
- Profound personality changes

Over the years, the brain of an older adult shrinks, or atrophies, leaving extra space between the dura mater and the brain itself. Because the extra space allows these tiny veins to stretch, they can more easily tear. Elderly people are therefore at increased risk for developing a subdural hematoma, even after seemingly minor head trauma.

Chronic alcoholics may suffer premature brain atrophy and are at similar risk, even at a young age.

EPIDURAL HEMATOMA

Another commonly seen intracranial hematoma is the **epidural hematoma.** This collection of blood is found outside the dura mater, just under the skull. The epidural hematoma is most often the result of a skull fracture with an arterial injury. The blood collection in this case is arterial in nature and typically accumulates quickly. Figure 34.11 illustrates this type of injury.

An epidural hematoma can expand and compress the adjacent brain tissue, causing injury in much the same way as does a subdural hematoma. Rapid identification of a significant head injury and appropriate treatment by the EMT with rapid delivery to definitive care can contribute to a good outcome.

INTRACRANIAL PRESSURE

Because the skull is a rigid container that does not expand, any increase in volume within it will result in an increase in pressure. The pressure inside the skull is called **intracranial pressure (ICP).** Elevated pressure within the skull results in compression of brain tissue and subsequent neurologic damage.

The brain has several complex compensatory mechanisms that can help prevent neurologic injury for a limited time. In the case of an expanding intracranial hematoma, the brain cannot compensate for long.

When the brain can no longer compensate for the extra volume of blood within the intracranial space, the pressure inside the skull begins to increase. This is referred to as a rise in ICP.

This rise in intracranial pressure damages brain cells and is evidenced by deterioration in the patient's neurologic status. Physical findings associated with such a rise in ICP are listed in Table 34-4. It is important to remember that not all symptoms may be present with an increase in intracranial pressure.

It is crucial that the EMT recognize these signs and take appropriate measures to attempt to lower the ICP. These measures are detailed later in this unit.

ASSOCIATED INJURIES

When considering the mechanism behind the head injury, the EMT should carefully consider the possibility of associated injury of other body parts.

NECK

Approximately 5% of patients suffering from severe head injury will also have a cervical spine fracture. A missed spinal fracture can result in serious neurologic injury and even paralysis.

It is generally accepted that if a patient suffers any significant trauma above the clavicles, injury to the cervical spine may also be present. This means that any movement of the patient should be done while keeping the

It is important for the EMT to realize that although trauma to the head is a common cause of brain injury, it is also possible to suffer intracranial bleeding without trauma. There are many different non–trauma-related brain injuries. Because the result within the brain may be similar, the patient presentation may also be similar to that of the head-injured patient. An example of a non-traumatic source of intracranial hemorrhage is a hemorrhagic stroke. This condition is discussed in Unit 27.

Management priorities for the patient with non–trauma-related brain injury are the same as those presented in this unit. The only exception is, of course, there is no need for cervical spinal immobilization unless trauma to the cervical spine cannot be ruled out.

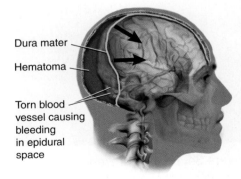

Figure 34.11 An epidural hematoma is often associated with a skull fracture and an arterial injury

Table 34-4 Physical Findings Associated with a Rise in Intracranial Pressure
Decrease in mental status
Persistent vomiting
Glasgow Coma Score <8
Unequal pupils
Seizure activity
Hypertension
Bradycardia
Altered respiratory pattern

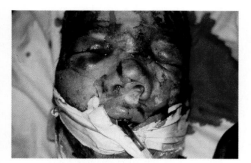

Figure 34.12 The presence of significant facial injuries is a contraindication to using a nasopharygeal airway (Courtesy of Kevin Reilly, MD, Albany Medical Center, Albany, NY)

cervical spine immobilized. The concepts of cervical immobilization are discussed in the Unit 35.

FACE

As discussed earlier, the face is a part of the head and the brain lies just behind the face. Despite the upsetting nature of facial injuries, the EMT must remain calm and remember the principles of treating the patient with potential head injury.

Patients with obvious injuries to their face should not have anything placed into their nose. The thin bones behind the nose may be easily broken, and a nasopharyngeal airway or soft suction catheter could easily penetrate into the brain itself. Figure 34.12 shows a patient with significant facial trauma in whom a nasopharyngeal airway would be contraindicated.

Patients with significant facial trauma should be assumed to have a head and neck injury until proven otherwise.

PATIENT PRESENTATION

It is easy to recognize that a patient has suffered a head injury when the injury is severe. Some patients may not have obvious findings. It will be up to the EMT to elicit important historical information and to observe physical findings to recognize the potential for serious head injury.

MECHANISM OF INJURY

To determine whether the patient is at risk of having a significant head injury, the EMT should carefully assess the mechanism of the injury. If anyone can provide the details of the injury, the EMT should document these details carefully.

If the patient was struck with an object, the EMT should determine what type of object and how many times the patient was struck. Did the patient fall and strike his head after being struck? If there was a fall, what type of surface was involved? How great a distance did the patient fall? What part of the body struck first?

If the mechanism was a motor vehicle collision, what parts of the vehicle sustained damage? Is there evidence of damage inside the car from the patient's head? A star pattern in the windshield is a classic sign of a person's head striking the glass forcefully. Figure 34.13 illustrates this important finding.

Seat belt restraint use inside a motor vehicle has been shown to significantly reduce the severity of injury in many cases. Properly used seat belt restraints prevent the person from being thrown about the vehicle in a crash. The EMT should determine whether the patient was wearing an appropriate seat belt restraint at the time of the accident.

If the patient was participating in a sport that usually requires a helmet, was a helmet used? If one was, looking at the helmet for damage can give the EMT an idea of the force of impact and the area of the head that received the force.

SIGNS AND SYMPTOMS

Trauma to the head is often apparent upon careful physical exam. During a detailed trauma assessment, the EMT should look for DCAP-BTLS on the head. If any of these indications of injury are present, the EMT should consider the patient to have sustained a head injury. Careful reassessment and examination looking for other evidence of serious head injury are indicated. Figure 34.14 illustrates some physical findings associated with a head injury.

If a patient suffered an injury to the head and has physical findings consistent with head injury but is awake with no apparent neurologic injury, then the head injury may be minor. Patients who are awake on first assessment and do not deteriorate have an excellent prognosis.

The patient who presents to EMS with signs of elevated intracranial pressure is considered to have a serious head injury. Depending on the type of intracranial injury, the prognosis may be quite poor.

HISTORY

It is important for the EMT to gather any available history from the patient or bystanders. The usual OPQRST and SAMPLE history is important to obtain, but in the case of head injury, there are additional points the EMT should attempt to elicit.

LOSS OF CONSCIOUSNESS

In addition to the mechanism of injury, bystanders can often provide valuable information regarding the patient's condition before the EMT's arrival.

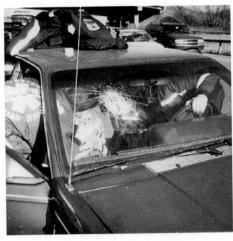

Figure 34.13 A starred windshield indicates that an object, likely a head, contacted it with great force (Courtesy of Deborah Funk, MD, Albany Medical Center, Albany, NY)

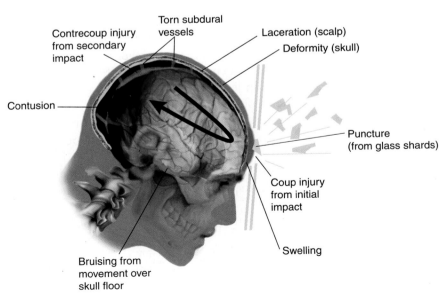

Figure 34.14 The EMT should look for physical findings that would indicate injury to the skull and brain

Torn subdural vessels
Contrecoup injury from secondary impact
Laceration (scalp)
Deformity (skull)
Contusion
Puncture (from glass shards)
Coup injury from initial impact
Bruising from movement over skull floor
Swelling

Street Smart

Remember that it often takes some time for obvious signs of trauma to develop. The EMT often must rely on tiny abrasions to provide clues to the possibility of head injury. It pays to watch these patients carefully and reassess them frequently. Head injury patients can quickly decompensate. The astute EMT will have picked up on minor signs of injury and will be prepared for such decompensation.

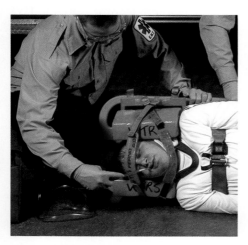

Figure 34.15 EMTs should be prepared to assist the head-injured patient in clearing her airway if vomiting occurs

Witnesses should be asked whether there was any loss of consciousness. It is not uncommon for a patient who has suffered an injury to the head to lose consciousness immediately after the incident. The length of the loss of consciousness should be determined if possible. The longer the loss of consciousness, the more significant the injury may be.

SEIZURE

Sometimes, after sustaining a head injury, a patient may suffer a seizure. A seizure that occurs immediately after a blow to the head is called a **post-traumatic seizure.** This type of seizure occurs in around 5% of patients sustaining blunt head injury. An immediate post-traumatic seizure does not necessarily mean that the head injury is severe. Often, the patient is awake by the time the EMT arrives.

The EMT should care for the patient in much the same way she would care for any other seizure patient, paying careful attention to the possibility of cervical spine injury. Careful reassessments and observation for deterioration are in order.

VOMITING

One sign of intracranial injury is persistent vomiting. It is not uncommon for a person who has sustained even a minor head injury to vomit; however, persistent vomiting is associated with more serious brain injury. Bystanders should be questioned about this symptom.

The EMT should ensure that the vomiting patient is able to clear his own airway. A backboarded patient may need to be lifted onto his side and assisted in clearing the airway with a large-bore suction catheter. Figure 34.15 illustrates this technique.

ASSESSMENT

In assessing the patient who has suffered a head injury, the EMT must pay careful attention to certain factors. The airway, breathing, and circulatory status are of key importance, as in any patient. There are also a few focused neurologic exam findings that will be useful. The EMT should become proficient in completing these.

PRIMARY ASSESSMENT

The most important thing an EMT can do to improve the outcome of a head-injured patient is to adequately assess and manage the airway, breathing, and circulatory status. The brain needs adequate perfusion with well-oxygenated blood. If the patient's airway is in jeopardy, there is no sense in proceeding with the assessment until that problem has been remedied.

After ensuring that an adequate airway exists, the EMT must address the effectiveness of the patient's own breathing. It is always appropriate to administer oxygen to a patient with a possible head injury during the "breathing" step of the primary assessment. After any issues related to adequacy of breathing have been dealt with, the EMT should turn her attention to the circulatory status.

Patients who have suffered traumatic brain injury may become hypertensive as ICP increases. This is considered to be a protective mechanism for the brain. If the brain is not getting sufficient oxygenated blood, raising the blood pressure will theoretically provide more blood to the brain. Low blood pressure in conjunction with a head injury is lethal. The EMT must recognize and address signs of hypoperfusion and hypotension rapidly to improve the outcome for a patient with serious head injury.

SECONDARY ASSESSMENT—RAPID TRAUMA ASSESSMENT

For the patient who has suffered a significant injury, after the primary assessment has been completed and any life-threatening problems have been addressed, the EMT should move on to a rapid trauma assessment.

This rapid trauma assessment will include a head-to-toe search for significant injury. For a high-priority patient, this assessment will be done immediately before or during transport.

A complete set of vital signs is needed as soon as possible and should be repeated as frequently as the patient's condition requires. Every 5 minutes is appropriate for the high-priority patient, less often for patients whose injuries are less severe.

PUPILS

During the rapid trauma assessment, check the pupils of the eye using a penlight. Normal pupils are equal in size and should react the same when the light is shined in only one pupil. This is a reflex known as a consensual response. One or both pupils fixed and dilated may be a sign of increased ICP.

Check eye movements in the conscious patient. Do both eyes follow the light, or is one eye position either downward or upward?

Finally, look for discoloration of the soft tissues around the eyes called *raccoon's eyes*. Raccoon's eyes are a delayed sign of a skull fracture that may also indicate an intracranial injury.

GLASGOW COMA SCALE

During the primary assessment and rapid trauma assessment, the EMT should be able to gather some important information about the patient's neurologic status. The patient's level of consciousness is the most important part of this neurologic exam. A reliable way to quantify this assessment is by using the Glasgow Coma Scale (GCS).

As discussed in Unit 33, the Glasgow Coma Scale is a method used to evaluate three aspects of a patient's responsiveness: eye opening, best verbal response, and best motor response. Each category has assigned values for different responses that, when totaled, are correlated with the degree of neurologic impairment.

The lowest score is 3, allowing one point for each category. The highest score is 15. A score of 8 or less defines a severe head injury; a moderate head injury is associated with a score of 9–12. Head-injured patients whose GCS score falls between 13 and 15 are considered to have a mild, although still significant, head injury.

The EMT must formally score the head-injured patient during the primary assessment and each reassessment. Any changes in the total score should be carefully noted and passed along to the staff at the hospital. It is not uncommon for a patient to either improve or deteriorate neurologically during prehospital care. This change can be easily measured using the GCS.

Table 34-5 outlines the point assignments in the Glasgow Coma Scale. A reproduction of this scale is useful for the EMT to keep in a pocket manual for easy reference.

VITAL SIGNS

As is done for every other patient, the EMT should initially measure the head-injured patient's baseline vital signs and reassess vital signs as often as is indicated by the condition. Certain characteristic findings may be seen with a serious head injury.

Table 34-5 Glasgow Coma Scale

	Best Response	Points
Eyes	Open spontaneously	4
	Open to verbal command	3
	Open to painful stimulus	2
	Do not open	1
Verbal	Oriented	5
	Disoriented	4
	Inappropriate words	3
	Incomprehensible sounds	2
	No response	1
Motor	Obeys command	6
	Localizes pain	5
	Withdraws from pain	4
	Shows abnormal flexion	3
	Shows abnormal extension	2
	No response	1
TOTAL		3–15

As previously discussed, the injured brain may induce an elevation in blood pressure in an attempt to improve its own perfusion. A reflex, called **Cushing's reflex,** results in a bradycardia in serious head injuries.

Another component to this reflex that is commonly seen is an alteration in the respiratory pattern. The normal, regular pattern of the respirations is no longer present. Respirations become irregular in any one of several patterns. **Cheyne-Stokes** respirations are one such irregular pattern associated with increased ICP. Cheyne-Stokes breathing is characterized by periods of shallow, slow breathing increasing to rapid, deep breathing and then returning to shallow, slow breathing followed by a short apneic period.

Hypertension, bradycardia, and an altered respiratory pattern are referred to as **Cushing's triad.** This triad of physical findings is indicative of a serious head injury.

MANAGEMENT

The priority in management of the patient with a head injury is to maintain an adequate supply of oxygenated blood to the brain without compromising the cervical spine. This goal can be achieved by following the same techniques of assessment and priorities in management that the EMT has learned in managing other high-priority patients.

THE ABCs

The primary assessment will reveal any problems related to the patient's airway, breathing, or circulation. The EMT must rapidly and proficiently gain control of the airway if needed. High-flow oxygen is always indicated for the head-injured patient. Ventilatory assistance may be needed if the patient is not effectively moving air.

Many patients who are involved in an incident that results in head injury may also have injury to other body systems. As a result, the EMT should identify signs of hypoperfusion and address them as appropriate. Adequate perfusion to the brain is critical to prevent worsening brain injury.

The EMT should remember to note the patient's initial mental status and, when time permits, calculate and document a GCS score. This can then be compared with scores obtained later in the management of this patient.

SPINE PRECAUTIONS

Because any significant trauma to the head may be associated with injury to the cervical spine, the EMT should always maintain immobilization of the spine of the head-injured patient. All management should be done with this principle in mind. A cervical collar should be applied to assist in keeping the neck immobilized. The details of this procedure are addressed in the next unit.

MAINTENANCE OF OXYGENATION

The injured brain has many compensatory mechanisms to maintain adequate oxygenation to itself. The EMT can assist in this effort by ensuring adequate oxygenation at all times. The use of 100% oxygen in the acute setting of a head injury will help reduce complications related to poor oxygenation.

VENTILATION

When serious brain injury exists and pressures within the skull are elevated, the EMT may be required to provide ventilatory assistance. The EMT should assist ventilations at the normal rates of 10 breaths/min for adults, 20 breaths/min for children, and 25 breaths/min for infants (Figure 34.16).

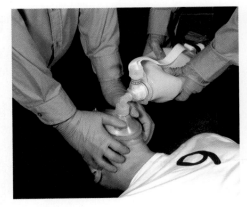

Figure 34.16 Assist ventilations to ensure adequate oxygenation of the brain

Hyperventilation will cause *hypocapnia* (low carbon dioxide) and underventilation can cause hypercapnia (high carbon dioxide) levels, both of which aggravate traumatic brain injuries. Falling carbon dioxide levels cause cerebral vasoconstriction that will lead to a decrease in cerebral oxygenation. For this reason, maintaining ventilatory rates within the normal range will provide for cerebral oxygen delivery and maintain appropriate levels of carbon dioxide.

CONTROL EXTERNAL BLOOD LOSS

For an adequate supply of oxygenated blood to the brain to be maintained, there must be a sufficient supply of blood within the vessels. The EMT should be sure to control any external blood loss during the initial assessment.

TRANSPORT

Once a patient has been determined to have a potential head injury, transport should not be delayed. The potential for decompensation always exists, and it is the job of the EMT to get the patient to the appropriate facility as soon as possible.

Many EMS systems have the option of several different modes of transportation for seriously injured patients. A ground ambulance is the most

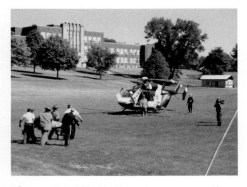

Figure 34.17 Helicopter evacuation may be necessary for some patients with serious head injuries (Courtesy of Deborah Funk, MD, Albany Medical Center, Albany, NY)

common means of transportation for injured patients. Some areas have the ability to use a helicopter, or air ambulance, to more rapidly transport a patient to the hospital (Figure 34.17). This option is obviously reserved for the most critical patients when ground transport would take an unacceptable amount of time. The use of such services is governed by local protocols.

High-priority patients should be transported directly to a hospital that is known to have the capability to care for such injuries. Usually the regional trauma center will be the choice hospital, but the choice may depend on local resources. The EMT should be familiar with the basic capabilities of surrounding hospitals. As with the use of helicopter transport, the EMT should always follow local protocols.

ONGOING ASSESSMENT

Just as it is important for the EMT to note any changes in patient condition during care, it is important to ask any witnesses to the event whether the patient's condition seems to have changed. Even untrained bystanders will be able to pick up on changes in mental status.

Any deterioration in mental status or neurologic function should be noted and considered to be an ominous sign of a serious head injury. The patient's vital signs and neurologic status should be reexamined frequently during transport. It is useful to repeat the GCS with each set of vital signs in the head-injured patient.

CONCLUSION

Head injuries account for many deaths and a significant amount of disability. Recognition of the potential for a serious head injury is the first step to providing appropriate care. Skilled assessment with efficient treatment provided by the EMT can help improve the outcome of patients with head injuries.

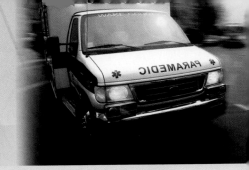

CASE STUDY Continued

Jose performs a quick trauma assessment, finding no additional injuries. The bartender states the patient had approximately six beers prior to the argument. He further states the patient was struck on the back of the head with a beer bottle and then fell off the bar stool, striking his head on the floor. He appeared dazed initially, then appeared to fall asleep and would not wake up.

Jose places a cervical collar while Roberto continues to maintain manual immobilization of the cervical spine. Jose, with the aid of law enforcement, logrolls the patient onto a long spine board and secures the torso and then the head with head blocks. Oxygen is administered via non-rebreather mask, and the team quickly moves the patient into the ambulance for transport to the trauma center. The patient groans when moved and continues to attempt to push the rescuers' hands away throughout packaging.

En route to the hospital, the patient remains responsive to painful stimuli. An ALS intercept is initiated

and Jose provides report to the medic stating the results of no additional injuries found after performing the secondary assessment and rapid trauma assessment findings. Baseline vital signs are a pulse of 110, respirations 16, and blood pressure 118/68. The patient's initial Glasgow Coma Scale is 7 (eyes-1, verbal-4, and motor-2). Jose states the patient has a gag reflex and ventilations have been adequate.

Later that night, Roberto and Jose run into the ALS crew and ask about the patient's outcome. The medic states the patient had a 4 cm laceration that was repaired with stitches. The CT scan showed no bleeding or hematoma. The patient regained consciousness at the hospital with a severe headache and no other signs or symptoms of a serious head injury. The doctor stated he had suffered a concussion, and the patient was admitted to the hospital overnight.

Key Concepts Revisited

- The brain controls all vital functions of life and is housed and protected within the skull.

- Injury to the skull and brain can be catastrophic, causing lifelong disability or death.

- Traumatic injuries to the face, including the eyes, nose, ears, and mouth, may include significant injury to the skull, brain, and cervical spine:

  ○ Facial injuries

    - Fractures, contusions, and lacerations to the upper and lower jaws and avulsion of the teeth

  ○ Impaled objects to the cheek

  ○ Fractures to the bones and cartilage and bleeding from the nose

  ○ Cuts, lacerations, bleeding, and avulsions of the ear

  ○ Eye

    - Foreign objects in the eye

    - Lacerations and burns to the eyelids

    - Lacerations, penetrations, chemical burns, impalements, and extrusion of the eyeball

- The mechanism of injury is the indicator for significant injuries to the head and affecting the face, cervical spine, and brain.

- Traumatic injury to the skull is either an open head injury where the brain is exposed or a closed head injury.

  ○ Basilar skull fracture—Closed head injury with fracture at the base of the skull, posterior to the face

  ○ Open skull fracture—exposing the brain to injury

    - Penetrating injury (knife or gunshot wound)

- Brain injuries can be divided into two categories: primary and secondary.
  - Primary—direct injury to the brain and associated vasculature
  - Secondary—injury extending from the primary brain injury, such as hypoxia due to inadequate oxygenation
- Skull fractures can cause bleeding between the meninges of the brain, increasing pressure within the brain and altering brain function.
  - Concussion—closed head injury caused by blunt trauma mildly tearing, stretching, and shearing brain tissue
  - Contusion—bruising and swelling of brain tissue
  - Subdural hematoma—collection of blood between the brain and dura mater
  - Epidural hematoma—collection of blood just under the skull, outside of the dura mater
  - Brain laceration—caused by a penetration in an open head injury or bone fragments in a closed skull fracture
- Elevated intracranial pressure causes compression of the brain and neurological damage.
  - The skull cannot expand, causing pressure to increase within the skull due to bleeding or swelling of the brain.
- Signs and symptoms of common head injuries are the same or similar, with one or two signs or symptoms specific to a particular type of head injury.
- Management of the patient with injuries to the head, face, and brain focuses on airway management, adequate oxygenation, and control of bleeding.

Review Questions

1. Why are head injuries relevant to the American public?
2. Describe the anatomy of the scalp, skull, and brain.
3. What injuries are commonly associated with head injuries?
4. What type of facial injury occurs from blunt force trauma?
5. What is the management for a chemical burn to the eye?
6. What are the two categories of brain injury?
7. Describe the management priorities of the patient with a scalp injury, a skull injury, and a brain injury.
8. What physical findings are associated with a scalp injury, a skull injury, and a brain injury?
9. What is the difference between a brain contusion and a concussion?
10. Discuss the consequences of raised intracranial pressure.
11. Identify the physical findings associated with increased intracranial pressure.
12. What are the management priorities for patients suffering a traumatic brain injury?

Key Terms

Acceleration/deceleration
Basilar skull fracture
Brain contusion
Cheyne-Stokes
Concussion
Coup-contrecoup
CSF otorrhea

CSF rhinorrhea
Cushing's reflex
Cushing's triad
Epidural hematoma
Hematoma
Intracranial pressure (ICP)
Mastoid process

Pia mater
Post-traumatic seizure
Primary brain injury
Secondary brain injury

Subarachnoid space
Subdural hematoma
Traumatic brain injury (TBI)

Further Study

Armstrong, J. "Bombs and Other Blasts." *RN* 61, no. 11 (1998): 26–35.

Badjatia, Neeraj, et al. "Guidelines for Prehospital Management of Traumatic Brain Injury 2nd Edition." *Prehospital Emergency Care* 12, no. S1 (2008): S1–S52.

Jastemski, C. "Trauma! Head Injuries." *RN* 61, no. 12 (1998): 40–44.

Murphy, P., and A. Heightman. "Head Injuries." *Journal of Emergency Medical Services* 23, no. 4 (1998): 66–70.

National Association of Emergency Medical Technicians. *PHTLS: Basic and Advanced PrehospitalTrauma Life Support.* 6th ed. Clinton, MS: Mosby/Elsevier, 2007.

Price, D., and B. Burns. "Brain Injuries." *Emergency Medical Services* 28, no. 6 (1999): 65–71.

Schultz, R. "Eggs and Brains." *Emergency Medical Services* 26, no. 4 (1997): 29–35.

UNIT (35) Spinal Injuries

Spinal cord injuries are devastating to the patient, the patient's family, and the community as a whole. The patient's entire lifestyle changes in the blink of an eye and life as he or she knows it changes forever. The effects to the community are in terms of lost productivity and health care costs. It has been estimated that costs exceed $1 million to care for a patient with a spinal cord injury in the first year alone.

New treatments offer hope for patients with spinal cord injuries. In addition, the rapid assessment and quick action of the EMT getting the patient to definitive care can make the difference between a good outcome and a less favorable outcome.

National Education Standard
The Emergency Medical Technician (EMT) will have a fundamental depth and foundational breadth of knowledge of the pathophysiology, assessment, and management of spine trauma.

Key Concepts

- Knowledge of the anatomy and physiology of the spinal column enables the EMT to better understand the causes of spinal column instability.

- Several common mechanisms of injury may lead to spine injury.

- Types of spinal cord injuries include compression, penetration, laceration, and transaction.

- Three life threatening complications of spinal cord injuries can occur.

- Neutral inline manual stabilization of the cervical spine is critical to prevent further injury.

- Proper application of the cervical immobilization device aids in the stabilization of the cervical spine.

- There are five key principles of spinal immobilization that must be maintained.

- The EMT must be able to apply the four long backboard techniques.

- Rapid extrication is an acceptable technique in limited circumstances.

- Short spinal immobilization devices are used as in interim device before the long backboard.

- Standing takedown is the preferred technique for patients standing or walking around with a possible spinal injury.

- Use of selective spinal immobilization depends on specific criteria.

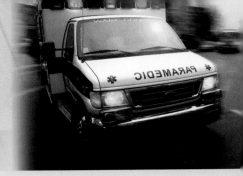

CASE STUDY

Officer Shulman knows as soon as he approaches the scene of a head-on motor vehicle collision that something is seriously wrong. As he approaches both vehicles, he notices the driver of one is already out of the car and rubbing his neck. "Not a good sign," thinks the police officer, as he asks, "Are you alright?" The driver insists he is fine but says his pregnant wife is still in the car and seems to be unconscious. That sends a shiver down Officer Shulman's spine. When his backup arrives, he directs her to the pregnant woman and turns his attention to the second car.

At this point only one ambulance has been dispatched, and Officer Shulman has not even gotten to the second car. "Dispatch, Unit 3. Please send additional EMS units and a paramedic supervisor to this location."

The other car is a mess, and the driver is still sitting in the front seat. Usually by the time the police arrive, all the drivers are out of their cars, or at least fumbling through their glove compartments looking for their insurance cards. This woman is sitting bolt upright, both hands on the steering wheel and staring straight out the window. She doesn't even turn her head as Officer Shulman approaches the car.

Officer Shulman introduces himself and says, "Good evening, ma'am." The driver of the car softly responds, "I can't feel my legs." Immediately recognizing the seriousness of the situation, Officer Shulman advises the driver not to turn or move her head. She whispers, "I know that. I heard something snap, and then I couldn't move my legs. I'm scared."

Officer Shulman tries to reassure her. "Ma'am, help is on the way. I am going to get into the backseat of your car and hold your head still. Don't answer me. Don't nod your head. Just be very still."

The police officer clicks his lapel mic and says, "Dispatch, Unit 3. Send a police supervisor to my location and a fire department response for a probable spinal injury from MVC, and tell them to expedite." He then climbs into the backseat of the car and manually stabilizes the patient's neck, telling her in a calm voice, "The ambulance is on the way."

The woman has a tear in her eye. Officer Shulman thinks for a moment to wipe the tear away but then he remembers how important it is to hold her head perfectly still. So he lets the tear drop run down her cheek.

Critical Thinking Questions

1. What is the care for an ambulatory patient with neck pain?
2. What techniques are used to extricate a seated patient?
3. What techniques are used to extricate a critical patient?

INTRODUCTION

An estimated 10,000 new spinal cord injuries occur in the United States each year. Spinal cord injuries can leave patients with an array of devastating neurologic injuries. These injuries can lead to permanent disability, paralysis, and even death. The impact of these injuries to patients, their families, and on society as a whole, is tremendous in terms of loss of quality of life and loss of productivity.

The immediate care provided by an EMT to the patient with a potential spine injury can have a crucial impact on the patient's long-term outcomes. An EMT is often the first health care provider that a patient who has sustained a suspected spine injury will encounter. The EMT's timely interventions can be truly lifesaving. The EMT must know how to recognize spine injuries and how to properly care for such patients.

ANATOMY REVIEW

The spinal column is actually made of three parts: the spinal vertebrae, the spinal cord, and the spinal ligaments. The heart of the spinal column is the spinal cord. The spinal cord is a collection of spinal nerves that receive input—that is, sensations—from the entire body and transfer them to the brain. This input is interpreted by the brain and another signal is sent down the spinal cord to direct the movements of the body, or to control motor function. The functions of these spinal nerves are explained in more detail shortly.

The purpose of the spinal vertebrae is to support and protect the all-important spinal cord. The spinal vertebrae are many individual bony structures aligned as a column and separated by soft cushions called *discs*. The different spinal vertebrae are named by segment, such as cervical, as well as their number in sequence. For example, cervical vertebrae one is referred to as C-1, second cervical vertebrae is C-2, and so on. Figure 35.1 illustrates both the segments and the numbering of the spinal vertebrae.

Finally, the spinal ligaments are bands of fibrous tissue that help the vertebrae support the spine and allow spinal column movement. During trauma these spinal ligaments can be injured.

The spinal column, including nerves, bones, and ligaments, can be thought of as a flexible long bone with many portions or segments, as shown in Figure 35.2. From between the vertebrae of each of these portions nerves leave and enter the spinal column. These nerves connect, or **innervate,** all of the muscles and organs of the body. The segments of the spinal column consist of the cervical spine, thoracic spine, lumbar spine, and sacral spine; the spinal column ends with the coccyx.

CERVICAL SPINE

Of all of the spine segments, the cervical spine is of greatest concern to the EMT because cervical spinal injury holds the most extensive consequences for the patient. Nearly 40% of cervical fractures have associated spinal cord injury. The cervical spine is relatively isolated from the rest of the body and is directly under the head, so sometimes keeping it motionless is difficult. The EMT's job is to prevent any movement of the cervical spine when an injury is suspected. In the United States, motor vehicle collisions (MVCs) account for a large number of cervical spine injuries.

The cervical spine is the uppermost portion of the spinal column. The first vertebra of the cervical spine is actually just under the skull and supports the entire skull. Because this first cervical vertebra supports the entire skull, the way that the Greek god Atlas supported the world on his shoulders, the first cervical vertebrae is sometimes called the *atlas*.

The next cervical vertebrae is sometimes referred to as the **axis** in reference to the bony projection, called the odontoid process, upon which the atlas sits. This connection allows the atlas to pivot and the entire head to turn. The spinal ligaments allow flexion, extension, and rotation of the head. This important vertebra is also protected by the skull. During a sudden deceleration, for example, during an MVC, the weight of the wildly swinging head is focused on this bony pivot. The analogy has been made to trying to balance a bowling ball on a broom stick. It is easy to understand how the upper cervical spinal vertebrae and ligaments can be injured. Figure 35.3 shows the all-important relationship between atlas and axis.

There are a total of seven cervical vertebrae. From between the 3rd, 4th, and 5th cervical vertebrae, several nerves leave the spinal column to form the

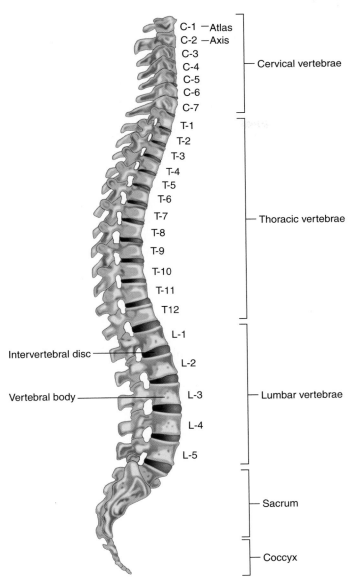

Figure 35.1 The spinal vertebrae are segments of bone, with a spinal lumen or canal for the spinal cord

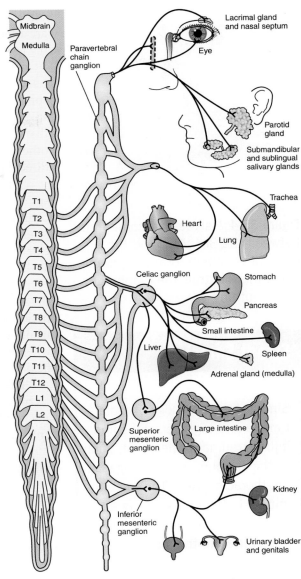

Figure 35.2 The spinal column is a series of vertebrae in a chain

phrenic nerve. The phrenic nerve is the nerve that controls the contractions of the muscular diaphragm. The saying goes "3 – 4 – 5 keeps a guy alive"; an injury to any of these nerves can lead to life-threatening paralysis of the diaphragm. The nerves that control the extremities also come from the same area of the spinal column and injury to these nerves can lead to paralysis of the extremities. For this reason, injury to the lower cervical spine, just where the neck joins the shoulders, can be devastating. Figure 35.4 shows how the nerves between the 3 – 4 – 5 cervical vertebrae come together to form the phrenic nerve.

SPINAL COLUMN IN THE TORSO

The spinal column in the torso starts with the twelve thoracic spinal vertebrae and ends with the lumbar—the sacral or lumbosacral—portion of the spine. The higher thoracic spinal vertebrae are attached to the ribs, or in

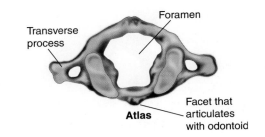

Figure 35.3 Atlas, holding up the skull, and axis, which allows the head to turn, have a delicate relationship that depends on the tiny bony thumb called the *odontoid process*

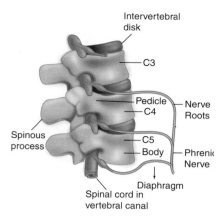

Figure 35.4 Nerves that come from between the 3rd, 4th, and 5th cervical vertebrae form the phrenic nerve that controls the diaphragm and breathing

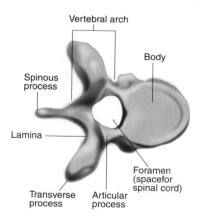

Figure 35.5 The heavy lumbar vertebrae, and accompanying intervertebral discs, support the entire weight of the torso

other words the ribs are attached to the spine. Because the thoracic vertebrae are attached to, and stabilized by, the rib cage, the entire vertebrae/rib assembly is rigid and less flexible than the cervical spine.

The thoracic spine is relatively immobile and therefore is not injured as often as the more mobile areas of the spine, such as the lumbar and cervical spine. When an injury does occur, however, it is more likely to involve the spinal cord because the **spinal canal,** the opening within the spinal vertebrae that the spinal cord occupies, is fairly narrow in this area compared with other areas of the spine. Thoracic spine injuries most often result from a direct blow to the back.

The spinal cord, housed within the spinal vertebrae, starts at the cervical spine. It might seem likely that it would end at the base of the spinal vertebral column, at the sacrum, but it does not. The spinal cord itself ends around the level of the first lumbar vertebrae, where it breaks up into multiple smaller extensions that resemble a horse's tail. This collection of nerve roots is known as the *cauda equine,* which literally translated means "horses tail."

The lower lumbar spinal vertebrae are not supported, or protected, by the rib cage. Lumbar spinal injuries may not be as evident on physical examination as other, higher cord injuries. The EMT should consider the mechanism of injury and the presence of pain in the low back area in determining whether injuries to this area may exist. These injuries are usually caused by a flexion/extension/rotational type of mechanism.

The final section of the spinal column, or the base of the column, is the sacrum and coccyx. These two bony portions of the spinal column are actually joined, or fused, with the pelvis. This allows the weight of the spinal column, and the torso, to be spread along the wide pelvis base.

The sacrum is a fairly strong collection of bones and is not often broken. Injury to this segment of the spine usually results from a direct blow. The bony tailbone, or coccyx, is commonly injured in a fall. While the pointy coccyx can be injured (i.e., a broken tail bone), this injury is more annoying than dangerous. Figure 35.5 shows the larger lumbar vertebrae that support the weight of the torso and that are prone to injury as well during am MVC.

SPINAL CORD

As previously mentioned, the spinal cord is composed of bands of nerve fibers that are found within the spinal canal and housed by the spinal vertebrae. Like the spinal vertebrae the spinal cord is divided into three portions: the anterior cord, the central cord, and the posterior cord.

The largest of these three cords is the anterior cord, which contains nerve fibers that bring signals, or sensations, to the brain and take instructions from the brain to the body. The tracts that bring signals up the spinal cord to the brain, or ascending tracts, start at the spine and end in the thalamus. The thalamus can be thought of as the switchboard of the brain, deciding which portions of the brain get which signal. For this reason, these ascending tracts are referred to as the **ascending spinothalamic tracts.** The spinothalamic tracts carry sensations of pain, such as a pinprick, hot or cold temperature, and touch.

Once the brain has received a sensation from the body, via the spinothalamic tract, the brain interprets that sensation and instructs the body on how to respond via the **descending corticospinal tract.** This motor tract starts at the cerebral cortex and descends down the spinal cord—hence the name *corticospinal tract.* The corticospinal tract controls the body's motor function of the body.

The central cord is actually part of the corticospinal tract, and its fibers are arranged in a pattern like the rings of a tree. The innermost ring contains the motor fibers for the hands and control the motor function, such as grasp, of the hands. The next set of rings, within the intermediate zone, control the movement of the upper extremities, and the outermost rings of the central cord control the movements of the lower extremities.

Finally, the posterior tracts of the spinal cord are part of the spinothalamic tracts and are therefore sensory fibers. These nerve fibers carry the sensations that sense vibration and the sense of position. The latter, the sense of position, allows the patient to stand upright and know that she is standing upright without looking at her feet. If the posterior cord is damaged, the patient will have trouble standing and walking. Figure 35.6 shows the tracts of the spinal cord.

NERVE ROOTS AND DERMATOMES

Spinal nerves called **nerve roots** exit and enter the spinal cord through the spinal column at various points. Some of these nerves are sensory nerves entering the spinothalamic tract, whereas others are motor nerves exiting the corticospinal tract to stimulate different muscles of the body.

If the spinal cord is injured by a crushed spinal vertebra—that is, the nerve is "pinched"—the corresponding motor/sensory nerves would also be affected. By a process of reverse assessment, and with knowledge of the different nerves that enter and exit the spinal column (the nerve roots), the EMT can roughly estimate where the spinal cord has been injured. Each spinal nerve has been traced from its origins to its end or terminus, and a map, called a **dermatome,** of the areas of sensation has been created. Table 35-1 cross-references these nerve roots to the corresponding areas, and Figure 35.7 illustrates the levels of sensation created by these nerve roots. Please note that nerve roots exit above their corresponding vertebra; an injury to the bony spinal column at C-7, therefore, would be expected to affect the C-6 nerve root.

Understanding where an injury has occurred can help the EMT care for the patient. For example, a patient may have sustained an incomplete spinal cord injury at level C-3, 4, 5. Initially, the patient may experience numbness along the top of the shoulders and down the arms, indicating an anterior cord injury. If the patient is mishandled, then the spinal cord injury could become worse, suffering a complete spinal cord transection, with loss of the spinal nerves at C-3, 4, 5 that control the diaphragm. Subsequently, the patient would experience respiratory distress and even respiratory arrest.

SPINAL COLUMN INSTABILITY

The EMT is primarily interested in spine injuries to the cervical spine, although injuries to the lumbar area can also be extremely painful. Injuries to the cervical spine can be potentially life threatening or have lifelong implications. These injuries usually occur when excessive force is applied to the cervical spine, such as forces that occur during a fall from a great height or during an MVC.

As a result of these forces, the neck can be hyperflexed. **Hyperflexion** is an excessive forward bending of the neck. This injury is seen when one car strikes another from behind. This bending may be so severe that the chin may

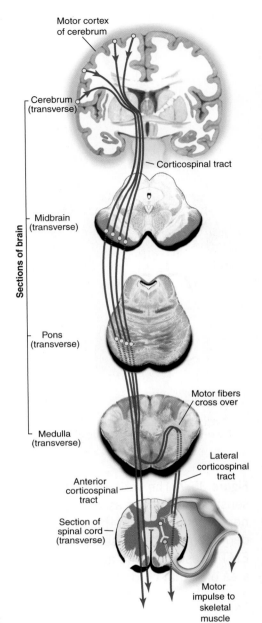

Figure 35.6 The ascending spinothalamic tract and the descending corticospinal tract combine to form the spinal cord

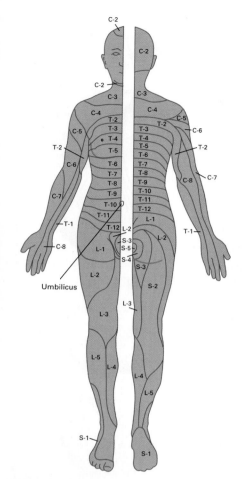

Figure 35.7 The various levels of sensation and their associated nerve roots shown in this dermatome can be used by the EMT to estimate the approximate area of spinal cord injury

Table 35-1 Dermatomes of the Body

Nerve Root	Motor	Sensory	Complication
C-3,4	Shoulder shrug (trapezius)	Top of shoulders	Quadriplegia
C-3,4,5	Diaphragm	Top of shoulders	Respiratory
C-5,6	Elbow flexion (Biceps)	Thumb	
C-7	Elbow Extension (Triceps)	Middle finger	
C-8/T-1	Finger abduction/ adduction	Little finger	Paraplegia
T-4		Nipple line	
T-10		Umbilicus level	
L-1,2	Hip flexion	Inguinal crease	
L-3,4	Quadriceps	Medial thigh/calf	
L-5	Great toe/foot dorsiflexion	Lateral calf	
S-1	Knee flexion	Lateral foot	
S-1,2	Foot plantar flexion		

touch the chest. In some extreme cases, if the person is wearing lipstick, there may be a smudge of lipstick on the front of the patient's shirt, which is called the *lipstick sign.* Figure 35.8 demonstrates hyperflexion.

If the force is from the front, as might occur during an explosion or front-end MVC, then there may be excessive backward bending of the neck, called **hyperextension** (Figure 35.9). This injury can be prevented by the use of a properly positioned headrest in a motor vehicle. However, an improperly positioned headrest can actually work as a fulcrum, causing increased neck injury from hyperextension (Figure 35.10).

Similar to hyperextension and hyperflexion, a force applied to the head can cause extreme **lateral bending.** Extreme lateral bending can occur as a result of a side impact during an MVC. The creation of side air curtains has helped reduce some of these cervical injuries because of lateral bending that occur in a lateral or T-bone MVC.

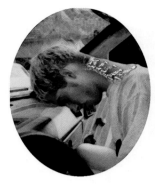

Figure 35.8 Hyperflexion, excessive forward bending of the neck, can cause spinal injury

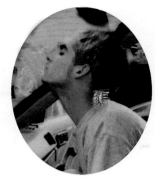

Figure 35.9 Hyperextension, excessive backward bending of the neck, can also cause spinal injury

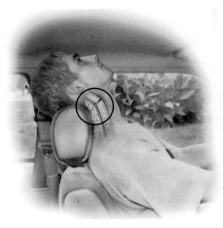

Figure 35.10 An improperly positioned headrest can actually work as a fulcrum, causing increased neck injury from hyperextension

If the force spins the patient's head around, the rotational force can injure the supporting ligaments. For example, a person struck in the face by a roundhouse kick or a hook punch could experience cervical spine injury from the rotational force to the head, neck, and spine.

If the force comes from above, as in the case of a falling object onto a hard hat, the sudden downward pressure along the length of the spine, called **axial loading,** could cause compression of the intervertebral discs, pinching the nerve roots and causing spinal cord injury. Axial loading can occur from force applied from above, or from forces applied from below (Figure 35.11). For example, the energy created from jumping from a great height can be transmitted up the legs and into the spinal column. This force can be so great that the vertebrae actually disintegrate in what is called a *burst fracture.*

The final type of cervical spine injury is called **axial distraction.** The opposite of axial loading, where the cervical spine is compressed, during axial distraction the cervical spine is pulled apart. While there are many causes for axial distraction, such as falling forward onto one's chin in what is termed a "dead man's fall," the classic cause of axial distraction is hanging. Normally there is a slight curvature of the cervical spine but when a sudden force is applied along the length, or axis, of the spine, a fracture can occur. Most typically, this fracture is at the level of C-2 and is known as a "hangman's fracture."

An injury to the spinal column poses a risk of damage to the sensitive spinal cord that lies within the spinal canal. Not all spinal injuries are associated with damage to the spinal cord, but when they are, the results can be devastating.

Some spinal injuries consist only of ligament or bone injuries. If the damage to these support structures does not compromise the patency of the spinal canal or directly traumatize the sensitive cord, neurologic injury will not be present. An isolated bone injury, however, can be unstable in its position. If the bone injury disrupts the supportive nature of the spinal column, any movement of the column can cause unnatural movement of the spine and compromise the spinal canal, thus injuring the spinal cord.

A patient who has sustained a possible spinal injury should not be allowed to move at all. Any movement can potentially cause injury to the spinal cord (Figure 35.12).

Some spinal injuries immediately cause injury to the spinal cord. Certain signs and symptoms indicate neurologic injury. These signs and symptoms, which result from an interruption in the normal message flow back and forth between the brain and the body, is discussed later.

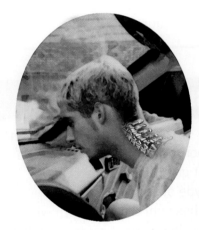

Figure 35.11 Axial loading can occur from force applied from above, such as when the top of the head impacts with the windshield of a car

Pediatric Considerations

A child's spinal column is more flexible than is an adult's. This can result in bending of the spine that does not result in a fracture but still causes injury to the spinal cord. This phenomena is called *spinal cord injury without radiologic abnormality* (SCIWORA) in that no fracture is actually seen on a radiograph. Children who have had a mechanism of injury that leads to suspicion of spine injury should be carefully assessed for symptoms of spinal cord injury.

Street Smart

A small percentage of children born with Down syndrome are at greater risk for a special type of spinal cord injury. These children are born with weaker spinal ligaments to help support the neck. As a result, extreme forces—during contact sports, for example—can lead to **atlanto-occipital dislocation.** Simply stated, the rear of the head, at the occiput, moves off the neck at the level of the atlas cervical vertebrae and can injure the spinal cord.

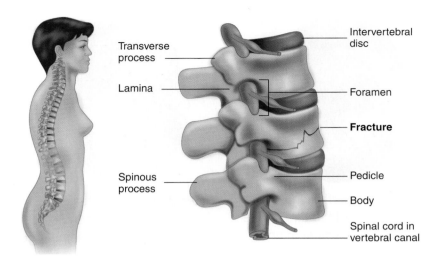

Figure 35.12 Some spinal injuries cause damage to the spinal cord that is immediately evident

MECHANISM OF INJURY

Any mechanism that involved a blow to the spine or created a severe flexion, extension, or rotation of the spine should be considered suspect. In addition, any significant injury to an adjacent body part, such as the head, chest, or abdomen, should create suspicion of spinal injury. It should be noted that the large majority of spinal cord injuries, approximately 82%, occur in males between the ages of 16 and 30 and are the result of MVCs, violence, or falls.

MOTOR VEHICLE COLLISION

The forces in an MVC often cause the neck to flex and extend forcefully as the vehicle comes to a stop, as explained by a fundamental physics concept known as Newton's second law. Any type of spinal injury is possible in an MVC, but the flexion/extension type is probably most common.

The spinal column is designed to allow a certain amount of flexion (forward movement of the upper body), extension (backward movement of the upper body), and rotation (side-to-side movement). If force, such as the force of an MVC, causes motion beyond that which is normally allowed, the spinal column may be damaged. The supporting ligaments may stretch or tear, and the vertebrae may crack or be dislocated from their normal position. When a significant disruption in the normal anatomy of the spinal vertebrae intrudes into the narrow canal, injury to the spinal cord may occur. (Figure 35.13)

FALLS

Falls may also cause injuries to the spine. As the force of fall is transmitted along the spinal column, the bones may fracture, or burst, resulting in an unstable spinal column and the potential for a spinal cord injury. A fall from any height can result in a broken bone, but falls from greater heights have a higher risk for creating such an injury. A fall of three times the patient's height is considered significant. However a fall from a standing position may cause spinal injury in an elderly patient with weak and fragile bones as a result of the disease osteoporosis. **Osteoporosis** is loss of bone strength, often due to a loss of calcium in the bones, which leads to brittle bones.

Victims who fall from a height and land on their feet, a phenomenon known as **Don Juan syndrome,** may experience significant spinal injuries

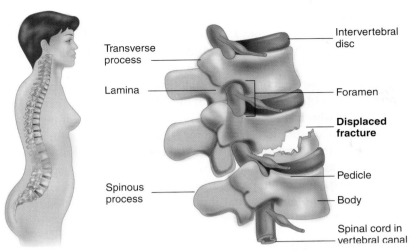

Figure 35.13 When supporting ligaments stretch or tear, the vertebrae may crack or be dislocated from their normal position and intrude into the narrow canal, causing significant injury to the spinal cord

secondary to axial loading. The force of the fall is transmitted from the feet, up through the legs, and into the spine. In this situation, broken bones in the patient's feet and injuries to the patient's lumbar spine and cervical spine are common. The spine injuries occur because the spine is curved in two places, at the lumbar and cervical segment, and the fall compresses these curves. See Figure 35.14 for an illustration of this concept.

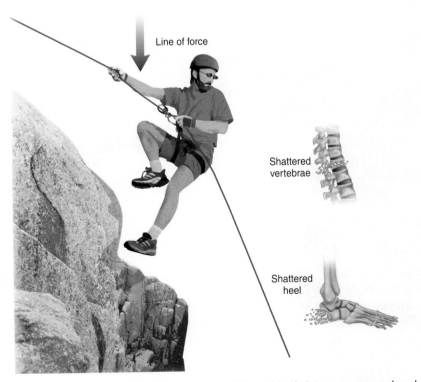

Figure 35.14 A jump or fall from a significant height can cause heel fractures and lumbar spine fractures

GUN SHOT WOUNDS

The projectile, or bullet, from a firearm has a considerable amount of energy. If a bullet were to strike the spinal column, that energy would be transferred to the spinal column, causing trauma and potentially causing spinal cord injury. Because the direction of internal travel of a bullet is often difficult to discern in the field, the EMT must not dismiss the possibility of spinal injury. Every patient who has suffered a gunshot wound to the midline torso or any region of the neck should be treated for a potential spinal injury.

Although less common than spinal injuries from gunshot wounds, sharp objects such as knives can cause injury to the spine and spinal cord. All patients who have suffered penetrating trauma near the back or neck should be treated for a potential spinal injury. Figure 35.15 depicts a penetrating injury resulting in injury to the spine.

SPORTS INJURIES

Recreational sports are usually a safe way to get exercise and keep healthy, but they can result in spinal injuries. Collisions that occur during sports can result in all types of forces—rotational, compression, and distraction—being applied to the neck and spine. These forces can cause considerable injury, particularly in football. Football injuries account for the largest number of spinal injuries during organized sports events. High school football results in 20 to 30 permanent spinal cord injuries annually in the United States. Diving and rugby also account for a significant proportion of spinal injuries from recreational sports.

Depending on the sport, the mechanism of the spinal injury may vary with each situation. The EMT must determine the exact mechanism of any

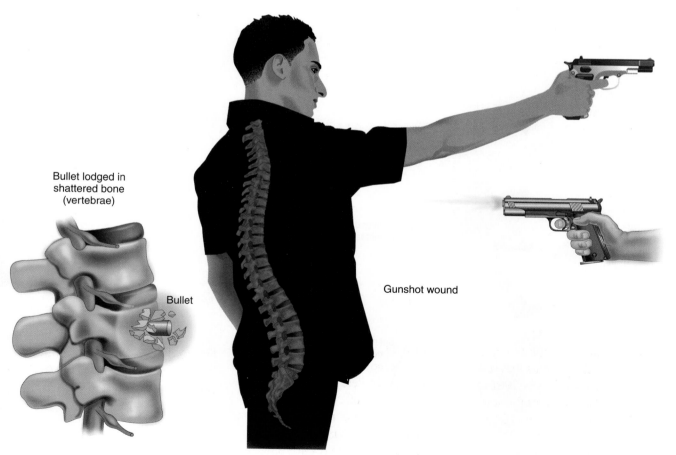

Bullet lodged in shattered bone (vertebrae)

Bullet

Gunshot wound

Figure 35.15 Penetrating injuries to the torso often cause spinal cord injury

Table 35-2	Causes of Spinal Cord Injury
Injuries	**Caused**
1. Motor vehicle crashes	36.0%*
2. Violence/crime	28.9%*
3. Falls	21.2%*

*Retrieved from Spinal Cord Injury Resource Center, http://www.spinalinjury.net.

injury from sport-related activity. If the patient may have experienced a direct blow or excessive flexion, extension, or rotation of the spine, the EMT should consider the potential for spine injury. Table 35-2 lists common types of incidents that may result in spinal injury.

ASSOCIATED INJURIES

Because the spine is located near many other body parts, an injury to other parts of the body can also cause injury to the spine. The EMT should maintain a high index of suspicion for spinal injury if any significant trauma is sustained by any part of the body that is close to the spine.

Twenty percent of patients who sustain significant cervical spine injuries also have facial injuries. Because the face is in such close proximity to the neck, the forces are easily transmitted to both, and coexisting injuries are frequently seen. The EMT should treat any patient with facial injuries as though the patient has a cervical spine injury. A good rule to follow is to assume that any significant trauma above the clavicles involves the cervical spine. Even if the patient denies any neck pain, it is always better to err on the side of treating for the possibility of spine injury if there is trauma above the clavicles.

The thoracic spine makes up the posterior support of the chest. If a patient sustains trauma to the chest, the potential for thoracic spine injury exists. The EMT should assume that any patient with significant chest injuries also has thoracic spine injuries and should treat the patient as though such injuries exist.

If any injury is sustained to the abdomen, the EMT should suspect lumbar spine injury as well. Proper treatment of the patient with a potential spine injury will reduce the possibility of complications and potential worsening of the injury.

TYPES OF SPINAL CORD INJURIES

Spinal cord injuries may be the result of compression of the vertebrae and subsequent compression of the spinal cord. Spinal cord injuries can result from penetration of the spinal cord by shards of bone, from a burst fracture, for example. Spinal cord injuries can result from overstretching or sprains of the supporting spinal ligaments that result in an unstable spinal column. Regardless of the cause, the result can be lacerations, including complete transection, of the spinal cord, compression of the spinal cord, or stretching of the spinal cord.

The injuries that occur at the time of incident such as penetrating trauma caused by a gun shot wound can cause **primary spinal cord injury.** These injuries result in an immediate and often irreversible loss of motion or sensation or both as seen in Brown-Sequard syndrome (Figure 35.16).

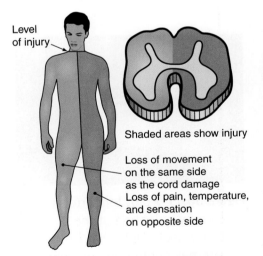

Level of injury

Shaded areas show injury

Loss of movement on the same side as the cord damage
Loss of pain, temperature, and sensation on opposite side

Figure 35.16 Primary spinal cord injuries such as those caused by penetrating trauma to the spine, may result in an immediate and often irreversible loss of motion or sensation or both (Brown-Sequard syndrome)

However, not all spinal cord injuries occur at the time of impact. Some spinal cord injuries, called **secondary spinal cord injuries,** are the result of improper handling of the patient with a potential spinal cord injury. For example, the patient may experience a **subluxation** of a spinal vertebrae, or a partial dislocation of the spinal vertebrae. Mishandling of a patient with a subluxation can convert the subluxation into a dislocation, with subsequent transection of the spinal cord. Prehospital spinal care has always focused on preventing secondary spinal cord injuries.

It is imperative that an EMT know the signs and symptoms of a spinal injury and to take into consideration the mechanism of injury, when deciding whether to immobilize a patient. The following section discusses the signs and symptoms of a spinal injury. The EMT should carefully assess the patient, looking for these signs and symptoms, to correctly identify those patients that need spinal immobilization.

SIGNS AND SYMPTOMS OF SPINAL INJURY

After considering the mechanism of the injury, the EMT should determine whether the patient has any signs or symptoms of possible spinal injury. The patient who has a mechanism of injury consistent with spinal injury along with signs and symptoms of that injury should be treated for spinal injury.

The classic triad of symptoms and signs of spinal injury include neck pain, tenderness along the spine, and obvious deformity of the spine. If the patient complains of neck pain, the EMT should take the patient at her word and treat her as if she has a spinal injury. There is no need for further examination. Needless palpation of the cervical spine could potentially worsen the spinal injury and therefore should be avoided.

If the patient does not complain of neck pain, the EMT should first examine the posterior neck along the midline. If visible deformity or soft tissue injury such as swelling is seen, the EMT should assume there is spinal injury and provide care accordingly.

Finally, if there is no concern of neck pain and no visible deformity or soft tissue injury, the EMT can gently palpate the midline posterior neck for **point tenderness,** or an exact place of reproducible pain. The EMT in Figure 35.17 is demonstrating an assessment for point tenderness. If the patient complains of point tenderness, the EMT should stop the examination, note the exact location of the point tenderness, and provide care accordingly.

Some patients may not have symptoms of spinal injury even though the mechanism of injury is one likely to cause such injury. These patients may be managed in a different manner than other patients, depending on regional protocols. This decision to not immobilize a patient is discussed in detail shortly, but an EMT who has any doubt whether a patient has a spinal injury should assume that is a possibility and treat the patient accordingly. Otherwise, the EMT should follow local protocol for patients who have no symptoms of spinal injury and a minor mechanism of injury.

Several signs and symptoms may be seen in the patient with a spinal cord injury. The EMT must be able to recognize these findings immediately, as they indicate possible spinal cord injury and the need for spinal immobilization. When the spinal cord is injured, the signs and symptoms—neck pain, deformity, or point tenderness—are usually evident soon after the incident. Some serious complications may also indicate a spinal injury. The following complications of spinal injury are listed in order of severity.

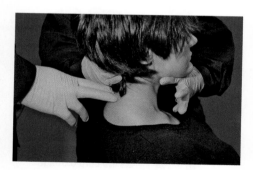

Figure 35.17 Point tenderness elicited by palpation of the posterior neck. Note that the patient has continuous manual stabilization

RESPIRATORY DISTRESS OR ARREST

The most severe complication of spinal cord injury is respiratory compromise. Without an intact spinal cord the body's lungs cannot function properly. The diaphragm, which controls inhalation, receives stimulation to contract from the brain via nerves that originate from the cervical spinal cord and go out the nerve roots. These nerve roots, which travel between the 3, 4, and 5 cervical vertebrae, must be intact for the diaphragm to function. Signals from these nerves stimulate the diaphragm, a muscle that is necessary for breathing. A good way to remember this important connection is the mnemonic "3, 4, and 5 keeps you alive." When the nervous control of the diaphragm is cut off, the diaphragm stops contracting, and the patient's breathing efforts become ineffective because the main muscle of breathing is no longer functioning. This may be evidenced by extreme shortness of breath, obvious respiratory difficulty, or apnea. The patient shown in Figure 35.18, who was involved in an MVC, is receiving assistance breathing using the jaw thrust airway maneuver and bag-valve-mask ventilation.

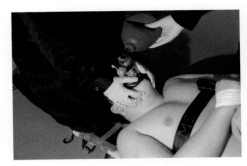

Figure 35.18 The patient with a high cervical injury, around the base of the skull, may have respiratory distress/arrest and need assisted ventilations

NEUROGENIC SHOCK

The next complication of a spinal cord injury can be sudden hypotension and *neurogenic shock.* Neurogenic shock is shock caused by the loss of nervous system control of the blood pressure. The nerves that control the constriction of blood vessels that keep the blood pressure up pass down the spinal cord and out to all of the arteries of the body. An injury to the spinal cord may interrupt the nervous system's control of these blood vessels and cause a general vasodilation of the blood vessels below the area of the spinal injury. This massive vasodilation of the blood vessels causes a relative blood loss and hypotension. A relative blood loss means that the container for the blood is larger than the volume of blood to fill it, and not the result of actual blood loss.

To understand what areas could be affected by this vasodilation, the EMT should use the dermatomes discussed earlier. The dermatomes correspond with the level of nervous control that the spinal cord and brain exert on the arteries. When that nervous system control is lost, the arteries naturally dilate and the blood pressure drops.

Externally, the vasodilation may cause the patient's skin to appear flushed as the arteries and arterioles under the skin dilate and move more blood to the skin's surface. Running the hand down the length of the patient's body, the EMT can feel a clear line of demarcation where the skin is cool and clammy above the level of the spinal injury and warm and flushed below it. Using the dermatome the EMT can estimate the level of the spinal cord injury.

For example, an injury to the lower thoracic spine, around T-10, would cause vasodilation below the umbilicus. The EMT running his hand down the chest would feel that the skin is cool and clammy up to the level of the umbilicus; then it would be warm and flushed.

Another sign of neurogenic shock is bradycardia. Normally, when blood pressure drops, the heart rate increases in response to compensate for the loss of blood pressure. This is part of the fight-or-flight response and requires communication between the brain and the heart. If a patient has a spinal cord injury, the communication between the brain and the heart may not be intact. If this is the case, the patient's heart rate will not increase despite a falling blood pressure.

The combination of hypotension with bradycardia and flushed, warm skin is characteristic of neurogenic shock and indicates that the patient may have a serious spinal cord injury. Figure 35.19 illustrates the triad of spinal paralysis, neurogenic shock, and bradycardia.

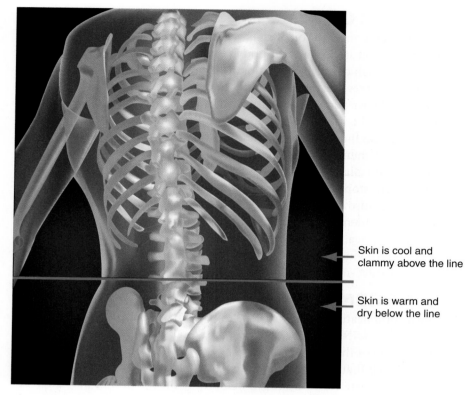

Skin is cool and
clammy above the line

Skin is warm and
dry below the line

Figure 35.19 Neurogenic shock is notable by distal vasodilation, manifest by warm and flushed skin, and bradycardia

PARALYSIS

Perhaps the most well-known and easily recognized complication of a spinal cord injury is the inability to move. This complication, known as **paralysis,** suggests that the patient may have a serious spinal cord injury.

Depending on the location of the spinal cord injury, the areas affected by paralysis differ. The nerves to the legs come from the lower parts of the spinal cord, while the nerves to the arms come from the higher parts of the spinal cord. If the cord is injured at a high level, however, all messages flowing through that area will be interrupted; this means that everything below the affected area may be paralyzed.

Again the EMT should refer to the dermatomes to determine at what level the spinal cord injury may exist. If the spinal cord injury is at the level of C-4, then all four extremities will be affected. A patient who has lost the use of both arms and legs is said to have **quadriplegia,** a term that refers to four extremities unable to function. A patient who has lost the use of only her legs is said to have **paraplegia,** a term that refers to loss of function in the lower part of the body.

The nerves that relay sensation usually are damaged when the nerves that control motor function, or movement, are damaged. Patients with spinal cord injuries may also not be able to feel their bodies below a certain level, depending on the level of the cord injury. The term used to describe a sensory problem is **paresthesia;** anesthesia is the absence of feeling sensations. Patients with paresthesia may complain of a feeling of numbness or tingling in their extremities. The EMT should check the arms and the legs for paresthesia during the trauma assessment. The EMT can test for paresthesia by asking the patient whether she can feel a particular physical stimulus, such as pinching a fingernail or a toe.

ASSOCIATED SIGNS OF SPINAL CORD INJURY

Another sign of spinal cord injury is the inability to control bowel function. Infants cannot control their bowel functions but learn bowel control—that is, potty training—as their spinal cord matures. If the spinal cord is injured, then the patient may lose control of their bowels and/or bladder. Although **incontinence,** the loss of control of bowels and/or bladder, can be caused by other illnesses, such as seizures, the presence of incontinence plus other symptoms or signs of spinal injury support a suspicion of spinal cord injury.

Another physical sign of possible injury to the spinal cord is **priapism.** This term refers to a painful penile erection that may be present when the nerves controlling this bodily function are injured. Table 35-3 lists some signs and symptoms that may be associated with a spine injury.

PRIMARY ASSESSMENT

After ensuring scene safety and personal safety, the EMT should ascertain the nature of the call. If the EMT suspects that the call involves trauma, he should take immediate manual cervical spine stabilization. Next the EMT should proceed with the primary assessment.

At one point, either during or at the end of the primary assessment, the EMT decides on the urgency of the patient's condition. Many traumatic injuries can make a patient a high priority. While treating these injuries is a priority, the EMT should always attempt to protect the spine from further injury, also referred to as *secondary injury*. Aggravating a spinal cord injury, while treating another serious injury, can only complicate care. For example, an aggravated spinal cord injury can lead to respiratory distress or even respiratory arrest, thus making a bad situation worse.

If the patient is a high-priority patient, then the EMT will have to move the patient to a long backboard for full spine immobilization and immediate transport to definitive care. If the patient is supine, then the EMT will have to lift or logroll the patient to a long backboard. If the patient is seated—in the front seat of a car, for example—the EMT will have to perform a rapid extrication to move the patient to a long backboard.

If the patient is low priority, or stable, the EMT may proceed to secondary assessment at a more measured pace and consider the best means of spinal immobilization. After completing the secondary assessment, the EMT may elect to move the patient to the long backboard by logrolling or lifting the patient if she is supine. If the patient is seated, the EMT may elect to use an intermediary transfer device such as short backboard to move the patient to the long backboard.

In some cases, and after a thorough examination, the EMT may even elect to not immobilize the patient. The decision to selectively immobilize those patients for whom immobilization may have the greatest benefit is discussed later in this unit.

CONSIDERATIONS WHEN DECIDING ON SPINAL IMMOBILIZATION

Several groups of patients may not notice or be able to describe symptoms of spinal injury even if such symptoms are present. These groups include patients who, for some reason, may not be able to feel pain and patients who are otherwise distracted.

Patients who are intoxicated may not feel even severe pain and, therefore, cannot be relied on to describe the symptoms of spinal injury. Intoxicated

Table 35-3 Signs and Symptoms of Spinal Injury

- Neck pain
- Tenderness along the spine
- Neck pain associated with movement
- Obvious deformity of spine
- Soft tissue injuries in proximity to spine
- Numbness, weakness, or tingling in the extremities
- Loss of sensation or paralysis below the suspected level of injury
- Loss of sensation or paralysis in the upper or lower extremities
- Incontinence
- Priapism

Street Smart

EMTs often treat patients for potential spine injuries when none exist, a practice that is acceptable. This practice of taking extraordinary precautions to possibly prevent an injury is called *over triage*. It is much better to immobilize too many people than to fail to immobilize one who really needs it.

patients who have a mechanism of injury consistent with a spinal injury should be treated as though a spinal injury is present.

The presence of another painful injury may distract a patient from the symptoms of a spinal injury. For example, a patient with pain from a broken leg may be distracted from the less severe pain of a spinal injury because the pain from the broken leg may be more intense. Any patient who has a significant mechanism of injury and a potentially distracting injury should be treated for a spine injury regardless of the presence of symptoms.

An unconscious patient, or a patient with an altered mental status, cannot relay symptoms of a spine injury to the EMT; therefore, the EMT should assume the patient has a spine injury if any potentially serious mechanism exists. For example, a patient who is found unconscious on a bed and whose family denies that any fall or other trauma occurred probably does not have a spinal injury. On the other hand, the EMT should assume that a patient who has fallen down a flight of stairs and has been found unconscious at the bottom has a spinal injury. The best rule is to assume spinal injury is present if the patient was found unconscious and no one witnessed what caused the patient's condition or can verify that the patient did not fall and strike her head.

MANUAL STABILIZATION

The main objective of spinal immobilization is to prevent further injury to the spine during treatment and transportation. While spinal immobilization must sometimes be done quickly, the principles of spinal immobilization should not be compromised in haste.

The first action of the EMT, after recognizing the potential for spinal injury given the presence of trauma and a significant mechanism of injury, is to manually stabilize the cervical spine. This action prevents further movement of an unstable or potentially unstable spine.

After taking standard precautions by donning gloves, the EMT should manually stabilize the cervical spine. The EMT needs to first control the movement of the head and neck by grasping the head at the base of the skull. If the patient is conscious, the EMT should explain to the patient what he intends to do. The patient should also be instructed to answer either yes or no to questions and not shake her head in response to questions.

Approaching from behind, the EMT cradles the occipital portion of the skull in his hands with fingers spread open, as shown in Figure 35.20. The EMT should avoid covering the patient's ears with the palms of his hands. Unable to hear instructions and other sounds, the patient may resist stabilization, risking further injury.

In some instances the EMT may approach the patient from the side—through a rolled-down window or open car door, for example. In those instances the EMT should place one hand on the occipital region and the other under the jaw, in a viselike manner, to stabilize the cervical spine, as shown in Figure 35.21.

On occasion it is necessary for the EMT to stabilize the cervical spine from the front, as in an entrapment. This anterior approach is the reverse of the posterior approach. With the EMT facing the patient, the EMT places one hand on either side of the face at the angle of the jaw as demonstrated in Figure 35.22.

NEUTRAL INLINE ALIGNMENT

While maintaining continuous manual stabilization, the EMT should attempt to move the patient's head into a neutral inline alignment. **Neutral inline alignment** is the natural anatomic position of the head and neck with the eyes looking forward and tilted chin upward. Generally speaking, returning any bone fracture to neutral inline alignment is considered safe and desirable.

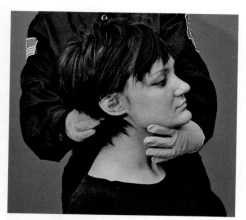

Figure 35.20 Manual head stabilization is the best way to keep a patient's head and neck in line

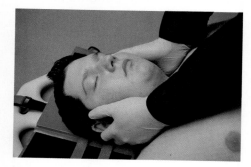

Figure 35.21 Lateral manual cervical stabilization

Figure 35.22 Anterior manual cervical stabilization

The neutral inline alignment affords the spinal cord the greatest opening in the spinal canal. A neck that is bent will necessarily limit the lumen, or opening, of the spinal canal and potentially compromise the spine. Figure 35.23 illustrates this point.

To attain neutral inline alignment, the EMT should move the head either forward, backward, or laterally, as the case may be, until the head is in the upright position. In neutral inline alignment the eyes should be looking forward and an imaginary line drawn between the eyes and the opening of the ears should be straight and zero degrees horizontal. Figure 35.24 illustrates this concept.

The EMT should always attempt to move the patient's head into neutral inline alignment unless the patient complains of sudden neck pain or tingling or weakness in the extremities. If this occurs, the EMT should immobilize the neck in the position found.

In some rare instances, the EMT will meet resistance when moving the head into neutral inline alignment. This is because the vertebrae may have been dislocated and locked into one another. The EMT should never attempt to overcome resistance with brute force but rather should immobilize the head and neck in the position found.

Manual stabilization is only a prelude to mechanical stabilization. Therefore, manual stabilization must be continuously maintained until full mechanical stabilization is complete.

DISTAL NEUROLOGIC FUNCTION

With manual cervical stabilization, the EMT should proceed with a focused examination that assesses the patient's peripheral neurologic function. The spinal nerves, emanating from the spinal roots between the spinal vertebrae, innervate the extremities. These sensory and motor nerves can be compromised during a spinal injury. Therefore, the EMT should check each extremity for movement (motor) and sensation (feeling).

The EMT should check both extremities for movement and sensation. These distal nerves tend to run along the shaft of long bones. If a long bone is fractured, the bone fragments can cut these nerves and leave the distal hand or foot without feeling. To ensure that the loss of distal nerve function is central—that is, secondary to spinal injury and not due to a fractured long bone—the EMT should check distal sensory and motor function in all extremities.

Some EMTs check the extremities for signs of distal circulation. This practice is consistent with principles of fracture management. Most arteries and veins, like nerves, tend to run next to the long bones. Therefore, if a long bone is fractured, the bony fragments could conceivably cut an artery or vein. However, this is not the case with a spinal injury. Because a pair of arteries, the spinal arteries, run parallel to the spinal cord, these arteries do not extend to the hands and feet.

However, checking distal circulation can be helpful in determining the absence or presence of neurogenic shock. As described earlier in this unit, during neurogenic shock, the blood vessels become dilated, because of loss of spinal nerve control, and the skin becomes warm and flushed below the level of the injury. The skin above the injury becomes cool and clammy as a result of the body's response to the loss of blood pressure. If the EMT finds that the feet are warm but the hands are cool, this might suggest that the patient has a spinal injury.

While there are several ways to check distal circulation, including capillary refill, peripheral pulses, and skin temperature, they all serve the same purpose, assessing distal circulation.

The EMT should minimally confirm distal circulation, sensation, and movement (CSM) before and after the patient is placed on a long

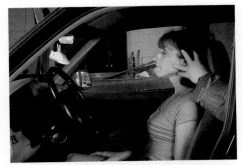

Figure 35.23 The spinal canal narrows when the spine column is bent

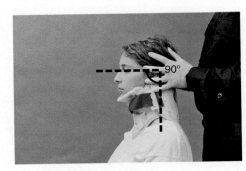

Figure 35.24 Neutral inline alignment of the cervical spine

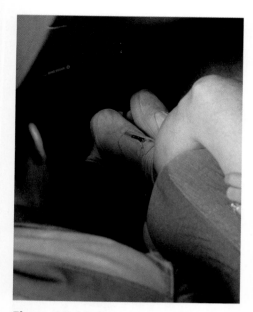

Figure 35.25 Checking for distal neurologic function

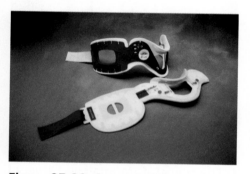

Figure 35.26 Several different sizes of cervical spine immobilization devices are available (Courtesy of Laerdal Medical Corporation, Wappingers Falls, NY)

backboard. Other times the EMT should consider checking for CSM during transfer from one spine immobilization device to another, as from short board to long board. Figure 35.25 shows an EMT checking distal neurologic function.

CERVICAL SPINE IMMOBILIZATION DEVICE

The best way to keep a patient's head and neck in a natural anatomic position, with neutral inline alignment, is to manually hold head stabilization. However, maintaining steady continuous manual stabilization can be tiring after awhile. As the EMT becomes fatigued, the risk for accidental movement increases. To aid the EMT, a tool called a cervical immobilization device (CID) is used. A **cervical immobilization device,** sometimes called a *cervical collar,* is a semi-rigid device used as an aid to help maintain neutral inline alignment of the cervical spine.

The CID is designed to fit around the patient's neck snugly enough to discourage movement, but not so tightly as to restrict breathing. There are many models of the cervical collar, but all of them operate on the same principle. The CID cups both the occipital area of the head and chin in a viselike fashion to prevent flexion, extension, lateral bending, or rotation of the neck. However, even when applied correctly, the CID does not provide complete restriction of motion. Therefore, the EMT must continue to maintain continuous manual stabilization.

The decision to apply a CID should be carefully considered. A CID, by design, prevents the jaw from moving. The proper application of CID can prevent the EMT from performing a jaw thrust to open the airway. Additionally, a CID can prevent the EMT from obtaining or maintaining a proper mask seal with a bag-valve-mask assembly. In those cases it may be in the patient's best interest to forego the CID and have the EMT maintain continuous manual stabilization.

Once the EMT has applied the CID, the EMT has committed to full spinal immobilization. Therefore, if there is any consideration that the patient may not need spinal immobilization, the EMT should maintain continuous manual stabilization until that decision is made. Figure 35.26 shows an example of a cervical immobilization device.

APPLICATION OF THE CERVICAL SPINE IMMOBILIZATION DEVICE

After instructing someone to maintain manual neutral inline alignment of the cervical spine, the EMT must choose a cervical immobilization device and measure the patient to determine the correct size of collar to use.

Different manufacturers have different methods of measuring their CID, but they all follow the same principles. First, the head must be held by the CID in a neutral inline alignment. This position is an eyes-forward, chin-up position with the imaginary line from the eye to the opening of the ear being 90 degrees horizontal. Furthermore, the opening of the ear should be directly over the midline of the shoulder, and the intersection of these two lines should make a 90-degree angle.

To apply the one-piece collar, the EMT should move the chin cup of the CID up the patient's chest until it traps the chin. With the chin firmly in the chin cup, the EMT should wrap the collar around the neck, through the space behind the neck, and around to the opposite side. This procedure is demonstrated at the end of the unit in Skill 35-1.

With the collar in place, the EMT should firmly attach the hook and loop fabric (Velcro®). There should be at least 70% adherence of the hook to the loop for adequate protection.

If a properly fitting cervical collar is unavailable, or if the patient's neck cannot be moved into the neutral inline position, the EMT can improvise with a towel wrap. A towel wrap is made by wrapping a rolled-up towel around a patient's neck and shoulders, as shown in Figure 35.27, and taping it like a horse collar.

In the worst-case scenario, when the CID will not fit and a towel wrap is inadequate, the EMT can maintain manual stabilization throughout transport. Cervical stabilization should not be released just because a CID is not available, nor should head stabilization be released because a CID is available. A cervical spine immobilization device is merely an aid to stabilization and not a definitive means of spinal immobilization. The EMT should assign a trained assistant to hold manual stabilization even after the collar has been applied. This stabilization should be maintained until the patient has been secured to a long backboard with full spinal immobilization.

SPECIAL PROBLEM OF HELMETS

As some spinal injuries are sustained during recreational sports or motorcycle riding, a patient may be wearing a helmet when the EMT arrives. It is important for the EMT to know whether it is safer to take the helmet off or leave it on.

A helmet may remain in place if it fits well and does not impede the EMT's ability to access and manage the patient's airway and breathing and to immobilize the patient. For example, football helmets, used during organized or professional play, are often custom fitted to the patient and permit limited movement. Furthermore, removing the helmet, while allowing the pads to remain in place, would cause the head to fall backward onto the long backboard. Thus, removing a football helmet requires that the player's pads be removed as well, which can be a time-consuming process. Because many football helmets are radio translucent, meaning that X-rays will penetrate the helmet, it is unnecessary to remove the helmet and pads.

In some instances, it is necessary to remove only the face shield to access the airway. These face shields are held in place by plastic flanges that can be easily cut with a pair of paramedic scissors or a Trainer's Angel. If the face shield is bolted directly to the helmet then the EMT should cut the face shield with small bolt cutters; often the T screws will only spin in the socket.

The EMT should take the time to remove face shields, helmets, and padding only when the access to the patient's airway is imperative, such as during a cardiac arrest. Especially if an EMT is assigned to stand by at athletic events, he should practice with a certified athletic trainer on helmet removal to perfect these techniques.

Other helmets, such as motorcycle helmets, hockey and lacrosse helmets, riding helmets, and other loose fitting helmets should be removed prior to immobilizing the patient to a long backboard. These helmets do not provide adequate cervical spine protection.

The removal of most helmets is basically the same process. First the EMT takes manual stabilization of the cervical spine from an anterior position. Next a second EMT grasps the helmet on either side and gently rotates the helmet forward, to slide it off the occiput, and then back to midline. With the helmet approximately half off the head, the second EMT continues to remove the helmet along the axis.

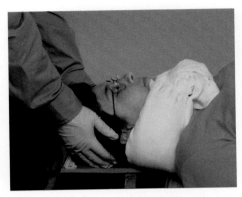

Figure 35.27 When a patient does not fit into a standard cervical collar, a towel may be used to help support the neck

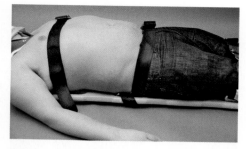

Figure 35.28 Application of the strap under the armpits, securing the shoulder girdle

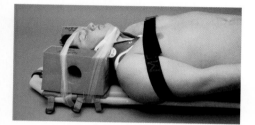

Figure 35.29 Inappropriate application of the strap over the shoulders, risking loss of immobilization if the strap slips

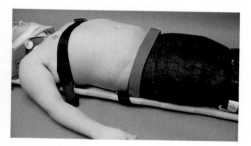

Figure 35.30 Application of the strap over the hips, securing the pelvic girdle

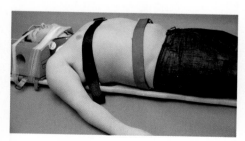

Figure 35.31 Inappropriate application of the strap over the abdomen, risking loss of immobilization

SPINAL IMMOBILIZATION PRINCIPLES

Splinting principles require that the joints above and below a fracture be immobilized to prevent movement of the bone fragments. Because the spinal column is one long series of joints, it is therefore necessary to treat the spine as a potentially unstable long bone fracture and immobilize the entire length of the spine. This is best accomplished using a long backboard, or spine board.

To fix the body to the long backboard, it is necessary to have firm anchor points. Placing a strap across the abdomen, for example, risks having the strap slip and the patient no longer immobilized. Straps should therefore be placed across the solid shoulder girdle and pelvic girdle. Strapping a patient at these two points provides a firm surface on which a strap can be tightened and the patient affixed to the long backboard.

The strap for the girdle should be placed under the arms and proximal to the clavicle, as shown in Figure 35.28. Placing the strap over the shoulders, as shown in Figure 35.29, risks having the strap slip off the shoulders and the patient would no longer be immobilized.

Similarly, the strap for the pelvic girdle should be placed over the iliac crests, in the same manner as a seatbelt, as shown in Figure 35.30. A pelvic strap that is too high may slip off the iliac crests and onto the soft abdomen, as shown in Figure 35.31.

There are several different strapping systems available to the EMT. Some use multiple straps that are attached to a long strap applied to the midline, called a "spider strap," as illustrated in Figure 35.32. Spider straps depend on loop and hook fabric (Velcro®) to secure the patient. Others are long 12- or 15-foot straps that have either a roller bar device or D ring to lock off the straps, as shown in Figure 35.33. These straps can be pulled very tightly across the patient. They are similar to seatbelts, with a metal snap that clips to the long backboard and a seatbelt clasp to secure the strap at the midline. Figure 35.34 shows one example of these straps. These seatbelt style straps can be attached very quickly and are sometimes called *quick straps*. Some EMTs still prefer the use of cotton muslin cravats or four-tail dressings tied to the board and to each other. Even duct tape has been used in an emergency. Regardless of the type of strap used, all straps must follow the same principle: immobilize the patient to the long backboard at the shoulders and pelvis.

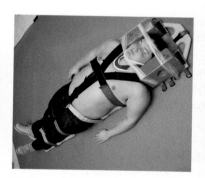

Figure 35.32 Use of a spider strap to immobilize a patient to a long backboard

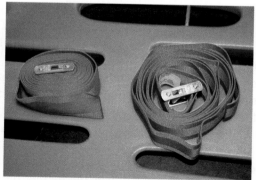

Figure 35.33 Use of a long strap to immobilize a patient to a long backboard. These straps are useful for the large patient

Considered by some to be a lost art, padding the voids between the patient and the long backboard prevents lateral movement of the patient under the straps. The EMT can use a rolled-up towel, short blanket, and even swimming noodles, like the one shown in Figure 35.35, to fill anatomic spaces and help maintain neutral inline anatomic position. Furthermore, use of padding allows the EMT to more firmly anchor the patient to the long backboard without causing undue pain.

The EMT should also consider using a blanket roll between the patient's legs. Placing a blanket roll between the patient's legs helps to relieve pain at sensitive pressure points where the bones of the ankles and knees touch. Figure 35.36 shows a patient properly immobilized with straps across the shoulder and pelvic girdle, shims under the straps, and a blanket roll between the legs.

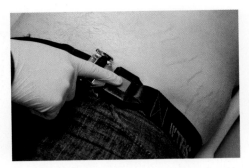

Figure 35.34 Use of a quick release strap to immobilize a patient to a long backboard

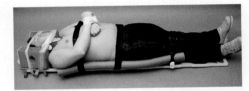

Figure 35.35 Use of swimming aid devices called noodles can help pad the patient's prominences so the restraints can be comfortably tightened

HEAD IMMOBILIZATION

After strapping the torso to the long backboard, the EMT must secure the patient's head. The patient's head is always secured last. This is done as a precaution. Some patients, for a variety of reasons, become nauseated and may suddenly vomit. The first reaction of the EMT should be to turn the patient onto their side to allow the vomit to drain naturally from the mouth and to prevent aspiration.

If the patient's head were immobilized first, then the entrapped head would act as a fulcrum—that is, a pivot point—upon which the body, as a lever, would turn. The result would be serious neck injury.

Alternatively, if the body is immobilized before the head and continuous manual stabilization has been maintained, then the body, as a unit, could be turned without compromising neutral inline alignment.

The EMT can choose from many "head immobilizers." Some are reusable, covered with an impervious plastic coating that allows cleaning, whereas others are disposable. In some emergencies, duct tape and rolled towels have been used to secure the patient's head to the long backboard.

All of these devices anchor the head to the long backboard by placing head blocks on both sides of the head and strapping the head at the forehead and chin to the long backboard. Many of these head blocks have holes on the side that permit the patient to hear and the EMT to assess the ears for leaking fluids, such as cerebrospinal fluid (CSF) See Figure 35.37.

The EMT should take care to ensure that the chin strap is accessible. The chin strap has a tendency to lock the jaw. The EMT must be prepared to quickly remove the chin strap if the patient should start to vomit. Otherwise the patient will not be able to vomit but will instead aspirate the stomach contents into the lungs.

Regardless of the tool chosen, the principles remain the same. The body, specifically the torso, must be immobilized to the long backboard before the head is immobilized. Figure 35.38 shows a patient completely

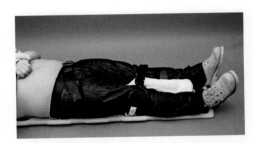

Figure 35.36 Placing a blanket roll between the patient's legs can relieve pain at the pressure points where the patient's bony prominences touch

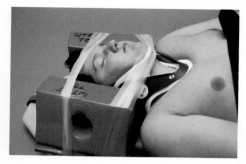

Figure 35.37 Many head blocks have holes on the side that permit the patient to hear and the EMT to assess the ears bleeding or leaking cerebrospinal fluid (CSF)

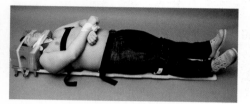

Figure 35.38 The patient is completely immobilized to the long backboard

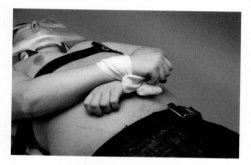

Figure 35.39 The use of a cravat to protect the patient's arms from injury

immobilized, rolled onto his side, chin strap removed, cervical collar opened, and the airway being suctioned, all the while manual stabilization is being maintained.

One final step is to secure the patient's arms across the body or to the long backboard. An unconscious patient's arms will naturally swing to the side when lifted, potentially injuring or even dislocating the patient's shoulders. Furthermore, unsecured arms, especially elbows, can be injured when they strike door jams, car doors, or even walls during transport.

There are several devices on the market that can quickly secure the patient's arms across her chest. Some EMTs prefer the use of muslin cravats (Figure 35.39), while others place an extra strap across the arms at the elbows and affix the strap to the long backboard. Regardless of the method used, it is important to secure the patient's arms before moving the patient.

After the patient has been completely immobilized, the EMT must recheck distal CSM. Loss of any distal neurologic function could have been the result of excessive cervical spine movement during immobilization or simply a worsening of the existing injury. Intact distal CSM reassures the EMT that the patient was properly handled during the immobilization. The EMT must always recheck distal circulation, movement, and sensation in all extremities following full board immobilization on to a long backboard. (Figure 35.40)

PEDIATRIC CHALLENGES

Children present unique challenges to the EMT who is attempting immobilization. The head of a child is relatively larger than that of an adult. As a result, when lying flat, the child's head forces the neck into a flexed position. This position compromises the inline stabilization of the cervical spine, which cannot be allowed to happen. This flexed position is illustrated in Figure 35.41

Pediatric immobilization boards are made specifically for smaller children to resolve this problem. These boards have a dip in the head section to make room for the child's larger occiput. Alternatively, the EMT can place padding under the child's body from the shoulders to the heels to maintain the child's neutral position on a long spine board (Figure 35.42). For older children, merely leaving out the padding that is normally on the head of the adult long spine board will likely solve the problem.

Once a child is placed on a long spine board, the EMT should carefully assess the child's position to ensure that the child's cervical spine is in an appropriate neutral position.

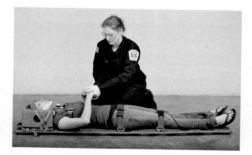

Figure 35.40 The last step in the spinal immobilization process is checking distal neurologic function

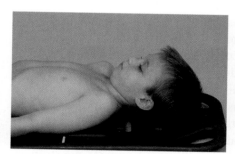

Figure 35.41 The prominent occiput of a child forces the neck into a flexed position when the child is lying flat

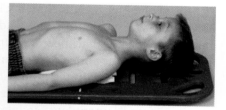

Figure 35.42 Padding behind the child's body from the shoulders to the heels puts the neck in a neutral position when the child is placed on a spine board

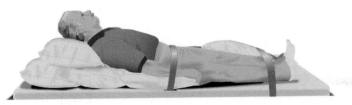

Figure 35.43 Padding the gaps around the elderly patient's spine makes immobilization more comfortable

GERIATRIC CHALLENGES

Some patients, especially elderly patients, have a condition in which the curvature of the spine is excessive. This condition is called *scoliosis* when the curvature is lateral and *kyphosis* when the curvature is in the anterior posterior dimension. Either condition presents a challenge for the EMT who needs to provide adequate immobilization on a long spine board.

The best way to provide immobilization for a patient with a curvature of the spine is to use a lot of padding. Placing the patient on the board and filling all the gaps with pillows, blankets, and towels, as shown in Figure 35.43, for padding will accomplish the goal of immobilization and will not create too much discomfort for the patient.

MOVING PATIENT TO LONG BACKBOARD

With the aforementioned principles in mind, the EMT still must move the patient to the long backboard. The first consideration in moving the patient is the position that the patient was found. If the patient is seated, the EMT must decide if the patient is in urgent or nonurgent condition. If the seated patient's condition is urgent, the EMT would elect to use the rapid extrication technique. If the condition is not urgent, the EMT may elect to use an intermediary device such as the short board before transferring the patient to the long backboard. These techniques are discussed later in the unit.

If the patient is prone when the EMT finds her, the patient is usually moved to the supine position. If the patient is supine, she can be moved to the long backboard by means of a four-person lift, long axis drag, or logroll.

PATIENT LYING DOWN

Upon discovering an injured patient in a prone position, the EMT should immediately gain control of the cervical spine by holding the head and neck, and then, with the help of other trained assistants, roll the patient into the supine position. The EMT should move the patient as a unit while keeping the patient's head and neck in line with the rest of her body. In the supine position, the airway can be more adequately managed and the patient may be fully assessed. It may be prudent to quickly check the patient's back and buttocks for evidence of bleeding or penetrating wounds before rolling the patient.

As stated under principles of immobilization, the EMT should first check circulation, sensation, and motor function in all four extremities before rolling the patient. Next the EMT should apply a collar and then move the patient onto the long spine board with the assistance of several trained assistants.

FOUR-PERSON LIFT AND SLIDE

The four-person lift, described in Unit 14 on lifting and moving, may be one of the safest means of placing a patient onto a backboard. After assessing distal CSM function and applying the CID, a team of EMTs position themselves

---

Street Smart

The long spine board can also be used to move patients who do not have spine injuries. The board is a firm surface on which patients can be supported as they are transferred. It is useful for carrying patients over distances and provides a firm surface on which cardiopulmonary resuscitation (CPR) can be performed.

astride the patient. One EMT is already maintaining manual stabilization while a second EMT is positioned at the shoulder girdle and, placing his arms under the armpits, is ready to lift the upper torso by lifting the scapulas. The third EMT also straddles the patient at the hips, and dropping the knee opposite the knee dropped by the second EMT, grasps the patient's hips at the iliac crest, holding the patient firmly. The fourth EMT places the long backboard under the patient's legs and firmly against the buttocks.

On the call of the EMT at the head, the team lifts the patient evenly for a distance of 2 inches while the fourth EMT slides the long backboard up to the top of the patient's head. On command the team then lowers the patient onto the long backboard and secures the patient's torso and head. Skill 35-2 at the end of this unit demonstrates a four-person lift of a patient onto a long backboard.

LONG AXIS DRAG

If the patient is too heavy for a four-person lift, or there is limited help on scene, the EMT should consider a long axis drag. A long axis drag is very similar to the four-person lift except the long backboard remains in place while the patient slides up the length of the long backboard. The advent of plastic/fiberglass long backboards has also made the long axis drag easier.

To start, the first EMT takes manual stabilization while the second EMT performs the assessment for distal CSM and applies the CID. The third EMT should be placing the long backboard at the patient's head, in line with the patient's midline.

Next the second and third EMTs position themselves as they would for a four-person lift, one at the shoulder girdle and one at the pelvic girdle. On command from the first EMT, the team slides the patient up the length of the long backboard. With the patient in position, the patient is immobilized to the long backboard with straps and head immobilization device. In Skill 35-3 at the end of the unit, several EMTs demonstrate the long axis drag.

MODIFIED LOG ROLL

Perhaps the most commonly used technique to move a patient to a long backboard is the logroll. However, studies have shown that the logroll permits more lateral movement and flexion of the cervical spine than does the four-person lift and slide or long axis drag. The advantage of a logroll is that it can be performed by as few as two people in an emergency. A logroll can also be performed in a more limited space, such as between a bed and a wall.

To start, the first EMT takes manual stabilization while the second EMT performs the assessment for distal CSM and applies the CID. The third EMT should be placing the long backboard next to the patient, in line with the patient's midline. The bottom of the long backboard should be at the back of the patient's knees.

The next two EMTs should position themselves, side by side, next to the patient, one at the shoulder girdle and one at the pelvic girdle. The EMT at the shoulder girdle should slip his hand under the armpit and grasp the scapula and then place the opposite hand low on the patient's pelvis. At this point the layout should be EMT, patient, and then long backboard, all lined up.

The third EMT should take a position at the pelvis. One hand should grasp the patient's knees, and the other should be able to grasp the backboard. In some instances it is helpful to bend the knees, provided there is no injury, in order to obtain a handhold behind the knee.

The patient is now ready to be logrolled. Some advocate placing the patient's arm over her head but studies suggest that leaving the arm next to the patient's body helps fill the voids and decreases lateral movement of the spine.

With everyone in place the first EMT, the EMT at the head, calls for the logroll. While the patient is up on her side, the third EMT may elect to assess the back and buttocks for signs of bleeding or trauma. With the assessment complete, the EMT grasps the far side of the long backboard and slides it up along the patient's back.

On command, the three EMTs logroll the patient back onto the long backboard. It is common for the patient to be slightly off midline of the long backboard. In those instances the patient should be slid down the backboard and then slid back up the middle of the board, in a manner similar to the long axis drag. The EMT should never push the patient sideways to place the patient on the long backboard. This lateral motion pushes the spine out of alignment and can potentially disrupt the spine or aggravate a spinal injury. Skill 35-4 at the end of this unit demonstrates the proper logroll technique.

ORTHOPEDIC STRETCHER

The orthopedic stretcher, also known as the *scoop stretcher*, can be used as an intermediate device to transfer the patient. Discussed in Unit 14 on lifting and moving patients, the orthopedic stretcher is useful in limited spaces and/or with limited number of EMTs.

The first EMT starts by taking manual stabilization of the patient's head and neck, while the second EMT performs the assessment for distal CSM and applies the CID. The second EMT then places the long backboard on the ground and breaks the orthopedic stretcher into two parts. After properly measuring the orthopedic stretcher, the two halves of the orthopedic stretcher are placed under the patient, the clasp closed, and the patient strapped into place. With the patient's head cradled in the orthopedic stretcher, the two EMTs lift the patient over the long backboard and gently lower the patient. With the patient in position the second EMT straps the patient to the backboard as usual.

SEATED PATIENT

Under some circumstances the patient may be found in a seated position, as in MVCs. Like with the patient found lying flat, the EMT must first decide, using the primary assessment, if the patient is stable or unstable. If the patient is stable, then an intermediate device, such as a short board, should be used to get the patient out of the vehicle without compromising the spine. These interim devices are discussed shortly.

If the patient is unstable, the EMT should immediately remove the patient from the motor vehicle. If the patient is in cardiac arrest, it may be necessary to use an emergency drag to remove the patient; emergency drags are discussed in Unit 14 on lifting and moving. If the patient is alive but unstable, a rapid extrication technique should be used.

RAPID EXTRICATION

Rapid extrication is a process whereby several responders can remove a seated patient from a motor vehicle quickly and without the use of intermediate devices such as a short board. Although the process is easy to learn, it is not without its hazards. Poorly performed rapid extrication can result in further spinal injury to the patient. For this reason the use of the rapid extrication technique should be limited to special emergencies where the patient's life may be in danger.

Rapid extrication may be used when environmental conditions are rapidly deteriorating. Examples of these conditions include fires, explosion hazards, danger from building collapse, or the potential for hazardous

Table 35-4 Patient Conditions That Might Require Rapid Extrication

1. Unconsciousness secondary to head trauma

2. Uncontrollable airway

3. Hypoxia/cyanosis in face of high-flow oxygen

4. Near respiratory arrest

5. Uncontrollable hemorrhage

6. Internal bleeding with decompensated shock

7. Patient is blocking access to a critically injured patient

materials exposure. These conditions are fairly rare, and the EMT should consider his own safety when deciding if there is time to perform a rapid extrication.

More customary reasons for rapid extrication are deteriorating patient condition. For example, a patient with an uncontrollable airway or hypoxia and/or cyanosis despite the administration of high-flow oxygen may be rapidly extricated. Table 35-4 lists some patient conditions that may necessitate the use of the rapid extrication technique. Rapid extrication should be used only when the patient's life is in immediate danger.

After ensuring that the scene is safe and the vehicle is stable, the EMT should gain entry into the vehicle and assess the patient for the presence of life-threatening injuries. Finding a life-threatening injury, the EMT should direct that rapid extrication be performed. Generally it takes four trained rescuers to perform a rapid extrication.

The first EMT should take immediate manual stabilization of the cervical spine and return the patient's head to the neutral inline position if possible. In some instances the EMT may have to use either a lateral or anterior approach to the stabilization; however, the preferred approach is for the EMT to maintain stabilization from the rear. The EMT must maintain continuous stabilization of the head in neutral cervical spine alignment until the patient is securely fastened to the long backboard with straps and head blocks.

A second EMT then applies a CID to the patient's neck, while a third EMT places the end of the long backboard under the patient's buttocks. It is possible to remove a patient either head first or feet first with rapid extrication. Both are effective. What is important is that the team understands the direction of movement. This decision is usually communicated by the EMT at the head.

Some EMTs prefer the long backboard be placed on top of a stretcher. Other EMTs prefer the end of the long backboard be placed on the ground. This leaves a slope and permits the EMT to use gravity to help move the patient onto the long backboard.

With the long backboard in place, the second EMT takes a position in the opening of the door and relieves the first EMT at manual stabilization. The first EMT is now free to enter the vehicle from the opposite side and help with moving the upper torso. A third EMT now stands in the door, opposite the second EMT and grasps the patient at the hips. At this point the three EMTs have the patient's head, chest/shoulder girdle, and pelvis girdle stabilized. It is helpful if the third EMT is able to pull the patient's legs free from under the dashboard. A fourth EMT should be standing by, just outside of the open doorway, to help grasp the legs and guide them onto the long backboard.

On command, from the EMT stabilizing the head, the EMTs should rotate the body, as a unit, while maintaining the patient in the seated position, until the patient is parallel to the backboard. The patient's head and back should continue to be straight.

With the patient on the long backboard, the four EMTs should, on command, pivot the patient to the long backboard, using the buttocks as the fulcrum. Next, the four EMTs should slide the patient, long axis down the backboard and secure the patient with straps and head blocks before moving the patient to the ambulance.

Although many EMTs have devised different methods of rapid extrication, the principles remain the same. The EMT needs to take immediate manual stabilization. The team of EMTs needs to immobilize and move the patient as a unit. The EMT needs to secure the patient to the long backboard. Skill 35-5 demonstrates one method of the rapid extrication technique.

SHORT SPINAL IMMOBILIZATION DEVICE

If a patient is seated and has a suspected spine injury, as would be the case in an MVC, a short immobilization device is used. A **short spine immobilization device (SSID)** is an interim apparatus that secures the spine while the patient is an upright position until the patient can be transferred to a long backboard. Several different types of short immobilization devices are available. Some are of the vest type with rigid slats or a plate to keep the spine straight, and others are just rigid boards. Each device has specific advantages in certain circumstances. For example, the vest style SSID is effective when the patient is seated in a bucket seat. Whatever their design, the purpose of all these devices is to maintain inline immobilization of the head, neck, and back while the patient is extricated from the vehicle and transferred to the long backboard.

Before placing a short immobilization device onto a patient, the EMT should place a CID to help maintain inline stabilization of the patient's neck. However, manual stabilization must be maintained until the patient is secured to the device.

The principles of using an SSID are the same as with a long board and application of an SSID follows the same sequence as applying a long backboard. In applying a short spine immobilization device, the EMT secures the torso prior to securing the head. The EMT uses the same anchor points for the straps—the shoulder girdle and the pelvic girdle. The EMT rechecks distal neurologic function, or CSM, before transferring the patient to the long backboard.

To place the SSID between the patient and the car seat, it is necessary to move the patient. There are two effective means of moving a patient so that an SSID can be placed behind her.

The first method is to bend the patient forward. While one EMT maintains continuous manual stabilization, another EMT stabilizes the torso. One method of doing this is to place one arm lengthwise along the midline at the sternum with the hand grasping the bottom of the CID. The other hand is slid into the hollow at the lumbar space and advanced along the long axis of the spine. This effectively braces the spine both front and back in a pincer maneuver. The third EMT stands by with the SSID. On the command of the EMT holding manual stabilization of the patient's head and neck, the second EMT bends the person forward and the third EMT slides the SSID behind the patient. Repeating the sequence in reverse, the patient is returned to a seated position and the second EMT removes his arms. The patient is then secured to the SSID and a distal check of CSM is performed. Bending the patient at the hips to place an SSID does not compromise the spine, as the spinal cord ends at the base of the thoracic cage. The advantage of this method is it can be done all from one side of the car. Figure 35.44 illustrates this method.

The second method involves sliding the patient forward and backward. As always, one EMT maintains manual stabilization of the head and neck while the second EMT applies the CID and performs distal checks for CSM. In this method two EMTs must be on either side of the patient. When in position, each EMT places one hand under the armpit of the patient and around to the scapula and then places the other hand under the buttocks at the bony prominence created by the ischial tuberosity of the pelvis. On the command of the EMT holding manual stabilization of the patient's head and neck, the team slides the patient forward as one unit. A fourth EMT then slides the SSID behind the patient, and the process is reversed to get the patient against the SSID. The patient is then secured to the SSID, and a distal check of CSM performed. The advantage of this method is that the EMTs needed to lift the patient out of the vehicle are already in place.

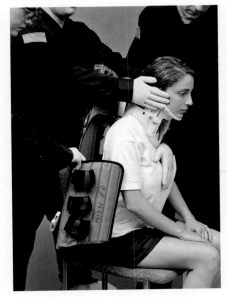

Figure 35.44 Moving the patient forward, as a unit, to place the SSID behind the patient

Once the patient is secured in a short immobilization device, the EMT should place the patient on a long spine board. This typically involves pivoting the patient on her buttocks. This motion can add a twisting force to the base of the spine. If resistance is met turning the patient, it may be advisable to lift and turn the patient using the technique just described. The long spine board provides support and immobilization of the entire spine and body.

Although some EMTs have learned certain sequences for strapping the patient's torso to the SSID, the principle remains the same regardless of the sequence of strapping: Always strap the body before the head. The next principle is to secure the entire length of the spine. Like the long backboard, the patient's shoulder girdle and pelvic girdle must be securely immobilized. Therefore, it is important to use the leg straps supplied with an SSID to secure the pelvic girdle. A complete application of the short immobilization device, from manual stabilization to removal to a long backboard, is detailed in Skill 35-6 at the end of this unit.

STANDING PATIENT

Upon arrival on the scene, the EMT may encounter patients who may have spine injury who are standing. A good example is an MVC in which less seriously injured patients may have gotten out of their cars and may be walking around the scene when the EMT arrives. These patients may be seen rubbing their necks or may complain of neck pain. In the worst-case scenario the patient may have gotten out of the car and collapsed to the ground with paralysis. If the crash is serious, the EMT should suspect spinal injury and should manually stabilize the patient's head and neck to protect the spinal cord immediately.

The problem is how to get the patient supine on a long backboard. Asking the patient to sit down or lie down on a long backboard could potentially injure or cause further injury to the spine. The best way to get the standing patient onto a long backboard is to perform the **standing takedown** technique. During a standing takedown, the long backboard is placed behind the patient and the patient is lowered to the ground, as a unit, with the backboard. This technique is an easy and safe way to have the standing patient become supine without compromising the patient's spine.

The standing takedown procedure is an effective way to immobilize the standing patient, but it can be quite frightening to the patient. The EMT should thoroughly explain the procedure to the patient and reassure the patient throughout the procedure that the patient will not be dropped. The patient must rest against the board as he is lowered to the ground. Patients will be able to do this with encouragement from the EMT.

To perform a standing takedown, the first EMT, preferably the tallest EMT, must take immediate manual stabilization of the patient's head and neck from behind the patient. The second EMT should then assess the patient's distal CSM and apply the CID. After the second EMT has applied the CID, a third EMT places a long backboard between the outstretched arms of the first EMT. The first EMT must maintain continuous manual stabilization throughout this process.

Next the second and third EMTs stand next to the patient, looking backward. Both EMTs slip their hands under the patient's armpits and grasp the long board at the highest handhold on the long backboard.

With the long backboard behind the patient, the two EMTs start to lower the long backboard. To prevent the long backboard from sliding, or "kicking out," both EMTs should brace the long backboard with their toes. It is important that the two EMTs bend at the knees as they lower the patient. The two EMTs are essentially kneeling, or more accurately, lunging. Stooping to lower the patient can cause a lower back injury. It is important that the two EMTs also communicate. One misstep can cause the patient to be off balance and cause the EMTs to drop the patient.

While the two EMTs are lowering the patient to the ground, the first EMT must maintain continuous manual head stabilization. This is maintained by rotating the wrists as the patient is lowered. Although it may appear that the long backboard might strike the EMT in the face, carefully lowering can avoid this problem. The standing takedown technique is demonstrated in Skill 35-7 at the end of this unit.

SELECTIVE SPINAL IMMOBILIZATION

Spinal immobilization can take a considerable amount of time and personnel on scene. Many of the procedures previously described require three or four EMTs working together. This can be problematic when on the scene of a multiple-patient incident where resources are scarce.

In some cases it is unnecessary to immobilize trauma patients. These patients have not experienced a significant mechanism of injury, and the likelihood of spinal injury is exceedingly low. Unnecessary immobilization of these patients results in unnecessary tests, such as X-rays, and increased costs to the patient.

Perhaps most importantly, spinal immobilization onto a long backboard is not without its hazards. Lying on a hard long backboard can be painful in and of itself. Although this risk is acceptable to protect the spine of a patient with potential spine injuries, it is unacceptable if the patient's risk of spine injury is remote at best.

This problem has been identified by physicians for more than two decades, and current emergency medicine has established protocols that dictate which patients need spinal immobilization. These protocols are based on multiple medical studies, such as the NEXUS (National Emergency X-Radiography Utilization Study) addressing cervical spinal immobilization in the prehospital setting. In some EMS systems, medical directors have authorized the EMT to use these protocols.

SELECTIVE SPINAL IMMOBILIZATION CRITERIA

To implement the selective spinal immobilization protocol, the patient must first meet preestablished criteria. Though the patient is a trauma patient, the mechanism of injury should be clearly negative or uncertain.

A negative mechanism of injury is one in which an EMT would reasonably believe that there is no possibility of spinal injury. Dropping a box on one's foot might be an example where it is reasonable to believe that no spinal injury occurred.

An uncertain mechanism of injury is more difficult to define. In the case of an uncertain mechanism of injury, it is difficult to determine whether the amount of violence or other forces were sufficient to cause spinal injury. For example, if an adult male slips on a throw rug and falls onto his buttocks, he may or may not have adequate mechanism of injury to require spinal immobilization. In those cases the EMT must resort to a careful assessment of the patient to make the decision. The easier decision in whether to immobilize is in those patients with a positive mechanism of injury.

All patients with a positive mechanism of injury should be considered for spinal immobilization. Positive mechanisms of injury include violent forces such as a high-velocity MVC or a fall from more than 20 feet. Trauma surgeons, in their Advanced Trauma Life Support (ATLS) course, have listed those mechanisms of injury that have been positively linked to spine injury.

Street Smart

When confronted with a patient with an uncertain mechanism, the EMT is well advised to take manual stabilization of the head and neck until the assessment is complete. However, some medical authorities consider application of the CID as the start of spinal immobilization and do not permit the EMT to remove the CID or to stop spinal immobilization once it has started.

However, some medical studies have shown that a positive mechanism of injury alone is insufficient criteria for spinal immobilization. In some EMS systems, the medical director has elected to remove a positive mechanism alone as sufficient criteria for spinal immobilization. EMTs must learn and know their EMS system's protocol for selective spinal immobilization.

ASSESSMENT BY CLINICAL CRITERIA

When confronted with a trauma patient who has experienced an uncertain mechanism of injury, the EMT must depend on the physical examination to help make the decision. There are three decision points during the physical examination that direct the EMT to take spinal immobilization.

Starting at the neck, the EMT should ask the patient if she has neck pain. If the answer is yes, the EMT should take spinal immobilization. If the answer is no, the EMT should proceed to the next step and palpate the posterior neck for midline point tenderness. The EMT should not palpate the posterior neck if the patient states that she has neck pain; the patient's statement is sufficient evidence of the need for spinal immobilization.

If the patient has posterior midline neck pain, her spine should be immobilized. If the patient does not have posterior midline neck pain, the EMT should go on to assess the distal neurologic function. That examination includes an assessment of the extremities for motor and sensory function. In some cases that examination is rudimentary. For example, the patient is asked if she can move her fingers and toes and if she can identify which finger and toe are being touched.

Other medical authorities advocate a more detailed neurologic examination, including finger and hand extension. The patient is asked to first hold her hands straight out from the body and resist the EMT who is pushing down on the hands. Next the patient is asked to spread her fingers and keep them spread while the EMT tries to squeeze them shut. Similarly, the EMT asks the patient to push her foot down, as if pressing on the gas pedal, and then dorsiflex the foot, or point the toes up toward the nose.

The EMT proceeds to test the patient's distal sensory function. First, the EMT asks the patient to close her eyes and then asks the patient which finger or toe he is touching. The EMT should assess all four extremities.

Any perceived weakness or numbness suggests spine injury, and the EMT should take spinal immobilization. If the patient, at any time, complains of tingling or numbness, suggestive of paresthesia, or weakness, suggestive of paralysis, the EMT should assume spine injury and take spinal immobilization.

UNRELIABLE PATIENT EXAMINATION

The assessment of the trauma patient with an uncertain mechanism depends on the patient's report being accurate and reliable. This best case is when patients are awake, alert, calm, sober, and cooperative. These patients can generally be considered reliable reporters. Some patient reports, owed to various conditions, are highly suspect and thus unreliable. These patients can be divided into three classifications: those with acute stress reaction, those with distracting injuries, and those with communication problems.

When a person first is involved in an MVC, for example, she can be very excited and anxious. In some cases the patient seems to react out of proportion to the trauma. These patients may be experiencing an **acute stress reaction**. An acute stress reaction is the result of sympathetic simulation, also known as the *fight-or-flight response*. An acute stress response can mask the patient's perception of pain. Given time, the patient will generally calm down, but in the interim the patient cannot be seen as a reliable reporter.

Similarly, a distracting injury can prevent the patient from noticing neck pain. The pain from a burn or broken bone can be more severe than the ache of a neck injury. As a result, the patient's mind ignores the neck pain and instead focuses on the distracting injury.

A final obstruction to assessment is communication difficulties. When a patient is hearing impaired or speaks another language, the EMT may not be able to communicate with the patient effectively. In those cases the EMT should err on the side of caution and immobilize the patient to protect the spine.

PREEXISTING MEDICAL CONDITIONS

Regardless of the assessment findings, certain trauma patients should be immobilized. Older patients often have brittle bones from loss of calcium and other minerals. A fall that seems insignificant to an EMT may easily result in a broken bone for an elderly patient. The EMT should be more suspicious of bone injury, including spinal injury, when the patient is elderly.

TRANSPORT

Usually the patient who has sustained a previous spinal cord injury not only has lost movement in the affected body part but also has lost sensation in that part. The EMT must pay special attention to handling the patient gently. Such a patient, for example, may not be able to feel her fingers get caught under the backboard, but the fingers will still be injured. The EMT also should provide extra padding to the patient's affected body parts during longer transports.

The final priority in managing the patient with a potential spinal injury is to get the patient safely to the most appropriate hospital in a reasonable amount of time. Some treatments for spinal cord injuries are time dependent. The sooner the patient gets to the appropriate hospital, the sooner the care can be given. The EMT should follow local protocols regarding the facilities to which these patients should be transported and the appropriate way to accomplish such transports.

The ongoing assessment of patients with potential spinal cord injuries must include a repeat of the initial assessment, vital signs, and an assessment for any of the findings of spinal cord injury discussed in this unit. The EMT should document any change in the patient's status and advise hospital staff of the change.

CONCLUSION

Many people in the United States sustain spinal cord injuries every year. The EMT's quick recognition of the potential for such an injury can help to prevent further damage from occurring to the sensitive spinal cord. Careful immobilization while maintaining inline stabilization is key in managing the patient who has sustained a spinal injury.

Street Smart

The intoxicated individual is generally considered an unreliable reporter. However, definitions vary for intoxication. Some medical authorities state that if the patient is able to answer questions intelligently and is generally cooperative with care, then the patient is not clinically intoxicated. However, this definition should be made by the EMS system's medical director.

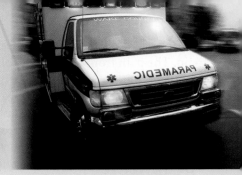

Thankfully, most of the ambulances are staffed today and respond promptly to the scene. The first arriving ambulance is directed by the EMS supervisor to the first car. The woman in the second car asks Officer Shulman, "Why aren't they coming to help me?" Officer Shulman explains that the passenger in the other car is a pregnant woman who is unconscious.

The second ambulance is directed to the woman with Officer Shulman. The EMT sticks his head in the car and says, "Good evening, ma'am. I will be right with you. Officer Shulman, will you be alright for a minute while I get the equipment ready?"

Looking over his shoulder, as he answers affirmatively, Officer Shulman notes that another ambulance crew has arrived and is assessing the first car's driver. They have already moved a long backboard behind him for the standing takedown.

Officer Shulman turns his attention back to the woman whose head he is holding in his hands and starts to explain the extrication procedure. He reassures her that she will be going to the trauma center shortly.

PURPOSE: To aid the EMT in stabilization of the cervical spine.

STANDARD PRECAUTIONS:

☑ Assortment of cervical spine immobilization devices (collars)

☑ Personal protective equipment

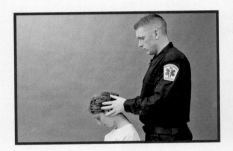

1 The EMT first moves the patient's head into neutral alignment. If the patient complains of pain or the EMT feels resistance, then the patient's neck should be splinted in position. The EMT should maintain continuous manual stabilization of the patient's head throughout the rest of the procedure.

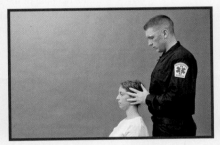

2 The EMT should maintain continuous manual stabilization of the patient's head throughout the rest of the procedure.

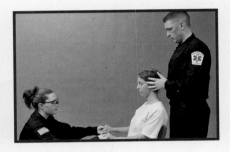

3 Next, a second EMT checks for distal pulses, movement, and sensation.

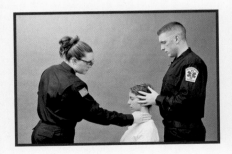

4 The second EMT then measures the patient's neck for a cervical collar, according to manufacturer recommendations.

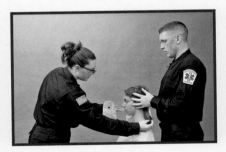

5 The second EMT then slides the posterior portion of collar in the void behind the neck.

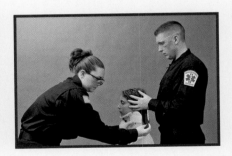

6 Cupping the chin piece in one hand, the second EMT slides the anterior portion of the collar up the chest until it captures the chin.

(Continued)

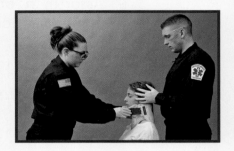

7 With collar in place, the second EMT fastens the Velcro securely.

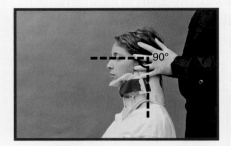

8 Checking for a proper collar fit, the second EMT mentally draws a line from the opening of the ear to the middle of the shoulder, and from the opening of the ear to the eyes. The imagined angle should be 90 degrees.

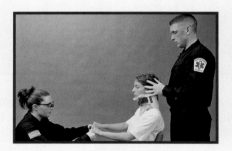

9 The second EMT finally rechecks for distal pulses, sensation, and movement.

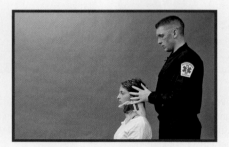

10 Continuous manual stabilization must still be maintained, despite the presence of the cervical immobilization device.

PURPOSE: To immobilize the spine of a supine patient who may have a spinal injury.

STANDARD PRECAUTIONS:

☑ Assortment of cervical spine immobilizations devices (collars)

☑ Long spine board

☑ Strapping system

☑ Head immobilization system

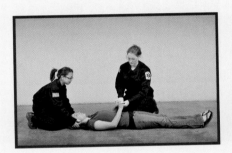

1 The first EMT kneels at the patient's head and immediately obtains manual stabilization. The second EMT checks the patient's distal pulses, movement, and sensation and applies a cervical collar.

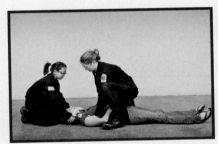

2 The second EMT then straddles the patient and drops one knee to the ground. Placing his hands under the patient's arms, he grasps the shoulder girdle.

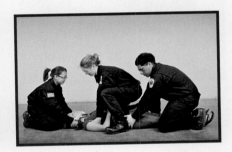

3 A third EMT straddles the patient, at the hips, and drops his opposite knee to the ground. He then grasps the patient around the hips.

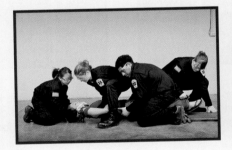

4 On command, all three EMTs gently and evenly lift the patient about 2 inches while a fourth EMT slides the long spine board under the patient.

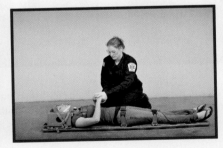

5 Once the patient is properly positioned, the EMTs proceed to immobilize the torso, and then the head, of the patient. Then the EMT rechecks distal pulses, movement, and sensation.

PURPOSE: To immobilize the spine of a supine patient who may have a spinal injury.

STANDARD PRECAUTIONS:

☑ Personal protective equipment

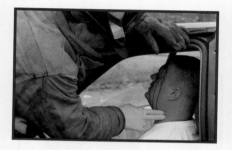

1 First, the EMT determines that the patient needs immediate extrication for some reason, for example, the patient is in cardiac arrest.

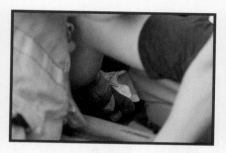

2 Opening the closest door and entering the passenger compartment, the EMT disentangles any extremities from pedals and other obstructions.

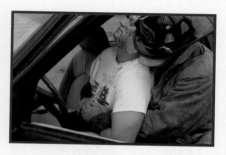

3 Then the EMT reaches behind the patient's back and under both of the patient's arms to grab the patient's wrists.

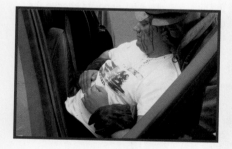

4 The EMT then rotates the patient, as a unit, and places the patient into a semi-inclined position.

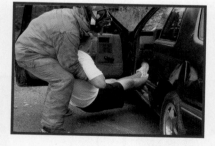

5 The EMT then drags the patient out of the motor vehicle with the patient's head resting on the EMT's forearms.

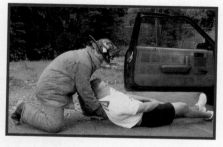

6 By dropping to his knees, the EMT can lower the patient and crawl backward with the patient, while performing a long axis drag.

Skill 35-4 Modified Logroll of the Supine Patient

PURPOSE: To immobilize the spine of a supine patient who may have a spinal injury.

STANDARD PRECAUTIONS:

☑ Selection of cervical collars
☑ Long spine board
☑ Strapping system
☑ Head immobilization system

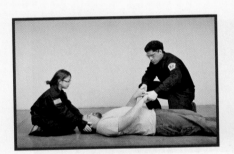

1 An EMT checks distal pulses, movement, and sensation of all four extremities while another EMT maintains manual stabilization.

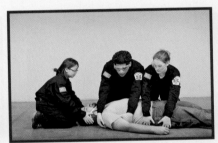

2 While one EMT holds manual stabilization, two more EMTs take positions at the patient's shoulders and pelvis, reaching across the patient and grasping the patient's shoulders and pelvis, respectively.

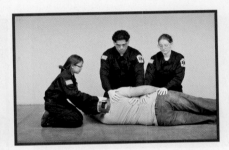

3 On command, the three EMTs roll the patient on his side. The patient's arms should be at his side.

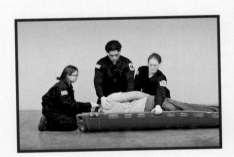

4 One EMT pulls the long spine board under the patient. The long spine board should end at the back of the patient's knees.

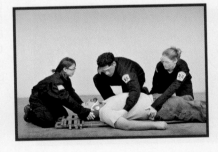

5 On command, the patient is rolled back onto the long spine board, and the patient is pulled up to the center of the board, using a long axis drag.

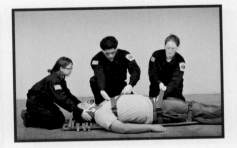

6 Once the patient is centered on the long spine board, the EMT secures the patient to the long spine board and reassesses distal pulses, movement, and sensation.

PURPOSE: To manually immobilize the spine of an unstable patient who may have a spinal injury as a result of a motor vehicle collision.

STANDARD PRECAUTIONS:

- ☑ Assortment of cervical spine immobilizations devices (collars)
- ☑ Long spine board
- ☑ Turnout gear
- ☑ Personal protective equipment

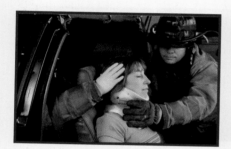

1 The EMT first checks distal pulses, movement, and sensation. Then the EMT moves the head to a neutral position and has another EMT apply a properly sized cervical collar.

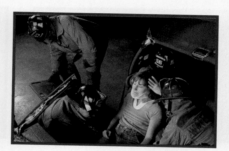

2 With an EMT on each side of the patient, the patient is gently lifted a couple of inches so that a long spine board may be inserted under the patient's buttocks.

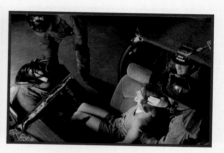

3 While an EMT continues to maintain manual stabilization of the spine, one EMT grasps the patient under the arms while another grasps the patient at the hips. Then, on command, the EMTs rotate the patient to the side about 45 degrees. At this point, the EMTs may need to switch places if the car's B post becomes an obstruction. After two or three small turns to rotate the patient, the patient should be parallel to the long spine board.

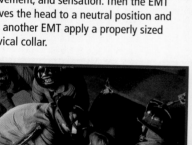

4 Once the patient is parallel to the long spine board, the patient is lowered, as a stiff unit, to the long spine board while the EMTs maintain inline stabilization.

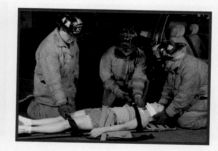

5 Once the patient is on the long spine board, first the body and then the head should be fastened securely, and the EMT should recheck the patient's distal pulses, movement, and sensation.

PURPOSE: To further immobilize the injured patient's spine after the application of the cervical collar.

STANDARD PRECAUTIONS:

☑ Assortment of cervical spine immobilization devices

☑ Short immobilization device

☑ Personal protective equipment

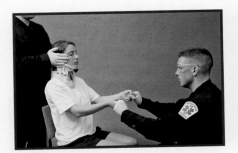

1 First, an EMT manually stabilizes the spine. A second EMT then applies a properly sized cervical spine immobilization device. Once the collar is secure, the second EMT checks distal pulses, movement, and sensation.

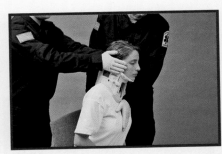

2 While a trained assistant maintains continuous manual stabilization, the EMT places his arms along the anterior and posterior thorax. The patient may now be moved forward as a unit, keeping the spine in line.

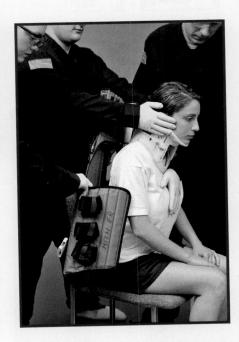

3 The device is then positioned behind the patient cautiously, and the patient is leaned back against the device.

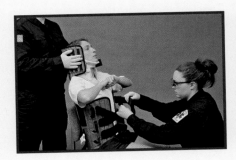

4 Next, the patient's torso, including the legs, is secured to the device.

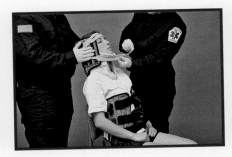

5 Finally, the patient's head is secured to the device. The EMT pads the void behind the head as needed.

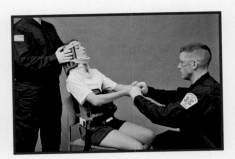

6 The EMT then reassesses distal pulses, movement, and sensory function of the patient before transferring the patient to the backboard.

PURPOSE: To immobilize the spine of a standing patient who has a potential spine injury.

STANDARD PRECAUTIONS:

☑ Assortment of cervical collars

☑ Long spine board

☑ Strapping system

☑ Head immobilization system

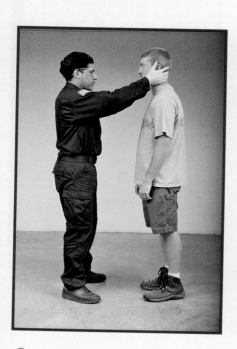

1 The EMT approaches the patient from the front and takes immediate anterior head stabilization.

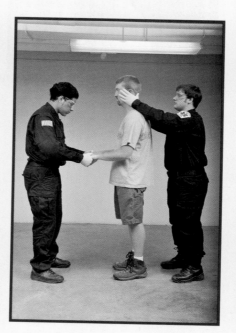

2 Another EMT takes head stabilization from the rear, while the first EMT assesses distal pulses, movement, and sensation.

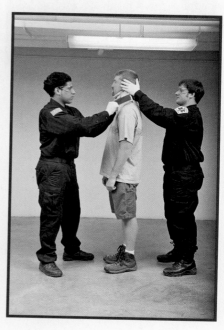

3 An appropriately sized cervical collar is applied to the patient.

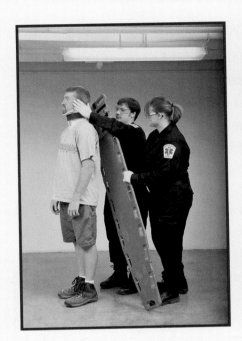

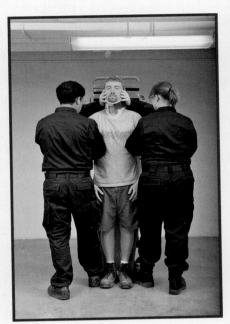

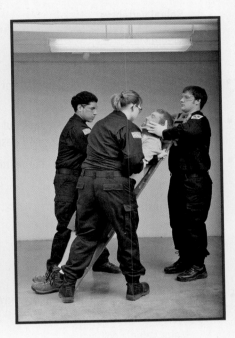

4 Another EMT places the long spine board upright behind the patient and between the arms of the EMT holding stabilization.

5 One EMT then stands on either side of the patient, holds the board under the patient's arms, and stabilizes the bottom of the board with a foot.

6 Slowly, the board and the patient are lowered to the ground, while the EMT at the head stabilizes the head and neck. The EMT then immobilizes the patient and rechecks distal pulses, movement, and sensation.

Key Concepts Revisited

- The spinal column consists of three parts.
  - Spinal vertebrae
  - Spinal cord
  - Spinal ligaments
- Possible injury to the cervical spine is of greatest concern to the EMT.
- Two nerve tracts containing sensory and motor fibers are in the spinal cord—the ascending and descending tracts.
- There are five causes of spinal column instability:
  - Hyperflexion
  - Hyperextension
  - Lateral bending
  - Axial distraction
  - Axial loading
- Three common mechanisms of injury may cause spine injury:
  - Motor vehicle collisions
  - Violence/penetrating trauma
  - Falls
- Three life-threatening complications can occur with spinal injury:
  - Respiratory arrest
  - Neurogenic shock
  - Paralysis
- Neutral inline manual stabilization of the cervical spine is critical to prevent further injury.
- Distal neurological function should be assessed before and after immobilization.

- A cervical immobilization device is an aid to manual stabilization.
- Key principles of spinal immobilization must be maintained:
  - Manual inline stabilization
  - Motor and sensory examination in all four extremities
  - Securing the shoulder and pelvic girdle
  - Securing the head
  - Repeating a motor and sensory examination
- There are four methods of moving a supine patient onto a long backboard:
  - Four-person lift
  - Long axis drag
  - Logroll
  - Orthopedic stretcher
- Rapid extrication is an acceptable technique in limited circumstances.
- Short spinal immobilization devices are used as an interim device before the long backboard.
- Standing takedown is the preferred technique for standing patients with spine injury.
- Use of selective spinal immobilization depends on certain criteria:
  - No major mechanism of injury
  - No neck pain
  - Absence of an acute stress reaction
  - No distracting injury
  - No intoxication

Review Questions

1. What are the three parts of the spinal column?
2. What relationship do atlas and axis have to one another?
3. What are the two main nerve tracts in the spinal cord, and what do they do?
4. Name three important nerve roots and their implication.
5. What are the causes of spinal column instability?
6. What are three common mechanisms of injury that lead to spine injury?

7. What is the difference between primary and secondary spinal cord injury?
8. What are the signs and symptoms of a potential spinal cord injury?
9. What is the primary mechanism of neurogenic shock?
10. What is neutral inline alignment of the cervical spine?
11. What are the spinal immobilization principles?
12. What are the four methods of moving a person to a long backboard?
13. What are three indications for rapid extrication?
14. What are the two methods of placing a short spinal immobilization device behind a patient?
15. What method is used to place a standing patient onto a long backboard?
16. What are the criteria for selective spinal immobilization?
17. What makes a patient unreliable, in terms of selective spinal immobilization?

Key Terms

Acute stress reaction
Ascending spinothalmic tracts
Atlanto-occipital dislocation
Axial distraction
Axial loading
Axis
Cervical immobilization device (CID)
Dermatome
Descending corticospinal tract
Don Juan syndrome
Hyperextension
Hyperflexion
Incontinence
Innervate
Lateral bending
Nerve roots

Neutral inline alignment
Osteoporosis
Paralysis
Paraplegia
Paresthesia
Point tenderness
Priapism
Primary spinal cord injury
Quadriplegia
Rapid extrication
Secondary spinal cord injury
Short spine immobilization device (SSID)
Spinal canal
Standing takedown
Subluxation

Further Study

Danziger, P. "Spinal Cord Injuries." Available online at http://www.spinal-cord.org
Hubble, M., and J. Hubble. *Principles of Advanced Trauma Care*. Clifton Park, NY: Thomson Delmar Learning, 2002.

Trauma.org. Available online at http://www.trauma.org

UNIT (36) Chest and Abdominal Injuries

What do motor vehicle collisions and gunshot wounds have in common? Both of these mechanisms of injury can result in injury to the chest and the abdomen. In fact, more than half of all serious trauma patients have chest and/or abdominal trauma.

The extent and severity of chest and abdominal trauma often is not immediately apparent as an external injury. It can often be overlooked as patients are distracted by the pain and dramatic appearance of fractures, lacerations, and abrasions.

The EMT must remember the chest and abdomen house the vital organs of the body and injuries can be life threatening.

National Education Standards
The Emergency Medical Technician (EMT) will be able to demonstrate a fundamental depth and simple breadth of understanding of the pathophysiology, assessment, and management of traumatic injury to the chest, abdominal, and genitourinary systems.

Key Concepts

- The most common consequence of chest trauma from any source is compromise of breathing and oxygenation resulting in hypoxia.

- Determination of the mechanism of injury will lead the EMT to find severe traumatic injuries to the chest that may not be immediately obvious.

- EMTs should have the ability to recognize the signs and symptoms and understand the initial management of specific traumatic injuries to the chest.

- The management of chest trauma is centered on ensuring adequate oxygenation and perfusion.

- The common mechanism of injury for abdominal organs, protected by the lower ribs and pelvis, is usually through blunt or penetrating trauma.

- Abdominal injuries are often initially overlooked by the patient and EMT due to more dramatic, distracting injuries that may be present.

- Specific abdominal organs are extremely vascular, and injury can produce life-threatening bleeding.

- Management of abdominal wounds often requires surgical intervention, and prehospital care focuses on assessment and management of hemorrhage and hypoperfusion with rapid transportation to a trauma center.

- Injuries to the organs of the pelvic and retroperitoneal cavities can involve significant hemorrhage.

- Injury to the genitalia can involve lacerations, penetrations, contusions, avulsions, and amputations.

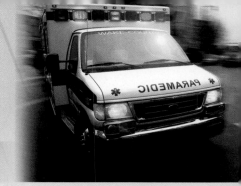

CASE STUDY

Dispatch advises, "Possible rollover, no victim found." The first deputy on scene knows someone had been driving the car recently, because the engine is still warm, but the driver is missing. When the state trooper and the county sheriff arrive, they started a search of the roads and local farmhouses while EMS stages on scene.

EMT Clayton decides to leave the ambulance and inspect the car in the ditch, looking for the mechanism of injury once the patient is located. He instructs his partner Avar to stay with the ambulance to monitor the radio and notify him when the patient is found.

The crushed roof indicates that the car may have rolled, and the starred windshield indicates that someone or something struck the windshield. The top half of the steering wheel is bent, and the directional signal is snapped in half at midshaft. Drops of blood are visible on the front and back seats. The rear window appears to have been kicked out, and blood is evident on the trunk lid and the ground behind the car.

The radio crackles to life, "Police Unit 4, report from the Everleigh farm, Route 11, possible prowler, man banging on the front door, appears to be bleeding stating he needs an ambulance because he can't breathe."

Clayton and Avar immediately respond with law enforcement to the farmhouse, suspecting this is the driver of the wrecked vehicle. Upon arrival the patient is seated on the front porch of the farmhouse, holding his right side. There is a laceration to the left side of his forehead with minor bleeding still present and dried blood below the patient's nose. The patient appears to have considerable blood on his clothes and hands, and states he thinks his nose is broken and it feels like his ribs are rubbing together each time he takes a breath.

Critical Thinking Questions

1. Based on the mechanism of injury, what injuries might an EMT suspect?
2. What are the assessment priorities for this patient?
3. What are the management priorities for this patient?

INTRODUCTION

Traumatic injuries to the chest can affect breathing, oxygenation, and circulation. Traumatic abdominal injuries can cause severe bleeding resulting in hypoperfusion and spillage of organ contents, causing life-threatening infections. The mechanism of injury will be the primary indicator of traumatic injuries to the chest and abdomen. Careful, complete assessment, including a thorough physical examination, will guide the EMT in providing the appropriate management of injuries of the chest and abdomen.

Prehospital care provided by EMTs has a positive impact on the survival of patients with chest and abdominal injuries. There are several basic principles regarding the management of these patients. This unit reviews those principles.

ANATOMY REVIEW

The thoracic cavity and abdominal cavity, located within the trunk of the body, contain some of the most important organs of the body (Figure 36.1). Vital activities, such as breathing, circulation, and digestion, occur within the

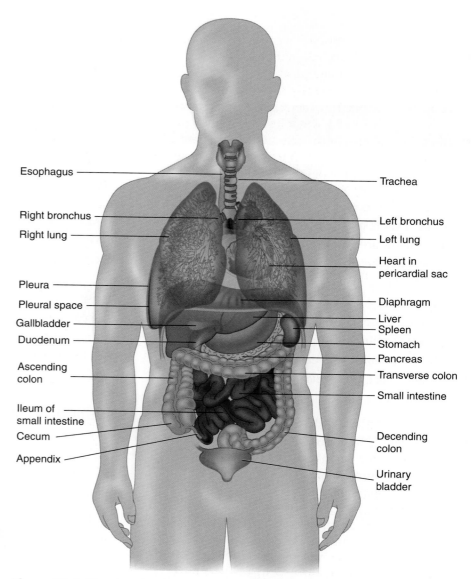

Figure 36.1 The trunk of the body contains the majority of vital organs

Esophagus

Trachea

Right bronchus

Left bronchus

Right lung

Left lung

Heart in
pericardial sac

Pleura

Pleural space

Diaphragm

Gallbladder

Liver

Duodenum

Spleen

Stomach

Ascending
colon

Pancreas

Transverse colon

Small intestine

Ileum of
small intestine

Cecum

Decending
colon

Appendix

Urinary
bladder

chest and abdomen. Unit 5 discusses the anatomy and physiology of the chest and abdominal organs and should be reviewed at this time.

CHEST TRAUMA

Injuries to the chest result in significant numbers of deaths each year. The chest contains organs that are essential to life. When these organs are damaged, life may be threatened. The most common consequence of chest trauma from any source is hypoxia. Injuries to the chest wall or internal organs can lead to ineffective ventilation and oxygenation. The job of the EMT is to recognize the presence of chest injuries, to quickly initiate the proper management, and to facilitate expedient transport to the most appropriate hospital.

MECHANISM OF INJURY

One of the first things an EMT will assess on the scene of an injured patient is the mechanism of injury. Knowing the forces that were applied to the patient will help the EMT to suspect and find even subtle injuries that may have significant consequences.

BLUNT CHEST TRAUMA

The most common cause of serious chest injuries is blunt chest trauma. Motor vehicle accidents, falls, direct blows, and crushing injuries are some of the ways that blunt chest trauma occurs. With this type of mechanism, the EMT may not immediately find evidence of a serious injury to the chest and underlying structures. Many of the findings on physical examination are somewhat delayed and may not be immediately apparent to the EMT. Nonetheless, failure to recognize a chest injury can have disastrous consequences.

Blunt trauma occurs when a force is applied to the chest wall. Depending upon the size of the object applying the force and the speed with which the force is applied, the injuries may be limited to the external chest wall or may extend deeper to involve internal thoracic organs. The more force that is applied to the chest, the deeper and more significant the injuries will likely be.

Upon arrival at the scene, the EMT should evaluate the forces that were applied to the patient. For example, in the case of a motor vehicle collision (MVC), the EMT should look at the vehicle the patient was in. Significant damage to the vehicle's exterior indicates high speed and a lot of force (Figure 36.2). Damage to the inside of the vehicle can further indicate the patient's potential injuries. A broken or bent steering wheel indicates that significant force was applied to the driver's chest.

The more significant the forces that were involved in the incident, the higher the EMT's suspicion should be for serious injury to the patient.

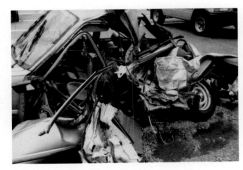

Figure 36.2 Major damage to a motor vehicle indicates that significant force was applied to the occupant's body during the collision (Courtesy of Craig Smith)

PENETRATING TRAUMA

Penetrating injuries to the chest are becoming increasingly common in today's society. Guns, knives, and other sharp objects can penetrate the chest wall and injure the underlying heart, lungs, and great vessels. The immediate result of penetrating injury can be severe bleeding or impaired breathing.

Although some penetrating chest injuries are certainly difficult to miss, others are quite subtle and may be easily missed without careful assessment. The key to proper management of the patient with penetrating chest trauma is to recognize that any wound to the chest can have associated underlying organ injury, no matter how superficial it may look at first glance.

The EMT can easily miss a tiny bullet entrance wound or small wound from a knife, or the EMT may assume that it is a minor wound. These mistakes will delay the proper treatment of a patient with a potential time-dependent injury. Injuries to the heart, lungs, and great vessels can quickly lead to shock and cardiac arrest. The EMT must find the wounds and be highly suspicious of the possibility of internal chest injury, no matter the size of the external wound. Figure 36.3 illustrates how a small wound can result in significant intrathoracic injury.

SIGNS AND SYMPTOMS

The most common symptoms seen in patients with chest injuries are pain and difficulty breathing. The pain is often centered in the area of the injury. Difficulty with breathing may be minor initially and may progress slowly or rapidly, depending on the injury.

Signs the EMT should look for include obvious injury to the chest wall. Using DCAP-BTLS during the chest assessment and remembering to look at both the front and back of the chest will lead the EMT to find any injuries.

Depending on the specific injury that is present, characteristic physical findings may be found on physical examination. When examining the patient's chest, the EMT should look specifically for any obvious deformities, contusions, abrasions, punctures, burns, tenderness, lacerations, or swelling

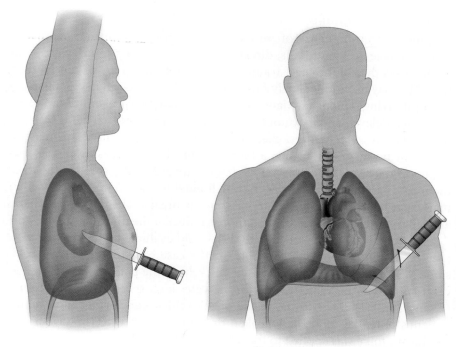

Stab wounds at nipple level or below frequently penetrate the abdomen

Figure 36.3 Despite small external wounds, penetrating chest trauma can be associated with serious organ injury

to the chest wall. Also, during palpation of the patient's chest, the EMT should note the presence of any subcutaneous air, or **subcutaneous emphysema.** Subcutaneous emphysema is air present under the skin; this air produces a palpable feeling like Rice Krispies as the EMT presses her hands against the patient's chest wall. This feeling is also known as *crepitus*.

The patient with significant chest injuries may have an elevated heart rate and respiratory rate, although the absence of these findings does not exclude injury. Vital signs should be monitored carefully.

ASSESSMENT

The patient who has suffered a potential chest injury should be assessed in the same manner as all trauma patients. The scene size-up allows the EMT to avoid any personal dangers and provides her with information regarding the incident. The primary assessment allows the EMT to find and treat immediately life-threatening injuries. The history and secondary assessment will be slightly different from patient to patient, depending on the severity of the mechanism of injury. Most patients having potential chest injuries require a rapid trauma assessment followed by vital signs and a SAMPLE history. A detailed physical examination may follow if time allows, and ongoing assessments are performed during transport to the hospital.

MANAGEMENT

The management of the patient with chest trauma is centered on ensuring the patient has adequate oxygenation and perfusion, which the EMT does by providing high-flow oxygen, ventilating when necessary, halting any obvious bleeding, supporting circulation when needed, and rapidly transporting the patient to definitive care. Treatment of specific injuries is addressed throughout this unit.

TRANSPORT

The patient with serious chest trauma must be seen at a hospital that has the capability to diagnose and treat serious traumatic injuries. The destination hospital is often guided by local protocols. In addition, if advanced life support (ALS) is available and indicated by local protocols, the EMT should arrange to intercept the unit while the patient with serious chest injuries is being transported.

The EMT should notify the receiving hospital early in the transport so the staff can prepare for the patient's arrival. Some systems require an EMT to obtain on-line medical control during the care of the seriously injured patient. The EMT should be familiar with and adhere to local protocols.

SPECIFIC INJURIES

Although the EMT is not expected to make a definitive diagnosis in the field, she can easily recognize several conditions that may affect the prehospital treatment of the patient. All EMTs should be able to recognize the signs and symptoms and understand the initial management of each of these conditions from the basic life support (BLS) perspective.

OPEN CHEST WOUNDS

A sharp object that penetrates the skin on the chest wall creates an open chest wound. Determining the deepness of a wound is difficult in the field; therefore, any wound on the chest caused by a penetrating object should be assumed to be serious, and the patient should be treated as a high priority.

Beneath each rib lies an artery. The middle of the chest contains the great vessels, the aorta, and the vena cava. If any of these blood vessels is lacerated, bleeding between the lung and the chest wall may occur. The accumulation of blood in the pleural space is called a **hemothorax.**

As much as 1,500 cc of blood can accumulate in the pleural space of each lung. The result of this massive blood loss is hypotension and shock. Eventually, the accumulation of blood can compromise breathing by crushing the air-filled lung. The EMT need not differentiate between a hemothorax and other life-threatening bleeding; instead, the EMT should concentrate on managing the hypotension and transporting the patient rapidly to the trauma center.

If a penetrating object has pierced the pleura, outside air can enter the thoracic cavity between the chest wall and the lung. As the volume of air between the chest wall and the lung expands, the lung starts to collapse. Air within the pleural space is called a **pneumothorax** (Figure 36.4).

As air passes in and out of an open chest wound, it can create a sucking sound. Whenever such a **sucking chest wound** is discovered, the EMT should consider the possibility of a pneumothorax.

The mechanism of injury should suggest to the EMT that a penetrating injury, and a pneumothorax, could be present. The signs of a pneumothorax include difficulty with breathing, cyanosis, and diminished breath sounds on the affected side.

After ensuring the patient has a patent airway, the EMT should proceed to examine the chest wall for holes, lacerations, or open wounds. Some chest wounds are very small, smaller than a dime; therefore, a careful inspection is needed. The EMT should look in the armpits (axilla) as well as under folds of skin.

MANAGEMENT

The EMT should immediately cover any open chest wounds with an occlusive dressing. An **occlusive dressing** prevents more air from entering the pleural space and enlarging the pneumothorax. A gloved hand, placed over the open

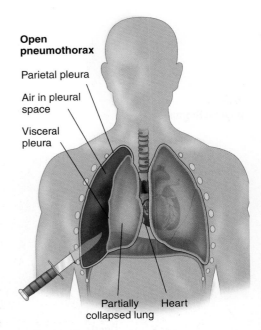

Open pneumothorax

Parietal pleura

Air in pleural space

Visceral pleura

Partially collapsed lung

Heart

- Chest wall defect
- Collapsed lung
- Ball valve effect

Figure 36.4 When air enters between the lung and the chest wall, pneumothorax is created

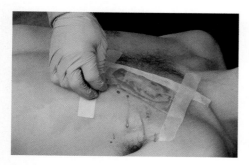

Figure 36.5 A sucking chest wound is covered with a 4- by 4-inch dressing that is secured on three sides; the fourth side is left open as a vent

wound, is an effective temporary occlusive dressing. A more effective dressing is usually prepared using clear plastic wrap placed over a 4- by 4-inch Vaseline gauze dressing or using a commercially prepared occlusive dressing.

To prevent the continued buildup of air in the pleural space during each breath, the EMT must create a dressing that does not allow air to enter the chest from the outside, yet still allows excess air to exit when necessary. This type of dressing can be created by securing an occlusive dressing on only three of the four sides (Figure 36.5). The fourth side acts as a flutter valve and allows air to escape if needed. When the patient breathes in, the negative pressure of inspiration draws the dressing against the wound, sealing the wound in the process. When the patient exhales, the positive pressure of exhalation allows excess air to escape from under the dressing.

High-concentration oxygen should be administered to the patient with an open chest wound, and the patient should be transported with the unaffected side slightly elevated. Elevating the unaffected side allows the uninjured lung to inflate maximally. A bedroll or a rolled blanket under the backboard can be used to accomplish this task. The patient should then be transported as soon as possible. An ALS unit should intercept the ambulance if possible.

TENSION PNEUMOTHORAX

Even with a flutter valve in place, air pressure can continue to build up inside the thoracic cavity, allowing a pneumothorax to enlarge. The increasing pressure from the expanding air pocket can eventually collapse the lung entirely and start to push the organs in the middle of the chest, the mediastinum, to the opposite side of the chest.

When organs are pushed to the opposite side of the chest, the great vessels that empty into the heart, the vena cava, are crushed. The resultant kinking of the vena cava prevents blood from returning to the heart. In addition, the heart itself is compressed. The pressure around the heart makes effective contraction of the ventricles more difficult. Without adequate blood to fill the ventricles, and with ineffective contractions, the blood pressure falls.

This buildup of pressure in the pleural space that results in a decrease in blood pressure is called a **tension pneumothorax** (Figure 36.6). A tension pneumothorax is a potentially life-threatening condition that must be treated immediately. A tension pneumothorax can occur in both penetrating chest wounds and blunt trauma.

The signs of a tension pneumothorax include all the signs of a pneumothorax. A patient with a tension pneumothorax may also have distended neck veins, called *jugular venous distention* (JVD), due to a backup of blood from the compressed heart and vena cava.

When a patient has a tension pneumothorax, his breathing may become so labored and rapid that the EMT is forced to assist his ventilation. When ventilations are delivered by bag-valve-mask, the EMT may note that ventilating the patient becomes increasingly more difficult. Increased difficulty with ventilation can be an indication of significant lung compression by the tension pneumothorax.

As a tension pneumothorax progresses, the organs in the mediastinum start to shift. Among these organs and structures is the trachea. Eventually the trachea shifts away from the affected side. **Tracheal deviation** is a late sign of a tension pneumothorax and may be seen by the EMT anteriorly in the neck, in the suprasternal area. The EMT may find it easier to feel than to see this movement of the trachea. The absence of tracheal deviation does not preclude the possibility of a tension pneumothorax. Signs of tension pneumothorax are outlined in Figure 36.7.

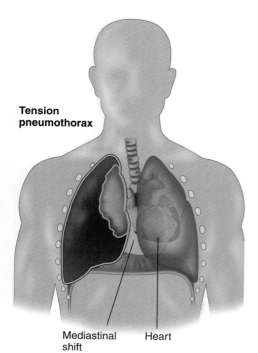

Tension pneumothorax

Mediastinal shift   **Heart**

Figure 36.6 Increasing pressure in the lung pushes the heart and great vessels to the opposite side of the chest

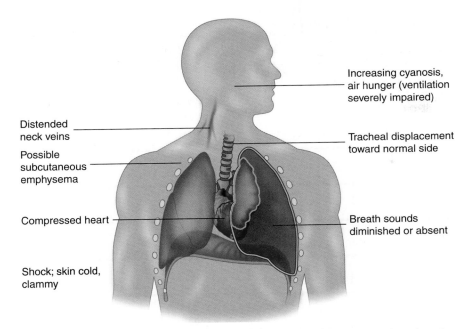

Increasing cyanosis, air hunger (ventilation severely impaired)

Distended neck veins

Possible subcutaneous emphysema

Tracheal displacement toward normal side

Compressed heart

Breath sounds diminished or absent

Shock; skin cold, clammy

Figure 36.7 A tension pneumothorax has all the findings of a simple pneumothorax as well as hypotension, JVD, tachycardia, and lack of breath sounds over the affected site

If a patient with an open chest wound becomes hypotensive, the EMT should immediately lift a corner of the occlusive dressing. Lifting a corner of the dressing may relieve the problem if the hypotension is being caused by an increase in pleural air pressure and a tension pneumothorax. A hissing sound from escaping air is sometimes heard. After releasing the corner of the occlusive dressing, the EMT should immediately recheck the patient's blood pressure.

If the patient's blood pressure has not improved, the EMT should transport the patient immediately. An ALS unit should be contacted and met en route to the hospital. ALS personnel have additional training with chest wound management. Table 36-1 summarizes the physical findings of pneumothorax.

RIB FRACTURES

The bony rib cage is intended to protect the vital organs within it. Trauma to the chest wall can result in broken or fractured ribs and injury to the underlying organs. Most rib fractures are the result of a large force being distributed over a small area. Ribs are interwoven with muscles and tendons. When a rib is fractured, these muscles and tendons help to maintain the ribs in alignment. Local swelling and tenderness may be the only outward sign that a rib is broken.

Rib fractures can be very painful. Any deep breath or cough grinds the bone ends together and creates a sharp pain. When an EMT assesses a patient with a possible fractured rib, she may note shallow breathing as well as guarding of the injured area (Figure 36.8).

A rib fracture, despite being painful, is not by itself life threatening, but the EMT should be concerned about whether the broken rib has damaged the underlying lung. Broken ribs can be forced inward, puncture the lung, and then spring back into alignment. The EMT should carefully listen to breath sounds near any suspected rib fracture. She should also be alert for signs of subcutaneous emphysema, which may indicate that the underlying lung has been injured.

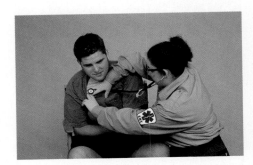

Figure 36.8 Breathing can be very painful with a fractured rib

Table 36-1 Signs of a Simple and Tension Pneumothorax*

Sign	Simple	Tension
Subcutaneous emphysema	+/−	+/−
Tachycardia	+	+
Tachypnea	+	+
Difficulty breathing (dyspnea)	+	+
Diminished breath sounds	+	+ (Absent)
Jugular venous distention	−	+
Loss of radial pulses	−	+
Decreased lung compliance	−	+
Hypotension	−	+
Tracheal deviation	−	+ (Late)

* Not all of these signs are present in every case.

MANAGEMENT

An EMT should move a patient with a rib fracture carefully to prevent the bone ends from puncturing a lung. Unlike other suspected bone injuries, the EMT cannot effectively splint a fractured rib. Instead, the EMT should administer oxygen and allow the patient to self-splint by assuming the most comfortable position possible. The patient should be encouraged to avoid any unnecessary movement.

FLAIL SEGMENT

When three or more ribs are broken in two or more places, a segment of the rib cage may be detached from the rest. This **flail segment** of the chest is a free-floating portion of the rib cage.

When the patient inhales, the rib cage expands and is pulled outward and upward by the muscles. The flail segment does not move together with the rest of the ribs. The negative pressure created inside the thoracic cavity during inspiration draws the free-floating segment downward and inward, in the opposite direction. This movement of a section of ribs in the opposite direction of the rest of the chest wall is called *paradoxical motion* (Figure 36.9).

Paradoxical motion can significantly impair breathing and cause injury to the underlying lung as the segment moves in and out. To prevent the painful grinding of the rib ends, the flail segment must be stabilized.

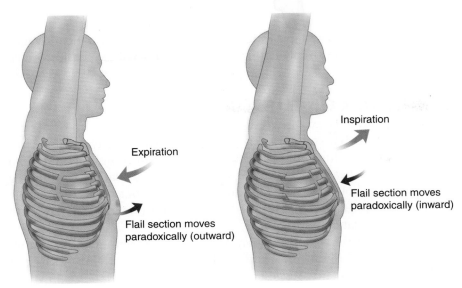

Figure 36.9 A flail segment impairs breathing because of its paradoxical motion

MANAGEMENT

The EMT can quickly stabilize a flail segment by placing a gloved hand(s) over the injured area. Once manual stabilization has been done, a folded universal dressing may be placed over the segment and taped securely in place. The dressing will help to prevent the segment from moving but will not restrict the patient's breathing. The EMT should be careful not to encircle the chest wall when taping the dressing in place, because that would restrict breathing.

A large flail segment can significantly impair the patient's ability to breathe. As the patient becomes increasingly tachypneic, the EMT may need to assist the patient's breathing. The positive pressure of the bag-valve-mask fills the lungs equally, expanding both injured and uninjured ribs together. In a sense, the positive pressure of assisted ventilation with a bag-valve-mask splints the flail segment internally.

Unless spinal precautions are needed, the patient should be transported on his side with the unaffected lung on top. Placing the patient on his injured side helps to stabilize the flail segment as well as decrease the pain the patient is experiencing from the moving bone ends.

PULMONARY CONTUSION

The lungs, like the skin, are rich with capillary beds. If blunt force is applied to the skin, a contusion (bruise) forms. Similarly, if a blunt force injures a lung, bleeding into the lung itself results. This condition is known as a **pulmonary contusion.**

The bleeding and associated edema impairs the lung's ability to exchange oxygen and carbon dioxide. If a large enough area of the lung is affected, the patient may have trouble breathing and become hypoxic. Like a bruise under the skin, a pulmonary contusion usually does not appear immediately but rather develops over a few hours.

Soft crackles may be heard over the site of the injury. Crackles can be an early indication of a developing pulmonary contusion. Chest pain, point tenderness, and localized swelling over the area of impact also suggest that the underlying lung might have sustained a pulmonary contusion.

When the alveoli are severely injured, bleeding can occur directly into the airway. The patient may cough up bright red, frothy blood. Coughing up blood, or **hemoptysis,** can be an indication of severe injury to the lungs.

Contusions to the chest, heart, and lungs take time to develop. At the scene, the EMT may not have any outward indications of the injury. Careful patient assessment, using DCAP-BTLS, may reveal tenderness and reproducible pain on deep inspiration; these symptoms, along with localized swelling, may lead the EMT to suspect a chest injury.

An EMT should be even more suspicious of a chest injury if a careful assessment of the interior of the motor vehicle reveals a bent steering wheel or a locked seat belt. These are indicators that a significant force may have been applied to the patient's chest.

MANAGEMENT

The care of pulmonary injuries focuses on supporting the patient's ventilation as needed and supplying high-flow supplemental oxygen to combat hypoxia.

CARDIAC CONTUSION

When a significant blunt force is directed toward the sternum, the heart can be bruised. A **cardiac contusion** can impair the heart's ability to pump, just as a pulmonary contusion impairs the function of the lungs. Bleeding into the tissue of the heart can cause the heart to beat irregularly. The resulting irregular pulse should alert the EMT to the possibility of a cardiac contusion. The irregular pulse caused by a cardiac contusion rarely deteriorates into ventricular fibrillation but it can.

A massive cardiac contusion may decrease cardiac output and can result in hypotension. A large bruise forming on the anterior chest, along with chest pain and tenderness, may suggest a cardiac contusion.

MANAGEMENT

The patient who is suspected of having a cardiac contusion has suffered significant blunt trauma to the chest. The management priorities are similar to those of any patient in this situation: high-flow oxygen, ventilation support when needed, and support of circulation if appropriate. Because the patient with a cardiac contusion can deteriorate quickly, transport should not be delayed, and ALS should be requested.

If the patient goes into cardiac arrest, cardiopulmonary resuscitation (CPR) and/or defibrillation may be needed. The EMT should follow local protocols regarding the care and transportation of a trauma-arrested patient.

PERICARDIAL TAMPONADE

Bleeding around the heart and into the pericardial sac that encloses the heart can lead to a condition called **pericardial tamponade.** This condition is usually a result of penetrating chest trauma with a laceration to the heart itself, although blunt trauma also can cause a tear in the heart and produce the same result. As with a tension pneumothorax, in which air fills the pleural space and compresses the lungs, blood filling the pericardial sac during pericardial tamponade can compress the heart.

As blood accumulates in the pericardial sac, the ventricles become compressed. Blood that cannot enter the ventricles backs up into the neck veins, causing JVD. As blood continues to accumulate in the pericardial sac, the ventricles cannot expand and contract effectively. The difference between the pressure created by the contraction (systole) and the resting pressure (diastole) starts to narrow. The **pulse pressure,** the difference between systolic and diastolic blood pressures, may approach zero.

For the EMT in the field, the most telling sign of cardiac tamponade may be the climbing heart rate, sustained above 120 beats per minute, and the weakening pulse, an indication of pulse pressure along with greatly distended neck veins.

The patient eventually becomes profoundly hypotensive and may go into cardiac arrest. Interestingly, the electrical system of the heart is usually unaffected, so although the patient may become pulseless, the electrical portion of the heart continues to function. Because this condition cannot be remedied by defibrillation, an automatic external defibrillator (AED) would likely indicate "no shock advised." Figure 36.10 summarizes the physical findings of pericardial tamponade.

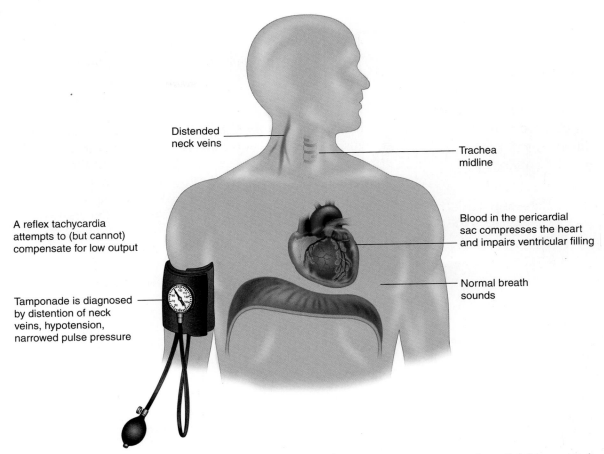

Figure 36.10 A narrowed pulse pressure and neck vein distention are signs of pericardial tamponade

MANAGEMENT

An EMT can do little in the field for patients with pericardial tamponade. The EMT should administer high-concentration oxygen, treat the patient for shock, and rapidly transport the patient to the emergency department. ALS personnel may have temporizing measures to offer and should be requested, but transport should not be delayed. Physicians may insert a needle into the pericardial sac to remove the blood that is compressing the heart. Early notification will help the hospital staff to properly prepare for the patient.

AORTIC INJURY

In sudden decelerations, such as a high-speed, head-on motor vehicle collision, the organs inside the body are thrown forcefully against the front of the body. When this occurs, tears may result to various organs. The most significant of these tears is probably one in the aorta. In a sudden deceleration, the heart and aorta are thrown forward into the anterior chest wall. However, a section of the aorta is well secured into the back of the chest by a ligament. As the rest of the aorta is forcefully thrown forward, a tear can result at the site where it is held back (Figure 36.11). If the tear is completely through the aorta, the patient will die in minutes, as all of the patient's blood will be pumped out of the torn aorta into the chest. If the tear is incomplete, severe bleeding can still occur, but the patient may not die immediately.

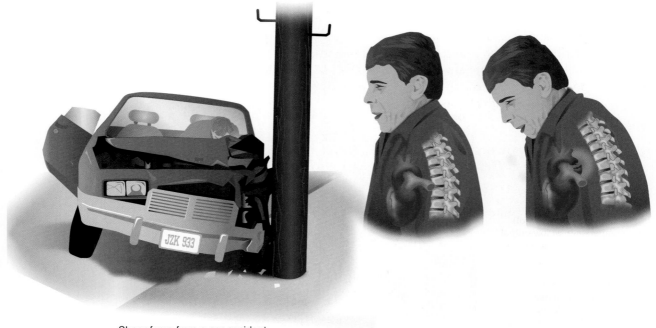

Shear force from a car accident
could result in this type of injury

Figure 36.11 The aorta can be torn during a sudden deceleration

MANAGEMENT

The EMT can recognize the potential for an aortic injury by identifying that a significant deceleration has occurred and noticing that the patient has chest discomfort or evidence of shock. An EMT in this situation should support the airway, breathing, and circulation as appropriate and should rapidly transport the patient to the most appropriate hospital. ALS care en route may be helpful, although transportation should not be delayed.

TRAUMATIC ASPHYXIA

When the chest is compressed rapidly, internal pressure increases dramatically, and blood is immediately forced out of the chest and into the vessels in the neck, head, and face. The neck veins instantly become distended (JVD). Cyanosis is apparent in the face, and bleeding into the sclera (white) of the eyes may occur. Small blood vessels in the cheeks and on the face may burst and bleed under the skin. These small red spots on the surface of the skin are called **petechiae.** The sudden increased blood flow to the brain also may result in brain swelling or bleeding.

Such a rapid ejection of blood and air out of the chest is called a **traumatic asphyxia.** Potential causes of traumatic asphyxia include being crushed or pinned between two objects.

MANAGEMENT

Crushing injuries to the chest may result in significant intrathoracic injury as well as injury to the brain, as described earlier. The injuries to the chest may result in hypotension and/or cardiac arrest. The EMT should address the airway, breathing, and circulation and should initiate rapid transport to the closest appropriate hospital.

ABDOMINAL TRAUMA

Although many of the abdominal organs are situated so that they are protected by the lower rib cage or the pelvis, injury to intra-abdominal organs can occur as a result of blunt or penetrating trauma. The EMT should be familiar with the location of the intra-abdominal organs and the principles of management of the patient with abdominal injuries.

MECHANISM OF INJURY

Although it is difficult to determine the exact extent of injury in the field, the EMT can expect certain types of injuries based on the mechanism.

PENETRATING ABDOMINAL TRAUMA

Although not as common as blunt abdominal injury, penetrating abdominal injury is often easier to recognize. A stab wound or gunshot wound to the abdomen, no matter how superficial it appears on the surface, can seriously injure internal organs. The EMT should gather as much information as possible regarding the mechanism to help her in identifying the injuries.

If the injury was caused by a stabbing, the EMT should attempt to determine what the patient was stabbed with. Was it a 3-inch switchblade or a 12-inch hunting knife? If the patient sustained a gunshot wound, what was the caliber of the weapon? How many shots were fired and from what trajectory? These questions often can be answered by law enforcement personnel at the scene.

BLUNT ABDOMINAL TRAUMA

When the abdomen forcefully strikes an object, such as the bottom of the steering wheel, the skin starts to stretch. If the skin remains intact, a contusion may result. The energy continues to be passed on to internal organs in the abdomen.

If the steering wheel strikes the lower ribs in the upper abdomen, the liver and spleen may be injured. If the force is directed toward the lower abdominal area, some of the intestine will be crushed, spilling its contents into the abdominal cavity.

Finally, as the abdominal organs are rocked violently, veins and arteries may be torn. Shearing forces can be so great that an organ, such as the liver, can be torn in half. These injuries can cause significant bleeding. Table 36-2 summarizes the types of injuries that can result from blunt trauma to the abdomen.

Although the external signs of injury may not be as impressive in blunt trauma as in penetrating trauma, the potential for injury is just as great. The EMT must assess the mechanism of injury and determine the likelihood of an intra-abdominal injury.

The potential for injury to intra-abdominal organs exists whenever a patient has experienced impact directly to the abdomen. The EMT must determine whether such an impact has occurred or may have occurred. Information about whether the patient was punched or kicked in the abdomen or flanks is often available in the history of the incident, but in the case of MVCs, the body parts that suffered impact must be inferred from the damage to the vehicle.

If the patient slid down and underneath the steering wheel, the bottom of the steering wheel may have struck the patient in the abdomen. The EMT should lift the deflated airbag and examine the steering wheel to determine whether it is bent along the bottom. A bent steering wheel is a good indicator of serious abdominal trauma.

Table 36-2
Intra-abdominal Injuries Sustained from Blunt Trauma

Abdominal contusions

Liver laceration

Splenic rupture

Mesentery artery tears

Intestinal rupture

Kidney contusion

Bladder rupture

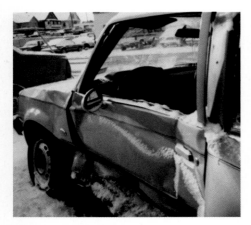

Figure 36.12 Side impacts can cause chest and abdominal injuries

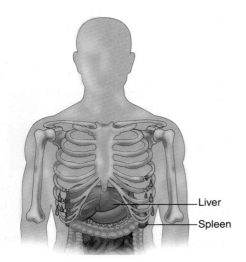

Figure 36.13 Lower rib fractures can result in injury to the liver or spleen

Liver
Spleen

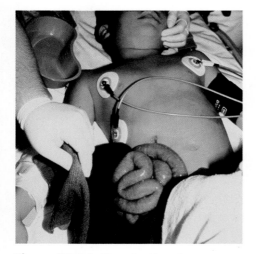

Figure 36.14 Penetrating trauma to the abdomen can result in evisceration of intestines (Courtesy of Deborah Funk, MD, Albany Medical Center, Albany, NY)

Although airbags, especially when coupled with use of a seat belt, have been very effective in preventing injuries and have saved countless lives, the EMT should keep in mind that in severe motor vehicle crashes, the patient may still sustain significant injuries. The patient can sustain serious abdominal injuries in a lateral impact. The door can be pushed into the passenger compartment, striking the patient from the level of the hip to the level of the lower ribs.

Side airbag protection is becoming available in more automobile models. Until side airbag protection is available in all cars, however, the EMT must be alert to the possibility of abdominal injuries in any side collision in which there is more than 12 inches of intrusion into the passenger side (Figure 36.12).

Patients who wear seat belts improperly, such as too high on the abdomen, may suffer injury to the abdomen in a collision. Young children who are not restrained appropriately in a booster seat are especially vulnerable to abdominal injury from ill-fitting seat belts. In addition, patients who do not wear seat belts at all will be thrown around the vehicle and perhaps ejected. Potential for serious abdominal injury is high in these situations.

SIGNS AND SYMPTOMS

Although pain is the most commonly found symptom in patients with abdominal injuries, there are many cases in which the patient is unable to express feeling pain or may simply fail to notice it because of other injuries or factors. The unconscious patient or the patient with an altered mental status will not be able to describe symptoms reliably. In such cases, the EMT has to rely upon sometimes-subtle physical findings and the mechanism of injury.

The EMT should assess for the following signs of abdominal injury: any evidence of deformities, contusions, abrasions, punctures, burns, tenderness, lacerations, or swelling to the lower chest, back, or abdomen.

Other signs of abdominal injury include abdominal wall rigidity, rebound tenderness, and abdominal distention. Abdominal wall rigidity can be the result of irritation of the peritoneal lining of the abdomen caused by the contents of rupture of hollow organs. This is often a late sign and may be confused with guarding, which can be involuntary tightening of the abdominal muscles or voluntary tightening (ticklishness). Rebound tenderness, another sign of peritoneal irritation, is pain that occurs as pressure is released by palpation. The EMT should focus on establishing point tenderness, the location of the discomfort, rather than establishing rebound tenderness or guarding. The third sign of abdominal injury is distention. Distention is the result of fluids, including blood, collecting in the abdominal cavity.

Abdominal distention can be difficult to detect because the abdomen is so distensible. However, during a trauma assessment, any palpable mass in the abdominal cavity should be assumed to indicate bleeding. The exact location of the mass should be noted and reported. These signs are generally less reliable in the field, and the EMT should focus on the patient's concerns of pain and assess for evidence of hypoperfusion.

The abdominal organs extend up into the lower chest, so lower rib injuries can often be associated with injury to the upper abdominal organs such as the liver and spleen (Figure 36.13).

Signs of penetrating trauma are often quite obvious to the EMT. Any puncture mark should be assumed to be associated with intra-abdominal injury. A larger opening in the abdominal wall may result in the internal organs, most often intestines, extruding out of the abdomen. The extrusion of intestines outside the abdomen as a result of penetrating trauma is called *evisceration* (Figure 36.14).

ASSESSMENT

The patient with abdominal injuries may have other injuries as well. The EMT must perform the usual assessment for a trauma patient in an orderly fashion, no matter how impressive a particular injury may seem. A scene size-up is needed to determine the safety of the area as well as the mechanism of injury. The EMT must complete the primary assessment quickly and address any immediately life-threatening conditions. The EMT also should complete the history and secondary assessment using the rapid physical examination to look for evidence of serious injury. The detailed physical examination may be done during transport if appropriate.

An orderly manner of assessment of the patient with serious injuries is the best way to find and manage the patient's most life-threatening injuries.

MANAGEMENT

Because the diagnosis of specific abdominal injuries often is not made in the field, the EMT should treat the patient who has potential abdominal injuries with several familiar principles in mind. The prehospital care of an abdominal wound should focus on assessment and management of hemorrhage and hypoperfusion with rapid transportation to a trauma center. Penetrating abdominal wounds frequently require surgical management.

The EMT should apply high-flow oxygen and support ventilation and circulation as necessary. One of the most important things an EMT can do for the patient with significant intra-abdominal injuries is to provide rapid transport to the closest appropriate hospital, usually a trauma center.

TRANSPORT

The greatest danger to the injured patient is excessive time spent on scene. The patient's best chance of survival depends on timely transport to a hospital capable of caring for the patient's injuries, along with appropriate emergency care while en route.

The EMT should continue care of the patient during transport by completing the ongoing assessment as often as is indicated by the patient's condition. ALS should be requested to assist in the management of the seriously injured patient, and the EMT should follow local protocols regarding need for medical control.

Early notification of the destination hospital will enable the staff to make appropriate preparations to best care for the seriously injured patient.

SPECIFIC CONDITIONS

Although the general management principles are the same for abdominal injuries, several specific conditions are worth addressing individually.

LIVER AND SPLEEN INJURY

The liver and spleen are the most commonly injured abdominal organs. Both are very vascular organs and have the potential to bleed into the abdomen, causing shock. The EMT who recognizes such injuries can provide the appropriate therapy and warn the receiving hospital staff of the situation.

Contusions and abrasions over the lower rib cage with upper abdominal tenderness are signs of liver or spleen injury. These findings may not be present on the first examination, so the ongoing assessment of the injured patient should include repeated abdominal examinations.

MANAGEMENT

There is nothing an EMT can do in the field aside from the usual airway, breathing, and circulation support that will benefit the patient with a liver or

Street Smart

An EMT may occasionally miss important physical signs if he fails to expose the patient properly. The abdomen starts just below the breasts and extends to well below the waist. The EMT must perform a complete assessment of the patient.

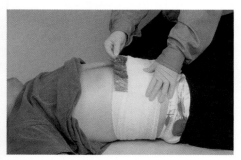

Figure 36.15 An evisceration should be covered with a moist sterile dressing and then a layer of aluminum foil to help retain the patient's body heat

spleen injury. Therefore, the best treatment the EMT can offer in this situation is rapid transport to the hospital.

EVISCERATION

A large abdominal wound may allow abdominal contents, such as the small intestine, to eviscerate through the wound opening. The EMT can recognize evisceration easily and should not let it distract her from addressing other potentially life-threatening issues.

MANAGEMENT

The EMT should never try to place the abdominal contents that have protruded from the abdomen back into the abdominal cavity once they have eviscerated. Instead, the EMT should cover the protruding abdominal contents with a dry sterile dressing; some EMS authorities advocate the use of a moist dressing. A non-adherent dressing is preferred. The entire dressing should be reinforced with a large dressing, usually an abdominal or universal dressing. Frequently, EMTs cover the moist dressing with a sheet of aluminum foil (Figure 36.15). The aluminum foil can be applied over the bandaging to help retain heat and protect the organs from further injury.

PELVIC FRACTURES

Fractures of the bony pelvis can result in injury to the underlying organs and vessels. A major problem with pelvic fractures is internal bleeding resulting in hemorrhagic shock. Fractures may be identified during the rapid trauma assessment by finding bony crepitus and tenderness during compression of the pelvic bones.

MANAGEMENT

If the EMT finds evidence of pelvic fractures on examination, she should consider using military anti-shock trousers (MAST) for stabilization, along with rapid transport to a trauma center.

GENITOURINARY TRAUMA

The primary male and female reproductive and urinary organs lie within the pelvic and retroperitoneal cavities of the abdomen. Injuries to the urinary bladder will spill their contents into the abdominal cavity, causing inflammation of the lining of the peritoneum called peritonitis. The kidneys are highly vascular, and lacerations to the kidney can cause life-threatening bleeding. Although injuries to the genitalia are not usually life threatening, they can cause severe pain and discomfort and are often embarrassing for the patient to discuss.

Injuries that can occur to the bladder include blunt force trauma causing a rupture or lacerations to the bladder from fractured pelvic bone ends. The kidneys can sustain serious tears, shears, and contusion from blunt trauma or penetrations, such as knife or gunshot wounds. Due to the rich blood supply through the kidneys, injuries can cause major hemorrhage and severe hypoperfusion. Management priorities are support of airway, breathing, and circulation; oxygen administration; and continuous assessment and management for shock.

MALE GENITALIA

Injuries to the male genitalia include lacerations, contusions, abrasions, penetrations, avulsions, and amputations. Injuries will cause severe pain in most cases and could produce excessive bleeding due to the vasculature of the penis.

Management of injuries to the penis or scrotum should be treated like a soft tissue injury. Place the patient on high-flow oxygen and transport. Cold packs can be applied to reduce pain and swelling and slow bleeding.

An avulsed or amputated penis will require direct pressure to control bleeding. Make sure to transport the avulsed or amputated part with the patient, wrapped in a moist sterile dressing in a plastic bag. Keep the part cool by placing the bag on a cool pack or on ice that has been wrapped in a towel and not directly touching the part. ALS intercept should be considered for management of severe shock and pain management.

FEMALE GENITALIA

The major female organs of reproduction are internal, in the lower abdominal cavity. However, injuries to the female genitalia can occur due to blunt trauma, sexual assault, abortion attempts, straddle injuries, lacerations from childbirth, and foreign objects inserted into the vagina. Injuries to this area will commonly cause severe pain. Additionally, injuries to the genitalia often cause great anxiety to the patient who fears long-term conditions such as the inability to reproduce, following a significant injury.

Management priorities include control of bleeding with direct pressure. Never pack the vagina, but place sterile sanitary napkins over the vagina. Place the patient on high-flow oxygen and monitor for signs and symptoms of shock throughout transport. ALS intercept should be considered for management of severe shock or pain management.

CONCLUSION

Serious trauma patients often have trauma to the chest and abdomen. Any major mechanism of injury has the potential to produce significant chest and abdominal trauma.

If the EMT suspects chest and abdominal injuries and assesses the patient with those suspicions in mind, she will have a greater chance of detecting life-threatening injuries, making the right decisions, and having a positive impact on the patient's outcome.

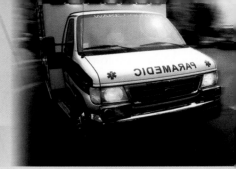

CASE STUDY Continued

Clayton instructs one of the deputies in establishing and maintaining cervical spinal stabilization, as he performs a primary survey, noting increased, shallow respiration and no life-threatening external bleeding. Oxygen via non-rebreather mask is applied.

After performing a rapid trauma assessment, Clayton determines the patient, Mr. Blencoe, has fractured ribs on the right side, with decreased breath sounds, a laceration to the scalp, and possibly a closed head injury. Mr. Blencoe is somewhat confused about the event and how he got hurt. Clayton determined he has a Glasgow Coma Scale score of 14 (eyes-4, verbal-4, motor-6). Baseline vital signs are pulse 110, respirations 24 (shallow), and blood pressure 130/88.

Mr. Blencoe is secured to a backboard, with a cervical immobilization collar in place and the head secured to the board. The laceration on his head is dressed and bandaged, with minor bleeding present at this time. There is no active bleeding from his nose. Clayton has requested an ALS intercept en route to the trauma center.

En route, Mr. Blencoe's respirations increase to over 30 per minute, with breath sounds no longer present on the right side and subcutaneous emphysema palpated in the right upper chest. Mr. Blencoe's level of consciousness decreases, and Clayton reassessed his GCS at 9 (eyes-2, verbal-3, motor-4). Reassessment of vital signs show a pulse of 120, respirations 32 and shallow, and blood pressure of 110/78.

As the ALS intercept arrives, Clayton has begun assisting respirations using a bag-valve-mask and oxygen. He reports to the medics there is resistance each time he squeezes the bag, and the chest is not rising on the right side. Clayton provides a complete report, including the extensive damage to the vehicle, as the medics on board start an IV and prepare to intubate Mr. Blencoe to secure the airway and provide more adequate ventilations during the rest of transport to the trauma center.

As Clayton is completing his documentation at the hospital, the emergency department physician reports to him Mr. Blencoe has four fractured ribs and a punctured lung on the right side, with a hemothorax. The results of the CT scan showed no skull fracture. Mr. Blencoe is doing well after a chest tube was placed to remove the blood from his chest cavity and the lung has reinflated. He has been admitted to the intensive care unit and is expected to recover nicely.

Key Concepts Revisited

- The most common consequence of chest trauma from any source is compromise of breathing and oxygenation resulting in hypoxia.

- Determination of the mechanism of injury will lead the EMT to find severe traumatic injuries to the chest that may not be immediately obvious:

  o Blunt chest injury results from falls, MVCs, direct blows, and crushing injuries.

  o Penetrating injury include gunshot and knife wounds and injury from other sharp objects.

- EMTs should have the ability to recognize the signs and symptoms and understand the initial management of specific traumatic injuries to the chest.
  - Open chest injuries
    - Hemothorax
    - Pneumothorax
    - Sucking chest wounds
    - Tension pneumothorax
      - Tracheal deviation
    - Rib fractures
      - Flail segment
    - Pulmonary contusion
    - Cardiac contusion
    - Pericardial tamponade
    - Aortic injury
    - Traumatic asphyxia
- The management of chest trauma is centered on ensuring adequate oxygenation and perfusion.
- The common mechanism of injury for abdominal organs, protected by the lower ribs and pelvis is usually through blunt or penetrating trauma.
  - Penetrating abdominal trauma
  - Blunt abdominal trauma
- Abdominal injuries are often initially overlooked by the patient and EMT due to more dramatic, distracting injuries that may be present.
- Specific abdominal organs are extremely vascular and injury can produce life-threatening bleeding.
  - Liver and spleen injury
  - Evisceration
  - Pelvic fractures
- Management of abdominal wounds often requires surgical intervention, and prehospital care focuses on assessment and management of hemorrhage and hypoperfusion with rapid transportation to a trauma center.
- Injuries to the organs of the pelvic and retroperitoneal cavities can involve signficant hemorrhage:
  - Urinary bladder spillage
  - Kidney hemorrhage
- Injury to the male and female genitalia can involve lacerations, penetrations, contusions, avulsions, and amputations.

Review Questions

1. What is the difference between blunt and penetrating trauma?
2. What differentiates a simple pneumothorax from a tension pneumothorax?
3. How does an EMT manage an open chest wound?
4. What are the signs of a fractured rib?
5. How does an EMT manage a flail chest segment?
6. What is evisceration?
7. How does an EMT manage an evisceration?
8. What injuries can be caused by blunt trauma to the lower ribs?
9. How does an EMT manage a closed abdominal injury?
10. What types of injuries can occur to the organs of the genitourinary systems?
11. What is the management for an amputation of the male genitalia?
12. What mechanisms of injury are commonly involved with trauma to the female genitalia?

Key Terms

Cardiac contusion

Flail segment

Hemoptysis

Hemothorax

Occlusive dressing

Pericardial tamponade

Petechiae

Pneumothorax

Pulmonary contusion

Pulse pressure

Subcutaneous emphysema

Sucking chest wound

Tension pneumothorax

Tracheal deviation

Traumatic asphyxia

Further Study

Hunt, D. "Thoracic Park Re-visited." *Emergency Medical Services* 26, no. 7 (1997): 47–57.

Keenan, D., and P. Phrampus. "Puncture Pathways." *Journal of Emergency Medical Services* 24, no. 9 (1999): 76–79.

Murphy, P. "Gunshot Wounds." *Journal of Emergency Medical Services* 22, no. 6 (1997): 74–79.

Phillips, K. "Prehospital Evaluation and Care of the Abdomen." *Emergency Medical Services* 26, no. 8 (1997): 37–40.

Rhodes, M., and A. Heightman. "Retroperitoneal Injuries." *Journal of Emergency Medical Services* 24, no. 4 (1999): 58–64.

Sahni, R. "Chest Trauma." *Journal of Emergency Medical Services* 23, no. 10 (1998): 86–90.

Stewart, C. "Prehospital Management of Cardiothoracic Trauma." *Emergency Medical Services* 28, no. 9 (1999): 37–45.

UNIT (37) Soft Tissue Injuries

Soft tissue injuries are rarely life threatening, unless there has been significant damage to the underlying blood vessels or organs. They can appear gruesome and may distract the EMT from recognizing a more serious internal injury. Emphasis for management of soft tissue injuries is on bleeding control, recognition and management of potentially serious underlying injuries, prevention or treatment of shock, and reducing the risk for infection.

National Education Standards
The Emergency Medical Technician (EMT) will demonstrate a fundamental depth and foundational breadth of understanding of the pathophysiology, assessment, and management of soft tissue injuries.

Key Concepts

- The severity of bleeding can be determined by the vessels that have been injured: arterial, capillary, or venous.

- The principles of bleeding control are to stop severe bleeding before it leads to hypoperfusion.

- The purpose of a sterile dressing is to prevent introduction of contaminants, such as dirt, into the wound, which can lead to infection.

- Soft tissue wounds may result from blunt forces or sharp objects.

- The type of dressing and bandages used on soft tissue injuries is determined by the need for additional control of bleeding and the type and location of the injury.

- Compartment syndrome can result from crush injury.

- The classification of burn injuries is based on the number of layers of skin and underlying tissues affected.

- Management of a burn injury begins by stopping the burning process; protecting from infections, fluid loss, and heat loss; and transporting to the appropriate facility.

- Chemical burns must be managed immediately by removing the chemical from the skin to prevent continuing tissue damage.

- An electrical shock can cause damage to the soft tissues, including entrance and exit wounds of the skin, and affect the function of the heart, possibly causing cardiac arrest.

- The management of an electrical injury begins with ensuring scene safety for the rescuers and administering CPR and AED if cardiac arrest occurs.

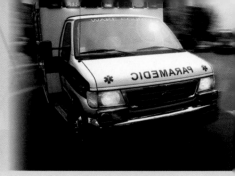

CASE STUDY

While reaching for the door upon leaving the house, Jannie misses the handle and puts her arm through the glass in the door. Instinctively, she pulls her arm back through, which results in a long cut down the length of her forearm. Now she is bleeding profusely.

Denise and Justin had just returned from a call to the local nursing home and were restocking the ambulance when the call came in for a "woman bleeding profusely from the arm." Denise quickly checks to make sure they have sufficient dressing and bandages for the wound, as well as cold packs for swelling and other potential soft tissue injury.

Upon arrival, Denise finds the patient, Jannie, sitting at her kitchen table with a large towel applied to her right forearm. The towel is heavy with bright red blood and there is a large puddle of blood on the floor next to the back door.

Jannie appears pale and states she has been trying to stop the bleeding for more than 10 minutes but it won't stop. She states it was spurting out of the part of the cut nearest her wrist.

Critical Thinking Questions

1. What are the immediate priorities in this case?
2. How would an EMT control this bleeding?
3. Is there a life threat here?

INTRODUCTION

An Emergency Medical Technician (EMT) seeing a pool of blood might be impressed by the apparent magnitude of the blood lost. Yet, the majority of people who are bleeding do not "bleed to death." That is not to say that bleeding cannot be fatal. Uncontrolled bleeding can lead to shock and even death. Fortunately, most external bleeding is easily controlled using some simple maneuvers. This unit reviews those methods as well as how to assess and treat other wounds.

ANATOMY REVIEW

The skin is a complex matrix of different cell types and specialized tissues. Together these cells protect the internal organs, regulate the internal environment, and allow us to sense our environment. The skin's cells and tissues constitute the largest organ system in the body, the *integumentary system*.

The integumentary system protects the body's internal organs from the outside environment. Bacteria and other infectious agents cannot penetrate healthy, intact skin. Thus, the skin protects the body from infection. The skin is also very resilient. It withstands constant wear and tear. The skin stretches to allow movement or prevent penetration.

The skin works in the opposite way as well—that is, the skin keeps all of the bodily fluids, including blood, inside the body. A break in the skin can result in bleeding that can ultimately lead to death.

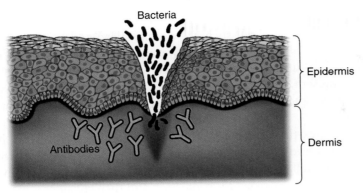

Figure 37.1 The body's response to injury is inflammation

INJURY TO THE SKIN

If the skin is damaged, the first and immediate sensation is pain. Pain warns the body that its protective barrier has been injured. Injury also sets off internal protective responses, called **inflammation.** This complex process is the body's attempt to prevent infection and begin healing (Figure 37.1).

Imagine the skin as a dam. When the dam is breached, a river (blood) pours through the break. The alarm is sounded (pain), and rescue workers swarm to the scene to seal the breach (clotting). Provided the rescue workers have the right tools in sufficient quantities, the dam's breach can be minimized and damage (infection) prevented. Any damage that remains will be repaired (scarring), and the dam will be as good as new.

BLEEDING

A **wound** is any break in the skin, and most wounds bleed. Some wounds bleed more vigorously than others. The amount of blood loss depends on how much skin is damaged and how much force is behind the bleeding. Of the two components of bleeding, the force behind the bleeding is the most important.

The blood in an artery is under a great deal of pressure (systolic pressure) when it leaves the heart. A cut to an artery can cause bright red blood to spurt across a room. (Oxygenated blood, on the arterial side, is generally bright red, whereas deoxygenated blood, usually on the venous side, is darker red.)

Capillary blood, on the other hand, is under very little pressure. This low pressure allows the blood to remain in the capillary beds while the cells extract the oxygen from the blood. As a result of this low pressure, when a capillary is cut, it oozes blood instead of spurting it.

The veins are at the end of the circulatory system. Usually a vein has been cut when serious bleeding is present. Because veins lie relatively close to the skin as compared to arteries, which usually lie next to bones, veins are at greater risk for injury. The blood returning to the heart in the veins is under low to moderate pressure. However, just because a vein does not spurt blood does not mean that a large amount of blood cannot be lost rapidly. Bleeding from a vein is usually constant, creating rivulets of blood that pour over the edge of the wound. The body's own protective mechanisms have difficulty controlling such bleeding. Figure 37.2 illustrates the different forms of bleeding.

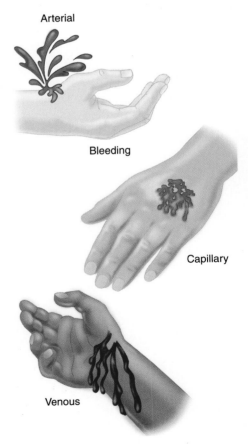

Figure 37.2 Arterial bleeding is bright red and spurts; capillary bleeding oozes; and venous bleeding is dark red and flows

ASSESSMENT

By the very nature of a call such as "woman bleeding," EMTs knows they will have to control bleeding when they arrive on the scene and will need to ensure there are sufficient bleeding control supplies on hand. When known bleeding is present, the first priority is for EMTs to protect themselves from possible exposure to blood and blood-borne infection by donning the appropriate PPE.

In most cases, the EMT only has to wear examination gloves, but in some cases, forceful bleeding can splash blood, and the EMT needs eye protection and a gown as well as gloves. The EMT should approach the scene wearing all the barrier devices needed for protection and then consider removing any unnecessary ones after the patient has been assessed.

SCENE SIZE-UP

A new EMT may feel overwhelmed when he sees a pool of blood next to a patient. His first instinct may be to spring immediately into action. Breaks and cuts in the skin, however, are usually caused by an object, such as a knife or machinery. The EMT should be mindful that the mechanism of injury can injure the EMT just as easily as it injured the patient. Therefore, the mechanism of injury should be assessed and rendered harmless before the EMT approaches the patient. Machines, for example, should be turned off and the power disconnected, and weapons should be removed from the area before the EMT approaches the patient.

The EMT is also responsible for seeing that no one else gets hurt. This responsibility includes preventing bystanders from becoming exposed to the blood at the scene. A perimeter should be established around the patient to prevent onlookers from becoming contaminated. Sometimes just placing the "jump kit," or first aid bag, in the way prevents well-meaning onlookers from trying to help.

PRIMARY ASSESSMENT

As with all patients, the EMT must first complete a primary assessment. The patient will be focused on the bleeding, but other problems, such as loss of the airway if the patient suddenly becomes unconscious, may be more important. The bleeding must be stopped, but the EMT must also constantly consider the patient's airway, breathing, and circulation.

In the past, ambulance drivers sometimes brought patients into the hospital with all the patients' wounds dressed perfectly, but the patients were dead. The EMT should always remember an essential fact: Bleeding itself is not fatal; hypoperfusion and resultant shock kill the patient. Effective patient care may mean simply holding a towel over a wound while rapidly extricating the patient rather than making sure that each minor wound is dressed.

The EMT should always expose the entire area around the wound. This exposure allows the EMT to better control the bleeding and to monitor the wound for further bleeding once bleeding is controlled. Typically, the EMT uses a pair of scissors to cut clothing, and then moves the clothing away from the wound.

MANAGEMENT

Once the scene has been made safe, the EMT's first concern is to control the bleeding. Fortunately, several means of bleeding control are available. In most cases, the EMT should begin with the easiest and safest techniques and then progress methodically through the other techniques, always mindful of the principles of bleeding control.

PRINCIPLES OF BLEEDING CONTROL

When an EMT discovers severe bleeding, the first question he must ask is, "Can this bleeding lead to shock and possibly even death?" If the bleeding is not immediately life threatening, the EMT should continue with the primary assessment of the patient. If the bleeding, or **hemorrhage,** is life threatening, it must be dealt with immediately. The following are some methods of controlling life-threatening bleeding.

First, the EMT should do nothing. The body does a good job of controlling hemorrhaging by itself. To stop bleeding, the body forms blood clots. Blood clots are made of clumps of cells, held together by strands of fiber. The clumps of cells eventually form an impenetrable barrier, and the bleeding stops. This process of blood clotting is called **coagulation.** For coagulation to occur, sufficient amounts of blood, with clotting factors, must be at the injury site. The process can be compared to building a dam. Without steel reinforcing rods, the concrete would crumble. Without concrete, the water would leak through the maze of rods. Together, the concrete and steel rods hold back the volume of water and create a dam.

To control active bleeding from a wound, the EMT should apply direct finger pressure to the bleeding site, exerting firm, constant force. This is referred to as **direct pressure** on the wound (Figure 37.3). The EMT's actions are intended to support the body's own clotting activities. Direct pressure helps to slow the bleeding by compressing the blood vessels, allowing the blood to clot. As the bleeding slows, the blood's clotting elements have time to clump together and form a clot.

If bleeding continues despite direct pressure on the site itself, the EMT should raise, or **elevate,** the wound above the level of the heart. Raising the wound above heart level helps to reduce the pressure at the wound site even more and allows blood to pool and clot.

If bleeding continues, the EMT should apply an absorbent cloth, called a **dressing,** to the wound and continue to apply pressure (Figure 37.4).

Finally, if bleeding still has not stopped, the EMT must physically occlude the artery that is supplying blood to the wound. By applying manual pressure to the artery where the artery lies next to a bone, or by using an arterial tourniquet, the EMT can stop blood flow to the wound (Figure 37.5).

Any point where a pulse can be obtained is a pressure point to control hemorrhage (Figure 37.6). Pressure on the radial pulse may help control bleeding of the hand, although the ulnar artery on the anterior lateral wrist can supply collateral blood flow. Firm, direct pressure to the brachial artery can help control bleeding of the forearm, and direct pressure to the femoral artery can control bleeding distal to it on the lower extremity.

Splinting can help to prevent or control bleeding by immobilizing the fractured bones and preventing the bone ends from damaging more tissue or blood vessels. Additionally, air or vacuum splints exert pressure on a wound, effectively acting like direct pressure or a pressure dressing. MAST pants can be used to control bleeding in the pelvis and lower extremities. Because the use of MAST pants in extremity fractures may potentially cause a complication called *compartment syndrome*, always follow local protocols and seek advice from medical control.

When bleeding is severe and the standard means of bleeding control—direct pressure, pressure point, elevation, and/or pressure dressings—are not effective in stopping bleeding quickly enough, an arterial-constricting band, called a **tourniquet**, must be applied (Figure 37.7).

When severe bleeding that is life threatening absolutely cannot be stopped by any other means, a tourniquet must be used. The situation, an

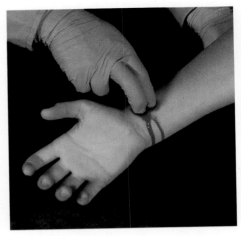

Figure 37.3 Firm direct pressure is effective in stopping bleeding

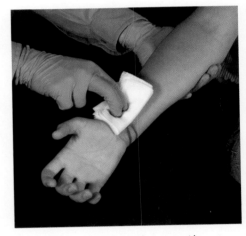

Figure 37.4 If bleeding continues, a dressing may be applied

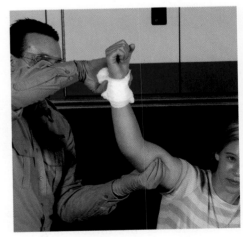

Figure 37.5 Manual pressure to a pressure point can limit blood flow to a wound

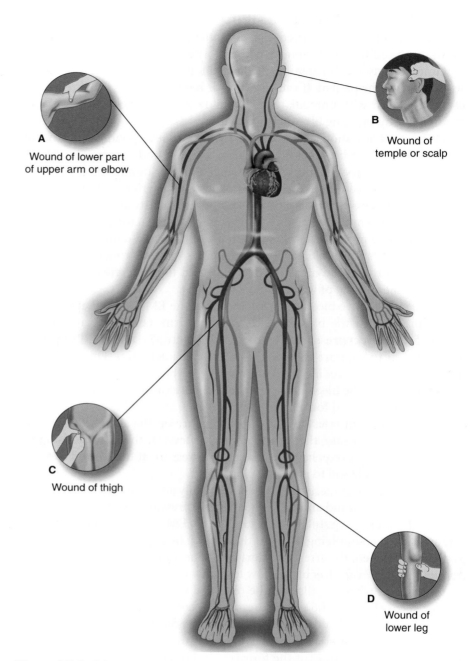

A
Wound of lower part
of upper arm or elbow

B
Wound of
temple or scalp

C
Wound of thigh

D
Wound of
lower leg

Figure 37.6 Direct firm pressure to a pulse point will help to control bleeding

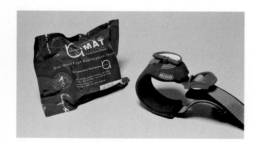

Figure 37.7 A tourniquet can be used to stop life-threatening bleeding such as from an artery when standard bleeding control methods are not effective

arterial bleed, clearly must be one of "life over limb" before the EMT applies a tourniquet.

Any tight, constricting band placed over an artery will function as a tourniquet. This type of tourniquet should not be confused with the venous tourniquet that paramedics use to distend veins. An arterial tourniquet eliminates any pulses distal to the tourniquet. Without pulses, the distal bones, muscles, and skin have a lack of perfusion with the associated tissue damage if it is left in place for a prolonged period of time.

The EMT should choose a wide-width material, no less than 2 inches. Nylon straps also can be used to make a constricting band. The EMT places the band between the heart and the wound. The constricting band is placed about 2 inches from the wound. A small padded board may be placed under the band and above the pulse to concentrate pressure on the artery supplying blood to the distal limb. Once the band is in place, the EMT ties a knot over the artery, places a stick in the middle of the knot, and finishes tying the knot. The stick can then be used like a Spanish windlass; each rotation of the stick will apply pressure to the tourniquet and make it tighter and tighter. When the bleeding has stopped, the ends of the windlass should be tied to the extremity with another cravat.

Once a tourniquet is in place, it should not be loosened or removed without a physician's order. If the tourniquet is prematurely released, blood clots may be liberated from the wound site to float upstream into the core circulation. The exact time that a tourniquet is applied should be noted. In some EMS systems, the practice is to write the time and the initials TK, for tourniquet, on the patient's forehead. Placing a piece of tape next to the tourniquet and noting the time on it is usually sufficient. Marking a tourniquet clearly makes the fact that the patient has a tourniquet more evident.

DRESSINGS

Once bleeding has been controlled, wounds are covered by a dressing that is intended to protect the wound from further injury, while supporting the clotting activity that is going on inside the wound. These dressings should not introduce contamination into the wound; ideally, a sterile dressing should be used. Unfortunately, in the field, maintaining sterility is difficult. However, the EMT should apply the cleanest dressing possible.

Dressings should be furnished in a sterile package, and the EMT should keep the dressing in the original packaging as much as is practical, removing the dressing from the package only while wearing clean gloves. Dressings should never be placed on the ground, on the crew bench, or on any other "dirty" surface. Opening the packaging and laying it flat provides a sterile surface on which to place the dressing. The EMT should lift the dressing by the corners and place it directly on the wound, and then apply pressure over the outside of the dressing. The EMT should never touch the side of the dressing that will lie next to the wound.

TYPES OF DRESSINGS

The most common type of dressing is a cotton weave cloth called a **gauze dressing.** Gauze dressings are remarkably flexible and absorbent. These two features allow gauze dressings to be wrapped around extremity wounds of any size. Gauze dressings also come in a variety of sizes, from the small 2- by 2-inch square (2 × 2) dressings, used for small puncture wounds, to the large trauma dressing. The **trauma dressing,** usually two layers of gauze with an absorbent cotton core, covers the majority of the abdomen, like a blanket.

Some dressings have a non-adherent material over the gauze to prevent the cotton from sticking to dried blood at the site of the wound. Some are self-adherent dressings, which means the dressing sticks to the wound by itself. A Band-Aid is an example of a self-adherent dressing. Others are called occlusive dressings. Occlusive dressings prevent the escape of air and moisture from the wound and are often impregnated with a petroleum gel, such as the Vaseline gauze dressing, or covered with a thin plastic film. Occlusive dressings are useful in several special situations, discussed elsewhere in this book.

The **universal dressing** is a large, 9- by 36-inch dressing with several layers of absorbent cotton inside. The universal dressing can be laid flat and

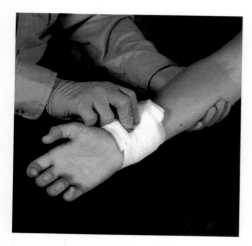

Figure 37.8 A pressure dressing helps to maintain constant pressure over the bleeding

used like an abdominal dressing, or it can be folded into halves or smaller to make a smaller dressing. Universal dressings are practical for mass casualty incidents when the EMT does not know what type or size of injury may be encountered.

Pressure Dressing   When bleeding continues despite direct pressure, a dressing, and elevation, then the EMT should use a pressure dressing. A pressure dressing, in effect, maintains continuous pressure over the wound edges and attempts to compress the surrounding blood vessels. In reality, the best pressure dressing that can be applied is the one that the EMT creates by using a dressing to apply manual pressure to the wound. It is not always practical, however, for an EMT to maintain constant pressure all the way to the hospital and applying a pressure dressing will relieve the EMT of this task.

To create a pressure dressing, the EMT starts by placing a roll of Kling or a roller bandage directly against the dressing over the wound. Then, using either a second roller bandage or cravat, the EMT ties down the rolled bandage firmly and tightly. Often the knot is placed over the wound site to help maintain the added pressure (Figure 37.8).

Street Smart

When an occlusive dressing is needed but is not readily available, the EMT can place a gauze dressing on the wound and wrap the dressing with a thin plastic wrap, the kind used to wrap sandwiches. The combination of plastic wrap and dressing makes an effective occlusive dressing.

Safety Tips

The EMT should consider all blood and body substances as being potentially dangerous and take appropriate protective measures. If there is any chance of arterial bleeding, the EMT needs to wear eye protection and some type of protective apparel, such as a gown. If arterial bleeding is not expected or, more commonly, the bleeding has stopped spontaneously, the EMT can wear just gloves while dressing the wound.

Hemostatic Dressings   Hemostatic agents are powders or substances inserted into wounds directly or impregnated into dressings that contain an agent that promotes clotting. These agents have been used by the military for years. Many treatments now employed by EMS began on the battlefield. **Hemostatic dressings** contain powders or substances that promote blood clotting when placed on an open would. They are another treatment that is gaining popularity in the prehospital setting. A variety of dressings and agents are available (Figure 37.9).

Hemostatic dressings being marketed for use in the prehospital setting are primarily one of two types: ground lava rocks or crustacean shells embedded in a dressing. One hemostatic dressing is a 4 × 4 dressing containing a chitosan (polysaccharide from ground crustacean shells) and vinegar mixture. The dressing has a polyester backing on one side and is glue-like on the other side. When applied to the wound, it creates a seal, like putting a patch on a tire. The chitosan granules are positively charged, attracting the negatively charged red blood cells to form a clot. These hemostatic dressings should be used only for heavy bleeding that is difficult to control, such as from an artery, and they should be used in conjunction with direct pressure. Because of the sticky nature of the dressing, it should be used with caution around the eyes.

Another hemostatic dressing is made from lava rocks ground into granules and either poured directly into the wound or incorporated into bandages.

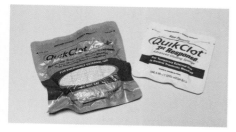

Figure 37.9 Hemostatic agents can be used along with direct pressure for severe hemorrhage to rapidly clot the blood

Some versions also contain antibiotic agents. Like all hemostatic dressings, use should be determined by heavy, hard-to-control bleeding and should always be used in conjunction with direct pressure. Always consult medical control or local protocols concerning the use of hemostatic dressings.

TRANSPORTATION

The priority of the patient's transport is not dictated by the type of bleeding but rather by the presence or absence of hypoperfusion. Therefore, a complete set of vital signs is critically important to the EMT's decision-making process. The EMT should ask, "Is this bleeding life threatening? Is the patient showing signs of hypoperfusion and going into shock?" The answers to these questions will help the EMT to determine the priority and destination of the patient.

TYPES OF WOUNDS

Injuries to the skin can result from either blunt force, like a baseball bat, or from sharp edges, like a knife. Each mechanism of injury leaves a break in the skin called a *wound*. The following is a review of common wounds and the mechanisms that might create them.

ABRASIONS

When the uppermost layer of skin is scraped away, minor capillary bleeding occurs, nerve endings are exposed, and an *abrasion* results. Abrasions are usually the result of the skin on an arm or leg being rubbed against a solid surface (Figure 37.10). If the skin is rubbed against a carpet, for example, an abrasion may result. The rub burn, like a thermal burn, removes the upper layer of skin, and the resulting abrasion is painful.

A fall forward onto outstretched hands can create abrasions on the palms of the hands. A cyclist who is thrown from his bicycle onto the asphalt roadway may acquire an abrasion called a "road rash." A wilderness EMT who slides down a rope bare-handed may develop a "rope burn." In fact, whenever a body in motion contacts a rough surface, an abrasion is a likely outcome.

LACERATIONS

When a large amount of force is applied to a small area of skin, the skin will tear. A skin tear that is the full thickness of the skin is called a *laceration*. Typically, the edge of a laceration is jagged and uneven.

Because a laceration is deep, it can involve veins and arteries, as well as bones. An EMT who observes a laceration should always be concerned about the tissues underneath. For example, a broken bone forced through the skin creates a laceration. Frequently, the bone ends fall back under the skin as the limb returns to its normal anatomic position. The only evidence of this bone injury may be the laceration. If the mechanisms of injury or the patient's symptoms support the possibility of an associated fracture, treatment should be appropriate for that diagnosis and a splint should be applied. Unit 38 details this management.

If the skin is struck with the straight edge of a surface, the laceration will be straight, or **linear.** If the skin is struck with a blunt force, such as the ground, the laceration may take on a starlike, or **stellate,** appearance (Figure 37.11).

INCISIONS

An **incision** is a full-thickness injury of the skin. Unlike a laceration, an incision is usually made by a knife, which goes through the full thickness of the skin. Also unlike a laceration, the wound edges are straight and the surrounding tissue has not been stretched or injured (Figure 37.12). An incision can

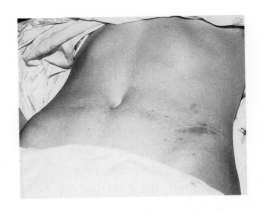

Figure 37.10 An abrasion usually oozes capillary blood (Courtesy of Deborah Funk, MD, Albany Medical Center, Albany, NY)

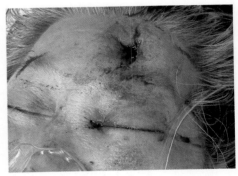

Figure 37.11 A blunt trauma can result in a stellate laceration (Courtesy of Ron Straum, MD, Albany Medical Center, Albany, NY)

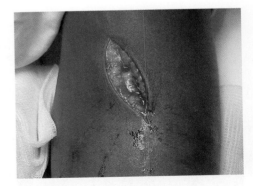

Figure 37.12 The small entrance wound of an incision can be deceptive. A larger area of injury can lie under the skin (Courtesy of Ron Straum, MD, Albany Medical Center, Albany, NY)

interrupt veins and arteries that lie immediately underneath the skin, causing potentially life-threatening bleeding.

PUNCTURES

A *puncture* is an incision made by a sharp, pointed object. The EMT should have the same issues and concerns about a puncture wound as he would have about an incision. The severity of a puncture depends on the depth and the location of the injury. Gunshot wounds (GSWs) are generally considered puncture wounds. Most of the damage done by a GSW is hidden under the skin and is not visible (Figure 37.13). Therefore, all GSWs should be considered serious.

A GSW typically makes an **entrance wound** that appears like a puncture and may leave a much larger **exit wound** as the blast creates an opening in the body. Every effort should be made to find all wounds associated with a GSW. If the weapon was discharged close to the patient, the entrance wound may have black speckles of partially burnt gunpowder on and around it. This phenomenon is called **tattooing.**

AVULSIONS AND AMPUTATIONS

The clean removal of a limb from the body, resulting in a clear line of demarcation, is called an **amputation.** A doctor surgically removes, or amputates, a lifeless extremity from the patient's body when there is no hope of recovery.

The forceful separation of a limb from the body because of trauma is called an **avulsion.** The forceful tearing of the skin leaves the wound margins ragged, and the remaining tissue may appear shredded. An avulsion can be either partial or complete.

EMTs commonly call a complete avulsion an amputation. Although not technically correct, this usage is widely accepted, and the two terms often are used interchangeably.

ASSESSMENT

The first order of business when approaching a patient who is bleeding is to don proper PPE. While gloves may be sufficient for capillary or even venous bleeding, arterial bleeding spurts and can quickly contaminate the EMT's uniform. In the case of suspected arterial bleeding, a gown and goggles are appropriate PPE.

Next, life-threatening arterial bleeding should be controlled. However, in most cases, although the bleeding may look significant, it is not truly life threatening, and the EMT should focus on performing the primary assessment.

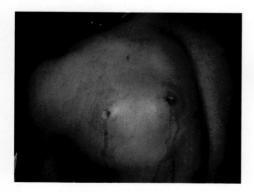

Figure 37.13 A gunshot wound (GSW) is a common puncture wound (Courtesy of Deborah Funk, MD, Albany Medical Center, Albany, NY)

SCENE SIZE-UP

The EMT should always be aware that the mechanism of injury can cause the EMT injury. Therefore, the EMT should identify the mechanism of injury and either render it safe by disabling it or by moving the patient away from the immediate danger to a safe location before proceeding with patient care.

It is fair to assume that if the patient is cut, she also may be bleeding. Standard precautions against blood should be taken by the EMT before approaching the scene. The EMT should carefully evaluate the scene as well as the patient for possible sources of blood contamination.

PRIMARY ASSESSMENT

Initially, the EMT may be absorbed by the gross appearance of the wound; however, he should remember that the external appearance of the wound is only part of the story. What has happened under the skin may be life threatening, and the EMT should focus on assessing for signs of hypoperfusion, such as tachycardia and tachypnea.

RAPID TRAUMA ASSESSMENT

Assuming that no life-threatening injuries have been identified, and deemed as appropriate for the situation, the EMT should proceed with a complete head-to-toe rapid trauma assessment while at the scene. The EMT should focus on the DCAP-BTLS to identify other injuries as well as other bleeding wounds.

MANAGEMENT

Once the bleeding has been controlled, the EMT's next priority in wound management is to protect the wound from further injury as well as contamination by applying a dressing and bandaging the wound.

BANDAGES

The primary purpose of a **bandage** is to hold a dressing in place. Bandages are strips of cloth or similar materials that serve this purpose. A bandage should be clean, but it does not need to be sterile as long as a dressing is against the wound. Bandages can also be used to apply pressure, over the dressing, to the wound site. This additional pressure can help to control bleeding.

A **roller bandage,** a cotton cloth rolled into a cylinder, is wrapped around and around the dressing until the dressing is held in place (Figure 37.14). Most roller bandages are one-headed, meaning that the bandage can be rolled in only one direction. Two-headed roller bandages are sometimes more convenient; they can be rolled in two directions at once, while still maintaining pressure on the dressing.

The military **compress** is a cotton dressing integrated into a two-tailed bandage or cravat (Figure 37.15). One provider can apply the dressing and wrap the bandage around the wound at the same time. Prepackaged for use in combat, these compresses are convenient for use in the field by civilian EMTs as well.

Some roller bandages have elastic fibers woven into the fabric. The result is a flexible, elastic bandage that applies constant pressure to prevent swelling. The Ace bandage is an example of an elastic bandage. Ace bandages are useful when the EMT wants to apply pressure to a wide area, such as an ankle, to prevent further bleeding and swelling.

The alternative to a roller bandage is the **triangular bandage.** The triangular bandage is made by cutting a 36- or 42-inch-square piece of muslin

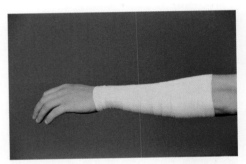

Figure 37.14 A roller bandage has a tail that can be anchored and then wrapped around the extremity

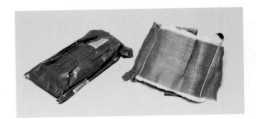

Figure 37.15 A military compress has a dressing integrated into the bandage, making it convenient to use in an emergency

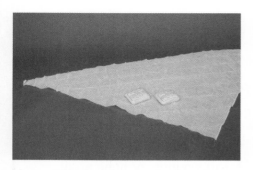

Figure 37.16 A triangular bandage was perhaps the most commonly used in the field before the development of roller gauze

cloth from corner to corner (Figure 37.16). The results are two triangular bandages. Triangular bandages have been used in many ways over the years. The first "Advanced First Aiders" were extensively trained in the application of the triangular bandage to every part of the body. The triangular bandage has fallen out of favor somewhat with EMTs, who prefer the shape-conforming, self-adhering gauze bandages available today.

Sometimes EMTs start at the apex of the triangle and fold the bandage into a strong belt. This belt, called a **cravat,** can be used instead of a roller bandage to tie dressings into place.

The saying "one size fits no one" often applies in EMS; sometimes the EMT must be creative with the application of EMS equipment. A cravat is often used to extend straps or adapt standard equipment, such as splints and backboards, to extremely small people, like children, and to extremely large people.

Although it is not frequently used in the field, an EMT might encounter a 12- to 18-inch-wide and 4-foot-long binder bandage. Binders wrap around the circumference of the patient's chest or abdomen to hold a dressing in place. Some binders are tied in place, whereas others use Velcro fasteners. Binders are usually used when trying to stabilize a large dressing. A large towel, wrapped around the abdomen like a binder, will hold several layers of abdominal dressings in place.

PRINCIPLES OF WOUND BANDAGING

Wounds can occur on the chest, back, on the abdomen, or on the extremities. Wounds can occur along flat skin, like the small of the back, or at joints, like the knees. All of these wounds are dressed somewhat differently. Several fundamental bandaging techniques help to reduce the confusion with wound bandaging. Whether used individually or combined, these bandaging techniques help the EMT to maintain bleeding control by effectively maintaining wound edges in close proximity, while keeping the dressing in place.

RECURRENT BANDAGE

A **recurrent bandage** is useful when the EMT is trying to hold a dressing down over a large area. Using a roller bandage, the EMT starts by anchoring the bandage with either one hand or a wrap around the narrowest portion of the limb. Then the bandage is passed over the dressing and anchored on the opposite side. The roller bandage is then passed back and forth over the dressing. Finally, the two anchors are wrapped securely, and the ends are taped or pinned (Figure 37.17).

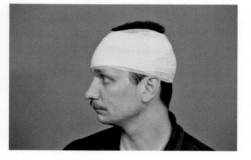

Figure 37.17 A recurrent bandage of the head holds a dressing in place

SPIRAL BANDAGE

Using a roller bandage, the EMT starts by anchoring the bandage, with a wrap, around the narrowest part of the limb. Then the bandage is wound around the limb in a corkscrew fashion. Each wrap should cover about half of the previous wrap to ensure complete coverage of the dressing. When completed, the **spiral bandage** looks like a barber's pole (Figure 37.18).

FIGURE-OF-EIGHT

In a **figure-of-eight,** the roller bandage turns across itself like a figure-of-eight. The end of the bandage is often just "tucked in" to the preceding winds of the bandage. The figure-of-eight is particularly useful for holding dressings on wounds in the joints (Figure 37.19).

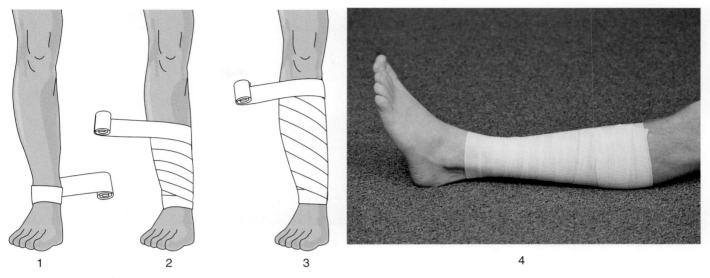

Figure 37.18 A spiral bandage is wrapped around the extremity, like the stripes on a barber's pole

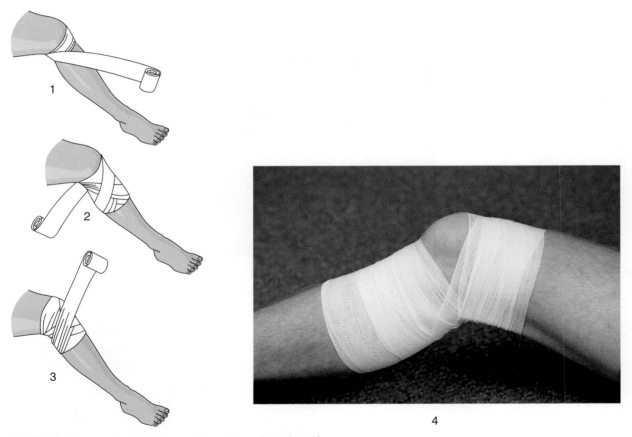

Figure 37.19 A figure-of-eight is anchored against itself

Figures 37.20 through 37.31 demonstrate how these three bandaging techniques are used, individually or in combination, on a large variety of wounds. EMTs are expected to be proficient at wound dressing. The key to success in wound bandaging is practice.

SPECIAL BANDAGES
Some wounds require special or unique bandages. The following is a review of some of those wounds and the bandages that would be used for them.

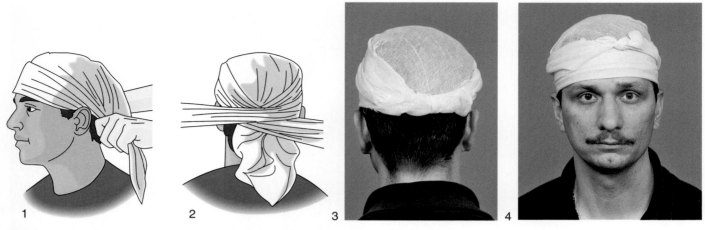

Figure 37.20 A triangular bandage has been applied over a head wound

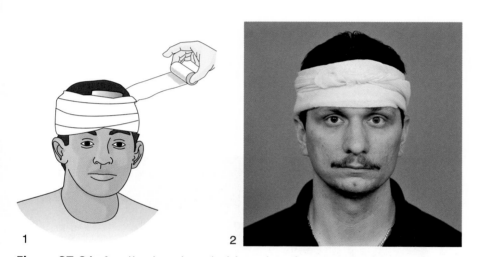

Figure 37.21 A roller bandage holds a dressing on a scalp wound

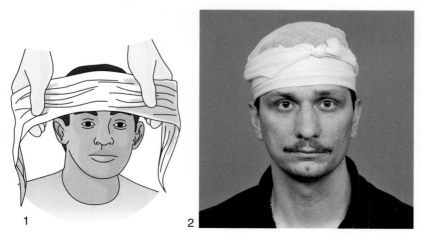

Figure 37.22 A cravat holds a dressing over a forehead wound

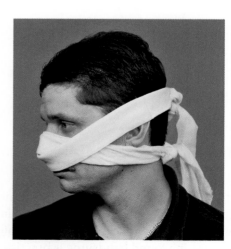

Figure 37.23 A four-tailed dressing created from two triangular bandages holds a dressing under a nose wound

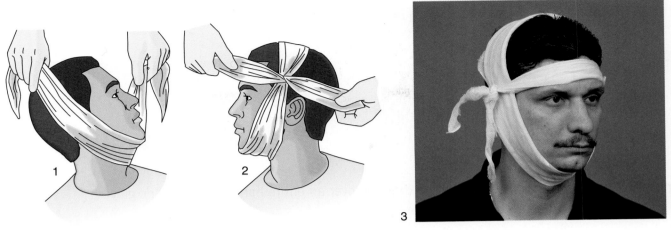

Figure 37.24 The juxtaposition of two cravats holds a dressing onto an ear injury

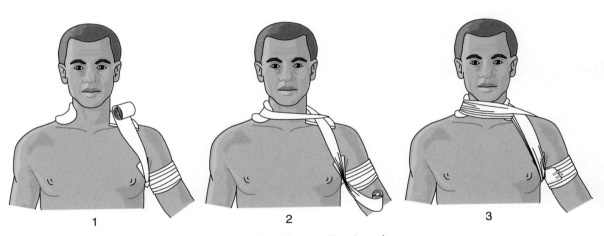

Figure 37.25 An occlusive dressing is held in place by a roller bandage

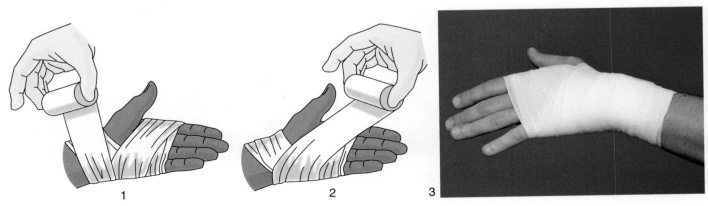

Figure 37.26 A figure-of-eight bandage holds a dressing on a dorsal hand wound

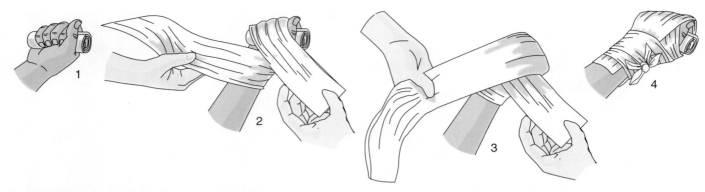

Figure 37.27 A triangular bandage holds a dressing over an entire hand, like a boxer's glove

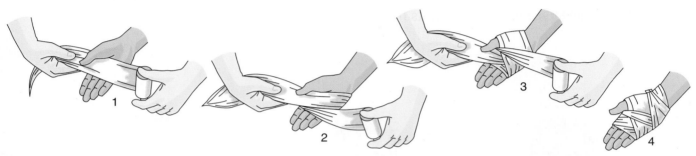

Figure 37.28 A triangular bandage across a palmer injury holds a dressing a place

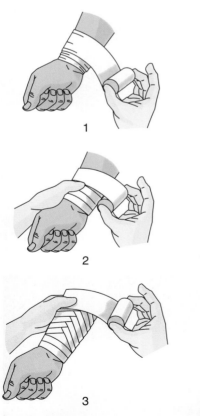

Figure 37.29 A reversed spiral roller bandage holds a dressing in place on a forearm

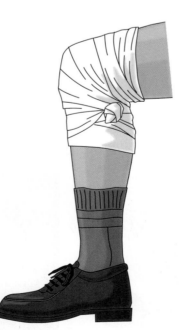

Figure 37.30 A triangular bandage holds a dressing in place on the knee

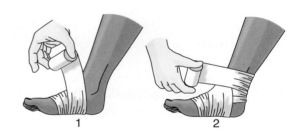

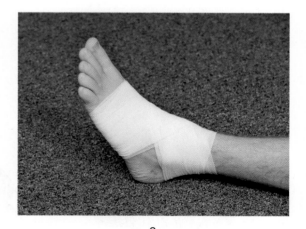

Figure 37.31 A foot wound is bandaged with a spiral roller bandage

Neck Wounds   A deep cut to the throat can lacerate a jugular vein. When the patient takes in a breath, negative pressure, created in the chest cavity, will draw air directly into the neck wound. This air creates a blockage, or **embolism,** that can occlude the vein and interfere with circulation.

To prevent an air embolism, an occlusive dressing must be immediately applied to any neck wound. Often a gloved hand is sufficient until a dressing can be assembled. Once the wound is properly dressed, the patient should be closely monitored for signs of hypoxia.

Sucking Chest Wound   When the chest wall is penetrated, air moves in and out of the wound. This type of wound is called a *sucking chest wound*. Whatever the cause of the injury, it is important to stop air from entering the chest cavity. An occlusive dressing is used for this purpose.

An occlusive dressing is applied, and three sides are taped down while the fourth side is left unattached so that it can operate as a flutter valve. Air that is escaping will lift the fourth side, but air is prevented from entering when the dressing is "sucked" into the wound. More details about a three-sided dressing are provided in Unit 36.

Evisceration   As discussed in Unit 36, an abdominal organ that protrudes through an open abdominal wound is called an *evisceration*. Although an evisceration may be gruesome in appearance, it is rarely immediately life threatening. Associated injuries to deeper internal organs may be more acutely dangerous.

Once any life-threatening conditions have been dealt with, the EMT should turn his attention to the evisceration. The EMT should not attempt to place the tissue back into the abdominal cavity. Any obvious gross contamination, such as glass fragments and the like, should be removed from the wound. The EMT should cover the protruding tissue with a dry, sterile dressing. The large trauma dressing was designed for this purpose. Some EMS authorities advocate the use of a moist dressing to keep the dressing from adhering to the tissue, and other EMS authorities advocate placing a layer of aluminum foil over the entire dressing to help retain heat. The EMT must follow the local medical protocols for the treatment of an evisceration. If the patient does not have any lower extremity injuries, having the patient flex her legs helps to relieve tension on the abdominal wall.

Straddle Injury   While riding a motorcycle, a bicycle, or a horse, the rider may be thrown forward and strike his genitals against a post or other fixed object. The resulting soft tissue injury is called a **straddle injury.** Cuts and injuries to the perineal area or the genitals can bleed profusely. The EMT should place an abdominal dressing or a universal dressing against the perineum first; then, using a cravat, the EMT should create a belt and tie it around the waist. Taking a second triangular bandage, the EMT should place it, apex forward, between the patient's legs. The EMT then secures the three corners of the triangular bandage to the belt/cravat in diaper-like fashion (Figure 37.32). This type of bandage effectively holds the dressing in place and helps to control the bleeding.

Impaled Objects   Any object that is discovered embedded in the patient is called an **impaled object** and should be stabilized in the position in which it is found. It is impossible to determine, in the field, the depth that the object may have penetrated and the internal organs that may have been injured. Therefore, it would be imprudent to remove the object. Rather, careful surgical extraction, with attention to bleeding control, is required; and this can be performed adequately only in the hospital.

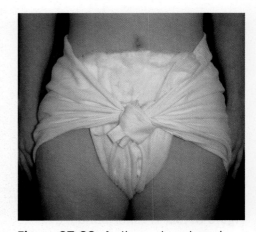

Figure 37.32 A diaper bandage is created to hold a trauma dressing in place in the perineal area

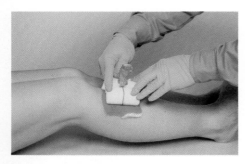

Figure 37.33 Two rolls of gauze can also help to stabilize an impaled object

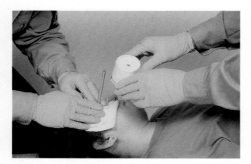

Figure 37.34 A cup helps hold an impaled object into the eye in place

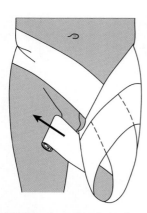

Figure 37.35 A roller bandage is applied to the stump remaining after an amputation, then held in place by a dressing

The EMT should first manually stabilize the object to prevent further tissue injury. Then the EMT should carefully expose the wound by cutting any clothing from around the object. The EMT should be careful not to cut through the hole, if possible. Law enforcement officers may need the clothing, including the intact hole, for evidence.

If copious bleeding is present, it can be controlled by applying direct pressure to both sides of the object at once. The EMT should avoid applying any lateral pressure to the penetrating object, as that could cause further tissue injury.

If the object is still part of a larger assembly—for example, a fence post—the EMT may need to separate the impaled section from the larger assembly. Once the patient and impaled object can be transported safely, the EMT should secure the impaled object with a large bulky bandage. A cravat can be rolled into a ring and placed around some narrow objects. Analogously, two rolls of gauze bandage can be placed on each side of the object to support it, and then a figure-of-eight bandage can be wrapped around the object and the extremity (Figure 37.33). Finally, a column of 4-by 4-inch (4 × 4) gauze pads, cut to the middle, can be stacked around the object to provide support as well as protection. Again, a figure-of-eight bandage is wrapped around the dressing to hold it in place.

If an object, like a pencil, is in the eye, a paper cup may be placed over the eye to stabilize the object (Figure 37.34). The EMT should puncture a hole in the bottom of the paper cup and slide the cup over the object, then tape the cup securely in place. Be sure to bandage both eyes due to sympathetic eye movement.

Avulsions and Amputations   A partially avulsed limb should be reaffixed to its natural position. Areas of the body that are commonly partially avulsed include the nose, toes, ears, fingers, and penis. The flap of skin holding the limb to the body may be supplying vitally needed blood to the avulsed limb.

Although amputations often stop bleeding spontaneously because the blood vessels contract into the stump and stop bleeding, avulsions tend to bleed vigorously because the blood vessels were torn, not cut. The first priority, in every case of amputation or avulsion, is to control the bleeding. Poor control of bleeding by the EMT may lead to life-threatening blood loss. Use of a tourniquet should be considered for avulsions.

The EMT's first action, after stabilizing the cervical spine, is to lay the patient down and elevate the stump above the level of the heart. Raise the long spine board to elevate the stump by placing blanket rolls or other materials under the foot section of the board.

If bleeding persists, the EMT should take a moistened dressing and place it directly against the end of the stump. It is important that the EMT maintain constant pressure on the dressing and not release the dressing. Premature release of a dressing can lead to further, perhaps uncontrollable, blood loss.

Once the bleeding is controlled, several layers of dressings, as well as pressure on a pressure point, may be needed to maintain control. The EMT uses a triangular bandage to secure the dressings in place. First, the EMT places the stump and dressing in the middle of the triangular bandage. The two corners along the base are then wrapped around the stump and tied on the opposite side. The remaining corner, or the apex of the triangular dressing, is then tucked into the band that has been created (Figure 37.35).

The EMT should administer oxygen, as per protocol, and monitor for signs of shock. The hospital should be alerted as soon as possible; surgeons should be on standby for the patient's arrival.

When the amputated part is found, it should be wrapped in moistened sterile gauze and placed in a plastic bag. A moist, but not wet, dressing is created by pouring sterile water over the sterile gauze dressing and then squeezing out the excess water. A moist dressing does not drip water when it is squeezed.

The EMT needs to keep the amputated body part cool, but not cold (Figure 37.36). Contact with ice, for example, can freeze the tissue. Frozen tissue cannot be reimplanted. Ice packs usually provide sufficient cooling.

Amputations of arms, hands, legs, and feet, unlike amputations of digits, are considered serious, and the patient with this type of amputation is high priority. Early notification of the hospital is important.

Degloving Avulsions Certain mechanisms, often high-speed spinning shafts such as the power takeoff on farm equipment, can rip the skin from the bone. When skin is completely torn from the shaft of an arm or leg, the wound is called a **degloving avulsion** (Figure 37.37).

Degloving avulsions should be treated in the same manner as any large wound. Great care should be taken in handling the extremity, as bone fractures often accompany a degloving avulsion.

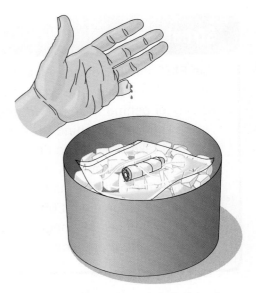

Figure 37.36 An amputated body part should be wrapped in moist gauze, placed in a plastic bag, then placed on an ice pack

TRANSPORTATION

A wound can be very painful; rough handling and even rougher roads can make even the most stoic patient cry out in pain. The EMT should carefully consider whether any true threats to the patient's life exist, based on assessment of the patient's perfusion. Often large wounds appear life threatening but in reality are not. If the patient does not have a life-threatening injury, the EMT should focus on caring for and comforting the patient, including driving carefully to the hospital.

ONGOING ASSESSMENT

All bandages must be carefully monitored. Often a bandage becomes slack and loosens its hold on the dressing. Subsequently, the bleeding may begin again. On the other hand, swelling under the bandage may cause the bandage to act like a tourniquet. If this effect is not desired, the EMT must frequently—every time he takes a set of vital signs, for example—check the distal pulses. If the pulses have become weaker or are absent, the EMT may have to loosen the bandage, after checking the patient's perfusion status.

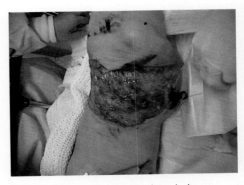

Figure 37.37 A degloving injury is seen most commonly around machinery (Courtesy of Kevin Reilly, MD, Albany Medical Center, Albany, NY)

BRUISING

When a force is distributed over a large area, the skin may remain intact, but bleeding can occur immediately under the skin, in which case a bruise will form. The medical term for a bruise is a *contusion*.

Contusions imply that there is a possibility of damage to deeper tissues and organs. When an EMT discovers a contusion over the right lower ribs, for example, he must suspect injury to the liver. Although an EMT cannot see internal injury, he can have a high index of suspicion that certain organs are injured, based on the location of the contusion.

HEMATOMA

At various points on the body surface, arteries and veins run close to the skin. If a force, from hitting the floor during a fall, for example, impacts on one of these points, the blood vessel can tear. Bleeding can quickly form a swelling under the skin called a **hematoma.** A hematoma on the forehead is often called an "egg" by laypeople. A considerable amount of blood can be lost in a hematoma that is the size of an egg. A hematoma the size of a person's fist can mean that as much as 250 cc of blood has been removed from circulation.

The EMT should not delay transportation of the patient with life-threatening injuries while searching for an amputated part. Life comes before limb. The EMT should transport the patient immediately, leaving personnel behind to search for the amputated part.

Personnel left behind to search for an amputated body part should organize a careful search of the area and take the time to find the amputated part. Snow blowers, chainsaws, and similar gas-powered devices can throw a body part a surprising distance; therefore, the search area should be generous.

When the body part is finally retrieved, it should be packaged and taken to the hospital quickly. Often a law enforcement officer can be enlisted to assist with transporting the body part to the hospital. The hospital should be advised immediately of the recovery and the impending arrival of the body part so that preparations can be made for reimplantation if possible.

CRUSH INJURY

Prolonged pressure on the skin and underlying tissue, from the weight of a body, for example, will eventually cut off circulation, compromise nerve function, and cause the tissue to die or become **necrotic.** The result of this sustained pressure is called a **crush injury.**

When tissues are crushed, they release toxic chemicals, including acids, from within the cells into the surrounding tissues and into the bloodstream. Some of these chemicals are toxic to the body, especially to the kidneys. Often these chemicals can cause kidney failure hours or days after a crush injury.

The body's chemistry changes when large amounts of acid are washed out from a crushed limb. The increased amount of acid in the blood, or acidosis, irritates the heart. If the heart becomes too irritated, it can go into ventricular fibrillation and cause sudden cardiac death.

COMPARTMENT SYNDROME

Muscles are enclosed and divided by thin sheets of fibrous tissue, called *fascia*, into individual compartments. If a limb is crushed under a large weight for a prolonged period, such as may occur in a cave-in, swelling within these muscular compartments results. As the swelling steadily worsens, the pressure within these compartments increases and compresses nerves and blood vessels. The result of compressed nerves and blood vessels is a loss of feeling, called *paresthesia*; a loss of motion, called *paralysis*; and a loss of circulation, or *pulselessness*. Together these three signs—paresthesia, paralysis, and pulselessness—indicate that the patient is experiencing **compartment syndrome.** Table 37-1 lists the mechanisms of injury that may result in compartment syndrome.

Compartment syndrome is a true surgical emergency. Treatment for compartment syndrome includes cutting through the skin and into the fascia to relieve the pressure. This surgical procedure is called a **fasciotomy.** In the field, treatment of the affected extremity includes splinting and transportation to the closest appropriate facility. En route to the hospital, the EMT also treats the patient for hypoperfusion.

ASSESSMENT

A contusion is slow bleeding under the skin. A visible bruise under the skin may take up to an hour to form. Therefore, an EMT must depend on other signs of injury to predict bleeding into soft tissues. Some of those signs include

Table 37-1 Mechanisms of Crush Injury/Compartment Syndrome

1. Prolonged immobilization
   Falls
   Alcohol
   Drug overdose
   Stroke
   Broken hip

2. Entrapment
   Building collapse
   Mud slides
   Trench collapse

3. Prolonged extrication
   Airplane crash
   Extensive driver compartment intrusion
   Vehicle rollover
   Entrapment under vehicle

abrasion marks, left by a seat belt, for example, and localized swelling. As the bleeding continues and the contusion enlarges, blood fills the spaces between the tissues, making the soft tissue feel denser. Using the uninjured limb for comparison, the EMT will note that a contused limb is slightly larger, asymmetrical, and firmer to the touch than the other limb.

This assessment is important. Bleeding into the thigh from a femur fracture, for example, can be serious. One liter of blood can be lost in each thigh. Similarly, bleeding from a pelvic fracture can be life threatening.

Bleeding from ruptured capillaries also may produce a large, irregularly shaped pool of blood under the skin that is larger than the margins of the point of contact. This skin injury is called **ecchymosis** (Figure 37.38). These areas of ecchymosis, like contusions, have a bluish tinge from the deoxygenated blood under the skin. Over time, the ecchymosis will turn black as the blood coagulates. (This is the origin of the term *black and blue* in reference to contusions.) Finally, a couple of weeks later, the ecchymosis will appear greenish-brown or yellow as the clot dissolves and the skin heals.

SCENE SIZE-UP

A confined space rescue is, by definition, a technical rescue that requires specialized equipment and specialized training. In many cases, however, the rescue team either consists of EMTs or is supported by a team of EMTs who can care for the patient once the rescue has been achieved.

An untrained and unequipped EMT should never enter into a potentially lethal confined space rescue. Instead, the EMT should stage in a convenient location that is proximal to the scene and observe the rescue, while asking, "What injuries could the patient have sustained?"

Confined space rescue is frequently a high-interest event, and onlookers tend to swarm around the rescuers. The incident commander ensures that an adequate perimeter is established, but every EMT is responsible for maintaining that perimeter, ever mindful of the dangers on the scene to onlookers.

PRIMARY ASSESSMENT

The priorities in a confined space rescue are the same as those used in other trauma cases. Patients who experience trauma need spinal immobilization and rapid primary assessment. The EMT needs to assess and treat any life-threatening injuries that the patient may have developed while entrapped and also should be mindful that hypothermia often occurs in these situations. The injury to the patient may not be clearly evident initially, so the EMT must be prepared to reassess the patient immediately if conditions change.

RAPID TRAUMA ASSESSMENT

It is critically important that the EMT completely assess the patient. No skin surface should remain untouched; every minor defect should be noted. A small hard area on the thigh may later turn into a large, swollen deformity.

MANAGEMENT

The management of the patient centers on the ABCs (airway, breathing, circulation) of the primary assessment and the provision of advanced life support (ALS). The EMT should ensure that the patient is cared for by an advanced EMT as soon as possible. As most of the injuries are internal, the patient should be promptly packaged for transportation. The EMT should spend little time at the scene trying to immobilize potential fractures; instead, the patient's entire body should be splinted on a backboard, and the patient transported immediately.

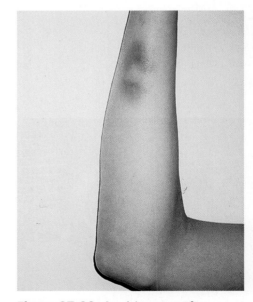

Figure 37.38 A wide area of capillary bleeding under the skin is called an ecchymosis

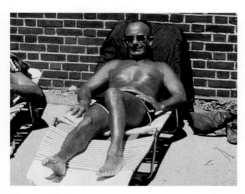

Figure 37.39 Sunburn is an example of a superficial burn (Courtesy of Phoenix Society for Burn Survivors, Inc)

TRANSPORTATION

These patients should be transported to a trauma center, where the patient's internal injuries can be properly assessed and treated. The decision of where and how to transport the patient should be made in compliance with local protocols as well as consultation with medical control.

ONGOING ASSESSMENT

The EMT should be prepared for the possibility of the patient going into shock. Repeated assessment of the vital signs, at least every 5–10 minutes, and continued assessment for hypoperfusion will ensure that the EMT identifies the impending shock and reacts correctly.

BURNS

Two million Americans suffer burn injuries annually. These burns result in more than 100,000 hospitalizations and approximately 8,000 deaths. Although the median age of a burn victim is 22 years old, those most in danger of dying are the elderly and the extremely young.

Over the short term, burns are painful and potentially life threatening. Over the long term, burns can be physically disfiguring and psychologically damaging. Prompt intervention by an EMT can decrease the patient's pain and suffering and increase the patient's chances of a full recovery.

There are four sources of burns. The majority of burns are caused by thermal energy or flame. Electrical burns, chemical burns, and radiation burns, however, make up a significant percentage of burns as well.

BURN TRAUMA

Open flame can be a source of a burn. A child pulling a pot of scalding hot water off the stove will be burned. Prolonged contact with a house radiator will create a burn. Superheated steam from a car radiator can cause a burn. There are numerous sources of burn injury. They all have the same impact, the destruction of the skin.

The skin provides protection against infections as well as protection and insulation of the body from the environment. The skin aids in the regulation of body temperature. Without skin, the patient is at risk for infection and hypothermia.

CLASSIFICATIONS OF BURN INJURY

Skin can be divided into three layers. The topmost, or superficial, layer is called the epidermis. The epidermis is largely dead cells that act as a barrier between the outside world and internal organs of the body. The middle layer, the dermis, contains live skin cells as well as nerve endings. Just below the dermis is the subcutaneous layer. The subcutaneous layer contains muscles, fat, and some shallow veins visible through the skin. For a more detailed description of the skin, refer to Unit 5.

Burns also can be divided into three classifications, each according to the layer of skin involved. A burn to the topmost, or epidermal, layer is called a **superficial burn** (first degree). Because most of the epidermis is dead, little physical damage is done. However, nerve endings just under the epidermis make the reddened skin feel very painful. Sunburn is a classic example of a superficial burn (Figure 37.39).

A **partial-thickness burn** (second degree) involves the dermal layer. Burn injury to the tissue causes swelling, blister formation on the surface, and vasodilation, which causes the skin to appear flushed (Figure 37.40). Severe scalds create a partial-thickness burn. The danger of secondary infections is greater in a partial-thickness burn than a superficial burn.

A **full-thickness burn** (third degree) involves all the layers of skin. The greatest risk presented by a full-thickness burn is the loss of the body's protective barrier. The skin acts as a barrier to keep bacteria out of the body and bodily fluids in the body. When the skin is no longer able to protect the patient from external contamination by bacteria, the patient is at risk for massive life-threatening infections that can lead to septic shock and death. When the skin can no longer keep bodily fluids from leaking out of the body, the patient is at risk for massive fluid loss, which can lead to hypoperfusion, hypovolemic shock, and death.

These consequences of burns, however, are seldom seen in the field. It takes days for an infection to set in or for a sufficient amount of body fluid loss to cause hypoperfusion. The more immediately pressing problems that occur along with the burn, such as inhalation of superheated air, are usually the cause of immediate death in the field.

With a full-thickness burn, nerve endings are all destroyed, creating a so-called *painless* burn. Muscle and fat also are destroyed, resulting in reduced movement and function in the affected area. The surface of a full-thickness burn quickly becomes hardened, inelastic, and almost leather-like and appears black, like charcoal and burnt (Figure 37.41).

BURN SEVERITY

A significant burn seldom has just one type of burn. A large area of superficial burn may be combined with areas of partial-thickness burn. Alternatively, an area of full-thickness burn, at a point of contact, may have concentric rings of partial-thickness burn around it.

A formula for estimating the percentage of burns over the body surface area has been developed. Called the **rule of nines**, the formula provides the EMT with a quick percentage of burn area. In an adult, each arm represents 9%, the head 9%, each leg 18%, the upper back and lower back together 18%, and the chest and abdomen together 18%. There are 11 areas that, when totaled, equal 99%. Refer to Figure 37.42 for a representation of all 11 areas in the rule of nines. The remaining 1% is assigned to the genitals.

The rule of nines is useful for large burns but is difficult to use with small burns or with burns that are spread across the body. A splash pattern from a scald injury can leave multiple small burns, for example. In those cases, the **palmar method** is more accurate. The palm of the patient's hand is estimated to be about 1% of the patient's body surface area. Therefore, the EMT can use the patient's palm to estimate the total percent of burn trauma.

CRITICAL BURNS

Patients with full- and/or partial-thickness burns benefit from the specialized burn care they would receive at a burn center. These patients, who are said to have critical burns, should be transported, by air or by ground, to the closest burn center. The EMT should refer to local protocol for guidance with this decision while in the field.

A full-thickness burn or a partial-thickness burn that is 10% or greater is considered to be critical.

Certain burns, regardless of area of body surface involved, are considered critical. A patient with such burns should be considered high priority, and transportation to a burn center should be considered.

Burns to the face are always considered critical. Burns of the upper or lower airway are one of the major causes of death from burns. If the patient experiences

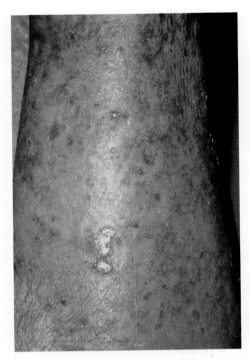

Figure 37.40 Blisters are the hallmark of a partial-thickness burn (Courtesy of Phoenix Society for Burn Survivors, Inc)

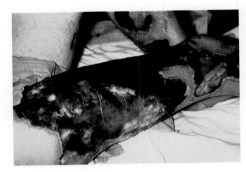

Figure 37.41 Full-thickness burns are frequently painless (Courtesy of Phoenix Society for Burn Survivors, Inc)

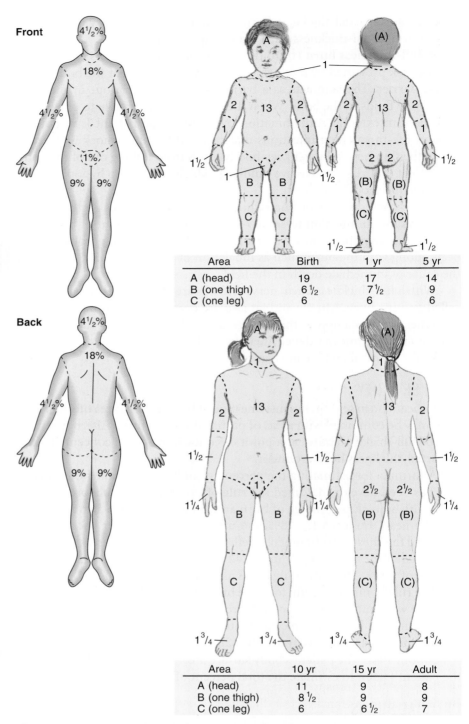

Area	Birth	1 yr	5 yr
A (head)	19	17	14
B (one thigh)	6 1/2	7 1/2	9
C (one leg)	6	6	6

Area	10 yr	15 yr	Adult
A (head)	11	9	8
B (one thigh)	8 1/2	9	9
C (one leg)	6	6 1/2	7

Figure 37.42 The rule of nines is used to estimate the percentage of body surface area burned

a loss of the airway in the field, immediate transportation to the closest facility, or ALS intercept, takes priority over transportation to the burn center.

Burns of the hands or feet also are considered critical. Burns of the hands or feet have significant long-term ramifications to the patient's productivity and quality of life. Similarly, burns to the genitals also are considered critical burns.

Table 37-2 lists the classification of patients with critical burns who may benefit from burn center management. Patients with critical burns should be

Table 37-2 Burn Unit Referral Criteria

A burn unit may treat adults or children or both.

Burn injuries that should be referred to a burn unit include the following:

1. Partial-thickness burns greater than 10% total body surface area (TBSA)

2. Burns that involve the face, hands, feet, genitalia, perineum, or major joints

3. Third-degree burns in any age-group

4. Electrical burns

5. Chemical burns

6. Inhalation injury

7. Burn injury in patients with preexisting medical disorders that could complicate management, prolong recovery, or affect mortality

8. Any patients with burns and concomitant trauma (such as fractures) in which the burn injury poses the greatest risk for morbidity or mortality. In such cases, if the trauma poses the greater immediate risk, the patient may be initially stabilized in a trauma center before being transferred to a burn unit. Physician judgment will be necessary in such situations and should be in concert with the regional medical control plan and triage protocols.

9. Burned children in hospitals without qualified personnel or equipment for the care of children

10. Burn injury in patients who will require special social, emotional, or long-term rehabilitative intervention

Source: Committee on Trauma, American College of Surgeons, Guidelines for the Operations of Burn Units, Resources for Optimal Care of the Injured Patient: 1999, 1998, 55.

transported to a burn center whenever possible. Local protocols may dictate that the patient be transported to a local hospital or regional trauma center, stabilized, and then transferred to the burn center.

ASSESSMENT

The assessment of the burn patient in many ways is no different from the assessment of any trauma patient. Yet, fires create special issues that are not typically seen with other trauma patients. For example, carbon monoxide poisoning makes the task of providing oxygen to these patients problematic. Still, the EMT should focus on the basics and care for the patient as if she were any other trauma patient.

SCENE SIZE-UP

The fire scene is inherently dangerous. The EMT must carefully assess the scene to ensure that an enlarging fire does not pose a hazard to the rescuers. Consideration must be rapidly given to the nature of the trauma and the ultimate destination to which the patient will travel. Early requests for assistance by an aeromedical mission, for example, can literally save a patient's life.

PRIMARY ASSESSMENT

Burns of the face are considered critical. Although the eyes and appearance are important, the loss of the upper airway can be fatal. The EMT must assess all facial burns for involvement of the airway. Singed nose hairs, circumferential burns of the mouth, and soot in the sputum are all signs of potential burns to the upper airway.

The EMT should examine the inside of the mouth, the oropharynx, for swelling. A hoarse voice may also indicate burns to the upper airway. Then the EMT should listen to the breathing by putting the stethoscope on the patient's throat. A narrowed airway in the throat makes a low-pitched inspiratory sound called *stridor*. Stridor that can be heard without the aid of a stethoscope indicates an airway about to close. Any audible stridor is a dangerous sign, and the patient should be transported immediately.

The EMT also should listen to, or auscultate, the lungs with the stethoscope at the apices of the lungs. Wheezes indicate narrowed airways, possibly secondary to inhalation of toxic or superheated gases.

RAPID TRAUMA ASSESSMENT

The burn trauma patient must have a complete head-to-toe examination. The intense pain from the burn may divert the patient's attention away from other more life-threatening injuries. The EMT must be aware that a burn is a distracting injury. He will have to depend on his assessment skills, and not the patient's responses, to discover other injuries.

MANAGEMENT

The EMT's first priority is to stop the burning. Smoldering clothing, grease, wax, and tarlike substances can continue to burn the skin long after the fire is out. The EMT should cool the area with sterile water and wash away excess debris, but should not attempt to remove material that is stuck to the wound. The EMT should then expose the burned area and examine the wounds, taking care not to break any blisters that have formed. Remove any jewelry the patient is wearing as the area around the burn will swell.

BURN FIELD DRESSING

The EMT should ensure that appropriate burn dressings or sheets are available. Universal dressings or burn sheets work well for large areas. Roller gauze works well for extremities. The EMT should never apply ointments or antiseptic lotions to either the bandages or the patient. If hands or feet are involved, the digits need to be separated with gauze dressings. Most medical authorities advocate dry dressings for all burn patients. Follow local medical protocols regarding proper burn care.

If the burn involves less than 10% of the body surface area and local protocols allow it, a wet dressing may be used. The EMT wets a gauze dressing, a 4 × 4, for example, with sterile water. After squeezing out excess water while the dressing is in the wrapper, the EMT then lifts the dressing by one corner and places the moist dressing(s) on the wound (Figure 37.43). Then the EMT wraps the dressing with a dry sterile bandage. Follow local protocols or medical control directions concerning the use of moist dressings on minor burns.

If the burn involves more than 10% of the body surface area, the EMT should apply dry sterile dressings only (Figure 37.44). Dry dressings have been used for major burns since 1957, when the American Red Cross first aid manual advocated dry dressings for major burns.

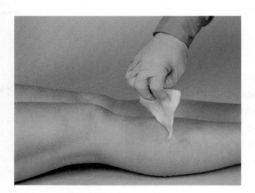

Figure 37.43 A wet dressing can be applied to a small burn

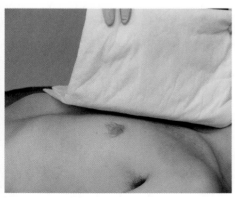

Figure 37.44 A dry sterile dressing should be applied to a large burn

Burn patients represent a challenge to the EMT. Beyond issues of wound management, the EMT is subjected to human disfigurement and witnesses much pain and suffering. Many EMTs complain of nightmares after a call to a burn patient. A call for a burn victim may be one of the most stressful calls in an EMT's career.

Critical incident stress debriefing (CISD) can help EMTs to deal with concerns and issues around the call. CISD can help prevent post-traumatic stress disorders.

Many plastics, acrylics, and compounds release carbon monoxide, cyanide, and other potentially lethal toxins when burned. Every patient suspected of smoke inhalation should be carefully monitored and transported for medical evaluation. Many of these patients will not manifest symptoms of poisoning on the scene. The EMT should contact medical control and ask for further instructions on how to proceed with patient care.

Hypothermia is a significant hazard to a major burn patient. Without skin, the body's heat escapes rapidly. The use of wet dressings only contributes to heat loss and hypothermia. Therefore, the EMT should minimize wet dressings, cover the patient, and use passive warming methods to treat the hypothermia.

TRANSPORTATION

Patients with critical burns should be transported to the closest appropriate facility. Specialized burn centers have specially trained physicians and special equipment to properly treat the critical burn patient. Air medical evacuation, in the field or from a local designated hospital's landing zone (LZ), provides rapid transportation to these regional burn centers.

CHEMICAL BURNS

Mishandling of chemicals and failure to wear proper protective apparel are frequent causes of chemical burns. Chemical burns can result from direct contact with strong acids or strong alkalis or from exposure to fumes. The injuries from chemical burns are similar to those from thermal burns. Chemical reactions between the skin and the acid/alkali can create heat as well. The depth of the burn is dependent on the amount of chemical spilled and the length of time that the chemical remains in contact with the skin. Removing the chemical from the skin quickly reduces the depth and percentage of burn.

SCENE SIZE-UP

By definition, a chemical spill is a hazardous materials incident. Specially trained personnel must respond to the spill. Routine protective equipment used by EMTs will not provide the level of protection needed. Further details regarding hazardous materials response are provided in Unit 50.

The hazardous materials team delivers the patient to the EMT in a safe area, called the **cold zone,** at the end of a decontamination corridor. The EMT should be wearing protective apparel, including gloves, mask, an impenetrable gown, and eye protection.

A victim of a very small chemical spill may be treated by an EMT, but caution is advised; the EMT should wear, at a minimum, eye protection and gloves. First the EMT removes the patient from the immediate vicinity of the spill and then treats the patient according to guidelines. If the EMT has any doubt about procedures, he should call the hazardous materials spill response team. Unless an EMT is trained for a hazardous materials incident, he should alert the appropriate authorities and remain out of immediate danger. Table 37-3 outlines some chemicals related to minor hazardous materials injuries.

Although it is important to remove clothing from a burn patient, the EMT must keep the patient's dignity in mind. Even a semiconscious patient realizes that she is being disrobed. The EMT should explain to the patient what he is doing and why, and cover the patient immediately after the assessment. A simple pillowcase over the groin, or a clean sheet over the body, can be a tremendous source of comfort to the patient.

Table 37-3 Minor Chemical Spills

Chemical	Source
Hydrochloric acid	Exploded battery
Lime	Dry cement
OCR	Pepper spray
Organophosphate	Garden fertilizers
CN/CS gas	Mace
Dry chemical	Fire extinguisher

PRIMARY ASSESSMENT

The primary assessment of the patient should focus on injuries to the airway and difficulty with breathing that could be life threatening. Seldom is there a problem of circulation and perfusion in these cases.

MANAGEMENT

Although there are literally thousands of types of chemicals, treatments for chemical burns are relatively similar. Once the patient has been decontaminated, basic medical care can begin. The first task is to identify the offending chemical. If a label is visible, the EMT can read the instructions on the label. If the patient is inside a storage or manufacturing facility, the EMT can refer to the **Material Safety Data Sheet (MSDS).** Federal safety regulations from the Occupational Safety and Health Administration (OSHA) require that employers keep copies of the MSDS readily available in case of emergency. The MSDS contains information about specific chemicals and how to treat an accidental exposure (Figure 37.45).

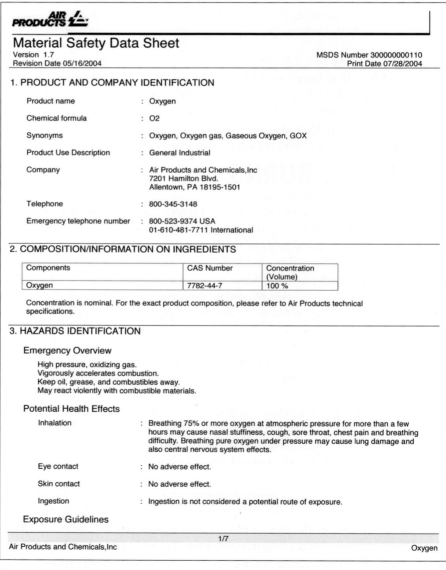

Figure 37.45 The Material Data Safety Sheet (MSDS) contains a great deal of information important to an EMT (Courtesy of Air Products and Chemicals, Inc)

If the patient is transporting the chemical at the time of exposure, the shipping papers, called the *manifest*, will list the name of the chemical(s). If the manifest is not available, the EMT should look for a diamond-shaped placard on the side of the truck and record the number on the placard. Then, using the **Emergency Response Guidebook (ERG),** a free publication of the federal Department of Transportation (DOT) that is available to all emergency response agencies, the EMT can cross-reference the chemical's number, or name, to the guide number (Figure 37.46). The guide provides detailed instructions on how to handle a chemical spill, including first aid.

If the hazardous materials (chemicals) that the patient is exposed to are being transported by air, rail, or road, it may be helpful to call CHEMTREC. CHEMTREC is a 24-hour emergency telephone number created by the American Chemistry Council (formerly known as the Chemical Manufacturers Association) that provides information on the materials and substances manufacturers have in transit to firefighters, EMS, and other emergency responders. The information provided includes first aid procedures in the event of accidental exposure. The toll-free number for CHEMTREC is 800-424-9300.

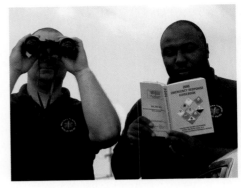

Figure 37.46 The Emergency Response Guidebook provides the EMT initial instructions at a hazardous materials incident

DRY CHEMICALS

Typically, dry chemicals have to be brushed off the patient, and clothing has to be removed before decontamination may begin (Figure 37.47). The EMT must, at a minimum, wear a dust/mist mask. Dry chemicals can become airborne and enter the EMT's airway. The EMT should flush the chemicals off the patient with copious amounts of water only if the MSDS, ERG, or similar authority indicates that this is the correct procedure. Some dry chemicals must be neutralized with oils or other substances. Other dry chemicals can react violently upon contact with water.

WET CHEMICALS

Typically, wet chemicals have to be washed off the patient after the patient's clothing has been removed. The EMT must wear a gown and eye protection. Splash from the patient can make the EMT a secondary victim.

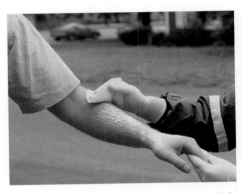

Figure 37.47 Dry chemicals should be brushed off first, then large volumes of water used to rinse the residue off the patient

The EMT should monitor the patient constantly when flushing chemicals off a patient as indicated by the MSDS, ERG, or other hazardous materials information source, using copious amounts of water. Although many experts advocate 20–30 minutes of flushing, continuous irrigation for as long as possible is preferred. Transportation should begin within 20 minutes, with continuous irrigation while en route.

A gentle irrigation is preferred to a forceful jet. Burned tissues are delicate, and further injury can occur when streams of water are used. The EMT should monitor the patient for hypothermia. The treatment of the mildly hypothermic patient is discussed further in Unit 39.

The EMT should carefully control runoff. If the patient is lying in a pool of runoff, she may experience secondary burns to her back and buttocks. The EMT needs to position the patient so that runoff does not flow into the patient's uninjured body areas.

EYE INJURY

Chemical burns to the eyes can be particularly distressing to the patient. The EMT needs to begin irrigation of the eyes, if indicated, as soon as possible. Irrigating an eye is difficult. The eye's protective reflexes want to close the eyelids. Often another EMT has to help keep the patient's eye open. Once the patient's eye is open, the EMT should keep the irrigation stream running continuously. Eventually, the eye becomes desensitized and will stay open on its own.

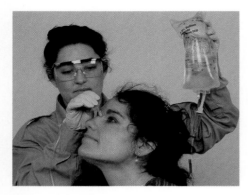

Figure 37.48 IV solution can be used to provide continuous eye irrigation

Street Smart

While awaiting the arrival of a hazardous materials team, the EMT should start the decontamination process. The EMT begins by having the patient remove all clothing. Spilled chemicals held in underwear material or against the skin by elastic bands will continue to burn. The patient needs to remove all watches, rings, and any other jewelry that could react with the chemical(s).

Following the instructions on the Material Safety Data Sheet or in the Emergency Response Guidebook, the EMT should encourage the patient to self-decontaminate. Garden hoses, emergency showers, and sinks all provide readily available water. If limited resources are available, the EMT should have the patient concentrate on decontaminating the eyes first.

A simple IV solution and tubing setup allows the EMT to irrigate one eye continuously for 20–30 minutes (Figure 37.48). The EMT must ensure that the drainage is running away from the unaffected eye. If both eyes need irrigation, the EMT can use an IV setup attached to a nasal cannula. The nasal prongs can be directed into each eye, and the drainage will be away from the other eye. Once both eyes have been sufficiently irrigated or the irrigation solution is gone, the EMT should bandage both eyes and notify the hospital early.

Once the patient has been properly decontaminated, the EMT's attention should turn to a complete assessment. Frequently, the chemicals on the skin are absorbed by the patient's body. The result is that the patient is poisoned as well as contaminated.

The EMT should monitor the patient's level of consciousness. Early contact with medical control can provide the EMT with much-needed instruction. All patients are routinely administered high-concentration oxygen. The EMT should complete a detailed physical examination, concentrating on hidden or concealed chemical burns in the folds of the skin. The pain from the burning chemicals may mask other injuries the patient has sustained. The EMT must be alert to the possibility of concurrent injury from falls, explosions, and fire. The EMT may need to protect the patient's spine, using a backboard and cervical immobilization device.

The EMT should cover any burned areas with a dressing, keep the patient warm, and transport the patient to an appropriate facility. The hospital needs early notification of a potential hazardous materials exposure. Early notification allows the hospital time to prepare for the patient and prevents secondary contamination of the emergency department.

ELECTRICAL BURNS

For electricity to pass through an object, or make a **current,** there must be a source and a ground. The source can be a high-powered electric line from a power pole. Ordinary house current, however, is sufficient to kill or injure a patient.

Some materials allow electricity to pass through them without any resistance. These materials are **conductors.** Water is an excellent conductor of electricity. Materials that resist the flow of electricity are called **insulators.** Skin and bones are excellent insulators. When electricity meets resistance in an insulator, heat energy is the by-product.

Finding a break in the skin, the electricity enters the body through an entrance wound. The electricity then flows through the path of least resistance toward a ground (Figure 37.49). The bloodstream offers the least resistance to electrical current. Therefore, electricity generally follows the blood vessels, looking for a ground.

Eventually electricity finds a ground. Once enough energy accumulates to overcome the resistance of the skin, the electricity literally explodes out of the body. This explosion creates an exit wound. Some exit wounds can be very deep, exposing bones and tendons.

SCENE SIZE-UP

Utility poles represent a serious hazard to all emergency responders. They line many of America's highways and are frequently involved during motor vehicle collisions. Some poles are broken, or even sheared off, at the base, and the only thing holding them is the power line. An average utility pole weighs between 800 and 1,200 pounds. That weight can quickly overcome the tensile strength of the power line.

Utility poles may drop power lines onto the ground. If the wire strikes the road surface, the asphalt may act as an insulator, preventing breakers

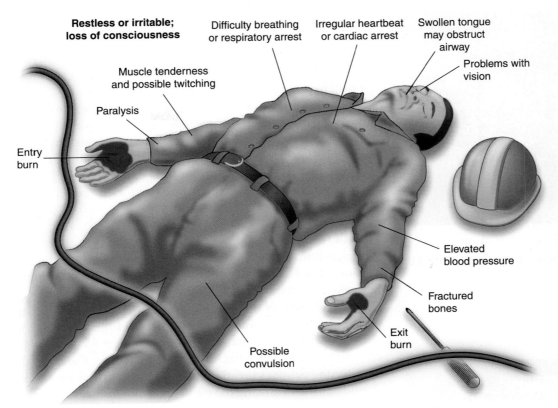

Figure 37.49 An electrical shock can cause a large number of injuries inside the body

Labels in figure:
- Restless or irritable; loss of consciousness
- Difficulty breathing or respiratory arrest
- Irregular heartbeat or cardiac arrest
- Swollen tongue may obstruct airway
- Problems with vision
- Muscle tenderness and possible twitching
- Paralysis
- Entry burn
- Elevated blood pressure
- Fractured bones
- Exit burn
- Possible convulsion

down the line from tripping and keeping the line energized. If the line falls across a guy wire, or a telephone line, it may energize those as well. The EMT should consider that all downed utility pole lines are dangerous until proven otherwise.

Many planned housing developments bury power lines underground. Often the only visible sign of a buried cable is the green splice box. Many homeowners conceal these splice boxes behind low bushes and shrubbery. When a motor vehicle travels across the lawn, it can come to rest on top of a splice box. The vehicle may become energized. Always look under, as well as above, a vehicle for electrical dangers.

Although a power line may appear to have insulation around it, the wrap on the line is primarily intended to prevent corrosion. An EMT should never touch a downed line or attempt to remove a charged power line with blocks and rope, "hot sticks," or any other apparatus. Instead, the EMT should call for assistance from the power company, have the fire department on scene, and leave the removal of power lines for the experts.

ASSESSMENT

Injuries from an electrical shock can be compared to an iceberg. While the tip of the iceberg is visible, the majority of the iceberg is under the surface. Similarly, the entrance wound can be small, but the internal damage created by the heat energy can be substantial.

The single most important factor in determining the degree of electrical burn injury is the duration of contact. At about 1.1 milliamperes (mA), the patient starts to feel an uncomfortable tingling. If the patient is holding the source, a wire, for example, she usually drops the wire immediately.

Street Smart

When the entire body is immersed in a conductive medium, such as a bathtub full of water, and a source, such as a hairdryer, is introduced, there may not be any entrance or exit wounds.

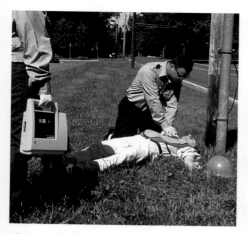

Figure 37.50 A heart stunned by an electrical shock may respond to CPR

When the energy increases to about 15 mA, the alternating current of the electricity paralyzes the patient, preventing her from dropping the wire. This is called the *let-go energy threshold*. Below that energy level, the patient can let go of the source, but above that energy level, the patient's muscles spasm and the patient is "frozen" to the electric source.

When a patient is unable to let go of the source, the electricity has ample time to create tremendous internal injuries. Frequently the diaphragm, the muscle that controls breathing, becomes paralyzed and the patient stops breathing. If the current continues to pass through the patient, the heart may fibrillate, and the patient may suffer a cardiac arrest. If the current stops, because of a circuit-breaker trip, for example, the patient may have a chance for recovery.

MANAGEMENT

Electrical burns should be treated like any trauma, starting with spinal precautions. The EMT should immediately check the ABCs and start cardiopulmonary resuscitation (CPR) as needed. The heart, stunned by the electrical shock, may respond quickly to CPR (Figure 37.50). Defibrillation should be performed, using an automated external defibrillator (AED), as indicated.

If the patient is breathing adequately, the EMT can administer high-concentration oxygen via a non-rebreather mask. The EMT should carefully monitor the patient's breathing. If the patient's breathing is erratic, the EMT should consider assisting the patient's ventilation with a bag-valve-mask. All entrance and exit wounds should be covered, and the electrical burns treated in the same manner as thermal burns.

All patients suffering an electrical shock require rapid transportation and evaluation by an emergency physician. The EMT should attempt to ascertain and report the energy (amperes and volts) encountered as well as the duration of the contact.

TRANSPORTATION

All electrical burns can create potentially serious internal injuries. Some EMS systems routinely transport all electrical burn patients to the regional burn or trauma center. The EMT should always refer to and follow local protocols.

ONGOING ASSESSMENT

The heart of the patient who has suffered an electrical shock can be very irritable, occasionally resulting in a "skipped beat." The EMT should constantly monitor the patient's pulse, particularly its rhythm, for these skipped beats and report them to either an ALS provider or the hospital staff. In rare circumstances, the heart may stop beating, and the patient may go into cardiac arrest. If this occurs, the EMT should follow standard cardiac arrest protocols. Nothing in the patient's condition prevents an EMT from using an AED to restart the heart of a patient who has suffered an electrical shock.

CONCLUSION

The EMT's first job is to prevent any further injury to the patient. After the EMT protects the patient with a soft tissue injury, the EMT must prepare expedient transportation of the patient to the most appropriate facility.

Although each type of tissue trauma is different, most are managed in the same, or a similar, way. Thus, the EMT can apply his knowledge of wound care in unique ways.

Street Smart

When approaching a scene, if an EMT starts to feel a tingling sensation in his legs, he should immediately stop. The EMT has entered an electric field. The tingling sensation indicates that the area is energized. Electricity fans out in ever-widening circles called gradients. The tingling sensation indicates that the EMT is on the edge of the first gradient.

Backing out of the danger can be more dangerous than standing still. By lifting one leg and then setting it down, the EMT creates a circuit. If possible, the EMT should wait until the all-clear sign indicates that it is safe to move. Otherwise, the EMT should shuffle backward, keeping both feet on the ground firmly, or hop out of the area. Whatever the EMT does, he should never run.

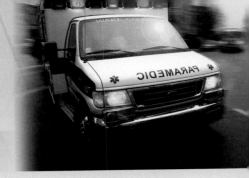

CASE STUDY Continued

Denise immediately applies a clean, sterile, universal dressing to the 3-inch laceration to Jannie's forearm and applies direct pressure. While she continues to hold pressure, she raises Jannie's arm above her head and holds it there.

Justin performs a quick primary assessment and history of the event. Jannie is able to provide all information without difficulty, but she states she is feeling weak and worries that she might pass out.

Jannie is transferred to the ambulance cot and placed in a supine position, with Denise maintaining direct pressure and elevation of the extremity. Using a roller bandage over the thick universal dressing, Denise applies a pressure dressing to the wound for the trip to the hospital.

Jannie states she feels better lying down. Denise applies oxygen via a non-rebreather mask at 12 lpm and takes a baseline set of vital signs: pulse 98, respirations 18, and blood pressure 118/68. Denise provides a report to the hospital and turns patient care over to the emergency department nurse, with a follow-up report given at the time of patient care transfer.

Key Concepts Revisited

- The severity of bleeding can be determined by the vessels that have been injured:
  - Arterial bleeding—pressurized (spurting) bright red, severe bleeding
  - Capillary bleeding—low pressure (oozing), usually minor
  - Venous bleeding—most common, low to medium pressure, dark red, potentially severe due to constant flow
- The principles of bleeding control are to stop severe bleeding before it leads to hypoperfusion:
  - Direct pressure at bleeding site
  - Elevate above the heart to slow bleeding
  - Dressings to absorb blood and apply pressure
    - Pressure dressings
    - Tourniquets—uncontrolled arterial hemorrhage
    - Hemostatic dressings—uncontrolled (arterial) hemorrhage not responsive to other methods
- The purpose of a sterile dressing is to prevent introduction of contaminants, such as dirt, into the wound, that can lead to infections.
  - Gauze dressings
  - Trauma dressings
  - Occlusive dressings
  - Universal dressings
- Soft tissue wounds usually result from blunt forces or sharp objects:
  - Abrasions—minor capillary bleeding
  - Lacerations—full thickness skin tears with minor to severe bleeding
  - Incision—full-thickness cut causing straight smooth cuts to the skin and severing underlying vessels; potentially life-threatening bleeding
  - Punctures—incision into the skin; heavy bleeding can occur inside the puncture wound with minimal external bleeding
  - Avulsions—forceful tearing of skin or body part leaving ragged wound margins; bleeding is usually somewhat controlled by the damaged vessel ends rolling up on themselves
  - Amputation—clean removal of a limb, resulting in a clean, straight line; bleeding can be severe; most amputations are surgical removals
- The type of dressing and bandages used on soft tissue injuries is determined by the need for additional control of bleeding and the type and location of the injury.

- o Bandages are used to hold a dressing in place.
  - Recurrent bandage—hold a dressing down over a large area
  - Spiral bandage—used mostly on extremity injuries
  - Figure-of-eight—roller type bandage that anchors against itself
  - Triangular bandage—can be used to anchor dressings over the hand, knees, nose, shoulders
- Compartment syndrome can result from crush injury and is characterized by three specific signs
  - o Paresthesia—loss of feeling
  - o Paralysis—loss of motion
  - o Pulselessness—loss of circulation
- The classification of burn injuries is based on the number of layers of skin and underlying tissues affected.
  - o Superficial burn—affects the epidermis, such as sunburn
  - o Partial-thickness burn—involves the dermal layer, causing tissue swelling and blisters and increased chance of secondary infection, such as severe scalds
  - o Full-thickness burns—involves all layers of skin, reaching to nerve endings, muscles, and fat; fluid loss and infection risks are great; hypoperfusion, hypovolemic shock, and death can occur
- Management of a burn injury begins by stopping the burning process; protecting from infections, fluid loss, and heat loss; and transporting to the appropriate facility.
  - o Initially cool with sterile water to stop the burning process if needed
  - o Dress with dry, sterile dressings or sterile burn sheet
  - o Prevent heat loss
  - o Transport to burn center
- Chemical burns must be managed immediately by removing the chemical from the skin to prevent continuing tissue damage.
  - o MSDS sheets for specific chemical treatments
  - o Emergency Response Guidebook (ERG)
  - o CHEMTREC
- An electrical shock can cause damage to the soft tissues, including entrance and exit wounds of the skin, and affect the function of the heart, possibly causing cardiac arrest.
- The management of an electrical injury begins with ensuring scene safety for the rescuers and administering CPR and AED if cardiac arrest occurs.

Review Questions

1. What are the principles of bleeding control management?
2. What are the types of bleeding?
3. What is the purpose of a dressing?
4. What are the indications and dangers of using a tourniquet?
5. What are the different bandages used?
6. What is the special danger of neck wounds?
7. What are the different types of wounds?
8. What is the field care of an evisceration?
9. What is the field care of an amputation?
10. What are the levels of burn injury?
11. What is the field care of a burn?
12. What danger do chemical burns represent to the EMT?
13. What injuries can occur from an electrical shock?
14. What is the field care of an electrical injury?

Key Terms

Amputation

Avulsion

Bandage

Coagulation

Cold zone

Compartment syndrome

Compress

Conductor

Cravat

Crush injury

Current

Degloving avulsion

Direct pressure

Dressing

Ecchymosis

Elevate

Embolism

Emergency Response Guidebook (ERG)

Entrance wound

Exit wound

Fasciotomy

Figure-of-eight

Full-thickness burn

Gauze dressing

Hematoma

Hemorrhage

Hemostatic dressing

Impaled object

Incision

Inflammation

Insulator

Linear

Material Safety Data Sheet (MSDS)

Necrotic

Palmar method

Partial-thickness burn

Recurrent bandage

Roller bandage

Rule of nines

Spiral bandage

Stellate

Straddle injury

Superficial burn

Tattooing

Tourniquet

Trauma dressing

Triangular bandage

Universal dressing

Wound

Further Study

Bozinko, G., K. Lowe, and C. Reigart. "Burns." *RN* 61, no. 11 (1998): 37–40.

Doyle, G., and P. Taillac. "Tourniquets: A Review of Current Use with Proposals for Expanded Prehospital Use." *Prehospital Emergency Care* 12, no. 2 (2008): 241–256.

Hansen, S., C. Paul, and D. Voigt. "Chemical Injuries." *Journal of Emergency Medical Services* 24, no. 8 (1999): 82–88.

National Association of Emergency Medical Technicians. *PHTLS: Basic and Advanced Prehospital Trauma Life Support.* 6th ed. Clinton, MS: Mosby/Elsevier, 2007.

Wiebelhaus, P. and S. Hansen. (1999). "Burns: Handle with Care." *RN* 62, no. 11 (1999): 52–58.

UNIT 38 Bony Injuries

Orthopedics, a term derived from a Greek word *ortho* meaning "straight" and pedics from the Greek *pais* meaning "children," is the study of the musculoskeletal system. In earlier decades, orthopedic doctors were involved in the treatment of crippled children, but orthopedics has expanded to include the management of a wide variety of musculoskeletal disorders and injuries in patients of all ages. Injuries to the bones, muscles, nerves, and joints are some of the most common emergency calls Emergency Medical Technicians (EMTs) will encounter during their career.

> ## National Education Standard
> The Emergency Medical Technician (EMT) will be able to demonstrate a fundamental depth and foundational breadth of understanding of the pathophysiology, assessment, and management of traumatic bone injuries.

Key Concepts

- The key to discovering bone injuries is a high index of suspicion that a bone injury may exist.

- The three mechanisms of force that can cause injury to a bone are direct, indirect, and twisting.

- Ligaments are sinewy tissue that connects bones together at the joint, and a tendon is connective tissue that attaches muscle to bones.

- A closed fracture, in which the bone ends remain within the skin, is the most commonly seen fracture, whereas an open fracture is characterized by bone ends erupted through the skin.

- The basic principles of splinting provide a foundation for the application of all splints.

- Distal pulses must be assessed prior to and following splinting.

- A dislocated or fractured bone is an extremely serious emergency when circulation and function distal to the joint are compromised.

- One attempt to realign the bones should be made when distal pulses are absent in an injured limb.

- The type of splint used in bone injuries is often dependent on the location of the injury.

- Traumatic bone injuries often include injuries to the structure surrounding the bone, such as the ligaments and tendons, and management should focus on stabilization and immobilization.

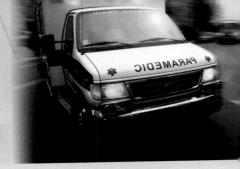

CASE STUDY

Brandon hears and feels a snap in his leg as he is tackled after making the catch in the end zone. As his teammates celebrate winning the game at the last minute, Brandon lies rolling around on the ground, holding his knee between both hands. Suddenly, the referee is there, asking him where he is hurt as he motions to clear the area and bring EMS onto the field.

Jeremiah and Jessie follow the athletic trainer onto the field, bringing the stretcher loaded with gear and a backboard. Once at Brandon's side, Jessie establishes and maintains manual stabilization of the player's helmet while the trainer asks, "Brandon, where do you hurt?"

"It is my knee," Brandon replies, "I think I dislocated or broke my knee." After a few more questions, both

Jeremiah and the athletic trainer are satisfied the injury is limited to Brandon's left leg in the area of the knee. Jeremiah immediately cuts the pant leg off the injured leg and notes deformity and blood just below the knee cap.

Critical Thinking Questions

1. Based on the mechanism of injury, what injuries might an EMT suspect?
2. What are the assessment priorities for this patient?
3. What are the management priorities for this patient?

INTRODUCTION

Many patients experience excruciating pain as a result of bone injury. Although most bone injuries are not life threatening, the event can be filled with visual and emotional drama. This may alarm the inexperienced EMT; however, knowing how to handle the situation can help calm the scene. The EMT should do her best to calm the patient, with the focus on carefully and methodically managing the injury.

When mistreated, bone injuries can result in permanent, lifelong disabilities. The EMT must pay careful attention to the important treatment of bone injuries; the reduction of suffering and prevention of further injury are the first steps in assisting the patient to return to health. This unit discusses the assessment and management of injuries to the musculoskeletal system.

ANATOMY REVIEW

As discussed in Unit 5, the body has three types of muscles: involuntary muscles, cardiac muscles, and voluntary muscles. This unit discusses voluntary muscles, those muscles that are under the patient's conscious control, and their responsibility in the movement of bones that permit locomotion. When a traumatic force is applied to a bone or a muscle, movement can be impaired, and an injury may result.

The bones of the body make up the skeletal system. The skeletal system can be divided into two subsystems. The bones of the spine and cranium are called the **axial skeleton.** The axial skeleton provides support for the muscles of the trunk and protection of the core organs, including the heart, lungs, and brain. The axial skeleton also allows movement, such as bending and lifting. Injuries to the head and spine have been discussed in earlier units.

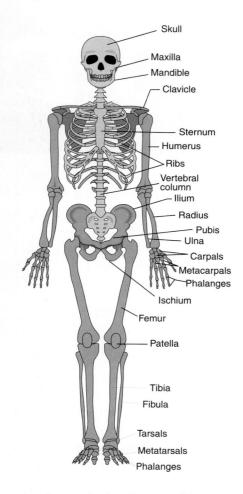

Appendicular skeleton (blue)
Axial skeleton (gray)

Figure 38.1 The appendicular skeleton consists of all bones outside of the axial skeleton

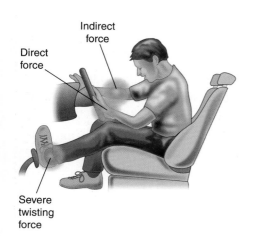

Figure 38.2 Direct, indirect, or twisting forces create bone injuries

The other bones, the bones of the extremities, form the appendicular skeleton (Figure 38.1). The appendicular skeleton allows the body to run, to shoulder a load, or to stand erect.

The bones of the **appendicular skeleton** can be further subdivided into two more groups of bones. The bones of the shoulder and arms make up what can be loosely called the **shoulder girdle.** The bones of the pelvis make up the **pelvic girdle.**

The advantage of putting these bones into groups is that it aids in understanding that force transmitted to one bone may be transmitted to adjacent bones as well. These bones work together, as a group, to effect motion; when one bone is injured, the range of motion of the bones in that group may be reduced.

INJURY

Injury to bones and muscles can occur from either a direct or indirect force. A **direct force,** such as a blow from a baseball, delivers energy immediately to the bone. An **indirect force** transmits energy, through either the shoulder or pelvic girdle, to a bone that is not in contact with the force. For example, when a person falls on an outstretched hand and injures the shoulder, the shoulder is injured by an indirect force.

Some forces, direct and indirect, can rotate along the axis of the bone. The result of this **twisting force** can be injury to both muscles and bones. The bones that are twisted may stay straight and inline, whereas the other mechanisms of injury often produce deformity. These three forms of force are illustrated in Figure 38.2.

MUSCULAR INJURIES

Muscles can be torn, crushed, bruised, and cut. Because of the attachment of muscles to bones, when a bone is injured, a muscle also may be injured. The connective tissue that attaches the muscle to the bone is called the **tendon.** Similarly, two bones are connected to each other at joints. These joints are held together by sinewy bands of connective tissue called **ligaments.**

These connective tissues provide stability to a joint. Tendons and ligaments in a joint allow a bone to move in certain directions within the joint's **range of motion (ROM)** (Figure 38.3). The tendons and ligaments also prevent the joint from moving beyond its normal ROM.

A violent force to a joint may force the joint beyond its normal ROM. When a joint is forced beyond its ROM, the tendons or ligaments can become stretched, torn, or **sprained,** resulting in tissue injury. For example, the knee normally moves forward and backward; that is the direction of the knee's normal ROM. When a severe force makes the knee twist laterally, the ligaments and tendons stretch, the knee fails (or buckles), and the knee is injured.

Because the tendons and ligaments are inserted into the bone itself, a tendon injury can also pull a piece of bone from the shaft. The EMT cannot determine whether the underlying bone has or has not been injured; therefore, she must treat all suspected sprains as though a bone injury is present as well.

JOINT INJURIES

A joint is usually stable as it moves through its normal ROM. When a person overextends the joint beyond the normal ROM, the bone ends can slip out of joint. When a bone slips out of joint and out of alignment, adjacent structures, including arteries, nerves, and veins, can be injured. The displacement of any bone from its normal position in a joint is called a **dislocation** (Figure 38.4).

When a dislocation occurs, adjacent muscles struggle to return the bone to the joint. A bone returning to its natural position within the joint without assistance is called a **spontaneous reduction.** The muscles around the joint will start to spasm from stress when the bone is **locked,** which means it is prevented from returning to the joint. This spasm can be very painful.

A dislocation can lock for a number of reasons. The bone's end may be broken. Tendons and ligaments may be torn or injured. The bone may be physically obstructed from returning to the joint.

A dislocated joint means that nerves, arteries, and veins may be injured. Arteries can be pinched in the joint, compromising distal circulation. Nerves can stretch beyond their physical limits, snapping and creating paralysis. Bleeding can compress surrounding soft tissues, further compromising distal function and movement.

The EMT must stabilize the joint to prevent further injury and transport the patient to the hospital. At the hospital, doctors can attempt to manually reduce the dislocation. In some cases, the patient may require surgery to have the reduction performed.

BROKEN BONES

When a great force is applied to a bone, the bone may break or **fracture.** Although an EMT usually cannot see the fracture, indirect signs of injury tell the EMT that the bone may be broken.

Fractures can be divided into two categories. If the force moves the bone out of line, the bone ends may erupt through the skin, lacerating the skin and creating an **open fracture** (Figure 38.5). If the bone ends do not break the skin, the fracture is called a **closed fracture.** Most fractures are closed fractures.

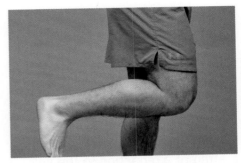

Figure 38.3 An injury to a joint can limit the patient's range of motion in that joint

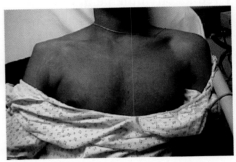

Figure 38.4 A dislocation is when a bone is forced out of a joint (Courtesy of Kevin Reilly, MD, Albany Medical Center, Albany, NY)

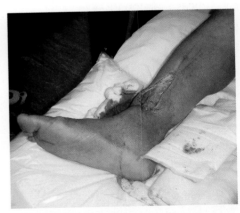

Figure 38.5 An open fracture occurs when the bone ends break through the skin (Courtesy of Deborah Funk, MD, Albany Medical Center, Albany, NY)

Street Smart

Injuries may occur during sporting events, such as football, soccer, and baseball games. EMTs are often called to respond to or stand by at athletic events. On the scene, the EMT may encounter a certified athletic trainer (ATC). Certified athletic trainers have undergone training in sports medicine. Sports medicine is the application of medicine to treat athletic injuries.

The athletic trainer is responsible for the care of the athletes and will request assistance from an EMT only when the trainer is unable to provide appropriate care on the scene. An ATC should be viewed as a fellow health care provider who is highly trained to treat athletic injuries.

An EMT working at a sporting event should identify the athletic trainer and verify his credentials before an athlete is injured. The EMT and the trainer must work together in the patient's best interest; cooperation, not competition, will ensure that an injured athlete gets the proper medical attention.

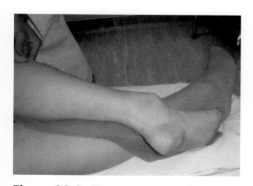

Figure 38.6 The area around a closed fracture may be painful, swollen, or deformed (Courtesy of Deborah Funk, MD, Albany Medical Center, Albany, NY)

ASSESSMENT

By its nature, a bone injury implies that a great deal of violence and resultant trauma has occurred. The appearance of a grotesquely deformed leg or arm may be sensational. The EMT must keep in mind that if there was enough force to break bones, then softer tissues are also likely to be injured.

SCENE SIZE-UP

The key to discovering bone injuries is a high index of suspicion that a bone injury may exist in the first place. The EMT should first consider carefully the mechanism of injury.

The mechanism of injury tells the EMT where the injury is likely to be found. By following the line of force, the direction of the violence, and the points of impact on the body, the EMT can suspect certain injuries. For example, if a person jumps from a significant height and lands on his feet, the line of force, through the body, will compress and crush bones in a predictable pattern, starting at the heels and proceeding up the axial skeleton.

GENERAL IMPRESSION

The EMT should carefully consider the patient next, stopping to listen to the patient. Bone injuries are painful. Often the patient's yelling will alert the EMT to the possible presence of a bone injury. Next the EMT should look at the patient's posture and demeanor. Patients often protect and even splint an injured limb rather than endure more pain. The patient's stance can say a lot about his injuries.

PRIMARY ASSESSMENT

Because of the proximity of bones and blood vessels, if one is injured, the other can be injured as well. An EMT who is assessing a patient should always remain focused on her priorities and not be distracted by the gross injury. Rarely does a broken bone cause death; however, bleeding from a broken bone, either internal or external, can lead to life-threatening consequences.

SECONDARY ASSESSMENT

Although individual bone injuries can have specific physical findings, an EMT can detect most bone injuries by simply focusing her attention on assessing DCAP-BTLS. A modified physical assessment can be quickly performed, focusing on the area of concern.

SIGNS AND SYMPTOMS

Next to most long bones lie an artery, a nerve, and a vein. Surrounding these bones are muscles, tendons, and other soft tissues. Covering all of this is the skin. When a bone is broken and moves out of alignment, the bone ends can damage these tissues. Rarely does an EMT see a broken bone unless the bone ends stick out of the skin. However, an EMT who is assessing a patient can detect the indirect signs of a broken bone and make an assumption, based on these findings, that the bone may be broken (Figure 38.6).

If the artery is pierced by sharp shards of bone, severe bleeding can occur. For example, if the femoral artery, which lies next to the femur, is cut by broken bone ends, the artery will bleed into the thigh. The soft tissues of the thigh will quickly become painful, swollen, and deformed. As the thigh fills with blood, as much as a liter in some cases, the thigh will feel firm to the touch.

If the artery is severed, distal circulation to the affected limb may be compromised. Distal pulses may become weak or absent. The limb may become bluish or cyanotic and pulseless.

Any injured extremity that is pulseless and cyanotic constitutes a serious medical emergency. Without medical treatment, the limb may have to be amputated. The EMT should promptly splint the limb and transport the patient to the closest appropriate facility.

A contusion, the blue-gray discoloration under the skin from bleeding, indicates that soft tissue injury may have occurred. Whenever a significant contusion is discovered overlying a bone, the EMT should suspect a bone injury.

Nerves provide pathways for signals to and from the brain. Some nerves, the **motor nerves,** affect muscles, causing them to contract and move. Other nerves, the **sensory nerves,** transmit feelings of pain and pressure to the brain.

If the sensory nerve is injured, the patient may complain of severe pain or no pain at all. A sensation of numbness or tingling, called *paresthesia,* may indicate that the sensory nerve has been injured (Figure 38.7).

If a motor nerve is injured, the patient may complain of weakness in the affected extremity. This weakness, called **paresis,** may be difficult to assess on the scene. An EMT should use extreme caution when asking the patient to move his hands or feet; one wrong move can move bone ends, causing more injury.

If the patient cannot move one of his extremities, a condition called *paralysis,* the EMT should quickly check the other extremity. If the patient cannot move either extremity, the EMT should suspect a possible spinal cord injury.

An elevated bone end may tent the skin. The EMT should carefully stabilize this injury. Sudden or improper movement of the limb may change a closed fracture into an open fracture. Open fractures frequently require immediate surgical repair and a longer recovery time.

If the bone breaks the skin, bone ends may be visible. The first priority is to control any bleeding. The EMT should cover any exposed bone ends with a dry sterile dressing and then splint the limb in the position found. The EMT should never push exposed bone ends back into the wound. If the bone ends fall back into the wound, the EMT needs to report and record this finding.

If the patient moves the injured extremity, a grating sound, called *crepitus,* may be heard. Crepitus is created when two bone ends grind against each other. An EMT should never move an injured extremity to try to hear crepitus.

When an EMT runs her fingers down the length of the shaft of the bone, feeling for injury, and contacts an injury, the patient may complain of sudden

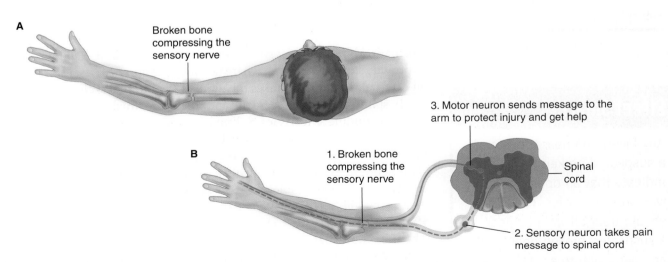

Figure 38.7 Broken bone ends can cut sensory and motor nerves, creating weakness or numbness below the injury

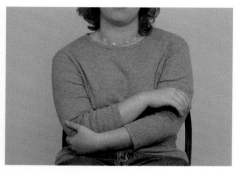

Figure 38.8 The patient may "self-splint" in an attempt to prevent further pain and injury

Table 38-1 Signs and Symptoms of a Suspected Fracture

Swelling

Pain

Deformity

Paralysis

Paresthesia

Pulselessness

Cyanosis

Crepitus

Point tenderness

Guarding

Self-splinting

Street Smart

Any laceration near the site of a suspected broken bone may indicate that an open fracture was present earlier. The EMT should treat all wounds near a suspected broken bone as if an open fracture exists.

pain. This sudden pain is called *point tenderness*. Once point tenderness has been established, the EMT need not repeatedly touch the area. The EMT should report point tenderness to the emergency department.

When a patient uses his own body to immobilize an injured extremity, he is attempting to **self-splint** the injured bone (Figure 38.8). When the EMT attempts to assess the patient, the patient will try to prevent the EMT from touching the injury. This behavior is called *guarding*.

In extreme cases, a patient may try to walk on a broken leg, to escape a fire, for example, and the bone will bend at an unnatural point. This new joint, or unnatural movement of the bone, is called **false motion** and is an indication of a severe fracture.

In short, DCAP-BTLS essentially covers all the physical findings that are typically found with a bone injury. Injuries to the muscles, tendons, ligaments, and dislocations of a joint can all present with the signs and symptoms of a fractured bone, which are summarized in Table 38-1. Therefore, any painful, swollen deformity is assumed to be a fractured bone until proven otherwise.

MANAGEMENT

An EMT's first priority is always safety. If the injury is an open wound, the EMT must take body substance isolation. Caution should be exercised when dressing the wound. Sharp bone ends can pierce the EMT's gloves and puncture the skin. A lacerated artery can spurt blood into an unsuspecting EMT's eyes. The EMT should wear eye protection if blood is present.

After performing a primary assessment and controlling any bleeding, the EMT should perform a focused history and physical examination. The EMT should concentrate on looking for DCAP-BTLS.

When a swollen, painful deformity is found, an EMT should immediately stabilize the injury. This is accomplished by placing a hand above and below the injury to prevent any further movement. The EMT should not release stabilization of the bone until after the limb has been properly immobilized.

Then a second EMT should expose the injury, cutting clothing away carefully, and control any bleeding. This EMT should then cover any protruding bone ends with a dry sterile dressing and proceed with splinting the limb.

Several different splints may be used on the limb, depending on the location of the injury. A variety of splinting techniques can be used for an injury in the same place on the same limb.

SPLINTING

Normally, a bone provides structure and support to a limb. A splint is designed to provide support to a limb where the bone is injured. In a sense, the splint is an external skeleton that takes the place of the internal skeleton.

A splint prevents movement and, therefore, further injury to the bone and surrounding soft tissues. Splints also reduce pain, because movement of bone ends against one another can be very painful. By preventing such movement, a splint reduces the pain the patient is experiencing.

Finally, splints help to control bleeding. A splint prevents bone ends from cutting soft tissues and blood vessels surrounding the injury site.

PRINCIPLES OF SPLINTING

There are more than 200 bones in the body. Each bone can be fractured—and splinted—in several different ways. The number of techniques used to splint fractures may seem endless, yet several basic principles provide a foundation for the application of all splints.

The first principle is life before limb. The EMT must never compromise a patient's survival just to splint an injured extremity. Life-threatening injuries must be dealt with first. If the patient needs immediate transportation and the possibility of bone injuries exists, the EMT should immobilize the entire body to a backboard.

Once life-threatening problems are appropriately managed, the EMT should immediately stabilize the injured limb to prevent further injury. The EMT should take a firm handhold above and below the injury and manually hold the bone in place until another EMT has a splint in place. The second EMT should always expose the wound and investigate the possibility of an open fracture. Bleeding control usually takes priority over fracture management. The techniques used to stop severe bleeding are described in Unit 37.

The second EMT should check for distal pulses, movement, and sensation before applying a splint. Pulselessness is always a medical emergency. Surgical intervention may be necessary. The EMT should contact medical control immediately for further instructions.

Some patients may want to try to walk (weight-bear) on the injured limb. The EMT should never allow the patient to walk on or use the extremity. Weight bearing can further aggravate the injury.

The EMT should attempt to splint the bones in the position found, if possible. Joints should never be straightened unless distal pulses are absent. Long bones should be straightened only when application of the splint in the position the bone was found is impractical. More information about straightening an extremity fracture is provided later in the unit.

The splint should immobilize the joints above and below the injury site. Movement of these joints can create movement of the bone ends. A splint should be chosen that is long enough to immobilize all three places.

Whenever possible, the patient's hands or feet should be placed in a natural position called the **position of function.** The position of function for the ankle is relaxed at a 90-degree angle. The hand should be splinted in a slightly closed position, as if the patient were holding an egg.

The EMT should pad the voids between the splint and the limb. This padding makes the splint more comfortable and improves stabilization by providing support along a wider surface. Towels, universal dressings, and foam are excellent materials to use for padding.

The EMT should avoid placing straps over the injury site. Pressure from a strap may displace bone ends and cause further injury. If pressure is needed at the site to control bleeding, a pressure bandage should be applied, and then the limb should be splinted.

The limb should be elevated above the level of the heart. Elevation of an injured limb helps to reduce swelling and pain. Application of ice or cold packs to the injury is also recommended.

Finally, the distal pulses, movement, and sensation should be reassessed and documented. Any change in the patient's condition should be noted. Loss of pulses may be caused by tight bandages. The EMT should loosen the bandages and recheck the pulses; if the pulse is still absent, the patient should be packaged and transported. Table 38-2 summarizes the principles of splinting.

DISTAL PULSES

Distal pulses should be assessed whenever a bone injury is suspected. The radial pulse is the distal pulse point for an arm. The radial pulse is located on the lateral wrist, proximal to the thumb.

The feet have several pulses an EMT can use to assess distal circulation. The pedal pulse (dorsalis pedis) is on the anterior surface of the foot, midline

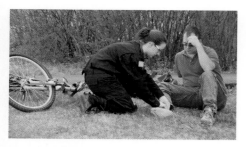

Figure 38.9 A pedal pulse is a positive sign of distal circulation

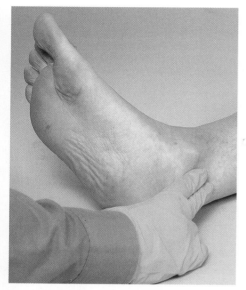

Figure 38.10 The posterior tibial pulse may be easier to palpate

Table 38-2 Principles of Splinting

1. Always consider life before limb.
2. Manually stabilize a suspected fracture.
3. Expose the injury.
4. Control bleeding. (Any life-threatening bleeding would have been dealt with during the primary assessment.)
5. Check for pulses, movement, and sensation distal to the injury.
6. Never allow the patient to bear weight on the injured limb.
7. Splint the injury in the position found.
8. Immobilize the joints above and below the injury. (If a joint is injured, then immobilize the bones above and below the joint.)
9. Elevate the injury above the level of the heart.
10. Pad the voids between the splint and the limb.
11. Avoid placing straps directly over the injured area.
12. Recheck distal pulses, movement, and sensation after the splint is applied.

and midway between the toes and the ankle. Figure 38.9 shows an EMT checking a pedal pulse.

At the distal tibia, on the inside of the ankle where the bone meets the ankle, is a bony protrusion called the **medial malleolus**. The posterior tibial artery runs just behind the malleolus, and a pulse usually can be palpated at that point. Figure 38.10 shows an EMT checking a posterior tibial pulse.

REALIGNING BONES

Pulselessness in an injured extremity is an ominous finding. If pulses do not return, tissue death may necessitate an amputation. In cases in which pulses are absent, the EMT should consider making one attempt to realign the bones and relieve pressure on the impinged artery. The EMT can call medical control for advice and direction and should always follow local medical protocols.

In attempting to realign the bones, the EMT grasps the limb firmly and exerts a continuous gentle pull, called traction, along the long axis of the bone. Slight rotation, back to a natural alignment, is sometimes needed as well. The EMT should stop applying traction once the bone is in line or resistance is met.

If pulses have not returned after the EMT's attempt to realign the bones, the patient should be packaged and transported immediately to the closest appropriate facility.

SPLINTING DEVICES

A large assortment of splinting devices and materials are on the market, but all of them serve the same purpose, to provide external support to an injured bone. These splinting devices can be grouped into five general classifications.

Street Smart

Often it is difficult to obtain a distal pulse in the feet. The patient may have poor peripheral circulation due to age, disease, or the cold. Many EMTs try to find the posterior tibial pulse because the landmark, the malleolus, is easy to identify. When a distal pulse is found, the EMT can lightly mark the pulse point with a pen. Pen ink can be easily washed off later, and the mark can save time when pulses are rechecked.

The **sling and swathe (S/S)** was probably the first splint ever used. An injured arm is suspended in a triangular bandage made into a sling, and then firmly anchored to the body's side using a cravat called a *swathe* (Figure 38.11). The body provides the external support and rigidity needed.

A **flexible splint** can be made from any material that can be formed to fit any angle and then made to be rigid. Aluminum ladder splints and structural aluminum malleable (SAM) splints are examples of flexible splints. Flexible splints are particularly useful for injuries in joints, including the joints in the hands and feet (Figure 38.12).

A **rigid splint** is made of any firm material that can be placed next to the limb to provide support. A padded board splint is commonly used as a rigid splint. Rolled newspapers and magazines, wooden spoons, and salad forks have all been used as rigid splints in an emergency. Some rigid splints are manufactured with an inflexible metal or wooden splint inside and a flexible canvas or plastic sleeve that can be closed with Velcro fasteners on the outside. Rigid splints are used whenever an injury occurs along the midshaft portion of the bone.

A splint that allows air to be pumped in or suctioned out of it is a **pneumatic splint** (Figure 38.13). The splint is placed around the limb and inflated/deflated until it becomes rigid. The military anti-shock trousers/ pneumatic anti-shock garment (MAST/PASG) used in the stabilization of pelvic fractures is an example of a pneumatic splint.

Femur fractures are stabilized with a splint that can maintain a continuous positive force, or traction, on the femur. **Traction splints** decrease muscular spasm and pain and prevent bone ends from overriding.

Some traction splints use just one pole for external support of the injured leg and therefore are referred to as **unipolar traction splints.** Skill 38-1 at the end of this unit demonstrates the use of this type of splinting device.

Another type of traction splint is the **bipolar traction splint.** The bipolar splint uses two external poles, one on each side of the leg, to provide external support for the injured leg. The bipolar splint is a direct descendant of the Thomas half-ring splint that was originally put into service in World War I. Skill 38-2 at the end of this unit demonstrates the use of this type of splinting device.

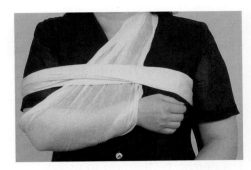

Figure 38.11 The sling and swathe, using triangular bandages, is commonly used to splint upper extremity injuries

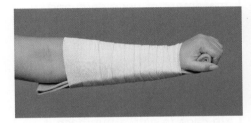

Figure 38.12 A flexible splint, like the SAM splint, is convenient for splinting a deformed extremity

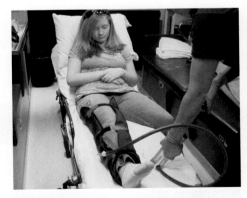

Figure 38.13 A vacuum splint is a type of pneumatic splint (Courtesy of Larry Torrey and MEDCU, Portland, ME)

Street Smart

A splint that was applied correctly on the scene can loosen with movement during transportation. The EMT should recheck the splint frequently, at least as often as she checks the vital signs, to ensure that the splint is doing what it was created to do—that is, splinting the injury. Failure to constantly monitor a splint can mean movement of bone ends, which can cut blood vessels and cause bleeding.

TRANSPORTATION

The EMT must always focus on the more important patient problems, such as hypoperfusion, and avoid being distracted by the dramatic appearance of grievous bony injuries the patient has sustained. The EMT's first priority is always life over limb. Sometimes a broken bone will not be individually splinted; rather, the patient's entire body will be splinted and the patient transported immediately. The EMT must make careful, appropriate decisions on when, where, and how to transport a trauma patient. A wrong decision may mean the difference between life and death.

In almost every case, from serious multisystem trauma with multiple broken bones to the simple twisted ankle, the patient is in pain. Advanced life support (ALS) can provide the patient with some relief from the sometimes excruciating pain due to traumatic injury. Pain management, including pain medicines such as narcotics, is a part of the expertise that an ALS provider can bring to the scene. The EMT should consider calling for ALS early during patient care.

ONGOING ASSESSMENT

Soft tissue injury almost always occurs with bone injury, resulting in tissue swelling that can cause bandages to become so tight they act like a tourniquet. For this reason, whenever an EMT checks the patient's vital signs, she should reassess the distal circulation of any extremity that is splinted.

INJURIES TO THE SHOULDER GIRDLE

Whenever an EMT is assessing for possible bony injury, she must be mindful of the possibility of a secondary associated injury. For example, a fractured forearm as well as an injured wrist are common in patients who have taken a fall.

INJURY OF THE CLAVICLE

The collarbone, or *clavicle*, is a long S-shaped bone located in the upper anterior chest wall. It is a part of the shoulder girdle. The clavicle, at its distal end, joins the shoulder blade, or *scapula*. Many of the accessory muscles of breathing are attached to the clavicle.

The clavicle is prone to injury because of its relatively exposed location. For example, any force on the arm may be transmitted to the clavicle, causing a fracture. An example of indirect trauma creating an injury of the clavicle would be when a child falls off a bicycle onto an outstretched hand, and a clavicular fracture occurs.

A direct force, such as a blow to the shoulder, can also fracture the clavicle. Likewise, compression of the thoracic cage and the shoulder girdle can produce a clavicular fracture. In fact, the clavicle is one of the most commonly fractured bones in the body.

Under the clavicle lie several major blood vessels, including the subclavian artery. For this reason, neurovascular injury may accompany a clavicular fracture.

SIGNS AND SYMPTOMS

The presentation of a patient with a clavicular injury is classic. At the site of the fracture, the skin is often tented, because the clavicle is just below the skin (Figure 38.14). Often the bone ends are displaced, leaving a distinctive "stepped off" appearance, like a bicycle's handlebar. Finally, the patient often holds the injured arm across the front of his body in an effort to self-splint the injury.

The shoulder girdle and clavicles are proximal to the rib cage and the lungs. A displaced bone can easily puncture a lung and cause a pneumothorax, discussed in Unit 36. The EMT should follow the standard order of assessment while remembering that a life-threatening injury to the lung may have occurred.

Once the EMT is satisfied that no immediate life threats exist, the EMT should continue with the modified physical examination as part of the secondary assessment, focusing on the signs and symptoms of a bone injury based on the chief concern.

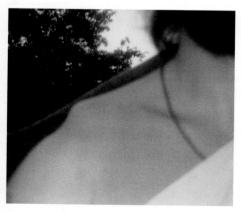

Figure 38.14 A fractured clavicle often has a classic handlebar shape that tents the overlying skin

MANAGEMENT

Before splinting a clavicle, the EMT must carefully assess the patient for any associated injury to adjacent scapula and humerus. Then, supporting the patient's efforts to self-splint, the EMT should use a sling and swathe. The sling supports the weight of the arm, while the swathe binds the arm to the body to prevent further movement. The EMT should keep the patient in a sitting position during transport.

INJURY OF THE SCAPULA

The scapula is a broad, triangular-shaped bone located in the upper portion of the back. Fractures of the scapula are rare. Thick, flat muscles overlying the scapula and elastic ribs underneath the scapula permit this bone to absorb a great deal of force without breaking. Consequently, when an EMT discovers a potential scapular fracture, she should have a high index of suspicion that other injuries also may be present.

SIGNS AND SYMPTOMS

The bone ends seldom displace in a scapular fracture; therefore, the classic "deformity" is not found. Often the only outward signs of a scapular fracture are point tenderness and a contusion at the site of injury.

MANAGEMENT

The patient's arm should be secured to the chest with a sling and swathe to prevent movement of the shoulder on the affected side.

INJURY OF THE ACROMIOCLAVICULAR (A/C) JOINT

The acromion process of the scapula and the clavicle join to form the shoulder joint. Inserted into this shoulder joint is the humerus. When the clavicle is forced downward, the tendons are torn. This movement of the clavicle out of the joint is called an **acromioclavicular (A/C) dislocation.**

A common mechanism that creates A/C dislocations is a blow from above directly onto the clavicle. Again, the patient will frequently self-splint to protect the injury. The EMT should apply a sling and swathe to prevent further movement of the bone.

INJURY OF THE SHOULDER

The shoulder has a great range of motion. When an arm is held overhead, or outreached, and a sudden force strikes it, the humerus can literally "pop" out of joint, resulting in a **shoulder dislocation.** The shoulder is one of the most commonly dislocated joints in the body.

SIGNS AND SYMPTOMS

A shoulder dislocation can be very painful. The powerful shoulder muscles spasm while attempting to get the humerus back into the joint. Any movement, even the vibration of the ambulance, can create severe pain.

The injured shoulder will appear "squared off," lacking its naturally rounded contour. The injured shoulder also will appear different, asymmetrical, when compared to the uninjured shoulder.

The majority of shoulder dislocations are anterior dislocations. The arm has been forced away from the body and is unable to return to its natural position. The patient, in an attempt to prevent further pain, will hold the arm out away from the body.

Pediatric Considerations

A child often has difficulty explaining exactly where the pain is located. Often the child will complain that an entire arm hurts. Observing the mechanism of injury may provide a clue to the injury. Falls from bikes or trees, for example, can cause wrist, elbow, shoulder, and clavicle injuries. If a clavicular injury is present, assessment of the child's clavicle will reveal point tenderness, swelling, and deformity of the clavicle.

Street Smart

Once injured, the shoulder is prone to injury again. The weakened ligaments allow the head of the humerus to "slip out of joint" easily. Many patients learn to reduce their own fractures. Eventually this approach fails, often after several dozen dislocations, and the shoulder becomes locked into position. When that occurs, the patient will call EMS.

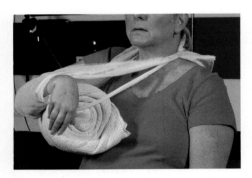

Figure 38.15 A bedroll, secured around the body by a cravat, maintains the arm in the position found

MANAGEMENT

A shoulder injury could be managed with a sling and swathe, but any attempt to move the patient's arm closer to his body usually elicits severe pain or discomfort. In addition, a nerve bundle runs over the top of the humerus, and the nerves occasionally become entrapped in the socket of a dislocated shoulder. Consequently, the patient may complain of numbness along the upper arm, near the deltoid muscle, or in the hands. Therefore, the EMT must be extremely cautious when splinting a potentially dislocated shoulder.

To splint a dislocated shoulder, the EMT may place either a pillow or a bedroll under the arm and secure the cushion in place with a cravat around the chest (Figure 38.15). Once the cushion is secured, the elbow may be flexed to a 90-degree angle and a sling and swathe applied. The EMT should carefully reassess distal pulses, movement, and sensation of the injured limb, and should place the patient in a seated position for transport.

INJURY OF THE UPPER ARM

The humerus is the long straight bone in the upper arm. Most injuries to the humerus occur after a large force has been applied to a small portion of the bone. Consequently, the bone ends may be displaced, and the injury appears swollen and deformed.

MANAGEMENT

In most cases, a fracture of the humerus can be splinted in the position found. In rare cases in which there is neurovascular compromise, the EMT may need to straighten the humerus before applying the splint.

After assessing distal pulses, sensation, and movement, the EMT grasps the patient's arm at the elbow and shoulder. Placing the thumb of one hand at the midline of the shoulder, the EMT then firmly grasps the upper arm, while her other hand grasps the elbow. By applying continuous downward pressure along the axis of the bone, the EMT may be able to realign the bone ends. The EMT should stop, however, if resistance is met or the patient complains of severely increased pain.

Once the arm is grossly in line, another EMT should place a padded board splint along the length of the upper arm and secure it. A sling and swathe can then be applied. The EMT should follow local protocols regarding straightening bone injuries or consider calling medical control for advice.

INJURY OF THE ELBOW

At the juncture of three bones, the ulna, the radius, and the humerus, is the elbow. Force applied to any or several of these bones can either fracture a bone or dislocate the elbow itself.

SIGNS AND SYMPTOMS

Typically, the elbow becomes locked into position and the patient complains of severe pain. The elbow will appear out of line and severely deformed.

MANAGEMENT

Blood vessels and nerves run through the elbow, as they do through the shoulder. Any movement puts these blood vessels and nerves at risk for further injury. For this reason, the elbow is usually splinted in the position in which it is found.

The EMT begins by assessing the distal pulse, movement, and sensation. Weak or absent pulses may indicate that a blood vessel has been crimped or severed. The EMT should contact medical control immediately for further instructions. Immediate transportation of the patient may be ordered. The

EMT also should follow local medical protocols regarding procedures for pulseless limbs.

If a pulse is present, the EMT places one padded board splint under the arm so that the ends are at the wrist under the forearm and at the shoulder. Then another padded board splint is placed on top of the first padded board splint. The EMT firmly secures the two ends of the board splints to each other. The elbow should be firmly immobilized between the two boards. A sling may be used to support the entire arm.

Flexible splints, like the wire ladder splint and the SAM splint, can be shaped to conform to the length of the limb (Figure 38.16). Once in place, the flexible splint should be secured with a roller bandage. A sling will help support the arm and relieve pressure on the elbow.

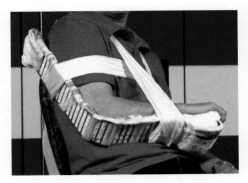

Figure 38.16 A ladder splint is effective when trying to splint a joint

INJURY OF THE FOREARM

Children commonly injure the forearm. Sports, horseplay, and falls account for a large number of these injuries. Typically, both the radius and the ulna are fractured. Without any bony support, the limb may move where there is no joint.

MANAGEMENT

Rigid splints, flexible splints, and pneumatic splints all can be used to splint the forearm. Before any splint is applied, the EMT must first manually stabilize the forearm.

Typically, a rigid board splint is applied to the underside of the forearm, and then the arm is secured, past the wrist to the fingertips, to the board splint with cravats (Figure 38.17). A sling and swathe is then applied to the patient's entire arm. The patient's fingers should be exposed so the EMT can easily access them for assessment, and the patient's hand should be elevated above the level of the heart.

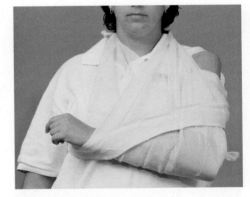

Figure 38.17 A padded board splint secures a forearm, and the sling and swathe stabilizes the joint above and below

INJURY OF THE WRIST AND HAND

The wrist and hand contain a complex collection of small bones that allow a deal great of motion. These bones are also prone to a great number of injuries.

SIGNS AND SYMPTOMS

When the distal radius bone is involved, the wrist takes on a characteristic deformity that looks like a silver fork. This silver fork fracture is also called a **Colles' fracture** (Figure 38.18).

Other injuries can result in rapid swelling, pain, and loss of function. The importance of properly caring for a wrist and hand injury cannot be overemphasized. Often the patient's ability to make a living is dependent on the hands. Serious hand injuries can lead to permanent disabilities. Any injury, whether a simple laceration or possible bone injury, should be treated as a serious condition.

MANAGEMENT

The EMT should first attempt to place the hand in the position of function. A 3-inch roller bandage placed in the palm of the hand works well. Then the EMT should place the entire forearm onto a padded board splint. Flexible splints, such as the wire ladder splint, can be useful for a severely deformed wrist.

When wrapping the forearm with a bandage, the EMT needs to make sure the fingers remain out in the open. The usual distal pulses will be covered by the bandage, so the EMT may need to depend on the presence of good capillary refill to verify distal circulation.

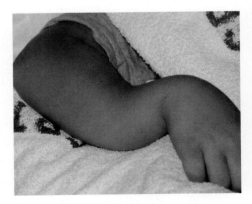

Figure 38.18 A Colles', or silver fork fracture, is very distinctive (Courtesy of Deborah Funk, MD, Albany Medical Center, Albany, NY)

The entire forearm should be placed in a sling and swathe, with the hand positioned above the heart. If this is not practical, then the forearm should be placed on a pillow to elevate it above the heart.

INJURIES TO THE PELVIC GIRDLE

The pelvic girdle contains some of the largest bones in the body. The pelvic girdle also accommodates some of the largest blood vessels in the body. When an injury occurs anywhere in the pelvic girdle, the possibility of serious internal bleeding must be considered.

The primary assessment must always be completed in order. If the EMT has a high index of suspicion, based on the mechanism of injury, that the patient may have sustained a pelvic girdle injury, the EMT should always keep in mind the possibility of internal bleeding and resultant systemic hypoperfusion.

INJURY OF THE PELVIS

The pelvis itself is made up of several flat bones that form a strong ring. Because of the strength of this ring, it takes extreme forces, usually a severe crushing force, to fracture a pelvis. When rings break, they usually break in two places opposite each other.

The broad wings, or crests, of the pelvis protect a large number of important organs. The bladder, the intestine, the uterus, the iliac arteries, and the sciatic nerve, to name a few, all reside within the pelvis. Injury to the pelvis may cause injury to those organs.

Open fractures of the pelvis are rare because the pelvis is surrounded by layers of large muscles and fat. The majority of bleeding from a pelvic fracture is internal, usually bleeding into the pelvis and the retroperitoneal cavity. The retroperitoneal cavity is found behind the abdominal cavity and contains the kidneys, aorta, vena cava, and other organs.

Bleeding into the retroperitoneal space is often obscure and thus goes undetected. Internal bleeding from a pelvic fracture into the retroperitoneal space can be life threatening. Over time, significant retroperitoneal blood collection can be seen as bruising at the flank (Figure 38.19). Several liters of blood can be lost, resulting in hypoperfusion and hypotension.

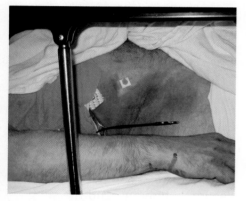

Figure 38.19 Significant retroperitoneal blood collection can be seen as bruising at the flank

SIGNS AND SYMPTOMS

Any patient who has been involved in a high-speed motor vehicle collision, a fall from a great height, or other similar high-velocity mechanism of injury, or who has been crushed between two objects, should be suspected of having a pelvic fracture.

Likewise, a patient who, after sustaining a serious trauma, complains of an ache or pain in the lower back should be suspected of having a pelvic fracture. The danger of serious life-threatening bleeding into the pelvic cavity is extremely high; therefore, any patient with significant, multiple traumas should be suspected of having a pelvic injury.

Perhaps the best indication of a pelvic fracture is a sharp pain or diffuse tenderness when the pelvic ring is lightly compressed. Gentle compression of the pelvis should be a part of every detailed physical examination. The **symphysis pubis,** the union of the two pubic bones found above the genitalia, also should be gently compressed. If the patient complains of pain to the pelvic area, this step should be avoided; no further assessment is needed, and a pelvic fracture can be safely assumed. The proper methods of assessing the pelvis are covered in Unit 19 and should be reviewed.

If sharp pain or point tenderness is noted upon gentle compression, a pelvic fracture should be suspected, and the EMT should assess for signs of hypoperfusion and shock.

MANAGEMENT

Fractures of the pelvis, also known as the pelvic ring, have been associated with a higher mortality. In any case of suspected pelvic instability, the fractured bones need external support. The EMT may elect to use the **pelvic wrap technique.** The pelvic wrap consists of a wide swath of material, generally cotton, which can be placed around the circumference of the pelvis and secured tightly.

The pelvic wrap, very similar to an abdominal binder that is used postoperatively to hold abdominal dressings in place, provides a gentle, circumferential pressure that keeps all of the bones of the pelvic ring in alignment. Keeping these bones in place will help to prevent lacerations of major blood vessels, such as the femoral artery, puncture of the bladder, or perforation of the colon and rectum.

The use of MAST has been somewhat controversial over the past several years, but this device has been shown to provide immobilization for unstable pelvic and lower extremity fractures. Consult medical control and local protocols concerning the use of MAST for unstable pelvic fractures.

Pelvic fractures can cause massive bleeding. The abdominal cavity and the retroperitoneal space can obscure and hide massive bleeding. Unfortunately, it is often late when an EMT discovers that the patient is experiencing massive internal bleeding from a pelvic injury. The EMT often attributes the sustained tachycardia and other signs of hypoperfusion that the patient is exhibiting to pain.

The key to early detection lies in careful reevaluation of the patient's vital signs and an analysis of the trend that is created. If the patient's heart rate is increasing steadily, instead of decreasing after splinting, and the blood pressure is starting to fall, the EMT should suspect internal bleeding and request an ALS intercept and ensure rapid transportation to a trauma center.

INJURY OF THE PROXIMAL FEMUR

The femur, the strongest bone in the body, provides the foundation for the muscles of the legs so that people can walk. Without an intact femur, walking is almost impossible.

When a powerful force is applied to the femur, either at the insertion of the femur into the pelvis or at the end of the femur proximal to the knee, the femur can either dislocate or break. The femur tends to break at the thinnest portion of the femur, called the surgical neck. The surgical neck is proximal to the head of the femur, which inserts into the pelvis.

SIGNS AND SYMPTOMS

Injury of the femur can be caused by indirect violence, such as when the knee is struck, which can drive the femur backward and dislocate the femur from the pelvis. The femur can be injured from direct trauma as well; for example, the door of a car may be driven into the hip of a patient in a motor vehicle collision. Regardless of the mechanism of injury, a hip injury can have serious complications.

The nerve that provides sensation and movement to the legs, the **sciatic nerve,** runs adjacent to the femur. A hip injury can injure the sciatic nerve, leaving the patient's leg numb (paresthesia) or unable to move (paralysis).

A subtle, yet easily detected, sign of sciatic nerve injury is **footdrop.** The sciatic nerve controls the elevation, or **dorsiflexion,** of the foot. A foot that

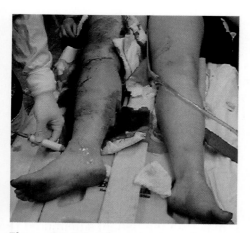

Figure 38.20 Often the leg of a broken hip will be shortened and rotated externally (Courtesy of Deborah Funk, MD, Albany Medical Center, Albany, NY)

cannot be lifted (dorsiflexion) is a sign that the patient's sciatic nerve and the hip may be injured.

The most dependable sign of a hip injury is severe pain with gentle compression on the femur's point of insertion into the pelvis. The EMT should place her hands on each side of the hip, with her palms on the firm portion of the lateral buttocks, and press gently. If the femoral head is broken or the hip is dislocated, the patient will experience severe pain.

Typically, when the hip is fractured, one leg will be shortened, compared to the other, and externally rotated, pointing away from midline (Figure 38.20). If the hip is dislocated, the injured hip will be flexed, and the leg internally rotated (pointing toward the midline).

MANAGEMENT

The EMT does not need to distinguish a hip fracture from a hip dislocation in the field. In both cases, the hip must be handled carefully to avoid further injury. The EMT should support the affected limb by putting either pillows or blankets between and under the legs. The patient's hip and leg should be securely fastened to a long backboard.

The EMT also must consider the possibility of concurrent spine injury. If the force was great enough to break a hip, it may have broken the neck as well. A detailed physical examination, with attention to peripheral pulses, movement, and sensation, should be performed before and after immobilization.

INJURY OF THE MIDSHAFT FEMUR

The femur is the longest bone in the body, almost 18 inches long in the average 6-foot-tall person. Powerful muscles in the thighs attach to the femur and, by contraction, move the leg forward, propelling the body along with it.

The middle portion of the femur, or the midshaft, is very strong and can resist injury. However, enough force, such as a fall from a significant height, can shatter even the strongest femur.

SIGNS AND SYMPTOMS

When the middle section of the femur is broken, the muscles contract and drive the bone ends together. The resulting spasm, as the muscle ineffectually strives to move the leg, is very painful.

Street Smart

A patient involved in a motor vehicle collision may complain that he simply cannot get out of the car. When the femur is driven backward and the hip becomes dislocated, the patient's hips will be locked into the seated position.

Careful examination of the crash bar under the dashboard may reveal damage from the patient's knee striking the crash bar. Palpation of the patient's knee may reveal swelling and tenderness over the kneecap, or *patella.* If the EMT palpates the posterior buttocks, she may discover a lump, which would be the head of the femur.

A hip dislocation is painful, and the patient may resist any attempts at moving the hip. The patient must be carefully moved as a unit, and the car may have to be dismantled before the patient can be lifted out. Fire-rescue and EMS must work together to create the easiest means of access to and exit for the patient.

Nearby blood vessels, as well as muscles, can be lacerated by the sharp bone shards. The result is significant bleeding into the thigh. As much as 1 liter of blood can be lost into each thigh from internal bleeding.

The effect of the muscles in spasm tends to cause the bone to become distorted and deformed. Severe deformity can result in an open fracture of the femur. If this occurs, the EMT should immediately control the bleeding and cover the wound with a dry sterile dressing.

MANAGEMENT

During World War I, Dr. Thomas, a noted orthopedic surgeon, realized that applying a gentle counterpressure against a muscle spasm relieved the spasm and prevented bones from lacerating blood vessels, thus preventing further bleeding. This finding was significant. At that time, there was a 50% mortality rate associated with a midshaft femur fracture. The Thomas half ring was an early medical device that provided the foundation for gentle counterpressure, or **traction,** to be applied to a broken femur.

Modern traction splints are easier to apply and operate than the early Thomas half ring with Spanish windlass. Some traction splints depend on two parallel bars, much like the early Thomas half ring. At the bottom of the device is a ratchet attached to an ankle hitch. When the ratchet is tightened, traction is applied to the ankle hitch and thus to the leg. See Skill 38-2 at the end of this unit for step-by-step instructions about application of a bipolar traction splint.

Another adaptation of the same idea uses a single pole, usually placed between the patient's legs, and a spring-loaded device that applies the traction. The advantage of the unipolar traction device is that the force is measurable. See Skill 38-1 at the end of this unit for step-by-step instructions about application of a unipolar traction splint.

When the traction device is in place and the traction is applied to the femur, the leg spasms less often, and the patient usually obtains noticeable relief of symptoms. The patient must be continually monitored for signs of hypoperfusion and transported to the closest appropriate facility.

INJURY OF THE PATELLA

The kneecap, or *patella,* is a flat triangular bone located anterior of the knee. It primarily protects the knee joint from injury, as when a person kneels on the knee.

SIGNS AND SYMPTOMS

Typically, the kneecap is injured when the knee is twisted. When the knee twists, the kneecap often shifts laterally and is then dislocated (Figure 38.21). Although a dislocated kneecap can be painful, it is not dangerous. Unlike other bones, there are no veins, arteries, or nerves near the kneecap.

A larger problem exists when the kneecap is actually fractured. Gentle palpation of the borders of the kneecap should reveal a single triangular-shaped bone. If the force against the kneecap was great enough, the kneecap may split into two or more pieces.

MANAGEMENT

An isolated injury to the kneecap should be treated with stabilization, immobilization, and transportation. Often the patient has already manually stabilized the knee by placing one hand on each side of the knee.

Immobilization can be accomplished with a pair of padded board splints in a manner similar to the way the elbow is immobilized. Immobilization also

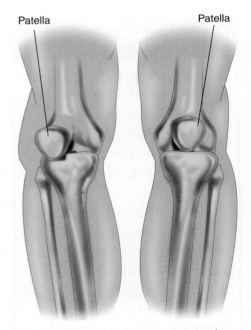

Figure 38.21 Kneecap dislocations usually shift laterally, appearing as a lump on the outside of the knee

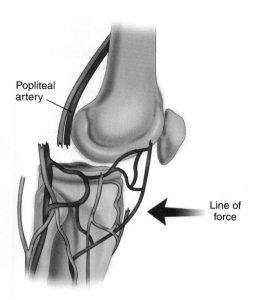

Popliteal
artery

Line of
force

Figure 38.22 A knee dislocation has a characteristic "stepped off" appearance

can be accomplished with a pillow placed under the knee and secured around the knee with cravats.

Local tissue swelling can be impressive. Ice or ice packs should be applied to the injury and the patient transported as soon as possible.

INJURY OF THE KNEE

As a joint, the knee consists of the femur, in the thigh, meeting the two bones of the lower leg, the tibia and the fibula. When a significant force is applied to either the femur or the tibia, the bone may move out of alignment. Frequently, the patient is unable to move his leg; the knee is said to be locked. The patient also may complain of severe pain. The knee is surrounded by many ligaments that are painful when injured. The leg also may appear grossly deformed, often with a distinctive drop, or "step off," in the skin's surface (Figure 38.22).

Behind the bones in the knee lie the major arteries of the lower leg. A disruption in the alignment of the bones may mean that distal circulation is disrupted. The EMT should check carefully for distal pulses. Pulselessness in the affected leg is a true medical emergency. Signs and symptoms of patella and knee dislocation are summarized in Table 38-3.

MANAGEMENT

In certain instances, medical control may advise the EMT to straighten the leg in an attempt to get pulses to return. The EMT should make only one attempt, being careful to monitor the pulses in the process. If pulses do not return after the leg has been straightened, the EMT should quickly package the patient for transportation. The EMT should call the hospital and advise the emergency department of the situation so that proper preparations can be made. In every instance, the EMT should follow local medical protocols.

INJURY OF THE LOWER LEG

The bone that is found just under the skin of the anterior leg is called the tibia; the lay term is shinbone. This bone is responsible for weight bearing. The smaller bone behind the tibia, the fibula, is fractured more frequently than the tibia. A fracture in the fibula has fewer consequences for the patient.

Table 38-3 Comparison of a Kneecap and a Knee Dislocation

Finding	Patella or Kneecap	Knee
Mechanism	Usually a fall or misstep	Major trauma
Deformity	Lateral	Anterior
Distal pulses	Present	May be absent
Severity	Low priority	High priority
Surgery	Rare	Common

MANAGEMENT

Because the tibia is so close to the skin, open fractures of this bone are common (Figure 38.23). The EMT should first control the bleeding and then bandage the injury with a dry sterile dressing.

The tibia and the fibula can be immobilized using padded board splints or a vacuum splint. Keeping the principles of immobilization in mind, the EMT can effectively splint this injury.

INJURY OF THE ANKLE

Ankle injuries frequently occur, whether from sports injuries, falls, or just stepping off a curb. The ankle, like the hand, is a collection of small bones. While the majority of ankle injuries are sprains of the ligaments, each bone is capable of being fractured.

MANAGEMENT

It is best if an ankle injury is treated like an ankle fracture. The ankle should be immobilized with an air splint, pillow splint, or a padded board splint (Figure 38.24).

INJURY OF THE FOOT

The heel is the most commonly fractured bone in the foot. The heel, or *calcaneus,* absorbs all the force of impact in a fall or a jump. If the force is great enough, the calcaneus usually swells immediately, and the heel becomes ecchymotic.

MANAGEMENT

A simple pillow splint is usually sufficient to immobilize the foot. The EMT should remember to leave the toes exposed so that distal circulation and capillary refill may be assessed.

The foot is very vascular, and swelling can be rapid. The EMT should place the foot on a pillow that elevates the foot above the level of the heart. Application of ice may also decrease swelling.

The EMT should be sure to assess all the joints immediately superior to the ankle. Injury from indirect trauma can impact the knee and the hip.

CONCLUSION

Given that more than 200 bones comprise the human skeletal system, it is logical to surmise a large number of bony injuries are possible. Treatment of bone injuries varies based on size, location, and proximity to other structures in the body; overall, treatments for all bony injuries are similar if the EMT keeps a few basic principles in mind. Often the EMT may need to use a little inventiveness to accommodate the different patients to the limited number of splints available. Using the basic principles learned in the management of bone injuries, the EMT will be able to immobilize the patient's injury and safely transport the patient for further treatment.

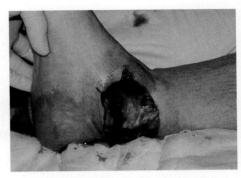

Figure 38.23 A tibia fracture is often an open fracture (Courtesy of Deborah Funk, MD, Albany Medical Center, Albany, NY)

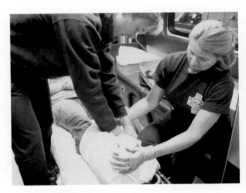

Figure 38.24 A pillow can serve as a splint for an ankle injury (Courtesy of Larry Torrey and MEDCU, Portland, ME)

Street Smart

When a heel injury occurs as a result of a fall or a jump, the EMT should suspect that there also might be a lumbar spine injury. The force of impact can drive the force up the legs and into the pelvis and lower back, injuring the lumbar spine.

If a lumbar spine injury is suspected, the EMT should use standard spinal precautions, including a long backboard and cervical immobilization collar.

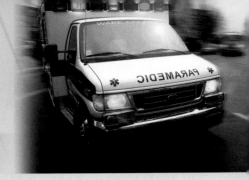

Jeremiah knows, based on the mechanism of injury and location of the open wound, there is a strong possibility this is an open fracture of the tibia. The athletic trainer has stabilized the fracture site by manually holding the leg just above the knee and below the wound site. Jeremiah checks for range of motion, sensation, and distal pulses, noting that all are present at this time.

Brandon's leg is splinted in the position found using a pneumatic vacuum splint. Jeremiah rechecks sensation, motion of the toes, and distal pulses following immobilization and documents left lower extremity function continues to be intact following splinting.

Brandon is logrolled onto a long spine board with padding placed to fill the voids under his neck and helmet. He is secured to the long spine board, taking all spinal precautions, and placed on the stretcher and into the ambulance.

En route to the hospital, baseline vital signs are assessed, and a complete secondary assessment is conducted with no additional injuries found. ALS intercept has been requested and is met en route. Jeremiah provides a report as an IV line is established, and the paramedic administers medication for Brandon's pain.

Later that evening, Jeremiah receives a phone call from Brandon's parents thanking him for his quick actions. Brandon's mother says he suffered an open fracture of the tibia, which has been repaired in surgery, and there was also some damage to the ligaments. He will be in a cast for 6 weeks and out for the rest of the football season.

PURPOSE: To apply a traction device to a possible midshaft femur fracture.

STANDARD PRECAUTIONS:

☑ Scissors
☑ Unipolar traction device
☑ Personal protective equipment

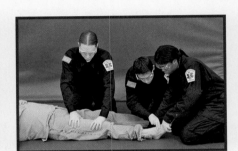

1 The EMT should manually stabilize the limb while instructing a trained assistant to grasp the leg and apply manual stabilization of the affected leg.

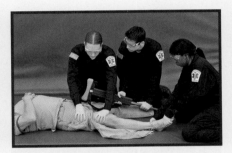

2 The EMT checks distal pulses, movement, and circulation in the affected leg.

3 The EMT then prepares the traction device, adjusting it to about 3 to 4 inches past the leg.

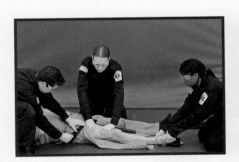

4 The EMT slides the traction splint between the leg and secures the ischial strap across the thigh.

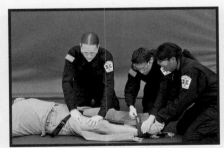

5 Next, the EMT applies the ankle hitch to the ankle and applies traction of the leg.

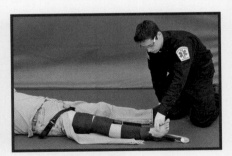

6 The EMT then puts the straps in place and rechecks distal pulses, movement, and sensation.

Skill 38-2 Application of a Bipolar Traction Splint

PURPOSE: To apply a traction device to a possible midshaft femur fracture.

STANDARD PRECAUTIONS:

- ☑ Bipolar traction splint
- ☑ Personal protective equipment
- ☑ Scissors

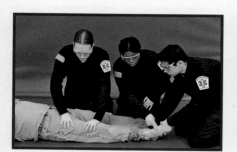

1 One EMT should manually stabilize the limb as another EMT checks for a distal pulse and exposes the wound.

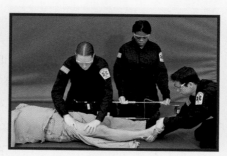

2 The EMT then prepares the traction device, adjusting it beyond the length of the uninjured leg, and moves the straps into place.

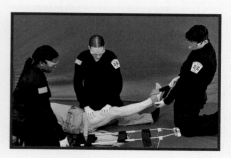

3 Next, the EMT applies the ankle hitch to the ankle and assumes traction of the leg.

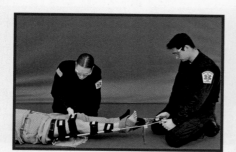

4 Then the EMT slides the traction splint under the leg and secures the straps.

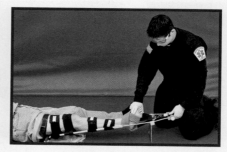

5 In the final step, the EMT applies the ankle hitch to the ratchet and applies mechanical traction. With the straps in place, the EMT rechecks distal pulses, movement, and sensation.

Key Concepts Revisited

- The key to discovering bone injuries is a high index of suspicion that a bone injury may exist.

- Ligaments are sinewy tissue that connects bones together at the joint; a tendon is connective tissue that attaches muscle to bones.

- A closed fracture, in which the bone ends remain within the skin, is the most commonly seen fracture, whereas an open fracture is characterized by bone ends that have erupted through the skin.

- A dislocated bone is a serious emergency when circulation and function distal to the joint are compromised.

- Bone injuries commonly present with deformity and swelling.

- The basic principles of splinting provide a foundation for the application of all splints.
  - Life before limb.
  - Stabilize manually.
  - Expose the injury.
  - Control bleeding.
  - Check distal pulses, motion, and sensation.
  - Immobilize joints above and below the injury.
  - Elevate above the heart.
  - Pad voids between the splint and limb.
  - Do not place straps directly over the injury.
  - Recheck distal pulses, motion, and sensation following splinting.

- Distal pulses must be assessed prior to and following splinting.

- One attempt to realign the bones should be made when distal pulses are absent in an injured limb.

- The type of splint used in bone injuries is often dependent on the location of the injury.
  - Sling and swathe
    - Shoulder girdle
      - Clavicle
      - Scapula
      - Shoulder A/C joint dislocation
  - Flexible splint
    - Pillows/padding
      - Hip
      - Knee
      - Ankle
      - Foot

- Ladder splints
- SAM splints
  - Elbow
  - Forearm
  - Wrist
  - Knee
  - Ankle
  - Foot
  - Rigid splints
    - Padded board
    - Inflexible metal
      - Upper arm/humerus
      - Forearm
      - Wrist
      - Knee
      - Ankle
      - Lower leg
      - Foot
  - Pneumatic splints
    - Air splint
    - Vacuum splints
      - Forearm
      - Ankle
      - Lower leg
      - Foot
    - MAST
      - Pelvic fractures
      - Lower extremity fractures
  - Traction splints
    - Unipolar traction splint
    - Bipolar traction splint
      - Femur

- Traumatic bone injuries often include injuries to the structure surrounding the bone, such as the ligaments and tendons; management should focus on stabilization and immobilization.

Review Questions

1. What are the three forces that can cause injury to a bone?
2. What are ligaments and tendons?
3. When does a dislocation become an emergency?
4. What is the difference between a closed and open fracture?
5. What are the common signs and symptoms of a bone injury?
6. What are the 12 principles of splint application?
7. What are the different techniques of splint application?
8. List some splint application techniques for the following bone injuries:
   Clavicle
   Humerus
   Wrist and hand
   Elbow
   Femur
   Patella
   Ankle
9. What is the importance of differentiating a knee dislocation from a kneecap dislocation?
10. When can an EMT straighten a fracture or dislocation?

Key Terms

Acromioclavicular (A/C) dislocation
Appendicular skeleton
Axial skeleton
Bipolar traction splint
Closed fracture
Colles' fracture
Direct force
Dislocation
Dorsiflexion
False motion
Flexible splint
Footdrop
Fracture
Indirect force
Ligament
Locked
Medial malleolus
Motor nerves
Open fracture
Orthopedics
Paresis

Pelvic girdle
Pelvic wrap technique
Pneumatic splint
Position of function
Range of motion (ROM)
Rigid splint
Sciatic nerve
Self-splint
Sensory nerves
Shoulder dislocation
Shoulder girdle
Sling and swathe (S/S)
Spontaneous reduction
Sprained
Symphysis pubis
Tendon
Traction
Traction splint
Twisting force
Unipolar traction splint

Further Study

National Association of Emergency Medical Technicians. *PHTLS: Basic and Advanced Prehospital Trauma Life Support.* 6th ed. Clinton, MS: Mosby, 2007.

Rizzo, D. C. *Fundamentals of Anatomy & Physiology.* Clifton Park, NY: Thomson Delmar Learning, 2006.

Skinner, H. B. *Current Diagnosis & Treatment in Orthopedics.* Columbus, OH: McGraw-Hill, 2006.

UNIT (39) Environmental Emergencies

The Emergency Medical Technician (EMT) will be called to care for patients who have been exposed to various environmental dangers. It is important that prehospital providers recognize when environmental factors, such as heat or cold exposure, cause a medical emergency. The principles of emergency medical care for environmental emergencies rely on the EMT recognizing what elements of nature have created the emergency.

National Education Standard

The Emergency Medical Technician (EMT) will demonstrate a fundamental depth and foundational breadth of understanding of the pathophysiology, assessment, and management of environmental emergencies.

Key Concepts

- Thermoregulation is the body's attempt to balance heat lost and heat gained to maintain a constant body temperature.

- Knowledge of the various mechanisms of heat generation and heat loss is vital to management of heat-related emergencies.

- Prolonged cold exposure leads to a wide spectrum of cold-related illness and injury.

- Management of cold exposure begins with removing the patient from the cold environment followed by determination of the best method of rewarming.

- Prolonged exposure to heat leads to a wide spectrum of heat-related injuries and illness.

- Hypoxia is the most common result of submersion emergencies, including diving emergencies.

- Altitude-related emergencies are related to hypoxia because of the partial pressure of oxygen being less than it is at sea level, creating a hypoxic environment.

- Lightning injuries can be separated into minor and severe injuries, including cardiac and respiratory arrest.

- Types of venomous bites and sting emergencies are specific to the area of residence.

- EMTs must be familiar with common environmental factors that may cause injuries and illness ranging from mild to severe and even life-threatening conditions.

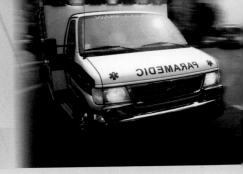

CASE STUDY

On Christmas morning Emergency Medical Services (EMS) are called to meet the local forest ranger. Herb the forest ranger tells the dispatcher he found a hunter who staggered out of the woods "acting drunk." Herb could detect no smell of alcohol, and the hunter was wet and shivering. Herb also noticed the hunter was not wearing a coat or gloves. Herb knew the hunter had to be suffering from hypothermia and called EMS.

When Montoya and Dave arrive, the hunter answers their questions but seems to be somewhat stuporous. He tells them he had been tracking deer and slipped, falling into the river. Montoya notices his speech is slurred. His only concern is pain in his feet and tingling in his hands.

Montoya notices that the patient's fingertips are blanched, almost white, and waxy looking, and his toes have the same appearance. His mental status is becoming more stuporous, and he keeps repeating that he is sleepy. Montoya also notes that the patient is not shivering, as one would expect of a person who is wet and cold.

Herb tells the EMTs he is familiar with the river the hunter must have fallen in and says the man must have walked, wet and exposed to the 20-degree temperature, for close to an hour.

Critical Thinking Questions

1. What are the priorities in management of this condition?
2. What additional signs and symptoms should the EMT attempt to assess?
3. What are the short- and long-term consequences of this condition?

INTRODUCTION

In addition to simple exposure to the elements, many outdoor activities may create other emergencies with which the EMT must be familiar. Water and altitude emergencies, lightning strikes, bites, and stings will be discussed in this unit so that the EMT may be better prepared to recognize and deal with problems related to these environmental issues.

TEMPERATURE REGULATION

The human body functions within a narrow range of temperature. If the body temperature is allowed to go outside of this narrow range, organ systems may malfunction.

A part of the brain called the hypothalamus is largely involved in temperature regulation. This centrally located part of the brain controls the body's set point, which can be thought of as the ideal temperature that the body wants to settle at for a particular time. For the most part, that temperature is within one degree of normal body temperature, 98.6°F, or 37°C.

The body is constantly faced with conditions that cause heat loss. On the other hand, many normal body activities generate heat that may need to be released. **Thermoregulation** can be thought of as an attempt to balance the amount of heat lost and heat gained to maintain a constant body temperature.

HEAT LOSS

The body generates heat with nearly every metabolic activity; therefore, it needs to get rid of excess heat. Heat can be removed from the body in four general ways: radiation, convection, conduction, and evaporation.

RADIATION

Radiation accounts for about 60% of the heat lost from the body at normal room temperatures. It is defined as the transfer of heat from the warm body into the cooler environment just by the fact that a temperature gradient exists. Warmth will leave the body and move into the cooler surrounding environment. Radiation is seen when a person who feels hot steps into an air-conditioned room and suddenly feels cooler. The excess heat is being dispersed into the cooler environment. Figure 39.1 illustrates this means of heat loss. Of course, when the ambient temperature rises, less heat will be dispersed in this manner.

CONVECTION

Air currents passing by a warm surface pick up heat and transfer it away from that surface. This means of heat loss, called **convection,** can be important to people out of doors. This concept is illustrated by a person who feels very

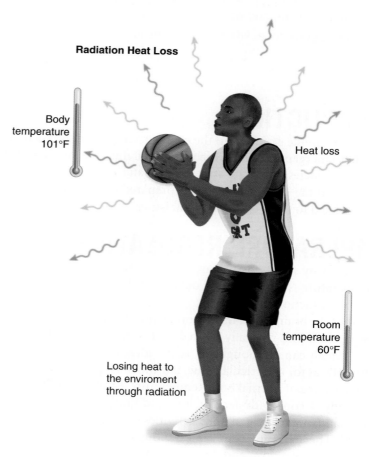

Radiation Heat Loss

Body temperature 101°F

Heat loss

Room temperature 60°F

Losing heat to the enviroment through radiation

Figure 39.1 Radiation is an important means of heat loss

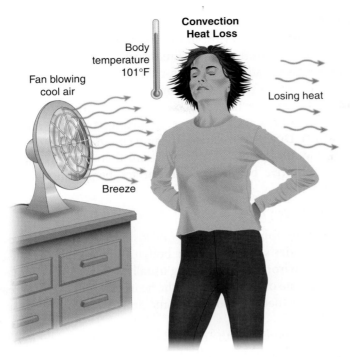

Figure 39.2 Convection is a mechanism that allows for heat loss

hot and cools off by standing in front of a fan. The excess heat is moved away from the person by the cooler currents of air moving past. Figure 39.2 depicts the concept of heat loss by convection.

CONDUCTION

If a warm object is in direct contact with a cooler object, heat will be transferred to the cooler object. This **conduction** of heat happens regularly when injured patients are left lying on the cold ground. It is important that EMTs be aware of this means of heat loss to prevent excess heat loss from occurring in their patients. Conduction is illustrated in Figure 39.3.

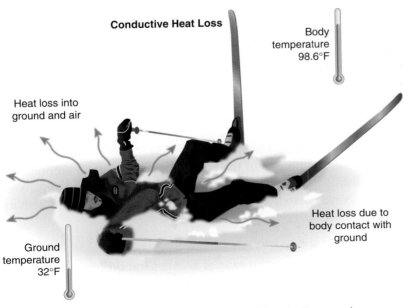

Figure 39.3 Conductive heat loss is a means of heat dispersal

Street Smart

The thermal conductivity of water is 30 times that of air; therefore, a person immersed in water will rapidly lose heat. The EMT should make it a priority to remove an even partially immersed victim from water as soon as possible to prevent rapid decline in body temperature.

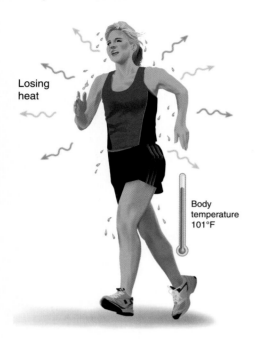

Evaporation of sweat into environment

Losing heat

Body temperature 101°F

Figure 39.4 Humans use evaporation to disperse excess heat from the body

EVAPORATION

Another major means of heat loss in warm environments is **evaporation.** This involves the transfer of heat into body fluids such as sweat, which then dissipates as it evaporates. Evaporation accounts for about 30% of the body's normal heat loss. If the humidity in the environment is high, the moisture on the body's surface will not evaporate; therefore, no heat loss occurs in this manner.

A large part of the heat lost by evaporation is via the moisture in the respiratory tract. During ventilation, the movement of air into and out of the lungs allows significant loss of moisture, and therefore of heat. Figure 39.4 illustrates evaporative heat loss from surface perspiration and from the respiratory tract.

MAXIMIZING HEAT LOSS

Understanding the four major means of losing heat from the body allows the EMT to consider several ways the body can maximize their use. In particularly warm environments, sweating usually occurs. The skin may become flushed, and the rate of breathing and the heart rate will likely increase. All of these are reactions that the body has to maximize heat loss by these different mechanisms.

Sweating and increasing the respiratory rate increase heat loss by evaporation. The flushed skin is a result of superficial vasodilation, which brings more of the blood up toward the surface, where it may come into closer contact with the cooler environment for additional loss of heat. Increasing the heart rate will increase the number of times the blood passes close to the surface of the body, where it can dissipate some excess heat.

HEAT GAIN

An understanding of how the body gains heat is necessary to maximize the use of the body's own mechanisms for getting rid of excess heat. Heat gain can be a desired increase in temperature to make up for heat loss somewhere else, or it can be an undesirable increase that must then be dissipated in some way.

As previously mentioned, the normal metabolism of the body produces heat. In particularly cold environments, the amount of heat lost may be greater than the amount generated with normal metabolism. In this case, the body must perform an about-face and figure out how to maintain its temperature or generate more heat.

INTERNAL SOURCES

Heat is generated inside the body by several means. These activities create a baseline level of heat production. This heat production may be increased as needed when the body requires additional heat. On the other hand, if these internal means of heat generation are diminished, the body will not have its usual amount of heat generation, and there may be a net loss in heat.

ROUTINE CELLULAR METABOLISM

The normal functioning of the body generates a certain amount of heat via metabolism. The minute-to-minute activity of cells and organs generates heat. Increased activity would create more heat. Decreased activity would generate less heat.

MUSCLE CONTRACTION

The other major internal means of heat generation comes from muscle contractions. As individual muscles contract, heat is produced. Heat generation by muscle contraction explains the rise in body temperature noted after heavy exercise or seizure activity. Both involve considerable muscle contraction.

The body may also create extra muscle contraction when a rise in temperature is desired. These extra muscle contractions are seen as shivering. Shivering is an effective means of increasing heat generation and creating a net rise in heat gain and therefore a rise in body temperature.

EXTERNAL SOURCES

Body heat can also be gained from external sources. Just as heat can be lost into a cooler environment, heat can be gained from a warmer environment. In extremely hot environments, such as in a sauna or hot weather, the body gains heat if the ambient temperature is higher than the body temperature.

PRESERVATION OF BODY HEAT

Just as the body has means of maximizing heat loss by vasodilation, sweating, and increased respiratory rate and cardiac output, heat gain can also be maximized in an attempt to preserve body temperature in a cold environment.

Vasoconstriction draws warm blood away from the surface of the skin to prevent heat loss to a cooler environment. *Piloerection* is a term that simply refers to hair standing up, essentially goosebumps. This primitive reflex is an attempt to maintain body heat.

Shivering in a cold environment increases the body's production of heat. Stimulation of the sympathetic nervous system results in an elevated heart rate and increases the body's metabolic rate, causing a greater amount of internal heat production.

Recognition of these signs of heat preservation may enable the EMT to more quickly identify a patient suffering from an environmental medical emergency.

INDIVIDUAL FACTORS

Individual factors may impair a person's ability to maintain body temperature within the ideal range.

EXTREMES OF AGE

Persons at extremes of age may be unable to protect themselves from extremes of heat or cold. This inability may be a result of physiologic issues, or these patients may simply not be able to remove themselves from the hot or cold environment or may not be capable of taking proper precautions, such as wearing protective clothing for the temperature. The EMT should be extra vigilant for temperature-related problems in infants and elderly patients.

MEDICAL CONDITIONS

In addition to extremes of age, any person who has chronic medical problems is likely to be at risk of having impaired thermoregulatory ability. Conditions such as diabetes, cardiac disease, thyroid disease, and many other chronic disease states put a patient at higher risk of suffering a heat- or cold-related illness due to an impaired ability to adequately balance heat loss and heat gain.

Acute medical problems such as shock, head injury, burns, generalized infections, injuries to the spinal cord, or hypoglycemia can also impair a patient's thermoregulatory ability. The EMT must therefore be attentive to maintaining body temperature in patients with problems such as these.

MEDICATIONS

Certain medications can decrease the body's ability to maintain an appropriate body temperature. Any medication that affects the sympathetic or parasympathetic nervous system or the metabolic rate has a chance of altering the patient's thermoregulatory ability.

Pediatric Considerations

Infants and young children are small and have a large body surface area relative to body mass or volume because they have a smaller muscle mass and less body fat. In addition, infants cannot shiver. Instead, they have a specialized adipose tissue, called *brown fat,* which is stimulated by cold to produce heat.

Geriatric Considerations

Elderly patients and patients with chronic medical illnesses are at increased risk for suffering cold emergencies. They may lose their ability to sense cold and to take appropriate protective measures. The ability to increase heat production and to conserve heat may be altered by age or by medical conditions.

Street Smart

Most acutely ill patients have trouble maintaining body temperature. It is therefore an important part of the management of the critically ill patient to prevent heat loss. Heat loss can easily be prevented by removing any wet clothing, moving the patient off any cold surface quickly, and covering the patient with a blanket as soon as the necessary assessment and treatment are completed.

EMTs should be aware that patients who are taking multiple medications are at high risk for being unable to adequately protect themselves from extremes of temperature by thermoregulation.

COLD EXPOSURE

Prolonged exposure to a cold environment can result in a wide spectrum of injuries and illnesses. The EMT must be familiar with the management of local cold injuries as well as systemic cold illness.

LOCAL COLD INJURIES

The spectrum of cold illness starts at a local level. Skin injury and musculoskeletal injury as a result of cold exposure are common and can be easily recognized and managed by the EMT.

CHILBLAINS

Chronic exposure of skin to cool, windy, damp weather can result in painful inflamed skin lesions called **chilblains.** These patchy skin lesions are often swollen and red to bluish and cause significant itching and burning. In longer-term exposures, the skin may blister or ulcerate. Symptoms of chilblains may develop up to 12 hours after the exposure.

The area of affected skin may be hypersensitive to cold after this injury, resulting in discomfort and increased chance of future cold injury. Women are particularly susceptible to this injury. The face and hands are the most commonly affected areas because they are often left exposed to the cool, damp wind.

TRENCH FOOT

Prolonged exposure of skin to cool, wet conditions can result in **trench foot.** Trench foot refers specifically to the injury seen after wearing wet footgear or being immersed in water for a prolonged period of time. This condition takes its name from military personnel who have spent a prolonged period of time standing in a trench full of water.

The injured extremity initially is cold, pale, and swollen and has diminished sensation and circulation. After it is rewarmed, the area becomes increasingly swollen, red, warm, and painful. This stage often lasts from 4 to 10 days. The patient is often left with some sensory deficit and local hypersensitivity to the cold.

FROSTNIP

When unprotected skin is exposed to freezing temperatures, local injury can occur that is similar to that seen in thermal burns. The mildest form of this local cold injury is called **frostnip.** Affected skin will be blanched and numb but can be easily rewarmed, leaving no permanent tissue damage.

FROSTBITE

Actual tissue damage that has occurred as a result of exposure to freezing and below-freezing temperatures is called **frostbite.** If the surface of the skin and superficial subcutaneous tissues are affected, the tissue appears white with blisters (Figure 39.5). Tissue affected by superficial frostbite feels soft and pliant and will flush as it is rewarmed. This type of injury is often quite painful as rewarming occurs.

When the tissue damage has extended deeper into the tendons, muscles, and nerves, the part is cold and hard with a classic wood-like feel. Tissues affected by deep frostbite are pale or mottled and do not regain circulation after rewarming. It is common for digits to become necrotic and be sloughed off (Figure 39.6).

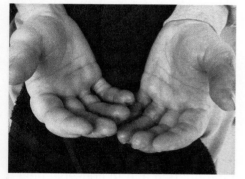

Figure 39.5 Superficial frostbite can be quite painful (Courtesy of Kevin Reilly, MD, Albany Medical Center, Albany, NY)

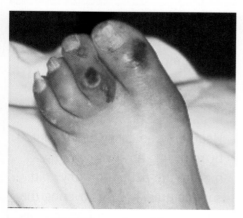

Figure 39.6 Deep frostbite results in permanent damage to tissue (Courtesy of Deborah Funk, MD, Albany Medical Center, Albany, NY)

MANAGEMENT OF LOCAL COLD INJURIES

The management for all local cold injuries is very similar. The priorities in management include removing the patient from the cold or wet environment, removing any cold and wet articles of clothing, and rewarming the injured part if there is no chance of reinjury.

Rewarming should involve immersion into tepid water (100 to 105°F) for up to 30 minutes. The less severe the injury, the less time it will take to warm it up. The EMT should attempt rewarming only if he can protect the patient from further cold injury and avoid refreezing the injured tissue.

When circumstances prevent immediate rewarming or when refreezing is a possibility, then the affected extremity should not be rewarmed. Instead, the area should be carefully bandaged and splinted to prevent further injury during transport.

Gentle handling of the injured tissue is important to prevent any further damage. After rewarming, the part should be carefully bandaged and splinted to avoid any rough movement. When the EMT is bandaging cold-injured skin, it is important not to allow contact with other skin. Gauze padding should be placed between fingers or toes to prevent the injured tissue from sticking to the opposing skin.

Finally, the patient suffering from a local cold injury should be evaluated in the hospital for evidence of any other injuries or effects from the exposure.

GENERAL HYPOTHERMIA

When net heat loss is greater than net heat gain, body temperature will fall, resulting in a condition called *hypothermia*. Hypothermia can be defined as a core body temperature of less than 95°F. The severity of hypothermia ranges from mild illness, when the temperature is just under 95°F, to severe hypothermia, when the body temperature is below 86°F.

Symptoms of hypothermia are related to failure of organ systems. The severity of the symptoms of this cold-related illness is directly related to the temperature. The signs and symptoms appear more dramatic as the body temperature gets lower. Decreasing mental status and motor function are well correlated with the increasing degree of hypothermia.

A patient does not necessarily have to be outside in subzero weather to become hypothermic. The exposure may be more subtle. Because patients with underlying illness have an impaired ability to thermoregulate, they can be in an environment that is cool, but not cold, and suffer from hypothermia. The EMT must keep this fact in mind when caring for ill and injured patients outdoors or in a cool indoor environment.

SIGNS AND SYMPTOMS

Some of the first signs seen in the hypothermic patient are poor coordination, memory disturbances, reduced sensation, mood changes, dizziness, and difficulty with speech. Patients suffering from early hypothermia may not realize that they are having a problem. Judgment is usually impaired, and often the hypothermic patient will begin taking off clothing, despite the cold weather. This is sometimes referred to as *paradoxical undressing*.

The mildly hypothermic patient will show signs of the body's attempts to maintain a normal temperature and decrease heat loss. Vasoconstriction results in pale, cool skin. Heart rate and respiratory rate are often increased. Shivering is common as the body attempts to generate additional heat.

As the body temperature falls, these signs become more pronounced. Muscles and joints become stiff, and below 86°F shivering no longer occurs. At these low body temperatures, organ systems do not function well. Breathing

It is important for the EMT to remember that in severe hypothermia, the pulse may be so slow and so weak that it may be nearly impossible to palpate. For this reason, it is important to assess pulses for 30–60 seconds before deciding to start cardiopulmonary resuscitation (CPR) in the hypothermic patient.

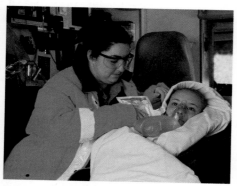

Figure 39.7 The EMT will likely treat patients suffering from hypothermia during cold weather

slows or even ceases; pupils no longer react; heart rate slows; and blood pressure falls. Eventually, if treatment is not provided immediately, the heart will stop completely and the patient will die.

MANAGEMENT

Management cannot start without recognition. The EMT should be sure to assess the skin temperature of every patient and determine whether the environment could have caused a low body temperature, given the patient's current health state. If mild hypothermia is clearly evident, the EMT must first remove the patient from the cold environment if possible. The patient should not be allowed to walk or exert herself and must be handled very gently.

The next priority in caring for the hypothermic patient is to prevent any further heat loss by removing any cold, wet clothing and covering the patient in warm blankets. Oxygen should be administered and should be warmed and humidified if available.

Treatment that is geared toward preventing further body heat loss is called **passive rewarming.** Actions taken to actually try to increase body temperature are considered **active rewarming.**

Active rewarming by the EMT consists of placing heat packs in the groin, axillary (arm pits), and cervical regions (corresponding to areas where major vessels come close to the surface) and increasing the heat inside the ambulance (Figure 39.7). Medical control may sometimes give specific instructions to give the patient warm, high-calorie liquids by mouth. The EMT is to give liquids only if specifically instructed to do so by medical control and only if the patient is awake and able to hold the cup and drink the liquid herself. The EMT should never administer anything by mouth to a patient who has a decreased level of consciousness. Every EMT should be familiar with local protocols regarding rewarming the hypothermic patient.

If a patient is hypothermic but awake and responding appropriately, the EMT should institute both passive and active rewarming measures. If the patient has a decreased level of consciousness, only passive rewarming should be attempted. External active rewarming in severe hypothermia can actually cause a drop in the core body temperature. This phenomenon is referred to as **afterdrop.**

Afterdrop results when peripheral vasodilation occurs and the cold blood from the surface and extremities is shunted into the core of the body, causing a drop in core body temperature. In severe hypothermia, it is better not to attempt to actively rewarm the patient but to simply prevent further heat loss, transport the patient, and support vital signs as necessary. Other, more invasive, techniques of active rewarming can be started at the hospital, so the EMT should not delay transport of the hypothermic patient.

The profoundly hypothermic heart is irritable and can easily go into ventricular fibrillation. At cold temperatures, defibrillation may not be effective. The EMT should always be gentle when handling the hypothermic patient to try to prevent the onset of ventricular fibrillation as a result of rough handling. When a patient is found in cardiac arrest, the EMT should follow protocols for CPR and defibrillation and should contact medical control as soon as possible (see Unit 24 for more details).

PREVENTION AMONG EMERGENCY WORKERS

As prehospital providers, EMTs commonly practice in environments that do not have controlled temperatures. Many emergencies require the EMT to work outside for prolonged periods, even in extremely cold or hot weather.

It is important that the EMT take steps to protect himself from adverse events related to extremes of temperature. Proper clothing for the weather is essential to working in the outdoor setting.

Several layers of clothing that can be taken off or put back on depending on the working environment are ideal for the prehospital health care worker. Gloves, hat, and face and ear protection are just as important as the heavy winter coat that keeps the body warm. Serious cold injury can occur rapidly and affects prehospital providers as adversely as it does the patient. Figure 39.8 shows an EMT dressed appropriately for working outdoors on a cold winter day.

HEAT EXPOSURE

When overall heat gain is greater than heat loss, the body temperature rises. This condition is called *hyperthermia*. Exposure to a hot environment does not always cause hyperthermia. Prolonged exposure to heat may result in a range of problems.

HEAT CRAMPS

One of the body's responses to a hot environment is perspiration. The perspiration will evaporate, and heat will be lost. Perspiration is made up of water and salts. In very hot environments, more than a liter of sweat can be lost each hour. A person can become quickly dehydrated and have significant electrolyte (salt) abnormalities.

When muscles become dehydrated and are deprived of certain electrolytes, they may spasm. These painful, involuntary spasms of muscles are called **heat cramps.** Heat cramps most often occur in the calf, thigh, or shoulder muscles and usually affect people who are not used to the heat.

MANAGEMENT

Heat cramps are uncomfortable but cause no permanent damage. A patient suffering from this condition should be removed from the hot environment and allowed to gently massage the painful area. Oral rehydration with water or an electrolyte solution will often result in complete recovery. Popular sport drinks are often given along with water for rehydration in a hot environment.

HEAT EXHAUSTION

As do cold-related illnesses, heat-related illnesses involve a spectrum of disorders that may begin as mild and without treatment may progress to a life-threatening condition. Some people who are exposed to heat compensate effectively; others have minor consequences such as heat cramps. Some patients cannot compensate for the excess heat and suffer a generalized heat-related illness.

One form of generalized heat-related illness is called **heat exhaustion.** This syndrome is characterized by symptoms such as dizziness, malaise, muscle aches, headache, fatigue, nausea, vomiting, and light-headedness. Often the patient suffering from heat exhaustion will have lost a great deal of fluid in sweat and may appear quite dehydrated or even have signs and symptoms of compensated shock.

The patient may have a normal or slightly elevated body temperature and elevated heart and respiratory rates and may have pale, clammy skin. The mental status in heat exhaustion is always normal. If the patient has an altered mental status, then she has a much more serious condition.

MANAGEMENT

Patients suffering from heat exhaustion should be removed immediately from the hot environment, and any excess clothing should be taken off. Because these patients are dehydrated, rehydration is a mainstay of therapy.

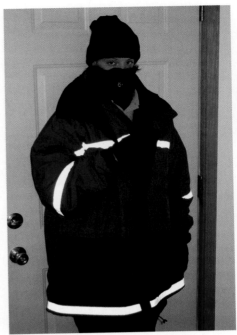

Figure 39.8 Proper dress can help prevent hypothermia in cold environments

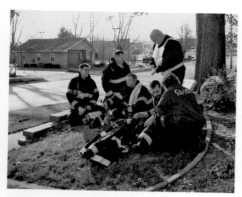

Figure 39.9 EMTs may be responsible for maintaining rehabilitation at the scene of a fire (Courtesy of Clive Fire Department, Clive, IA)

Oral rehydration with water and electrolyte solutions is possible if the patient is not nauseated or vomiting. Sometimes intravenous hydration is necessary and must be provided by advanced-level providers or by hospital staff.

Patients suffering from heat exhaustion will usually fully recover after adequate hydration, although this illness may aggravate other underlying medical conditions such as diabetes or heart disease. The EMT should be alert for such complicating factors in caring for these patients.

The EMT will encounter many situations in which heat exhaustion is common, one of which is standing by at the scene of a fire. Firefighters wear heavy, restrictive protective clothing. Even when the weather is not hot, firefighters are often exposed to extremely hot temperatures while fighting a fire.

It is crucial that appropriate rehabilitation be provided for firefighters on a regular basis to enable them to cool off and rehydrate themselves (Figure 39.9). EMTs are often responsible for this type of "rehab station" and must be able to properly care for firefighters and recognize the signs of a serious heat illness.

Many areas have a recommended protocol for managing patients in such a situation. Other situations in which frequent assessments of persons involved in strenuous physical activity in a hot environment might be necessary include marathons and outdoor concerts or other events. The EMT should be familiar with local protocol for such situations. An example of such a protocol is seen in Table 39-1.

HEAT STROKE

A life-threatening form of heat illness is present when the heat-exposed patient is found to have an altered mental status. Altered mental status indicates brain malfunction. This condition is called **heat stroke.** The patient suffering from heat stroke may have been exposed to high temperatures for a short period of time or may have been exposed to moderate temperatures for a prolonged period of time. Alternatively, exposure to moderate temperatures combined with intense exertion and internal heat generation will have the same result.

For heat stroke to occur, the overall heat gain must greatly exceed heat loss, and the body temperature must rise considerably. Temperatures exceeding 106°F are not uncommon in this condition.

The EMT must be able to recognize the signs of heat stroke and rapidly initiate therapy because more than 70% of patients with heat stroke will die if the body temperature is not lowered within 2 hours.

The signs of heat stroke include hot skin, with or without associated sweating; elevated body temperature; and altered mental status with a history of heat exposure. The progression of the disease may include seizures, coma, and eventually death.

MANAGEMENT

Removal of the patient from the hot environment and aggressive cooling measures should be initiated as soon as heat stroke is suspected. The EMT should carefully monitor the airway, breathing, and circulation and be prepared to support them if necessary. Oxygen should be administered as for any patient with an altered mental status.

The most effective means of cooling victims of heat stroke is to completely undress them, then spray them with tepid water, and allow fans to blow over the body. Alternatively, cold packs can be placed in the groin, armpit, and neck regions.

Table 39-1 Emergency Incident Rehabilitation

The following guidelines are intended for use at events where fluid loss is a concern for participants or spectators. These guidelines may also be used at fire scenes to treat firefighters.

The use of this protocol assumes that the person has no significant concern. If a person arrives at the rehab area complaining of chest pain or shortness of breath or has an altered mental status, keep the patient NPO (nothing by mouth) and follow the protocol appropriate to the patient's concern.

At fire scenes, the "rehab area" should be located near the self-contained breathing apparatus (SCBA) bottle-changing, triage, or staging area.

1. When the person arrives in the rehab area for the first time:
    A. Encourage the person to drink at least 8 ounces of fluid.
    B. An EMT should do a visual evaluation (the look test) for signs of heat exhaustion or fatigue.
    C. If vital signs are not within the criteria listed in this table, protective gear should be removed, and the person should rest for at least 15 minutes and be given continued oral rehydration.
    D. If vital signs return to criteria limits, the person can be released to return to duty.
    E. If vital signs are still beyond the limits, continue rehab for another 15 minutes and determine whether further intervention may be needed.
    F. If after 30 minutes the vital signs are still beyond the limits, advanced life support (ALS) transport to the hospital should be initiated.

2. When a person arrives in the rehab area a second time:
    A. Protective gear and constrictive clothing should be removed, and the person given at least 8 ounces of fluid to drink.
    B. An EMT should do a visual evaluation for signs of heat exhaustion and fatigue.
    C. If vital signs are not within criteria limits, further hydration should be provided and the person should rest for 15 minutes.
    D. Continue procedure 1F as above.

3. Vital signs criteria:
    A. Blood pressure: systolic <150 mmHg or diastolic <100 mmHg
    B. Respirations: <24 per minute
    C. − Pulse: <110 per minute (An irregular pulse mandates ALS intervention, electrocardiogram (EKG) monitoring, and removal from active duty or the event.)

4. Other considerations:
    A. Names and vital signs for each patient should be recorded on a log sheet for the incident.
    B. A full patient care report (PCR) should be written on any transported person.
    C. Electrolyte solutions are encouraged.
    D. More aggressive treatment should be used during extremes of temperature.
    E. Consider carbon monoxide poisoning during prolonged exposure to smoke.
    F. Other agency procedures may be used in place of these guidelines as appropriate.

If any questions exist regarding the treatment of a patient according to this protocol, contact medical control for advice.

(Adapted from 2008 REMO ALS Treatment Protocols, New York, Hudson-Mohawk Region. Courtesy of the Regional Emergency Medical Organization, Albany, NY)

Ice-cold water should not be used to cool victims of heat stroke. The icy water may induce shivering, which would result in an increase in body temperature—exactly the opposite outcome of the goal of therapy.

The EMT should initiate transport as soon as possible. An advanced life support (ALS) intercept should be requested, and transport to the closest hospital, in accordance with local protocols, should be initiated.

PREVENTION AMONG EMERGENCY WORKERS

EMTs often work in hot environments. It is vitally important that they realize they are susceptible to heat-related illnesses. Proper clothing and adequate hydration with frequent breaks from intense heat or exertion are important to keep the rescuers healthy.

WATER-RELATED EMERGENCIES

Nearly 8,000 people die each year in the United States as a result of drowning. More than 40% of these drowning deaths are children under 5 years of age, followed by teenagers and the elderly. Approximately 85% of drownings victims are male.

The bathtub is the most common location of drowning in children less than 1 year of age. Incidences of drowning in teenagers and young adults often occur in ponds, lakes, oceans, and rivers.

Alcohol and drug use are often involved in drowning incidents, placing teenagers and young adults at higher risk. Additional factors that increase the risk for drowning include patients with a history of diabetes and related hypoglycemia, cardiac history, seizure disorders, behavioral disorders (depressions, anxiety, suicidal ideology), and neuromuscular disorders causing poor body control.

NEAR-DROWNING

The term *drowning* refers to submersion in water resulting in death within 24 hours. If death does not occur in this time period, the term used to describe the event is near-drowning.

Although **near-drowning** by definition does not cause death, it is nonetheless a devastating event. If the brain is left without oxygen for a period of time, severe neurologic injury will result. It is the job of the EMT to quickly evaluate and provide emergency medical care to victims of near-drowning. Early rescue and resuscitation will improve the prognosis of the near-drowning victim.

SERIES OF EVENTS

The series of events occurring in a drowning incident is somewhat variable, although the final result is always hypoxia. Upon submersion, victims may hold their breath, causing blood oxygen levels to fall and carbon dioxide levels to rise. They are eventually forced to take a breath by the rising carbon dioxide levels in the blood.

Upon inhalation, water entering the airway will cause laryngospasm and bronchospasm. Often, this airway spasm will prevent any further water from entering the lungs, called aspiration. Water may also is swallowed, often in large amounts, resulting in stomach distension.

As blood oxygen levels continue to fall, the heart rate slows. As the heart rate slows, the blood pressure falls. If rescue does not occur at this point, the victim will suffer a cardiopulmonary arrest. The speed with which rescue occurs often determines how likely resuscitation is to be successful.

SALTWATER VERSUS FRESH WATER

Although there are differences between saltwater aspiration and fresh-water aspiration, resuscitation of the patient is conducted the same way for either incident. Both fresh water and saltwater affect the lungs by washing away surfactant, the substance that keeps the alveoli of the lungs from collapsing.

COLD WATER

When submersion occurs in cold water, the resulting hypothermia, for reasons that are unclear, seems to have a protective effect on the patient's organs. Survival of cold-water drowning victims has been recorded after even 40 or more minutes of submersion. The EMT should keep this fact in mind when resuscitating patients who have been submerged in cold water for any length of time.

MANAGEMENT

The first priority of management of the near-drowning victim is to remove the patient from the water. The EMT should be sure he and his crew are not in danger during this rescue. Only persons trained in water rescue should venture into water after a submerged victim.

A good rule of rescue to remember when dealing with water rescues is "reach, throw, row, then go." This is to remind the rescuer to try as many techniques as possible to help the victim that do not involve going into the water. Figures 39.10 through 39.13 depict this series of rescue techniques. The EMT who is likely to encounter water emergencies frequently in his job should consider further training in water rescue. A rescuer who enters the water with no training in water rescue has a good chance of becoming a victim. It will have served no purpose other than to distract further rescue efforts from the initial victim as rescuers attempt to rescue the EMT.

When rescuing a victim from the water, the EMT should consider the possibility of spinal injury. If there is any likelihood that spinal injury exists, as might happen in a dive into a shallow pool or onto rocks, careful attention to spinal immobilization must be a priority.

Upon removal of the victim from the water, the EMT should perform a primary assessment and treat any cardiac or respiratory compromise. There is no need to attempt to remove water from the patient's lungs, although vomiting is common as water returns from the stomach after having been swallowed. The EMT should have suction readily available.

All near-drowning victims should be transported to a hospital. Delayed respiratory difficulty can occur as a result of exposure of the airways to water. Near-drowning victims who are awake on rescue from the water generally have a good prognosis if proper treatment is provided.

DIVING EMERGENCIES

Diving emergencies an EMT encounters most often involve someone diving into a shallow pool, pond, or lake. In the case of submersion emergencies involving patients diving into the water from a diving board, shore, boat, or dock, head, neck, and spinal injuries must always be assumed. Additional injuries from diving into a shallow pool or pond can include fractures to the arms, legs, and ribs.

Although submersion emergencies involving scuba diving certainly are not common throughout the country, EMTs in some areas may be called on to care for patients suffering complications of deep water diving. It is important for the EMT to understand a few basic points about diving emergencies.

BOYLE'S LAW

A quick lesson in physics can improve an EMT's understanding of diving emergencies. One primary concept on why divers get into trouble, known as **Boyle's law,** holds that the volume of a gas varies inversely with the surrounding pressure. This concept is more easily understood with examples.

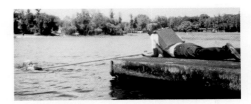

Figure 39.10 In any attempt to rescue a patient from a body of water, the first technique used is to reach out while maintaining a secure hold on a stable object

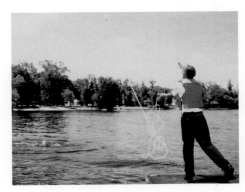

Figure 39.11 If the EMT is unable to reach a victim in the water, the next step is to throw a rescue rope or flotation device for the patient to hold onto

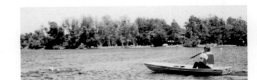

Figure 39.12 If the rescuer has been unable to reach the victim by reaching or throwing, he should use an appropriate watercraft to reach the patient if he is trained to do so

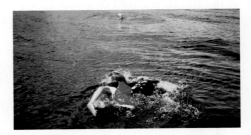

Figure 39.13 Only if all other methods have failed or are not available should a rescuer enter the water to go after a water-bound victim, and only if he is properly trained to do so

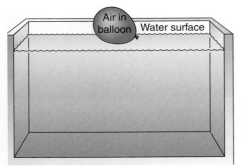

A.

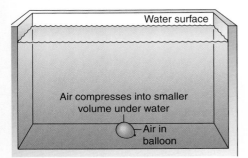

B.

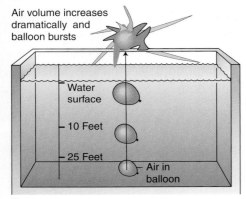

C.

Figure 39.14 A. Air takes up a defined volume of space at sea level B. The same amount of air is compressed into a smaller volume when under 25 feet of water C. As air is brought from a depth back to sea level, the amount of space it takes up will increase

Consider a bag of air that is put under 25 feet of water. The water exerts pressure on that bag of air. The pressure compresses the air into a smaller volume, allowing it to fit into a smaller bag.

Take that small bag of air from under the 25 feet of water and bring it back up to the surface. As the pressure around it is removed, the air expands back to its original volume. If left in the small bag, it may pop the bag as it expands. Figure 39.14 depicts this concept.

This concept of Boyle's law explains diving-related emergencies. This section discusses the most commonly seen diving emergencies related to pressure problems with which the EMT should be familiar.

DESCENT

Divers can have complications upon descent due to the compression of air in enclosed body spaces. These conditions are appropriately called "squeeze-related problems".

SQUEEZE

As you might expect, the term *squeeze* refers to the compression of a volume of air in an enclosed space as the diver goes farther down under water and the pressure of the surrounding water increases. There is often a pocket of air in a diver's ears and sinuses that can be compressed with the increase in pressure during a dive.

Divers often employ a technique of breathing that equalizes the pressures in these spaces as they descend in the water. If the pressures are not equalized, the air enclosed in these spaces will be "squeezed," causing pain and even damage to the area. The eardrum may even perforate with the increased pressure.

Symptoms of ear squeeze or sinus squeeze are pain during descent that often will force the diver to ascend immediately. If squeeze occurs, the diver should not be permitted to dive again until she has been examined by a physician at a hospital. EMTs should facilitate this exam by transporting the patient to the hospital for evaluation.

MANAGEMENT

Management of ear and sinus squeeze is generally limited to pain medicines prescribed by a physician. The EMT should advise the patient not to dive and to be examined by a physician to determine the extent of any injury. If the eardrum ruptures in this manner, permanent hearing loss may result.

ASCENT

Just as divers can have problems with compression of air in enclosed spaces on the way down, they can have problems with expansion of air on the way up. Some of these ascent-related emergencies can actually be life threatening.

DECOMPRESSION SICKNESS

A commonly known diving injury occurs during a rapid ascent as the pressure on the diver decreases. The gases that were used for breathing during the dive are compressed and can become trapped in tissues. If the diver ascends too rapidly to allow proper decompression of these gases, they can expand, forming bubbles. These bubbles can become stuck in joint spaces and in various tissues such as muscles, lung tissue, the brain, or the spinal cord. This condition is known as **decompression sickness.** This condition can occur if the patient takes an airplane flight within 24 hours of a dive, when returning home from vacation, for example.

Symptoms often do not occur for 1 to 6 hours after the dive has been completed and consist of pain in the areas listed previously. The most common concern is severe aching joint pain, although neurologic problems such as paralysis can occur as can respiratory problems if the lungs are involved. The classic joint pain is likely the origin of the term *the bends*.

PULMONARY OVERPRESSURIZATION SYNDROME

Another emergency of ascent is related to expanding air within the lungs as pressure decreases and the volume of air proportionally increases. A diver should always ascend slowly and exhale constantly during this time to allow the excess volume of air to escape.

If an ascent is too rapid or if the diver does not exhale, the volume of air in the lungs increases and can actually cause the tiny alveoli in the lungs to rupture. This so-called **pulmonary overpressurization syndrome (POPS)** will result in immediate symptoms of chest pain and difficulty breathing. Figure 39.15 illustrates this process.

AIR EMBOLISM

If a diver has sustained alveolar rupture during POPS, the air may actually rupture into a pulmonary blood vessel. Air that enters the bloodstream can travel wherever that blood vessel goes. The air bubble will become lodged in a small vessel and cause an inflammatory reaction that will result in a rapidly forming blood clot. Air that is traveling through the bloodstream is called an **air embolism.**

Because the vessels most commonly affected by this condition are the pulmonary capillaries, the air bubbles will follow the pulmonary vessels into the left heart. From there, they will then be sent to any organ in the body along the arterial system. The bubbles will travel in the arteries until they reach a small vessel that they cannot pass through. The resulting blood clot will occlude blood flow and cause severe pain, ischemia, and infarction of the tissue.

The symptoms of this air embolism are evident immediately upon ascent and may consist of severe pain, paralysis, or even unconsciousness or stroke-like symptoms, depending upon the location of the embolism.

MANAGEMENT

The management of all emergencies of ascent involves support of the airway, breathing, and circulation as appropriate. In addition, 100% oxygen should be administered to all patients who have symptoms of ascent emergencies. The patient should be placed in a supine position and transported immediately to a hospital for treatment.

Definitive treatment of these types of emergencies involves placing the patient in a specialized type of device called a **hyperbaric chamber.** These hyperbaric chambers create a simulated dive and allow recompression of air. Only specialized hospitals have hyperbaric chambers. The EMT who works in an area where scuba diving is common should be familiar with surrounding hospitals and know where the closest chamber is located.

NITROGEN NARCOSIS

One additional diving-related emergency the EMT should be familiar with is **nitrogen narcosis.** Sometimes called "rapture of the deep," this illness is a reversible condition caused by the anesthetic effect of nitrogen at high partial pressure. Nitrogen is one of the gases present in a diver's air bottle.

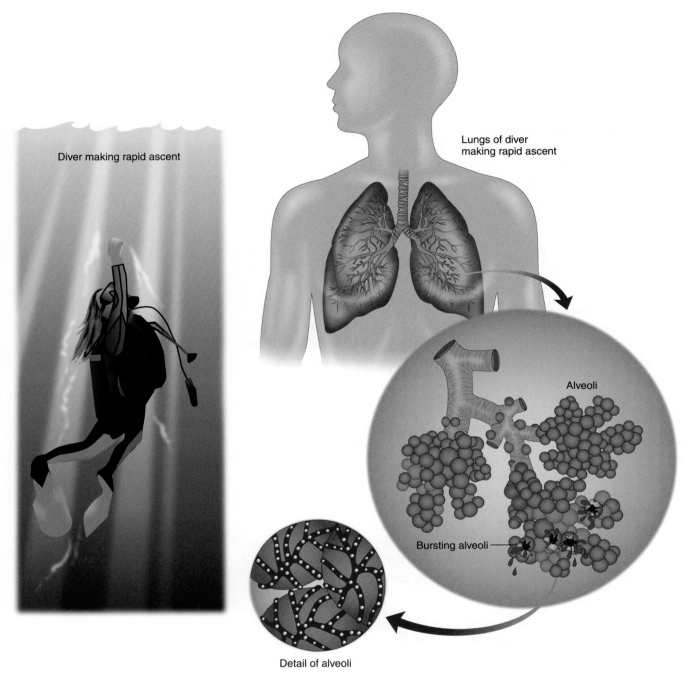

Figure 39.15 Expanding air can rupture a lung if not allowed to properly escape during ascent from a dive. Air can rupture into a pulmonary blood vessel during ascent from a dive

The patient suffering from nitrogen narcosis will appear as though he is intoxicated during the dive. The incidence increases with the depth of the dive and completely resolves with ascent.

MANAGEMENT

It is uncommon to see the residual sign of nitrogen narcosis after the diver has surfaced. If signs of intoxication or other mental status changes are present after a dive, air embolism to the brain or other, non–dive-related, medical illnesses should be suspected.

ALTITUDE EMERGENCIES

At high elevations, the partial pressure of oxygen is less than that at sea level, essentially creating a hypoxic environment. It makes sense, then, that altitude-related emergencies are related to hypoxia.

People who live at high altitudes have grown accustomed to, or acclimated to, the lower oxygen levels. Those who are not acclimated to this environment can become ill.

Altitude-related emergencies are a spectrum of illnesses that begin with a mild disease called *acute mountain sickness* and progress to a life-threatening emergency known as *high-altitude pulmonary edema*. The EMT who practices in an area that services high altitudes should be familiar with these illnesses.

ACUTE MOUNTAIN SICKNESS

Persons who are not acclimated to a high altitude can suffer from **acute mountain sickness (AMS)**. It is usually seen during a rapid ascent above 2,000 meters, or 6,600 feet, above sea level.

Symptoms of AMS begin with light-headedness and mild breathlessness. After a period of around 6 hours, other symptoms may occur such as headache, nausea, weakness, and fatigue. These symptoms will progress to severe headache, vomiting, and weakness if treatment is not provided.

HIGH-ALTITUDE CEREBRAL EDEMA

If left untreated, AMS can progress and may result in cerebral edema. This condition is called **high-altitude cerebral edema (HACE).** Altered mental status, trouble walking, decreasing level of consciousness, and focal neurologic weakness can all be symptoms of this extreme progression of mountain sickness.

HIGH-ALTITUDE PULMONARY EDEMA

The most lethal complication of mountain sickness is **high-altitude pulmonary edema (HAPE).** Early symptoms of this very serious condition include dry cough and dyspnea on exertion.

If the condition is allowed to progress, the patient will become weak and will have dyspnea even while at rest. Crackles will be clearly heard in the lungs as fluid builds up in the alveoli. Without treatment, this condition may become fatal.

MANAGEMENT

The management of any of the altitude-related emergencies involves oxygen and descent. Mild mountain sickness may be treated with oxygen and special medications to help the body more rapidly acclimate to the altitude. More severe symptoms of AMS, HACE, or HAPE should be taken seriously, and descent should be initiated immediately while oxygen is administered to the patient.

LIGHTNING STRIKES

Each year there are 300 fatalities and 1,500 injuries in the United States related to lightning strikes. Most deaths are due to immediate cardiac arrest. Among survivors, 75% sustain some sort of significant permanent disability or complication.

A direct lightning strike involves the instantaneous delivery of 100 million volts that usually rapidly pass over the victim's body. People who are not directly struck by lightning can still be injured as a result of a side splash of current from the initial impact site. Lightning injuries can be separated into minor and severe injuries.

MINOR INJURIES

Minor injuries from a lightning strike result in a stunned patient. Confusion, amnesia, and short-term memory difficulties are common. Other common symptoms may include headache, muscle pain, numbness, and temporary visual or auditory problems. Most patients with minor lightning injuries gradually improve and do not generally have long-term problems.

Common findings after lightning strikes are that more than 50% of people struck have ruptured eardrums. Superficial skin burns are fairly common but are usually not serious.

In addition to electrical injury, blunt trauma is common as a result of the force from the strike or secondary to a fall afterward. The EMT should be alert for possible traumatic injury such as broken bones and an injured spine. It is always a wise idea to assume the presence of traumatic injury and immobilize the patient to prevent any worsening of injuries.

SEVERE INJURIES

In severely injured people, the electricity produces a sudden direct current (DC) countershock that results in a halt in all cardiac electrical activity, and cardiac arrest results. After a few minutes, the heart may spontaneously resume its electrical activity. The lungs, on the other hand, may still be stunned as a result of the high-voltage shock and may not allow breathing to begin again. Persistent respiratory arrest will result in hypoxia. Hypoxia to the irritated heart may result in ventricular fibrillation. The state in which the severely injured patient is found depends on the timing of the rescuer arrival.

Early in this sequence of cardiac arrest, good airway and ventilatory management will likely result in a reversal of cardiac arrest and a favorable outcome. The longer the heart goes without oxygen, the less likely resuscitation is to be successful.

Even without causing cardiac arrest, a lightning strike results in a loss of consciousness in more than 70% of victims. Permanent neurologic injury to the brain or spinal cord may result.

MANAGEMENT

The first priority in the management of the victim or victims of a lightning strike is scene safety. The EMT must be sure that it is safe to allow the crew to approach the victims. It may be necessary to enlist the assistance of the fire department or power company if there is still a risk of electrical injury in the vicinity owing to downed power lines or other damage caused by the storm.

The next important consideration is to decide who should be treated first if there are multiple victims. In the case of lightning strikes, the principles of triage are reversed. People who are not in cardiac arrest upon the arrival of the rescuers will likely survive, and the people in cardiac arrest will likely be easily reversed. If personnel are limited, it may be reasonable to expend the limited resources in attempting to resuscitate the cardiac arrest victim. Unit 49 discusses the usual methods of triage.

Understanding the physiology of lightning injuries, the EMT should provide support for the airway, breathing, and circulation as needed and immobilize patients who may have suffered a blunt traumatic injury.

All victims of lightning strikes should be evaluated at the hospital because some of the consequences of a lightning strike can be delayed hours to days.

BITES AND STINGS

The EMT may get called to treat victims of envenomations from a variety of sources. Types of bite and sting emergencies are specific to the area of residence. It is useful for prehospital providers to be familiar with the most serious and common varieties they may be called to treat.

SNAKES

The venomous snakes native to the United States are rattlesnakes, copperheads, and water moccasins (all pit vipers) and coral snakes. Although there are nearly 8,000 reported venomous snake bites each year, the reported mortality rates are low. Despite the low number of deaths due to snake bites, the EMT who practices in an area where these snakes are found is likely to be called to treat a victim of a bite. It is therefore important to recognize the venomous nature of the snake and be knowledgeable about the effects of the bite and the appropriate prehospital treatment.

The degree of poisoning after a bite may range from a completely dry bite (25% of bites) to a severe envenomation, with symptoms evident immediately after the strike. The symptoms seen with each type of snake bite vary slightly, so they will be covered individually.

PIT VIPERS

A **pit viper** can be recognized by its two movable fangs and the depression (pit) that is seen in front of each eye (Figure 39.16A). The typical pit viper bite will have two fang marks with local pain and swelling (Figure 39.16B).

In severe envenomations, the patient develops extensive edema and systemic symptoms such as nausea and signs such as tachycardia. In very severe envenomations, the patient will appear acutely ill, with hypotension, tachycardia, altered mental status, respiratory distress, and spontaneous bleeding.

CORAL SNAKE

"Red on yellow, kill a fellow; red on black, venom lack." This rhyme can be recalled when identifying a true coral snake. **Coral snakes** can be recognized by their brightly colored body with red and yellow bands directly opposed in addition to black bands (Figure 39.17).

The bite of the eastern coral snake is toxic and causes neurologic decompensation in its victims. Tremor, salivation, respiratory paralysis, seizures, and other neurologic problems can occur after a significant bite.

MANAGEMENT

Every patient who is bitten by a snake should be evaluated in the hospital. The patient should be kept calm. The bitten extremity should be immobilized and kept below the level of the heart.

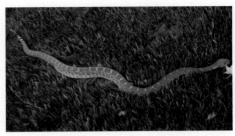

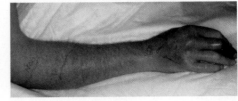

Figure 39.16 A. A pit viper can be recognized by the sunken pit in front of each eye B. The bite produces local pain and swelling

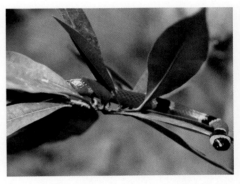

Figure 39.17 Despite its beautiful coloring, the coral snake is quite venomous (Courtesy of PhotoDisc)

Street Smart

The EMT should obtain a description of the snake but should never attempt to capture the snake to identify it. It is useful for the hospital staff to know the species of snake that bit the patient, but not at the expense of the EMT's safety. Most areas will have an animal control officer who can come and capture or identify the snake.

Safety Tips

In the past, it was taught to cut the snake bite and attempt to suck out the venom. This treatment is no longer practiced and is not appropriate prehospital management because it tends to cause more tissue damage than the bite itself and places the EMT at risk.

If the patient has any symptoms other than local pain and swelling, oxygen should be administered and the EMT should consider an ALS intercept. Transport should not be delayed in an attempt to find or identify the snake.

SPIDERS

Most spider bites are harmless, but bites from two species of spider may result in some long-term consequences. The brown recluse and black widow spiders are the offending arachnids.

BROWN RECLUSE SPIDER

Most commonly found in the south central and midwestern to western United States, the **brown recluse spider** is about 1/4 to 3/4 inch long (6–20 mm). Its brown body has a violin-shaped mark on the back, and the spider may be referred to as the "fiddle-back" (Figure 39.18).

The brown recluse usually resides outdoors under rocks, woodpiles, and other debris. They are not aggressive, and bites usually occur only if the spider becomes trapped against the skin. Brown recluse spiders have small fangs that cannot penetrate clothing; therefore, bites are usually found on areas of the body not commonly covered by clothing, such as the hands or exposed feet or ankles.

The bite of the brown recluse may go initially undetected and then appear a few hours later as a mildly red lesion that can develop with severe pain into a blister and bluish discoloration (Figure 39.19).

The severe form of the spider bite may become necrotic, appearing as a red halo or "bull's-eye" pattern and result in large areas of skin and tissue being damaged. A rare systemic reaction to this envenomation may occur 1 to 2 days after the bite. In rare instances, these bites are fatal.

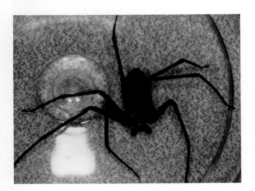

Figure 39.18 The venomous brown recluse spider is found most commonly in the southern and western United States

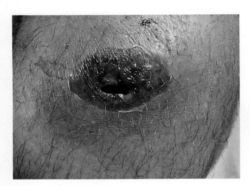

Figure 39.19 A characteristic wound from a brown recluse spider (Courtesy of Deborah Funk, MD, Albany Medical Center, Albany, NY)

Street Smart

Methicillin-resistant *Staphylococcus aureus* (MRSA) is a bacteria that typically causes skin infections and may form a collection of pus under the skin, called an abscess. The appearance of this abscess may look very much like a spider bite. If an EMT encounters a patient with what he believes to be a spider bite, it is imperative that the EMT keep in mind the potential infectious nature of the condition and use appropriate personal protective equipment.

BLACK WIDOW SPIDER

The female **black widow spider** is a jet-black spider, around 1 inch (25 mm) long, with a red hourglass mark on the abdomen (Figure 39.20). The male is much smaller and does not bite. This spider is found throughout the United States in crevices, woodpiles, stables, and garbage piles. More frequent encounters are reported in the warmer months.

The black widow spider is the leading cause of death from spider bites in the United States. Children under 16, adults over the age of 60, and individuals with chronic health issues, including hypertension, are at a greater risk for developing a severe reaction to a black widow spider bite. However, the black

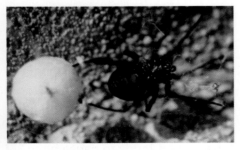

Figure 39.20 The black widow spider has been found throughout the United States in crevices, woodpiles, stables, and garbage piles

widow spider commonly avoids humans, and the females usually bite only if they are hungry, agitated, or protecting their egg sac.

The black widow spider bite is initially painful, and within 1 hour the patient may have redness, swelling, and generalized painful muscle cramping. This severe muscular pain can last for several days and may result in muscle weakness that lasts for weeks to months. Although less common, other serious complications of the black widow spider bite include severe hypertension, respiratory failure, shock, and coma.

MANAGEMENT

The emergency treatment of these spider bites is merely supportive: bandaging of the site and transport of the patient to the hospital where specific medications may be administered for the more serious symptoms. Although most spider bites will not result in serious symptoms, some can be fatal and all patients encountered by the EMT should be transported to the hospital for complete evaluation.

SCORPIONS

Scorpions are most frequently encountered in the southwestern United States and very rarely cause fatal injury in adults (Figure 39.21). A scorpion sting most commonly occurs to the hands and results in a slightly reddened area and a stinging or burning feeling. Occasionally, local tissue damage can occur.

Severe reactions more often occur in children and can consist of hypertension or hypotension, heart arrhythmias, throat spasms, muscle twitching, abdominal pain, and respiratory trouble.

MANAGEMENT

Most scorpion stings will require only pain medication; however, patients with severe reactions can decompensate quickly. Patients who were stung by a scorpion and call EMS should be transported to the hospital for further evaluation.

Patients whose sting is limited to localized symptoms can be transported without any specific treatment. Patients who have any evidence of symptoms in addition to local stinging and pain should be placed on oxygen, and an ALS intercept should be considered. The EMT should carefully monitor the airway, breathing, and circulation during transport of these patients.

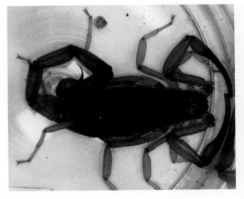

Figure 39.21 Scorpion bites rarely cause significant illness

FIRE ANTS

Fire ants are most commonly found in the southern United States and get their name from the intense burning pain, often described as "fiery" caused by their bite. Fire ant bites produce a circular pattern bite caused by their pivoting on the skin while stinging downward, producing excruciatingly painful, fluid-filled vesicles. The fluid in the vesicles is initially clear, then turns cloudy. The reaction from the fire ant bite is usually local, but it can affect the entire extremity and produce swelling, pain, and redness.

Although fire ant bites are not commonly the reason EMS is called, the EMT should treat any bites encountered using general wound care procedures, always following local protocols.

MARINE ANIMALS

The variety of injuries the EMT may see as a result of encounters with marine animals will vary depending on their area of practice. These injuries may vary from a shark bite to a jellyfish sting, and each is treated differently. Some marine injuries can be extremely painful and are potentially fatal.

MANAGEMENT

The EMT who regularly cares for patients exposed to such marine animals should seek further specific training to help recognize and treat such injuries. In general, the EMT should assess the patient as he would any other patient and support the vital signs as appropriate.

CONCLUSION

EMTs will encounter many patients throughout their career who have been exposed to a variety of environmental factors. Many of these may cause a life-threatening problem. It is the responsibility of the EMT to be familiar with common environmental emergencies.

Further training is encouraged for those EMTs who will be called on routinely to treat patients who suffer from other specific types of environmental injuries or illnesses.

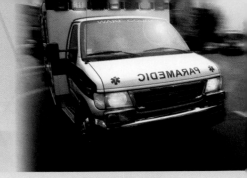

CASE STUDY Continued

Montoya and Dave prepare the hunter for transport, first removing all remaining wet clothing and wrapping him in warm blankets. Dave places him on humidified oxygen while Montoya begins to place warm packs under his armpits, on his neck, and in his groin area. The heat in the back of the ambulance has been turned up high and as they begin transport, Dave lets Montoya know ALS is en route for an intercept.

Montoya conducts the secondary assessment with no additional injuries found. She obtains a set of baseline vital signs with a pulse of 63, respirations of 16, and blood pressure of 118/68. She then gently applies dry dressings to the hunter's fingers and toes, making sure to place gauze between each finger.

Upon arrival with ALS, Montoya notes the patient's level of consciousness has improved and he is able to state his name is Kalvin. He states he remembers tracking a deer through the woods and then slipping and falling into a shallow stream. He remembers that he removed his heavy, wet coat and began walking back to where he left his car, but doesn't remember anything after that.

During the rest of the trip to the hospital, an IV is started by the ALS crew using warm IV fluids. Kalvin states he is feeling much warmer and no longer feels sleepy and confused; however, he has pain in his fingers and toes. He is assured his cold injuries will be further evaluated and managed at the hospital.

Key Concepts Revisited

- Thermoregulation is the body's attempt to balance heat lost and heat gained to maintain a constant body temperature.

- Knowledge of the various mechanisms of heat generation and heat loss is vital to management of heat-related emergencies.
  - Heat loss
    - Radiation—transfer of heat from a warm body to a cool environment
    - Convection—air passes over a surface, cooling it
    - Conduction—warm body transfers heat by being in direct contact with a cold surface
    - Evaporation—heat transfers into liquid that dissipates into the air
  - Heat gain
    - Internal sources
      - Routine cellular metabolism
      - Muscle contraction
    - External sources
      - Environment

  - Individual factors
    - Age
    - Medical conditions
    - Medications

- Prolonged cold exposure leads to a wide spectrum of cold-related illness and injury.
  - Local cold injuries
    - Chilblains
    - Trench foot
    - Frostnip
    - Frost bite
  - General hypothermia

- Management of cold exposure begins with removing the patient from the cold environment followed by determination of the best method of rewarming.

- Prolonged exposure to heat leads to a wide spectrum of heat-related injuries and illness.
  - Heat cramps

- o Heat exhaustion
- o Heat stroke
- Hypoxia is the most common end result of submersion emergencies, including diving emergencies.
  - o Near-drownings
    - Saltwater versus fresh water
    - Cold water
  - o Diving emergencies
    - Diving into a shallow pond or pool
    - Deep scuba diving
      - o Descent
        - Squeeze (compression) of air volume
      - o Ascent
        - Decompression sickness
        - Pulmonary overpressurization syndrome (POPs)
        - Air embolism
    - o Nitrogen narcosis
- Altitude-related emergencies are related to hypoxia due to the partial pressure of oxygen being less than it is at sea level, creating a hypoxic environment.
  - o Acute mountain sickness
- o High-altitude cerebral edema
- o High-altitude pulmonary edema
- Lightning injuries can be separated into minor and severe injuries. including cardiac and respiratory arrest.
  - o Minor injuries such as ruptured eardrums, minor burns, and blunt trauma causing falls
  - o Severe injuries—disruption of heart rhythm and breathing
- Types of venomous bites and sting emergencies are specific to the area of residence.
  - o Snakes
    - Pit vipers (rattlesnakes)
    - Coral snakes
  - o Spiders
    - Brown recluse spider
    - Black widow spider
  - o Scorpions
  - o Fire ants
  - o Marine animals
- EMTs must be familiar with common environmental factors that may cause injuries and illness ranging from mild to severe, even life threatening.

Review Questions

1. What are the various mechanisms by which the body loses heat?
2. What are the various mechanisms by which the body generates heat?
3. What are local cold injuries and the proper treatment for these conditions?
4. What are the signs and symptoms of generalized hypothermia?
5. What is the appropriate emergency medical care of the patient with generalized hypothermia?
6. What are signs and symptoms and management of heat exhaustion and heat stroke?

7. What are the complications of near-drowning?
8. What are signs and symptoms and emergency management of diving-related emergencies?
9. What are signs and symptoms of altitude emergencies?
10. What is the emergency medical care of altitude emergencies?
11. What are the priorities in caring for the victim of a lightning strike?
12. What is the emergency medical care of a victim of a bite or sting?

Key Terms

Active rewarming

Acute mountain sickness (AMS)

Afterdrop

Air embolism

Black widow spider

Boyle's law

Brown recluse spider

Chilblains

Conduction

Convection

Coral snake

Decompression sickness

Evaporation

Frostbite

Frostnip

Heat cramps

Heat exhaustion

Heat stroke

High-altitude cerebral edema (HACE)

High-altitude pulmonary edema (HAPE)

Hyperbaric chamber

Near-drowning

Nitrogen narcosis

Passive rewarming

Pit viper

Pulmonary overpressurization syndrome (POPS)

Radiation

Thermoregulation

Trench foot

Further Study

Mahadevan, S. V., and G. M. Garmel. *An Introduction to Clinical Emergency Medicine: Guide for Practitioners in the Emergency Department.* New York: Cambridge University Press, 2005.

National Association of Emergency Medical Technicians. *PHTLS: Basic and Advanced PrehospitalTrauma Life Support.* 6th ed. Clinton, MS: Mosby, 2007.

National Ski Patrol and Warren D. Bowman, eds. *Outdoor Emergency Care: Comprehensive Prehospital Care for Nonurban Settings.* Sudbury, MA: Jones and Bartlett, 2002.

CHAPTER 7

Maternal Health

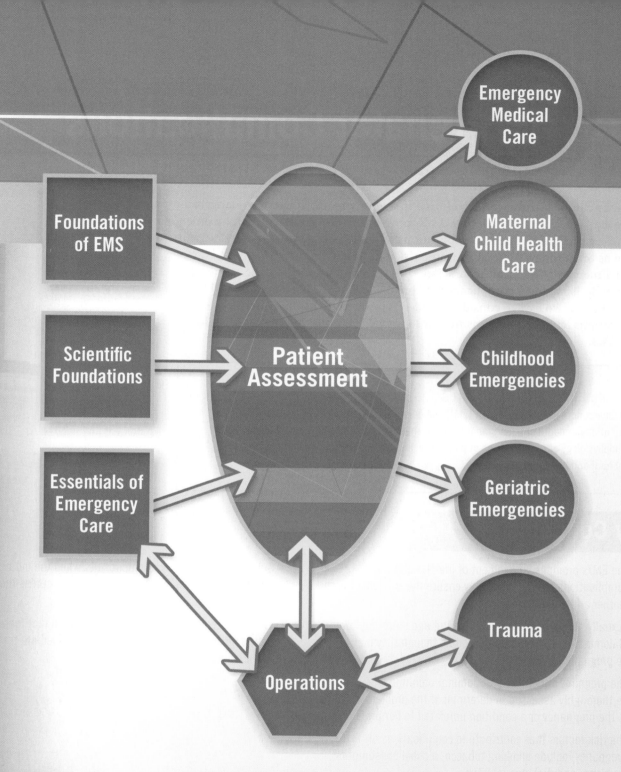

Maternal Health

Although childbirth heralds the start of a new life, it also can be the harbinger of disaster if something goes wrong. The EMT's role in childbirth is usually one of an assistant as the mother gives birth.

However, the EMT must constantly assess both mother and child for signs of distress and be prepared to support the mother throughout the pregnancy as well as during childbirth.

This section reviews the special problems that can occur with pregnancy, the role of the EMT in emergency childbirth, and care of the newborn.

UNIT (40) Prenatal Complications

Pregnancy can be a truly wonderful time in a woman's life. It can be a dangerous time in her life as well. In the late 19th and early 20th centuries, many women died during pregnancy due to complications of childbirth. Although that does not happen as often today, some of the same risks still exist.

An Emergency Medical Technician (EMT) may be called to the scene of a woman who is having a complication of pregnancy. At those scenes, the EMT has not one life but two lives to consider. An EMT's prompt attention to life-threatening complications can help to ensure the survival of both mother and child in many cases.

National Education Standards

The Emergency Medical Technician (EMT) will demonstrate a fundamental depth and foundational breadth of understanding of the anatomy and physiology of pregnancy, pathophysiology of complications of pregnancy, and the assessment and management of normal and abnormal delivery.

Key Concepts

- The EMTs prompt management of life-threatening complications of pregnancy may ensure the survival of both mother and child.

- Sexually active women of childbearing age suffering lower abdominal pain should be treated as though they may be pregnant.

- The pregnant patient with abdominal pain must be thoroughly assessed to determine if the problem is related to the pregnancy or a condition unrelated to her pregnancy.

- The risk factors that contribute to complications of pregnancy include smoking tobacco, alcohol consumption, drug use, and diabetes mellitus.

- Complications of early pregnancy include bleeding and possible loss of the fetus.

- Vaginal bleeding late in pregnancy should be considered serious and potentially life threatening.

- Toxemia of pregnancy leads to coma and death if untreated.

- The fetus is protected internally against most blunt trauma.

- Supine hypotension syndrome results when the mother is laid flat, causing the weight of the uterus to compress the vena cava.

- The management of complications of pregnancy focuses on the ABCs, treatment for shock, and immediate transport to the appropriate facility.

Candice and Jacob respond to the local urgent care clinic for severe bleeding. Upon arrival, the receptionist escorts them to the end of the hall where they are met by a nurse attending an obviously pregnant young woman in the exam room.

Candice enters the room while Jacob stays with the stretcher in the hall outside. Candice introduces herself to the patient. The patient is quiet, tearful but calm, stating her name is Cindy and she is 36 years old. She further states this is her first pregnancy and reports that she experienced a little bleeding during the first couple of months of pregnancy, but none since then until today.

The nurse provides the patient's current history, which includes 30 weeks of pregnancy and heavy, painless vaginal bleeding for the past 2 hours.

Candice and Jacob manage to get the stretcher into the cramped exam room, knowing it is important to keep the patient in a supine position. They gently lift her to the cot. They place Cindy on oxygen by non-rebreather mask at 12 lpm and help her shift onto her left side on the cot as they prepare for immediate transport.

Critical Thinking Questions

1. Based on the patient presentation, what prenatal emergency might exist?
2. What are the assessment priorities for this patient?
3. What are the management priorities for this patient?
4. How could this patient deteriorate?

INTRODUCTION

Childbirth is a natural event normally filled with anticipation and joy. However, when a patient is experiencing an emergency involving the pregnancy or delivery, anxiety and fear of losing the child will present the EMT with additional challenges. The EMT must be prepared to provide professional, effective, and compassionate care. This unit discusses assessment and management of the prenatal patient as well as prenatal problems the EMT may encounter in the prehospital setting.

ANATOMY REVIEW

The *uterus,* also called the womb, is a muscular chamber that holds the products of conception until birth. The nonpregnant uterus looks like an inverted bottle and is located inside the pelvis. The superior portion of the uterus, or the bottom of the bottle, is called the **fundus.** At the inferior portion of the uterus, or the neck of the bottle, is the **cervix.** The cervix is a ring of muscle that closes the uterus to the outside world. Through this small muscular opening, a baby is carried, or born, into the vagina. The baby then travels down the vagina, or birth canal, in a process called **childbirth.** The anatomy of the female reproductive system is illustrated in Figure 40.1. Further review can be found in Unit 5.

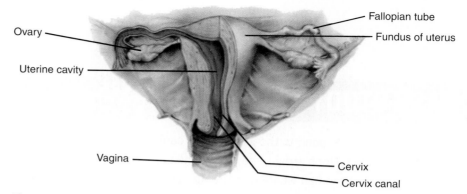

Figure 40.1 The female reproductive system

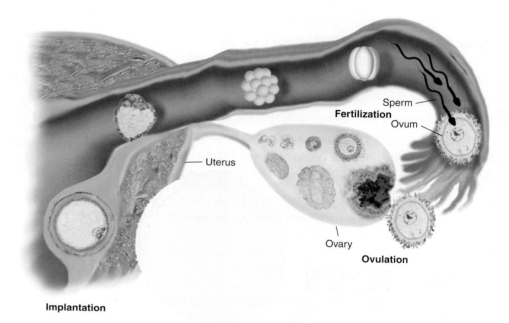

Figure 40.2 The fertilized egg becomes an ovum and is implanted in the uterine wall

CONCEPTION AND PREGNANCY

Attached to either side of the uterus are two tubes, called *fallopian tubes*. The fallopian tubes lead to the *ovaries*. The ovary is the source for a woman's lifetime supply of eggs. When an egg is released from an ovary, during a process called **ovulation,** it travels down the thin-walled fallopian tubes. (The fallopian tube has the same diameter as the lead of a pencil.) Once inside the fallopian tube, if sperm is present, fertilization of the egg may take place. The fertilized egg, called an **ovum,** travels into the uterus where, under normal circumstances, it will implant into the uterine wall on the uterine lining (Figure 40.2). Once the ovum is implanted in the uterine wall, it begins to grow, first into an embryo and then a **fetus.**

Early in fetal development, a bridge is created from mother to infant called the **placenta.** The lay term for placenta is the *afterbirth.* The placenta is important to the developing fetus. The placenta carries oxygen and nutrients from the mother to the fetus (Figure 40.3). Without a placenta firmly attached to the uterine wall, the fetus is at risk for hypoperfusion and hypoxia.

Figure 40.3 The anatomy of a pregnant uterus

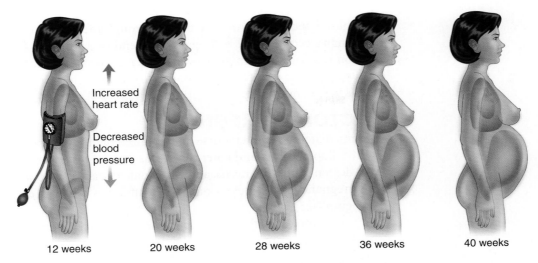

Figure 40.4 Breathing, heart rate, and blood pressure all change in pregnancy

THE CHANGES OF PREGNANCY

Pregnancy begins when the fertilized ovum implants in the uterine wall and continues to grow and develop for 37–40 weeks. The 9-month pregnancy is divided into three time periods, or trimesters. The first trimester is when implantation occurs and organs first start to appear in the fetus. The second trimester is a period of rapid growth and development for the fetus. During the third and final trimester, the fetus completes development.

Following fertilization, in the first trimester, powerful hormones are released that have a dramatic impact on the woman's body, preparing it for the rest of the pregnancy. Blood flow is increased to the uterus in anticipation of the demands of the placenta and the needs of the fetus. The blood volume in the body increases about 30% to 35%. Because of this, more blood can be lost before the pregnant patient shows signs of hypoperfusion. The increased blood volume also leads to an increased heart rate, on average 10–15 beats per minute. However, the baseline blood pressure normally drops approximately 10–15 mmHg during pregnancy. The changes in vital signs during pregnancy are illustrated in Figure 40.4.

As the uterus expands, it presses against the mother's diaphragm and makes breathing more difficult. The mother starts to breathe more rapidly and to take more shallow breaths. On average, the mother gains between 2 and 3 pounds of weight for every month of pregnancy. This weight gain represents the weight of additional fluid, such as blood and amniotic fluid, as well as the weight of the baby.

ABDOMINAL PAIN IN WOMEN OF CHILDBEARING AGE

There are many different reasons for a woman to have abdominal pain. Some are related to pregnancy; most are not. Abdominal pain due to a complication of pregnancy, however, can be life threatening. Because a woman may not know she is pregnant early on, any sexually active woman of childbearing age with lower quadrant abdominal pain is treated as though she were pregnant. The childbearing years start when a female has her first menses at menarche. Some females start their menses as early as 8 or 9 years of age, although 11 is the average age of menarche in the United States.

Menses, the root of the word "menstruation," is the periodic discharge of blood and tissue from the uterus through the vagina, commonly called a woman's *period*. Until menopause, the end of a woman's fertility, menstruation occurs approximately every 28 days when a woman is not pregnant. Menarche, represented by a woman's first menses, is the beginning of a woman's period of fertility.

ECTOPIC PREGNANCY

Immediately after intercourse, the fertilized ovum is supposed to travel down the fallopian tubes and enter the uterus. In rare instances, the ovum may fail to descend into the uterus, and a pregnancy may develop outside the uterus. A pregnancy that develops outside the uterus is called an **ectopic pregnancy** (Figure 40.5).

In some cases, the ectopic pregnancy develops in the fallopian tube. The fallopian tubes are very thin, and the developing ovum eventually ruptures the fallopian tube. The rupture of a fallopian tube from an ectopic pregnancy can cause significant internal bleeding. Unchecked, the bleeding can eventually lead to shock, and even death. A woman is at greatest risk for a ruptured ectopic pregnancy between her 6th and 12th week of pregnancy. Ectopic pregnancies are the leading cause of maternal death occurring in the first trimester.

ASSESSMENT

The symptoms of an ectopic pregnancy include lower abdominal pain and possibly even scant vaginal bleeding. The abdominal pain may be described as crampy or achy. If internal bleeding is significant, the patient may have symptoms consistent with hypoperfusion such as dizziness, thirst, and anxiety.

The signs of an ectopic pregnancy are similar to the signs of any severe hemorrhage. Tachycardia, tachypnea, pallor, and other signs of hypoperfusion will be present. Hypotension is a grave indication of severe internal bleeding. Lower abdominal tenderness to palpation is also usually found.

Street Smart

Despite the denials of the patient or the results of home pregnancy tests, an EMT should always consider the possibility of pregnancy in a woman of childbearing age with a concern of lower abdominal pain. Accordingly, the EMT must err on the side of caution and treat every female of childbearing age who has a concern of lower abdominal pain as if she may have an ectopic pregnancy.

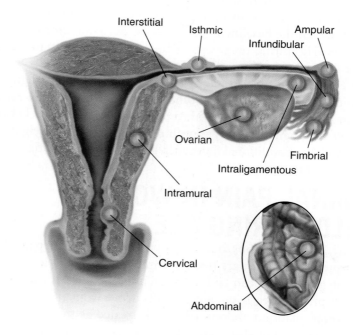

Figure 40.5 An ectopic pregnancy can occur at many sites outside the uterus

MANAGEMENT

The focus of prehospital care of the pregnant woman who may have an ectopic pregnancy is to treat for hypoperfusion (shock). The EMT should always provide high-concentration oxygen, reassess vitals signs every 5 minutes, keep the patient warm, and provide immediate transport.

TRANSPORTATION

If the patient presents with clear signs of hypoperfusion, she should be transported immediately. An advanced life support (ALS) intercept should be arranged if possible so that intravenous (IV) lines can be established. It is important to transport the patient to an appropriate facility that is capable of dealing with hemorrhage and can provide blood if the need should arise.

COMPLICATIONS EARLY IN PREGNANCY

Prenatal care can help to reduce the risk for complications of pregnancy and to ensure the delivery of a healthy baby. Young females such as teenagers may be in denial of the pregnancy or will attempt to hide their pregnancy from parents or peers as long as possible. Some women may not realize they are pregnant until after the first trimester, a time when some of the greatest risks for complications exist.

Women who smoke tobacco products or who drink alcohol are at greater risk for prenatal complications. Women who suffer from diabetes before pregnancy experience more complications of childbirth. Some women develop diabetes during pregnancy because of the pregnancy. This type of diabetes is called *gestational diabetes* and may spontaneously resolve with the completion of the pregnancy. Women who decide to become pregnant later in their reproductive lives are also at greater risk for complications of pregnancy.

SUBSTANCE ABUSE

"You are eating for two" is a common phrase many pregnant women hear or say themselves. The pregnant woman is not only "eating for two," she is "drinking and breathing for two." Any substance that enters the woman's body can have an effect on the baby; therefore, the pregnant woman who drinks alcohol, smokes, or otherwise ingests recreational drugs or medications is giving those substances to her baby.

Women who continue to use drugs such as cocaine, methamphetamine, and heroin are at a greater risk for prenatal problems, including premature labor, bleeding, spontaneous abortion, placental abruption, and prenatal trauma. Additionally, some over-the-counter medications should not be taken during pregnancy. Labels of over-the-counter medications that pose a risk to the pregnant and/or developing fetus list warnings stating they should not be taken during pregnancy.

Babies exposed to drugs during pregnancy often have low birth weight, which puts them at risk for health complications early in life and developmental delays. They may go through withdrawal from the drug the mother used, and have lifelong health and learning disabilities.

Management includes high-flow oxygen, management for shock if bleeding is present, and immediate transport to the appropriate facility. ALS intercept should be requested. Contact medical control and follow local protocols for more specific management guidelines.

GESTATIONAL DIABETES MELLITUS

Sometimes pregnant women with no history of diabetes will develop diabetes during pregnancy, called **gestational diabetes mellitus (GDM).** Gestational diabetes is comparable to Type II non–insulin dependent DM that occurs most often in mothers over 30 years of age, who may have maternal obesity and a family history of diabetes. Other risk factors include having previously given birth to an infant weighing more than 4,000 grams (8 pounds, 13 ounces) and experiencing excessive weight gain (over 40 pounds) during pregnancy.

Prenatal complications for women with gestational diabetes include preterm labor, preeclampsia, and increased risk for kidney and bladder inflammations. There can be complications with the fetus, including shoulder dystocia (discussed in Unit 41), stillbirth, cesarean section birth, and excessive birth weight.

Management for the pregnant woman with diabetes (Type I, II, or gestational) is the same as for nonpregnant diabetic emergencies. Administer high-flow oxygen and check glucose levels if possible. ALS intercept should be requested and met en route to the hospital. Transport the patient on her left side. Always follow local protocols and consult medical direction for more specific management.

BLEEDING DURING EARLY PREGNANCY

A woman may experience light bleeding early in her pregnancy. Many of these pregnancies will be normal; however, any bleeding during pregnancy should be seen by a physician because it is impossible to know what the bleeding means without an evaluation.

SPONTANEOUS ABORTION

Many pregnancies are not completed, or carried for the full term. A pregnancy may end prematurely for a variety of reasons. The termination of a pregnancy before a fetus reaches the stage of viability, at about 20 weeks, is termed an **abortion.**

If the embryo is imperfect or conditions are not right, the woman may lose the fetus very early in the pregnancy. The woman may experience what is called a **spontaneous abortion.** A spontaneous abortion, also called a **miscarriage,** occurs in 1 out of every 200 pregnancies.

Usually a spontaneous abortion occurs in the first 6–12 weeks of pregnancy. A woman who is unaware that she is pregnant may spontaneously abort the pregnancy without her knowledge. The only change she might note is that her menstrual flow, her period, is heavier than normal. Today, home pregnancy tests can determine that a woman is pregnant within the first few days. A woman who knows she is pregnant may interpret any bleeding as a spontaneous abortion, or miscarriage.

A spontaneous abortion may be accompanied by abdominal pain. It is difficult to differentiate between a spontaneous abortion and an ectopic pregnancy without an ultrasound. Because an ectopic pregnancy is potentially life threatening and a spontaneous abortion usually is not, the EMT should treat for the worst possibility. Any woman of childbearing age with lower abdominal pain should be assumed to be having an ectopic pregnancy and treated accordingly.

ELECTIVE ABORTION

A woman may elect to terminate the pregnancy, for a variety of personal reasons, by having an elective abortion. Most often these procedures are done in a hospital or clinic by trained medical practitioners. However, the EMT

Street Smart

An EMT cannot determine whether a woman has had a spontaneous abortion. It is possible to bleed during pregnancy and still carry to full term. Therefore, an EMT should treat every pregnancy as though the fetus is alive and the pregnancy still viable.

Street Smart

Any pregnancy is a highly emotional event. Emotional support for the patient is important. Pregnancy is a private condition, and the EMT should be kind and considerate of the patient's rights to privacy.

The EMT must ask the patient sensitive questions about the pregnancy as a part of the history gathering during the assessment. A female EMT attending the patient may make the situation more comfortable.

may be called for a woman with vaginal bleeding who has attempted to abort the fetus at home using crude methods. Treatment will focus on management of shock, including high-flow oxygen and immediate transport with ALS intercept.

ASSESSMENT OF THE PREGNANT WOMAN

The assessment of a pregnant woman should begin the same way as for any other patient, with a scene size-up and primary assessment. Any life-threatening problems found in the primary assessment should be addressed at this time. The history and secondary assessment of the pregnant woman who is responsive should be based on her presenting concern. Additional factors that are important to obtain as part of a pregnant woman's history, regardless of her concern, are how far along she is in her pregnancy; whether she has had prenatal care; whether she has had any complications with the pregnancy; and how many times she has been pregnant before this pregnancy. This information, along with the usual SAMPLE history and a history of the present illness, will be useful in the care of the patient.

When measuring vital signs, the EMT should remember the expected slight elevation in heart rate and respiratory rate and drop in blood pressure that is found toward the end of pregnancy. The remainder of this chapter covers other specific assessment techniques and the management of conditions related to pregnancy.

SIGNS AND SYMPTOMS

The EMT should ask the patient whether there is any pain or cramping associated with the bleeding. If the answer is yes, the EMT should ask when the pain began and have the patient characterize it. The EMT should also ask when the bleeding started. A rough estimate of blood loss can be determined by asking for a pad count. A pad count is the number of sanitary napkins that the woman has used since the bleeding began.

The other physical signs found in the woman who may be miscarrying are the same signs and symptoms of hypoperfusion from hemorrhage. The EMT should assess the patient for signs of pallor, tachycardia, and tachypnea.

MANAGEMENT

Care of the patient who is having, or may have had, a spontaneous abortion is largely supportive. The EMT should complete a primary assessment and gather the SAMPLE history. High-concentration oxygen should be administered and the patient prepared for immediate transport. Occasionally, a patient may show the EMT a sanitary pad. The EMT should note the color and consistency of the blood on the pad. It is not necessary for an EMT to ask to see a sanitary pad; it is enough that the patient said she is bleeding. The EMT should try to save any blood clots or tissue that may be found (Figure 40.6). Any plastic cup with a lid is an acceptable container for this material, which should be given to hospital staff so they may examine it.

COMPLICATIONS OF PREGNANCY

Once a woman has passed the sixth month of her pregnancy and entered the final trimester, the chances of successfully completing the pregnancy are greatly increased. By the third trimester, the infant may survive even if it is born early. Some risks to the mother, however, still exist. The EMT should recognize the risks involved with complications in the third trimester and transport the mother and child immediately to an appropriate facility.

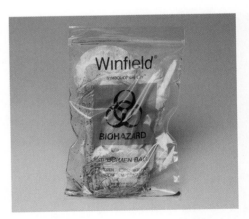

Figure 40.6 Blood clots and tissue should be collected and delivered to the emergency department

BLEEDING LATE IN PREGNANCY

Any vaginal bleeding during pregnancy should be considered serious. Vaginal bleeding can be life threatening to both the mother and the fetus. Any vaginal bleeding during pregnancy should be evaluated by a medical provider as soon as possible. Sudden vaginal bleeding, especially in the third trimester of pregnancy, may indicate a problem with the placenta.

PLACENTAL ABRUPTION

Vaginal bleeding may indicate that the placenta has prematurely detached from the uterine wall, a condition called **placental abruption.** *Placentae abruptio* (placental abruption) results in a decreased blood flow to the fetus and significant blood loss for the mother.

This condition most commonly follows some kind of trauma. Even minor falls can be the inciting factor for an abruption; therefore, every woman in her third trimester of pregnancy who suffers even a minor injury should be evaluated at the hospital in a timely fashion. Other predisposing factors for placental abruption include hypertension or diabetes in the mother, preeclampsia, previous abruption, smoking, premature rupture of the amniotic sac, use of drugs such as cocaine, and a short umbilical cord.

There are two types of placental abruption: a complete separation of the placenta from the wall of the uterus and a partial abruption, where the placenta is only partially torn from the uterine wall.

The woman with a placental abruption (Figure 40.7) may complain of abdominal pain followed by vaginal bleeding. Vaginal bleeding may not be present if the bleeding is contained behind the placental barrier and does not leak out of the uterus through the cervical opening.

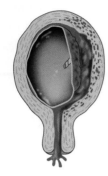

Figure 40.7 A detached placenta is called a placental abruption

PLACENTA PREVIA

Another major cause of third trimester vaginal bleeding occurs when the placenta is placed abnormally low in the uterus and the placenta has grown over the opening of the uterus, or the cervix (Figure 40.8). This condition, which is known as a **placenta previa,** results in significant vaginal bleeding without any associated pain and can rapidly result in hemorrhagic shock for the mother and lack of blood flow to the fetus. Placenta previa occurs on average once in every 200 pregnancies, usually in first-time mothers.

Placenta previa can be total, when the placenta completely covers the *os,* or opening of the uterus, blocking the birth canal and preventing delivery. When the placenta only partially covers the os, it is considered a partial previa. A partial previa can also prevent delivery. A marginal previa occurs when the placenta is implanted near the neck of the cervix. In a marginal placenta previa, the placenta will partially tear as the cervix thins and effaces (discussed further in Unit 41).

The existence of placenta previa is greater in women who are over 35 years of age and who have had a rapid succession of pregnancies, more than two previous deliveries, a history of early vaginal bleeding during the pregnancy, bleeding immediately after intercourse, and previous placenta previa.

MANAGEMENT

An EMT should not perform an external vaginal examination of a pregnant woman in the field unless anticipating imminent delivery of the infant. The EMT can study the signs of an imminent birth in Unit 41.

The EMT need not distinguish between the conditions causing bleeding in the third trimester. Instead, the EMT should consider the patient to be having a complication of pregnancy and transport immediately.

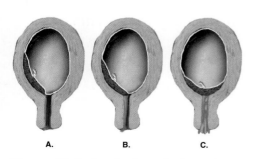

A.   B.   C.

Figure 40.8 A misplaced placenta is called placenta previa

The bleeding can be profuse and life threatening to both mother and fetus. The mother should be assessed and reassessed for signs of hypoperfusion. It stands to reason that if the mother is hypoperfused, then the fetus will be in distress. The mother should be transported on her left side, kept warm with a blanket, and given continuous high-concentration oxygen via a non-rebreather facemask. ALS intercept should be requested and met while en route to the appropriate facility.

TOXEMIA OF PREGNANCY

During her pregnancy, a woman may develop a condition called *toxemia of pregnancy*. Toxemia of pregnancy literally means the "poisoned pregnancy." If left untreated, toxemia can lead to coma and death. The cause of toxemia is not known, but the condition occurs more commonly in women during their first pregnancy. Women who are very young, less than 17 years, or older, more than 35 years, are at greater risk for developing toxemia. Toxemia of pregnancy is more commonly called **eclampsia.** Eclampsia can be divided into two stages: preeclampsia and eclampsia.

PREECLAMPSIA

A woman with preeclampsia may experience a variety of symptoms, including mild to severe hypertension and edema of the face and hands. Some patients with preeclampsia complain of severe headaches and visual disturbances.

The woman with preeclampsia should be transported quietly to the hospital with oxygen in place. Bright lights and loud sirens may induce a seizure and should be used only if the mother is unconscious. ALS intercept and medical direction should be obtained as indicated by local protocol.

ECLAMPSIA

The hallmark that separates eclampsia from preeclampsia is a seizure. The seizure indicates severe brain irritation. If the eclampsia is not treated, the patient will lapse into a coma. The EMT should initiate rapid transportation to the closest ALS unit or hospital while managing the airway, breathing, and circulation (ABCs) of mother and ultimately the infant. Intravenous medications are used in the treatment of eclamptic seizures; therefore, the most definitive treatment the EMT can provide is immediate transport.

BLUNT ABDOMINAL TRAUMA

The developing fetus has a number of protections from outside forces. In the early stages of pregnancy, the pelvis provides a bony shield against blunt and penetrating trauma. As the fetus develops and enlarges, outgrowing the confines of the pelvis, amniotic fluid is produced in larger and larger quantities. Almost 500–1,000 cc of this almost-clear fluid can be found in the amniotic sac within the uterus and surrounding the fetus as a protective cushion or shock absorber.

At about the 12th week of pregnancy, the uterus expands outside the protective confines of the pelvis. In the third trimester, the pregnant uterus markedly protrudes past the rest of the body's silhouette and, thus, becomes more prone to injury.

In severe cases of blunt trauma, the force can be so great that the uterus actually ruptures. This rupture is more common in women who previously had a cesarean section because of the weakened uterine wall. A uterine rupture can quickly lead to serious life-threatening internal hemorrhage.

ASSESSMENT

The assessment of the pregnant patient who has experienced a blunt trauma is no different than that of any other patient except that the EMT must remember it is not one patient but two being treated. The second patient, the fetus, is much more sensitive to changes in blood volume. Therefore, the EMT must have a heightened awareness and a higher index of suspicion that bleeding may be occurring internally.

SCENE SIZE-UP

The mechanism of injury is the key to understanding why a pregnant woman who has sustained a blunt trauma may be bleeding internally. A variety of mechanisms, from assaults to vehicular collisions, can cause blunt trauma, and the severity of the trauma depends on the force involved. How fast was the vehicle moving? How many stairs did she fall down? These are an example of the questions the EMT must ask while approaching the scene and conducting the scene size-up.

FALLS

The additional weight of the infant shifts the woman's center of gravity forward. This change makes a pregnant woman prone to falling forward. This condition, a forward center of gravity and a resultant tendency to fall, makes the uterus prone to injury from blunt trauma. Injury to the uterus can occur from some common mechanisms of injury. For example, the expectant mother may trip on a curb she cannot see and fall forward, striking her abdomen and suffering blunt trauma.

It is important that the EMT document not only the fall but also the height from which the patient fell, as well as the type of surface on which the patient landed. The EMT also needs to perform a thorough assessment for head and spine injury.

INTENTIONAL TRAUMA

Some women, including those who are pregnant, are victims of domestic violence. Spouses and fathers of unexpected babies may be angry about the pregnancy. The pregnant abdomen then becomes the target of the attack. Pregnant women have been shot in the abdomen, pushed down a flight of stairs, and punched or kicked in the abdomen. The attackers may intend to cause a miscarriage and/or punish the woman for the pregnancy.

MOTOR VEHICLE COLLISIONS

Pregnancy doubles the chance for injury in a motor vehicle collision. As the body is thrown forward, the bulging abdomen becomes the area of first contact. Both mother and child can be adversely affected. Restraint devices, like seat belts and padded steering wheels, can help to lessen the blow. Yet, some women fail to wear their seat belt properly. Saying that the seat belts are "uncomfortable," they wear the seat belts higher on the abdomen and not across the pelvis where the seat belt is supposed to be (Figure 40.9). Some expectant mothers think that wearing a seat belt will actually increase the chance for injury to their unborn baby. Research has shown that seat belts, a lap belt with a shoulder restraint, actually decrease the rates of maternal mortality and uterine injury. EMTs should encourage all pregnant women to wear their seat belts when driving.

ASSESSMENT

After the scene size-up and consideration of the mechanism of injury, the EMT should proceed with the primary assessment. The treatment priorities for a pregnant patient are the same as those for a nonpregnant patient. The

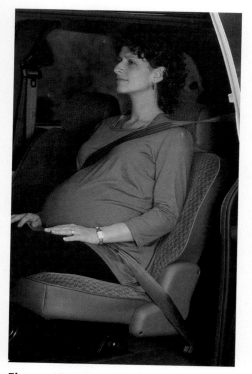

Figure 40.9 A properly worn seat belt can decrease injuries sustained by a pregnant woman in a motor vehicle collision

EMT should secure the airway, assess and assist respiration, control bleeding, and rapidly transport high-priority cases.

The EMT also should ask the mother whether she felt a gush of fluid from her vagina. If she did, then her membranes may have ruptured. Fluid leaking from the vagina may be amniotic fluid, or it may be blood. The presence of blood should lead the EMT to suspect either placental abruption or possibly a ruptured uterus. In both cases, the patient needs rapid transportation to the closest appropriate facility.

At or before the 20th week of pregnancy, a mother may feel fetal movement, called **quickening.** The EMT should ask the mother whether she can feel her baby move. The fetus is usually more active after trauma. However, a still baby may just be a quiet baby. The EMT should take care not to alarm the mother by making any rash statements about the baby not moving.

The EMT should carefully palpate the pregnant woman's abdomen to assess for tenderness (Figure 40.10). A pregnant uterus normally feels firm and should be non-tender. The abdomen should be examined for signs of trauma. Reddened areas, abrasions, contusions, and point tenderness may indicate the place where the force struck the abdomen.

It is difficult to assess fetal heart sounds in the field, so the EMT should not spend time trying to ascertain whether these sounds are present. Instead, the EMT should advise the hospital about the situation so that a fetal heart monitor will be ready when the patient arrives.

The EMT should ask the mother whether she is feeling any cramps or labor pains. Have her make a comparison between her present level of discomfort and that caused by her worst menstrual cramps. Usually labor pains are worse than the patient's worst menstrual cramps.

The EMT should ask the mother whether she was wearing her seat belt at the time of the accident and should examine the car for air bag deployment. If the air bag has been deployed, the EMT should look at the steering wheel under the air bag for deformity.

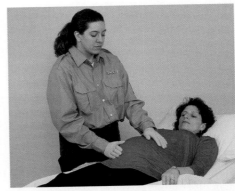

Figure 40.10 The EMT should feel for point tenderness as well as fetal movement

MANAGEMENT

When trying to manage the pregnant patient who has suffered a traumatic injury, the EMT is faced with not one, but two, patients. How does the EMT manage both? Although the concept of caring for two seriously injured patients may be daunting, the EMT need only concentrate her skills on the mother. The infant's survival is tied to the mother's survival. Simply stated, "Save the mother to save the baby."

The EMT should concentrate on the ABCs. High-concentration oxygen is always appropriate. Even if the mother is well oxygenated, the fetus may not be because of vasoconstriction and shunting. As with any other injured patient, the pregnant trauma patient should have spinal immobilization if appropriate. Oxygen should be administered if it is indicated by the injury. Any pregnant woman with abdominal pain after trauma should receive high-flow oxygen.

HYPOPERFUSION IN PREGNANCY

When the body loses blood, vasoconstriction of selected organs occurs, shifting or shunting blood to more vital organs. The skin is usually the first organ to shunt blood, followed by muscles, gut, kidneys, heart, lungs, and lastly, brain. The pecking order of hypoperfusion is different during pregnancy. When the pregnant body loses blood, the placenta is the first organ to vasoconstrict, shunting blood away from the fetus to the mother's vital organs.

It is difficult for an EMT to assess fetal distress. However, an EMT can assess the mother and indirectly infer the fetal condition. When the mother's skin is pale and clammy, that would imply that the placenta is vasoconstricted and the fetus is in distress.

Because of the changes of pregnancy, the traditional signs of hypoperfusion may not be as reliable. A pregnant woman's resting heart rate is naturally higher than usual, and her resting blood pressure is slightly lower than usual. These findings should not be mistaken as signs of hypoperfusion and impending shock. The EMT should remember that the increased blood volume, about 35% more blood volume than normal, will allow for more blood loss before a significant drop in blood pressure occurs. The EMT should take repeated vital signs during an ongoing assessment and report any changes immediately.

TRANSPORTATION

The patient should be transported to the closest appropriate facility. When the EMT considers transportation destinations, she should consider the fetal-monitoring capabilities of the hospitals. The EMT should follow local triage protocols regarding destination hospitals.

Typically, a trauma patient is immobilized to a backboard supine to protect the spine. A pregnant trauma patient should also be immobilized to the backboard; however, the weight of the uterus, when the mother lies flat, compresses the vena cava and stops blood from returning from the lower extremities to the heart. Immediately the patient's heart receives about 30% less blood return than is normal. The patient's blood pressure will drop suddenly, and the patient may even lose consciousness. The sudden loss of blood pressure when a pregnant woman lies flat is called **supine hypotensive syndrome.**

Supine hypotensive syndrome happens more commonly in the third trimester and is easily treated. Once the patient has been immobilized, head and body, to the backboard, the backboard is tilted onto the left side at about a 15-degree angle. A bedroll or rolled blanket placed under the backboard works well to maintain this position (Figure 40.11). If tilting the backboard is not possible, an EMT can take two hands and manually shift the uterus to the left side, off the vena cava. After either technique is used, the blood pressure should immediately return.

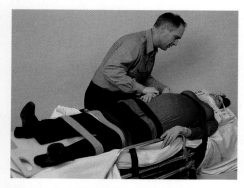

Figure 40.11 Tilting the backboard as little as 15 degrees can prevent supine hypotensive syndrome

CONCLUSION

The changes of pregnancy present many challenges to the EMT who is trying to manage the complications that can occur during a pregnancy. By providing competent, professional prehospital care, however, the EMT can be part of helping to bring a new life into the world.

Candice and Jacob gently place Cindy in the ambulance and prepare to transport her to the hospital. Candice notes that Cindy's vital signs at the clinic were a heart rate of 110, respirations 22, and blood pressure 112/72.

Cindy continues to deny any abdominal pain but states it feels like there is a gush of something whenever she moves. The clinic had placed several pads over the vagina and Candice ensured there are clean, absorbent towels in place under the patient.

During the short trip to the hospital, Candice reassesses Cindy's vital signs, showing no significant change with a heart rate of 114, respirations 22, and blood pressure 108/70.

Cindy continues to be tearful, stating she and her husband have been trying to have a baby for the past 6 years. Candice provides emotional support, offering reassurance and stressing to Cindy the need to remain calm.

Candice and Jacob take Cindy up to the Childbirth Center at the local hospital, where she is met by her obstetrician. Candice provides a full report of the short transfer from the urgent care clinic and turns over the documentation the clinic sent along. Cindy's vital signs had remained stable throughout transport and were unchanged at the time Candice turned patient care over to the OB staff.

Key Concepts Revisited

- The EMT's prompt management of life-threatening complications of pregnancy may ensure the survival of both mother and child.

- Sexually active women of childbearing age suffering lower abdominal pain should be treated as though they may be pregnant.

- The pregnant patient with abdominal pain must be thoroughly assessed to determine if the problem is related to the pregnancy or a condition unrelated to her pregnancy.
  - Ectopic pregnancy

- The risk factors that contribute to complications of pregnancy include smoking tobacco, alcohol consumption, drug use, and diabetes mellitus.
  - Substance abuse
  - Gestational diabetes

- Complications of early pregnancy include bleeding and possible loss of the fetus.
  - Spontaneous abortion
    - Elective abortion

- Vaginal bleeding late in pregnancy should be considered serious and potentially life threatening.
  - Placental abruption
  - Placenta previa

- Toxemia of pregnancy leads to coma and death if left untreated.
  - Preeclampsia
  - Eclampsia

- The fetus is protected internally against most blunt trauma.
  - Falls
  - Intentional trauma
  - Motor vehicle collisions

- Supine hypotension syndrome results when the mother is laid flat, causing the weight of the uterus to compress the vena cava.

- The management of complications of pregnancy focuses on the ABCs, treatment for shock, and immediate transport to the appropriate facility.

Review Questions

1. What are the components of the female reproductive system?
2. What changes occur in the body of a pregnant woman?
3. What are several factors that increase a woman's risk of a complication during pregnancy?
4. What effects does the mother's use of drugs have on the fetus?
5. What is gestational diabetes?
6. What conditions can cause bleeding in early pregnancy?
7. What are the signs of placenta previa?
8. How does the EMT differentiate between placenta previa and placental abruption?
9. What mechanisms protect the fetus from blunt trauma?
10. Why is the pregnant woman more susceptible to falls?
11. How would an EMT treat preeclampsia?
12. What differentiates preeclampsia and eclampsia?

Key Terms

Abortion
Cervix
Childbirth
Eclampsia
Ectopic pregnancy
Fetus
Fundus
Gestational diabetes mellitus (GDM)
Miscarriage

Ovulation
Ovum
Placenta
Placenta previa
Placental abruption
Quickening
Spontaneous abortion
Supine hypotensive syndrome

Further Study

Bledsoe, B. E., and R. W. Benner. *Critical Care Paramedic.* Upper Saddle River, NJ: Pearson/Prentice Hall, 2006.

Johansson, Helgi, Gubby Ayida, and Chris Sadler. "Faking It? Simulation of the Training of Obstetricians and Gynaecologists." *Current Opinion in Obstetrics & Gynecology* 17, no. 6 (December 2005): 557–561.

Littleton, L. Y., and J. Engebretson. *Maternity Nursing Care.* Clifton Park, NY: Delmar Cengage Learning, 2005.

UNIT (41) Emergency Childbirth and Newborn Care

Most women deliver their infants within a hospital or other health care facility. Some women, however, choose to deliver their infants at home, with or without professional assistance. Although childbirth is not common in the field, the Emergency Medical Technician (EMT) may be called to assist with a delivery, in the case of complications or simply because the mother cannot get to the hospital before the birth occurs. In these situations, the EMT is called on to assist with rapid transport and, if necessary, to facilitate the delivery and care of the newborn.

National Education Standards

The Emergency Medical Technician (EMT) will be able to demonstrate a fundamental depth and foundational breadth of understanding in the anatomy and physiology, assessment, and management of emergency childbirth and newborn care.

Key Concepts

- The EMT must be familiar with the three distinct stages of labor.

- The EMT must be able to recognize the signs of impending delivery.

- The brief predelivery history is important to establish a controlled delivery.

- The EMT must able to recognize and manage complications of delivery.

- The proper care of the mother postdelivery focuses on the assessment and management of excessive bleeding if it should occur.

- The primary assessment of the newborn is conducted through the Apgar score.

- The first priority of management of the newborn focuses on the airway and breathing.

- The detailed physical examination of the secondary assessment is to assess for normal and abnormal characteristics beyond the ABCs.

- Babies with large birth weights can experience trauma during delivery.

- Resuscitation of the newborn follows standard CPR guidelines with just a few modifications.

Juanita and Dawn are watching the snow fly by the window in the stationhouse, thankful their shift would be over soon. They had been fortunate not to have any calls requiring them to go out into the blizzard. Suddenly, the tones go off: "Medic 6 from dispatch: respond to a woman in labor, contractions less than 5 minutes apart. Time out 18:45."

The county Juanita and Dawn work for always keeps a county snowplow standing ready in case the ambulance has to go out in a snowstorm. The snowplow clears a wide path in front of the ambulance doors and then proceeds down the road clearing a path as the ambulance follows.

Upon arrival at the residence, Juanita grabs the obstetrics kit as well as the first-in bag and is met at the door by a middle-aged man who ushers the crew to the bedroom down the hall. Lying on the bed in a knees-to-chest position is a woman in her mid-30s. She is panting, but appears calm.

Juanita introduces herself and Dawn and asks the patient her name. The patient replies, "My name is Erin

and the nurse-midwife was supposed to be here by now." Juanita explains the roads are covered with snowdrifts and they were able to get there because they had a snowplow clearing a path for them.

Juanita begins conducting a history by asking Erin how long she has been in labor. Erin replies she had been having contractions for the past 4 hours, and this was her fourth baby. Juanita asks how Erin felt with each contraction and Erin replies:

"I feel like pushing!"

Critical Thinking Questions

1. What are the signs of impending delivery?
2. What should be included in the assessment of a woman in labor?
3. What should the EMT do for the mother after the delivery?
4. What should the EMT do for the infant after the delivery?

INTRODUCTION

Because EMTs do not frequently encounter an emergency involving childbirth, they should review the basic principles of childbirth often. Such review and continuing education are important with this and any other conditions the EMT may infrequently encounter.

Although most deliveries are without complications, in the first hour of life, a newborn is at high risk for a number of potentially serious problems. An EMT may be caring for the newborn and mother during that first hour. This unit discusses the EMT's role in the assessment and management of prehospital emergency childbirth and newborn care.

ANATOMY REVIEW

A review of relevant anatomy aids in a discussion of the process of childbirth. As a pregnancy progresses, the uterus enlarges in the abdomen, pushing other structures aside. Inside the uterus, the fetus grows and develops over the course of the pregnancy.

The fetus receives all necessary nutrients via the placenta, which is firmly adhered to the uterine wall. The umbilical cord is the connection between the placenta and the fetus.

The fetal-placental unit is surrounded by a membrane called the **amniotic sac.** This sac encloses the growing fetus and the amniotic fluid that serves as a protective cushion. Figure 41.1 illustrates this anatomy.

As the pregnancy nears its conclusion, the lower uterine segment, or cervix, begins to thin out. This thinning of the cervix is referred to as **effacement.** As the fetal head descends into the pelvis, it slowly stretches the cervix open. This progressive opening of the thinned cervix is called **cervical dilation.** This process can be seen in Figure 41.2.

NORMAL CHILDBIRTH

In most circumstances, childbirth is accomplished without complications. However, the EMT needs to be familiar with the normal progression of childbirth to assist in delivery if needed.

STAGES OF LABOR

The term **labor** refers to the process by which the uterus expels the products of conception, namely, the fetus and placenta. For purposes of discussion and management, this process can be divided into three separate stages. The EMT must be able to recognize which stage of labor an expectant mother is in, because this may alter management decisions.

STAGE ONE: DILATION

Toward the end of pregnancy, as the fetal head moves down into the pelvis, the cervix thins and begins to dilate. When this occurs, a collection of mucus is expelled from the cervix. This expulsion of a small amount of bloody mucus is known as the **bloody show.** The bloody show does not indicate labor has begun; it is merely a sign of cervical thinning.

When a pregnancy reaches its full term, usually around 40 weeks, the uterus begins to contract. The contractions become increasingly frequent and intense as the uterine muscle attempts to force the baby out.

The organized uterine contractions push the fetal head down into the pelvis, causing further effacement and dilation of the cervix. For the fetus to exit the uterus, the cervix must be completely effaced and dilated to 10 centimeters. This process of cervical effacement and dilation is known as the **first stage of labor** and takes a few hours to upward of 30 hours. Usually, women who have had children before progress through this stage more rapidly.

At some point during the first stage of labor, the amniotic sac usually ruptures, resulting in expulsion of amniotic fluid. Normally amniotic fluid is fairly clear. Any odor or color to the fluid should be noted, because it may influence later management.

Occasionally, the amniotic sac does not rupture spontaneously during this stage of labor. In such cases, if delivery begins and the sac has not

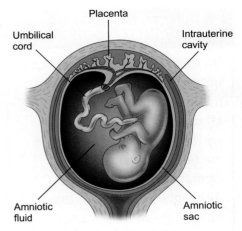

Figure 41.1 Amniotic fluid surrounds the fetus, providing a physiologic cushion

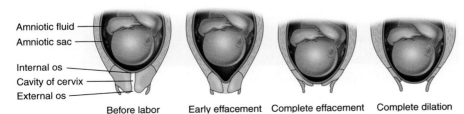

Figure 41.2 As the fetal head descends, the cervix thins and opens to allow the baby to pass through

ruptured, the EMT will have to actually open the sac as the infant's head delivers. The sac can be opened easily by pinching the membrane and twisting or pulling it away from the infant's presenting part.

STAGE TWO: DELIVERY

After the cervix is completely dilated, the **second stage of labor** begins. During this stage, more coordinated uterine contractions force the fetal head through the uterine opening and into the vaginal canal.

As the fetal head descends and pushes against the rectum, the mother may have an intense feeling of the need to move her bowels. This feeling is followed by increasing vaginal pressure as the infant continues his descent.

Impending delivery is evident as the fetal head becomes visible at the perineum. The fetal head pushes through the vagina and forms a bulge at the vaginal opening, stretching the perineum. This appearance of the fetal head at the vaginal opening is called **crowning.**

Crowning is initially evident during forceful uterine contractions. The infant's head bulges at the perineum between contractions as the head pushes further into the birth canal. At this point only a few more coordinated contractions are needed for delivery to occur.

At this stage, the mother should be encouraged to inhale, hold her breath, and bear down steadily for as long as she can with the onset of each contraction. This pushing helps to bring the baby through the birth canal.

Because the space for the infant to come through is relatively small, the infant makes a series of natural movements on descent through the birth canal. These movements are known as the **cardinal movements of labor** and are pictured in Figure 41.3. The EMT who is familiar with these movements can assist an infant through these maneuvers during an emergency delivery to bring the infant through the easiest path to the outside world.

The second stage of labor ends on delivery of the infant. This stage of labor lasts an average of 30–60 minutes, although it can occur very quickly. The EMT must be able to recognize the woman who is in this stage of labor so that he can prepare for an emergency delivery.

STAGE THREE: PLACENTAL

After delivery of the infant, the uterus rapidly decreases in size. With the change in shape of the uterus, the placenta separates from the inner uterine wall and is expelled through the vagina. This usually happens within 30 minutes of delivery of the infant. The delivery of the placenta is the **third stage of labor.** Transport usually can be accomplished safely during this stage of labor.

Placental delivery is often accompanied by a gush of blood, because the placenta is a vascular organ. From 250 to 500 cc of blood loss is expected. The increase in maternal vascular volume helps the mother's body compensate for this loss.

The placenta should be delivered into a container or bio bag so that it can be taken to the hospital with the patient. The obstetrician will examine the placenta to make certain that it has been entirely expelled. In rare

Safety Tips

Childbirth always involves splashing blood and body fluids. The EMT should use proper personal protective equipment, including, at a minimum, gloves, goggles, and a gown.

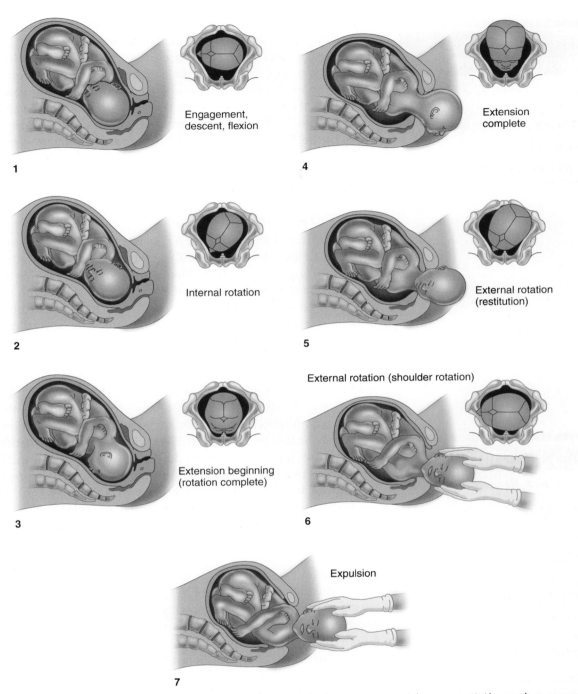

Figure 41.3 The infant makes a series of natural movements to maneuver his way out through a narrow birth canal

cases, a piece remains inside the uterus and may continue to bleed or become infected. A physician who finds that a piece of placenta is missing may need to check the patient for retained placental tissue inside the uterus.

EMERGENCY CHILDBIRTH

Childbirth that takes place in the field is an emergency the EMT may be faced with due to a complication that caused premature labor or a mother who unexpectedly delivers before safe transport can be accomplished. The EMT must recognize this situation when it happens and be prepared to facilitate a controlled delivery and newborn care in the field.

When an EMT is called to care for a woman in labor, the best course of action is to rapidly evaluate the patient and begin transport expediently. Delivery by an obstetrician in a hospital is always a better prospect than delivery by an EMT on the living room floor or in the back of the ambulance.

If the EMT believes that delivery is imminent, he must prepare for delivery in the field. A decision must be made, based on the progression of labor and signs of imminent delivery, where the delivery will take place—in the location the mother is found or in the back of the ambulance. Table 41-1 lists some signs of impending delivery.

HISTORY

Despite the rapid progression of a delivery, the EMT should attempt to ask the patient a few relevant historical questions. The answers to these questions may have a large impact on the management of the upcoming delivery.

The due date is an important piece of information for the EMT. If a delivery is occurring more than 4 weeks before the due date, it is considered to be premature. The EMT must be aware of some special considerations when delivering a premature infant. This topic is covered in more detail later in this unit.

Any known complications with the pregnancy should be elicited. If the mother has had no prenatal care or doctor's attention prior to the delivery, it is unlikely that she will be aware of any problems. On the other hand, the mother who has been under a doctor's care during the course of the pregnancy may be able to provide the EMT with valuable information. The presence of twins, for example, is certainly a relevant factor that the EMT should know about prior to the actual delivery so that appropriate preparations can be made for two infants rather than one.

If the amniotic sac has already ruptured, the color of the amniotic fluid should be noted. The presence of a green tinge is indicative of meconium and will have implications for the immediate care of the infant on delivery. This topic is discussed in more detail later in the unit.

If the time is available, the EMT may initiate a more detailed focused history during transport. The EMT should question the mother about the timing of her contractions. Knowing when they started, how much time is between them, and how long each one lasts will give the EMT an idea of how far the labor has progressed.

The longer the contractions last and the closer together they become, the closer the patient is to delivery.

Past pregnancy history can be detailed with the total number of pregnancies, including the current one, being noted. In addition, the number of live children born should be determined. These numbers can be expressed by a commonly used convention: the total number of pregnancies is referred to as **gravidity,** and the number of live children born is referred to as the **parity.**

The initials "G" and "P" are often used to represent the gravidity and the parity. A woman who is pregnant with her first child is G1P0 because she is with her first pregnancy and has yet to deliver a child. A woman who is in her third pregnancy and has delivered two previous live infants is G3P2.

These numbers can be broken down further and detailed, but for the purposes of an initial history, the EMT should report the gravidity and parity as described. Table 41-2 lists the questions the EMT should ask to gather pertinent history prior to childbirth.

ASSESSMENT

The primary assessment and measurement of baseline vital signs should be performed, as they would be on any patient. The modified physical assessment during secondary assessment should be based on the concern. If the patient is complaining of contractions or describes rupture of her membranes, the EMT should briefly examine the perineum for signs of crowning or any abnormality.

When performing an examination of the perineum, the EMT should make every attempt to respect the mother's privacy by doing the examination in a private area and keeping the mother covered as much as possible. A sheet draped over the mother's lower body will provide some privacy, although the examining EMT obviously needs to look beneath the sheet. The best position to facilitate the examination is with the mother lying on her back with her heels drawn up toward her buttocks and her knees allowed to fall to the sides.

The EMT should visually inspect the perineum during and between contractions. Any evidence of bulging or obvious crowning should be noted. The presence of amniotic fluid should be noted, along with its color. Anything protruding from the vaginal opening should be noted.

The EMT has no need to touch any part of the mother's genitalia and should never perform an internal vaginal examination to determine the position of the fetal head. The EMT should also perform this visual inspection of the perineum with another health care professional present if possible, to avoid any allegations of inappropriate behavior.

When this examination has been completed, if imminent delivery is not expected, the mother may be prepared for transport. Supplies should be readily available during transport to facilitate delivery and care of an infant if needed.

This examination should be repeated only if the patient's symptoms change and the EMT suspects that an examination might reveal a change. For example, if the contractions have become more frequent and the mother feels an urge to move her bowels, the perineum should be reassessed.

PREPARATION FOR DELIVERY

The EMT should be prepared for a delivery to occur at any time. The first and most important thing to do is to apply appropriate personal protective equipment. Childbirth can be quite messy, so the EMT should apply gloves, face and eye protection, and a gown.

The remaining supplies needed to facilitate a delivery come packaged in commercially available kits. The contents of such a kit are listed in Table 41-3 and shown in Figure 41.4.

An EMT who plans to facilitate a delivery should consider contacting medical control. Many regional protocols require a medical control decision to attempt a delivery on the scene. It is helpful to have the medical control physician on the telephone or radio during the delivery to help with any unforeseen complications.

At least two EMTs should facilitate a delivery if possible, which allows one EMT to attend the mother, while the second EMT can care for the newborn.

Creating a calm and efficient atmosphere is the best way to accomplish an emergency delivery in a controlled manner. A controlled delivery is healthier for both the mother and the infant. Uncontrolled expulsion of the infant can result in severe tears to the mother's perineum and in injuries to the baby.

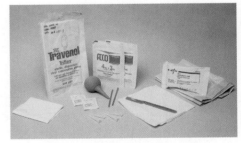

Figure 41.4 The EMT should be familiar with the contents of an OB (obstetrics) kit

Table 41-3 Contents of a Typical Obstetrics Kit

Supply	Use
Surgical scissors	To cut the umbilical cord
Clamps	To clamp the umbilical cord
Bulb suction	To suction the infant's mouth and nose
Towels	To dry and warm the infant, to drape over the mother's perineum
Gauze sponges	To apply pressure to the perineum
Gloves	To protect the EMT's hands
Baby blanket	To wrap the infant
Sanitary napkins	To place over the vagina after delivery of the placenta
Plastic bag	To contain the placenta after delivery

NORMAL DELIVERY

Because EMTs infrequently deliver babies, they will find it helpful to review this skill in a step-by-step manner. Skill 41-1 at the end of this unit presents the steps involved in an emergency delivery. Most deliveries are completed without any difficulty, but the EMT should know about potential complications and how to manage them.

SPECIAL DELIVERY SCENARIOS

Unfortunately, every delivery does not go as smoothly as planned. The presence of complications during childbirth can be dangerous to both mother and infant. The EMT should be familiar with the more common special delivery situations and be prepared to manage them appropriately.

PROLAPSED UMBILICAL CORD

Occasionally, during the fetal movement down into the birth canal, the umbilical cord becomes lodged between the birth canal and the fetus's head. In this case, the umbilical cord may exit the birth canal before the fetal head. This condition is called **prolapsed umbilical cord** and is depicted in Figure 41.5.

A prolapsed umbilical cord results in the fetal head compressing the blood supply that passes through the cord as the fetus descends in the canal. This condition can be life threatening to the infant and, therefore, must be quickly recognized and managed by the EMT.

SIGNS AND SYMPTOMS

The mother with a prolapsed umbilical cord often presents with contractions like any other laboring mother. Sometimes she will be aware of something coming out of her vagina. Upon initial perineal examination, the EMT will see the silvery-white umbilical cord coming from the vaginal opening.

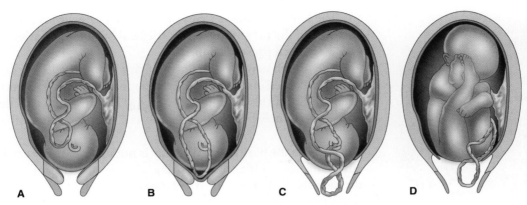

Figure 41.5 If the umbilical cord precedes the infant's head, the head will compress the cord as it descends into the birth canal

Because the umbilical cord carries the blood flow to the infant, it normally pulsates with the beat of the mother's heart. If the cord is not pulsating, it is probably being compressed inside the birth canal and all blood flow to the infant has been cut off.

MANAGEMENT

Management by the EMT of a mother with a prolapsed umbilical cord begins with the discovery of the condition on visual perineal examination. The mother should be immediately placed on 100% oxygen and put into a head-down, buttocks-raised position to allow gravity to lessen pressure in the birth canal.

The EMT should insert a sterile gloved hand into the vagina and push the fetal presenting part (usually the head) away from the cord. If blood flow is reestablished, pulsations of the cord should be visible. This technique is demonstrated in Figure 41.6.

The mother should be rapidly transported in the head-down, buttocks-up position with the EMT constantly maintaining pressure on the infant's head to keep it from compressing the umbilical cord. Medical control should be contacted as soon as possible during transport.

BREECH PRESENTATION

The majority of infants are delivered head first, but occasionally the fetus fails to rotate into a head-down position prior to the onset of labor. When the fetal buttocks or lower extremities are low in the uterus at the time of labor, these parts exit the birth canal first.

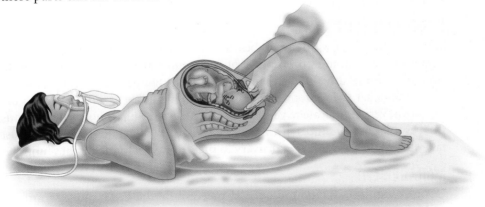

Figure 41.6 The EMT can help to prevent complete compression of the umbilical cord and the vessels within it by holding the infant's head away from it during contractions

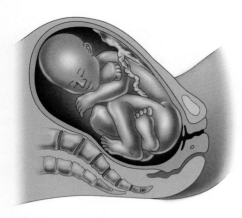

Figure 41.7 Because the breech newborn is at greater risk for injury during delivery, physicians often choose to perform a cesarean section

The fetal part that is first visible at the perineum is called the *presenting part.* When the presenting part is the fetal buttocks or lower extremities, it is called a **breech presentation.**

The breech newborn is at greater risk for injury during delivery. In addition, a prolapsed umbilical cord is seen more often with a breech presentation. Recognition of this condition by the EMT is imperative so that appropriate management may be initiated. Figure 41.7 illustrates this difficult position of the infant.

Because the position of the baby is not ideal, delivery can be complicated and dangerous. Often obstetricians choose to perform a surgical delivery through the abdomen, called a **cesarean section,** to avoid injury to the infant during a vaginal delivery.

SIGNS AND SYMPTOMS

The mother who has a fetus in the breech position experiences labor like any other mother. As the fetus descends in the birth canal, the buttocks or legs rather than the head become visible at the perineum.

MANAGEMENT

Once the breech presentation has been recognized, the EMT should place the mother on 100% oxygen and position her head down with her pelvis elevated. This position may help to slow delivery. Transport should be initiated immediately to the closest appropriate hospital. Medical control should be established while en route according to local protocols.

MECONIUM

During the normal course of labor, the amniotic sac breaks, allowing the amniotic fluid to be expelled from the vagina. This fluid is normally clear and watery. Occasionally, however, the fluid has a green tinge. This color is due to the presence of meconium in the fluid.

Meconium is the term for newborn feces. The very mature fetus or the distressed fetus may expel some meconium into the amniotic fluid. Because he is completely bathed in this fluid on delivery, the infant may have amniotic fluid in his mouth and nose. If the infant were to breathe in, or aspirate, the meconium, it would be potentially harmful.

Aspiration of meconium into the lungs can result in serious infection and injury to the newborn's lung tissue. Recognition of the presence of meconium is crucial so that appropriate steps may be taken to prevent its aspiration by the infant.

SIGNS AND SYMPTOMS

When evaluating a woman in labor, always question her regarding the color of the amniotic fluid upon rupture of her membranes. The EMT also should note the color of any fluid present during the initial perineal examination.

The thicker the meconium is in the fluid, the more hazardous it is to the newborn. Very thin, watery, yet slightly green-tinged fluid is not as big a risk as fluid as thick as pea soup. Regardless of the viscosity of the fluid, the EMT must take special measures during delivery to prevent injury to the infant's lungs.

MANAGEMENT

Upon recognition of the presence of meconium, the EMT should immediately make preparations for its management. Transport should be initiated so that the newborn may be cared for by advanced medical personnel as soon as possible. The delivery should be allowed to progress in as controlled a manner as possible.

As soon as the infant's head has been delivered, the EMT should ask the mother to stop pushing. It is often helpful to ask her to concentrate on her breathing to overcome the urge to push the baby out completely. The infant's nose and mouth must be suctioned several times to remove any meconium present. Once this has been accomplished, the EMT should encourage the mother to continue to push and deliver the infant.

Upon delivery, the infant should not be immediately stimulated, but should be placed on a firm surface where the EMT can again suction the infant's mouth and nose. The infant should then be assessed and resuscitated as appropriate. Involving advanced life support (ALS) providers in the care of the newborn with meconium aspiration is often helpful.

NUCHAL CORD

Immediately following delivery of the head, it is important to check the position of the umbilical cord. The cord can become wrapped around the baby's neck, called a *nuchal cord,* and must be removed before allowing the delivery to continue.

MANAGEMENT

When the cord is around the infant's neck, the mother must stop pushing while the cord is being removed. To remove the cord, use two fingers and carefully slip the cord over the infant's shoulders and head. If the cord is too tight to unwrap, place two clamps 2 to 3 inches apart, then cut between the clamps.

MULTIPLE GESTATION

One in 90 pregnancies in the United States results in twin births. A twin birth is the delivery of two infants during one pregnancy. Complications of pregnancy and delivery are increased with multiple gestations.

A single-infant pregnancy usually delivers at 40 weeks; however, twins tend to deliver at an average of 37 weeks, triplets at 33 weeks, and quadruplets at 29 weeks. Earlier delivery means that the infants have less time in utero for development. The special considerations associated with premature deliveries are discussed later in this unit.

SIGNS AND SYMPTOMS

The mother who is carrying more than one fetus often knows this and can share the information if specifically asked. A mother who has not had prenatal care may not realize that she is carrying more than one fetus. The EMT should specifically question the mother regarding this issue prior to delivery.

If this history is not obtained or not known, the EMT will become aware of the presence of more than one infant when the uterus does not decrease in size significantly after delivery of one infant. Often the second infant is not in a head-first position.

MANAGEMENT

Because the risk for complications is increased in delivery of multiple gestations, the mother laboring with multiple gestations should be transported immediately in hope that delivery can occur at the hospital. When caring for the mother, the EMT should prepare multiple delivery kits. A twin delivery will require two complete delivery kits and two complete infant resuscitation setups. Ideally, additional trained providers should be available if delivery is to occur in the field.

PREMATURE DELIVERY

As previously stated, most normal pregnancies end at an average of 40 weeks. This length of a pregnancy allows complete development of the fetal organs. One of the last organ systems to mature is the pulmonary system. Infants who are born prematurely can be underdeveloped with immature lungs. The earlier the delivery, the more likely it is that complications will occur.

A delivery that occurs prior to 36 weeks of gestation is considered to be a **premature delivery** and ideally would not be attempted in the field. The premature infant is especially prone to injury during delivery and may require extensive resuscitation that is available only at the hospital.

SIGNS AND SYMPTOMS

When caring for the woman in labor, the EMT should always determine the gestational age or the due date of the pregnancy. If the due date is more than 4 weeks away or the estimated gestational age is less than 36 weeks, the labor is premature.

MANAGEMENT

If a mother presents in labor prior to 36 weeks of gestation, the EMT should initiate transport as soon as possible. The destination hospital should be notified, and medical control should be established if recommended by local protocol.

If delivery is imminent, the EMT should prepare for it. A smaller infant usually is delivered much more quickly than a full-term baby. Care should be taken to cover the premature newborn to prevent loss of body heat. The premature infant is at great risk of developing hypothermia.

Any necessary resuscitation should be performed unless the small size of the very premature newborn makes this resuscitation physically impossible. Infants born prior to 24 weeks generally do not survive because of inadequately matured organ systems.

PRECIPITOUS DELIVERY

A **precipitous delivery** occurs when the birth of the fetus takes place less than 3 hours after labor begins. It is seen most often in mothers who have delivered several children (multipara). There is a higher risk for traumatic injury to the fetus, mother, and umbilical cord when a precipitous delivery occurs.

MANAGEMENT

The EMT should be prepared for the possibility of a precipitous delivery based on the past history of the multipara mother. The delivery will be conducted as for any other normal delivery; however, it may occur very quickly, with little to no warning.

INTRAUTERINE FETAL DEMISE

Intrauterine fetal demise is the term used for a fetus who has died while still in the uterus, occurring after the 20th week of gestation and/or a fetal weight of 500 grams (1.1 lb). Fetal demise occurs in approximately 5 in 1,000 in normal, uncomplicated pregnancies.

SIGNS AND SYMPTOMS

There are no specific signs and symptoms for fetal demise as it is usually determined through the absence of fetal heart tones, lack of uterine growth, and ultrasound examination during a prenatal visit. In later pregnancy the mother may state the absence of fetal movement.

MANAGEMENT

The EMT will rarely be called to assist with a fetal demise delivery. Often the fetus will spontaneously abort within two weeks of demise. If the EMT should be called, the mother should be managed with high-flow oxygen and hypoperfusion if heavy bleeding is present.

If possible, any tissue that has delivered should be placed in a container and transported with the patient to the hospital for examination by a physician. One of the most important elements of management in this case will be a caring, empathetic manner and emotional support for the parents.

POSTDELIVERY CARE

After delivery is completed, the EMT should transport the mother and the infant to the hospital in a timely fashion. If she is able, and the infant is healthy, the mother should be allowed to hold the infant unless the infant must be placed in a car seat according to local law or protocol. The EMT should frequently reassess the flow of vaginal bleeding. Excessive bleeding is defined as greater than 500 cc or if the mother exhibits signs or symptoms of hypoperfusion.

MOTHER

After the placenta is delivered, the uterus normally contracts, which slows bleeding. If the uterus does not contract, the uterus may continue to bleed heavily. If excessive bleeding occurs, the EMT can attempt to cause contraction of the uterus.

Uterine contraction can be stimulated by firmly massaging the uterus, called *fundal massage*. The EMT should place a hand on the lower abdomen just above the pubis and firmly knead the area. The massage may be uncomfortable for the patient but will help to slow the bleeding. Figure 41.8 demonstrates this technique. Uterine massage should continue until the bleeding stops.

If excessive bleeding has occurred, the EMT should treat the mother for shock by applying high-flow oxygen, closely monitoring vital signs, and immediately transporting to the closest appropriate facility. The EMT should reassess frequently and arrange for an ALS intercept if possible.

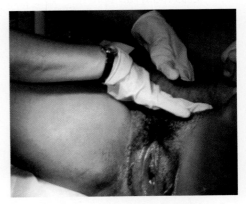

Figure 41.8 Firm massage of the empty uterus helps to stimulate uterine contraction

INFANT

The initial resuscitation of the newborn is centered on a primary assessment of activity, color, breathing, pulse, and tone. It is helpful to have a second EMT care for the infant. If the newborn is sick and requires active resuscitation, the infant may need to be transported in a separate ambulance so that adequate room is available for care.

NEWBORN CARE

Immediately after a prehospital delivery, the EMT is faced with caring for two patients. Ideally, one EMT is assigned to care for the mother, while another takes responsibility for the care of the newborn.

A newborn, up to 1 month of age, is called a *neonate*. The most stressful period in life for the neonate may occur immediately following birth. The newborn must quickly adjust to life outside the womb or he will not survive.

The EMT's role is to support the newborn's first steps in meeting the demands of life. The EMT is primarily interested in preventing complications such as hypothermia and alerting the hospital of any difficulties.

PRIMARY ASSESSMENT OF THE NEWBORN

The **Apgar score** was developed in 1952 by Dr. Virginia Apgar as a standard tool for measuring the health of a newborn. The Apgar score has become the tool, like the Glasgow Coma Scale in trauma, used as a means of communication of the infant's health between healthcare professionals.

Table 41-4	Apgar Score

A = Appearance

2—Completely pink

1—Cyanotic extremities

0—Central cyanosis

P = Pulse

2—Greater than 100 bpm

1—Less than 100 bpm

0—No pulse

G = Grimace

2—Cough or sneeze

1—Grimace

0—Unresponsive

A = Activity

2—Active

1—Flexion

0—No motion

R = Respiration

2—Good respiration, strong cry

1—Slow or irregular respiration, weak cry

0—Apneic

The Apgar score measures heart rate, respiration, muscle tone, response to stimuli, and color. The Apgar score is based on the newborn's condition at 1 minute after birth and 5 minutes after birth. Table 41-4 details the point assignments associated with this well-known scoring system.

The EMT should integrate the Apgar scoring tool into the primary assessment of the newborn. The primary assessment of a newborn starts with an assessment of level of consciousness. Although newborns are not expected to interact with the environment, they should be awake and active.

The EMT should attempt to straighten the legs (Figure 41.9). If the newborn is active and kicking, the newborn is awarded 2 points. If the newborn slowly/weakly flexes the legs back into the fetal position, 1 point is awarded. If no motion is detected, no points are given.

Proceeding to the airway, the EMT should take the bulb syringe and again suction the nostrils (Figure 41.10). If the newborn coughs or sneezes, a strong protective reflex, the EMT awards 2 points. If the newborn merely grimaces, the EMT awards only 1 point. If the newborn does not react to this noxious stimulus, no points are awarded.

Next, the EMT assesses the newborn's breathing. The strong cry of a newborn is an excellent indication of good respiratory effort (Figure 41.11). A strong cry is awarded 2 points. If the newborn's breathing is shallow or irregular, only 1 point is awarded. If the newborn is apneic, no points are awarded.

Circulation is assessed using both pulses and color. The EMT may attempt to obtain a brachial pulse in the newborn's upper arm. If the brachial pulse is difficult to palpate, then the EMT should count the apical pulse (Figure 41.12). The EMT places the stethoscope over the newborn's heart

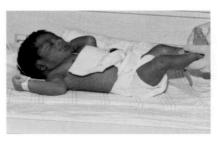

Figure 41.9 An active, kicking newborn is awarded 2 points on the Apgar score

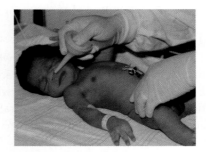

Figure 41.10 If the newborn sneezes when his nostrils are suctioned, he is awarded 2 points on the Apgar score

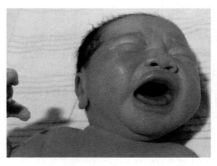

Figure 41.11 The newborn with a strong cry is awarded 2 points on the Apgar score

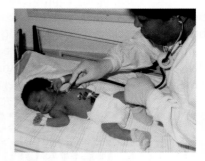

Figure 41.12 A newborn with a heart rate greater than 100 beats per minute is awarded 2 points on the Apgar score

and then counts an apical pulse. An apical pulse is counted by listening to the heartbeat at the apex, or bottom, of the heart.

Immediately after childbirth, it is sometimes possible to gently palpate the umbilical cord and feel the pulsation of the heart. A pulse may be also counted in this manner.

A newborn's heart rate should be very fast, greater than 100 beats per minute. If the pulse rate is greater than 100 beats per minute, two points are awarded. If the pulse rate is less than 100 beats per minute, 1 point is awarded. If no pulse is present, no points are awarded.

Another indicator of good circulation is capillary bed perfusion. A hearty circulation will flush the capillary beds of the hands and feet, making them appear pink. If the palms of the hands or the soles of the feet are pink, 2 points are awarded (Figure 41.13). If cyanosis, a bluish or gray pallor, is present in the feet and hands, 1 point is awarded. If the newborn is centrally cyanotic, as well as peripherally cyanotic, no points are awarded. A bluish or gray pallor to the chest is called central cyanosis.

The newborn's level of consciousness, airway, breathing, and circulation (ABCs) are all assessed using the Apgar tool. Each should be awarded points, and the infant assigned a total Apgar score.

Most newborns lose at least one point in color/appearance in the initial 1-minute assessment. **Acrocyanosis,** cyanosis of the extremities, may be normal in the newborn within the first hour after birth.

An Apgar score of 7 to 10 points usually indicates that the newborn is having no difficulty adjusting to life outside the womb. A score between 4 and 6 points indicates that the newborn is moderately depressed. Several actions the EMT can take to stimulate a moderately depressed newborn are discussed later in this unit.

A score of 3 or less indicates a high-priority newborn who will require vigorous resuscitation in the field and probable admission to a neonatal intensive care unit. Despite vigorous resuscitation, newborns with a 1- and 5-minute Apgar score of 3 or less have a 50% chance of survival.

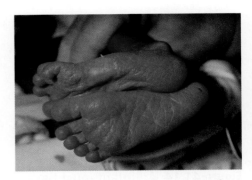

Figure 41.13 If the soles of the feet and the palms of the hands are pink, the newborn is awarded 2 points on the Apgar score

MANAGEMENT OF THE NEWBORN

The first priority of management of a newborn, as with any other patient, is maintaining the airway. Newborns are obligatory nose breathers. When at rest, a newborn will naturally choose to breathe through the nose. This is an important protective function of the body.

The nose not only heats and humidifies the air that is inhaled but also filters the air, trapping bacteria in mucus. In the first 30 minutes to an hour after birth, the newborn produces large amounts of mucus.

The EMT must keep the newborn's nostrils clear of mucus. A bulb syringe is convenient for this purpose. First, the newborn should be placed head down to facilitate drainage. Picking up the syringe, the EMT should compress the bulb to express the air within the bulb. Keeping the bulb compressed, the EMT should place the tip of the syringe gently into the nostril. Once the tip is within the nostril, the bulb is released and the mucus is suctioned into the bulb. The bulb is emptied onto a 4 × 4 pad, and the process repeated with the other nostril.

If the mucus is thick and tenacious, a flexible French suction catheter may need to be used. A great deal of caution must be observed because the suction can injure tender tissues within the nostrils. The suction should be set at the lowest setting on the suction machine. The tip of the French catheter should be gently inserted no more than one-half inch into the nostril. Low-pressure suction should be applied, as the catheter is withdrawn, for no more than

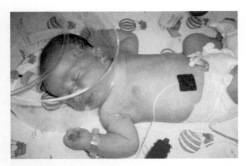

Figure 41.14 An infant must be watched carefully for signs of respiratory distress (Courtesy of the Nicholas Scadden Family)

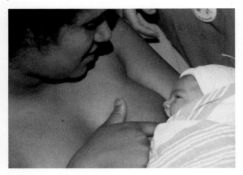

Figure 41.15 Breast-feeding helps the mother's uterus contract and return to normal

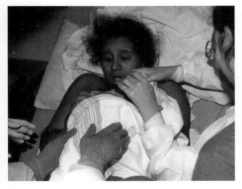

Figure 41.16 Placing the newborn against the mother's body will help to maintain body temperature

3–5 seconds. The process should be repeated for the other nostril. Always follow local protocol and consult medical direction regarding use of low-pressure suction in the newborn.

If the newborn's respirations are still depressed or irregular, oxygen should be gently administered. Oxygen tubing, connected to an oxygen regulator turned to 4 liters per minute, is held about 1 inch away from the newborn's mouth and nose. If the infant does not immediately improve, or "pink up," from this blow-by oxygen, the liter flow can be increased.

After about 30 seconds the newborn should be reassessed. If the newborn still has poor respiratory effort or is bradycardiac (heart rate less than 100), the newborn's respiration must be assisted with a bag-valve-mask (BVM) and high-concentration oxygen.

Indications that an infant may be experiencing respiratory distress include seesaw respirations, marked chest retractions, and audible grunting. Seesaw respiration is the result of an exaggerated paradoxical movement of the chest and the abdomen as the infant uses abdominal muscles to assist the weak diaphragm to breathe.

As the diaphragm tries to draw in more air, the skin between the ribs is also drawn in, causing the skin to retract. This sign of respiratory distress is called *intercostal retractions*. With intercostal retractions, the outline of each rib becomes more prominent. When the newborn is in serious distress, sternal retraction also may be observed (Figure 41.14).

Respiratory failure is more commonly seen in the premature newborn and the newborn with congenital heart defects. Eventually, these newborns may go into respiratory arrest.

If the newborn shows signs of respiratory distress or failure, the EMT should transport the newborn immediately. In some cases, an additional ambulance may be requested if the mother's transportation is delayed to rapidly transport the newborn.

If the mother permits, a newborn who is healthy can be put to the mother's breast (Figure 41.15). It is a good sign if the newborn appears interested in suckling, because this indicates that the newborn is stabilizing and is ready to take nourishment.

Breast-feeding is also good for the mother. Stimulation of the nipple in turn stimulates hormones that increase uterine contractions. The uterus contractions aid in delivery of the placenta and slow bleeding.

A newborn is very prone to hypothermia. The EMT can take several steps to ward off heat loss and hypothermia. A great deal of heat is lost via the evaporation of the amniotic fluid that once bathed the infant. To prevent this heat loss, the newborn should be immediately dried with a clean towel.

The newborn should not be placed directly on a table or other solid surface for assessment, because the heat loss from conduction, or contact on a cold surface, can lead to hypothermia. Initially, the newborn should be placed on a blanket while being assessed. When the EMT is done with the assessment, the newborn should be placed on a surface close to body temperature, such as in the mother's arms (Figure 41.16).

SECONDARY ASSESSMENT OF THE NEWBORN

After completing the newborn's primary assessment and assigning an Apgar score, the EMT should perform the secondary assessment. This detailed physical examination is conducted to assess for normal characteristics and note any abnormalities.

GENERAL APPEARANCE

The newborn is typically found in a fetal position, with the knees flexed and the chin resting on the chest. Premature newborns and hypoxic newborns take a more relaxed posture, with legs and arms extended.

The newborn's skin should be red and flushed when he is crying. The hands and feet may be cyanotic. Hypothermia may increase the degree of acrocyanosis that is seen. Cyanosis may be transient, lasting only seconds, as the lungs are exercised and eventually begin to function properly all the time.

The EMT may notice a white, cottage-cheesy substance on the newborn's skin. This substance is called **vernix caseosa,** sometimes referred to as "nature's cold cream." It is thought to help protect the newborn from heat loss. The EMT need not remove it.

At first glance, the newborn's head may appear to be misshapen. A misshapen head after a vaginal delivery is a natural finding, a result of the molding process, which compresses the newborn's skull during delivery. The head will return to its normal shape in approximately 1–2 days.

The EMT should observe for the soft spots, or *fontanels*. The fontanels are the junction of the bones of the skull. Eventually, the fontanels close as the infant matures. Usually there are only two fontanels that can be seen, one anterior and one posterior. Crying, coughing, and lying down may cause the newborn's fontanels to bulge temporarily. If a fontanel is depressed, the child may be dehydrated.

Light-skinned newborns usually have dark blue eyes, while dark-skinned newborns have brown eyes. The newborn's eyes commonly appear to lack focus, scanning back and forth. The EMT may also notice some blood in the sclera; this is a result of the newborn's compression during delivery and is not significant.

As was previously mentioned, the nose may contain a large amount of mucus and need to be suctioned frequently. Nasal flaring is a sign of air hunger. The EMT should assess the newborn to determine whether further treatment is necessary.

The newborn's chest should be assessed for signs of respiratory distress. The respiratory findings should be reported to a physician.

The umbilical cord should be carefully inspected. Immediately after birth, the umbilical cord should appear bluish-white. Any odor or drainage should be reported.

Finally, the EMT should assess the extremities for movement. Almost every new mother wants to know whether the newborn has 10 fingers and 10 toes. The EMT should check the fingernail beds for capillary refill. Persistent cyanosis may indicate either hypoxia or hypothermia.

BIRTH TRAUMA

Birth trauma is usually associated with a difficult delivery. Babies with above-average weight commonly suffer some birth trauma.

At times when the shoulders are larger than the fetal head, they become wedged against the pubic bone and sacrum during birth. This impaction of the fetal shoulders is called **shoulder dystocia.** Shoulder dystocia usually requires delivery to take place in the hospital because there are specific methods needed to deliver the shoulders, possibly including a cesarean section. However, if the shoulders do deliver in the field, the EMT should be aware that traumatic injury to the newborn's shoulder region may occur.

The EMT may notice that the newborn is not moving the arms symmetrically. This could indicate that the clavicle has been fractured. The EMT need not splint the clavicle but should simply handle the newborn gently and report any deformity or loss of motion to the physician.

Street Smart

The new mother may be concerned about oxygen being administered to her new baby because she may have heard that oxygen can affect an infant's vision. Oxygen toxicity leading to visual impairment occurs only after prolonged exposure to high concentrations of oxygen, so concerns about vision should not affect the EMT's decision to use this lifesaving drug. The EMT should explain to the new mother that the lowest concentration of oxygen that is effective is being used, and only for a very short amount of time.

Street Smart

The newborn radiates a great deal of heat into the atmosphere from the large head. To reduce this type of heat loss, a cap or bonnet should be placed on the neonate. Additionally, to prevent further heat loss, the newborn should be swaddled in a warmed cotton blanket or the receiving blanket supplied in the emergency OB (obstetrics) kit from the ambulance.

BIRTH DEFECTS

One of the first questions an EMT may have to answer from a mother is, "Is my baby all right?" If the answer is no, the mother has to immediately deal with the loss of the "perfect baby."

Mothers sometimes react emotionally, displaying anger and grief. Other mothers go into denial. The EMT must be prepared for these possibilities and deal with his own emotions while helping the mother to cope with hers.

Usually a physician is responsible for explaining the circumstances to the new parents; however, when EMS is involved in the delivery that may not be possible. If the mother asks the EMT whether her baby is all right, it is probably best to briefly explain to the mother what has been found, in simple terms she can understand.

Parents attach a great deal of meaning to the behaviors and facial expressions of caregivers. The EMT must remain professional and nonjudgmental at this time. The EMT should present the newborn as something precious and emphasize the well-formed portions of the body.

The EMT should defer any questions about the deformity to the physician but try to be open, caring, and honest.

Table 41-5 High-Risk Pregnancy
Premature delivery
Multiple births
Prolapsed umbilical cord
Severe maternal bleeding
Meconium aspiration

NEWBORN RESUSCITATION

When a newborn is in cardiopulmonary arrest, the EMT must react quickly. Otherwise, the newborn may suffer permanent brain damage and possibly even death. Fortunately, the EMT can use some basic procedures that should be familiar. These basic procedures will be effective in the majority of cases. The EMT need only modify these procedures somewhat, based on the size of the newborn (see Figure 41.17).

Not all newborns breathe spontaneously at birth; some need assistance. The EMT can identify early those newborns that are more likely to need resuscitation by taking an accurate history. Newborns of high-risk pregnancies, listed in Table 41-5, are the most likely to require some assistance.

A newborn depressed from hypoxia will be bradycardiac and may even be pulseless. To reverse this condition, the EMT need only reverse the hypoxia

---

Street Smart

In some cases, a newborn is not born alive. Newborns can be stillborn for a number of reasons. Prolonged compression of the umbilical cord or hypotension of mother or child are two common reasons that a newborn can be stillborn.

Whatever the explanation, the newborn will be unresponsive, apneic, and pulseless. The EMT should begin resuscitation unless there are signs of prolonged fetal demise. Although the effort may appear to be fruitless, the mother and the EMT need to know that all that could have been done for the newborn was attempted. When the mother and child arrive at the hospital, professional counselors will be available to help the family cope with the loss.

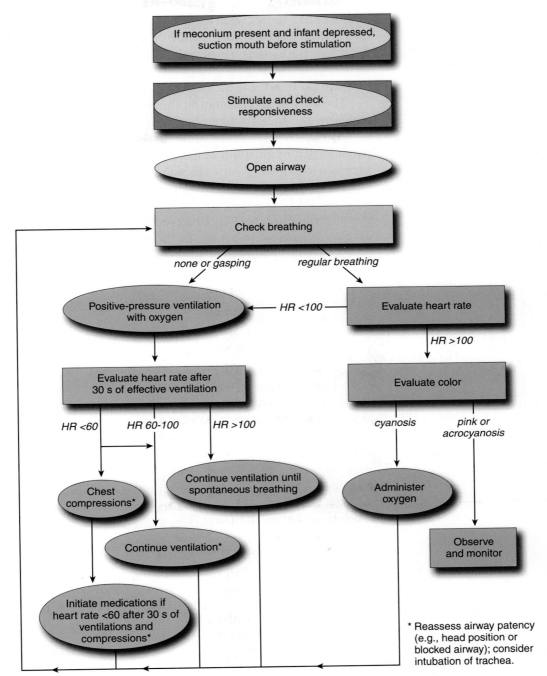

Figure 41.17 Algorithm for advanced life support of the newborn (Reprinted courtesy of the American Academy of Pediatrics)

in the majority of cases. Therefore, the EMT should focus his attentions on the newborn's breathing.

Some newborns need only a little encouragement to breathe better. The EMT should lay the newborn on his back and vigorously dry in a circular motion using a clean towel (Figure 41.18). This is often all it takes to stimulate the newborn to breathe.

If drying does not stimulate the infant to breathe, the EMT must proceed to the ABCs. The cornerstone of newborn resuscitation is attention to airway and breathing. In fact, 80% of apneic newborns can be resuscitated with basic management of the airway and breathing alone.

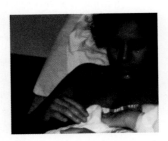

Figure 41.18 Stimulation, such as a back rub, is all that is needed to help a newborn breathe better

The EMT should open the newborn's airway, using a modified jaw thrust. Care should be observed to ensure the head is not tilted back. Overextension of the newborn's neck can actually close off the airway. The newborn's head should be in a neutral position. Often padding under the newborn's shoulders will aid in keeping the head in a neutral position.

The nostrils and the mouth should be suctioned clear of mucus, blood, and other fluids. Suctioning should not last longer than 5 seconds.

A newborn has a much shorter airway and therefore larger tongue compared to that of an adult. Maintain the airway in a neutral position and be prepared to provide positive pressure ventilations as needed.

When the newborn remains bradycardiac (less than 100 bpm) or becomes pulseless, the EMT must proceed to positive pressure ventilation. It is important that the EMT carefully observe ventilation technique. Overly aggressive ventilation can lead to hyperinflation of the lungs and stomach. A distended stomach reduces lung expansion and risks regurgitation. An overinflated lung can burst, creating a pneumothorax.

Ventilation should continue at a rate of between 40 and 60 breaths per minute or a breath every second. The volume of each breath should be only enough to see the chest rise.

If the heart rate is below 60 beats per minute despite positive pressure ventilation, then cardiac compressions should be started. For cardiopulmonary resuscitation (CPR) to be effective, the spine must be supported during compressions. A newborn's chest usually can be encircled by the EMT's hands. The EMT's interlocked fingers on the newborn's back provide a platform for compressions. The EMT's two thumbs can then compress the chest.

If the newborn is small or premature, the EMT may have to overlap his thumbs before beginning compressions. If the newborn is large, which is often the case with newborns of diabetic mothers, or if the EMT's hands are compromising chest expansion, then two fingers should be placed on the chest over the midsternum. Compression should be about one-third the depth of the chest and be maintained at a rate of 120 times per minute.

Two EMTs can perform effective ventilation and compression provided they work together. One EMT is at the head of the patient providing one ventilation at the end of the every third compression as the other EMT continues to deliver chest compressions, pausing only briefly for each ventilation. Figure 41.19 shows the inverted pyramid developed by the American Heart Association as a guideline for neonatal resuscitation.

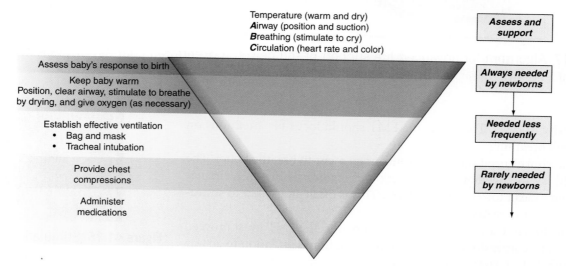

Figure 41.19 The resuscitation triangle starts with the basics and ends with the advanced life support procedures

MECONIUM ASPIRATION

Meconium is the first feces (bowel movement) of a newborn. It is made up of bile and mucus and has a greenish color to it. Meconium may pass into the amniotic sac during delivery if the newborn is distressed.

Aspiration of meconium by a newborn can cause difficulty in the newborn's ability to breathe. If the EMT observes meconium, proceed with the newborn's resuscitation, as previously described, and transport the newborn immediately. The EMT should give more attention to clearing the airway with suction and should consider providing supplemental oxygen as needed. If possible, ALS providers should be intercepted.

CONCLUSION

Childbirth is a natural process that the EMT does not often encounter in the field. However, when called for an emergency delivery, the EMT should keep in mind that most deliveries will be uncomplicated and the EMT will merely facilitate the process. However, complications during childbirth do occur and can be devastating for both the mother and the baby.

The EMT should be familiar with normal labor and delivery and must also be able to recognize and appropriately manage patients with complicated deliveries or special delivery considerations. Because EMTs do not handle deliveries often, they should review the procedures frequently.

By applying their understanding of newborns to previous knowledge of prehospital emergency care, EMTs can competently manage the newborn.

Juanita knows Erin's desire to push means delivery is imminent, and she explains to Erin she needs to check to see if the baby is crowning. Erin states she feels a lot of pressure, like the baby is coming out and Juanita coaches her to pant while she checks her and they prepare for delivery.

Because Erin had planned to give birth at home with a midwife present, the room and bed are already prepared for a birth. Dawn helps Erin to roll onto her back so Juanita can check for the baby's head. Erin advises she is starting another contraction, and Juanita observes the head beginning to bulge from the perineum. Juanita knows the infant is ready to be born and with the next contractions, Juanita assists the infant as she leaves her mother's womb.

Immediately after the baby delivers, Dawn wipes the newborn with a dry towel. This is the first delivery Dawn has ever assisted with, and she is quietly amazed by the tiny human being in her arms. The baby is perfect. She has tiny hands that were a little blue, with perfect, tiny little fingers. She has a hearty wail that indicates she is moving good air, and she is just kicking, kicking, kicking. She is extremely active and seems a little unhappy to be out here in the big world.

Dawn refers to the laminated card she has taken out of the birth kit and informs Juanita the baby has an Apgar of 9 at 1 minute following delivery.

Juanita looks up, smiling at Erin who has relaxed back on the bed following delivery. "She looks very healthy, but sounds a little unhappy right now."

Erin smiles, telling Juanita and Dawn that she and her husband have three boys and had been hoping for a girl. They are naming her Marisa Ann, and she can't wait to hold her daughter.

Juanita explains that Dawn must finish wrapping the baby up in a warm blanket and placing a little pink stocking hat on her head. In the meantime, Erin needs to let her know when she feels the additional contractions that would deliver the afterbirth. Juanita has a bag positioned below Erin to place the placenta in for transport to the hospital.

Once Erin delivers the placenta and has little Marisa Ann safely cuddled in her arms, Juanita and Dawn prepare to transport them to the local hospital. The delivery and birth have been without complications and Marisa Ann's second Apgar score is a 10. She is happily snuggled against Erin and will be kept warm during the trip to the hospital.

Erin agrees to be transported to the hospital after Juanita explains that as a precaution, both Erin and Marisa need to be evaluated by a physician. Dawn assures her the back of the ambulance will be kept very warm and the snowplow will be leading the way.

Erin smiles, telling Juanita, "Marisa will have a wonderful story to read in her baby book someday about the day she was born during a snowstorm with two wonderful EMTs named Juanita and Dawn!"

Skill 41-1 Emergency Delivery

PURPOSE: To assist the mother in the natural delivery of a newborn infant.

STANDARD PRECAUTIONS:

☑ Surgical scissors or cord clamps
☑ Bulb suction device
☑ Towels
☑ Gauze sponges
☑ Baby blanket
☑ Sanitary napkins
☑ Plastic bag or bucket
☑ Personal protective equipment

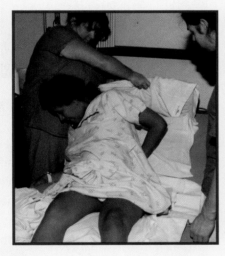

1 The EMT should position the mother supine with knees drawn up and spread apart and can assist the mother by helping her to elevate her buttocks on a pillow or blankets.

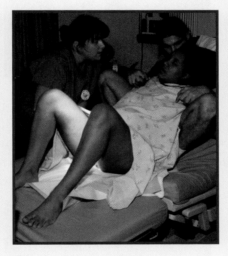

2 The EMT should create a clean area around the vaginal opening with clean towels or paper barriers.

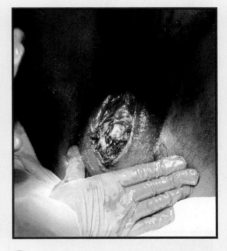

3 As the infant's head appears during crowning, the EMT should place her fingers gently on the skull and exert very gentle pressure to prevent explosive delivery.

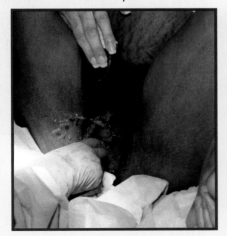

4 If the amniotic sac has not broken, the EMT should use her thumb and forefinger, or a clamp, to puncture the sac and push it away from the infant's head and face.

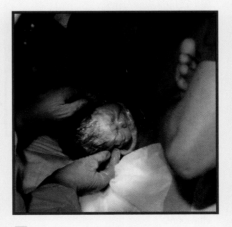

5 As the infant's head is delivered, the EMT should determine whether the umbilical cord is around the neck and, if it is, slip it over the infant's head or shoulder. If it is not possible to slip the cord, the EMT should clamp the cord in two places, cut the cord between the clamps, and unwrap the cord from the infant's neck.

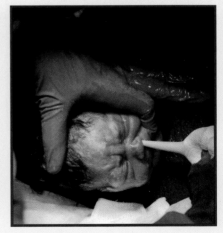

6 After the infant's head is born, the EMT supports the head and suctions the newborn's mouth and then the nose several times with the bulb suction device.

(continued)

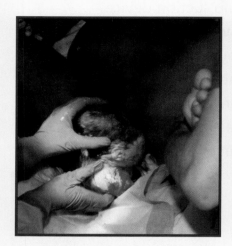

7 As the torso and full body are born, the EMT supports the infant with both hands. As the feet are born, the EMT should grasp them firmly.

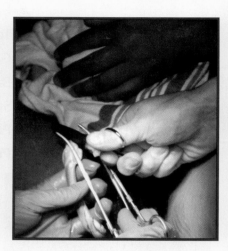

8 After pulsations cease in the umbilical cord, the EMT should clamp the cord in two places, with the closest clamp about four fingers' width away from the infant, and then cut the cord between the clamps.

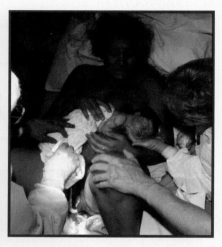

9 Then the EMT should gently dry the infant with towels and wrap the infant in a warm blanket. The infant should be placed on his side, preferably with the head slightly lower than the trunk.

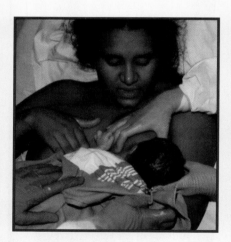

10 Another EMT should monitor the infant and complete initial care of the newborn.

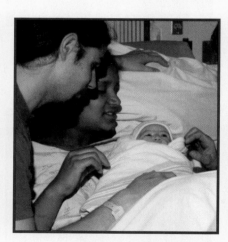

11 The EMT should place a sterile sanitary napkin between the mother's legs and have her close her legs. The EMT should also comfort the mother and monitor vital signs.

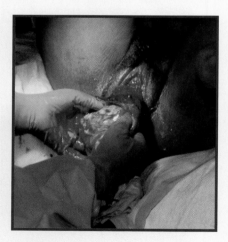

12 While preparing the mother and infant for transport, the EMT should watch for delivery of the placenta. When the placenta is delivered, the EMT wraps the placenta in a towel, places it in a plastic bag or container, and transports it to the hospital with the mother.

Key Concepts Revisited

- There are three distinct stages of labor:
  - First Stage
    - Dilation of the cervix
  - Second stage
    - Delivery of the fetus
  - Third stage
    - Delivery of the placenta
- The EMT must be able to recognize the signs of impending delivery:
  - Crowning
  - Feeling need to move bowels
  - Increasing vaginal pressure
  - Increased need to push
- The brief predelivery history is important to establishing a controlled delivery:
  - Have you been pregnant before and, if so, how many times?
  - How many pregnancies resulted in live births?
  - Have you had prenatal care?
  - Were there any complications during this or past pregnancies or births?
  - Are you having pain or discomfort? What does it feel like?
  - Does the pain come in regular intervals?
  - How long does the pain last, and how often do the contractions occur?
  - When is your due date?
- The EMT must able to recognize and manage complications of delivery:
  - Prolapsed umbilical cord
  - Breech presentation
  - Meconium

- Nucal cord
- Multiple gestation
- Premature delivery
- Precipitous delivery
- Intrauterine fetal demise
- The proper care of the mother postdelivery focuses on the assessment and management of excessive bleeding, if it should occur.
- The primary assessment of the newborn is conducted through the Apgar score.
  - Appearance
  - Pulse
  - Grimace
  - Activity
  - Respiration
- The first priority of management of the newborn focuses on the airway and breathing:
  - Cyanosis
  - Retractions
- The detailed physical examination of the secondary assessment is to assess for normal and abnormal characteristics beyond the ABCs.
- Babies with large birth weights can experience trauma during delivery:
  - Shoulder dystocia
  - Fractured clavicle
- Resuscitation of the newborn follows standard CPR guidelines with just a few modifications:
  - Reversed triangle
  - 30 second reassessment
  - 3:1 compression to ventilation ratio

Review Questions

1. What changes take place in female anatomy during pregnancy?
2. What are the components of the three stages of labor?
3. What are signs and symptoms of impending delivery?
4. What is the importance of a brief predelivery history?
5. What is the proper care of the mother postdelivery?
6. What are the special considerations with the passage of meconium-stained amniotic fluid?
7. What are the signs of a newborn in respiratory distress?
8. What are the elements of the Apgar score?
9. What unique features does an EMT look for in the focused physical examination of the newborn?
10. What are "high-risk" pregnancies?
11. What are the steps of resuscitation of a newborn?
12. At what rate should the EMT do CPR compressions on a newborn?

Key Terms

Acrocyanosis
Amniotic sac
Apgar score
Bloody show
Braxton Hicks contractions
Breech presentation
Cardinal movements of labor
Cervical dilation
Cesarean section
Crowning
Effacement
First stage of labor
Gravidity
Intrauterine fetal demise

Labor
Meconium
Molding
Multiparous
Parity
Precipitous delivery
Premature delivery
Primiparous
Prolapsed umbilical cord
Second stage of labor
Shoulder dystocia
Third stage of labor
Vernix caseosa

Further Study

Bledsoe, B. E., and R. W. Benner. *Critical Care Paramedic*. Upper Saddle River, NJ: Pearson/Prentice Hall, 2006.

International Liaison Committee on Resuscitation. "Consensus on Science with Treatment Recommendations for Pediatric and Neonatal Patients: Pediatric Basic and Advanced Life Support." *Pediatrics* 117, no. 5 (May 2006) e955–e977.

Kattwinkel. J. *Neonatal Resuscitation Textbook*. 5th ed. Elk Grove Village, IL: American Academy of Pediatrics and American Heart Association, 2006.

Littleton, L. Y., and J. Engebretson. *Maternity Nursing Care*. Clifton Park, NY: Delmar Cengage Learning, 2005.

CHAPTER 8

Childhood Emergencies

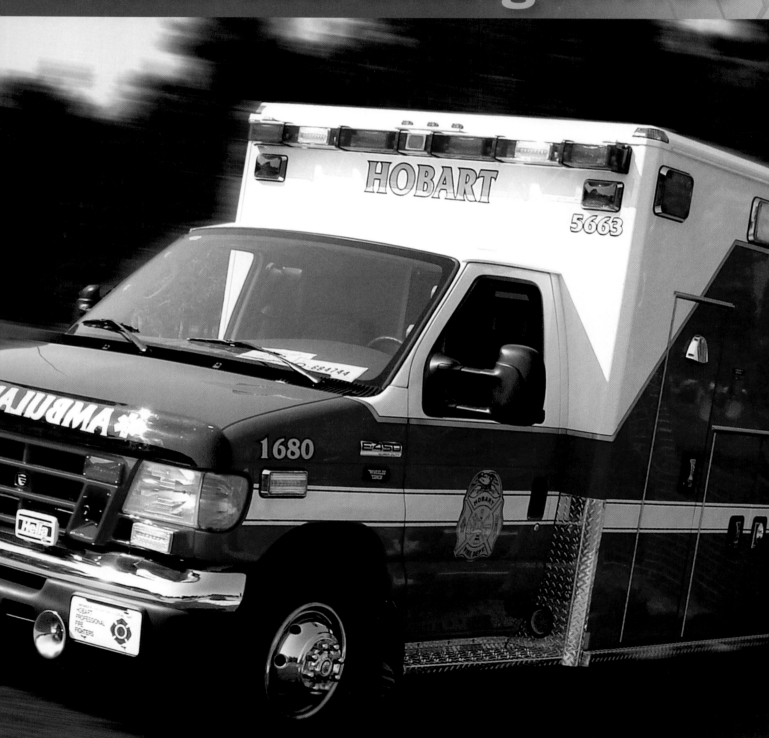

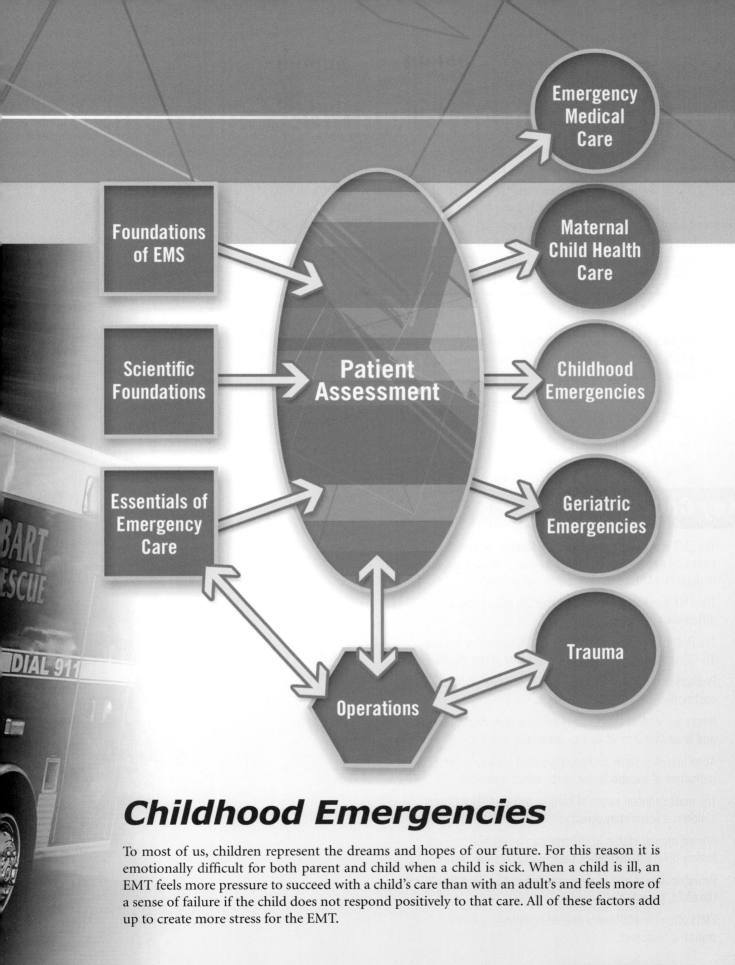

Childhood Emergencies

To most of us, children represent the dreams and hopes of our future. For this reason it is emotionally difficult for both parent and child when a child is sick. When a child is ill, an EMT feels more pressure to succeed with a child's care than with an adult's and feels more of a sense of failure if the child does not respond positively to that care. All of these factors add up to create more stress for the EMT.

Caring for ill or injured children can be a stressful situation for an Emergency Medical Technician (EMT). Care is based on the age of the child. Children of different ages are susceptible to different types of illnesses. Familiarity with general techniques of pediatric assessment and with the common illnesses in each age-group can help the EMT to feel more comfortable when faced with an ill or injured child.

National Education Standards

The Emergency Medical Technician (EMT) will demonstrate a fundamental depth and foundational breadth of understanding in the anatomy, physiology, pathophysiology, assessment, and management of medical emergencies affecting children.

Key Concepts

- The EMT must understand the developmental considerations based on age-groups to provide appropriate assessment and management of medical emergencies in children.

- The EMT must understand age-specific developmental differences in children.

- The Pediatric Assessment Triangle (PAT) provides a quick 15–30 second assessment of the severity of the illness.

- Pediatric airway emergencies range from foreign body obstruction to obstructive diseases.

- Increased work of breathing is evidenced by physical signs and is an indicator of illness severity.

- Abnormal skin signs and capillary refill are two reliable indicators of hypoperfusion in the infant and child.

- The most common cause of cardiac arrest in infants and children is respiratory arrest.

- Altered mental status in children can be verified through history taking to determine their normal mental status.

- Pediatric illness and injuries can be emotionally difficult for the child, parent, and provider.

- EMTs often benefit from a debriefing following a difficult pediatric transport.

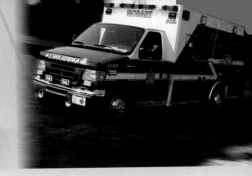

CASE STUDY

Gordy and Kerry are just sitting down to supper when the tones go off: "Unit 68-dispatch. Please respond to an 18 month old having a seizure. Time out 17:45."

Gordy has been an EMT for more than 20 years, and he still gets that queasy feeling in the pit of his stomach whenever they get a call for a sick or injured child. He has experienced a lot of calls involving children over the years, with the majority of them having a good outcome. However, the calls that always come to mind first when dispatch indicates a sick or injured child are the few really bad ones.

Upon arrival Gordy and Kerry are met at the door by a distraught teenager. "Mom said to hurry, my little sister is having some kind of fit in the living room, and she doesn't think she's breathing." Gordy and Kerry glance at each other, glad they grabbed the pediatric jump kit with all the equipment designed for children of various ages.

As they enter the living room, they see a small child lying still on the sofa, covered in heavy blankets. A woman turns toward them, stating, "This is my daughter Mackenzie, and she is 18 months old. She has been really quiet, not active at all today and then tonight when I tried to get her to eat some soup, her eyes went back in her head and she started shaking all over. She just finally stopped when you walked through the door."

Critical Thinking Questions

1. What are some causes of altered mental status in a child?
2. What other potential causes, besides seizures, are there for an altered mental status in children?
3. How should the EMTs manage care of this child?

INTRODUCTION

Children present special challenges to the EMT because children are, after all, not little adults. By understanding the special developmental considerations of children as well as the importance of parenting to the child's total care, the EMT may feel less anxiety about caring for a child. This unit discusses the developmental considerations of children and how they relate to the assessment and management of children with medical emergencies.

NORMAL CHILDHOOD DEVELOPMENT

Although every child is not the same, children of the same age share some well-known developmental characteristics. It is important for an EMT to understand some of these characteristics. Understanding these similarities, as well as the differences, should guide an EMT's care of a pediatric patient.

NEWBORN

Although it is somewhat uncommon for the EMT to be called to care for a newborn, or *neonate* (0 to 1 month of age), it is important to be familiar with the normal developmental characteristics of these infants. Even though it may not seem that a neonate interacts much with his environment, these tiny babies have very well-developed senses of smell and hearing. Early in life, they tend to recognize the smell of their mother and the sound of her voice.

The EMT should allow the newborn's mother to hold the newborn during the assessment and care, as much as possible given the newborn's condition

If newborns are to be transported, it is important they are adequately and safely secured in the ambulance. It is recommended that any newborn be transported in an approved infant car seat appropriately strapped into the ambulance stretcher or bench unit. If the ambulance does not have an appropriately sized car seat for the neonate, the parents likely will.

and the mother's emotional state. If the mother is calm, having her hold the newborn may calm the newborn and allow a more accurate examination. When the neonate is quiet, the EMT can do the parts of the examination that require quiet, such as listening to lungs, counting respiratory rate, observing the work of breathing, and noting skin color. These signs can be difficult to assess in the screaming newborn.

Many congenital illnesses are discovered in the first month of life. A congenital illness is a condition with which the child is born. The signs and symptoms of the illness may not have been evident immediately at birth but may begin to show up as the child grows and develops.

Common conditions that may develop during this time in life are jaundice, vomiting, respiratory distress, and fever. Some of these illnesses are discussed later in this unit.

YOUNG INFANT

The young infant, aged 1 to 5 months, is growing rapidly. Babies usually double their birth weight during this period. The visual acuity of young infants is improving, and they begin to follow objects with their eyes. Curiosity and amazement are predominant findings in infants as they observe their environments. Typically, verbalization, such as cooing, begins in this time period.

Common illnesses and injuries seen in this age range, which are discussed more throughout this and the next unit, include sudden infant death syndrome, vomiting, diarrhea, meningitis, child abuse, and accidents. Examination techniques for this age-group are similar to those used with the neonate. These infants are becoming curious and will definitely watch all movement around them intently. Slow movements and gentle handling are the keys to the successful assessment of the young infant.

When examining an infant of any age, the EMT should remember that the child is at increased risk for hypothermia. The EMT should keep the infant covered as much as possible and try to warm her hands and stethoscope prior to coming into contact with the infant. Much of the primary assessment can be done without even touching the infant. Observing the infant's mental status (alertness), airway patency, respiratory rate, and skin color is easily done without actually touching the infant.

OLDER INFANT

The older infant, from 6 to 12 months of age, is becoming more active and is likely to begin standing and walking. This increased mobility will lead to an increased risk for injury during exploration. Infants in this age-group sometimes do not like being around strangers. The stress they feel in this situation is referred to as *stranger anxiety*. The EMT can help to alleviate this anxiety by gaining the parent's confidence first and allowing the infant to remain as close to the parent as possible.

Common presenting problems in this age-group are febrile seizures, vomiting, diarrhea, dehydration, bronchiolitis, motor vehicle collisions, croup, child abuse, poisonous ingestion, and falls.

TODDLER

The 1- to 3-year-old age-group is often called the toddlers. At this age, children are constantly moving around. They often are becoming increasingly independent. The do not like to be touched, and despite their apparent desire for independence, toddlers do not like to be separated from their parent or caregiver. They should be allowed to remain close to a parent or caregiver whenever possible during emergency care.

This increase in mobility and perception of independence can lead to more accidents. The most common emergencies seen in this age-group are motor vehicle accidents, vomiting, diarrhea, febrile seizures, ingestions, falls, child abuse, croup, meningitis, and ingestion of foreign bodies.

When examining the toddler, it is important to remember that the child will need encouragement and reassurance. Toddlers do not like to be undressed; therefore, only undress what is necessary, immediately redressing them after the examination. Enlisting the help of the parent or caregiver can help calm the child and made the examination easier.

The child may believe his illness or injury is a punishment and is often afraid of the possibility of pain. Toddlers do not like needles, and something as simple as a blood pressure cuff on their arm or an oxygen mask over their face can be frightening. Demonstrating the use of equipment by placing it on a parent or another EMT before it is applied to the fearful toddler will go a long way in calming those fears.

The toe-to-head approach for an assessment is useful in this age-group. Involving the child in the examination with constant reassurance is helpful. Making a game out of the exam is often a good way to gain the child's cooperation.

PRESCHOOL

As the child gets older and enters the preschool age (3 to 6 years), motor development continues. These children have concrete thinking skills and interpret everything they hear literally. They also have active imaginations and can tend to dramatize an illness or injury. They are often very attached to parents and personal belongings. A teddy bear will go a long way in gaining the confidence of this child.

It is important to provide simple and honest explanations to the preschool child for every part of any examination. This will help to alleviate some of the fear of the unknown and fear of pain the child may be experiencing. Making the examination a game is also useful in this age-group.

Common presenting problems in the preschool age-group include croup, asthma, ingestions, motor vehicle collisions, burns, child abuse, foreign body ingestions, drownings, epiglottitis, febrile seizures, and meningitis.

SCHOOL-AGE

School-age children (6 to 12 years old) are usually curious, able to rationalize, and more cooperative because they have a fundamental understanding of what an EMT is and what they do. These children are generally very active and go through rapid growth periods. The combination of rapid growth and high levels of activity can result in clumsiness and an increase in injuries. In a child this age, it is important to take the history directly from the child, confirming only important information with an adult. The child will have more confidence and respect for the EMT if it is clear that he is being listened to and taken seriously.

During the assessment, it is often helpful for the EMT to share findings and to provide reassurance. Protection of modesty during an examination is also important at this age. The child should be moved into an environment away from friends so he can feel free to express his feelings and pain without fear of embarrassment. Fear of permanent injury or disfigurement is a very real concern to these children. Common occurrences in this age-group are drowning, motor vehicle collisions, bike accidents, fractures, falls, sports injuries, child abuse, and burns.

ADOLESCENT

From the ages of 12 to 18 years, adolescents are undergoing various degrees of growth and development. They are concrete thinkers and at a point at which abstract thinking skills are being developed. Teenagers also tend to believe nothing bad can happen to them, and they will take risks that can lead to increased possibility of trauma. Most likely because they believe themselves to be invincible, when they are ill or injured, they can have a dramatic reaction. The teenager places a great deal of importance on body image and can be temporarily devastated by what seems to the EMT to be a minor illness or injury.

In the teen years, peers become more important in the child's life, and the child becomes much more independent. Risk-taking behaviors such as drug- and alcohol-related emergencies are increasingly common in the teen years. Despite their apparent lack of concern for injury, adolescents are often afraid of permanent disfigurement once they have sustained an injury. Other common emergencies in this age-group are mononucleosis, asthma, motor vehicle collisions, sports injuries, suicide gestures, sexual abuse, and pregnancy.

ANATOMICAL DIFFERENCES

There are significant anatomic differences between a child and an adult that the EMT must take into consideration during the assessment and management of pediatric illness. Although most medical emergencies are handled the same as for the adult, the EMT will need to make adjustments to the treatments based on these differences in anatomy and physiology of the child.

AIRWAY

Children, especially younger infants, have proportionately larger heads than an adult and are more prone to head trauma. The large occipital (back) of the child's head causes the neck to flex forward when lying supine. This flexion, combined with proportionately large tongue and smaller, less rigid trachea can lead to increased chances of an airway occlusion.

BREATHING

Children naturally breathe faster than adults. The EMT should know the normal pulse, blood pressure, and respiratory ranges for children of each developmental age. The lung tissue is more fragile and the ribs are more pliable than in adults. For these reasons, a healthy child's chest may show minimal movement with respirations, and the abdomen may rise and fall. The chest muscles are also underdeveloped, causing the use of accessory muscles and visible intercostal retractions when breathing becomes difficult.

CIRCULATION

Children's heart rates are naturally rapid at birth, slowing over the course of their development until they reach adolescence, when they fall into the same normal ranges as adults. A child can have a normal heart rate of 110 at the age of 2 that will increase in response to fear, fever, hypoxia, hypovolemia, and activity. The EMT must be familiar with the normal ranges of children's heart rates, based on their age. Bradycardia in children is a late sign in response to hypoxia. Children have a smaller volume of circulating blood, because of their smaller size, and hypotension can be a sudden sign that compensation has failed after 30% of their blood volume has been lost.

METABOLISM

Children have higher metabolic rates than adults; therefore, their cells use oxygen and glucose out of their bloodstream at a faster rate than adults. When a child experiences periods of poor oxygenation due to respiratory distress or even arrest, damage to the central nervous system can quickly occur. Serious injury can affect respiratory function and ultimately result in poor ventilation and oxygenation.

ABDOMEN

The child's abdomen can appear large and round. The muscles of the abdomen are not as well developed as those of an adult, and the internal organs are more vulnerable to damage from blunt force trauma. The liver and spleen especially are more exposed until the child reaches the age of puberty.

SKIN

The child's body surface area is larger and covered by skin that is thinner with less subcutaneous tissue than an adult. The child also has an underdeveloped hypothalamus, which helps to regulate body temperature and can lead to greater incidences of hypothermia.

EXTREMITIES

Children's bones are very flexible, often referred to as "green." When the bones of the extremities are stressed by trauma, they will often fracture due to extreme bending or splintering, called a *greenstick fracture*. Additionally, motor skill development begins at the head and works it way to the toes as children grow. The head is larger, as discussed previously, and is therefore the first thing an infant learns to control. Children have tenuous coordination during this head-to-toe development, leading to an increased frequency of injuries due to falls.

GENERAL CONSIDERATIONS

When caring for infants and children, the EMT must first remember that these patients are not small adults. They are people with many age-specific differences about their bodies and age-related illnesses of which an EMT must be aware.

The EMT may face a significant challenge when called to care for a pediatric patient. The child may not be able to provide an account of the illness or injury as well as an adult. The child also does not have as much experience with illness or injury. In addition, the EMT may not have a lot of experience caring for children.

When treating a pediatric patient, the EMT also has to care for the child's parents. With experience, the EMT will learn that in many situations, the care provided to the parent through careful explanation and compassionate support will be instrumental in successful management of the child's illness. If the EMT can keep the parents calm and gain their confidence, she will be much more successful in obtaining a history and performing a physical examination on the child (Figure 42.1).

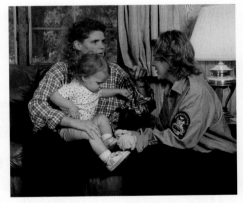

Figure 42.1 Many times when an EMT is called to care for a child, she must also care for the parent by providing reassurance

INITIAL APPROACH

As the EMT initially approaches the pediatric patient, she should immediately place herself at the child's eye level. If the child is seated, the EMT should kneel beside the child, rather than stand and tower over them. This simple act puts the child more at ease and gives the parent the sense that the EMT is comfortable with the situation.

It is helpful for EMTs to introduce themselves to the child as well as to the parent. From this position the EMT establishes a calm presence and begins the process of building trust with the child and parent. The EMT can then conduct the primary assessment quickly and efficiently with the cooperation of both the child and parent.

PEDIATRIC ASSESSMENT TRIANGLE

Many components of patient assessment can be performed by the EMT through observation of the child as the EMT enters the scene. The **Pediatric Assessment Triangle (PAT)** provides a quick 15- to 30-second assessment of the severity of the illness. This assessment tool is used prior to addressing the ABCs and does not require touching the patient. The three components of the PAT—appearance, work of breathing, and circulation to the skin—can be used in forming a general impression of the child.

APPEARANCE

When determining the severity of the illness or injury, management criteria, and response to treatment, the general appearance of the child is one of the most important factors. Adequate ventilation, oxygenation, brain perfusion, central nervous system function, and homeostasis of the body are all reflected in the child's appearance. The mnemonic TICLS defines the most important characteristics of appearance the EMT should assess (Table 42-1).

Abnormal appearance may be indicating inadequate oxygenation, ventilation, and brain perfusion or systemic abnormalities such as poisoning or infection or hypoglycemia. Abnormal appearance is the first component to establishing severity of the illness or injury.

WORK OF BREATHING

The work of breathing for a child, as demonstrated by respiratory rate and breath sounds, is a more accurate measure of oxygenation and ventilation than the standard methods of evaluation in adults. How hard the child is working to breathe is an indicator of the child's attempt to compensate for inefficient oxygenation and ventilation.

The EMT should listen carefully as she enters the room for abnormal sounds, such as crowing or grunting, and look for any signs of increased work to breathe, such as retractions and nasal flaring. Is the child seated in a sniffing position in an attempt to draw more air into his lungs?

Table 42-1 Characteristics of Appearance: TICLS

Characteristic	Features to Assess
Tone	Is the child moving or resisting vigorously? Does the child have good muscle tone, or is he limp, listless, or flaccid?
Interactiveness	How alert is the child? Can the child be distracted or his attention drawn by a person, object, or sound? Does the child reach or grasp and play with a toy or instrument? Is the child uninterested in playing or interacting with the parent or EMT?
Consolability	Can the child be consoled or comforted by the parent or caregiver? Is the child crying or displaying agitation unrelieved by reassurance?
Look/Gaze	Does the child make eye contact, or is there a "nobody's home," glassy-eyed stare?
Speech/cry	Is the child's cry strong and spontaneous, weak, or high-pitched? Is the content of speech age-appropriate, or confused or garbled?

Combine the assessment of appearance and work of breathing to further determine the severity of the child's illness or injury. As an example, if a child's appearance is normal, but the child is seated forward in a tripod position, the child is experiencing respiratory distress. If the child's appearance is abnormal and there is an increased work of breathing, the child may be going into respiratory failure.

CIRCULATION TO SKIN

Adequacy of the child's cardiac output and perfusion to the vital organs is the purpose of this rapid circulatory assessment. From across the room, look for pallor, mottling, or cyanosis, all indicators of reduced circulation. Pallor may indicate the child is in compensated shock, but may also be a sign of hypoxia or anemia. Mottling is a sign of poor skin perfusion indicating abnormal blood vessel tone in the capillary beds. It is important for the EMT to remember that mottling may also be present in a child exposed to cold environments.

Cyanosis is an extreme indicator of poor perfusion or poor oxygenation and is a late sign usually seen when the child is in respiratory failure. Acrocyanosis, or blue hands and feet, is a normal finding in a newborn less than 2 months of age who has been exposed to cold (see Unit 41).

The three components of the PAT work together in determining the severity of the child's illness, with abnormalities of all three components indicating a critically ill child.

PRIMARY ASSESSMENT

The PAT can be conducted as the EMT enters the scene and observes the child from across the room. The PAT should take no more than 15 to 30 seconds of observation, to be immediately followed by the primary assessment and management of the child's airway, breathing, and circulation. A child who has an abnormal finding of any of the components of the PAT should be placed on high-flow oxygen, with transport priority determined immediately following the PAT and primary assessment. The child with abnormal PAT findings should have all further assessment and management conducted en route to the appropriate facility.

GATHERING A HISTORY

When gathering a history regarding a child's illness, the EMT may need to alter the technique used based on the child's age. If the child is old enough to respond to any sort of question, the EMT should question the child in a friendly manner. If the child is too young or too ill to speak, the parent is the primary source of information. If the original questions are asked of the child, the parent should be asked for confirmation. Often the parent will add useful details. However, the EMT must remember to ask the child the questions first.

SECONDARY ASSESSMENT

When performing the secondary assessment on an infant or child, the most important part of the examination is sometimes gained by careful observation. Observing children's interaction with the environment, the comfort with which they speak and breathe, and the way they hold and move their body will tell the EMT how sick the child may be. The child who is talking a mile a minute and running back and forth in a room is not likely to be in danger of losing his airway or requiring ventilatory support.

Simple observation can tell the EMT a lot about the patient, and because it involves no touching or hurting, the child will not mind that it is being done. After allowing the child to become accustomed to her presence, the EMT should initiate the necessary physical examination. Different examination techniques can be used for each age-group, based on the child's expected response or level of interaction. However, some general points about the examination of the infant or child will be helpful to the EMT.

The EMT should always try to gain the child's confidence before attempting to physically touch the child. The EMT should be honest about examination requirements and should move slowly and gently. If it is possible, allowing the child some control during the examination may help the child to feel more in control of the entire situation and, for that reason, less afraid. For example, asking the child which body part should be examined next or what he thinks will be found there can give the child a sense of control and lessen any fear he may have.

The EMT who is trying to gain the child's acceptance so that physical examination may be performed should consider placing simple assessment tools, like a stethoscope, within reach of the child so that the child is not afraid of the equipment. Similarly, using the equipment on mom or dad before using it to assess the child may help lessen the child's anxiety (e.g., listening to dad's lungs first).

Any part of the examination that is expected to cause pain should be done last. If a painful, swollen, deformed extremity is manipulated before any other examination is done, the child will not be likely to allow the EMT to perform any further examination without a fight.

It is helpful for the EMT to remember the normal physical findings for each age-group. Infants and children have ranges for normal vital signs that differ from those of the normal adult. Table 42-2 lists the normal pediatric vital signs by age. The EMT should be familiar with these ranges and may want to carry a card or other reference that lists these important numbers.

COMMON PEDIATRIC ILLNESSES

Although children can suffer from illnesses that are common to adults, there are some unique differences about how a child presents with the same illness. There are also some illnesses typically found only in children. It is useful for the EMT to be familiar with the clinical presentation of illnesses in children.

Table 42-2 Normal Pediatric Vital Signs by Age

Age	Respiratory Rate	Heart Rate	Systolic BP
Newborn	30–60	100–160	50–70
1–6 weeks	30–60	100–160	70–95
6 months	25–40	90–120	80–100
1 year	20–30	90–120	80–100
3 years	20–30	80–120	80–110
6 years	18–25	70–110	80–100
10 years	15–20	60–90	90–120

AIRWAY PROBLEMS

Children have relatively small airways when compared to those of an adult. The child's smaller upper airway can become more easily blocked by secretions or foreign bodies. For this reason, airway problems are more common in children than in adults.

FOREIGN BODY OBSTRUCTION

The curious nature of children often results in them getting into places that a parent may have never imagined. Younger children, especially, tend to put every new object in their mouth for a taste test. This investigative nature can and does often lead to airway obstructions by foreign bodies.

A typical story would be of a child playing with some small object. The child suddenly becomes quiet, with or without associated coughing. A parent who discovers the child immediately may realize what has happened. If the parent does not find the child until after the airway has been occluded for a few minutes, the parent will likely find the child unconscious.

The progression of events in an airway obstruction in a child is for the object to be inhaled into the airway. When the inhaled object reaches an airway that is too small to get through, it becomes lodged and blocks any further airflow in or out. If this airway is a proximal airway, such as the trachea, the child will not be able to breathe in or out at all. After a short period of time without oxygen, the blood will become low in oxygen, causing the brain to malfunction, and the child becomes unconscious. If the condition is not remedied quickly, the heart will begin to slow as a result of the low oxygen levels and will eventually stop. This progression of events from airway obstruction to cardiac arrest can happen in as little as a couple of minutes.

INCOMPLETE OBSTRUCTION

If an airway obstruction is not complete, evidenced by the ability of the child to cry, speak, or cough, the EMT should encourage the child to cough. Oxygen should be applied, and the EMT should calmly but quickly initiate transport. As long as the child can still verbalize and move enough air to keep his chest rising and skin a well-oxygenated pink color, the EMT should take no action other than to initiate transport. If at any point the obstruction becomes complete, it should be managed as described in this unit.

ASSESSMENT

The primary assessment of the child with a foreign body in the airway often reveals the source of the problem. If the object has completely occluded the airway, the child will likely be unconscious by the time EMS arrives. The initial management involves opening the airway and checking for breathing. When no breathing is noted, two breaths are given. In the case of a complete airway obstruction, the EMT will be unable to get a breath into the child. Just as the child was unable to breathe spontaneously because of the obstruction, air cannot be forced through by the EMT.

The next step is to reposition the child's airway. The pediatric patient has a relatively large tongue that can create an airway obstruction. With a slightly different airway position, the rescue breath may be effective. If still no effective ventilations are provided, the EMT should assume a complete airway obstruction and proceed with foreign body airway obstruction procedures.

MANAGEMENT

The appropriate management of a complete airway obstruction depends on the child's age. The following section is an overview of the procedures for

Street Smart

Remember that the infant's airway is narrow and flexible. The proper position for opening the airway is neutral. If the head is hyperextended, the airway can be kinked like a straw and occluded. Careful attention should be paid to the position of an infant's airway. The child's head should be placed in the neutral-plus position.

Neck flexion may be avoided by placing a small towel or other material for padding under the child's shoulders, lifting the body even with the relatively larger head.

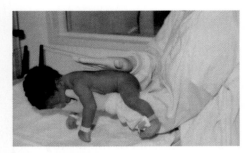

Figure 42.2 Back slaps alternating with chest thrusts are the appropriate treatment for a foreign body airway obstruction in an infant

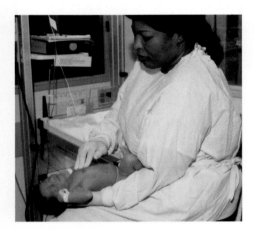

Figure 42.3 The positioning for chest thrusts on an infant is one finger width below the nipple line

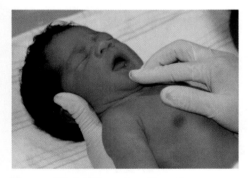

Figure 42.4 When treating the infant with a foreign body airway obstruction, the EMT should never reach into the airway with his fingers unless the object is actually seen

relieving an obstructed airway. The EMT should refer to manuals on emergency pediatric care by the American Red Cross or the American Heart Association for further details (see "Further Reading" at the end of this unit).

INFANT

The infant under 1 year of age can be lifted into the EMT's arms, turned face downward, with the head lower than the chest. In this position, the EMT delivers five **back slaps** between the infant's shoulder blades. Figure 42.2 demonstrates this technique.

These five back slaps are then followed by turning the child over to a faceup position, in which **chest thrusts** can be performed. These chest thrusts involve placing two fingers one finger width below the nipple line and thrusting inward one-third the depth of the chest as shown in Figure 42.3. The combination of these two maneuvers will hopefully generate enough intrathoracic pressure to result in the foreign body being expelled.

If the infant remains conscious, the cycle should continue with back slaps being followed by chest thrusts until the object is expelled or the infant becomes unconscious.

If the infant becomes unconscious, the EMT should open the infant's airway using the head-tilt, chin-lift and look into the infant's mouth to see whether the foreign body is visible when opening the airway, as illustrated in Figure 42.4. If it is, it should be removed with the EMT's little finger. The EMT should never perform a blind finger sweep, because this may push an unseen object farther into the infant's throat.

Provide two breaths over a 1-second period. If there is no chest rise with ventilation attempts, begin chest compressions, by placing two fingers just below the nipple line and compressing approximately one-third to one-half the depth of the chest. Provide chest compressions at a rate of 30:2, looking in the mouth for the obstruction after each set of chest compressions, prior to ventilations, until the foreign body is removed. Transport the patient immediately and call for an ALS intercept en route.

CHILD

In a child aged older than 1 year, an airway obstruction is managed in much the same way it is in the adult patient, with a few important differences.

Once the complete obstruction has been recognized in the conscious child, the EMT should initiate abdominal thrusts until the object is expelled or the child becomes unconscious (Figure 42.5).

In the unconscious child, the EMT should open the airway using the head-tilt, chin-lift and look into the mouth to see if the object can be visualized. If the object is visible, use a finger sweep to remove it. Do not use a blind finger sweep as it may push the object further into the airway. Give two breaths over a 1-second period looking for chest rise. Using one or two hands placed on the lower half of the sternum, compress approximately one-third to one-half the depth of the chest at a rate of 30 compressions to 2 ventilations, checking for the obstruction after each set of 30 compressions before breaths. Only if the object is visible in the pharynx should the EMT attempt to remove the object. Continue this cycle of CPR, checking for the object before breaths until the foreign object is removed. Once the object is removed, attempt ventilations and reassess the need for continued CPR.

TRANSPORTATION

If the ventilation is unsuccessful, the EMT should immediately prepare for transport. ALS personnel should be requested. ALS personnel have advanced airway skills and equipment and may be able to use this equipment, such as a laryngoscope and Magill forceps, to remove the foreign body.

If the ventilation is successful and the apparent source of the obstruction recovered, the child should still be transported to the emergency department for evaluation. Trauma to the soft tissues of the throat can lead to swelling and more airway difficulty.

TROUBLE BREATHING

The single most common medical emergency for a child is trouble breathing. Small airways can become narrowed and occluded for a number of reasons. Regardless of the cause, the result is the same—breathing difficulties. Common childhood illnesses that can lead to breathing difficulties include croup, bacterial tracheitis, epiglottitis, pediatric asthma, and respiratory infections.

CROUP

One illness that can result in airway narrowing and trouble breathing in a child is croup. Croup is a viral illness that causes swelling of the upper airways, specifically the larynx, the trachea, and the bronchi. This infection is most commonly seen in the fall and winter. It often begins with usual upper respiratory infection symptoms such as cough, runny nose, and sore throat, and then progresses to troubled breathing. Croup commonly lasts several days and is not usually associated with a very high fever, although a low-grade fever is possible. Children ages 6 months to 4 years are typically affected by this illness.

BACTERIAL TRACHEITIS

Bacterial tracheitis is a bacterial infection that often follows a viral upper respiratory infection. It appears to affect mostly small children, whose small trachea can easily become blocked by swelling. Signs and symptoms include a high fever; deep cough, similar to the "seal bark" croup cough; and increasing respiratory difficulty. The child will look very ill, with intercostal retractions and stridor on inhalation.

Management is high-flow oxygen and support of ventilations with immediate transport to an appropriate facility, such as a pediatric hospital. ALS intercept should be requested and met en route because the child with bacterial tracheitis often needs to have an advanced airway, such as an endotracheal tube, inserted to maintain a patent airway and assist breathing. The child will require hospitalization for oxygen and antibiotic therapy and monitoring for airway obstruction.

EPIGLOTTITIS

Another condition that affects a child's airway is a bacterial infection of the epiglottis, called *epiglottitis*. Epiglottitis is far less common than croup, but it is more likely to cause life-threatening airway obstruction. Because this condition is most commonly caused by bacteria, children are routinely vaccinated against the bacterium that causes it. Children who have not been vaccinated are at increased risk of epiglottitis.

Epiglottitis involves an inflammation of the epiglottis, the floppy piece of tissue that covers the tracheal opening during swallowing. The normal epiglottis serves a protective purpose by covering the tracheal opening into the lungs and preventing aspiration when swallowing occurs; but when the epiglottis becomes swollen and inflamed, it can cover the tracheal opening, block the airway, and create an airway obstruction.

ASSESSMENT

Croup is characterized by a harsh-sounding cough that has been likened to a seal bark. This harsh sound is created by a forceful expelling of air through a swollen

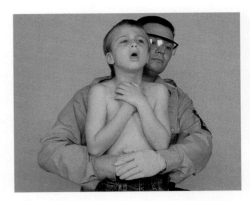

Figure 42.5 A child who is choking but conscious should have the abdominal thrust maneuver performed on him to relieve the upper airway obstruction

Street Smart

If humidification of oxygen is not possible, the EMT can take the child suffering from croup outside into the cooler night air; this often decreases the symptoms. Another helpful technique is to turn on the shower in the bathroom, close the door, and have the parent sit in the bathroom with the child. The mist from the shower also helps to relieve the symptoms. If these techniques do not help, the child should be transported rapidly to the hospital.

and irritated airway. If the swelling is severe, the child can develop inspiratory stridor. Symptoms of croup usually are worse at night than during the day.

The child with epiglottitis will present with the sudden onset of a high fever and brassy cough. A sore throat is a common concern, and the child often breathes shallowly with obvious dyspnea, stridor, and an inability to handle secretions, visibly drooling in some cases.

MANAGEMENT

The most severe cases of epiglottitis can result in a complete airway obstruction. In this case, the foreign body removal techniques will not be effective. The EMT has to do her best to ventilate the child with a bag-valve-mask and quickly transport the child to the closest appropriate hospital.

Complete airway obstruction happens rarely with croup. Management of the patient with croup involves calm transport to the hospital with delivery of humidified oxygen. Humidification of the inspired air often helps air to pass more easily through the child's narrowed airway.

TRANSPORTATION

During transport, the child with respiratory distress should be allowed to sit in whatever position is most comfortable for the child. The parent should be allowed to sit close to the child to help calm the child. Blow-by oxygen may be helpful, as long as it does not agitate the child. When agitated, the child with croup often experiences an increase in symptoms, and a child with epiglottitis can develop a complete airway obstruction.

Some EMTs are taught to use a nebulizer system for administration of certain inhaled medications. Several milliliters of sterile saline may be placed in a nebulizer and with oxygen applied, held near the child's mouth and nose. If the child tolerates this technique, the mist of the saline and oxygen create the necessary humidification needed to ease the child's work of breathing somewhat.

The EMT should never attempt to visualize the oropharynx of any child who has symptoms that sound even remotely like epiglottitis. Any pharyngeal manipulation can result in a complete airway obstruction. If a complete airway obstruction does occur, despite the EMT's careful avoidance of the airway, the EMT should ventilate the child with a bag-valve-mask and transport the child quickly to the closest hospital. Advanced life support may be helpful but should be intercepted while en route to the hospital.

PEDIATRIC ASTHMA

Asthma is a common disease state that involves reversible spasm of the smaller airways in the chest. In addition, there is a component of inflammation that serves to further narrow the airways. Asthma is a very common disease in children. Some children actually outgrow the disease as they grow older. Asthma is also commonly seen in adults and is addressed in Unit 26. Asthma can be caused by many factors as outlined in Table 42-3.

RESPIRATORY INFECTIONS

Although asthma is certainly a common disease in children, it does not account for all episodes of respiratory distress in children. Probably one of the most common causes of respiratory difficulty in children is an upper respiratory infection. Infections of the upper respiratory tract, such as a simple cold, can cause enough inflammation and secretions in the child's airway to cause difficulty breathing. Clearing of the secretions often helps to ease the child's breathing.

BRONCHIOLITIS

Bronchiolitis is a viral respiratory infection caused when the mucosal layer of the bronchioles in the lungs become inflamed. The infectious form of

Table 42-3 Common Triggers of Asthma

Cold

Exercise

Animal dander

Dust

Smoke and other airborne irritants

Respiratory infections

bronchiolitis prehospital providers are more familiar with is **respiratory syncytial virus (RSV).**

Bronchiolitis is sometimes confused with asthma because wheezing during exhalation is present. Additional symptoms include fever, tachycardia, and tachypnea, shortness of breath, chest tightness, and cough. Assessment for bronchiolitis is performed in the same way as for asthma, and management is the same as for other respiratory infections, as discussed in the following sections.

PNEUMONIA

Pneumonia is an infection of the lungs that may be seen in patients of any age. The elderly and children tend to be more susceptible to the pathogens that cause pneumonia, whether viral or bacteria, with viral pneumonia being the most common in children. The elderly are more susceptible to a specific type of pneumonia called *aspiration pneumonia,* discussed in the next chapter.

The symptoms of pneumonia in children include high fever or a history of fever at some point in the illness, chills, tachypnea, lethargy or irritability, poor appetite, and occasionally chest pain. Bacterial pneumonia in children can cause a fluid buildup in the lungs or pleural space that produces rales or decreased breath sound, increased work of breathing.

Management for pneumonia will focus on supporting oxygenation and ventilation as needed and the same management criteria as for other respiratory infections.

PERTUSSIS

Pertussis the highly contagious infectious disease caused by a bacteria, more widely known as "whooping cough" as it is characterized by a severe, hacking cough followed by an intake of breath that makes the sound "whoop." In infected babies and small children, the sound is described as a high-pitched whoop.

Pertussis is a preventable disease affecting both adults and children who have not been immunized against it. It is one of the leading causes of vaccine-preventable deaths worldwide with most deaths occurring in young infants who have not been vaccinated or have not finished the three doses of vaccine necessary for complete protection against pertussis.

The history of illness is an important factor when determining the possibility of pertussis infection. Pertussis in infants and children is characterized by common symptoms seen in other mild respiratory infections such as coughing, sneezing, and runny nose. One to two weeks later the cough changes, increasing in occurrence with a "barking" sound followed by the "whoop" with inhalation. The coughing can become violent and induce vomiting, which can become significant and cause dehydration.

Management for pertussis begins with the EMT taking full infectious disease precautions if responding to a residence where pertussis may be suspected. High-flow oxygen should be administered and transport immediately initiated to the appropriate facility. The EMT should be alert and prepared for vomiting if the child has a coughing fit en route. ALS intercept should be considered and met in route. Children suffering from pertussis will require antibiotic and intravenous (IV) fluid therapy in the hospital. The management for EMS will be primarily supportive during transport.

ASSESSMENT

Asthma is characterized by periods in which the child is well and periods in which the child is in bronchospasm. The bronchospasm is often brought on by a recognized trigger, such as those listed in Table 42-3. This bronchospasm causes the child to feel short of breath. Severe bronchospasm can sometimes generate a

Table 42-4 Signs of Respiratory Difficulty in a Child

Increased respiratory rate
Shallow respirations
Intercostal retractions
Accessory muscle use
Nasal flaring
Sternal retractions
Noisy respirations

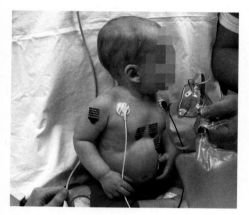

Figure 42.6 The child in respiratory distress often has intercostal retractions that are visible to the EMT if he looks for them

Table 42-5 Signs of Respiratory Failure in a Child

Cyanosis
Altered mental status
Abdominal breathing
Decreasing respiratory rate
Bradycardia

cough as well. Listening through the stethoscope on the patient's chest, under the clavicles, the EMT will hear the characteristic wheezing sound of asthma.

The child suffering from an asthma flare-up, or exacerbation, often describes his chest as feeling "tight." This is because the airways are in spasm and it is difficult to breathe air in and out through such narrowed passages. A cough is sometimes a predominant feature of this condition. Signs of respiratory difficulty in a child are listed in Table 42-4.

These signs of increased respiratory difficulty are evidence of the increased work the child is putting into getting air into and out of the chest. Increasing the rate of breathing brings in more air, and usually the volume of each breath is less than the volume of a normal breath.

The use of thoracic muscles to help the diaphragm in creating an effective breath is evidenced by visualization of the outline of each rib with each breath. This obvious retraction of the skin between each rib is called **intercostal retraction** and is a fairly reliable sign of respiratory distress in a child (Figure 42.6). In more severe cases, the sternum is actually pulled inward with all of the effort to breathe. This **sternal retraction** is a sign of severe respiratory distress in a child.

When a child is trying to increase the amount of air he pulls into his lungs, often the mouth is open and the nares flare widely to allow for more air entry. It takes a lot of energy to breathe when all of the airways are narrowed to near-collapse.

The child who is in respiratory distress for a protracted period of time may become physically exhausted. When the child is no longer able to maintain the extra work of breathing, he will experience a respiratory failure. Signs of respiratory failure are listed in Table 42-5.

MANAGEMENT

The signs of respiratory failure, listed in Table 42-5, may indicate that the child is in need of immediate ventilatory support. The EMT must recognize these signs and provide such support or the child will progress to cardiac arrest. Methods for ventilation are described in Unit 10.

The child suffering from asthma often has bronchodilating medication prescribed by his physician. The EMT can assist a child with the metered dose inhaler just as she assists the adult patient with an inhaler. Unit 13 describes the use of the metered dose inhaler. (Figure 42.7) The EMT should refer to local protocols before assisting a child with a metered dose inhaler.

Very small children who cannot cooperate with the administration of a metered dose inhaler can be given the same medication via a special apparatus called a nebulizer (Figure 42.8). Parents are often prescribed a small air compressor that blows air into a small medication-filled chamber.

Street Smart

Some pediatric bag-valve-mask devices come with an additional valve called a *pop-off valve,* which are designed to release pressure when the lungs become full. Sometimes these valves prematurely release because of back-pressure from a collapsed airway or a kinked trachea. For this reason, the EMT should disable the pop-off valve and pay close attention to airway position as well as lung inflation to ensure that the child is receiving adequate ventilatory volumes.

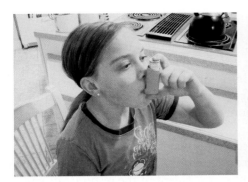

Figure 42.7 Pediatric metered dose inhaler (Photo Courtesy of Larry Torrey, Portland, ME)

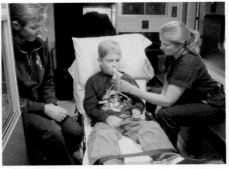

Figure 42.8 Children may require the use of a special apparatus called a nebulizer (Photo Courtesy of MEDCU & Larry Torrey, Portland, ME)

This creates an aerosol that may then be inhaled by the small child. Figures 42.9 A-D illustrates the use of such a device. The EMT should follow local protocols regarding medication administration.

HYPOPERFUSION

There are several causes of hypoperfusion in the pediatric patient. One of the most common causes of hypoperfusion is a large fluid loss resulting in hypovolemia. The blood volume of a child is much smaller than that of an adult; therefore, a child cannot afford to lose much fluid before experiencing hypovolemia and hypoperfusion. Common causes of pediatric fluid loss include dehydration and blood loss from trauma.

Vomiting and diarrhea from common viral illnesses can cause massive fluid losses in a child. If a child is not given enough to drink to replenish the fluid lost, the child will become dehydrated. Dehydration from nausea and vomiting can quickly lead to hypoperfusion and hypovolemia in small children.

ASSESSMENT

It is important that the EMT recognize signs of hypoperfusion in the pediatric patient. A child generally can compensate for volume loss fairly well by increasing the heart rate and shunting blood away from the skin and abdominal organs. These compensatory mechanisms lead to tachycardia, pale skin, delayed capillary refill, and nausea. Decreased urine output from poor kidney perfusion is evidenced by a decrease in the number of wet diapers.

If the volume loss continues or the child is not treated, compensation will fail and the heart will no longer be able to adequately perfuse the brain, resulting in an altered mental status. The child who does not recognize her parents or who does not act appropriately should be considered to be extremely sick.

A final sign of decompensation in the pediatric shock patient is a fall in blood pressure. When the heart is no longer able to generate enough forward pressure to allow a normal blood pressure, the blood pressure falls. A falling blood pressure in a child is a bad sign. The heart then begins to fail, resulting in a slower heart rate. Unless treated quickly, the child will die.

MANAGEMENT

The EMT must recognize the early signs of hypoperfusion to initiate proper treatment and begin transport of the child to the most appropriate facility. Waiting for a falling blood pressure and hypotension before diagnosing hypoperfusion is a mistake.

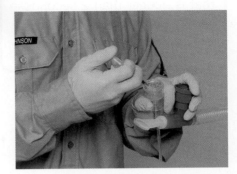

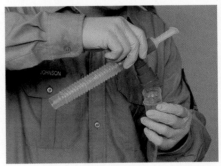

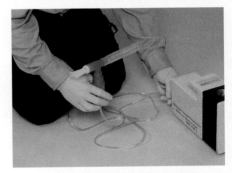

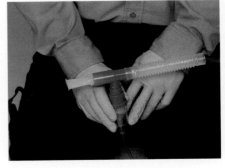

Figure 42.9 The prescribed liquid medication is placed into the nebulizer, and either the compressed air or oxygen is turned on to 8 lpm

CARDIAC ARREST

The most common cause of cardiac arrest in children is respiratory arrest. Children do not often have a cardiac event that leads to cardiac arrest. More often what happens is the child goes into respiratory failure that leads to profound hypoxia. In turn, profound hypoxia leads to cardiac failure and then cardiac arrest. The next most common cause of cardiac arrest in children is hypoperfusion.

The EMT's priority in pediatric cardiac arrest is to provide good ventilation with 100% oxygen, along with cardiac compressions. Good ventilation in the pediatric patient is essential. Often, treatment of the respiratory arrest will lead to a reversal of the cardiac arrest.

Signs of cardiac arrest in children are the same as found in adults. Positive pressure ventilations should be started if breathing is inadequate or absent, and chest compressions should be started if the heart rate drops below 60 with signs of poor perfusion or is absent. Transport rapidly to the appropriate facility and request ALS intercept to be met en route. Review Unit 24 for the steps of infant and pediatric cardiopulmonary resuscitation.

SIDS

The sudden, unexplained death of an infant in the first year of life is known as *sudden infant death syndrome (SIDS)*. This somewhat mysterious syndrome occurs at a rate of 2 in 1,000 live births and is the leading cause of death in children 1 week to 1 year of age. The peak incidence is from 2 to 4 months of age and usually occurs during the infant's sleep. Males are more commonly affected than females. The winter months also seem to account for more cases of SIDS than other times of the year.

Although it is not known exactly what the cause of death is in these otherwise healthy infants, several risk factors have been associated with its occurrence. Infants of mothers of low socioeconomic groups are at increased risk as well as infants of low birth weight.

An EMT may be called to the scene of a family who is unable to wake an infant from a nap. If the child is found to be in cardiac arrest, the EMT should initiate resuscitative efforts and transport the infant to the closest appropriate hospital if the infant is not showing signs of being deceased for an extended period. Emotional support must be provided to the parents as well. The EMT must avoid making any comments that might suggest blame to the parents. The cause of death in SIDS is unknown, but parents often blame themselves.

During the resuscitation, it is probably helpful for the EMT to explain to the parents each intervention. Explaining that the infant is not breathing, that the heart is not beating, and that those things are being supported during transport will inform the parents about what is being done for their child. If the resuscitation is not successful, the parents will have seen firsthand the work that went into trying to save their infant.

Because the death of an infant is such a difficult situation to deal with, both for the parents and for the providers, an extra provider may need to be present to help support the parents while the primary EMT cares for the infant.

ALTERED MENTAL STATUS

There are several causes of an altered mental status in a child. The EMT must first focus on the child's ABCs. If the EMT finds that all of these are normal, he must investigate other possible causes. This section discusses the most common causes of an altered mental status in the pediatric patient.

SEIZURES

Many children suffer a seizure at some time in their childhood. Probably the most common type of seizure seen in children is called a **febrile seizure.** This type of seizure is caused by a rapid increase in body temperature. Usually associated with some type of infection, this fever causes the brain, in effect, to short-circuit, resulting in a seizure.

A febrile seizure usually does not last more than a few minutes, although rarely it can last longer. The child has a brief period of lethargy and confusion followed by a return to a more normal mental state, just as is seen after a nonfebrile seizure.

A child who has had a febrile seizure is at higher risk for having future such events whenever the child experiences a rapid onset of fever, but the child is not at increased risk for chronic seizures like epilepsy.

When the EMT is called to treat a child who has had a seizure, if the child feels hot to touch, the EMT should perform the usual primary assessment and manage the airway and breathing as appropriate. Usually manual repositioning of the airway and some simple suctioning solve any airway issues after a seizure. The application of 100% oxygen by mask is usually appropriate.

The history of an infection or fever is usually obtained. The child should be undressed from any bulky clothing, and moistened washcloths or towels should be wiped over the child's body to moisten the child's skin. A fan should then be applied to the child so that evaporation may allow a decrease in body temperature.

DIABETES

Diabetes is a condition of altered glucose utilization that can affect children as well as adults. Unit 27 discusses this condition in more detail. The EMT should realize that the child who has a history of diabetes and who has an altered mental status may be suffering from low blood sugar, or hypoglycemia.

If the child is able to maintain his own airway and swallow on command, the EMT may give the child some sugar by mouth. If the child is unconscious or cannot effectively handle airway secretions, nothing should be placed in the mouth, and transport should be initiated immediately. An ALS intercept should be requested.

BEHAVIORAL

Although not very common, children can suffer from behavioral disorders that result in abnormal behavior. If there is a known history of such a disorder, the EMT should consider it. In the absence of a history of a similar reaction because of a behavioral disorder, the EMT should assume that any abnormal behavior is the result of a medical illness and should treat the child as a medical emergency.

POISONING

Because of their inquisitive nature, children are at high risk for being poisoned. Children who can get into household cleaners, cosmetic products, and medications may become poisoned. The first indication of such a poisoning may be an altered mental status. Earlier signs of poisoning may include the presence of a spilled bottle of some chemical or medication, smells on the child's breath, discoloration of the mouth or lips, and vomitus with pill fragments or a chemical smell.

Street Smart

While application of cold cloths might seem wise when dealing with a febrile child, the cold cloths can actually induce shivering. Shivering actually generates body heat and can raise, instead of lower, the body temperature. Gentle cooling with moist, tepid hand towels will help to reduce the fever without inducing shivering. Often all that is needed is disrobing the child and letting the heat dissipate naturally.

If a poisoning is suspected, the EMT should maintain the child's airway and breathing and then follow local protocol. Some regions advocate calling a Poison Control Center, whereas others require the EMT to contact local medical control first. Regardless of protocol, the child who is poisoned is in need of rapid transport to an appropriate hospital.

It may be useful to the hospital staff if the EMT brings any potential containers so that the poison may be more rapidly identified and appropriate treatment started.

INFECTIONS

Because children play in close contact with many other children, they are susceptible to contracting many infectious diseases that are spread by casual contact. Some common infectious diseases spread from child to child include colds, the flu, gastroenteritis (stomach bug), strep throat, mononucleosis (a viral infection), and chickenpox.

Many of the illnesses spread among children are not life threatening. Meningitis, on the other hand, is an infectious disease that can be caused by a virus or bacteria and is transmitted by coughing and sneezing. It is an infection of the lining surrounding the brain and spinal cord, and it can be very serious, especially when it is caused by particular types of bacteria. A child with meningitis may have a fever, headache, stiff neck, rash, and altered mental status. A child with meningitis may have a seizure. A child with these symptoms should be considered to have a potentially serious illness and should be transported to the hospital immediately.

The EMT who recognizes the signs of any infection in a child should wear a mask. Whether the illness is a minor cold or potentially deadly meningitis, EMTs should protect themselves from contracting any airborne disease while caring for the patient (Figure 42.10). Often a mask can be used with children as an object for fun and attention as well.

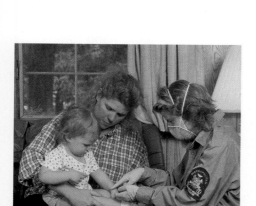

Figure 42.10 It is a good policy for the EMT to isolate herself from any potentially infectious respiratory secretions

ASSESSMENT

The focus of assessment for any child with an altered mental status remains on the ABCs. Treating a child's troubled breathing, for example, improves the child's mental status.

Every child is different. If the EMT is unsure about whether the child's mental status is normal, he should ask the parent or caregiver. The parent will be able to ascertain whether the child has returned to baseline.

MANAGEMENT

A number of minor treatments can be offered by the EMT in the instances described earlier. The most common treatment, however, is simply caring support of the child and family and transportation to the hospital.

STRESS IN CARING FOR CHILDREN

The EMT should recognize that caring for sick and injured children can be quite stressful, not only for the EMT, but for the child, the parents, and other health care providers as well.

CHILD

An ill or injured child is often forced to endure examination by a complete stranger who is sometimes dressed in a scary uniform. This may happen without the benefit of having a parent nearby. The illness itself is frightening to the child, and the fact that a stranger is doing strange things to him is even scarier.

The EMT should realize the potential for such fear and do everything in her power to reduce the child's anxiety. Knowing the normal stages of development and the needs of a child of a particular age-group can be helpful. Probably the best way the EMT can put a child at ease is by being honest and calm and by enlisting the aid of the parent or caregiver to keep the child calm.

EMTs should never lie to a child if they expect that child to trust them. If a procedure will hurt, the EMT should tell the child that it will hurt and also how long it will hurt and what will happen when it is over.

FAMILY

The family of a sick child is under a great deal of stress. The EMT must not only care for the sick child but must make time to care for the anxious parents as well. Keeping the parents informed and allowing them to participate when that is appropriate will help to reassure them. If the parents are calm, the chances of keeping the child calm are increased.

Occasionally, a parent will be unable to be calm and quiet. If attempts to put the parent at ease are unsuccessful, the best plan of action is to separate the child from the parent. A parent who is hysterical only worsens the child's anxiety. The EMT might have better luck with the child alone in this case. If a parent is separated from the child, a separate provider should be assigned to the parent and should continue trying to calm and support the parent.

PROVIDER

Perhaps because EMTs do not care for children often, caring for a sick child is nearly always stressful for the EMT. It is important to realize in advance that feelings of fear and anxiety when faced with an ill child are normal. These feelings must be put aside at the time of the incident so that appropriate care may be given.

Later, after the call, EMTs should take a moment to allow their feelings to surface. Talking about the situation with coworkers is often helpful. This type of informal debriefing after a stressful call is necessary to prevent a buildup of such feelings of stress and anxiety.

CONCLUSION

Caring for an ill child is often an anxiety-producing event for the EMT. Knowledge of normal child development and the common illnesses affecting the pediatric population can help the EMT to feel more at ease with the situation.

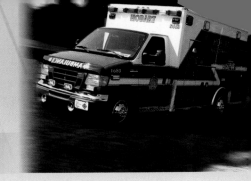

CASE STUDY Continued

As Gordy listens to Mackenzie's mother, he determines through the use of the Pediatric Assessment Triangle that the child is seriously ill. Mackenzie's appearance is lethargic, and she does not make eye contact with anyone in the room. Her work of breathing is see-saw breathing with intercostal retractions present. Her skin is flushed and hot to touch.

As Gordy removes the numerous blankets and clothing from Mackenzie, he gathers a history from her mother. Mackenzie had been experiencing a runny nose and cough and began running a temperature earlier today. She was drinking normally; however, she had not eaten much today and had vomited a couple of times from coughing. Mackenzie's mother states she was getting ready to take her to the hospital for the sudden fever when she started having convulsions.

Kerry places high-flow oxygen on Mackenzie through a pediatric non-rebreather mask as the EMTs place her on the cot. Gordy continues to bathe her with a washcloth dipped in tepid water. Mackenzie starts to cry weakly as they begin transport to the hospital, with an ALS intercept requested to meet them en route, in case of a recurrent seizure.

Mackenzie's skin temperature is cooler, and she becomes interactive with Gordy, grabbing the stethoscope as he listens for abnormal lung sounds, finding diminished lung sounds with some wheezing present.

Baseline vital signs are obtained: blood pressure of 90/58, respirations 36, heart rate 126, pulse oximeter reading 95% with oxygen. Gordy conducts a thorough secondary assessment with injuries noted.

Gordy provides a complete report to the ALS crew they meet en route, turning patient care over to the paramedic, who administers an albuterol treatment for her breathing and started an IV on the way to the hospital.

Key Concepts Revisited

- Developmental considerations for children are differentiated by placing them into age-groups:
    - Newborn 0 to 1month
    - Young infant 1 to 5 months
    - Older infant 6 to 12 months
    - Toddler 1 to 3 years
    - Preschool 3 to 6 years
    - School age 6 to 12 years
    - Adolescent 12 to 18 years
- The EMT must understand age-specific developmental differences in children.
    - Large head
        - Smaller airways
    - Breathing
        - Rapid rate, undeveloped chest muscles
    - Circulation
        - Rapid rate, lower circulating blood volume
    - Metabolism
        - Greater use of oxygen and glucose
    - Skin
        - Larger surface area, greater chance of hypothermia
    - Extremities
        - Pliant bones, greenstick fractures
- The Pediatric Assessment Triangle (PAT) provides a quick 15- to 30-second assessment of the severity of the illness:
    - Appearance
    - Work of breathing
    - Circulation to skin

- Pediatric airway emergencies range from foreign body obstruction to obstructive diseases:
  - Foreign body airway obstruction
  - Croup
  - Bacterial tracheitis
  - Epiglottitis
  - Asthma
  - Respiratory infections
    - Pneumonia
    - Pertussis
- Increased work of breathing is evidenced by physical signs and is an indicator of illness severity.
  - Nasal flaring
  - Intercostal retractions
  - Sternal retractions
  - Increased respiratory rate
  - Shallow breathing
  - Accessory muscle use
  - Noisy respiration

- Abnormal skin signs and capillary refill are two reliable indicators of hypoperfusion in the infant and child.
  - Dehydration
- The most common causes of cardiac arrest in infants and children is respiratory arrest.
- Altered mental status in children can be verified through history taking to determine their normal mental status.
  - Seizures
  - Diabetes
  - Behavioral
  - Poisoning
  - Infections
    - Meningitis
- Pediatric illness and injuries can be emotionally difficult for the child, parent, and provider.
- EMTs often benefit from a debriefing following a difficult pediatric transport.

Review Questions

1. List some general techniques useful in history taking and performing a physical examination on a pediatric patient.
2. List some developmental considerations for infants, toddlers, preschool children, school-age children, and adolescents.
3. What are some of the anatomic and physiologic differences in the infant, child, and adult patient, and how do they affect emergency care?
4. What is the Pediatric Assessment Triangle?
5. What physiologic systems are assessed using the components of the PAT?
6. List several causes of pediatric airway emergencies. How are they managed?
7. What pediatric respiratory emergencies are commonly seen, and how are they managed?
8. What are the signs and symptoms of hypoperfusion in the infant and child?
9. What are the most common causes of cardiac arrest in infants and children, and how do they impact emergency management?
10. What is SIDS?
11. What are some common causes of pediatric altered mental status, and how are they managed?
12. Why does an EMT need to debrief following a difficult pediatric transport?

Key Terms

Back slaps

Chest thrusts

Febrile seizure

Intercostal retraction

Pediatric Assessment Triangle (PAT)

Respiratory syncytial virus (RSV)

Sternal retraction

Further Study

American Academy of Pediatrics. *Pediatric Education for Prehospital Professionals (PEPP)*. Sudbury, MA: Jones and Bartlett, 2006.

American Heart Association. *Handbook of Emergency Cardiovascular Care*. Dallas, TX: Author, 2008.

Wertz, E. M. *Emergency Care for Children*. Clifton Park, NY: Thomson Delmar Learning.

UNIT (43) Pediatric Trauma Emergencies

Pediatric trauma is the number one killer of children over 1 year of age. In fact, trauma accounts for more pediatric deaths in the United States than all other causes of pediatric death combined. Many more children are permanently disabled.

Pediatric trauma death is largely preventable. The majority of these deaths occur in motor vehicle collisions. If everyone transporting children used properly worn restraints or appropriately installed child safety seats, the number of fatalities would be far fewer.

When a collision does not end with a fatality, it often results in an injury that causes permanent disability or disfigurement. This lifelong affliction influences the child's development, both mentally and physically.

National Education Standards
The Emergency Medical Technician (EMT) will demonstrate a fundamental depth and foundational breadth of understanding of the anatomy, physiology, pathophysiology, assessment, and management of pediatric traumatic injuries.

Key Concepts

- Trauma is the leading cause of pediatric mortality.

- A child's head is proportionately larger, leading to a greater risk for head injury.

- Children have a higher ratio of body surface area to mass, making them more susceptible to hypothermia.

- Children have a natural inclination to explore their world without thought of consequences, putting them at a higher risk for serious injury or death from trauma.

- The Pediatric Glasgow Coma Scale can be used to more thoroughly assess the neurologic system in children suffering head or spinal injury.

- The injuries sustained if struck by a motor vehicle are reflective of the height of the child and the height of the car.

- A child's body will compensate for blood loss by shunting blood to the vital core organs for a time before decompensated hypoperfusion occurs.

- Severe underlying internal injuries to organs may exist due to the flexibility of a child's ribs.

- Children are at greater risk for neck and spinal injury due to their relatively larger and heavier heads.

- The EMT must immediately assess and treat for possible inhalation of smoke, heat, and toxins when managing a child with burns.

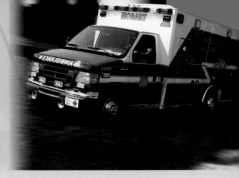

CASE STUDY

Anton and Elise had been running all day on both transfers and 9-1-1 calls. They have just returned to quarters after the eighth call of their 12-hour shift, hoping the last two hours will be quiet. Instead, the tones sound:

Dispatch to Unit 42—Respond to the intersection of Highway 20 and County Road C28. Child hit by a car. Time out: 1705.

As Anton and Elise leave the station, their emotions are high. They had worked a pediatric trauma call 4 months ago, car versus tree, and the child had not survived. Now they are responding to another pediatric trauma call involving a motor vehicle on one of the busiest highways.

The local fire department has also been dispatched as is the policy for all motor vehicle collisions (MVCs). Elise knows that at least two of the guys on the truck today were also on that call 4 months ago. It is going to be a difficult call for them all.

Upon arrival they see an approximately 8-year-old boy lying on the road being attended by his mother and the driver of the pickup truck. As they approach the scene, the driver says, "I didn't see him, he ran up out of the ditch, and I couldn't stop in time."

Anton directs one of the firefighters, who is also an EMT, to take manual stabilization of the boy's cervical spine. The mother is crying, "Wake up, Billy. Please wake up for mommy." The boy is unconscious, but breathing. There is some bleeding from an exposed cut on his left lower leg. A large hematoma is starting to form on his left temple. Anton knows this is a high-priority transport patient.

Critical Thinking Questions

1. What are the most common causes of pediatric trauma?
2. What are the indications for transporting this child to a pediatric trauma center?
3. What additional injuries should the EMT suspect based on the mechanism of injury?

INTRODUCTION

One of the most anxiety-producing emergencies for an Emergency Medical Technician (EMT) is pediatric trauma. Fortunately, an EMT does not need to learn a new set of skills. For the majority of pediatric trauma cases, the EMT need only integrate a few new facts into an already developed skill set. With practice, an EMT can become as comfortable with pediatric trauma care as with adult trauma care. This unit addresses the assessment and management of pediatric traumatic injury.

PEDIATRIC TRAUMA ASSESSMENT

The maxim "children are not small adults" is particularly applicable to pediatric trauma care. Children have significant anatomic and psychological differences compared to adults. These differences make children more prone to certain injuries. The EMT must consider these differences when assessing a child.

ANATOMIC DIFFERENCES

The anatomic differences between a child and an adult are directly related to the child's physical development. As a child matures, the body is constantly changing to more adult-like proportions. During that period of growth, the child can be categorized into several groups, usually based on age.

Nevertheless, the EMT should remember that every child is an individual and should seek to address that child's specific needs. For example, the EMT may treat a large 12-year-old as an adolescent and a small teenager as a child.

Some anatomic differences are common among children of all age-groups and diminish as the child gets older. These differences should be taken into account when an EMT is assessing and treating a child.

For instance, a child's head is proportionally larger than an adult's head, which makes the child more "top heavy" and more prone to head injuries (Figure 43.1). Children who are unrestrained in an MVC can suffer head and neck injuries.

The "head leads." In other words, the head will often be the first point of contact in a collision or fall. Children who are passengers in the front seat can sustain neck, face, and chest injuries from the deployment of the airbag because of their size and position in the seat. Additionally, the child who is improperly restrained in a car can sustain abdominal and lumbar injuries.

A child also has a higher ratio of body surface area to mass, which means a child has more skin per pound of body weight. Therefore, a child loses heat faster and is more prone to hypothermia than an adult under similar circumstances.

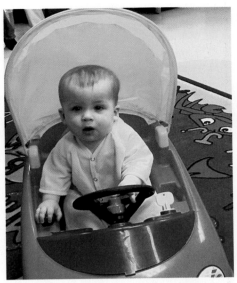

Figure 43.1 Children's heads are proportionately larger than adult's heads (Courtesy of the Nicholas Scadden Family, Illinois City, IL)

MECHANISM OF INJURY

Why is death from trauma more prevalent in children? The very nature of children put them at a higher risk for death from trauma. Each age range, from mobile toddlers to adolescents, has unique psychological characteristics that put children at risk for different types of trauma.

Small children are curious. A child learns a great deal about the world by exploring it. During infancy they begin to explore the world with their mouths. The older infant and toddler will put small objects into the mouth to taste them and, therefore, are at risk for foreign body airway obstruction.

School-age children play with implements of daily living, such as matches, in which case the result may be burn trauma. Sometimes children sense that something, like a gun, is forbidden and test the boundaries of adult tolerance (Figure 43.2). These children do not understand that serious injury or even death can result from mishandling a weapon.

In general, a child is less likely than an adult to understand that certain acts can result in serious injury. Children do not give thought to the consequences of actions ahead of time; for example, they do not consider the potentially disastrous results of running into the road to get a ball. They are focused on the need of the moment; they have to get the ball to continue to play the game.

Adolescents, on the other hand, understand these risks, and many choose to take them anyway because they have an unrealistic belief that nothing bad will happen. Adolescent risk-taking behavior, such as drinking and driving, all too often results in death or serious injury. Adolescents are still curious, but in different ways than toddlers. An adolescent is more willing to experiment,

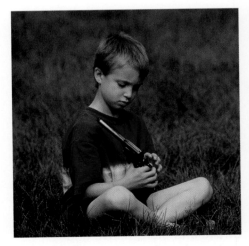

Figure 43.2 Children do not understand the consequences of their actions

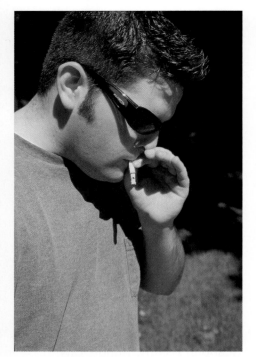

Figure 43.3 Adolescents are likely to experience problems from their experimentation

Table 43-1	Pediatric Trauma by Age Category	
Age Category	**Types of Trauma**	**Examples**
Toddlers	Blunt trauma	Motor vehicle collision
	Drowning	Pool and bucket
	Burn trauma	Scalding
	Poisoning	Household cleaners/pills
School-age	Blunt trauma	Motor vehicle collision
	Falls	Bicycle
	Burn trauma	Intentional fires
Adolescents	Blunt trauma	Motor vehicle collision
	Penetrating trauma	Suicide/homicide
	Poisoning	Overdose

by using alcohol or illicit drugs, for example (Figure 43.3). Table 43-1 relates common types of trauma to the age of the child.

PRIMARY ASSESSMENT

After conducting a scene size-up and determining the mechanism of injury, the EMT should perform the quick observational assessment using the Pediatric Assessment Triangle (PAT), discussed in Unit 42, immediately followed by the primary assessment and management of any life-threatening injuries. Chapter 4 discusses the phases of assessment, and Chapter 6 details trauma care; both should be reviewed prior to this discussion of special considerations during pediatric trauma assessment.

GENERAL IMPRESSION

As the EMT approaches the child, he should form a general impression and immediately try to ascertain the degree of the child's distress based on the PAT. Is the child in severe distress, apparent distress, or somewhere in between? An EMT does not need a great deal of experience with injured children to make this decision. This can be accomplished by comparing the way the injured child is acting with how a normal child acts.

MENTAL STATUS

A normal child is active, almost constantly moving. An injured child is often inactive, keeping unusually still due to pain, fear, and/or respiratory or circulatory difficulty. A normal child's eyes are bright, attentive, and constantly scanning the environment (Figure 43.4). An injured child appears self-absorbed, either quietly working to compensate for the injury or loudly seeking comfort from caregivers.

When children are hurt, they usually seek the comfort of their parents through crying, kicking, and other attention-getting behavior. The EMT should determine whether these are age-appropriate behaviors or are due to their injury. If the child appears distracted by an injury or, worse, disinterested in her parents' attention, she probably has significant injuries.

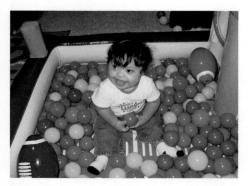

Figure 43.4 A normal child is awake and alert, active and interactive with his environment (Courtesy of the Paul Nyane Family, Iowa City, IA)

PEDIATRIC GLASGOW COMA SCALE

A child with a traumatic injury may have an abnormal appearance according to the PAT due to a variety of reasons that do not pertain to their brain or spinal cord function. In fact, a child's appearance may be abnormal, but she may be assessed as "alert" if using the AVPU scale discussed in Unit 16. A form of the adult Glasgow Coma Scale (Unit 27) modified to assess neurological injury in children, the **Pediatric Glasgow Coma Scale (PGCS)** can be used in place of the AVPU scale (Table 43-2). It is important to pay close attention to the motor component of the PGCS in predicting the neurologic outcome of a traumatic brain injury.

AIRWAY

In general, a child's airway is smaller and more prone to obstruction than an adult's airway. A blockage can be life threatening in many cases. An EMT should carefully assess a child's airway and take pains to keep it clear.

Normally, a child breathes through her nose. Infants are natural, or obligatory, nose breathers. When a child is breathing through her open mouth, the child either is in pain or has "air hunger."

BREATHING

The muscles in a young child's chest wall are not well developed. To breathe deeply, tight the child uses her abdominal muscles to help the diaphragm muscle. When the child is breathing fast and deep, a kind of seesaw breathing motion is seen.

Table 43-2 Pediatric Glasgow Coma Scale

Score	Child	Infant
Eyes		
4	Opens eyes spontaneously	Opens eyes spontaneously
3	Opens eyes to speech	Opens eyes to speech
2	Opens eyes to pain	Opens eyes to pain
1	No response	No response
Motor		
6	Obeys commands	Spontaneous movement
5	Localizes	Withdraws to touch
4	Withdraws	Withdraws to pain
3	Flexion	Flexion (decorticate)
2	Extension	Extension (decerebrate)
1	No response	No response
Verbal		
5	Oriented	Coos and babbles
4	Confused	Irritable cry
3	Inappropriate words	Cries to pain
2	Incomprehensible words	Moans to pain
1	No response	No response
_____ = Total Score (Eyes, Motor, Verbal—range 3–15)		

A child's sternum is very soft, still largely made of cartilage. With a very deep inhalation, sternal and intercostal retractions may both be seen. These signs—mouth breathing, sternal and intercostal retractions, and seesaw respiration—are all signs of a child having severe difficulty breathing. Unit 42 offers more information on pediatric respiratory medical emergencies.

CIRCULATION

Even a small amount of blood loss can be significant to a child. Comparatively, a child's blood volume is much smaller than an adult's. Loss of as little as 12 ounces (350 cc), or the amount in a soda can, can be life threatening.

HISTORY AND SECONDARY ASSESSMENT

Units 18, 19, and 33 discuss history taking and secondary assessment in detail. The specific techniques used in assessing children of different ages should also be reviewed in Unit 42. The priorities in the pediatric trauma assessment, as with adult assessments, are based on the injuries found in the primary assessment and on the mechanism of injury. Table 43-3 lists injuries and mechanisms of injury that are considered high priority in a child. These criteria can be used to triage a pediatric patient to the most appropriate hospital, according to local protocols.

BLUNT TRAUMA

Anybody struck by a motor vehicle has the potential for being seriously injured. A car weighing as much as a ton can transfer a great deal of energy and create significant injuries. The injuries a child may sustain, if struck by a motor vehicle, are a function of the height of the child and the height of the car.

When a sports car strikes a teenager, the direct trauma from the bumper can cause lower leg injuries. When the teen is thrown, chest and head injuries also can occur. If a truck strikes a school-age child, the direct injury may cause immediate head injuries.

In most cases of accidents with motor vehicles and pedestrians, some blunt trauma occurs. Blunt trauma can result in internal bleeding, hypoperfusion, and shock.

Sometimes assessing injuries from blunt trauma in a child is difficult. There may be outward signs of deformity, contusions, abrasions, and burns, but sometimes these signs are initially quite subtle. When an EMT relates the size and age of the child to the specific mechanism of injury, he can predict the area of injury and may be better able to discover these subtle signs.

HYPOPERFUSION

A child's body has a wonderful capacity to compensate for blood loss. Shunting blood to the vital core organs, the child is able to mobilize lifesaving stores of blood from the skin and abdominal organs.

Outwardly, the child becomes very pale and diaphoretic. The child's capillary refill becomes increasingly prolonged, beyond the normal 2 seconds. The child may even complain of nausea.

During this time, the heart continues to pump adequate amounts of blood to the vital organs, keeping them alive. The child's body is able to compensate in this manner up to a certain point.

However, at the point at which a significant volume of blood is lost, the child rapidly decompensates. The child's peripheral pulses become weaker, as the body shifts, or shunts, blood from the extremities to the vital organs.

Table 43-3 Pediatric Transport Criteria

Trauma triage—Child should be transported to a Level One pediatric trauma center.*

Vital Signs

> Signs of severe hypoperfusion
>
> Sustained tachycardia
>
> Bradycardia
>
> Hypotension

Presenting Injury

> Uncontrolled airway†*
>
> Severe difficulty with breathing
>
> Uncontrollable bleeding
>
> Paralysis or paresthesia
>
> Open fracture
>
> Penetrating trauma
>
> Head injury
>
> Severe facial trauma

Mechanism of Injury

> Pedestrian struck at speed greater than 20 mph
>
> Dragged by a motor vehicle
>
> Fall three times or greater than child's height
>
> Unrestrained passenger in a rollover
>
> Ejected from motor vehicle
>
> Restrained passenger in high-speed crash (>50 mph)
>
> Passenger where another passenger died

* If a level one trauma center is within a reasonable distance. The EMT should always follow local protocols.

† The child should be taken to the closest available hospital, preferably a trauma center.

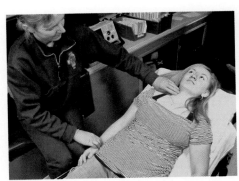

Figure 43.5 Pulse differences between central and peripheral pulses may indicate hypoperfusion (Courtesy of Larry Torrey and MEDCU, Portland, ME)

The EMT can feel the result of this shunting of blood by comparing radial pulses and carotid pulses (Figure 43.5). In the presence of hypoperfusion and shunting, the radial feels weaker than the carotid. This comparison of pulses confirms that the child is shunting blood to the vital organs and may be in danger of decompensation.

As the bleeding continues, the child's capillary refill times increase and the child becomes less responsive (Figure 43.6). These signs—weaker peripheral pulses, delayed capillary refill, and lethargy—and the other signs of hypoperfusion in the face of trauma are indications that the child has likely lost a significant amount of blood.

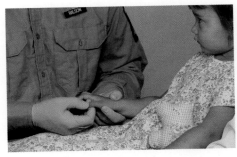

Figure 43.6 Capillary refill is a dependable indicator of perfusion in children

A loss of consciousness and a slow, or bradycardiac, heart rate may be signs of imminent cardiac arrest. Any child who is unconscious or bradycardiac is a high priority.

MANAGEMENT

The principles of management of hypoperfusion are similar whether the patient is an adult or a child. The EMT must realize, however, that the signs of hypoperfusion in a child are not as obvious as those in an adult, and the child may decompensate quickly.

Ensuring adequacy of oxygenation and circulation is the basic goal in the management of the pediatric patient suffering from hypoperfusion. Unit 11 discusses hypoperfusion and its management in more detail.

CHEST INJURY

A child's rib cage has a large amount of soft cartilage that makes it very flexible. When a blunt force is applied, the rib cage will bend inward, and then spring back to its original position.

The possibility of a severe underlying injury requires the EMT to understand the internal injuries that may exist due to these flexible ribs. When an EMT observes an abrasion or contusion on a child's chest, he should have a high index of suspicion that internal organs may have been injured.

It takes a great deal of force to break a child's ribs. Severe internal injury is usually associated with a pediatric rib fracture.

MANAGEMENT

The management of pediatric chest injuries is similar to that described in Unit 36. Oxygenation, ventilation when needed, and stabilization of obvious chest injuries should be accomplished during the primary assessment.

The EMT must keep in mind that fewer signs of external trauma will be evident in the small child, despite potential serious internal injuries. Evidence of difficulty breathing or circulatory compromise in the child, along with an appropriate mechanism of injury, should prompt the EMT to suspect chest injury.

ABDOMINAL INJURY

Unlike those of an adult, a child's liver and spleen are only partially protected by the rib cage. That leaves these solid, blood-filled organs more susceptible to injury. Blunt trauma to the child's abdomen may tear, or lacerate, a child's liver or spleen.

An EMT should have a high index of suspicion that if a child was struck in the abdomen and has signs of hypoperfusion, then the child may have internal bleeding from abdominal organ injures.

MANAGEMENT

A child with signs of abdominal injury, such as tenderness or bruising, should be carefully monitored for signs of hypoperfusion and shock. The principles discussed in Unit 36 should be reviewed. A child with potential intra-abdominal injuries should be transported, if possible, to a hospital that is capable of managing pediatric surgical emergencies.

HEAD INJURY

The signs and symptoms of a pediatric head injury are similar to those of an adult. Loss of consciousness, headaches, and blurred vision are all examples of signs of head injury. Unit 34 should be reviewed for further signs and symptoms of head and traumatic brain injury.

Children are more likely to experience nausea and subsequently vomit from a head injury than an adult. Nausea and vomiting are so common with a pediatric head injury that an EMT should suspect a head injury in a traumatized child who has nausea or vomits.

The EMT must be prepared to turn a head-injured child quickly onto her side and suction the airway clear if the child should vomit while supine on the long backboard. For this reason, a suction device should always be ready for use.

A child may experience a seizure after trauma. These post-traumatic seizures may be caused by a serious head injury that is not immediately evident. The first concern when the child seizes is to maintain the airway without compromising the child's spine. The child should be protected from further injury during the seizure. Remember that a postictal period of decreased level of consciousness is common after a seizure. The EMT should continue to support the child's airway and breathing as needed during this period.

MANAGEMENT

The management of the child with a head injury is also based on adequacy of oxygenation, ventilation, and circulation. The injured brain is dependent on receiving an adequate supply of oxygenated blood. Unit 34 reviews the details of management of head injuries.

SPINAL INJURY

In any deceleration injury, such as a fall or MVC, there is potential for neck injury. Children are perhaps at greater risk for this type of injury given their relatively larger and heavier heads. The large head is thrown forward in the incident, forcibly flexing or extending the neck. This mechanism can result in injury to the spine. Unit 35 discusses spine injuries in detail. Table 43-4 summarizes mechanisms of injury related to spinal trauma.

Table 43-4 Causes of Pediatric Spinal Trauma by Classification

Motor vehicles
- Motor vehicle collisions
- Motor vehicle versus pedestrian
- Motorcycles—on and off road
- All-terrain vehicles
- Snowmobiles

Sports
- Swimming/diving
- Football
- Rock climbing
- Downhill skiing/snowboarding

Crime
- Gunshot wounds
- Knife wounds
- Blunt trauma—assault

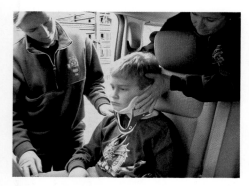

Figure 43.7 Manual stabilization may be held from a superior position (Courtesy of Larry Torrey and MEDCU, Portland, ME)

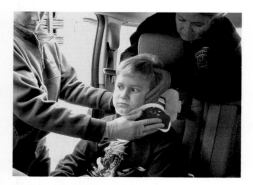

Figure 43.8 Pediatric cervical immobilization collars must fit the patient (Courtesy of Larry Torrey and MEDCU, Portland, ME)

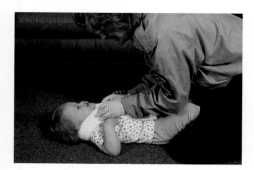

Figure 43.9 A cervical immobilization device may be improvised from a rolled towel

MANAGEMENT

Management of any spinal injury always begins with ensuring the spine is in a neutral alignment and maintaining manual stabilization of the head and neck. The EMT may need to take anterior stabilization when a child is in a car seat. The EMT should avoid covering the child's ears; loss of hearing can be frightening to a child.

If the EMT can get above and behind the car seat, manual stabilization can be held from above, as demonstrated in Figure 43.7. The EMT needs to explain to the child what is going to happen before it happens to reduce the child's apprehension and improve her cooperation.

A primary assessment of the child should be performed, including oxygen administration as indicated. If the child is high priority, she should be removed from the car seat quickly.

Car seats are not designed as pediatric immobilization devices. It is difficult to manage an airway, suction a child, or even splint an injured extremity while the child is still in the car seat. The EMT should remove any child showing signs of serious or potentially life-threatening trauma from the car seat to immobilize the spine and manage life threats. If a pediatric immobilization device is not available, an adult long spine board can be used. The EMT must make sure to keep the airway and spine in a neutral position by placing padding under the child's shoulders and padding all additional voids.

Small children can be transported in their car seats after an MVC under certain circumstances. If the car seat's plastic shell is not damaged, there are no jagged metal edges exposed and the patient is not in need of resuscitation, the EMT can consider immobilizing the child in her car seat. There are several advantages to leaving a child in a car seat. One benefit is that the child may be more comfortable and cooperative if she is left in the familiar surroundings of her car seat.

Another advantage is convenience; it is easier to move a child from the motor vehicle to the ambulance gurney if the child is in a car seat. If a child can be reasonably immobilized in the car seat, leave the child in the seat and pad as necessary to immobilize the head, neck, and spine in alignment. If this is not possible, the child must be removed and immobilized in a pediatric immobilization device.

A cervical collar should be applied as soon as practical. A variety of pediatric cervical collars are available on the market, and children come in a variety of sizes. The EMT should carefully match the right size collar to the patient (Figure 43.8).

In some cases, especially in the case of infants, it is difficult to find a properly fitting cervical collar. In those cases, a rolled towel can be placed around the neck, in the form of a horseshoe collar, and then secured at the chest. Figure 43.9 demonstrates the use of a towel as a cervical immobilization device.

Throughout the process of applying a cervical collar and afterward, the EMT must maintain continuous manual stabilization.

IMMOBILIZATION IN CAR SEAT

While maintaining manual stabilization, the EMT should consider whether it is necessary to pad behind the child's thorax. When a child is flat, her large head can lift the cervical spine out of alignment. It may be necessary to pad behind the child's thorax to move the cervical spine back into alignment.

If it is necessary to pad the thorax, the EMT must first release the restraint straps and/or lift the front guard from the child. The EMT then gently slides a folded blanket, towel, or foam pad into place behind the child (Figure 43.10).

The child is properly immobilized, and in neutral spinal alignment, when the opening of the ear is directly over the middle of the shoulder. The EMT should then resecure the restraint straps or replace the front guard, immobilizing the torso before proceeding to immobilize the head.

The head may be immobilized in the car seat by placing two rolled towels on each side of the child's head. The head and towels can then be secured by placing a length of tape around the car seat, as demonstrated in Figure 43.11. Sandbags are not acceptable for use as head blocks. If the child must be turned suddenly, to clear the airway, for example, the sandbags would act like a counterweight to the body, forcing the neck out of alignment.

The child, immobilized securely in the car seat, should be placed on and fastened to the ambulance gurney. When the gurney is secured in the ambulance, the EMT should sit where the child can see him without turning her head.

REMOVING A CHILD FROM A CAR SEAT

Sometimes it is necessary to quickly remove a child from a car seat, if the child is in respiratory and/or cardiac arrest or has an uncontrolled airway, for example. Using a backboard (long or short), several EMTs can quickly remove a child from a car seat. Commercial pediatric immobilization devices are also available. If using such a device, the EMT should follow the manufacturer's recommendations regarding proper use.

If a backboard is to be used, one EMT must first maintain manual stabilization of the spine. Another EMT then places a backboard at the head of the car seat. It may be necessary to place a mat or block under the backboard to make it level with the lip of the car seat. Another EMT removes, or cuts, the restraint straps on the car seat and then quickly applies the properly sized cervical immobilization device.

Slowly tilting the seat backward, while maintaining manual stabilization of the head and spine, the EMTs should center the top of the car seat with the bottom of the backboard.

The EMT at the head maintains stabilization while the other EMT grasps the child under the arms and slightly lifts and slides her, along her long axis, onto the backboard. It may be necessary to lift the child onto padding placed on top of the backboard.

Once the child is on the short backboard, her torso should be immobilized to the board. The spaces between the straps and the child may need to be padded. Straps should be placed under the arms, at the top of the chest, as well as across the hips. The restraint straps should not severely restrict the child's breathing.

BONY INJURY

A child's bones are somewhat flexible and seldom break. It takes a great deal of force to create a fracture of the bone of a child. An EMT should have a high index of suspicion that there may be other more significant injuries if a fracture is indicated.

MANAGEMENT

Any painful, swollen deformity needs to be immobilized and then evaluated by a physician. However, the EMT should not be distracted by painful bony injuries and ignore more life-threatening injuries.

It is important to use the appropriately sized splinting or immobilization equipment. Unless there is severe pain or an extremity shows signs of circulatory or neurologic impairment, a dislocated or fractured bone should be immobilized in the position found (Figure 43.12). As with adults, never try to push an exposed bone back under the skin.

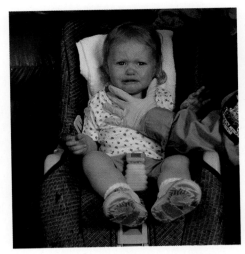

Figure 43.10 Padding behind the thorax helps to maintain neutral cervical spine alignment

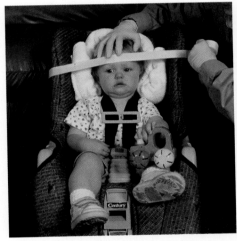

Figure 43.11 Rolled towels may be used as head blocks and the entire assembly taped into place

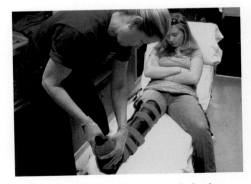

Figure 43.12 Splint bone injuries using the appropriately sized splint or materials (Courtesy of Larry Torrey and MEDCU, Portland, ME)

BURNS

The thought of a child with severe burns makes the most experienced EMT anxious. By applying the basic principles of adult burn care, reviewed in Unit 37, and modifying them to accommodate the pediatric patient, the EMT can provide effective patient care and help improve the patient's outcome.

Children become burn victims for a variety of reasons. A child playing with matches may unwittingly start a house fire. A toddler exploring her world may unintentionally pull a pot of hot water off the stove. A burn may also be a result of child abuse; an adult may inflict a burn on a child.

ASSESSMENT

Assessment should begin with a scene size-up, using the mechanism of burn injury to determine risk factors for the airway and breathing. The child who has been pulled from a fire should lead the EMT to a high index of suspicion for smoke inhalation and thermal burns of the airway. Additionally, the EMT should always suspect the presence of carbon monoxide, cyanide, or other toxic fumes released from burning substances the child has inhaled.

The EMT should perform a rapid physical examination looking for hidden injuries of the bones or organs of the abdomen due to a fall or explosion.

A quick estimation of the body surface area that has been burned is important information to provide the receiving facility and estimate the severity of the burn. The "rule of nines" used for the adult is modified for the child based on age. Figure 43.13 shows the modified anatomic diagrams of children per age to calculate the extent of a burn. If the modified rule of nines cannot be used, use the "rule of palms." It is important to remember the palm (child's palm, not the EMT's) is equal to 1% of the body surface (Figure 43.13 and 43.14).

MANAGEMENT

The EMT is immediately concerned about maintaining an open airway. Inhalation of smoke and superheated air can cause upper airway swelling. The pediatric airway is narrow. A small amount of swelling, or edema, can completely close off the airway in a matter of minutes.

The EMT should listen for the sounds of stridor, a low-pitched inspiratory sound created in the throat as air rushes through a narrowed airway. The EMT should then look into the mouth for evidence of burn injury. A reddened throat, soot on the tongue, and singed nose hairs are all signs of potential burn injury to the airway.

Toxins, such as carbon monoxide, may have been inhaled by the child. Carbon monoxide interferes with oxygen absorption and can lead to hypoxia. High-concentration oxygen should be administered via a pediatric mask as soon as possible for every burn victim (Figure 43.15).

Children have a relatively large surface area compared to weight ratio, making them more prone to hypothermia. Hypothermia is a major concern for the pediatric burn patient. An EMT must be cautious that the use of local irrigation does not create hypothermia, further complicating the patient's situation. Unit 37 should be reviewed for further specific details of burn care.

CHILD ABUSE

Whenever the pattern of injury does not match the reported mechanism of injury, an EMT must consider the possibility of child abuse. Between 500,000 and 4 million children are abused each year in the United States, and some of these children present for emergency medical care. Unit 44 discusses child abuse in more detail.

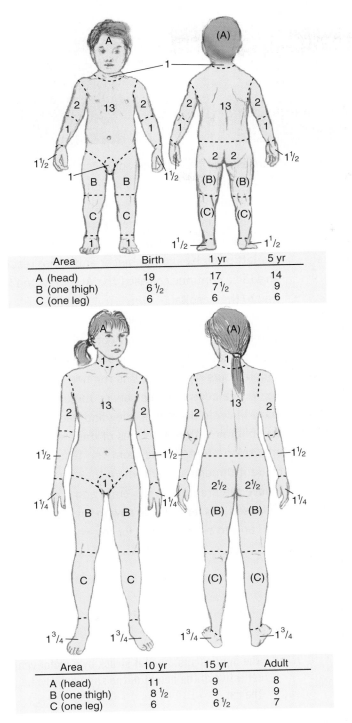

Area	Birth	1 yr	5 yr
A (head)	19	17	14
B (one thigh)	6 ½	7 ½	9
C (one leg)	6	6	6

Area	10 yr	15 yr	Adult
A (head)	11	9	8
B (one thigh)	8 ½	9	9
C (one leg)	6	6 ½	7

Figure 43.13 Modified "rule of nines" in children of different age-groups

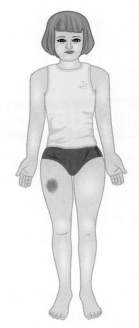

Figure 43.14 The rule of palm is approximately 1% of the body surface area

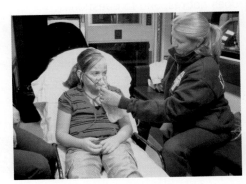

Figure 43.15 Children showing indications of inhalation burns need immediate high-flow oxygen (Courtesy of Larry Torrey and MEDCU, Portland, ME)

CONCLUSION

Pediatric trauma care is challenging for an EMT. The added emotional component makes the EMT's job that much harder. However, if an EMT remembers basic care principles and modifies them to accommodate the pediatric patient, he can render competent pediatric emergency care.

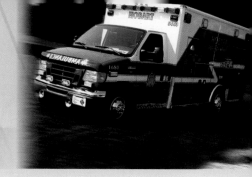

CASE STUDY Continued

Anton and Elise, with the help of the firefighters on scene, place a cervical collar and logroll Ben to the long spine board. Elise places padding in the voids to ensure Ben is secure. Ben's head is secured to the board using head rolls and tape. High flow oxygen at 15 lpm via non-rebreather mask is in place. Ben is breathing adequately at this time.

Elise has one of the firefighters drive so she and Anton can both work on helping Ben en route to the pediatric trauma center. His level of consciousness continues to be altered. ALS intercept has been requested because Ben's Pediatric Glasgow Coma Score is 7 (eyes-1, motor-4, verbal- 2). Ben's left pupil looks bigger and doesn't respond to the light as quickly as the right pupil.

Baseline vital signs show a blood pressure of 92/60, pulse 120, respirations 26. Ben occasionally moans but does not respond to questions.

A rapid physical assessment shows a hematoma to the left temple and a small laceration to his left knee that is no longer bleeding. His chest and abdomen both have

bruises, and his chest is not rising equally on both sides. Breath sounds are diminished on the left side.

Anton instructs Elise to begin assisting ventilations as Ben's breathing becomes labored and irregular. Just as the ALS intercept arrives and takes over care, Anton notes the left pupil has gotten bigger and is not reacting. Anton and Elise continue to assist the ALS crew the rest of the way to the hospital.

Later that night, Anton, Elise, and the two firefighters who had been with them on both calls await word from the hospital on Ben's condition. They have spent the last couple hours discussing this run and the run 4 months ago with a counselor the service director called. They know they did everything they had been taught to do for children with these types of traumatic injuries. The counselor returns to the room and tells them Ben has made it through surgery where they put in a drain to relieve the pressure in his brain and a chest tube for his collapsed left lung. He is now in the pediatric intensive care unit to be monitored for the next few days.

Key Concepts Revisited

- Trauma is the leading cause of pediatric mortality.

- A child's head is proportionately larger, leading to a greater risk of head injury.

- Children have a higher ratio of body surface area to mass, making them more susceptible to hypothermia.

- Children have a natural inclination to explore their world without thought of consequences, putting them at a higher risk for serious injury or death from trauma.

- The Pediatric Glasgow Coma Scale can be used to more thoroughly assess the neurologic status in children suffering head or spinal injury.

- The injuries sustained if struck by a motor vehicle are reflective of the height of the child and the height of the car.
  - Head
  - Chest
  - Abdomen
  - Legs (long bones)

- A child's body will compensate for blood loss by shunting blood to the vital core organs for a time before decompensated hypoperfusion occurs.

- Severe underlying internal injuries to organs may exist due to the flexibility of a child's ribs.
  - Lungs
  - Liver
  - Spleen
- Children are at greater risk for neck and spinal injury due to their relatively larger and heavier heads.
  - Traumatic brain injury
    - Head is point of first contact because of size and weight
  - Cervical spine
    - Forced flexing or extension of the neck due to the larger, heavier head

- Immobilization decisions
  - Immobilize in car seat
  - Removal from car seat
- The EMT must immediately assess and treat for possible inhalation of smoke, heat, and toxins when managing a child with burns.
  - Airway damage for inhalation burns
  - Structural damage to burned skin
  - Hypothermia due to large surface area skin loss

Review Questions

1. What is the leading cause of pediatric mortality?
2. How does pediatric anatomy alter an EMT's patient assessment?
3. What is the Pediatric Glasgow Coma Scale?
4. How does pediatric anatomy relate to chest trauma?
5. How does pediatric anatomy relate to abdominal trauma?
6. How does pediatric anatomy relate to head injuries?
7. What are some causes of pediatric spinal trauma?
8. What is the treatment for pediatric spinal trauma?
9. How does pediatric anatomy relate to bone injury?
10. What pediatric trauma cases are considered high priority?
11. How would an EMT care for a pediatric burn patient?
12. What types of burns should raise an index of suspicion for child abuse?

Key Term

Pediatric Glasgow Coma Scale (PGCS)

Further Study

American Academy of Pediatrics. *Pediatric Education for Prehospital Professionals (PEPP)*. Sudbury, MA: Jones and Bartlett, 2006.
National Association of Emergency Medical Technicians. *PHTLS: Basic and Advanced PrehospitalTrauma Life Support*. 6th ed. Clinton, MS: Mosby, 2007.
Wertz, E. M. *Emergency Care for Children*. Clifton Park, NY: Thomson Delmar Learning, 2002.

UNIT (44) Child Abuse and Neglect

Every EMT has a duty to protect the weak and vulnerable from abuse and mistreatment. This duty is exemplified by the fact that an EMT is a mandated reporter of child abuse. This duty should be looked on as both a responsibility and an honor. It is to the credit of the Emergency Medical Technician (EMT) that the public looks on Emergency Medical Services (EMS) as a trusted guardian and protector of children.

National Education Standard

The Emergency Medical Technician (EMT) shall have a simple depth and simple breadth of knowledge regarding recognizing, reporting, and understanding the health care implications of child abuse and neglect.

Key Concepts

- The EMT is a mandated child abuse reporter in all 50 states and territories of the United States.

- Child abuse can be act or a failure to act to protect a child from physical or psychological harm.

- An EMT must be alert to indicators of child abuse during the assessment of the child.

- The EMT's documentation is important to proving child abuse and to potentially preventing future abuse.

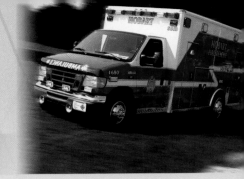

CASE STUDY

"Infant seizing." The radio report sends shivers up Carney's spine. As his mind races, he recalls that many children seize because of fever, and he remembers the case of the immigrant family who tried cooling their infant down with rubbing alcohol, poisoning him in the process. Although it was originally investigated as a case of possible child abuse, it was later found that the family was merely following telephone instructions, albeit bad instructions, from a grandmother in the old country.

As the ambulance responds to the scene, fire department EMTs are already on scene and report that the seizure had stopped, but the child remains unconscious and unresponsive. Carney grabs the jump bag while his partner starts to unload the stretcher. Meeting at the back of the ambulance, Carney places the bag on the gurney, and together they head into the house.

The baby is in the living room, and the firefighters are assisting ventilation with a bag-valve-mask assembly. Carney asks the firefighters if the child has a fever, as he puts on his N95 mask. The Captain barks, "No fever." As Carney removes his mask, he notices an adult male, the apparent boyfriend, and an adult woman, the infant's mother, arguing in the corner. She is wearing a waitress uniform, and it appears that she has just returned from work. The obviously pregnant woman keeps trying to pull away to go to her baby, but the boyfriend keeps pulling her back to him to continue the argument. The hair on the back of Carney's neck stands up, but he knows he must focus on the infant.

Critical Thinking Questions

1. What are some reasons an infant would seize?
2. Why would an infant go into respiratory arrest?
3. Why is Carney concerned about the boyfriend?

INTRODUCTION

Child abuse and neglect are tragic realities the EMT may encounter on the job. The EMT must recognize signs of abuse and to report it to the proper authorities so that action can be taken to protect the child from further harm.

The first step in recognizing child abuse is the suspension of disbelief. The EMT must suspend disbelief that child abuse could have occurred. Most EMTs, and most people, cannot imagine a parent harming a child. It is important for the EMT to suspend that disbelief to have a suspicion of child abuse when injuries do not match the stated mechanism of injury or when the EMT witnesses unacceptable living conditions.

While the EMT is required to report suspected child abuse, she should not accuse the parents of child abuse. It is important that the EMT maintain a nonjudgmental attitude toward the parent or caregiver. The EMT's first priority in the case of suspected child abuse is to care for and protect the child. If the EMT appears to condemn the parents, they may withdraw their consent for the EMT to treat the child. Therefore, criticism and judgment of the parent or caregiver would be counterproductive to the end goal of caring for and protecting the child from further harm.

Although parents, adult family members, and caregivers directly involved in the care of children are all potential perpetrators of child abuse, the majority of perpetrators are parents. Therefore, the term *parent(s)* will be used throughout this unit, and the reader should understand that it includes all adult parties with custodial responsibilities.

CHILD ABUSE

Every child in the United States has a right to grow up in an environment without fear, especially fear of harm from loved ones and caregivers. When a child appears fearful of those loved ones or caregivers, then child abuse should be suspected. The term *child abuse* encompasses acts of violence and willful acts of neglect. Using the term more narrowly, child abuse involves nonaccidental injury to a dependent person. Child abuse actually encompasses both physical abuse and neglect. Therefore, child abuse can occur as either an act (i.e., a commission) or a failure to act (i.e., an omission, also referred to as *neglect*).

ACTS OF COMMISSION

Acts of commission are deliberate and intentional acts that result in harm to the child, even though harm may not have been the intended consequence. For example, a caregiver may intend to hit a child as punishment for misbehavior but did not intend to cause the child to have a concussion.

Federal law defines *child abuse* as any act, or failure to act, on the part of responsible adults that results in death, serious physical or emotional harm, sexual abuse or exploitation, or an act or failure to act that presents an imminent risk of serious harm (Child Abuse Prevention and Treatment Act, 42.U.S.C.A. §5106g).

INDICATORS OF PHYSICAL ABUSE

Several specific behavioral indicators are suggestive of child abuse. Both the parent(s) and the child will manifest these behaviors. Careful observation of parent and child for the presence of these indicators during the course of the EMT–parent–patient interaction should alert the EMT to the potential of child abuse.

PARENTAL BEHAVIOR

Certain parental behaviors should alert the EMT to possible child abuse. For example, it is natural for a parent to be concerned about his or her child. Therefore, it is abnormal for a parent to appear indifferent or unconcerned about the welfare of the child. This indifference may be demonstrated by a delay in seeking medical attention. Or it may be apparent during the course of the child's care. In either case, indifference is abnormal and should be reported.

Inconsistency between parents or the parent and the child's story is another red flag. The EMT should be concerned if the parent gives an inadequate explanation of the child's injury, or the parent's explanation conflicts with the child's story.

All too often alcohol abuse and illicit drug use occur concurrently with child abuse. Parental intoxication, or signs of intoxication such as empty alcohol bottles or visible drug paraphernalia, should alert the EMT to the possibility of child abuse.

Acts of anger toward the child while in the presence of an EMT are particularly worrisome and may require immediate action and police intervention. Whether these acts are statements of shame in which the parent describes the child as evil or bad or attempts at physical discipline in the presence of the EMT, these acts can demonstrate poor impulse control. Table 44-1 is a short list of parental indicators of child abuse.

Street Smart

In order to avoid suspicion, some parent(s) will ask to have the child taken to different hospitals for each injury. So-called "doc shopping" is another indicator of potential child abuse. The most common factors in those cases is dispatch, who may notice several calls to a single address with transport to different hospitals and EMS. An EMT who observes this behavior should consider reporting it to authorities.

Table 44-1 Parental Indicators of Child Abuse

- Delay in seeking medical attention for ill or injured child
- Parental indifference to child's illness or injury
- Alcohol abuse and illicit drug use while caring for child
- Conflicting history about cause of injury

CHILD BEHAVIOR

A child's fear of adults, especially their parents, suggests that the child may have been abused. Abused children may be wary or fearful of adults, including their parents, and will cower and may even physically tremble around adults. The child may also express dread about going home, fearing a beating when they get home. These behaviors are suspicious, and child abuse should be suspected.

An abused child may also demonstrate extremes of behavior, one moment being aggressive and the next moment withdrawn. These behaviors may be inappropriate to the situation. Of particular concern is when the child appears apprehensive when other children in the room, particularly siblings, cry.

Alternatively, the child may attempt to endear himself to adults, any adult, seeking the adult's sympathy and protection. Attempts at affection should be viewed cautiously. Any sexual talk from the child is a red flag to the EMT, and sexual acting out is even more alarming. Sexual acting out can be subtle, such as inappropriate touching, or as brazen as exposure of the genitals and even public masturbation. If the EMT observes any of these behaviors, firm boundaries should be immediately established and another EMT asked to accompany the EMT and the child to help witness behaviors.

SPECIAL CASE OF SHAKEN BABY SYNDROME

A crying infant can test the nerves of even the most patient person. Unfortunately, some parents act out in frustration to an infant who cannot be soothed and shake the baby violently to try to get the baby to stop crying. If an infant is violently shaken to and fro, the baby can experience **shaken baby syndrome.** During shaken baby syndrome the violent forces created by swinging the baby tear fragile bridging veins from the skull to the brain and cause subsequent bleeding in the skull. These forces may even cause hemorrhages in the blood vessels in the eyes. As a result of the bleeding in the brain, the infant may become unresponsive (i.e., comatose) or have a seizure.

When this occurs, the alarmed parents call EMS and may report that the infant fell from a changing table or from a bed, for example. Falls from a height of less than 4 feet are unlikely to cause bleeding in the brain, which results in seizures or coma. Under these circumstances the EMT must consider the possibility of child abuse and shaken baby syndrome.

After completing the primary assessment of the unresponsive infant, the EMT should perform a thorough head-to-toe examination. Close inspection of the scalp may reveal contusions or lacerations from impact of the head against hard surfaces. The cranium should be palpated for an uneven surface, especially along the sutures, that would suggest a "step–off" from a displaced fracture. The ears and nose should be examined for signs of leaking clear fluid, or cerebrospinal fluid.

It is important for the EMT to report her suspicions of shaken baby syndrome immediately. Up to 50% of deaths attributed to child abuse are from shaken baby syndrome. Other complications associated with shaken baby syndrome include blindness from retinal detachment and hemorrhage in the eyes, cerebral palsy, and long-term mental impairment.

SEXUAL ABUSE

Sexual abuse is a subcategory of physical abuse. It has been estimated that one of every four girls and one out of every ten boys will be sexually abused in their childhood. Sexual relations with a parent, relative, or caregiver before the age of consent is considered **sexual abuse.**

Sexual abuse includes the traditional definitions of rape and sodomy. Sexual abuse also includes the vaginal or rectal penetration of the child with any body part or object, including the mouth, finger(s), or penis. Another definition of child sexual abuse is offered by the American Professional Society on the Abuse of Children:

> "Child sexual abuse involves any sexual activity with a child where consent is not or cannot be given. This includes sexual contact that is accomplished by force or threat of force, regardless of the age of the participants, and all sexual contact between an adult and a child, regardless of whether there is deception or the child understands the sexual nature of the activity. Sexual contact between an older and a younger child also can be abusive if there is a significant disparity in age, development, or size, rendering the younger child incapable of giving informed consent. The sexually abusive acts may include sexual penetration, sexual touching, or non-contact sexual acts such as exposure or voyeurism." (CDC 2007)

Sexual molestation is another form of sexual child abuse that is performed for the sexual gratification of the parent or caregiver. Key to the description of sexual molestation is unwanted or improper sexual contact. Examples of sexual molestation include permitting a child to watch adults having intercourse or masturbating in front of a child or having a child touch an adult's genitals.

It has been suggested that the shame and guilt associated with these sexual acts experienced by the victim has led to underreporting. Referred to as the "conspiracy of silence," adults convince impressionable children that reporting such acts to others would harm the family. Alert EMTs looking for subtle signs or behavioral indicators may be able to detect suspected sexual abuse. Table 44-2 lists the forms that sexual abuse can take.

ACTS OF OMISSION

The failure to provide for a child's basic physical, emotional, or educational needs or to protect a child from harm or potential harm (i.e., an act of omission) is also a form of child abuse called *neglect*. Like acts of commission, harm to a child may or may not be the intended consequence. Whether the failure to act was unintended is immaterial. An adult is responsible to act in the child's best interests. All types of neglect, shown in Table 44-3, involve acts of omission (i.e., a failure to provide).

INDICATORS OF CHILD NEGLECT

Typically child abuse is thought of as an act of violence against a child. However, the most common form of child abuse is not the result of an action but of inaction. **Child neglect** occurs when an adult with custodial responsibilities fails to provide legally mandated care for the child. Parents and custodial caregivers are obligated to provide food, clothing, shelter, medical, surgical,

Table 44-2 Sexual Abuse

- Penetration
  - Oral–penile
  - Anal–either penile or digital
  - Genital–either penile or digital
- External manipulation (Fondling)
  - Breast
  - Anal
  - Genital
  - Buttocks
- Indecent exposure
- Exploitation
  - Prostitution
  - Pornography

Table 44-3 Acts of Omission

- Failure to provide
  - Physical neglect
  - Emotional neglect
  - Medical/dental neglect
  - Educational neglect
- Failure to supervise
  - Inadequate supervision
  - Exposure to violent environments

and dental care, and compulsory education to children. Failure to meet these responsibilities risks charges of child neglect. To be actionable, or to permit the intervention of the courts in the child's care, the neglect must result in physical and/or psychological impairment of the child.

Whereas physical neglect, such as the lack of clean clothes or provision of medical care, may seem more obvious, many cases of neglect stem from the lack of supervision of minor children. Supervisory neglect can lead to juvenile delinquency. For example, an EMT responding to care for an unlicensed underaged driver at the scene of a motor vehicle collision, whose act of driving was illegal, might suspect the parents of supervisory neglect; therefore, the parents could be arrested for child abuse.

One area of concern is supervision, daycare, and babysitters. Parents make decisions as to whether a child is responsible enough to be left alone every day. That decision to leave a child alone should be made after careful consideration of the quality of previously demonstrated independent judgments of that child and his physical, cognitive, and emotional capabilities. The decision should be tempered with contemplation of potential dangers the child could face. Parental decisions that put a child at risk for physical, emotional, or psychological harm constitute supervisory neglect, and supervisory neglect is another form of child abuse.

PARENTAL BEHAVIOR

Two key attitudes can be used to sum up the behavior of parents who neglect their children: hopelessness and helplessness. Parents who neglect their children often have disorganized home lives and may express feelings of apathy. Often the parent is isolated, without the support of an extended family or friends. The parent's statements may express a sense of helplessness and hopelessness.

CHILD BEHAVIOR

A child's behaviors may also be indicators of child neglect. For example, because of constant hunger the child may resort to begging for food on the street, stealing food in the market, or picking food out of the cafeteria garbage. Similarly, because of a lack of shelter, particularly on hot, humid days or cold, frigid days, the child may arrive early or stay late at school.

SPECIAL CASE OF ABANDONED INFANTS

Some young women do not realize they are pregnant until after they deliver the baby. Others are not prepared for the arrival of the baby and panic. Overwhelmed by the sudden appearance of a baby and all of the life-changing events that surround parenting, these women may choose to abandon or even kill their babies.

To protect the lives of these infants, many states have enacted an **abandoned infant protection act**. These acts permit the young women, or a concerned adult, to relinquish care of the newborn to others at a "safe haven," such as a fire station or rescue squad building, without fear of criminal prosecution.

Typically the individual is not asked for the name of the mother or any other identifying information. However, the EMT should ask the person leaving the baby, in a nonjudgmental manner, if there is medical information that would help in the care of the infant.

PHYSICAL EXAMINATION

While trying to appear unobtrusive, so as to not alarm the patient or alert the parent, the EMT should assess, in a head-to-toe fashion, for signs of physical abuse. After a proper introduction and age-appropriate explanation of the examination, the EMT should begin the examination by starting at the head.

Approximately 50% of child abuse victims have injuries to the head and face; therefore, a careful examination of the head and face is appropriate.

The EMT should examine the head for missing patches of hair or hairline bleeding beneath the scalp. These findings are suggestive of hair pulling and traumatic hair loss. If the child is an infant, the EMT should observe the posterior and the anterior fontanels for bulging. A bulging fontanel may be indicative of increased intracranial pressure, possibly secondary to bleeding within the skull (see "Special Case of Shaken Baby Syndrome").

The EMT should examine both eyes for evidence of bilateral periorbital eccyhmosis, or raccoon's eyes. Bruising around the eyes is suggestive of a basilar skull fracture, which may occur when a child is thrown to the floor or his head is struck against a solid object. The EMT should also observe for bruising behind the ear, called Battle's sign, another indication of potential head injury.

Next the EMT should observe for lacerations or abrasions to the lips and gums. Lip tears may occur because of a direct blow to the mouth, by a fist, for example, or forced feeding from an infant's bottle. Looking into the mouth, the EMT should observe the frenulum, the short flap of tissue that attaches the lips to the gums and the tongue to the floor of the mouth, to see if it is torn. Normally it is difficult to tear the frenulum, but forced bottle feeding can cause a laceration to this tissue.

After finishing the assessment of the child's head, the EMT should perform a complete examination of the body, with the exception of the genitals, observing for bruises and other signs of child abuse. Table 44-4 lists some of the physical signs that suggest child abuse. The following sections on bruising, bites, burns, and broken bones describe these signs in detail.

BRUISING

The single most significant indicator of physical child abuse may be bruises in unusual places, unexplained bruises, or bruises in various stages of healing. A bruise, also known as a contusion or ecchymosis, is a collection of blood under the skin that occurs as a result of trauma. Bruises typically heal in approximately one week.

During the healing process the bruise changes colors. Initially, and for the first few days, the bruise is a deep purple, referred to as a *black and blue*. By week's end the bruise usually lightens to become brown and then eventually becomes greenish. After the first week the bruise becomes yellow or tan and heals. The presence of multiple bruises in various stages of healing suggest repeated trauma and should be viewed suspiciously.

Similarly, bruises in unusual places should also be cause for concern. Usual locations for bruises are the knees and the elbows, as a result of a fall, for example. Unusual places for bruises include the inside of the upper arm, the ribs, or the inner thighs. These bruises may be the result of forceful grabbing of the child. This nonaccidental distribution of bruises is suggestive of child abuse.

Finally, bruises are usually the result of trauma, and therefore an event, or mechanism of injury, can be linked to each bruise. In the case of child abuse, the mechanism of injury that supposedly caused the bruise often does not match the location of the bruise, or the healing of the bruises, by staging, does not match the timing of the incident.

The EMT should also make note of the time and date of the incident and which adult was responsible for the child at the time of the incident. Bruises that appear after the noncustodial parent has had visitation, such as weekends or vacations, may be cause for concern.

Bruises to the face are of particular concern. Eye injuries, resulting in a loss of vision, loss of teeth, and traumatic brain injury can result from facial

Table 44-4 Physical Examination Findings Suggesting Child Abuse

1. Bruising
   a. Bruising inconsistent with mechanism of injury
   b. Atypical locations for bruise
   c. Bruises in multiple stages of healing
2. Bite
   a. Back
   b. Arms
   c. Thighs
   d. Genitals
3. Burns
   a. Cigarette
      i. Palms of hands
      ii. Soles of feet
   b. Hot water immersion
      i. Stocking burn
      ii. Glove burn
      iii. Donut burn
   c. Stoves
      i. Grill marks
4. Broken bones
   a. Multiple fractures
   b. Spiral fractures

trauma, and all of these injuries have lifelong implications. Bruises of the face, lips, and mouth can be the result of a fall, but also can result from a slap or a punch. Slap or punch injury may reflect a parent's problem with anger control and inappropriate coping mechanisms when dealing with frustration over the child's behavior. Figure 44.1 shows bruises around a child's mouth suggesting the child was gagged.

Of special concern are bruises that are clustered and/or that form regular recurrent patterns. These regular recurrent patterns can reflect the shape of objects that were used to inflict trauma. Objects used as a whip or switch may leave a distinctive mark that helps identify what was used. For example, electrical cords will leave loops of bruise on the skin, as seen in Figure 44.2, or the buckle of a belt may leave a squared bruise on the skin.

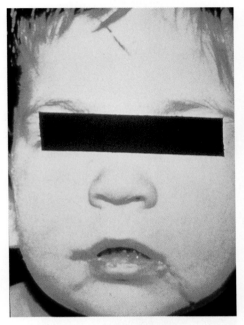

Figure 44.1 Odd bruises are an indication of child abuse

BITES

Many parents have experienced the dismay of finding out their child has bitten someone else's child. Although this behavior is natural, it is not acceptable and the child is quickly corrected. However, an adult biting a child is never acceptable.

Adult bite marks are distinguishable from a child's bite marks because they form a larger semi-circle of puncture marks than a child's. The shape of the punctures also helps to differentiate adult human bite marks from other puncture wounds. Adult incisors leave a narrow rectangular puncture mark whereas a child's canines leave a triangular puncture mark.

Again, the location of the bite mark may help distinguish accidental from intentional injury. Children typically bite each other on the hand or forearm. Bites on a child's shoulders, back, or inner thighs would be suspicious.

BURNS

A child may, by accident, pull a hot sauce pan from the stove and receive a scalding burn or may run hot water into the bathtub and then get burned when he steps into the tub. These unfortunate burns are an experience of youth. Burns of concern are nonaccidental burns, such as those caused by cigarettes, immersion burns, and pattern burns. These burns should never be part of a childhood.

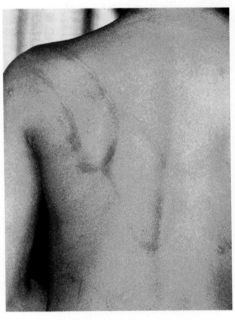

Figure 44.2 Pattern bruises are suggestive of child abuse

A cigarette burn leaves a characteristic small round burn that is distinctive and cannot be easily confused with other burns. A parent, in a moment of rage, will often use any convenient object to inflict pain on the child. In some cases the object is the lit cigarette in the parent's hand. Using the cigarette like a brand, the parent burns the child's palms, back, buttocks, or soles of the feet.

A scald burn also has a characteristic pattern. When a child sticks a foot into scalding hot water, there is splashing as the child reflexively pulls the limb out of the water. As a result the accidental scald burn has an irregular border and associated smaller "splash" burns.

A nonaccidental immersion scald occurs when a parent forcibly holds a limb underwater. A nonaccidental immersion scald is the result of a forceful restraint of the child, because even infants will reflexively withdraw their legs. Burns from a forced immersion in scalding hot water will leave a characteristic dunking pattern. There is a clear line of demarcation where the burn ends. If just the hands or feet are immersed, then the burn will have a glove-like or sock-like appearance. Since the child cannot pull away or kick, there are not burns from side splash.

If the child's entire torso is immersed in scalding hot water in the bathtub, a characteristic "donut" burn may occur. As the child's buttocks rests on the bottom

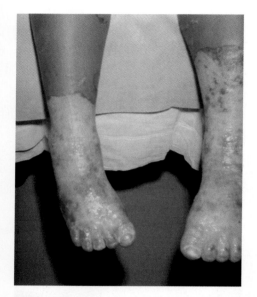

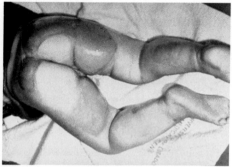

Figure 44.3 Burns in a pattern are suggestive of child abuse

of the bathtub, and away from the scalding hot water, the genitalia are spared. This action leaves a characteristic bull's eye or donut appearance to the burn.

Another burn of concern is a patterned burn. These burns are the result of forced contact with an object, such as a hot curling iron, stove burner, or a hot water radiator. These burns have a characteristic striped or circular pattern. Figure 44.3 shows burns suggestive of child abuse.

BROKEN BONES

Broken bones can be the result of trauma, and certain fractures are indicative of certain types of trauma. For example, a spiral fracture, a fracture that runs up the shaft of the bone like the ribbon on a barber's pole, is the result of a twisting action. A spiral fracture may occur when a limb is caught in a machine. However, a spiral fracture can also occur from child abuse.

A spiral fracture occurs when a parent grabs a child by the arm and applies a twisting action around the arm to inflict pain on the child. Although an EMT would not be expected to diagnosis a spiral fracture, which would require an X-ray, an EMT should suspect child abuse when she sees bruises in the pattern of a hand print on the child's inner arms and a swollen painful limb, particularly if the stated mechanism of injury, such as a fall, does not match the injury pattern.

Other fractures of concern are skull fractures, nasal fractures, and multiple long bone fractures. Although some children play "hard" and fall, breaking bones in the process, children who have a history of repeatedly breaking bones should be examined carefully.

SPECIAL CASE OF SUDDEN INFANT DEATH SYNDROME

When an infant dies unexpectedly and without apparent cause, the patient's death may be labeled *Sudden Infant Death Syndrome (SIDS)*. SIDS is not due to child abuse. However, child abuse can result in the death of an infant. Regardless of the cause of death, the EMT should proceed with routine care, including CPR if necessary, focusing on the emergency at hand and providing compassionate care to the parents for the loss of their child.

ASSESSMENT

Although physical signs of child abuse certainly are indicative of child abuse, parents may go to great lengths to conceal the abuse. Instead of looking for signs of abuse, the EMT should observe the child for unusual or suspicious behavior. Behavioral signs of possible child abuse include visible apprehension when other children are crying and inappropriate fear of the EMT. The child could also display an inappropriate affect or demonstrate extreme mood swings, for example, changing from tearfulness to elation in a matter of minutes. The EMT should also watch the parent's behavior. The parent may display agitation over the EMT's questioning or a complete indifference to the plight of the child. These observations are important to note on the patient care record, and the suspicion of child abuse should be reported to authorities.

SEXUAL ABUSE

A suspicion of child sexual abuse cannot be confirmed in the field, but sexual abuse may be suspected based on observation. For example, an EMT may observe, and thus suspect sexual abuse, if a child has difficulty in walking or sitting; the child cannot walk or sit because of the trauma to the genitals. The EMT may also observe blood in the child's pants. Bleeding from the genitals is not normal and suggests sexual abuse. The child may also complain of pain or itching in the genitals. These findings all suggest that sexual abuse may have occurred.

Generally it is inappropriate for an EMT to perform an external examination of the genitalia for contusions, lacerations, or bleeding. Instead, the EMT should report her suspicions of child sexual abuse to authorities. If the EMT is given torn, stained, or bloody underclothing from a child by a parent, it should placed in a paper bag and provided as evidence to a law enforcement officer.

TREATMENT

Treatment in the case of suspected child abuse should proceed as normal, focusing on the child's presenting problem and transporting the patient to the hospital for further treatment. It is not the place of the EMT to accuse a parent of child abuse even when child abuse is suspected.

EXCITED UTTERANCE

Sometimes, during the course of providing patient care, the child may make statements that incriminate the parents. If the EMT reports these statements, it is not hearsay.

Hearsay is reporting of one person's statement by another. Under the rules of law, hearsay testimony is generally not admissible in a court of law because hearsay is not considered to be direct evidence of the truth of a matter. However, there is an exception to that rule made in certain situations, such as child abuse.

When a person, such as a child, makes a spontaneous statement during a stressful time, called an **excited utterance,** the statement may be allowed into evidence. For example, if a distraught child said, "Mommy whipped me with a spoon," that might be considered an excited utterance and the EMT's documentation of that statement may be admitted into court as evidence that the child was beaten with a spoon.

Not only is the verbal utterance considered an admissible statement in court but the child's behaviors, observed and documented by the EMT, may be introduced as evidence in court. For example, a child responds emotionally to a question such as "Did Daddy touch you where your bathing suit covers?" and points at his genitals, that reaction and finger pointing would be considered a statement, and the EMT's documentation of the behavior may be admissible in court. These behaviors are taken into account because it is understood that a child may not be able to express himself in words but does have other means of expression. Therefore, an EMT should note all of the child's responses, such as trembling, crying, or pressured speech, when asked specific questions.

DISPOSITION AND DOCUMENTATION

After turning the child over to the hospital, the EMT should report the suspicion of child abuse. Every state and territoy has a mandated child abuse reporter law. **Mandated child abuse reporters** are certain groups of individuals, such as educators, law enforcement, day care workers, and EMTs, who are in a position to observe a child and report suspected child abuse.

As mandated reporters, EMTs must document (usually on a state-approved form) and report (usually on a special telephone line) their suspicions of child abuse. Generally that report must include the basis for the suspicion, actions taken to protect the child, the identity of the child, and often the location of other children who may be at risk.

In many states the failure to report suspected child abuse can expose the EMT to both criminal and civil penalties that include imprisonment and/or fines. However, to encourage child abuse reporting, the courts provide the EMT with protection from frivolous or unwarranted lawsuits brought by the parent.

Cultural Considerations

Every culture has common folk remedies that originated in earlier times before Western medicine was widely practiced. These traditional forms of healing include some practices that an EMT might perceive as child abuse.

For example, some Southeast Asians practice cao gio, or coin rubbing, to relieve pain, fever, abdominal pain, and even the cough from a common cold. Usually oil, such as tiger balm, containing camphor, oil of winter green or peppermint, or similar aromatic solution is applied liberally over the person's back and then a coin is rubbed repeatedly in a linear pattern until blood raises to the surface. This dermal abrasive technique leaves a distinctive striped pattern on the patient's back.

It should be emphasized that cao gio is not child abuse. The purpose of the use of cao gio is well intentioned and is not intended to cause injury or harm to the child. False claims of child abuse can lead to alienation of this population and seed distrust of EMS among people of this culture.

An EMT who, in good faith, reports suspected child abuse is granted immunity from lawsuits for reporting the suspected child abuse, even if it eventually is discovered that child abuse did not occur and that the allegation was false.

It is important for the EMT to report suspected child abuse. The National Child Abuse and Neglect Data System (NCANDS) reports that two thirds of cases of reported child abuse are investigated and approximately 30% of reported cases of child abuse are true. Furthermore, the vast majority of child abuse cases, more than 80%, involve children less than 4 years old. If it were not for the EMTs reporting their suspicions, these cases of child abuse might go undetected until the child is either seriously injured or dies.

ELEMENTS OF PROPER DOCUMENTATION

It is critical that the EMT accurately document her observations and the child's and parent's statements. An abusive parent may collaborate with others, or even with the child, to fabricate a story to "explain away" the injuries. This deceit is often discovered when the physician compares the EMT's written report to the parent's explanations. For this reason the EMT should try to document the parent's explanations of the cause of the injury as accurately as possible, using the parent's own words whenever possible.

The EMT should first start by describing the scene, then documenting the history, using the parent's and child's own words and setting direct quotes off in quotation marks whenever possible.

The EMT should also take time to exactly describe the physical assessment findings. When documenting, for example, an intoxicated parent, the EMT should avoid judgmental terms, such as "mother was drunk," in favor of descriptive terms, such as "half-empty beer bottles were strewn around the floor and the smell of an alcoholic beverage was on the mother's breath." These descriptions should be as specific and objective as possible.

Next the EMT should state what led her to suspect child abuse. The EMT should provide as much detail as possible. Some EMTs even use human body outlines to mark the exact placement of bruises, bites, burns, and broken bones.

Finally, the EMT should note all protective actions taken to prevent further harm to the child, including calling for law enforcement, if needed. The EMT should document that the child was transported to the safety of the hospital. Next, the EMT should document on the patient care report that the suspicion of child abuse was reported and was also reported to other mandated reporters, such as the emergency doctors and nurses.

In many instances the EMT must also complete a special child abuse reporting form as well as the patient care report. These forms should be filled out completely and with as much detail as possible before leaving the hospital. It is unprofessional and unacceptable to report suspicions to another mandated reporter and expect the mandated reporter to report the child abuse for the EMT. EMTs have a duty to report child abuse and cannot reassign that responsibility to others.

CONCLUSION

An EMT has a duty to report suspected child abuse to the proper authorities and to protect the child from any further harm. The EMT must keep her duty to the patient foremost in her mind and not let emotions interfere with the provision of emergency medical care to the child. It is not the place of the EMT to accuse the parent of child abuse. Rather, through a combination of careful assessment and proper documentation, the EMT can help prevent future child abuse by reporting suspicions of child abuse to the proper authorities.

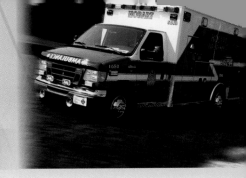

CASE STUDY Continued

Carney later hears that the infant died in the hospital and that the boyfriend has been arrested on suspicion of child abuse. Following his suspicions, Carney had elected to report that he suspected child abuse, and he was glad he did. Carney knows there is another child at home and the mother is pregnant. A few days later, police detectives knock at the ambulance bay door looking for the crew that took care of the infant. Apparently the boyfriend had violently shaken the baby to get it to stop crying. Now the police detectives want a statement from the EMS crew.

Key Concepts Revisited

- Child abuse can be an act of commission or an act of omission.

- Child abuse can be physical and/or sexual.

- Child abuse can also be the result of neglect.

- Lack of parental supervision can be a form of child neglect.

- Juvenile delinquency can be a sign of child neglect.

- Injuries that do not match the mechanism of injury may indicate child abuse.

- Particular types of bruises, bites, burns, and broken bones may indicate child abuse.
  - Bruising
    - Bruising inconsistent with mechanism of injury
    - Atypical locations for bruise
    - Bruises in multiple stages of healing
  - Bite
    - Back
    - Arms
    - Thighs
    - Genitals
  - Burns
    - Cigarette
      - Palms of hands
      - Soles of feet
    - Hot water immersion
      - Stocking burn
      - Glove burn
      - Donut burn
    - Stoves
      - Grill marks
  - Broken bones
    - Multiple fractures
    - Spiral fractures
- Accurate documentation of events is important in a case of child abuse.

Review Questions

1. What is the definition of child abuse?
2. What are some parental indicators of child abuse?
3. What is shaken baby syndrome?
4. What is sexual abuse?
5. What is sexual molestation?
6. What are the four forms of neglect?
7. What are the provisions of the abandoned infant protection act?
8. What are some signs of a head injury in a child?
9. What are some signs of child abuse?
10. Why are EMTs mandated reporters of suspected child abuse?

Key Terms

Abandoned infant protection act
Child neglect
Excited utterance
Mandated child abuse reporter

Sexual abuse
Sexual molestation
Shaken baby syndrome

Further Study

Centers for Disease Control and Prevention (CDC). National Center for Injury Prevention and Control. Division of Violence Prevention. Atlanta, Georgia: 2007.

Child Abuse Prevention Network. Available at http://www.child-abuse.com (information about child abuse and neglect and how the EMT can report it).

Crosson-Tower, Cynthia. *Understanding Child Abuse and Neglect.* Boston: Allyn & Bacon, 2008.

Tennyson Center for Children. Available at http://www.childabuse.org (excellent site for information about the signs of child abuse and mandated reporting of child abuse).

UNIT (45) Children with Special Challenges

An estimated 12 million children in the United States have special health care needs. **Children with special health care needs (CSHCN)** are defined as those who have or are at risk for having chronic physical, developmental, behavioral, or emotional conditions that require health and other related services not routinely required by children who are developing normally. In the past, most children with special challenges did not survive past infancy, many never leaving the hospital. Today, medical advances in science and technology have allowed these children to survive for years at home, usually under the care of parents or other caregivers who have been trained to manage their daily care.

In the course of their practice, Emergency Medical Technicians (EMTs) will encounter children who have some sort of physical or mental disability. Some of these children with disabilities are dependent on advanced technology for survival. These children frequently require emergency medical services, and the EMT should be familiar with some of the more common tools used to help these children live comfortably.

National Education Standards
The Emergency Medical Technician (EMT) will demonstrate a simple depth and breadth of understanding of the health care implications, anatomy, physiology, assessment, management, and technology of children with special challenges.

Key Concepts

- EMTs are called to care for children with special challenges because of equipment failure, exacerbation of their condition, or onset of a new medical condition or injury when the parent or caregiver can no longer manage alone.

- The EMT's knowledge of normal baseline mental status and vital signs in children must be modified for children with special challenges.

- Assessment and management of children with special challenges require communication and partnership with the parents or caregivers of these children.

- The Pediatric Assessment Triangle can be modified for use with the AVPU scale in assessment of children with special challenges.

- The EMT should be familiar with the special medical needs and equipment of children who are technologically assisted.

- Children with special challenges include those with physical disabilities.

- Children with hearing impairment communicate through a variety of methods.

- Cognitive impairment in children with special challenges such as Down syndrome can range from mild to profound.

- Behavioral disabilities affect how the child interacts with people and present unique challenges for the EMT.

- Children with special challenges requiring transport should be transported to a facility that is familiar with the children, their conditions, and ongoing treatments whenever possible.

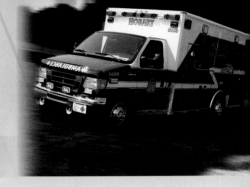

CASE STUDY

"Unit 16 from dispatch: Respond to infant having difficulty breathing. Time out: 11:45."

Mariah and Kelsey look at each other with dread. Whenever a call for a child comes in, they know it will either be minor or really bad. An infant having difficulty breathing sounds bad. While en route to the scene, they discuss the pediatric equipment they need to take into the house with them and the possible need for an ALS intercept.

Upon arrival they are met at the door by a man who appears to be calm as he directs them back to the baby's room. As Kelsey enters the room, she is met by the infant's mother, Katarina, who is holding the baby. Katarina explains Wyatt is 6 months old and was born with a heart problem. He has been having increasing trouble breathing since last night. His breathing has gotten faster as the morning has progressed, and he has not been interested in eating today, which is very unusual for him.

Wyatt is quiet, watching his mother talk, and obviously working hard to breathe, with retractions between his ribs. As his mother continues to provide Kelsey with the baby's history, Wyatt turns to look at Kelsey and Mariah as they move about his room. Mariah

attempts to place an oxygen mask over Wyatt's face. Katarina offers to hold the oxygen in front of Wyatt's face, as she explains he never leaves the mask on anyway.

As Kelsey continues to make a visual assessment, using the Pediatric Assessment Triangle, she determines his appearance is normal for his age. He is making eye contact, but he is quiet, not cooing or crying. His work of breathing is abnormal with retractions and audible wheezing. His skin is pale, with some cyanosis present around his mouth.

Kelsey also notices that Wyatt has familiar characteristics: a flatter face, slanted eyes, and tongue protruding out of his mouth. Kelsey is not surprised when Katarina adds, "Oh, and Wyatt has Down Syndrome." Kelsey's nephew also has Down Syndrome.

Critical Thinking Questions

1. What is Kelsey's next step in assessment?
2. What congenital heart defects are associated with Down syndrome?
3. What physical characteristics of Down syndrome might make managing Wyatt's respiratory difficulty more challenging?

INTRODUCTION

Emergency Medical Services (EMS) is most often called for children with special challenges when there is a crisis the parent or caregiver cannot handle on her own. This crisis can be an equipment failure, a sudden onset of an illness or injury that may be unrelated to the child's normal condition, or an exacerbation of a condition the child already has, such as respiratory compromise. EMTs can also sometimes be called because the caregiver is new at caring for a special child.

CHILDREN WITH SPECIAL CHALLENGES

When assessing a child who has special challenges, the EMT must realize that his idea of a normal baseline for mental status or vital signs may not be that child's baseline. The EMT should realize that many of the children with chronic medical conditions or who rely on technologic equipment have vital signs outside the normal range for their age. The parents or caregivers usually have a clear understanding of what is normal and abnormal for the child. The EMT should rely on the information provided by the caregiver.

The techniques used for assessment and management of the airway, breathing, and circulation are often the same as those used for other children, except in certain circumstances where technologic equipment alters the management.

ASSESSMENT

When assessing a child with special challenges, the parents or caregivers are the most important resource for the EMT. They are familiar with the daily mental, physical, and behavioral condition of the child and their equipment. They are also the first ones to recognize when something is abnormal in the child's daily routine. They are the single best source for providing the EMT with the child's baselines, general appearance, oxygen saturation, vital signs, medical history, medications, and allergies.

The EMT will need to use his knowledge of pediatric assessment and then modify those assessments to the child's developmental level. The caregiver will be able to provide the child's developmental age, weight, and baseline vital signs, as well as troubleshooting the equipment. It is vital that the EMT use the assistance of the child's caregiver.

BASELINE ASSESSMENT

The modifications the EMT must make when assessing children with special challenges begins with establishing the normal baseline for the child. The EMT should always perform common assessment elements, such as looking for a medical alert bracelet, form, or card that provides important information about the medical problems, normal baselines, and medications that some states require caregivers of children with special challenges to have available. Table 45-1 lists additional important modifications in the assessment of children with special challenges.

PEDIATRIC ASSESSMENT TRIANGLE

The Pediatric Assessment Triangle (PAT), introduced in Unit 43, is a quick, observational tool to assess the severity of a child's condition and help form a general impression (Figure 45.1). However, the PAT has several limitations and needs to be modified because of the altered baseline physiology of children with special challenges.

APPEARANCE

Appearance, which reflects the adequacy of oxygenation, ventilation, perfusion, and mental status of the patient, is the element of the PAT that may need the most modification in children with special challenges. These children often have muscle tone abnormality, such as spasticity seen in cerebral palsy (Figure 45.2), or decreased interactivity, as seen in children with brain injury or developmental delays. However, children with special challenges can usually recognize their caregivers by look or by hearing their voice. The EMT should focus on the strength and quality of the child's cry or her facial expression as a sign of distress.

WORK OF BREATHING

Chronic respiratory problems are often commonly seen in children with special challenges. All children with fever or with a respiratory illness or injury, such as pneumonia or chest trauma, will exhibit an increase in respiratory rate in an attempt to compensate. Children with special challenges have less oxygen reserves and decompensate far more quickly than other children. They

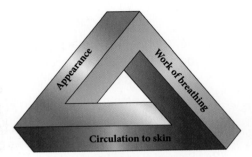

Figure 45.1 Pediatric Assessment Triangle

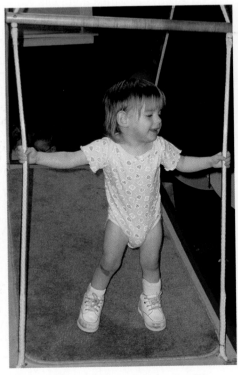

Figure 45.2 Some children with special challenges have abnormal muscle tone (Courtesy of KatyBeth Grayson Family)

1. Baselines: Ask the caregiver for the baseline vital signs, as well as the medical, physical, and behavioral conditions for the child.

2. Ask the caregiver what she thinks is wrong. The caregiver deals with the child on a daily basis and is usually the person who called for help. Ask specifically how the child is "acting differently today"?

3. If the child is stable, obtain the history on scene, allowing the caregiver to guide the EMT in the approaches she knows work best in managing the child's care.

4. Always talk directly to the child, giving her ample time to respond. Stable specially challenged children may be slow to answer, but that does not mean they cannot answer. When communicating with children who are able to speak, use developmentally appropriate language, gestures, and techniques.

5. Children with special challenges may have little reserve when faced with what would normally be considered a minor illness. The common cold can become a life-threatening condition for some children with special challenges.

6. Remember the normal baseline vital signs may be outside the "normal range" when compared to children who do not have special challenges. Vital signs in specially challenged children may have a limited value, and the observations of the caregiver and the pediatric assessment triangle often have far more value than the vital signs.

7. Never assume a child with physical disabilities, such as spasticity seen in cerebral palsy, is also cognitively impaired. It is important to establish with the caregiver the child's cognitive ability and then assess and manage the child accordingly.

8. Be professional and polite, keeping in mind the families of children with special challenges have extensive experience with the health care system, some of which may have left them suspicious and initially untrusting of the ability of a health care provider to care for their child.

9. Always ask the caregivers what therapies or interventions have already been attempted to manage the child's emergency.

10. Always transport the child to the facility that is familiar with the child and her condition, if possible. Follow local protocols if unsure of destination and transport decisions.

show increased work of breathing much more quickly in the early stages of an acute illness or injury.

Assess for abnormal breath sounds such as stridor, wheezing, or grunting, keeping in mind that some children with special challenges, such as those with tracheostomy tubes, may have noisy breathing, which is normal for them.

Abnormal positioning, such as the tripod position or head bobbing, are visual signs of respiratory distress in all children. Some children with special challenges will normally present with mild retractions. The EMT should ask the caregiver if the retractions are baseline or more severe than normal. Nasal flaring is not a baseline condition, even in children with special challenges. Any child with nasal flaring is exhibiting an extreme work of breathing suggestive of potentially severe disease.

CIRCULATION TO SKIN

Children with special challenges often have skin color that may appear abnormal when compared to that of other children. For example, children with cyanotic congenital heart disease or chronic lung disease often have bluish lips, mucous membranes, fingernail beds, and extremities, all of which are normal for them. Children with liver disease may appear to have a yellow tint to their skin, and those with cancer may be chronically pale. When assessing the circulation to skin element of the PAT in a child with special challenges, it is necessary to establish what the child's baseline skin color is by asking the child's caregiver.

PRIMARY ASSESSMENT

Once the PAT has been completed, the primary assessment should be performed, adjusting for the normal baseline airway, breathing, circulation, and mental status of the child with special challenges.

AIRWAY

The airway of a child with special challenges may be more difficult to keep open because of poor muscle tone and head control or because of secretions the child cannot manage. Place padding under the shoulders to keep the head in a neutral position and align the airway. Use the chin lift or jaw thrust maneuver to open the airway and always have suction available. ALS intercept should be requested for children with special challenges experiencing airway compromise.

BREATHING

Assessment of breathing follows the same process as for any other patient. Establish the respiratory rate and quality, and listen for abnormal breath sounds, keeping in mind that the child with special challenges may have noisy breathing or not be able to sit still during the assessment.

Obtain a pulse oximetry reading, establishing from the caregiver the baseline, and compare. Give supplemental oxygen to any child with signs of increased work of breathing and respiratory distress. In the child with special challenges, if the caregiver is able to provide a baseline oxygen saturation level, attempt to provide oxygen to achieve or maintain that baseline.

CIRCULATION

Assessment of the pulse (rate and quality), skin temperature, and capillary refill time do not usually differ in children with special challenges. Once the EMT has established the baseline circulatory status from the caregiver, he can accurately interpret the assessment finding through comparison.

Abnormal findings in circulatory status may indicate the presence of hypoperfusion, and the EMT must keep in mind that children with special challenges have a lower threshold for compensation. The management of hypoperfusion is no different than it is for normal children; oxygen, positioning, and ventilatory support.

MENTAL STATUS

The baseline mental status of children with special challenges is often abnormal when compared to other children. The child's caregiver will be the best resource for the EMT in establishing the child's baseline mental status. The EMT should use the appearance element of the PAT and assess the level of consciousness using AVPU (alert, verbal, painful, and unresponsive), then compare his findings with the child's baseline mental status to determine any true abnormalities. When assessing the child's motor activity, look for purposeful movement of extremities, seizures, posturing, or abnormal flaccidity. Any change from her baseline mental status should be treated immediately.

HISTORY AND SECONDARY ASSESSMENT

When assessing children with special challenges, listening to the caregiver is essential. The caregiver is the best resource for establishing the child's baseline status, as well as providing information as to the best methods of approach in direct interaction with the child.

> **Street Smart**
>
> Use of the Pediatric Glasgow Coma Scale in children with special challenges is not applicable for children whose baseline cognitive and physiologic problems may affect the score. The EMT should simply describe the child's mental status as being different from her baseline mental status.

Table 45-2 Transport Considerations for Children with Special Challenges

1. Children who are dependent on home oxygen should be kept at the same rate of oxygen flow as they use at home, providing there are no signs of respiratory distress, during transport.

2. A child on a home ventilator should be transported using her personal ventilator as long as there is no equipment failure or difficulty involved. If the potential for ventilator (equipment) failure is present, ventilate the child with positive pressure ventilations using a bag-valve-mask (BVM). Always transport the home ventilator with the child, even if ventilations are being administered by BVM, so the ventilator can be evaluated by the hospital for problems or setting adjustments.

3. Immobilize the child in the position of comfort if the child has poor muscle control or increased muscle tone. Transport any special equipment (wheelchair, special seat, feeding pump, suctioning device) to the hospital with the child if possible.

4. Transport the child to the facility that is familiar with the child's special challenges and ongoing care whenever possible.

When performing a secondary assessment, inspect the child's entire body, but do not allow the child to become chilled. Children with special challenges often have minimal body fat and are at a higher risk for developing hypothermia. As with all patients, make sure to respect and protect the child's modesty during the physical examination.

TRANSPORT

EMTs may be faced with additional challenges when transporting children with special challenges, especially those who rely on technology assistance. All children should be secured in the ambulance, using accepted restraint systems. Children with special challenges often require special transport considerations based on their specific needs, such as oxygen delivery systems, ventilators, and positioning. Table 45-2 lists some transport considerations for children with special challenges.

TECHNOLOGY-ASSISTED DEVICES

One group of children with special challenges are those requiring *technology-assisted devices* such as tracheostomies, mechanical ventilators, central venous access devices, feeding tubes, and cerebrospinal fluid shunts. It is important for EMTs to be familiar with these children and their special medical needs, as well as their specialized types of equipment and the types of interventions required in an emergency.

TRACHEOSTOMIES

A tracheostomy or *stoma* is an opening in the front of the neck that has been surgically created to allow for the placement of a rigid tube, called a **tracheostomy tube.** Children who require this rigid tube all suffer from a condition that requires the need for an artificial airway to maintain adequate oxygenation and ventilation. Table 45-3 lists several reasons a child may require a tracheostomy. Figure 45.3 shows an illustration of a child with a tracheostomy tube in place.

ASSESSMENT

The child with a tracheostomy may encounter problems related to the tracheostomy tube. The tube can become obstructed by foreign bodies,

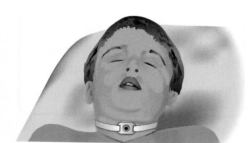

Figure 45.3 A tracheostomy tube creates an open airway for a child who may have difficulty maintaining one on his own

Table 45-3 Examples of Conditions Requiring a Tracheostomy

1. Children with head injuries causing unconsciousness for a prolonged period or who are unable to breathe independently
2. Muscular or neurologic disease or injury causing paralysis
3. Children who require assistance with removal of secretions from the trachea (cerebral palsy)

secretions that are difficult to clear, improper positioning, a kink in the tube itself, or incorrect insertion of the tracheostomy tube.

The EMT should look for signs and symptoms of hypoxia, including a change in the child's baseline level of consciousness; restlessness, cyanosis, tachypnea, tachycardia, intercostal muscle use, sternal retractions, increased work of breathing, absent or decreased breath sounds, or lack of chest rise and diaphoresis.

MANAGEMENT

Airway and breathing compromise is a life-threatening situation that will quickly lead to death if not immediately managed. If secretions are present, the EMT can use a small French suction catheter to clear out the tracheostomy tube to help the child breathe more easily.

If oxygen delivery is necessary, the oxygen mask should be directed over the tracheostomy. If ventilations are necessary, the EMT can accomplish this by attaching a bag-valve-mask directly to the tracheostomy tube (most will fit; others may require an adapter that the parents will often have) and ventilate as usual. Alternatively, the EMT can ventilate the patient with a mask over the mouth and nose while sealing the tracheostomy site with a finger and looking for the rise and fall of the chest with ventilation (Figure 45.4).

If an EMT is having difficulty managing a child with a tracheostomy, he should arrange for an advanced life support (ALS) intercept while beginning transport to the closest appropriate hospital.

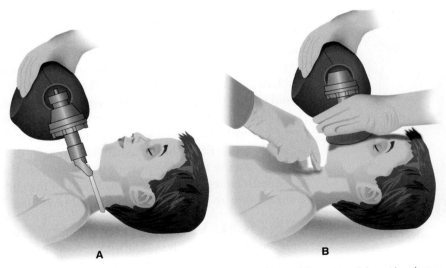

Figure 45.4 A. The child with a tracheostomy tube can be ventilated by attaching the bag-valve-mask directly to the tracheostomy tube. B. The child with a tracheostomy may also be ventilated by sealing the tracheostomy with a finger and providing mask ventilation over the mouth and nose

Table 45-4 Conditions Requiring Ongoing Mechanical Ventilator Support
1. Chronic lung disease (bronchopulmonary dysplasia, or BPD)
2. Weakened respiratory muscles (muscular dystrophy)
3. Cervical spinal cord injury
4. Traumatic brain injury

MECHANICAL VENTILATORS

Some children who have problems breathing adequately on their own are dependent on machines to breathe for them. These machines are called **mechanical ventilators** and can be very small and portable. Home ventilators assist children to breathe through positive pressure ventilation that pushes the air in with each breath at the appropriate tidal volume and pressure. Examples of conditions that may require mechanical ventilator use at home are listed in Table 45-4.

EMS may be called to respond for a child who is dependent on a mechanical ventilator, usually due to a diminished oxygen supply or malfunction of the ventilator. Home ventilators have back-up batteries; however, they have a relatively short life. Therefore, a sustained power outage can become a dire emergency for a child dependent on a mechanical ventilator to breathe.

ASSESSMENT

Ask the child's caregivers if there has been a change in the child's condition and baseline. Does the child have the signs and symptoms of a new illness, increased seizures, or decreased level of consciousness, or is the child taking any new medicines? If a child who is dependent on technology to breathe appears cyanotic, has an increased work of breathing, or is showing other signs of respiratory distress, immediately check the equipment after assessing the child.

MANAGEMENT

The parent or caregiver will know how to operate the child's ventilator, and the EMT should not attempt to manipulate it. If the child is having respiratory difficulty while on the ventilator, the EMT should disconnect the child's tracheostomy tube from the ventilator tubing, suction the tube as necessary, and use a BVM to assist the child's ventilations. If the child's respiratory distress improves after several ventilations with BVM and high-flow oxygen, the problem may be a faulty ventilator. The EMT who is providing ventilation to a child should arrange to intercept with an ALS provider.

If the child who is dependent on a mechanical ventilator requires transport for another reason, the parent may choose to bring the ventilator if it is portable. The EMT should assist the parent in this situation. Alternatively, the EMT can use a BVM to provide ventilation for the child during transport. Any questions regarding the management of the child on a ventilator should be directed to an on-line medical control physician.

CENTRAL VENOUS CATHETERS

Children who require frequent intravenous medications or frequent blood sampling often have a **central venous catheter** in place. This is an intravenous catheter that is placed in one of the large vessels, often in the upper arm or the upper chest (Figure 45.5). Some of the common reasons for a central venous access device are listed in Table 45-5.

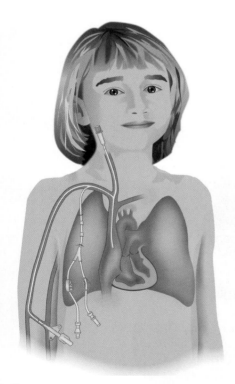

Figure 45.5 Central venous catheters are used to administer intravenous medications or to withdraw blood samples from the venous system

Table 45-5 Reasons for a Central Venous Access Device

1. Repeat blood sampling
2. Administration of blood products
3. Administration of large concentrations and/or quantities of fluids
4. Administration of medications (chemotherapy)
5. Administration of drugs that cause damage to small veins if given peripherally (potassium and some chemotherapy drugs)
6. Total parenteral nutrition (TPN)

ASSESSMENT

EMTs called to assess a child with a central venous access catheter may find the child is showing signs and symptoms of infection, including redness, swelling, tenderness, and drainage at the insertion site; fever and chills; and possibly circulatory compromise as seen with sepsis. If the caregiver indicates the EMT was called because the catheter appears to be plugged, the EMT should explain he is not trained in managing the line and call for ALS assist.

MANAGEMENT

Because the EMT does not administer intravenous (IV) medications or draw blood samples, the focus of care will be on managing any conditions the child may be experiencing as a result of an infected or plugged catheter. Manage any problems with airway, breathing, and circulation, as with any other emergency.

If there is bleeding from the catheter, the EMT should kink the tubing and then find a clamp to close off the tubing to prevent further bleeding. Follow local protocols or on-line direction regarding the management of bleeding directly from the catheter. If the bleeding is from the site of entry, direct pressure with a sterile dressing may be applied while the child is being transported to the closest appropriate hospital.

FEEDING TUBES

Feeding tubes are soft, flexible tubes that are placed into the stomach, either through the nose or through the anterior abdominal wall. These tubes are used to provide liquid nutrition to children who are otherwise unable to obtain nutrition. The tube placed through the nose is called a *nasogastric tube,* while the tube that is surgically placed through the anterior abdominal wall is called a *gastrostomy tube* (Figure 45.6).

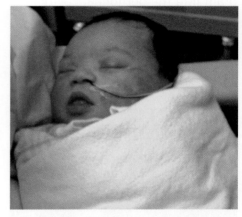

Figure 45.6 Nasogastric and gastrostomy tubes can be used to supply nutrition to a child who cannot eat by mouth (Courtesy Paul Nyane Family)

ASSESSMENT

Children with feeding tubes may require assistance from EMS because of tube-related problems such as dislodgement of the tube due to trauma, inadvertent balloon deflations or rupture of the internal balloon. Usually, the caregiver has been trained to reinsert a nasogastric tube.

The EMT may also be called because of illness caused by the feeding tube. Gastric irritation may occur in patients with gastrostomy tubes, leading to ulceration of the stomach. Children with gastric ulcer because of mechanical trauma from gastrostomy tubes will present with the same signs and symptoms as seen in any patient with ulcers, including abdominal pain, irritability, bright red blood in the emesis, coffee-ground gastric drainage from the G-tube lumen, or tarry stools. Look for additional signs of pain, including increased pulse and respiratory rates, discomfort with abdominal palpation, and decreased activity to avoid pain with movement.

Stoma-related problems include skin irritation around the stoma from leakage of gastric fluid around the tube that can progress into an infection (cellulitis). Signs and symptoms of infection of the stoma include a red, warm, tender, swollen area around the stoma, discomfort associated with manipulation of the tube or button, and resistance to feedings due to pain.

MANAGEMENT

Rarely will a feeding tube contribute to an emergency situation, but an ambulance may be called to transport a child who has such a tube. The EMT should take care to keep the site of the tube clean and avoid any pulling of the tube. Occasionally the child will need transport to the hospital if a feeding tube has been accidentally removed. The EMT should never attempt to replace the tube, but should bring the tube with the child to the emergency department where a physician can manage the problem.

CEREBROSPINAL FLUID (CSF) SHUNTS

A **cerebrospinal fluid (CSF) shunt** is a special catheter that is used to drain excess CSF off the brain and into the abdomen, where it can be easily absorbed. There are several conditions that do not allow adequate drainage of CSF from the brain and thus require this therapy. These shunts, also called **ventriculo-peritoneal (VP) shunts,** are under the skin and extend from the ventricles of the brain down the side of the neck and chest wall and into the peritoneal cavity (Figure 45.7).

An EMT may be called to care for a child who is suffering from a complication of her primary disease or as a result of the shunt itself. Infection is a common reason for emergency evaluation. Fever in a child with a shunt must be evaluated immediately. Infection of the shunt can result in brain infection.

Failure of the shunt to work also may result in a rise in intracranial pressure if CSF is unable to adequately drain. This condition is evidenced by vomiting, altered mental status, seizures, or cardiorespiratory compromise.

ASSESSMENT

When CSF shunts malfunction, the result is an increase in intracranial pressure (ICP). The signs and symptoms are the same as increased ICP in any patient. Look for a change in the level of consciousness, including irritability, unusual sleepiness, lethargy, and eventually coma. Additional signs and symptoms include headache, nausea, and vomiting, bulging fontanels in infants; difficulty walking in children who are mobile; and periods of apnea and seizures. If infection is present, the child may have fever and general malaise in addition to the signs and symptoms of increased ICP.

MANAGEMENT

The EMT should treat the child with a CSF shunt for the presenting problem as indicated. Airway, breathing, and circulation management is done in the same manner as for any other child. The child with possible shunt failure or infection should be evaluated immediately by a physician. Transport should be to a facility capable of providing pediatric neurosurgery.

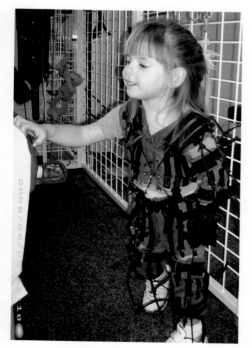

Figure 45.7 A cerebrospinal shunt allows drainage of CSF from the brain into the peritoneal cavity

Ventricular catheter

Ventriculoatrial (VA) shunt

Ventriculoperitoneal (VP) shunt

Figure 45.8 Children with special challenges include those with physical disabilities (Courtesy of KatyBeth Grayson Family)

PHYSICAL DISABILITIES

Children with special challenges include those with physical disabilities caused by congenital birth defects, premature or traumatic birth deficits, or traumatic injury (Figure 45.8). EMTs should have an understanding of a child's disability, even when they are called for an unrelated emergency.

CONGENITAL HEART DEFECTS

Congenital heart defects (CHD) are any structural or functional anomaly of the heart or great vessels present at birth. Congenital heart defects are some of the most common birth defects, occurring in an estimated 4/1,000 to 50/1,000 live births. CHDs are considered the leading cause of death in neonates due to any congenital abnormality, even with a decline in recent years due to advances in medical technology, early detection, and better management. Table 45-6 lists the types of CHDs.

ASSESSMENT

Signs and symptoms of congenital heart disease are somewhat dependent on the location of the anomaly of the heart. Commonly these children are small for their age and have normally increased baseline heart and respiratory rates. Those with cyanotic heart disease, such as tetralogy of Fallot, will appear pale or with a bluish tint to their skin and baseline pulse oximeter readings in the low 80s. Many children with congenital heart disease can develop congestive heart failure.

Children who have progressed to congestive heart failure (CHF) have the same signs and symptoms as adults with this condition, including increased respiratory rate, tachycardia, subcostal and intercostal retractions, cyanosis or pallor, poor perfusion, delayed capillary refill, extremity edema, poor feeding, and/or sweating with feeding.

The parents or caregivers are the EMT's best resource in establishing which type of congenital defect exists, the progress or interventions that have taken place, and the child's baseline.

MANAGEMENT

Children with CHDs who are being managed at home prior to corrective surgery will often be on medications to control CHF. Some of these children will be small because they are not able to feed well. These children require supplemental feedings, and some may have feeding tubes as they await the definitive surgical procedure to correct the defect. As soon as the child is deemed big and strong enough, the surgical procedure to correct the defect will be performed.

The EMT's management will focus on management of the airway, breathing, and circulation; placing the child in the position of comfort; keeping her calm; and providing oxygen to maintain the child's baseline oximetry. Medical direction should be consulted and local protocols followed.

HEARING IMPAIRMENT

One of the most common disabilities in the United States is **hearing impairment,** the reduction in the ear's responsiveness to loudness and pitch. **Deafness** typically refers to a child who could not hear before she learned to talk, whereas **hard of hearing** indicates a child who has some hearing ability, usually with the use of hearing aids. Approximately 1 million children from birth to age 21 are affected by hearing impairment. Of those, an estimated one third has additional disabilities, including cognitive or visual challenges. Hearing impairment presents many challenges for the patient and the EMT during a medical emergency.

ASSESSMENT

Children with hearing impairments are often frightened during an emergency. Their ability to communicate through different methods can cause frustration and raise anxiety for both them and the EMT. The situation can become emotional and result in the child becoming uncooperative.

Table 45-6 Types of Congenital Heart Disease

Heart Defect	Description	Common Associated Conditions
Ventricular septal defect (VSD)	Opening in the wall (septum) between the ventricles Most common defect	Down syndrome Fetal alcohol syndrome
Pulmonic stenosis	Narrowing of the pulmonary artery	Rubella syndrome Noonan syndrome
Patent ductus arteriosus	Opening between the pulmonary artery and aorta that fails to close following birth	Rubella syndrome Down syndrome
Atrial-septal defect (ASD)	Opening in the wall (septum) between atria	Noonan syndrome Down syndrome Fetal alcohol syndrome
Coarctation of the aorta	Localized narrowing of the aorta Increased pressure before defect Decreased pressure past the defect	Turner syndrome Apert syndrome
Tetralogy of Fallot	Four defects include: Pulmonic stenosis (narrowing of the pulmonary artery) Ventricular septal defect Malposition of the aorta (arises from septal defect or the right ventricle) Right ventricular hypertrophy (enlarged right ventricle)	Down syndrome Fetal alcohol syndrome
Atrioventricular canal defect	Opening in the wall (septum) between the atrium and ventricles Tricuspid and mitral valve abnormalities Oxygenated blood mixes with deoxygenated blood	Down syndrome
Atrioventricular valve defect	Defect in valve in which blood flows from the atria to the ventricles Left atrium to left ventricle → mitral valve Right atrium to right ventricle → tricuspid valve	Down syndrome
Tricuspid atresia	Failure of the tricuspid valve to develop No communication from right atrium to right ventricle	
Hypoplastic left heart syndrome	Incomplete or underdeveloped left side of the heart	
Transposition of great vessels	Pulmonary artery arises from the left ventricle Aorta arises from the right ventricle	Diabetes Prediabetes in mother

The EMT must maintain a calm demeanor, using the parent or caregiver as the bridge of communication.

The child's level of hearing impairment can range from a small decrease in hearing usual sounds to a complete loss of hearing all sounds. Children may wear hearing aids that improve their hearing levels; however, most who have had hearing impairment have learned to use sign language or read lips to communicate. It is important for the EMT to recognize that children who are lip reading may only understand a small amount of what is being said. The EMT must make sure he is down on the child's level, facing her and presenting the child with a clear view of his mouth, while speaking normally at all times.

Some children may have undergone a procedure that surgically placed a device, called a **cochlear implant,** which converts sounds to electrical impulses, sending them directly to the auditory nerve. Cochlear implants have helped many children and adults improve hearing loss and their communication abilities (Figure 45.9).

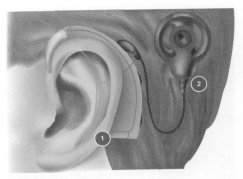

Figure 45.9 Cochlear implant

MANAGEMENT

Children with hearing impairments may present a larger challenge of communication, but their medical emergencies are treated the same as any other patient's. Enlist the aid of family and friends who are familiar with the child's communication methods to explain to the child what treatments will be applied, especially if it is a procedure that may cause anxiety or discomfort.

COGNITIVE DISABILITY

Cognitive is the term that refers to the mental processes of comprehension, judgment, memory, and reasoning. **Cognitive impairment** refers to an alteration in any of these processes. Several types of cognitive disabilities can affect children. Cognitive impairment can be caused by infections or exposure to toxins, trauma, metabolic disorders, nutritional inadequacy, chromosome abnormality, psychiatric disorders, environmental factors, and unknown prenatal influences.

Children with cognitive impairment commonly have some form of physical disabilities or impairment. These disabilities may be a congenital defect or due to trauma, infections, or diseases that occurred anytime during their development following birth.

The child's level of impairment can range from mild (the child may be slow to develop and require specialized education to acquire practical skills of living) to profound (the child has gross delay, requires total care, and usually never develops beyond the mental age of a young infant).

The EMT may not be able to immediately discern cognitive impairment in a child with mild disability. The parents or caregivers will be able to establish the child's baseline abilities and health issues. It is important for the EMT to be sensitive to the parent's feelings when asking questions or referring to the child. Many parents do not approve of the use of the word *retarded* in reference to their child. The EMT may find that parents and caregivers prefer health care professionals to refer to the child as *special* and verify the child's disability by specifically asking about the child's level of *cognitive impairment.*

DOWN SYNDROME

Down syndrome is a congenital condition occurring in 1 in 800 to 1,000 live births. Most children with Down syndrome have some level of cognitive impairment ranging from mild to profound. Down syndrome was once believed to occur mostly in children born to mothers over the age of 35;

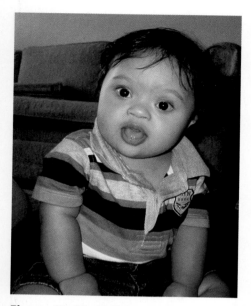

Figure 45.10 Child with Down syndrome (Courtesy of Paul Nyane Family)

in fact, in women over age 35, the chances of Down syndrome increase to 1 in 100 births. Research also shows the incidence drops to 1 in 1,500 births in women 30 years of age. However, despite these statistics, the majority of children with Down syndrome are born to women under the age of 35.

This condition is commonly referred to as Trisomy 21, because the most common of the three types of Down syndrome is caused by an additional or third 21st chromosome. The other two types of Down syndrome are translocation and mosaicism. Regardless of the type of Down syndrome, these children all share similar physical characteristics, and many live well into adulthood (Figure 45.10).

Children with Down syndrome are at an increased risk for medical complications, including congenital heart defects in the form of septal defects discussed previously. Respiratory infections are also common and, when combined with the heart defects, are the most common cause of death in these children during infancy.

Children with Down syndrome also have some physical deficiencies that can affect emergency treatments. The EMT should be familiar with these deficiencies. These children are normally short in stature and are prone to being overweight. Table 45-7 lists common physical characteristics found in children with Down syndrome.

ASSESSMENT

Children with Down syndrome are at a high risk for developing serious medical conditions, including lifelong heart conditions stemming from CHDs. They are also susceptible to respiratory problems and airway compromise

---

Table 45-7 Common Physical Characteristics of Down Syndrome

- Eyes slanted upward and outward
- Skin folds on the inner side of the eye (epicanthal fold)
- Eye slit narrow and short
- Small, white patches on the edge of the iris
- Face appears flat
- Head smaller than average
- Fontanels (soft spots) larger than normal and do not close as soon because of the infant's slower growth and development
- Ears smaller and lower-set
- Small mouth with thin lips resulting in the tongue sticking out due to the smaller-sized inside of the mouth
- Neck appears slightly short, and loose folds of skin are seen at the back and sides (disappear as the child grows)
- Legs and arms short in relation to the body
- Hands broad and flat with short fingers; little finger slanted inward
- Single crease across the palm
- Broad feet with short toes with a larger space between the big toe and the other toes
- Poor muscle tone (hypotonia) and loose-jointedness (hyperflexibility)
- Weaker reflexes and cry

---

because of the structure of their oral cavities, which can also make airway management and assisted ventilations challenging.

Children with Down syndrome are susceptible to orthopedic conditions because of **hypotonia,** or poor muscle tone, and **hyperflexibility,** loose-jointedness; dental problems; developmental delays; seizures; infections; gastrointestinal disorders; and childhood leukemia.

MANAGEMENT

Management will be the same as for most children, with a special focus on the airway. Fifteen to 20 percent of children with Down syndrome have **atlantoaxial instability** in which the first two cervical vertebrae are unstable due to weak ligaments. Atlantoaxial instability can cause neck pain and weakness and places these children at a risk for spinal cord compression if the head is hyperextended.

Airway maneuvers in children with Down syndrome should focus on keeping the head and neck in a neutral position, and avoiding hyperextension. Any child with Down syndrome who is unconscious or awake and complaining of neck pain or weakness, even when there is not evidence of cervical trauma, should have her head and neck immobilized.

BEHAVIORAL DISABILITIES

Children with behavioral disabilities present unique challenges for EMTs. These **behavioral disabilities** commonly affect how the child interacts with people, things, and the general environment. Behavior problems in children can be due to a disorder or can arise following traumatic brain injury, exposure to toxins or poisoning, and psychiatric conditions that appear as they grow and develop.

AUTISM

Autism, sometimes called *classical autism,* is the most common form of a group of developmental disorders called autism spectrum disorders (ASDs). **Autism** is characterized by social interaction deficit; impaired communication, both verbal and nonverbal; and severely limited range of activities and interests of play with repetitive behaviors.

Research estimates that 3 to 6 of every 1,000 children will be diagnosed with autism, with males being four times more likely than females; however, females are more severely affected. There is no definitive known cause for autism, but there may be a higher incidence of autism in children who have a sibling who is autistic. Most children with autism will require lifelong assisted living and adult supervision.

ASSESSMENT

The parents or caregivers are vital during the assessment and management of children with autism. Children with autism have an inability to maintain eye contact with other people. Although the signs and symptoms of autism do not usually begin to appear until the child is around 30 months to 2 years of age, infants showing early signs of autism may not want to be cuddled or touched and show limited social interaction normally associated with older infants. Often toddlers and older children with autism seem to be unaware of other children or appear to not pay any attention to them. Autistic children do not adapt well to changes in their routine or environment and can act out, sometimes violently when their immediate surroundings or routine change.

Autistic children have a higher incidence of traumatic injuries due to extremes in behavior, banging their heads on objects or other self-inflicted injuries, as well as due to their inability to recognize the consequences of their behavior. As an example, an autistic child may play with or grab a knife by the sharp blade without realizing she could cut herself by doing so.

Children with autism display repetitive behaviors, including rocking, spinning in circles, flipping switches on and off, spinning the wheels on a truck, or lining up pieces of paper or toys over and over again. If they have verbal abilities, they may repeat what they have heard on a radio or television or what another person says. Some repetitive behaviors, called **stimming** or *stereotyping*, can be characterized by prolonged humming or repetitive body movements, such as hand flapping. Stimming is believed to self-stimulate one or more senses in a form of self-regulation. The humming creates vibration in the child's inner ear and is believed to be a "self-soothing" behavior.

MANAGEMENT

Management of children with autism can be challenging for the EMT. It is important to remember that although the child may not be able to verbally communicate, that does not necessarily mean she does not understand verbal communication. It is also important for the EMT to be prepared for the child to have a sometimes violent response to the changes in her routine or environment. Injury or illness in the autistic child creates the same fear and anxiety as for any other child; however, autistic children have more extreme responses to fear and anxiety.

Enlist the help of the parent or caregiver. Explain all treatments to the child and family. The EMT should expect the autistic child to resist being touched and may need to have the parent or caregiver aid in assessments and treatments that require physical interactions.

Do not attempt to stop the child who is stimming unless her repetitive behaviors are destructive, and be prepared to restrain the child to ensure safety of the crew and the child. ALS intercept should be considered if sedation will be needed to provide treatment. Transport decisions should be discussed with the family. Autistic children should be transported to the facility that is familiar with them whenever possible. The family will be the best resource to the EMT concerning transport and the need for ALS assistance in the child requiring sedation to facilitate treatment.

CONCLUSION

Children with special challenges may also have medical and physical conditions the EMT may not be familiar with. The EMT may be called for children with technology-assisted devices because of a malfunction of the equipment they need to maintain health or due to an unrelated medical condition.

Children with physical, cognitive, and behavior impairments present the EMT with challenges in assessment and management. Through modification of the EMT's assessment and management skills, some basic knowledge of technologic equipment, and the parents' or caregivers' familiarity with their children's needs, the EMT will be able to effectively assess and manage children with special challenges and provide transport to the appropriate facility.

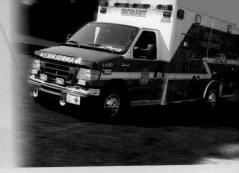

CASE STUDY Continued

Kelsey's assessment determines Wyatt has an open airway at this time, an increased work of breathing, and abnormal skin signs. As Mariah obtains baseline vital signs—pulse 140, respirations 44, pulse oximeter reading 84%—Wyatt's father, Kalvin, comes into the room and hands Kelsey an information card as he collects Wyatt's favorite stuffed animal and blanket to take to the hospital.

The information card explains that Wyatt was born with an AV-canal heart defect and is taking medications to support his heart function until he has the surgery to repair the hole. Wyatt has a normal baseline pulse oximeter reading of 88%, respirations that run from 30 to 40 breaths a minute, and a heart rate of 110 that increases to the 130s when he eats.

Kelsey compares her assessment findings with the normal baselines for Wyatt and determines that he is in respiratory distress and needs to be transported to the hospital with oxygen support. Kelsey knows that children with Down syndrome have small airways and oral cavities that cause the tongue to be proportionately larger, creating a potential airway obstruction. Katarina states she has learned to hold Wyatt in the current position, which helps him to breathe easier and keep his airway open.

En route to the hospital, Wyatt's pulse oximeter increases to 86%; however, the retractions continue to be present. Wyatt's appearance continues to be normal as he makes eye contact and looks around the ambulance. His work of breathing continues to be abnormal, with retraction around his ribs and coarse breath sounds. He continues to be pale with cyanosis around his lips; however, Katarina states the bluish tint is normal for him when he has respiratory difficulty.

ALS intercept had been requested, in case further airway management is needed and is met en route. Wyatt and his mother are transported to the Children's Hospital where Wyatt is scheduled to have heart surgery in a couple weeks.

Key Concepts Revisited

- EMTs are called to children with special challenges due to equipment failure, exacerbation of their condition, or onset of a new medical condition or injury when the parent or caregiver can no longer manage alone.

- The EMT's knowledge of normal baseline mental status and vital signs in children must be modified for children with special challenges.

- Assessment and management of children with special challenges requires communication and partnership with the parents or caregivers of the child to be effective.
  - Determination of the child's baseline conditions and vital signs are required for effective clinical interpretation of assessment findings.

- The Pediatric Assessment Triangle can be used with the AVPU scale in assessment of children with special challenges with modification.
  - Appearance is determined on the strength and quality of the child's cry or facial expression compared to the child's baseline appearance.
  - Work of breathing assessment of the severity of retractions is compared to the presence of baseline retractions.
  - Circulation to skin assessment is determined after establishing the child's normal skin color and condition.

- The EMT should be familiar with the special medical needs and equipment of children who are technologically assisted.
  - Tracheostomies are artificial airways to maintain adequate oxygenation and ventilation.
  - Mechanical ventilators provide positive pressure ventilations at the appropriate tidal volume and pressure.

- Central venous catheters provide a route for intravenous medications and blood sampling in children with chronic conditions requiring frequent venous access.
- Feeding tubes provide a route, either through the nose or anterior abdominal wall, for liquid nutrition to children who are not able to obtain nutrition normally.
- Cerebrospinal fluid (CSF) shunts are used to drain excess CSF off the brain and into the abdomen to be absorbed.
- Children with special challenges include those with physical disabilities.
  - Congenital heart defects are structural anomalies of the heart or great vessels.
  - Hearing impairment reduces the child's ability to hear sound.
- Children with hearing impairment communicate through a variety of methods.

- Cognitive impairment in children with special challenges such as Down syndrome can range from mild to profound.
  - Children with Down syndrome commonly have mild cognitive impairments but also have physical conditions and are at a higher risk for medical illnesses.
- Behavioral disabilities affect how the child interacts with people and present unique challenges for the EMT.
  - Autism is the most common form of a spectrum of developmental disorders characterized by social interaction deficit, impaired communication, and repetitive, obsessive behaviors.
- Children with special challenges requiring transport should be transported to a facility that is familiar with the children, their conditions, and ongoing treatments whenever possible.

Review Questions

1. What are some considerations for assessment and management of children with special health care needs?
2. What is the primary resource the EMT must depend on when assessing and managing children with special challenges?
3. Name some of the technological devices a child with special challenges will depend on to live.
4. What is a cerebrospinal fluid shunt and what does it do?
5. What are congenital heart defects?
6. What is the difference between hard of hearing and deafness?
7. What are two methods children with hearing impairment use to communicate?
8. What are some of the causes of cognitive impairment?
9. What physical characteristics are common in children with Down syndrome?
10. What is autism?
11. What challenges will the EMT face in the assessment and management of a child with autism?
12. What is the definition and purpose of stimming?

Key Terms

Atlantoaxial instability

Autism

Behavioral disabilities

Central venous catheter

Cerebrospinal fluid (CSF) shunt

Children with special health care
  needs (CSHCN)

Cochlear implant

Cognitive

Cognitive impairment

Congenital heart defects (CHD)

Deafness

Down syndrome

Feeding tube

Hard of hearing

Hearing impairment

Hyperflexibility

Hypotonia

Mechanical ventilator

Stimming

Tracheostomy tube

Ventriculo-peritoneal (VP) shunt

Further Study

Adirim, T. A., and E. Smith. *SCOPE: Special
  Children's Outreach and Prehospital Education.*
  Sudbury, MA: Jones and Bartlett, 2006.

American Academy of Pediatrics. *Pediatric
  Education for Prehospital Professionals (PEPP).*
  Sudbury, MA: Jones and Bartlett, 2006.

Wertz, E. M. *Emergency Care for Children.* Clifton
  Park, NY: Thomson Delmar Learning, 2002.

CHAPTER 9

Geriatric Emergencies

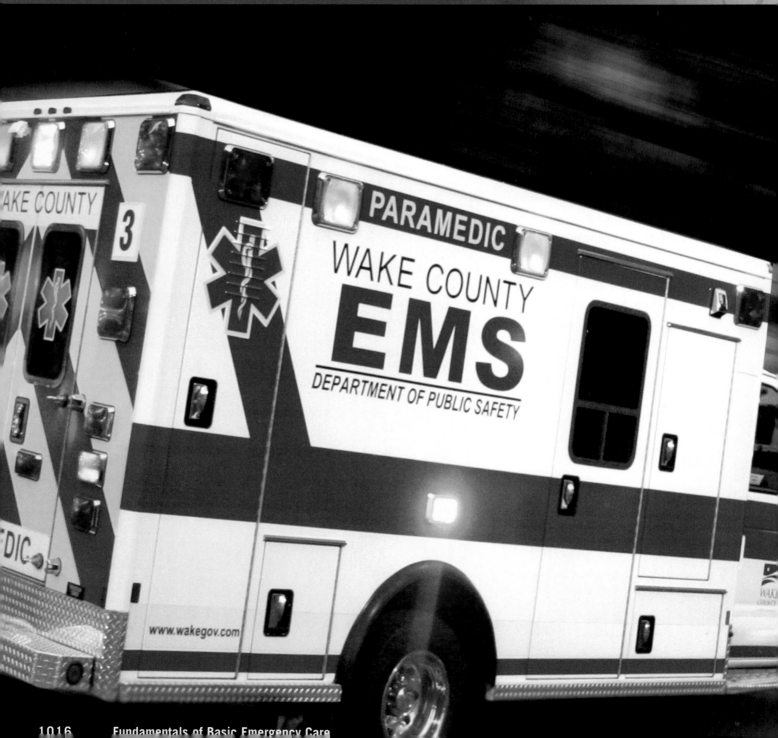

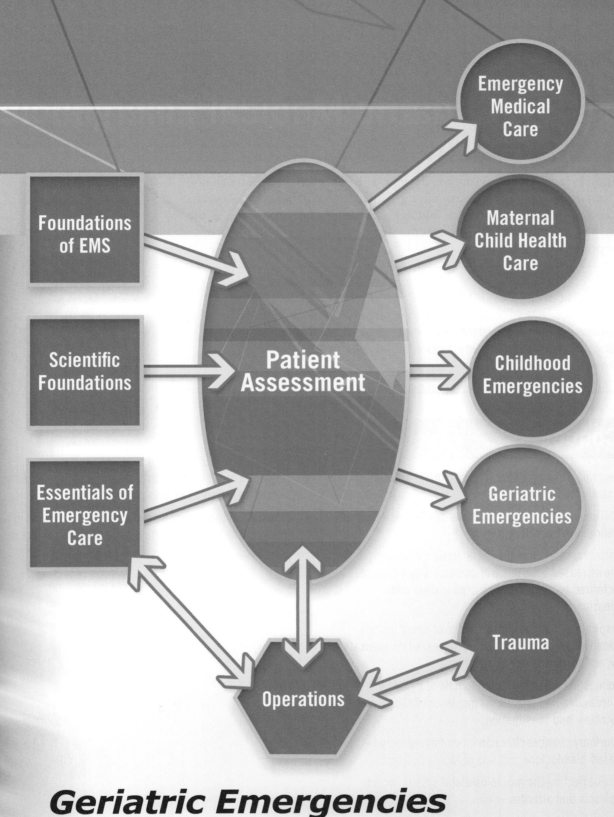

Geriatric Emergencies

In a phrase, America is graying. On average, Americans are getting older, and this fact represents a special challenge to the Emergency Medical Technician (EMT).

An EMT must understand the changes that occur with aging and the particular health problems that accompany those changes. This section helps the EMT understand those changes and thus manage the resulting medical problems.

UNIT (46) Geriatric Medical Emergencies

Today, advances in medicine, sanitation, hygiene, and control of infectious disease have led to an increase in life expectancy in the United States to more than 75 years. Our concept of what age constitutes "old age" has significantly changed. As the body ages, there are characteristic changes that leave people susceptible to particular disease processes.

National Education Standard

The Emergency Medical Technician (EMT) will be able to demonstrate a fundamental depth and foundational breadth of understanding the changes associated with aging, including age-related assessment and treatment of major or common geriatric diseases and emergencies.

Key Concepts

- The neurologic changes characteristic of aging include decreases of the senses.

- The EMT must understand the differences between dementia and delirium in the elderly patient.

- The cardiovascular changes characteristic of aging include increased occurrence of coronary artery disease, characterized by stiffened, restricted vessels and hypertension.

- The respiratory changes characteristic of aging include decreased elasticity of lung tissue, decreased compensatory ability, and increased risk of infections.

- Gastrointestinal changes characteristic of aging include tooth decay, leading to a higher incidence of choking, malnutrition, and constipation.

- Genitourinary changes characteristic of aging include decreased bladder tone and loss of kidney function.

- Diseases affecting the musculoskeletal system include osteoporosis and arthritis.

- Soft tissue injuries and higher incidence of hypothermia are the result of changes to the integumentary system due to aging.

- Medication use by the elderly often results in polypharmacy, increasing chances of adverse reactions.

- The EMT's rapid recognition of potential for serious illness or injury in the elderly leads to greatly improved outcomes.

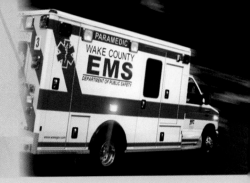

CASE STUDY

Ian and Carlotta are just beginning their shift. As they are in the process of conducting equipment checks, the pager goes off. The first call of the day is for an elderly woman complaining of weakness and fever.

Upon arrival to the scene, they are greeted at the door by an elderly woman in her late 70s. She introduces herself as Emily Carlyle as she turns to walk back into the kitchen, where Ian and Carlotta can hear the distinct whistle of a tea kettle.

As they follow Mrs. Carlyle into the kitchen, Carlotta notices there are three cups and saucers on the kitchen table and a small plate of cookies. The kitchen appears clean and well kept, with no dirty dishes in the sink and a tea pot and two medicine bottles the only items on the counter.

"Would you like some tea?" Mrs. Carlyle asks.

"No, thank you, ma'am," Ian replies. "Can you tell us why you called EMS today, ma'am?"

Mrs. Carlyle sits down at the table, indicating that Ian and Carlotta should also be seated and proceeds to list about a half-dozen concerns, including trouble breathing whenever she walks out to the mailbox, a sore hip from a fall several days ago, and a general allover ache she believes is from her arthritis.

"Mrs. Carlyle, what specifically is bothering you today, that you want checked out at the hospital?" Carlotta asks, as she attempts to determine the patient's medical need.

Critical Thinking Question

1. What physiologic changes are common as a person ages?
2. How does this affect a person's health?
3. How might this impact the EMT's care?

INTRODUCTION

Geriatrics is the study of the diseases of elderly adults. The elderly have physiologic differences from other adults. The methods of assessment and management are largely the same; however, those physiologic differences necessitate a few modifications. Geriatrics is the largest growing age-group in the population and represents the majority of EMS calls. This unit discusses the physiologic differences and types of emergencies affecting the geriatric population as well as assessment and treatment modifications the EMT should use for effective care of the geriatric patient.

THE AGING OF SOCIETY

People ages 85 and older are the fastest growing age-group in the United States. The U.S. Census Bureau estimates the older-than-85 age-group will double in size by the year 2025. Chronologic age does not determine a person's state of health. Every person ages differently. Elderly people as a group have more health problems than younger people do. Studies have shown that geriatric patients use EMS three to four times more frequently and require more advanced life support (ALS) care than younger adults. Emergency department (ED) usage shows similar increasing trends in patient population. Furthermore, this group accounts for nearly half of all hospital and intensive care admissions from the ED. The more complicated nature of an elderly person's medical problems often requires more time and resources to manage effectively.

It is important for the EMT to be familiar with the normal changes associated with aging and the disease processes most commonly found in the elderly.

PHYSIOLOGIC CHANGES ASSOCIATED WITH AGING

From the moment we are born, our bodies start to age. This aging process is inevitable. Some changes, such as hair loss or graying, may be obvious, but others may be more subtle until they lead to a problem. This section discusses some of the more subtle changes that occur in each organ system as a body ages.

NEUROLOGIC

Some changes that occur in the neurologic system become more obvious as a person ages. Visual acuity notably decreases, as evidenced by the need for glasses as one gets older. The senses of hearing, taste, and smell also become less acute.

These changes are not only an inconvenience; they can sometimes have devastating effects on the geriatric patient. Poor vision can lead to an increased risk for falls and subsequent injuries. Loss of hearing and sense of smell can take away the ability to recognize warning signals such as smoke alarms or the smell of smoke or gas.

Many times, the progressive decline in these sensory abilities is not noticed by the person, but by family members. Glasses and hearing aids may help to reduce the effects of this aging process. The EMT should make an effort to bring any such physical aids with the patient to the hospital. This will facilitate patient comfort and communication in the hospital.

When caring for an elderly patient, the EMT should determine whether any sensory deficits are prominent and be sure to accommodate for the problem. On the other hand, the EMT should also not assume that every elderly person is hard of hearing or cannot see. Each patient should be individually assessed and treated.

If a hearing deficit is present, the patient is sometimes described as hard of hearing. Several techniques may be used to improve effective communication between the EMT and the patient who is hard of hearing. These techniques are listed in Table 46-1. Be sure to make the hospital staff aware the patient has a hearing deficit. If the patient has hearing aids, have the patient put them in to make communication easier.

CARDIOVASCULAR

As vessels age, their elasticity decreases, resulting in stiffening. This stiffening can result in higher blood pressure. In addition, the buildup of fatty deposits

Street Smart

When communicating with the person who is hard of hearing, the EMT can place a stethoscope in the patient's ears and speak into the head. This may allow some magnification of the sound for the patient and may improve his ability to hear.

Table 46-1 Communication Techniques for Patients with Hearing Deficits

Directly face the patient when speaking.

Be sure the patient is looking at you when speaking.

Speak slowly and clearly.

Stand close to the patient when speaking, and speak in a loud, clear tone of voice. Yelling is not necessary.

inside the blood vessels throughout life results in a decrease in the size of the inner lumen of the vessel.

These changes in the vessels lead to a decreased ability to change the amount of blood flow to a particular area based on need. The person's tolerance for exercise decreases. As the heart continues to pump against these stiffening vessels, it becomes less and less efficient as a pump, further decreasing the individual's exercise ability.

These changes in the cardiovascular system put elderly people at increased risk of a heart attack or heart failure. The incidence of these two conditions increases as they continue to age. These conditions are discussed in Units 25 and 26.

RESPIRATORY

Decreasing elasticity in the chest wall and lung tissue also results in decreased lung volumes. The alveoli and the cilia that clear the lungs of unwanted particles also become less efficient.

This results in increased risk for infection in the lungs and a decreased ability to compensate for it. Elderly patients with respiratory infections such as pneumonia can become very ill very quickly. Unit 26 reviews the common respiratory diseases.

GASTROINTESTINAL

One of the most obvious findings in old age is the loss of teeth. Although this may seem merely an inconvenience, it does limit the food a person can eat, which can potentially lead to malnutrition.

Decreased motility of the gastrointestinal system results in less efficient absorption of nutrients and problems with elimination. Constipation is a common problem among the elderly.

GENITOURINARY

A loss of bladder tone and a decrease in the bladder's capacity can result in embarrassing incontinence and also increase the risk for urinary tract infection.

Progressive decreases in blood flow to the kidneys results in a decline in kidney function. This can result in difficulty maintaining an appropriate fluid and electrolyte balance, as this is primarily regulated by the kidney. Dehydration is common in the elderly.

Many medications are eliminated by the kidney. If the kidney function is decreased, medications may not be eliminated as quickly as expected. If medication doses are not appropriately decreased, this can lead to a buildup in the body. This buildup can have harmful effects on the patient.

MUSCULOSKELETAL

A progressive loss in the calcium content of the bones, called *osteoporosis*, occurs more commonly in women than in men as they age. This loss of calcium leaves the bones weaker and increases the risk of bone fractures. Sometimes even minor trauma can result in bone fractures in an older patient. A decrease in the flexibility of joints, together with an inflammation within those joints, called **arthritis,** can lead to decreased mobility.

Falls are quite common in elderly patients. EMS may be called when an elderly patient has fallen and is unable to get up (Figure 46.1). When evaluating these patients, the EMT must remember that even a minor fall can result in broken bones. Before allowing the patient to stand, a thorough assessment should be performed to ensure that no bones are painful, swollen, or deformed. The management of bony injuries is discussed in Unit 38.

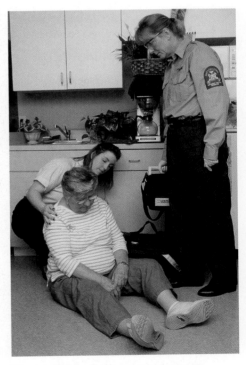

Figure 46.1 Falls are common among the elderly. A detailed assessment should be performed to ensure no bones have been broken

INTEGUMENTARY

Integumentary refers to the skin and the structures immediately underlying it. A loss of subcutaneous fat and water content leaves an elderly person's skin dry and wrinkled. It is at increased risk of tearing and does not heal as quickly as younger skin. Care should be taken during movement and transport to avoid damage to an elderly patient's sensitive skin.

The loss in the fatty layer under the skin leaves the elderly person much more susceptible to hypothermia in the cold. Elderly people are unable to insulate themselves as well as younger persons. In addition, the decrease in water content and declining function of the sweat glands leave the elderly patient unable to effectively dissipate heat, leading to heat-related illnesses as well.

Finally, as the body ages, the hair loses color, becoming gray or white. Hair also does not grow as quickly and becomes less prevalent on the body. Figure 46.2 summarizes the physiologic changes that occur as the body ages.

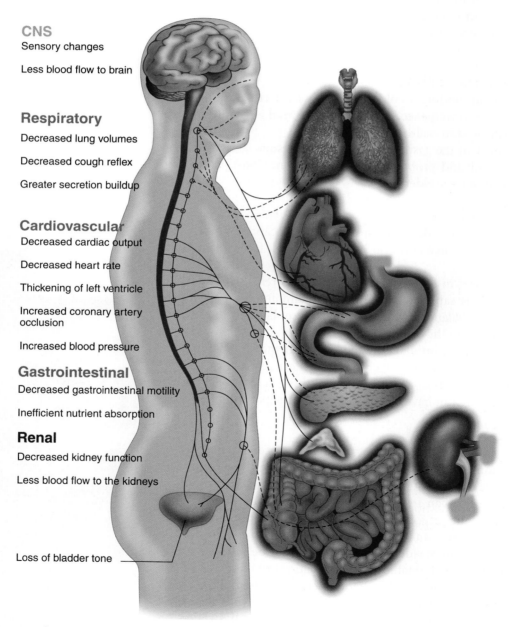

CNS
Sensory changes

Less blood flow to brain

Respiratory
Decreased lung volumes

Decreased cough reflex

Greater secretion buildup

Cardiovascular
Decreased cardiac output

Decreased heart rate

Thickening of left ventricle

Increased coronary artery occlusion

Increased blood pressure

Gastrointestinal
Decreased gastrointestinal motility

Inefficient nutrient absorption

Renal
Decreased kidney function

Less blood flow to the kidneys

Loss of bladder tone

Figure 46.2 Changes in nearly every organ system become evident as a person ages

ASSESSMENT OF THE ELDERLY PATIENT

Although the steps in assessing the elderly patient are the same as those used to assess any other patient, there are some special considerations in the assessment of this population.

SCENE SIZE-UP

When going into a patient's home, an EMT has a unique opportunity that the hospital staff will not have. The EMT can observe the patient's living conditions. As people age, they sometimes find it increasingly difficult to do the things that they once were able to do without difficulty, such as cook, clean, or shop for necessities. If the patient does not have family or friends to help perform these duties, the home may not be in a healthy, livable condition for an elderly person.

The EMT should take time to look around the room and note the general condition of the home. When looking for the patient's medications, the EMT may have occasion to enter the kitchen. She should take a moment to look around the kitchen to see how well it is stocked with nutritional food. Are there several days worth of dirty dishes in the sink or empty medication bottles sitting around? The general appearance of the home should give the EMT an idea of the patient's ability to care for himself or how long he may have been ill.

If there is a possibility the patient is unable to adequately manage alone, ask the patient whether there are any resources available to come in and help. Many older patients have family, friends, or visiting health care personnel who help them manage. If the EMT finds that a patient seems unable to care for himself adequately based on the condition of the home, receiving hospital personnel should be notified of the situation. Hospital personnel can involve a social work team to determine whether the patient needs further assistance.

PRIMARY ASSESSMENT

The principles of the primary assessment remain the same no matter what the age of the patient. Assessing mental status and ensuring an adequate airway, breathing, and circulation are the priorities in elderly patients as well as younger patients. Unit16 reviews the principles of the primary assessment.

HISTORY AND SECONDARY ASSESSMENT

Based on whether the patient is suffering from a medical or traumatic problem, the EMT will follow the assessments that are detailed previously in Chapter 4.

Obtaining a history from an elderly patient may present challenges. Communication difficulties may contribute, and the complexity of the problem may be hard to communicate in an efficient manner. The EMT should make the effort to obtain an accurate and thorough history when the patient's condition and time permits. It is not uncommon for family, friends, or others to have significant contributions to the history of the patient's illness or injury. If these people do not accompany the patient to the hospital, the EMT is the only person who can obtain such information. It is crucial that any such information obtained is well documented and relayed to the receiving staff.

TRANSPORT

During transport of the elderly patient, the EMT should remember the changes in the body that occur in this age-group and protect the patient from further harm. Careful transferring will avoid further injury to fragile skin and bones. Adequate protection from excessive heat or cold is important to prevent hyperthermia or hypothermia.

It is a good practice to gather all the patient's medications into a container and bring them along to the hospital for review by the receiving staff. However, the EMT must realize that these medications are often quite costly. Special care should be taken to ensure that these items do not get misplaced.

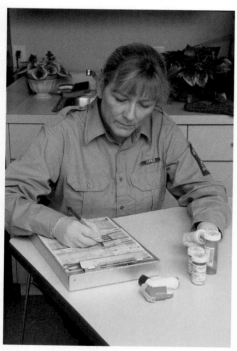

Figure 46.3 Many elderly adults are prescribed multiple medications; during history taking, the EMT should note the medications used

REASSESSMENT

As reviewed in Unit 20, reassessment should be performed during transport to find any changes that may be occurring during this time.

GENERAL MEDICAL CONSIDERATIONS IN THE ELDERLY

The EMT will frequently be called to care for an elderly patient. It is important to be familiar with some of the general considerations that may affect the health of these patients.

MEDICATION USE BY THE ELDERLY

As adults get older, they are more likely to have medical problems. Medications are usually prescribed to help the person deal with these problems. If more than one illness is present, more than one medication will probably be prescribed (Figure 46.3). The average elderly American takes more than four prescription drugs and two or more over-the-counter drugs.

The use of multiple medications by a single patient is known as **polypharmacy.** Polypharmacy, while sometimes necessary to treat multiple disease processes, increases the risk of medication side effects. If one medication has two possible side effects and another medication has another two possible side effects, that leaves the patient with four possible side effects. The elderly patient's body responds to medications in different ways.

In addition, the more medications that are prescribed, the more difficult it becomes to remember when to take each one. Medication compliance decreases with every drug that is added to the list of prescriptions. The use of multiple medications can be fraught with complications.

Each of these factors leads to up to one third of elderly persons developing adverse effects to medications. Furthermore, they are at least twice as likely to have undesirable side effects of medications as younger adults. In fact, 1 in 20 hospital admissions among the elderly is thought to be due to adverse reactions to medications.

It is important that the EMT carefully document each of the patient's medications and pass that information on to the receiving staff at the hospital. A complete knowledge of the patient's medication history may help the physician to appropriately manage the patient.

SUSCEPTIBILITY TO DISEASE

The physiologic changes associated with aging leave the elderly person at increased risk for multiple illnesses and injuries. Table 46-2 lists some medical problems that become more prevalent in the elderly.

ALTERED PRESENTATION OF DISEASE

Along with the increase in incidence of illness, elderly patients present health care workers with a challenge. Because of the changes associated with normal aging, they may not present with the concerns EMTs typically see for a specific illness. Disease states are more often discovered in advanced stages in elderly patients because their presence may not have been obvious earlier.

An example is a heart attack. Perhaps because of alterations in nerve stimulation, an elderly patient who is suffering from a myocardial infarction may not experience chest pain. The patient's perception of any discomfort may be greatly altered. The symptoms in the elderly patient may be atypical or absent altogether. The occurrence of a heart attack without the presence of the classic pattern of chest pain is called a **silent myocardial infarction.** A silent myocardial infarction is more likely to occur in an elderly patient.

The index of suspicion for serious disease in the elderly patient has to be even higher than it is with a younger patient because of elderly patients' altered presentation patterns.

MISTREATMENT OF THE ELDERLY

In other countries, elderly people are considered to be wise and are held in a position of respect. The young routinely care for their parents and elderly relatives until they die. In the United States, the philosophy of caring for the elderly is a little different.

Many families choose to place elderly relatives in a facility where they can receive care from trained staff. The industry of assisted living and skilled care facilities is growing daily as our society makes arrangements to care for its elderly. Nevertheless, many elderly people continue to live on their own, receiving assistance from special programs for meals, transport, and daytime activities.

Their dependence on others for help places elderly people at risk for mistreatment. Mistreatment of an elderly person is known as *elder abuse* and is unfortunately prevalent in the United States today. General estimates of elder abuse in this country suggest that it may affect 10% of the elderly population. With more than 1 million victims reported annually and with gross underreporting assumed, EMTs must be aware of the possibility the elderly patient they are caring for may have been abused.

Elder abuse can consist of physical or psychological abuse as well as neglect or exploitation. The elderly person who is living with family is often at greatest risk, although patients in nursing homes have been victims as well.

Just as in other forms of abuse, the EMT is often the first health care provider to become aware of the possibility of abuse. Any suspicions the EMT has based on what is seen in the home should be communicated to hospital staff so that further investigation can take place.

COMMON ILLNESSES IN THE ELDERLY

Although any illness can occur at nearly any age, some illnesses occur more commonly or require unique considerations in an elderly population.

ALTERED MENTAL STATUS

Elderly patients may develop an altered mental status that is subtle and only recognized by family members. This altered mental status may have a dramatic disturbance in their level of consciousness, prompting a call to EMS. The causes of an altered mental state in an elderly patient are many and often involve multiple factors. Many issues inherent to the elderly make assessment of altered mental status difficult. Several disease states cause an altered mental status that are worthy of review here.

DEMENTIA

A common illness seen in the elderly is dementia. *Dementia* is a syndrome that is characterized by a progressive decline in intellectual function that usually leads to deterioration of occupational, social, and interpersonal functions. The incidence of dementia increases with age; in the United States dementia is estimated to affect 5% of people between the ages of 72 and 80, increasing to affect more than 37% in people over age 90.

Difficulties with memory are often the first symptoms or signs of dementia. The onset of this disease process is usually subtle. A gradual progression over a period of years is characteristic of this syndrome. Often the patient does not even notice the symptoms. Many times this illness goes unrecognized for a significant period of time. It may become apparent during a period of stress,

Table 46-2 Prevalent Medical Conditions in the Elderly
Hypertension
Heart attack
Heart failure
Kidney disease
Complications of diabetes
Stroke
Dementia
Falls
Infections
Fractures

when the symptoms of dementia may be acutely worsened. Any additional medical or psychological stress can temporarily worsen the condition.

Loss of memory may lead the patient to wander away from home and then not remember where he lives. The patient with dementia may not even recall his name.

There are many different causes of dementia, some of which are reversible. The most common cause of dementia in the United States is Alzheimer's disease.

ALZHEIMER'S DISEASE

Alzheimer's disease is the most common form of dementia in the elderly. The incidence of this condition increases sharply with age. The cause of the disease is unknown, but it has been found to be somewhat genetic in nature, although with variable expressions. Many people who have been diagnosed with Alzheimer's disease are hardly symptomatic, especially in the early stages, whereas others are completely nonfunctional, relying on others for all of their activities of daily living.

The clinical presentation of this disease is dementia of varying degrees. Subtle changes are found in the brain tissue of patients who suffer from Alzheimer's disease. Not much is known about the etiology of the disease; therefore, treatments are largely experimental.

DELIRIUM

Delirium can be defined as an acute change in mental status occurring secondary to a potentially reversible medical condition. Although delirium can exist in conjunction with dementia, it is important to realize the acute nature of the process in this case. Elderly patients are at high risk for delirium during the course of even minor illnesses because of physical sensitivity to illness and to medications prescribed for those illnesses. Medications are the most common reversible cause of delirium, even when they are used appropriately.

Rather than a disease process on its own, delirium can be thought of as a marker for another disease. Often the underlying disease is one that may pose a serious threat to life, such as myocardial infarction, stroke, pneumonia, gastrointestinal bleeding, overwhelming infection, traumatic brain injury, or pulmonary embolus. Classic symptoms and signs of these conditions may be absent in the elderly patient with the only sign of illness being a confused state.

Because patients suffering from delirium may not be able to provide an adequate history, EMTs may not have historical clues to guide management of such conditions. For this reason, the elderly patient with an acutely altered mental status should be treated as if a potential life threat existed.

When possible, the EMT should attempt to obtain a history from family, friends, caregivers, or other personnel who might be able to provide clues to the patient's current condition. Of key importance is a description of the patient's baseline mental status and how the current presentation differs. Additionally, symptoms of recent illness or any medication changes, whether over the counter or prescription, should be elicited.

DEPRESSION

Many elderly patients suffer from some degree of depression. In one study of nonhospitalized patients, nearly a third had some symptoms of mild depression, with 6% classified as severe. Not unexpectedly, the rates are higher among hospitalized patients. Depression in the elderly can present to the EMT in several ways. In some cases, the patient can become confused as a result of the depression. The EMT may be called for an altered mental status. Alternatively, patients may not be able to care properly for themselves because of their depressed state, resulting in a call for EMS. At the extreme, EMS may be activated for a suicide attempt. The suicide risk is highest among elderly men. While the depressed mood of the patient may be obvious to the EMT, there is often a coexisting medical condition that results in a need for EMS.

ALCOHOL ABUSE

Abuse of alcohol is exceedingly common in the elderly population in the United States. It is estimated that more than 2.5 million elderly people abuse alcohol. In this age range, women seem to be affected more than men. Chronic alcohol use can lead to a number of serious medical problems, especially in an elderly person. Gastrointestinal bleeding, injury from falls, and other trauma can be related to the abuse of alcohol. More details regarding the presentation and management of alcohol abuse can be found in Unit 28.

STROKE

Stroke can occur in any age-group, but advancing age is a significant risk factor, and the majority of strokes occur in the elderly population. Elderly patients may delay accessing EMS and often have higher rates of death and significant disability after a stroke. The EMT may be able to impact these statistics through early recognition and expedient transport to an appropriate hospital.

ACUTE MYOCARDIAL INFARCTION (AMI)

The risk for cardiovascular disease increases as people age. In fact, more than half of myocardial infarctions happen in elderly persons. It is important for the EMT to remember that elderly patients often do not have the classic symptom complex expected with an AMI, as described in Unit 25. The presence of atypical or no apparent symptoms can lead to a delay in presentation and treatment. Perhaps for this reason and due to multiple coexisting medical conditions, elderly patients have double the risk of dying from a heart attack as does someone younger. AMI is the leading cause of death in the over-65 population, accounting for two thirds of deaths in this age-group.

The EMT must vigilantly consider the possibility of AMI in elderly patients who have concerns such as shortness of breath, nausea, dizziness, weakness, sweating, syncope, and altered level of consciousness (LOC), even without the presence of chest pain. Proper treatment and transport decisions as discussed in Unit 25 can have an impact on the outcome of the elderly patient with an AMI.

CONGESTIVE HEART FAILURE

Congestive heart failure is another commonly seen cardiac condition in the elderly. Because the heart weakens as a result of the physiologic changes with aging, the elderly are susceptible to higher blood pressure (hypertension), plaque buildup in their arteries, and damage to heart valves. As a result, the heart no longer pumps effectively, causing blood to back up into the lungs and peripheral circulation.

Elderly patients may have been previously diagnosed with CHF and call EMS when their symptoms become unmanageable at home. Some patients call EMS because they are experiencing symptoms such as swelling in their extremities, especially the feet and ankles, fatigue, and difficulty breathing and have never been diagnosed with congestive heart failure. The EMT may find additional signs of jugular vein distention, crackling (rales) in the lungs, and wheezing during assessment.

Management for CHF, whether previously diagnosed or a suspected new onset, includes high-flow oxygen, placing the patient in a position of comfort that facilitates breathing, such as Fowler's, and immediate transport.

The EMT should consider ALS intercept en route and be prepared to assist ventilations if breathing becomes inadequate because of fatigue.

DIFFICULTY BREATHING

Difficulty breathing can result from a number of conditions common in the elderly. CHF causes fluid to back up into the lungs, resulting in difficulty breathing; however, difficulty breathing may be the primary symptoms of a pulmonary problem. It is important for the EMT to remember the elderly have diminished respiratory function and therefore have less oxygen reserve and capability to compensate for inadequate oxygenation.

PULMONARY EMBOLISM

A respiratory emergency seen more often in the elderly than younger adults is a **pulmonary embolism** or blockage of the arteries of the lungs. In fact, aging is one of the predisposing factors to a pulmonary embolism, along with smoking, cancer, fractures of large bones, major surgery, heart disease, prolonged bed rest, and trauma. The emergency usually occurs when the blockage breaks free from a lower extremity and is transported to the right side of the heart, eventually lodging in the arteries of the lungs.

Signs and symptoms include a sudden onset of difficulty breathing, with chest discomfort that does not radiate. The patient may or may not experience a syncopal (fainting) event. The blockage causes an inadequate exchange of oxygen and carbon dioxide, causing the respiratory distress. Therefore, management for pulmonary embolism includes high-flow oxygen, assisted ventilations for inadequate breathing, and rapid transport to the appropriate facility. The EMT should consider ALS intercept en route to the hospital.

ABDOMINAL PAIN

The concern of abdominal pain in a patient over the age of 65 is much more likely to result in hospital admission, need for surgery, and significant morbidity and mortality than in any other age-group. The EMT should take note of the likelihood of a serious condition existing when abdominal pain is the concern in the elderly patient. This is true even in the absence of classic physical findings. The elderly patient may not exhibit guarding or rigidity due to relatively thin abdominal musculature and other anatomic changes associated with aging. Unit 29 discusses specific causes of abdominal pain and the treatment of each.

UNDERNUTRITION

For a multitude of reasons, nearly one fifth of elderly patients presenting to emergency departments in the United States are undernourished. It is thought that depression, lack of money, lack of transportation for shopping, inability to manage cooking, and problems with chewing and swallowing all contribute to this important issue. Undernutrition can lead to immune compromise and resultant infections. Additionally, worsening of chronic medical conditions can be seen. If an EMT identifies any of these problems in an elderly patient, it would be appropriate to report such concerns to the receiving staff at the hospital so that appropriate referrals can be made to assist the patient with his nutritional needs.

INFECTION

For a multitude of reasons, elderly patients are more susceptible to infection and, as with many other disease processes in this age-group, will often present atypically. Many elderly patients with severe infections do not even have a fever. The presenting concern may be as nonspecific as a poor appetite, feeling tired, or confusion. Respiratory infections, urinary tract infections, intra-abdominal infections, and soft tissue infections are the most common sources for serious infection in the elderly population. Many times, an elderly patient with a particular infectious problem will require hospitalization when a similar disease in a younger person would be easily treated at home.

RENAL FUNCTION

The elderly are susceptible to a variety of conditions affecting the renal system due to the aging process. The kidneys lose mass, becoming smaller in size and weight, as they lose **nephrons,** the functional parts of the kidney. The loss of surface area of the kidneys as they shrink causes a decrease in surface area available to filter blood. Combined with the loss of circulation to the kidneys due to the aging cardiovascular system, the decreased function of the kidneys can lead to fluid buildup and toxicity from inadequate filtration of medications.

Urinary tract infections, including bladder and kidney infections, are seen with more frequency in the elderly. Chronic kidney failure develops as the kidneys decrease in size and the function of cleansing the blood of waste continues to fail. The elderly often require an external method to clean the body of its waste products to avoid a buildup of ammonia, leading to toxicity. Dialysis is the process that "washes" the blood of waste products the kidneys have failed to filter.

Renal failure usually presents with signs and symptoms of toxicity, including mental confusion, drowsiness, visual disturbances, nausea, vomiting, diarrhea, and a urine smell to the breath, and can lead to seizures and coma. Immediate dialysis is needed to remove the toxic waste until the kidneys begin to function again. The EMT should apply high-flow oxygen and transport immediately to the appropriate facility with dialysis capability. ALS intercept should be considered en route. Always follow local protocols.

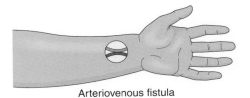
Arteriovenous fistula

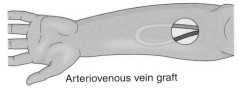
Arteriovenous vein graft

Figure 46.4 Hemodialysis AV shunt sites

TRAUMA

In the over-65 population, trauma is the fifth leading cause of death. This population accounts for 20% of all trauma patients and nearly 30% of fatalities. Injuries that might be easily survived by a younger adult may be fatal in an elderly person. Furthermore, those who survive their injury will often require long-term care. The EMT should be aware of the high morbidity and mortality associated with even seemingly minor trauma in this patient population and take care to provide expedient transport to a facility capable of managing geriatric trauma. When assessing the elderly trauma victim, the EMT must also remember that the physiologic changes associated with aging result in subtle visible physical findings, even when significant disease is present. For example, the elderly patient can lose a significant amount of blood before showing any signs of shock. Rapid decompensation, once a critical threshold is reached, is classic. The EMT must look carefully for those subtle signs, such as confusion, and treat aggressively to prevent further decompensation.

Regional trauma protocols often have special considerations for elderly patients, many times mandating treatment at a trauma center following a significant mechanism of injury even when no physical abnormalities are noted. While an EMT will not be in a position to diagnose specific injuries definitively, it is worthwhile to review the unique factors associated with specific injuries in the geriatric population.

FALLS

Falls account for the most significant injuries in the elderly, although motor vehicle accidents, pedestrian accidents, violent assault, and burns contribute to the numbers of injured elderly adults as well.

Falls occur in nearly one third of adults over age 65 living independently and at an even higher rate in institutionalized adults. One in 10 falls result in an injury that requires emergency department care. The frequency of falls and severity of injuries sustained increases with each decade of life.

There are many reasons for falls in the elderly, and these can be separated into several categories. It is useful for the EMT to consider these factors while obtaining a history and observing the patient's home environment. The first category is environmental objects that contribute to a fall. Poor lighting, lack of handrails, loose floor coverings, and unstable furniture are a few examples of how environmental issues in the patient's home can lead to a fall.

Physiologic factors can also lead to a trip, slip, or fall. Degenerating vision, poor balance, decreasing strength, and slower reaction times are among the physiologic changes associated with aging that frequently contribute to falls. It is obvious that physiologic factors can add to environmental objects and create a fall. If the EMT notes things in the patient's home environment that seem a likely contributing factor to a fall, this should be reported to hospital staff. It may be useful for a social worker to visit the patient's home and assess the safety of the environment to prevent further injury.

The final category of factors leading to falls in the elderly is pathologic processes that result in the patient falling down. Acute neurologic conditions, cardiac conditions, and other potentially serious disease processes can lead to a loss of consciousness and a fall. In obtaining a history, it is important for the EMT to question the patient regarding symptoms that preceded the fall, such as palpitations or dizziness. Additionally, witnesses to the incident should be questioned about any noted loss of consciousness, seizure activity, or other obvious sign of illness.

HEAD INJURIES

Traumatic brain injury is one of the leading causes of trauma death in the elderly population. In the elderly patient, a Glasgow Coma Scale of 8 or less is associated with a mortality of greater than 90%. Subdural hematomas are seen with three times the frequency as in a younger population. This is due largely to the normal shrinkage of brain tissue within the skull, known as atrophy, resulting in more movement of the brain with sudden movements of the head. Violent movement of the brain within the skull can lead to tearing of veins and subsequent bleeding into the subdural space.

The addition of medications that are meant to thin the blood and prevent clotting can worsen this condition. Elderly patients are more often prescribed such medications. Even minor head trauma can lead to a significant injury. Often the bleeding is slow in nature and results in a delay in the onset of any symptoms. Subtle symptoms such as confusion or headache may occur several days to weeks after an injury. The EMT should specifically ask the patient if she has sustained any injury in the weeks preceding the current problem. Unit 34 reviews the management of the patient with a head injury in detail.

CHEST AND ABDOMEN

Aging, brittle bones are more susceptible to fracture. An elderly patient may sustain a fractured rib with a mechanism as benign as a strong cough or sneeze. A careful physical exam may reveal point tenderness over a fracture site or even crepitus as a result of bone ends rubbing together. Rib fractures may be associated with significant internal organ injury.

Mortality from intra-abdominal injury can exceed four times that seen in younger patients. Additionally, the physical exam of the elderly adult's abdomen may be falsely reassuring due to the altered response to peritoneal irritation. The classic rigid, tender abdomen may not be present despite significant intra-abdominal injuries. Unit 36 discusses the assessment and management techniques used in the case of chest and abdominal injury.

SPINE

Many elderly adults have chronic degenerative changes in their spines that result in pain. After sustaining trauma, it may be difficult to determine whether any pain in the neck or back is due to previous disease or to new injury. It is best for the EMT to treat for a new injury and take precautions to prevent further injury by providing spinal immobilization in any case in which significant trauma exists or even in the case of minor trauma with neck or back pain. Unit 35 discusses spine injuries in detail.

EXTREMITIES

Fractures to extremities can occur with minor trauma or even with no noted trauma in the elderly population. Bones are more susceptible to injury due to the normal aging process, and the presence of abnormality in a bone causing a spontaneous fracture is more common in this population. The EMT should be vigilant to the possibility of a fractured bone even when a history of trauma is not clear. Any extremity pain should be suspicious and treated as a possible fracture as described in Unit 38.

CONCLUSION

The aging of our society makes it necessary for the EMT to become familiar with the normal changes associated with aging as well as the common illnesses encountered in this age group. The EMT's rapid recognition of the potential for serious illness or injury can lead to greatly improved outcomes for elderly patients.

Street Smart

Due to degenerative arthritis in the neck in many elderly patients, caution must be used when maneuvering the neck to maintain airway patency. Additionally, when packaging an elderly patient on a long spine board, severe kyphosis (curvature of the spine) requires the EMT to place padding such as rolled-up towels, in voids along the board to achieve appropriate immobilization and avoid tissue injury.

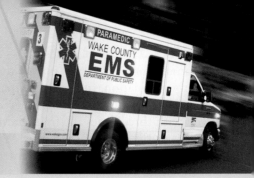

CASE STUDY Continued

Carlotta sits down at the table next to Mrs. Carlyle, and taking her hand, does a quick pulse check. Mrs. Carlyle's pulse is slow and steady, and her respirations are shallow at 16. Mrs. Carlyle does not seem to be in acute distress; however, Carlotta believes she is not feeling herself and being alone scared her into calling for the ambulance.

Ian listens to Mrs. Carlyle's lungs, after asking her permission to touch her and notes her lung sounds are diminished with some crackles in the left side. Ian places Mrs. Carlyle on oxygen by nasal cannula at 3 lpm and obtains a set of baseline vital signs: blood pressure 110/78, pulse 54, respirations 16.

Carlotta gathers a history from Mrs. Carlyle, who states she has been feeling weak today and sometimes a little short of breath. She is allergic to penicillin and

takes medicine for hypertension and fluid in her lungs. She was in the hospital for a few days 3 months ago with pneumonia and sometimes has swelling in her feet and ankles, as she does today. She ate some toast this morning around 7 a.m. and felt weak when she got out of bed. Mrs. Carlyle denies any falls or injuries over the past several weeks.

Carlotta and Ian assist Mrs. Carlyle onto the stretcher. En route to the hospital, Mrs. Carlyle continues to visit about her family to Carlotta, occasionally stopping to take a deep breath. Carlotta gives a radio report of Mrs. Carlyle's condition to the receiving hospital and turns patient care over to the staff RN in the ED upon arrival with a follow-up report. Mrs. Carlyle's condition had not changed throughout transport.

Key Concepts Revisited

- The neurologic changes characteristic of aging include physical shrinking of the brain and decreases of the senses.
  - Diminished visual acuity increases potential for falls.
  - Loss of hearing and smell decreases the ability to recognize warning signs.
  - Impaired communication may result from hearing loss.
- The EMT must understand the differences between dementia and delirium in the elderly patient.
  - Dementia is a progressive decline in intellectual function usually leading to deterioration of occupational, social, and interpersonal functions.
    - Gradual onset
    - Loss of memory
  - Delirium is an alteration in the level of consciousness usually caused by an acute medical problem.
    - Sudden onset
    - Usually reversible once the medical problem is corrected

- The cardiovascular changes characteristic of aging include increased occurrence of coronary artery disease; stiffened, restricted vessels; and hypertension.
  - Increased risk of heart attack
  - Increased risk of stroke
  - Increased risk of congestive heart failure
- The respiratory changes characteristic of aging include decreased elasticity of lung tissue, decreased compensatory ability, and increased risk of infections.
  - Pneumonia
  - Pulmonary embolism seen more often in the elderly than younger adults
- Gastrointestinal changes characteristic of aging include loss of intestinal mobility and increased tooth loss
  - Malnutrition
  - Choking
  - Constipation

- Genitourinary changes characteristic of aging include decreased bladder tone and loss of kidney function.
  - Urinary tract infections
  - Bladder infections
  - Renal failure
    - Dialysis
- Diseases affecting the musculoskeletal system include osteoporosis and arthritis.
  - Loss of bone density makes bones fragile and easily fractured.
  - Decreased flexibility in joints with inflammation decreases mobility and increases the risk for falls.

- Soft tissue injuries and higher incidence of hypothermia are the result of changes to the integumentary system due to aging.
  - Thinner skin
  - Less subcutaneous fat
- Medication use by the elderly often results in polypharmacy, increasing chances of adverse reactions.
  - Use of multiple medication by a single patient
    - Decreases compliance with medication use
    - Increased risk of multiple drug reaction
- The EMT's rapid recognition of potential for serious illness or injury in the elderly leads to greatly improved outcomes.

Review Questions

1. What are the neurologic changes characteristic of aging?
2. Explain the differences between dementia and delirium.
3. What cardiovascular changes are characteristic of aging?
4. What respiratory changes are characteristic of aging?
5. What are the signs and symptoms of a pulmonary embolism?
6. What gastrointestinal changes are characteristic of aging?
7. What genitourinary changes are characteristic of aging?
8. Why are the elderly susceptible to renal failure?
9. What is dialysis?
10. What musculoskeletal changes are characteristic of aging?
11. What integumentary changes are characteristic of aging?
12. Describe the problems that can occur with polypharmacy.

Key Terms

Arteriorvenous (AV) shunt
Arthritis
Geriatrics
Nephrons

Polypharmacy
Pulmonary embolism
Silent myocardial infarction

Further Study

Bledsoe, B. E., and R. W. Benner. *Critical Care Paramedic*. Upper Saddle River, NJ: Pearson/ Prentice Hall.

National Association of Emergency Medical Technicians. *PHTLS: Basic and Advanced Pre-hospitalTrauma Life Support*. 6th ed. Clinton, MS: Mosby/Elsevier, 2007.

Nixon, R. G. "Geriatrics and Their Meds: Problems and Perils." *Emergency Medicine Service* 32, no. 2 (February 2003): 35–38, 40–42.

Plassman, B. L., K. M. Langa, G. G. Fisher, et al. "Prevalence of Dementia in the United States: The Aging, Demographics, and Memory Study." *Neuroepidemiology* 29, No. 1–2 (2007): 125–132.

UNIT (47) End of Life Issues

Advances in medicine have created opportunities for people to live longer and more productive lives. Advances in medicine have also made it possible to delay the inevitable, death. As medicine and society struggle with this life-or-death contradiction, patients have tried to assert their right to make the decisions about their own lives, to decide when they want to be allowed to die.

National Education Standard
The Emergency Medical Technician (EMT) will demonstrate a fundamental depth and foundational breadth of understanding of end of life issues in the geriatric patient.

Key Concepts

- Advance directives allow a patient's wishes about resuscitation to be known to family and health care providers before a patient becomes incapacitated.

- Advance directives allow the EMT to take the patient's wishes into consideration at the end of life.

- Living wills are legal documents directing a patient's care if the patient becomes unable to do so.

- A durable power of attorney designates a person who makes decisions on behalf of another who is incapacitated.

- A do not resuscitate (DNR) order is a physician order to withhold CPR in a patient in cardiac arrest.

- The Patient Self-Determination Act is a federal law that provides protections to a patient's right to decide end of life issues.

- A health care proxy is a person chosen to make medical decisions on behalf of the patient.

- Out-of-hospital DNR is binding in the prehospital setting, specifying that lifesaving measures should not be started.

- Hospice is a team of health care professionals who care for dying patients.

- In appropriate circumstances, not performing CPR is providing the best care for the patient.

Lou and Gary had just sat down for coffee when the pager goes off for an unresponsive male, unknown respiratory status. Lou makes sure their resuscitation equipment is handy as he gets into the truck.

Upon arrival, they are met at the door by a distraught young woman who points to the hospital bed in the corner of the living room. "I think my grandfather is dead. Please do something."

The patient, an elderly man lying in bed, is not breathing. The man's wife, Eunice, is standing next to the bed, holding his hand. She looks up as Lou approaches the bed, saying there is nothing to be done and that her husband should be left alone to "die in peace. That's what he would have wanted."

Shantelle tearfully tells Gary that her grandfather was gasping for breath and she got scared, so she called 9-1-1. Her grandfather has had a long history of Alzheimer's disease and was diagnosed with lung cancer 3 months ago. The doctors have told Eunice that there is nothing more that can be done for him.

Looking down at the elderly man, Lou notices the patient looks oddly at peace.

Critical Thinking Questions

1. Is the EMT obligated to start CPR?
2. Is there any order or directive that could have an impact in this case?
3. Would medical control help in this situation?

INTRODUCTION

In the past, decisions about end of life were typically made in the hospital. Increasingly, however, these decisions are now being made by and for patients who are out of the hospital and in the community. Emergency Medical Technicians (EMTs) are increasingly confronted with end of life issues in the prehospital setting. This chapter discusses the situation in which an EMT is faced with an order to not start cardiopulmonary resuscitation (CPR) on a patient in cardiac arrest and various other legal documents dealing with end of life issues.

ADVANCE DIRECTIVES

When EMTs are called to care for terminally ill patients, they may also be confronted with a potential role conflict. The EMT is typically seen and may see himself in the role of lifesaver—a person who would make a valiant effort to save another human's life regardless of how futile that effort may be. However, the EMT may also be faced with a patient who is asking that he not fulfill that lifesaving role. Instead, the patient may be asking the EMT to fulfill his role as a compassionate caregiver, a person who understands the patient's pain and suffering and would do nothing to prolong it. The patient may even ask the EMT not to start CPR if he should suffer a cardiac arrest.

This conflict is not unique to EMTs. Physicians and nurses—in fact, all health care professionals—have had to grapple with this life or death decision. Should they start CPR on a terminally ill patient when they suspect it may cause needless pain or, worse, is contrary to the patient's wishes?

Advances in medicine have made it possible to substantially prolong life. However, the issue that arises is quality of life. Some patients have decided they do not want heroic efforts made to save their lives. They state that they have lived long enough and do not want to live life if they must suffer from an illness that cannot be cured. They would rather die than continue a prolonged struggle with a painful and debilitating illness. Other elderly patients are concerned that if they survive after resuscitation, they will become a burden on their families.

These patients have used a variety of methods to make their wishes known before they die and to prevent the interference of health care providers in what is seen as a natural act, the act of dying. Collectively these efforts to express patients' wishes before they become incapacitated are called *advance directives.*

This unit does not attempt to answer the moral and ethical questions surrounding decisions regarding advance directives or to definitively answer the complex legal questions that surround the issue. The intent of this discussion is to provide EMTs with a basic foundation for understanding advance directives and their impact on the practice of Emergency Medical Services (EMS).

GENERAL PRINCIPLES OF CONSENT AND REFUSAL

The foundation of the advance directive is the fundamental principle that every patient has a right to control his or her own body. Control means the patient must consent before a health care professional may begin any treatment. Logically, if the patient can consent, the patient can refuse treatment as well. It is an established fact in American jurisprudence that a patient may refuse treatment, even if the foreseeable outcome will be death.

What if the patient becomes unconscious and is unable to consent or refuse? The legal principle of implied consent assumes that the patient could have changed her mind at the last moment and wanted treatment. In other words, the dying patient might have wanted to be resuscitated but was unable to express her wish. Therefore, it is common practice to start resuscitation of the unconscious patient, based on the principle of implied consent.

PATIENTS AFFECTED BY ADVANCE DIRECTIVES

Advance directives are not restricted for use only by the elderly. Persons with profound disabilities may, for legitimate reasons, decide not to have extraordinary measures taken to prolong their lives, despite the fact that technology is available to prolong life.

An EMT should never think that a person who is physically disabled has a decreased mental capacity. The two are not directly related. Similarly, patients with incurable diseases also may decide to stop or restrict treatment that they view as a futile delay of the inevitable.

Finally, the treatment of a disease that has afflicted a patient may reach the limits of modern technology. Medicine cannot offer these patients any more hope. These patients are at the end of their disease; in other words, their condition is **terminal.**

TYPES OF ADVANCE DIRECTIVES

Many instruments—some legal documents and others that are medical orders—have been used to prevent someone from being resuscitated. The single unique characteristic of these advance directives is that they enable health care professionals to follow a patient's expressed wishes after her death.

LIVING WILLS

Living wills may represent one of the oldest forms of advance directive. *Living wills* are documents that specifically address the wishes of the patient in

Pediatric Considerations

Discussions of consent and refusal assume that the patient has the legal capacity to consent, by virtue of age and competency, and to make decisions. In the case of children and others who are legally incompetent, it is the responsibility of the family, physician, and courts to make that determination. If a decision, an advance directive, is made in this fashion, it is legally binding on all health care providers who care for that patient.

regard to resuscitation. The instructions in a living will are meant to be followed by the patient's physician and other health care providers if the patient is unable to express these instructions.

In most cases, living wills are created by the patient with the assistance of a lawyer and without input from a physician. An example of a living will can be found in Figure 47.1. A patient's living will is witnessed by adults and signed by the patient in the same manner as other wills. However, a living will does not designate or rely on an agent to enforce it. An agent is usually a family member or friend entrusted with making decisions on behalf of the patient. Rather, a living will assumes that the physician or health care provider will accept the document as being the patient's last request and will abide by that decision.

Therefore, there is an implicit understanding within a living will that a physician will comply with the patient's final wishes. But a living will is not legally binding; and on occasion, especially during emergencies, the patient is treated by an emergency physician or other health care provider who is not the patient's primary or attending physician. This person may not know the circumstances surrounding the decision to create the living will and may not agree with the patient's decision. In addition, some physicians believe that a patient who is not a physician is not capable of making a wise medical decision alone. They contend that living wills should not be recognized as a matter of principle.

DURABLE POWER OF ATTORNEY

A **power of attorney (POA)** allows a designated person to make decisions on behalf of another who is unable to make decisions. This decision-making authority is usually restricted to business or personal matters. Seldom is a durable power of attorney used to make medical decisions. Typically, a patient assumes that a physician will make the best decision on her behalf and that a POA is not necessary.

Ordinarily, a power of attorney expires when the patient expires. The unique quality of a durable power of attorney for health care (DPOA-HC) is that it outlasts the patient. A durable power of attorney allows a patient to designate an agent, frequently a spouse or offspring, to make life-and-death decisions on her behalf in the event she cannot make those decisions on her own. A sample durable power of attorney can be found in Figure 47.2.

A durable power of attorney, like a living will, is a legal document, and not a medical document. Because this document is prepared without advice or recommendations from a medical professional, some physicians prefer to make the decisions they consider to be best for the patient regardless of the presence of such a document. Occasionally, when a physician disagrees with the family and proceeds with treatment despite the family's protest, conflicts erupt between family members and physicians.

DO NOT RESUSCITATE ORDERS

In some cases, the judgment of physicians attending the patient is that, in their medical opinion, any efforts at resuscitation will be futile. These physicians can write a medical order to be followed by all health care providers to prevent further life-preserving therapies, up to and including CPR.

This medical order will state that if the patient's heart and/or breathing should stop, no attempt should be made to revive the patient. This order to not resuscitate a patient is called a *do not resuscitate order (DNR)* (Figure 47.3).

A DNR order is usually written after the physician has spoken to the patient and family and all have agreed that resuscitation will not be in the patient's best interests.

Declaration

Declaration made this _____day of _____(month, year).

I, _____, being of sound mind, willfully and voluntarily make known my desire that my dying shall not be artificially prolonged under the circumstances set forth below and do hereby declare:

In the absence of my ability to give directions regarding the use of such life-sustaining procedures, it is my intention that this declaration

If at any time I should either have a terminal and irreversible incurable injury, disease, or illness or be in continual profound comatose state with no reasonable chance of recovery, certified by two physicians who have personally examined me, one of whom shall be my attending physician, and the physicians have determined that my death will occur whether or not life-sustaining procedures are utilized and where the application of life-sustaining procedures would serve only to prolong artificially the dying process, I direct that such procedures be withheld or withdrawn and that I be permitted to die naturally with only the administration of medication or the performance of any medical procedure deemed necessary to provide me with comfort care.

In the absence of my ability to give directions regarding the use of such life-sustaining procedures, it is my intention that this declaration shall be honored by my family and physician(s) as the final expression of my legal right to refuse medical or surgical treatment and accept the consequences from such refusal.

I understand the full import of this declaration and I am emotionally and mentally competent to make this declaration.

Signed:_____

City, Parish, and State of Residence_____

The declarant has been personally known to me and I believe him or her to be of sound mind.

Witness:_____

Witness:_____

Figure 47.1 The living will was one of the first advance directives (Courtesy of the Louisiana Hospital Association, Baton Rouge, LA)

Part I. Durable Power of Attorney for Health Care

• If you do NOT wish to name an agent to make health care decisions for you, write your initials in the box

[Initials]

This form has been prepared to comply with the "Durable Power of Attorney for Health Care Act" of Missouri.

1. Selection of agent. I appoint:
Name:_____
Address:_____

| It is suggested that only one Agent be named. However, if more than one Agent is named, anyone may act individually unless you specify otherwise. |

Telephone:_____
as my Agent.

2. Alternate Agents. Only an Agent named by me may act under this Durable Power of Attorney. If my Agent resigns or is not able or available to make health care decisions for me, or if an Agent named by me is divorced from me or is my spouse and legally separated from me, I appoint the person(s) named below (in the order named if more than one):

First Alternate Agent

Name:_____
Address:_____
_____
Telephone:_____

Second Alternate Agent

Name:_____
Address:_____
_____
Telephone:_____

| This is a Durable Power of Attorney, and the authority of my Agent shall not terminate if I become disabled or incapacitated. |

Part I. Durable Power of Attorney for Health Care (Continued)

3. Effective date and durability. This Durable Power of Attorney is effective when two physicians decide and certify that I am incapacitated and unable to make and communicate a health care decision.

• If you want ONE physician, instead of TWO, to decide whether you are incapacitated, write your initials in the box to the right.

[Initials]

4. Agent's powers. I grant to my Agent full authority to:

A. Give consent to, prohibit, or withdraw any type of health care, medical care, treatment, or procedure, even if my death may result;

• If you wish to AUTHORIZE your Agent to direct a health care provider to withhold or withdraw artificially supplied nutrition and hydration (including tube feeding of food and water), write your initials in the box to the right.

[Initials]

• If you DO NOT WISH TO AUTHORIZE your Agent to direct a health care provider to withhold or withdraw artificially supplied nutrition and hydration (including tube feeding of food and water), write your initials in the box to the right.

[Initials]

B. Make all necessary arrangements for health care services on my behalf, and to hire and fire medical personnel responsible for my care;

C. Move me into or out of any health care facility (even if against medical advice) to obtain compliance with the decisions of my Agent; and

D. Take any other action necessary to do what I authorize here, including (but not limited to) granting any waiver or release from liability required by any health care provider, and taking any legal action at the expense of my estate to enforce this Durable Power of Attorney.

5. Agent's Financial Liability and Compensation. My Agent acting under this Durable Power of Attorney will incur no personal financial liability. My Agent shall not be entitled to compensation for services performed under this Durable Power of Attorney, but my Agent shall be entitled to reimbursement for all reasonable expenses incurred as a result of carrying out any provision hereof.

Part II. Health Care Directive

• If you DO NOT WISH to make a health care directive, write your initials in the box to the right, and go to Part III.

[Initials]

I make this HEALTH CARE DIRECTIVE ("Directive") to exercise my right to determine the course of my health care and to provide clear and convincing proof of my wishes and instructions about my treatment.

If I am persistently unconscious or there is no reasonable expectation of my recovery from a seriously incapacitating or terminal illness or condition, I direct that all of the life-prolonging procedures which I have initialed below be withheld or withdrawn.

I want the following life-prolonging procedures to be withheld or withdrawn:

| • artificially supplied nutrition and hydration (including tube feeding of food and water) . . . . [Initials] |

• surgery or other invasive procedures. . . . . [Initials]

• heart-lung resuscitation (CPR) . . . . [Initials]

• antibiotic. . . . . [Initials]

• dialysis. . . . . [Initials]

• mechanical ventilator (respirator). . . . . [Initials]

• chemotherapy. . . . . [Initials]

• radiation therapy. . . . . [Initials]

• all other "life-prolonging" medical or surgical procedures that are merely intended to keep me alive without reasonable hope of improving my condition or curing my illness or injury. . . . . [Initials]

However, if my physician believes that any life-prolonging procedure may lead to significant recovery, I direct my physician to try the treatment for a reasonable period of time. If it does not improve my condition, I direct the treatment be withdrawn even if it shortens my life. I also direct that I be given medical treatment to relieve pain or to provide comfort, even if such treatment might shorten my life, suppress my appetite or my breathing, or be habit forming.

IF I HAVE NOT DESIGNATED AN AGENT IN THE DURABLE POWER OF ATTORNEY, THIS DOCUMENT IS MEANT TO BE IN FULL FORCE AND EFFECT AS MY HEALTH CARE DIRECTIVE.

Part III. General Provisions Included in the Directive and Durable Power of Attorney

YOU MUST SIGN THIS DOCUMENT IN THE PRESENCE OF TWO WITNESSES.
IN WITNESS WHEREOF, I have executed this document this_____day of
_____, year____.

_____
Signature

Print name _____
Address _____

The person who signed this document is of sound mind and voluntarily signed this document in our presence. Each of the undersigned witnesses is at least eighteen years of age.

Signature_____   Signature_____
Print name _____   Print name _____
Address _____   Address _____

| ONLY REQUIRED FOR PART I — DURABLE POWER OF ATTORNEY |

STATE OF MISSOURI   )
) as
_____OF_____   )
On this_____day of_____, year_____, before me personally appeared to me known to be the person described in and who executed the foregoing instrument and acknowledged that he/she executed the same as his/her free act and deed.

IN WITNESS WHEREOF, I have hereunto set my hand and affixed my official seal in the County of _____, State of Missouri, the day and year first above written.

_____
Notary Public

My Commission Expires:_____

Figure 47.2 The durable power of attorney gives legal authority to someone to make health care decisions after death (Reprinted with permission of the Missouri Bar)

DNR DOCUMENTATION FORM #1

CONSENT FOR DNR ORDER
BY ADULT PATIENT WITH CAPACITY

PATIENT IDENTIFICATION PLATE

The patient's consent to a DNR order must be obtained at or about the time the order is issued. The patient's consent may be **either** oral or written.

ORAL CONSENT must be given in the presence of a physician and another witness.

Physician's Statement
I have provided the patient with information about his/her diagnosis and prognosis, the reasonably foreseeable risks and benefits of CPR, the range of available resuscitation measures, and the consequences of a DNR order. The patient has expressed the decision to consent to a DNR order orally in my presence.

_____   _____
Physician Signature   Date

Witness' Statement
The patient has expressed the decision to consent to a DNR order orally in my presence.

_____   _____
Witness Signature   Date

_____
Print name

ALTERNATIVELY, WRITTEN CONSENT may be given, and signed by the patient and two adult witnesses. If written consent is obtained, a copy must be placed in the chart.

After consent is obtained, the DNR order is to be issued by the attending physician, and entered on the Physician's Order Sheet.

If the attending physician objects to a DNR order, he/she must either:
— transfer the patient to another attending physician, or
— notify the Medical Director that dispute mediation is required

REMINDER: The DNR order must be reviewed by the attending physician at least **every three days,** to determine if the order is still appropriate in light of the patient's condition. A notation must be made in the chart to reflect that review. It is **not** necessary to repeat the consent process when the order is reviewed.

Figure 47.3 A do not resuscitate order is a physician's order to not revive the dying patient

THE PATIENT SELF-DETERMINATION ACT

In 1991, Congress sought to enact a body of law that would protect the rights of the patient as well as provide some direction to physicians on how to react to patient requests for advance directives. That law was the **Patient Self-Determination Act of 1991.**

The Patient Self-Determination Act is binding on any institution or organization that accepts Medicare or uses federal funding. It was specifically directed toward the population of patients that were already in health care institutions.

HEALTH CARE PROXY

The Patient Self-Determination Act also created a new entity, the *health care proxy*. The health care proxy is a person who is appointed by the patient to make decisions on behalf of the patient. The health care proxy is similar to a DPOA-HC, except that an attorney need not be involved in the process.

The health care proxy can make broad decisions, including decisions about resuscitation, for the patient. The health care proxy can also make specific decisions about tube feedings or machine ventilation, for example. A sample health care proxy can be found in Figure 47.4. In some states, the decision of a health care proxy is not binding on an EMT in the out-of-hospital environment. The exception may be when an EMT is transferring a patient from one health care facility to another. The EMT should follow local protocols regarding health care proxies, DNR orders, and interfacility transfers.

OUT-OF-HOSPITAL DNR ORDERS

In some circumstances, a patient who is not in a health care institution may wish not to be resuscitated. The patient may have been discharged for home care, for example, yet still desire the protection a health care proxy or a DNR order offers from unwanted intrusions into her private life by well-meaning EMTs. Physicians and EMS authorities have sought a way to provide such patients the same rights out of the hospital as they would have within the hospital.

The **out-of-hospital DNR** provides the means and is used in some states to give direction to EMTs faced with a dying patient. The out-of-hospital DNR is a binding medical order issued by the physician attending the patient that prevents the EMT from starting lifesaving measures such as CPR.

An out-of-hospital DNR should be written either on the physician's letterhead or on a preapproved DNR form (Figure 47.5). It should be clearly written, leaving no room for ambiguity. A statement such as "no heroics" can be meaningless. On the other hand, a statement specifying "no CPR or defibrillation" leaves little doubt about the patient's or the physician's wishes.

Frequently, a standard legal form is used that EMTs can quickly identify as a legitimate medical order. In some states, a specified state form must be used.

PROBLEMS WITH OUT-OF-HOSPITAL DNRS

Problems have arisen in the field with out-of-hospital DNRs. In an emergency, family members may be confused and forget where the DNR is located. In some cases, family members may not be present to produce the document at the time the patient expires.

To help with this problem, some states are using DNR bracelets or necklaces. These bracelets minimally have imprinted on them the patient's name and the words "Do Not Resuscitate." EMTs should review the local medical protocols before accepting a DNR bracelet or necklace as a directive to be followed.

Advance Directive

Part A

APPOINTMENT OF HEALTH CARE AGENT

(Optional Form)

(Cross through if you do not want to appoint a health care agent to make health care decisions for you. If you do want to appoint an agent, cross through any items in the form that you do not want to apply.)

1. I, _____, residing at

   _____

   _____ appoint the following individual as my agent to
   make health care decisions for me _____

   _____

   _____ (Full Name, Address, and Telephone Number)
   Optional: If this agent is unavailable or is unable or unwilling to act as my agent, then I appoint
   the following person to act in this capacity _____

   _____

   _____ (Full Name, Address, and Telephone Number)
2. My agent has full power and authority to make health care decisions for me, including the
   power to:
   a. Request, receive, and review any information, oral or written, regarding my physical or
   mental health, including, but not limited to, medical and hospital records, and consent to
   disclosure of this information;
   b. Employ and discharge my health care providers;
   c. Authorize my admission to or discharge from (including transfer to another facility) any
   hospital, hospice, nursing home, adult home, or other medical care facility; and
   d. Consent to the provision, withholding, or withdrawal of health care, including, in appropriate
   circumstances, life-sustaining procedures.
3. The authority of my agent is subject to the following provisions and limitations:
   _____

   _____

   _____

   _____

   _____
4. My agent's authority becomes operative (initial the option that applies):
   _____ When my attending physician and a second physician determine that I am incapable of
   making an informed decision regarding my health care;
   or
   _____ When this document is signed.
5. My agent is to make health care decisions for me based on the health care instructions I give in
   this document and on my wishes as otherwise known to my agent. If my wishes are unknown

Figure 47.4 A health care proxy was created by the federal Patient Self-Determination Act of 1991

or unclear, my agent is to make health care decisions for me in accordance with my best interest, to be determined by my agent after considering the benefits, burdens, and risks that might result from a given treatment or course of treatment, or from the withholding or withdrawal of a treatment or course of treatment.

6. My agent shall not be liable for the costs of care based solely on this authorization.

By signing below, I indicate that I am emotionally and mentally competent to make this appointment of a health care agent and that I understand its purpose and effect.

_____   _____
Date   (Signature of Declarant)

(Signature of Declarant) The declarant signed or acknowledged signing this appointment of a health care agent in my presence and based upon my personal observation appears to be a competent individual.

_____   _____
Signature of Witness 1   Signature of Witness 2

Figure 47.4 (Continued)

State of New York
Department of Health

Nonhospital Order Not to Resuscitate
(DNR Order)

Person's Name _____

Date of Birth ___/ ___/ ___

Do not resuscitate the person named above.

Physician's Signature_____

Print Name _____

License number _____

Date ___/ ___/ ___

It is the responsibility of the physician to determine, at least every 90 days, whether this order continues to be appropriate, and to indicate this by a note in the person's medical chart. The issuance of a new form is **NOT** required, and under the law this order should be considered valid unless it is known that it has been revoked. This order remains valid and must be followed, even if it has not been reviewed within the 90 day period.

Figure 47.5 Some EMS systems use a special out-of-hospital DNR form (Reprinted with permission of the New York State Department of Health)

RESUSCITATION DECISION MAKING

An out-of-hospital DNR is effective only if it is accepted by medical control and meets all the criteria that have been established by medical control. The medical directors in some communities have chosen not to allow an EMT to accept an out-of-hospital DNR. Although this decision may seem to eliminate the issue of out-of-hospital DNRs, in reality, the problem is often not that simple.

Family members may become agitated if CPR is started and may feel they have the right to decide the patient's treatment. The EMT should try to explain to the family that the EMT is under medical orders to start CPR. If the family becomes hostile, the EMT should either move the patient to the ambulance quickly or make a tactful retreat and call for law enforcement officers.

If an out-of-hospital DNR is accepted by medical control, it must meet a few basic conditions before an EMT can accept it as legitimate. An out-of-hospital DNR should clearly state the name of the patient and the limitations for care. For example, the out-of-hospital DNR may state that no external chest compressions may be done or that the EMT may not assist ventilation. Some out-of-hospital DNRs are effective only for a specified period of time. State law may stipulate that an out-of-hospital DNR is effective for only 30 or 60 days. The EMT must know the local protocols regarding DNRs.

Some opponents of out-of-hospital DNRs argue that an EMT has to be a "street lawyer" to be able to react correctly when confronted with a pile of "legal papers" and a dying patient whose treatment decisions are in question.

When in doubt and without further guidance, if an EMT is unsure of how to proceed, the EMT should always err in favor of helping the patient through the emergency. If EMS was called, it can be assumed that an emergency existed and that the patient would have wanted resuscitation under the principle of implied consent; therefore, routine patient care is in order. The EMT should then immediately contact medical control for further instructions on how to continue or discontinue treatment.

STANDARD COMFORT MEASURES

Despite having a valid DNR order, a patient's family may decide to call EMS for a variety of other good reasons. The family may be unsure of how to react to the situation, such as the patient's choking, so they call EMS. Alternatively, the patient may be extremely uncomfortable, and the family may think that EMS can provide pain medication. For all these reasons and more, EMS is called to the home of a patient with a DNR.

A DNR means that an EMT should not start CPR on a pulseless patient. A DNR does not mean that the EMT should not provide care for the patient who is not in cardiac arrest. Supportive care designed to ease the patient's suffering is called **standard comfort measures.** Examples of standard comfort measures include suctioning the patient's airway clear of secretions and the administration of oxygen if the patient's breathing is labored.

Ventilating the nonbreathing patient, however, is not a standard comfort measure. It is a part of resuscitation. An EMT should consult with his medical director, before the call, about what procedures fall under standard comfort measures and what procedures are considered resuscitation.

HOSPICE

An EMT may encounter hospice staff while on the scene of a terminally ill patient. **Hospice** programs provide supportive care to dying patients and their families both in special hospice centers and at home. A hospice nurse may call EMS to help transfer a patient to a hospice center or for assistance with patient care in a crisis.

Hospice nurses provide care that is outlined in a predetermined set of medical orders. These medical orders may differ from those of an EMT. These differences may lead to conflicts on the scene. The EMT should meet with hospice staff in their community to discuss these differences beforehand in order to prevent conflict and ensure a seamless provision of care between patient care providers. If a hospice nurse is on scene and there is a question regarding treatment, the EMT should contact medical control for direction.

CONCLUSION

At first glance, advance directives can appear confusing. EMTs have felt that they are in the unenviable position of having to make snap decisions about life and death. For this reason, it is important that an EMT knows his local medical protocols regarding out-of-hospital DNRs. Moreover, whenever an EMT is in doubt, he should contact medical control for advice and direction.

The core issue with an out-of-hospital advance directive often comes down to performing CPR or not performing CPR. In some cases, it may not be in the patient's best interest to have CPR performed. The EMT who does not perform CPR may, in appropriate circumstances, be providing the best care for the patient.

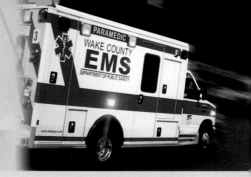

CASE STUDY Continued

Gary calls medical control, explaining the patient has no pulse or respirations, noting his medical history and the presence of a durable power of attorney designating his wife, Eunice, as the person to make medical decisions on his behalf. Gary also relates that Eunice has informed them her husband had a "Do Not Resuscitate" (DNR) document signed by him and his doctor. Medical control confirms no CPR is to be attempted.

Lou gently directs Shantelle into the kitchen, giving Eunice some time to finish her goodbyes. Gary has taken the equipment back out to the ambulance and called into dispatch this was a DOA and they would be spending a few minutes on the scene helping the family.

Gary asks Eunice if there is anything they can do for her, such as call the funeral home or family, before they leave. Eunice sighs tiredly and shakes her head. Shantelle continues to weep softly from the kitchen where Lou is doing his best to provide some comfort for the loss of her grandpa.

Eunice finally gets up and walks to the kitchen, where she takes Shantelle into her arms. She looks at Gary and Lou with a sad smile and states, "There is a copy of the DPOA and DNR sitting on the table next to the door. Please take that for your records."

Gary and Lou get up to leave, conveying condolences for the family's loss. Eunice takes Gary's hand and thanks them both for respecting her husband's wishes, as well as their kindness, compassion, and professionalism.

Key Concepts Revisited

- Advance directives allow a patient's wishes about resuscitation to be known to family and health care providers before a patient becomes incapacitated.
  - Potential role conflict for EMS switching roles from lifesaver to end-of-life caregiver
- Advance directives allow the EMT to take the patient's wishes into consideration and without CPR.
  - Negates implied consent
  - Directs others on the patient's behalf
- Living wills are legal documents directing a patient's care if the patient becomes unable to do so.
  - Attorney created
  - Dependent on the physician's goodwill to carry out the patient's wishes
- A durable power of attorney designates a person who makes decisions on behalf of another who is incapacitated
  - Attorney created

- A do not resuscitate (DNR) order is a physician order to withhold CPR in a patient in cardiac arrest
  - Physician created
  - Binding in the hospital
- The Patient Self-Determination Act is a federal law that provides protections to a patient's right to decide on end of life issues.
- Health care proxy is a person chosen to make medical decisions on behalf of the patient.
  - Created by the Patient Self-Determination Act
  - Delegates authority for all medical decisions to another person
    - May or may not be binding to EMTs
- An out-of-hospital DNR is binding in the prehospital setting specifying lifesaving measures should not be started.
  - Problems with out-of-hospital DNRs
    - Sometimes ambiguous wording

- Resuscitation decision making
  - Must be familiar with local protocols
  - Medical control

- Hospice is a team of health care professionals who care for dying patients.
  - Organized supportive care for dying patients
- In appropriate circumstances, not performing CPR is providing the best care for the patient.

Review Questions

1. What is an advance directive?
2. What is meant by terminal?
3. What are the types of advance directives?
4. What is a durable power of attorney?
5. How is a health care proxy different from a durable power of attorney?
6. What is a do not resuscitate order?

7. What is a comfort measure as opposed to a resuscitation treatment?
8. What should an EMT do if a terminal patient does not have an advance directive?
9. What should an EMT do if the advance directive is incomplete?
10. What is the role of the hospice team?

Key Terms

Hospice
Out-of-hospital DNR
Patient Self-Determination Act of 1991

Power of attorney (POA)
Standard comfort measures
Terminal

Further Study

Fuster, Valentin, Robert O'Rourke, Richard Walsh, and Philip Poole-Wilson. *Hurst's the Heart.* 12th ed. Columbus, OH: McGraw-Hill, 2008.

Paradis, N. A., and H. Halperin. *Cardiac Arrest: The Science and Practice of Resuscitation Medicine.* New York: Cambridge University Press, 2007.

Stone, C., K. Stone, and R. Humphries. *Current Emergency Diagnosis and Treatment.* Columbus, OH: McGraw-Hill, 2004.

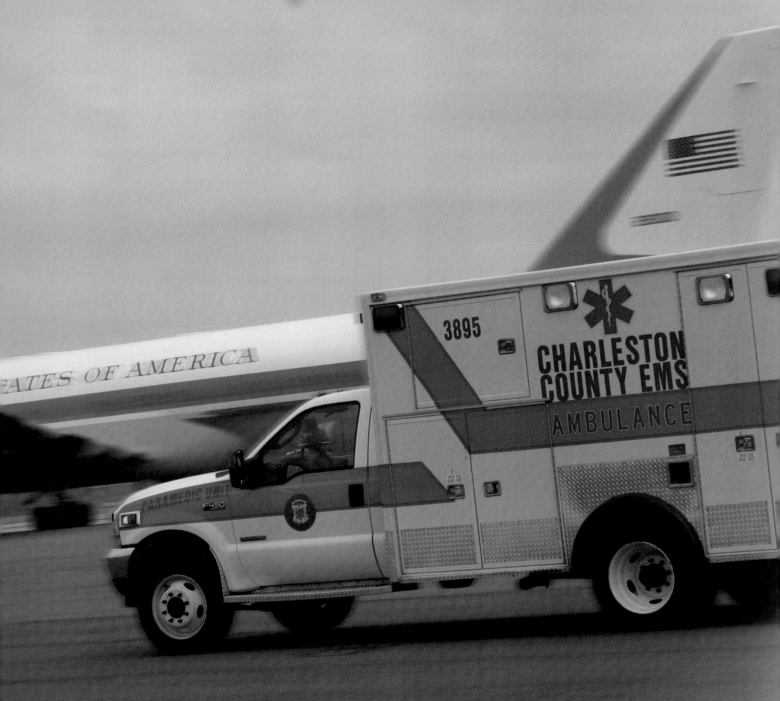

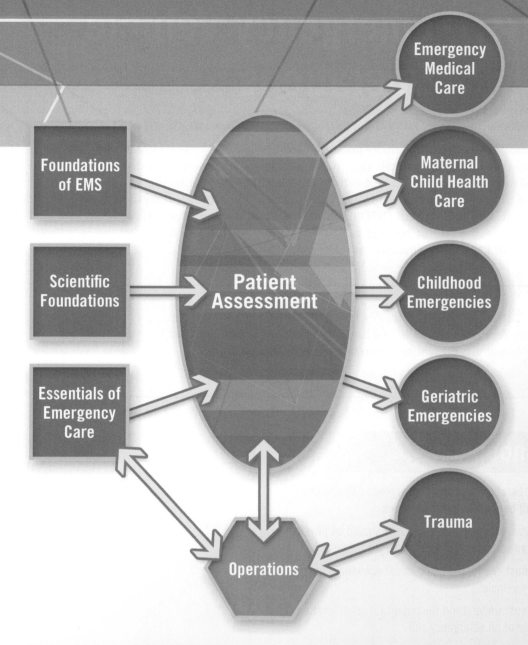

EMS Operations

One of the more exciting and stressful times in the career of Emergency Medical Technicians (EMTs) is when they are faced with a special situation, such as a hazardous materials spill or multiple patients.

These emergencies can occur during times of natural disaster or in the calm of night. Whenever they occur, the EMT must be prepared to respond to the emergency quickly and appropriately.

This section on Emergency Medical Services (EMS) operations details what actions an EMT should take at the scene of a special situation as well as how the EMT should respond to everyday emergencies.

UNIT (48) Emergency Vehicle Operations

Ambulance crashes are one of the many potential hazards faced by EMTs. In fact, studies are showing EMS professionals face the same risks for injury or death due to vehicle collisions as law enforcement officers and firefighters. Due to the rising number of motor vehicle crashes involving ambulances, the National Institute for Occupational Safety and Health (NIOSH) began researching ambulance safety, including the types of restraint systems needed in the back of the ambulance to prevent injuries to EMTs in the patient compartment of ambulances.

National Education Standards

The Emergency Medical Technician (EMT) will be able to demonstrate a simple depth and foundational breadth of understanding of the risks and responsibilities of emergency transport.

Key Concepts

- Proper preparation prior to an emergency call ensures the vehicle will be roadworthy at all times.

- The emergency vehicle operator (EVO) should be physically and mentally prepared for emergency responses.

- The EVO must ensure the mechanical soundness of the emergency vehicle.

- The EMT must understand the important considerations of each phase of an emergency call.

- The EVO has several specific considerations during an emergency response.

- Controlled intersections are the most common place for a crash involving an emergency vehicle.

- The EVO should be familiar with local laws and regulations governing the use of emergency warning devices and operation of emergency vehicles.

- The EVO must properly position the emergency vehicle on every scene.

- The emergency vehicle must be cleaned, decontaminated, and restocked in preparation of the next call.

- Failure on the part of an EVO to anticipate, recognize, and respond appropriately to the dangers of the road is what leads to many ambulance collisions.

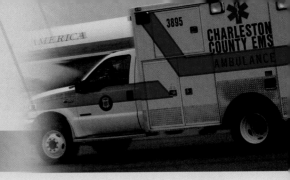

CASE STUDY

As their morning shift begins, Tru, the new EMT on crew, and her partner Barney are discussing the responsibilities for the day as they walk to the ambulance to begin the vehicle and equipment checks. This is Tru's third full-time shift since being hired last week. She has not been assigned emergency vehicle operations duties on the ambulance yet and is anxious to get the opportunity. When she asks Barney if today would be a good day for the first emergency vehicle operations training assignment, he replies, "The roads are wet from last night, and the temperature is supposed to stay around 30 degrees. Since there is a good chance of the roads icing up, I think it would be best to wait."

Noting that his new partner looks a little dejected, Barney adds, "Tru, it is not that I doubt your ability to drive, but we have a policy, as you know, that new employees will be orientated to driving during a day shift,

when the weather is generally good. No adverse weather, if possible. Your next shift is Saturday, and the weather is supposed to warm up and be nice. We'll tentatively plan for that to be your first EVO assignment. Why don't you ride in the back today, and I'll drive."

Picking up the vehicle checklist, Barney starts to perform a routine vehicle inspection while Tru inspects the equipment in the rear of the ambulance.

Critical Thinking Questions

1. What is necessary preparation for duty as an EMT?
2. Why is it necessary to perform an equipment check at the beginning of every shift?
3. Why is it necessary to perform a vehicle inspection at the beginning of every shift?

INTRODUCTION

For obvious reasons, the ambulance is a crucial part of the EMS system. It is the vehicle that transports the patient to definitive care. It should be a safe, clean, and comforting environment where patients can feel confident they are getting the best care by professionals. It is imperative that EMT education makes learning to skillfully and safely operate the ambulance as high a priority as all other aspects of patient care. The EMT must know the laws, regulations, and service policies before climbing into the driver's seat of an ambulance. This unit discusses emergency vehicle operations, including vehicle and equipment readiness, emergency response, and transportation of the sick and injured.

READINESS

The best way to do a job well is to be well prepared to do the job. The EMT will have a hard time caring for a patient who is ill or injured if the ambulance will not run, the equipment is defective, or needed medical supplies are missing. Before the alert is sounded and the pager tones go out, EMTs must check both the medical supplies and equipment completely and ensure the readiness of their emergency vehicle.

EMERGENCY VEHICLE CLASSIFICATIONS

Wherever someone gets hurt or is ill and calls for help, EMS must be able to respond to the scene, regardless of where that scene may be located. EMS responds in a wide variety of environments, and frequently each environment

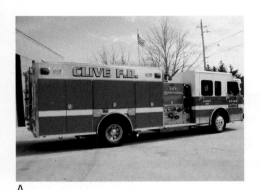

A

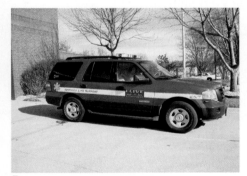

B

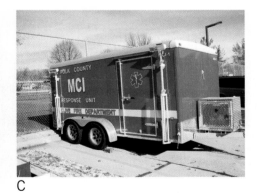

C

Figure 48.1 (A, B, C) Many types of vehicles are used for emergency response (Courtesy of Clive Fire Department, Clive, IA)

Table 48-1 EMS Vehicles

Condition	Vehicle
1. Snow and ice	Ice rescue platforms and sleds
	Snowmobiles
	Snow tractors
2. Off road	Dirt bikes
	Four-wheel all-terrain vehicles
	Four-wheel trucks
3. Water	Airboats
	Aluminum boats
	Deep submergence rescue vehicles
	Hovercraft
	Personal watercraft
4. Mass gatherings	Bicycles
	Buses
	Motorcycles
	Motorized carts
5. Remote wilderness	Fixed-wing aircraft
	Helicopters

requires a specialized vehicle. Table 48-1 lists just a few specialized vehicles used by EMTs to respond to the scene of a medical emergency.

Every EMS call has two components: the emergency response phase that brings both medical personnel and equipment to the scene and the transportation phase in which the patient is taken to the emergency department. Police cruisers and fire apparatus are two examples of an **emergency services vehicle (ESV)** typically used to quickly get equipment and trained personnel to the scene but not capable of transporting the patient to definitive care. Figure 48.1 shows examples of these vehicles.

Emergency ambulances are designed for both emergency response and patient transportation. There are several different types of ambulances, each with its own distinctive features and advantages.

The van style type II ambulances are often preferred by urban EMS systems because they are easier to handle on narrow city streets. Modular type III ambulances are often preferred by paramedic systems for the roominess of the patient compartment.

Many fire-based EMS systems prefer the truck style type I ambulances because of their additional compartment space and load-carrying capacity. Figure 48.2 shows examples of two types of ambulances commonly used in the United States.

MEDICAL SUPPLIES

To care for an ill or injured person, the EMT needs certain basic medical supplies and equipment. The specific medical equipment that is required onboard an ambulance is often regulated by state or local agencies. This equipment can be divided into equipment needed on scene and during transport.

PORTABLE MEDICAL SUPPLIES

Once EMS has arrived on scene, the medical supplies must be carried to the patient's side. Typically, these medical supplies are carried in durable bags referred to using a variety of names; first-out bags, first-in bags, medic bags, or jump kits.

All of these portable medical kits must minimally contain the medical supplies needed for performance of immediate lifesaving treatments. An **emergency ambulance service vehicle (EASV)** should minimally carry the equipment that is dictated by state or regional medical authorities. These legally mandated minimal stocking regulations exist to protect the public and may come with substantial penalties or fines for noncompliance. Table 48-2 shows a typical equipment list for a portable medical kit.

EMERGENCY AMBULANCE SUPPLIES

A well-stocked emergency ambulance is a minimal expectation of the public. Every EMT should know where each piece of equipment is in the ambulance. During an emergency, there is no time to refer to a checklist or search through compartments. Further guidance on minimal emergency ambulance supplies is provided by the American College of Emergency Physicians in its position paper titled "Guidelines for Ambulance Equipment."

All the supplies and equipment in an EASV should be securely fastened or stored within a compartment. In the event of a collision, unsecured equipment can become a projectile, injuring the patient or the crew. A simple seat-belt style restraining belt will secure a 10-pound automated external defibrillator (AED), for example, and prevent it from becoming a danger to the crew. Many ambulances have rolling or sliding doors that allow easy access to equipment within the compartment while preventing the equipment from shifting during a crash. Table 48-3 lists the general medical supplies that might be required to be onboard an ambulance.

SAFETY EQUIPMENT

Proper preparation and familiarity with safety equipment are essential to prevent the EMT from becoming ill or getting injured (Figure 48.3). Personal protective equipment is discussed in detail in Unit 8. Other safety equipment that may be necessary includes protective helmets, coats, and gloves. Additional equipment, such as fire extinguishers, flares, traffic cones, and reflective safety vests, is also useful and may be required by local or state regulation.

MAPS

Regardless of how well an **emergency vehicle operator (EVO)** knows an area, it is always wise to have local maps readily available in the emergency ambulance service vehicle. Knowing the quickest way to get to a patient and to get the patient to a hospital is important. A quick look to confirm the location on a map before starting the response will confirm the appropriate route (Figure 48.4).

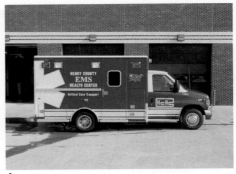

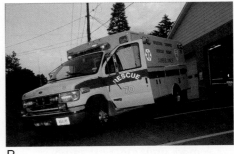

Figure 48.2 Several types of ambulances are commonly used in the United States (A. Courtesy of Henry County Health Center EMS, Mt. Pleasant, IA. B. Courtesy of Western Turnpike Rescue Squad)

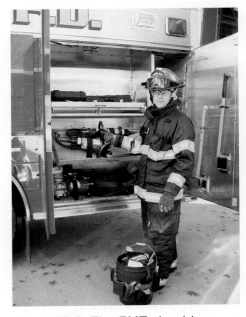

Figure 48.3 The EMT should use whatever safety equipment is appropriate for the specific emergency situation (Courtesy of Clive Fire Department, Clive, IA)

Table 48-2 Onboard Patient Care Equipment

Action Wall—Interior

- ❐ Bag-valve-mask with tubing
- ❐ Suction onboard/test at 300 mm Hg
- ❐ Yankauer tip and tubing
- ❐ Goggles
- ❐ Oxygen regulator—wall
- ❐ Onboard oxygen—500 psi minimum
- ❐ Latex gloves—small/medium/large/extra large
- ❐ Nonlatex gloves—small/medium/large/extra large
- ❐ Penlight

Vital Signs Supplies

- ❐ Blood pressure cuff—adult
- ❐ Blood pressure cuff—large adult
- ❐ Blood pressure cuff—pediatric
- ❐ Stethoscope/bell and diaphragm
- ❐ Spare tips and diaphragm
- ❐ Trauma scissors

Airway Supplies

- ❐ Suction tubing
- ❐ Suction canisters
- ❐ Yankauer tips
- ❐ Water for suction—500 cc
- ❐ Cups for sterile water
- ❐ Nasopharyngeal airways (2 each) size 30, 32, 36, French
- ❐ Oropharyngeal airways (2 each) size 04, 06, 08
- ❐ Emesis basins

Breathing Supplies

- ❐ Adult bag-valve-mask with tubing
- ❐ Facemask—small adult
- ❐ Facemask—adult
- ❐ Facemask—large adult
- ❐ Flow-restricted oxygen-powered ventilation device
- ❐ Pediatric bag-valve-mask
- ❐ Pediatric mask
- ❐ Spare oxygen regulator
- ❐ Spare oxygen rings/tips
- ❐ Non-rebreather masks
- ❐ Nasal cannula
- ❐ Pediatric oxygen masks
- ❐ Pediatric nasal cannula
- ❐ Oxygen humidifier

Circulation Supplies

Sterile Dressings

- ❐ 2 × 2 dressings
- ❐ 4 × 4 dressings
- ❐ 5 × 9 dressings
- ❐ Ace bandages

Clean Bandages

- ❐ Gauze dressings
- ❐ Gauze roller 2-inch
- ❐ Gauze roller 4-inch
- ❐ Gauze roller 6-inch
- ❐ Kerlix roller 6-inch
- ❐ Tape 1-inch
- ❐ Tape 2-inch

- ❐ Tape 3-inch
- ❐ Military compress
- ❐ Binder bandage

Major Wound Dressing

- ❐ Trauma/universal dressing
- ❐ Aluminum foil—nonsterile
- ❐ Sterile water—1,000 cc
- ❐ Tape 4-inch

Burn Care

- ❐ Sterile water for irrigation
- ❐ Sterile sheets
- ❐ Sterile facemasks
- ❐ Prefabricated wet dressings

Fracture Management

- ❐ Trauma scissors
- ❐ Sports "shark" cutting tool
- ❐ Cravats
- ❐ Ice packs
- ❐ Tape 1-inch
- ❐ Tape 2-inch
- ❐ Tape 3-inch

Splints

- ❐ Prefabricated arm short splint
- ❐ Prefabricated leg short splint
- ❐ Prefabricated leg long splint
- ❐ Ladder splint
- ❐ Padded board splint—short
- ❐ Padded board splint—medium
- ❐ Padded board splint—long
- ❐ Unipolar traction splint

Table 48-2 Onboard Patient Care Equipment (Continued)

- ❏ Bipolar traction splint
- ❏ Pediatric traction splint

Hazardous Materials Supplies

- ❏ Nitrile gloves
- ❏ Nitrile booties
- ❏ Duct tape
- ❏ Tyvek one-piece suit
- ❏ Goggles
- ❏ Dust mask
- ❏ Disposable stethoscope
- ❏ Disposable blankets

Childbirth Supplies

- ❏ Sterile obstetrics (OB) kit
- ❏ Silver swaddler
- ❏ Sterile sheets
- ❏ Sterile aprons—cloth
- ❏ Goggles
- ❏ Large sealable bags for placenta

Infection Control Supplies

- ❏ HEPA/N95 masks—small
- ❏ HEPA/N95 masks—medium
- ❏ HEPA/N95 masks—large
- ❏ Dust mist mask
- ❏ Goggles

- ❏ Red bags—small
- ❏ Clear garbage bags—small
- ❏ Red bags—extra large
- ❏ Spray bottles (empty)
- ❏ Bleach (small bottle)
- ❏ Nitrile gloves—small, medium, large
- ❏ Spill kits

Patient Comfort Supplies

- ❏ Bedroll (blanket and sheet)
- ❏ Pillow
- ❏ Blanket
- ❏ Sheets
- ❏ Pillowcases
- ❏ Towels
- ❏ Face towels
- ❏ Bedpan—fracture
- ❏ Toilet paper
- ❏ Urinal
- ❏ Paper chux

Patient Carrying Devices

- ❏ Long backboards
- ❏ Stairchair
- ❏ Flexible stretcher
- ❏ Portable stretcher

- ❏ Extrication collars
- ❏ Straps
- ❏ Short backboard
- ❏ Flexible spinal immobilization device
- ❏ Head immobilization device
- ❏ Rescue basket
- ❏ Webbing

Advanced Life Support (ALS) Supplies

- ❏ Electrocardiogram (ECG) electrodes
- ❏ IV solution—1,000 cc saline solution
- ❏ IV solution—250 cc saline solution
- ❏ Microdrip IV tubing
- ❏ Macrodrip IV tubing
- ❏ Extension tubing
- ❏ Pressure bag

Many services have installed Global Positioning Systems (GPS) in ambulances. GPS allows the EMT to enter the address from dispatch, and a map is displayed on the screen directing the EMT to the scene. Most GPS units also have voice prompts that can be turned on, giving directions along the route on when and where to turn, allowing the EMT driving the ambulance to keep her eyes on the road. GPS is becoming a popular tool in emergency response, especially in rural areas (Figure 48.5).

Table 48-3 Rescue Equipment for Ambulance

Incident Management

- ☐ Triage tags with pencils
- ☐ EMS command vest
- ☐ Triage vest
- ☐ Staging vest
- ☐ Transportation vest
- ☐ Treatment vest
- ☐ Clipboards
- ☐ Multiple casualty incident (MCI) plan

Rapid Vehicle Rescue

- ☐ Step-blocks
- ☐ Cribbing
- ☐ Toolbox
  - ☐ Phillips screwdriver

- ☐ Standard screwdriver
- ☐ Mallet
- ☐ Claw hammer
- ☐ Hacksaw with blades
- ☐ Oil can
- ☐ Can of oil
- ☐ Bolt cutters
- ☐ Gloves—leather
- ☐ Goggles
- ☐ Vise grips
- ☐ Lineman's pliers
- ☐ Channel pliers
- ☐ Duct tape
- ☐ Orange surveyor's tape
- ☐ Window punch

- ☐ Razor
- ☐ Cold chisel
- ☐ Linoleum cutter
- ☐ Contact paper
- ☐ Tarp—blue
- ☐ Disposable blankets

Shore-based Water/ Ice Rescue

- ☐ Rope in a bag
- ☐ Personal flotation device (PFD)
- ☐ Whistles
- ☐ 200 feet of nylon rope
- ☐ Carabiners
- ☐ Loops of webbing
- ☐ Basket stretcher
- ☐ 30 feet of webbing

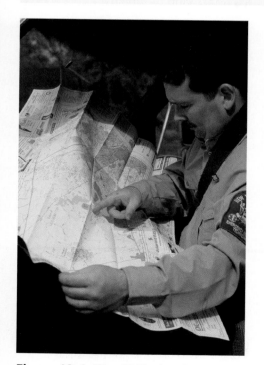

Figure 48.4 The EVO should take a few moments to confirm the location of the incident and the appropriate route to take

The term *ambulance driver,* as used in the past, failed to fully explain the role of an EMT or other designated individual who was part of the EMS team. The term *emergency vehicle operator* more fully encompasses the EMT's many responsibilities, which include driving the ambulance, helping to establish scene safety, assisting with the patient's packaging and transportation, and decontaminating the emergency vehicle. Furthermore, the term *ambulance driver* is based on the assumption that the EMT will always be operating an ambulance. The various vehicles listed in Table 48-1 demonstrate the large variety of emergency vehicles an EMT might be called on to operate.

MOBILE WORK STATION (MWS)

A **mobile work station (MWS),** sometimes called a *mobile computer terminal* (MCT) by fire departments, is a computerized device that has been used in police cars, taxicabs, courier vehicles, military logistics, and emergency vehicles, to name just a few, to communicate with a central dispatch or communications center. Mobile work stations (once known as mobile data terminals, or MDTs) have become more popular in EMS over the years as an extension of the Ambulance Computer Aided Dispatch (CAD) system. CAD is used by many emergency services, including ambulance, police, and fire operations around the world.

Mobile work stations usually consist of a screen mounted in the driver's compartment of the ambulance on which information about the response is displayed. The screen can be a touch screen with a keyboard or keypad also available for entering information. MWS may also be connected to various peripheral devices, including a mobile computer that may be placed in the patient compartment.

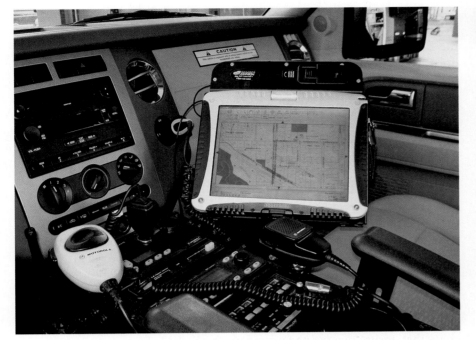

Figure 48.5 GPS mapping (Courtesy of Clive Fire Department, Clive, IA)

The MWS provides relevant dispatch information on the location of the emergency as well as patient information to EMTs and EVOs. Mobile work stations often include mapping tied to the GPS system with route suggestions built in. They are also often used for more than just dispatch. CAD systems include the ability for unit-to-dispatch or unit-to-unit text messaging. Many MWS systems incorporate GPS technology, enabling communication or operation centers to locate or track a vehicle's position on a mapping screen.

Mobile computers are also used for the documentation of patient contacts through electronic patient care reporting. This enables the EMT to work on or complete an electronic patient care report (ePCR) from the ambulance or hospital immediately following patient contact without having to return to the station.

Mobile computers and the MWS can be a distraction to the EVO if not used properly. The EVO should make all appropriate responses required by the MDT prior to going en route.

PROTOCOLS/PROCEDURES MANUAL

Most EMTs operate under a set of protocols. These protocols and any relevant standard operating procedures are often in writing. These documents should be in a place that is readily available to the EMT. For example, the recommended procedure for what to do if the ambulance is involved in an accident should be in the vehicle, where the EVO can refer to it when needed. Treatment protocols can be referenced if needed while providing patient care.

COMMUNICATIONS DEVICES

As discussed in Unit 21, emergency personnel need to be in constant communication with their emergency communications center. Communication is usually done by radio. Most vehicles have a mounted mobile radio, and portable radios are often used by the providers outside the vehicle (Figure 48.6). The EMT should be familiar with the operation of all communications devices prior to responding to any emergency call.

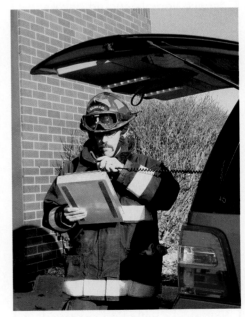

Figure 48.6 The EMT must be familiar with the use of different types of communication devices (Courtesy of Clive Fire Department, Clive, IA)

Cellular or wireless telephones are often used by emergency personnel in place of or in addition to radios. If a portable telephone is to be used, the EMT should know where it is located, how it is charged, and how it is operated. Keeping a list of commonly needed telephone numbers with the telephone is useful.

DAILY PREPARATION

The EMT should make a number of routines a part of her daily work routine. These routines help to ensure the EMT is prepared to respond at all times.

PERSONNEL

The personnel expected to respond to emergency calls should not only be properly trained, but well rested and physically and mentally prepared for an emergency operation. The work environment should support these requirements. Unit 4 discusses the EMS work environment in more detail.

Staffing for ambulances is often guided by local regulation. Usually at least one EMT is required to be in the patient compartment. Two trained providers are often preferred, especially with high-priority patients who may need multiple interventions performed simultaneously. Some systems require crews that ensure two trained providers are available for patient care.

EQUIPMENT PREPAREDNESS

At the start of their daily duties or at the beginning of their tour of duty, EMTs should carefully check all the equipment they may need to use during the shift. They should check to be sure that all the required items are where they belong and are functioning appropriately. Any equipment that requires an electrical charge should be tested to ensure that it is charged. Any battery-operated equipment should be tested to ensure a full charge on the batteries. Oxygen tanks should be tested and filled as needed.

Everything should be clean and in working order. If anything is not functioning properly, the EMT should take steps to fix the problem prior to receiving an emergency call.

EQUIPMENT FAILURE

Every EMS service should have a policy and a procedure for reporting defective equipment. Reporting defective equipment ensures that patient care will not be compromised while permitting corrective action to be taken by the service. The United States Food and Drug Administration (USFDA) may require an EMT to report any medical equipment failures under its mandatory medical device reporting regulations as well (Figure 48.7).

VEHICLE PREPAREDNESS

The EVO should carefully check the EASV at the start of her shift and follow a mechanical checklist to ensure that the vehicle is sound and fully operational. Table 48-4 lists items that should be inspected in the EASV at the start of every shift. Properly checking the EASV at the start of a shift will uncover potentially dangerous mechanical problems. These issues should be properly dealt with prior to taking any emergency calls.

RESPONSE

During a call, the EMT can think about several different phases of emergency operation. Each phase has specific considerations that must be acknowledged by every member of the crew.

Street Smart

Every emergency ambulance service vehicle should have a backup communication system. This planned redundancy is critical to ensure that EMS will be ready and available in time of disaster. It is not unusual for downed trees to block microwave links or for radio towers to be struck by lightning, both of which can cause communication problems, especially if a service depends on cellular telephone technology. Past experience demonstrates that during times of natural disaster and public emergencies, a large number of cell phone calls by concerned civilians can quickly tax and then overwhelm the available cellular system.

Equipment Failure Report

NEW YORK STATE DEPARTMENT OF HEALTH
Emergency Medical Service Program

Date Problem Reported:

Month	Day	Year

Type of Failure

☐ Vehicle

☐ Vehicle's Radio

☐ Portable Radio

☐ On-board Equipment

Vehicle # _____ Mileage _____

Vehicle # _____

I.D. # _____

Type _____

Vehicle/Equipment Failure Discovered   (Check only one box in this section)

☐ While completing ambulance daily/shift inspection

☐ Enroute to a call or hospital

☐ On scene of a call

☐ Other (describe) _____

Was patient on board?   ☐ Yes   ☐ No

Time Crew Affected

Time failure discovered:	
Time failure reported:	
Time taken out of service:	
Time put back in service:	
Total out of service time:	

Did the crew go back into service with:

☐ Same equipment   ☐ Different equipment

Was anyone injured by the failure?   ☐ Yes   ☐ No

If yes, report all accidents to the supervisor.

Description of Problem: _____

_____

_____

_____

Impression of Problem Cause: _____

_____

_____

_____

Reporting Crew Member's Signature

DOH-2502 (11/88)   p. 1 of 2

(continued)

Figure 48.7 An EMT should report and fill out an equipment failure report as needed (Reprinted with permission of New York State Department of Health)

Mechanic's Report on Vehicle Failure/Supervisor's Report on Equipment Failure

Description of problem and/or part(s) found defective: _____

_____

_____

_____

_____

Description of repairs/replacement solving problem: _____

_____

_____

_____

☐ Internal repair   ☐ Outside vendor repair

Name   Date repairs
                                     completed: /   /

....
Mechanic's Signature   Ambulance Supervisor's Signature

Comments: _____

_____

_____

_____

_____

Once actions are completed on this report, it should be filed in either the individual vehicle's maintenance file, the communications equipment repairs file, or the equipment repair file.

DOH-2502 (11/88) p. 2 of 2

Figure 48.7 (Continued)

Table 48-4 Inspection of Emergency Ambulance Service Vehicle

Safety Check	Front Compartment
❑ Tires (soft or flat?)	❑ Portable radio
❑ Leaks under vehicle	❑ Radio
❑ Front radio mic	❑ Hazardous materials book (ERG)
❑ Turn signals	❑ Binoculars
❑ Reverse lights	❑ Clipboard with:
❑ Headlights high/low	❑ Patient Care Report (PCR)
❑ Light bar front	❑ Pens
❑ Light bar rear	❑ Special Incident Report (SIR)
❑ Red corner flashers	❑ Protocol manual
❑ Scene light left	❑ Map book
❑ Scene light right	❑ Spotlight
❑ Siren wail	❑ Safety vests
❑ Compartment lights	❑ Fire extinguisher
❑ Portable radio	

ALARM AND ALERT

The crew must be notified of an EMS call in some fashion. Notification of a call is usually accomplished by the communications center setting off a pager or direct communication via radio or telephone. The communications specialist at the center is notified of the need for medical assistance either directly by the patient or through another dispatch center. Many systems provide communications specialists with special emergency medical dispatch (EMD) training so that they know how to obtain critical patient information for responding EMS units.

INITIAL INFORMATION

Initially, the communications specialist provides the EMT with the information necessary to find the patient and to consider what equipment will likely be needed to care for the patient. This information should include the nature of the call, the location of the patient, the presence of more than one patient, and any special problems such as limited access. Additionally, the communications specialist should have the name, location, and telephone number of the caller so that if any further information is needed, the caller can be called back.

DEPARTURE

Once the nature and location of the call have been given, the EVO should look up the location of the incident on a map and decide on the most appropriate route to take or program it into the GPS. Also, the EVO should ensure that any **shorelines,** electrical power sources from the building to the ambulance, have been removed and that crew members are wearing safety belts. Only after these things have been done should the vehicle be put into drive gear.

DRIVING

Many times the priority of a response, based on preapproved guidelines, is assigned by the communications specialist. A high-priority call, sometimes called a *priority one response* or a *Delta response,* is likely to require a response with red lights and sirens being used. Lower-priority calls should be responded to at normal speed while observing usual vehicle and traffic laws.

EMERGENCY VEHICLE OPERATOR

Although anybody with a driver's license can drive an ambulance in most states, possession of a driver's license should not be the minimum standard. The person who is entrusted with the lives of the patient and the crew should be appropriately trained to drive an emergency vehicle. Many states mandate that the EVO attend an approved **Emergency Vehicle Operators Course (EVOC).**

EVOs should be physically and mentally prepared for emergency responses. They should be capable of performing calmly under stress. Tolerance of other motorists and a positive attitude about their abilities as an EVO are essential. There is no place for road rage behind the wheel of an emergency vehicle.

The EVO also should be given time to become familiar with the characteristics of the vehicle she will be driving. The new EVO should not drive an emergency vehicle for the first time with lights and siren or in bad weather conditions to respond to an emergency. The EVO should drive the emergency vehicle under normal operating conditions and on dry roads on several occasions before driving it to an emergency.

DRIVING SAFETY

Safe driving is an essential part of every emergency response. With the amount of time the EMT will spend in a moving vehicle during the course of her job, eliminating the practice of unsafe driving habits is critical. Safe habits that begin early in an EMT's career will serve her well throughout the course of that career.

The EVO should always adjust the driver's seat as well as the mirrors when entering the vehicle. The mirrors are particularly important in an ambulance. The interior driver's mirror is useful for observing the patient's compartment. With one less mirror, the EVO is dependent on the two outside mirrors. The EVO should be aware that the passenger-side mirror, the one the EVO must depend on while proceeding through stopped traffic, often has a limited view.

The EVO must be properly restrained in the vehicle with a seat belt while the vehicle is in motion. The use of seat belts protects vehicle occupants from serious injury in many motor vehicle crashes. Since 1987, the National Fire Protection Association (NFPA) has advocated the use of seat belts for all fire department vehicles, including fire department ambulances. The EVO also must remain attentive to all surroundings. It is important to always maintain a safe following distance and avoid situations that could result in the ambulance being blocked in.

WARNING DEVICES

Bells, whistles, lights, and sirens do not give the EVO the right-of-way on the road. The **right-of-way,** a legal right for passage ahead of someone else, must be given by other drivers on the road. Even when the right-of-way is given to the EVO, she must exercise **due regard** for other drivers on the road, practicing good judgment and not endangering other motorists needlessly.

Failure to exercise due regard for other motorists may result in collisions, injuries, and legal complications, including criminal charges. While the Good Samaritan law can provide the EMT with some protection while the EMT is rendering medical care, the EVO does not have any similar protection and must accept full responsibility for her actions.

To improve safety and to alert other drivers, elaborate markings, flashing lights, and sirens have been created. None of these improvements, however, can replace good judgment when the EVO is driving.

Markings   Almost 30 years ago, the U.S. federal government attempted to standardize ambulance markings for a number of reasons. One reason was that if ambulances were similar in appearance, the public could more readily identify them on the road. Subsequently, the federal government advanced what has become the standard for ambulance construction, the Federal Specification for the Star-of-Life Ambulance (KKK-A-1822E). The original federal specifications called for all ambulances to be white and have a broad Omaha Orange stripe around the entire ambulance.

White was believed to be the most visible color to other motorists. However, the EVO should be aware that white blends in more easily with snow, fog, smoke, and haze. Therefore, the EVO must be more vigilant of other drivers in such conditions.

Many EMS systems initially adopted the standard orange stripe but eventually abandoned it in favor of more distinctive coloring. This decision involves no potential harm in view of the fact that the National Research Council has reported that there was no special research to support the choice of Omaha Orange.

Most ambulances also display the word *ambulance* and the blue star of life prominently on the sides of the ambulance. To enhance recognition of the ambulance in the rearview mirror, the word *ambulance* is reversed and in capital letters on the hood of the ambulance.

Many ambulances have a highly reflective tape placed around the entire vehicle to enhance visibility at night. The EVO should remember that this reflective tape is visible only when light strikes it directly. Therefore, reflective tape does not add any special protection when the ambulance crosses an intersection at an angle to the headlights of other vehicles.

Emergency Warning Lights   There is no standardization of the color of emergency warning lights across the United States. Many states have chosen red lights, the original emergency color recognized by a majority of the public as signifying emergency. Blue lights have become more popular due to the belief blue light is more visible, particularly at night when the danger to emergency workers is greatest. Finally, many states and EMS systems have put white light into the combination of emergency warning lights that are displayed.

Studies have shown that white light is highly visible during both day and night operations. Many emergency service providers have equipped emergency ambulance service vehicles with alternating headlights, also referred to as **wig-wags.**

Recently, the Federal Specification for the Star-of-Life Ambulance added one yellow light, midship and rear facing. Research has shown that a yellow light can be seen for a great distance. Yellow is now identified as the standard "warning" color; it warns motorists of an impending danger ahead. To prevent or reduce the number of rear-end mishaps at motor vehicle collisions, a blinking yellow light has been added.

Safety Tips

The vehicle's headlights should be on whenever the vehicle is in motion. Studies have shown that even during daylight hours, the use of headlights can reduce the chances of a collision by more than 15%. The headlights permit other drivers to recognize the ambulance sooner as another vehicle in motion.

Three types of emergency lights, sealed beam, LED, and strobe, are used on emergency vehicles. Each type has its advantages. The long, steady flash of a sealed beam allows drivers visual reaction time to identify the light and determine its location. The bright flash of the strobe allows the light to be seen for great distances but has the drawback of flashback during snow or rainstorms. **Flashback** occurs when the bright light of a strobe bounces off the rain or snow and back into the EVO's eyes. The newest emergency warning lights are light-emitting diodes (LED). The LED, a small semiconductor device that emits light when charged with electricity, does not tend to fail when hit, and it is visible over greater distances than standard emergency lighting. As an added bonus the LED has a greater useful life, 100 times greater, than an incandescent bulb and uses 80–90% less energy than an incandescent bulb. LED studies performed at the Lighting Research Center of the Rensselaer Polytechnic Institute, New York, have demonstrated the utility of LED in many applications, including emergency vehicle lighting. Current experience with LED emergency lights for emergency vehicles suggests that, in the future, LED may be the primary emergency light system.

Light Patterns   The number of light pattern configurations rivals the number of light combinations. However, there are a few constants in every light pattern. At least one forward-facing flashing light is placed in the grill of the ambulance. This light permits drivers who are immediately in front of an ambulance and unable to see the lights on the roof to recognize that an emergency vehicle is behind them.

When on the scene of a road call at night, the EASV needs to have its outline illuminated so that other drivers can discern its location in the dark. This is usually accomplished by placing a flashing light in each corner of the roof.

Finally, most emergency ambulances have additional scene lights affixed to the ambulance compartment. Some of these scene lights help to illuminate the scene, and the rear-facing scene lights illuminate the crew as they load the patient into the ambulance.

Emergency warning lights have long been recognized as important to the on-scene safety of emergency personnel. Yet despite the ever-increasing variety and patterns of emergency warning lights on emergency vehicles, a number of firefighters, law enforcement officers, and EMTs are killed every year while on American highways by other motorists. Twenty-five percent of all firefighter fatalities are the result of crashes with other vehicles while either responding to or returning from an emergency.

In an effort to reduce the number of emergency vehicle–related fatalities in the United States, the United States Fire Academy (USFA), together with the United States Department of Transportation (USDOT) and the Society of Automotive Engineers (SAE), have established the Fire Service Emergency Vehicle Safety Initiative. Part of that initiative is to study the effect and effectiveness of emergency lights, including incandescent lights, strobe lights, LED lights, light patterns, and light colors. The results of these studies will be forwarded to the NFPA, a national fire consensus group whose recommendations are widely accepted by the fire and EMS communities.

Audible Warning Devices   The earliest emergency vehicles used a bell that rang loudly to announce the vehicle's presence and provide a warning of danger. Modern electronic sirens are a far cry from the distant ancestor, yet they accomplish essentially the same task. Most emergency ambulances in the United States have two basic **siren modes.** These siren modes are characteristic patterns of sound designed to alert other motorists.

Street Smart

The use of lights and sirens on a limited-access highway is highly questionable. The time saved by going over the posted speed limit is often insignificant and not worthwhile when compared to the risks of high-speed driving. Some states and highway authorities forbid the use of lights and sirens by emergency vehicles on superhighways.

The first siren mode is the **wail.** The wail is a long unwinding of the sound after it reaches a peak. This monotonous up-and-down sound travels well over long distances and is almost universally perceived by drivers as an emergency alert. The other sound, called a **yelp,** is a short staccato sound that almost chirps at other motorists. The yelp is more effective than the wail in shorter distances and around obstacles.

Some newer electronic sirens have other tone patterns beyond the traditional wail siren and yelp siren. One of those new sirens, the hi-lo siren, is frequently added to the collection of sirens. The hi-lo is the primary siren sound for emergency vehicles in Europe and has been gaining in popularity in the United States. The hi-lo takes advantage of a wider spectrum of sound across the audible frequencies. Its sound more readily overcomes environmental noises, has better penetration of enclosed vehicles, and has a rapid cycling time. Better penetration allows more rapid identification of the sound—alerting—and the rapid cycling of the siren allows drivers to better locate the source of the sound, a result of comparing the tonality of two sounds and establishing their location and movement, called Doppler shift.

However, there is some controversy about the hi-lo siren. The more traditional siren mode, the wail, created by the Q mechanical siren, a trademark of the Federal Signal Company, has been in existence for 50 years, and American drivers have been conditioned to associate that sound with an emergency vehicle. Some EMS authorities believe that the unfamiliar hi-lo siren would not alert drivers to the presence of an emergency vehicle as quickly as the traditional wail siren sound.

At times this difference may be used to an advantage for the EVO. If one emergency vehicle unavoidably must follow another emergency vehicle, from a safe distance, the presence of another siren sound, hi-lo, for example, may alert motorists that once one emergency vehicle has passed, another emergency vehicle is approaching.

In the past, sirens were mounted on the roof with the lights, which meant that the driver had to listen to this almost deafening noise for prolonged periods. Today, almost all sirens are mounted ahead of the driver in the grill, where the sound is less deafening.

Although technology has improved sirens, it has not improved their effectiveness. Soundproofing built into new cars can reduce outside noise interference, including sirens, by as much as 40%. The volume of high-powered car radios and speakers also can mask outside sounds. These factors, combined with the fact that there are more hearing-impaired drivers on the road today, create a dangerous driving environment for the EVO.

Drivers who do not hear and recognize the siren until the last moment may react suddenly and unpredictably when they finally hear the siren. The EVO must drive defensively to avoid collisions with these drivers. Methods of defensive driving are discussed later in this unit.

Some emergency ambulances come with either mechanical or electronic airhorns. These devices can be effective for alerting motorists ahead of the impending arrival of an emergency ambulance into an intersection. The EVO should use the airhorn to direct other motorists to bear right and give up the right-of-way if it appears they have not heard the sirens. Some EMS services require the airhorn be used at each intersection as an added safety measure.

Most siren systems also contain a public address (PA) system. This system is useful in times of disaster when public notification of evacuation, for example, is needed. The PA system is seldom used when the ambulance is in emergency response mode. However, when an emergency ambulance is entrapped by other vehicles in a gridlock, the EVO can use the PA system to

Street Smart

New ambulances also are soundproofed, potentially preventing the EVO from hearing other emergency vehicles as well. It may be a good driving practice to operate the ambulance with the driver's-side window rolled down a few inches, regardless of the weather. This affords the EVO a better opportunity to hear other emergency vehicles and to respond appropriately. It also helps to prevent driver fatigue by allowing fresh air to circulate through the driver's compartment.

The mere sound of a siren causes an individual's adrenaline to rise; often becoming anxious. This response may not be beneficial to a patient, particularly a cardiac patient. Many EMS systems transport their conscious chest pain patients without lights or siren. If the siren is used, the EVO should first alert the patient and the patient's family that she will be using it. This warning can help to reduce the anxiety the siren creates.

give directions to the other drivers. This is effective only if the other drivers understand. Therefore, the EVO should slowly and clearly describe any vehicle about which she is giving directions. For example, "The gray car with Florida license plates, please move to the shoulder of the road." The EVO should not be surprised if drivers do not immediately react. The PA system is seldom used, and drivers are often confused about the "voice" they hear.

PRIORITY RESPONSE

Red lights and sirens should be used with caution, if used at all. In the past, most emergency vehicles routinely used red lights and sirens as warning devices for every response and for every patient transport to the hospital. This is no longer the case.

The use of red lights and sirens tremendously increases the risk of collision and subsequent personal injury. The EVO and EMT must always question the use of red lights and sirens before proceeding on an EMS call. Advances in the field of prehospital medical treatment as well as the widespread use of emergency medical dispatch have made these red lights and siren responses unnecessary in many cases.

Furthermore, in many jurisdictions there is no immunity from liability for driving with red lights and sirens. The burden of the safe operation of the emergency vehicle lies with the EVO. In fact, the largest percentage of lawsuits against EMTs are directly related to the operation of the emergency vehicle.

Laws and Regulations   Every state has laws and regulations governing the use of emergency warning devices and the operation of emergency vehicles. The EVO should be familiar with local laws and regulations related to each of the issues listed in Table 48-5.

DRIVING CONDITIONS

Every EVO should adjust her driving to the conditions of the road. Any changes in weather or road conditions should be noted and dealt with appropriately.

Adverse Weather   Driving in poor road conditions is a way of life for the EVO and EMT. When others will not drive, the EMT and all other emergency services providers have no choice. When an emergency arises, EMS must make a reasonable effort to respond regardless of the conditions.

Table 48-5 Motor Vehicle Laws Pertaining to Ambulance Operation

Vehicle parking or standing

Procedures at red lights, stop signs, and intersections

Regulations regarding speed limits

Direction of flow or specified turns

Emergency or disaster routes

Use of audible warning devices

Use of visual warning devices

School buses

However, the EVO and EMT can maximize the chance of success by thinking ahead and being proactive instead of reactive to the driving conditions.

For example, when heavy snowfall and drifting conditions make roads almost impassable, the assistance of a county snowplow, to lead the way, can be invaluable. Similarly, the EMT should monitor both highway department radio traffic as well as National Weather Service reports for information about flash floods and road closings.

If compelled to drive in bad conditions, the EVO must exercise extreme caution. For example, the speed should be reduced, and the vehicle should be driven in a lower gear if needed. Asking communications to recontact the residence and explain the delay to the patient is helpful.

Street Smart

When approaching an intersection, most EVOs switch from the wail siren mode to the yelp siren mode. However, some less-experienced EVOs rapidly switch between different siren modes, assuming that this makes the emergency vehicle more noticeable. This assumption demonstrates a fundamental misunderstanding of siren operation.

For a siren to be effective, the listener/driver must first hear it, identify from which direction the sound is coming, and visually confirm the source—in this case, an ambulance. Rapidly changing sounds do not permit the listener/driver to identify the direction of the sound and only serve to confuse and frustrate the listener/driver. Changing the siren mode at about 100 feet from the intersection and then leaving it in one single mode for at least 60 seconds is the most effective method.

Heavy Traffic   Heavy traffic is a fact of life for many EMTs operating in suburban and urban systems. Drivers on the way to or from work may not be willing to grant the emergency ambulance the right-of-way. Other drivers may attempt dangerous maneuvers like the squeeze play. The squeeze play occurs when a driver on the right of the ambulance tries to move in front of the ambulance, around another car, and then back into the traffic. This maneuver can result in a rear-end collision for the ambulance.

The EVO should avoid weaving in and out of traffic in order to make progress. Instead, the ambulance should wait for the traffic to yield the right-of-way, keeping in mind that drivers will be pulling over to the right side of the road.

Whenever the EVO is negotiating the ambulance through heavy traffic, consider **covering the brake**. By putting one foot over but not on the brake, the driver effectively reduces her reaction time for emergency braking and may prevent a collision.

Controlled Intersections   **Controlled intersections** are intersections with traffic signal devices and are the most common place for a crash involving an emergency vehicle. Other motorists may not hear or see the approach of the emergency vehicle in time to stop. Extreme care must always be used when passing through intersections. When going against the red traffic light,

Street Smart

When an ambulance stops for a flashing red light of a school bus, the EVO should wait for the school bus to turn off the flashing lights prior to attempting to pass it. This will decrease the chance of misunderstood hand signals and minimize the chance of inadvertently striking a child.

Street Smart

Inexperienced EVOs and EMTs think that using the lights and siren during bad weather will improve their response times. Research, however, has shown that EVOs drive the ambulance 15 miles per hour faster when the lights and siren are used than when they are driving without lights and siren. This increased speed may be inadvisable during poor weather and even poorer driving conditions. It is better to arrive safely a few minutes later than not to arrive at all.

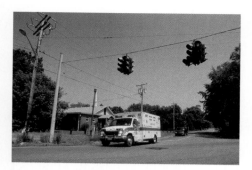

Figure 48.8 A complete stop at a red light gives the EVO time to be sure that all other vehicles in the intersection know of his intention to drive through it

the emergency vehicle should come to a complete or near-complete stop depending on state laws (Figure 48.8). The EVO should try to make eye contact with each of the drivers in the other vehicles before proceeding through the intersection cautiously.

Many driving authorities advocate that the driver look right, then left, and then right again before proceeding. This routine encourages the EVO to always scan the intersection for dangerous situations.

When multiple emergency vehicles are traveling the same route, the EVOs must use extreme care. The presence of more than one emergency vehicle can be confusing to motorists and is extremely dangerous. Once one emergency vehicle passes, the motorist may not realize that another is coming and might not appropriately yield to it.

Because of the associated danger, multiple emergency vehicles that must travel the same route should maintain a wide following distance and should be extremely attentive to surrounding traffic. Multiple vehicles on the same route, however, should be avoided when at all possible.

Braking   The EVO should always consider the impact that braking will have on the patient. If the patient has a broken leg, for example, a sudden unexpected stop can violently force the bone ends together, causing more injury and significant pain. Therefore, the EVO should anticipate stops and start to slow while approaching the stop. For example, a prolonged or stale green light indicates the EVO can anticipate that it will change to a red light in just a moment.

The first action in slowing an ambulance is to take the right foot off the accelerator. This allows the engine to slow the vehicle. Then the EVO should gently start to depress the brake pedal. A quick jab at the brake pedal will cause the ambulance to lurch forward and potentially cause more injury to the patient.

To avoid **panic stops**—fast, unexpected braking—the EVO should maintain a safe traveling distance that allows time to react if the situation should suddenly change. The **four-second rule** is often recommended by expert drivers and Emergency Vehicle Operators Course instructors. To follow the four-second rule, the EVO need only pick an object, like a sign on the side of the road, and count the time between when the vehicle in front of her passes it and when she passes it. The total elapsed time should be greater than 4 seconds.

Often new EVOs have a difficult time estimating the distance it will take to stop the ambulance. Part of the reason is because their normal driving and braking experience is with a standard automobile. The average emergency ambulance is actually as heavy as a light truck (about 10,000 pounds) and thus takes more time to stop and covers more distance in the interim. Table 48-6 shows the braking distance of a light truck at various speeds. Note that as the speed increases, the braking distance increases at a much greater rate.

In the past, ambulance drivers were taught to "pump the brakes." Pumping the brakes has been a questionable practice for some time. The theory states that a steadily applied brake will heat up to about 700 degrees and then fail or "lock up." Hypothetically, the pumping action of the driver allows the brakes time to cool and thus grip better.

New brakes are made of composite materials that resist overheating, and most ambulances have antilock braking systems (ABS) that automatically pump the brakes for the driver. Therefore, the EVO must apply the brakes in a steady and forceful fashion, and the ambulance will do the rest.

Sometimes, panic stops are unavoidable. Panic stops occur when something, such as a dog or a child running after a ball from between two parked cars, suddenly and unpredictably moves in front of the ambulance. The EVO

Table 48-6 Braking Distance—Light Truck (10,000 pounds)

Speed (mph)	Reaction Time (ft)		Braking (ft)		Total Distance (ft)
10	11	+	7	=	18
20	22	+	30	=	52
30	33	+	67	=	100
40	44	+	125	=	169
50	55	+	225	=	280
60	66	+	360	=	426

should simultaneously warn the occupants to brace for impact while applying the brake, if there is time. This warning may give an EMT who is standing in the patient compartment time to sit down.

Whenever the ambulance comes to a complete stop, the EVO should be able to see the rear wheel of the vehicle in front of her. In this position, if the ambulance needs to pull out to respond to a call or the vehicle in front should stall, there is room to evade the vehicle ahead and proceed. Many EMS systems encourage their EVOs to drive in the outside or passing lane at all times. Then if the ambulance needs to "light up" to respond to a call, it does not need to wait for traffic to clear in front of it before it can respond.

Crew   During an emergency response, the crew should behave in a manner that will not distract the EVO. The crew should be constantly on the lookout for potential dangers and should immediately, but calmly, relay them to the EVO if found. The crew should remain restrained in their seats until the vehicle has come to a complete stop and the EVO has indicated it is safe to unbuckle seat belts and exit the vehicle.

ARRIVAL

On arrival at the scene, EVOs have much to do aside from actual patient care. The EVO must always think about the positioning of the vehicle, placement of lights, possible destinations, and routes to those destinations.

EMERGENCY LIGHTS

When arriving at a residence for a house call, the EVO should consider turning off or reducing the number of flashing lights. Flashing lights in residential neighborhoods tend to attract children, adding to the danger present when operating an emergency vehicle.

When the ambulance arrives at the scene of a roadside call, the EVO should consider shutting down the headlights to prevent them from blinding oncoming traffic. Furthermore, on the scene of a motor vehicle collision, the large number of flashing lights from multiple emergency vehicles serves only

Street Smart

It is the complacent EVO who gets into a crash with the ambulance. Failure on the part of an EVO to anticipate, recognize, and respond appropriately to the dangers of the road is what leads to ambulance collisions. This assertion is supported by the well-established fact that the majority of ambulance collisions occur on clear days with good visibility. This fact should be a sobering thought for an EMT.

to confuse the other drivers in traffic. Therefore, the EVO should consider leaving only the corner flashers lighted on the ambulance to illuminate its position for other drivers.

POSITIONING

The emergency vehicle should always be positioned in a place that is safe for the emergency crew. It should always be uphill and upwind from any potential hazards. Generally, staying 100 feet from any wreckage is a good idea at a motor vehicle crash.

When arriving on the scene of a traffic accident, if no police or other units have arrived yet, the ambulance should park 100 feet in front of the wreckage and leave all emergency warning lights on. The headlights should be shut down, unless they are needed to illuminate the scene, to avoid the blinding of oncoming traffic. This protective positioning serves to block the crew and the patients from passing traffic (Figure 48.9). It is important to remember to set the parking brake.

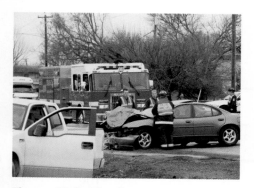

Figure 48.9 The first vehicle to arrive at a motor vehicle crash should be used to shield the accident scene from passing traffic (Courtesy of Clive Fire Department, Clive, IA)

If other units have arrived and taken up the protective position, the ambulance should proceed approximately 100 feet past the wreckage (Figure 48.10). This positioning will leave the vehicle free for easy egress from the scene when it becomes necessary.

On the scene of an incident at which multiple emergency vehicles are arriving, the EVO is wise to stay with the ambulance at all times. She can then move the ambulance if necessary to prevent it from becoming blocked in. A path of exit must always be available for the ambulance so that it may leave expediently once a patient is loaded. A more extensive discussion of vehicle positioning and scene safety considerations is contained in Unit 15.

BACKING AND PARKING

A large percentage of ambulance collisions involve the rear passenger section, the portion of the ambulance that cannot be seen by the EVO. Emergency vehicles have unintentionally backed over and injured or killed civilians and fellow emergency service providers. By following a few simple rules, the EVO can avoid a backing collision.

First, backing the ambulance or any emergency vehicle should be avoided whenever possible. The EVO's careful consideration of scene location and probable direction of travel to the hospital will help make the decision concerning the best approach to the scene to avoid the need to back up.

Whenever backing is unavoidable, a **spotter** or backer should be used. A spotter is a person who observes the ambulance as it is in reverse and directs the EVO to avoid obstacles. Note the use of the phrase "avoid obstacles"; every time an ambulance is backing up, there are obstacles and potential collisions. A spotter extends the EVO's perception of right, left, and rear space.

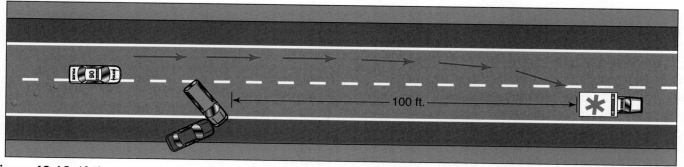

Figure 48.10 If the scene is already shielded on arrival, the ambulance should be positioned just beyond the accident scene to allow for an easy exit

The spotter should be clearly visible in the EVO's mirrors, standing about 10–15 feet to the left rear of the ambulance. Spotters should never be allowed to ride on either the tailboard or running boards. One bump and a fall could be disastrous for the spotter.

With the spotter in sight, the EVO should start to move the ambulance slowly in reverse, with one foot covering the brake. The EVO should always keep the spotter in sight. If the EVO loses sight of the spotter, she should stop immediately.

The spotter should signal the driver which direction the vehicle should turn, using standard signals. To direct the ambulance straight back, the spotter would put one hand above his head and wave the ambulance back. To direct the ambulance to turn in one direction or another, the spotter should point with both hands in the direction of travel. To direct the ambulance to come to a complete stop, the spotter would cross his arms and clench his fists while simultaneously yelling "stop."

Backing in the dark can be more difficult. When possible, the EVO should use the rear scene lights to illuminate the spotter. If the ambulance or emergency vehicle is not equipped with functional rear scene lights, the spotter should use two flashlights. A flashlight with a traffic wand attached can be useful. Under no circumstances should the spotter point the flashlight at the ambulance mirrors. The bright light could blind the EVO.

In certain situations, the ambulance is staffed with only an EVO. All other personnel are actively engaged with rescue. In those rare instances, the EVO should attempt to use any available on-scene personnel. If this is not possible, the EVO should stop the ambulance, proceed to the rear, and perform a complete survey of the area behind the ambulance.

Whenever the ambulance is parked, the emergency brake should be engaged as a precaution. At every EMS call, sooner or later, an EMT and the patient will be behind the ambulance. Therefore, it is only prudent to maximize the crew's safety and engage the emergency brake.

SCENE SIZE-UP

On arrival at the scene, the EVO should advise the communications specialist they have arrived. It is important to keep the communications specialist up to date on locations and activities. The first-arriving crew should immediately perform a scene size-up and relay key information back to dispatch.

Appropriate personal protective equipment should be put on prior to any emergency personnel entering any scene. The safety of the scene must be immediately assessed. Any dangers to incoming crews should be quickly reported. The safety of the vehicle positioning should again be confirmed.

The mechanism of injury or nature of illness should be quickly apparent during this initial scene survey. If there are multiple patients, the initial crew should immediately assess the need for additional resources and advise the communications specialist, and then begin appropriate triage. Mass casualty incidents are discussed in detail in Unit 49.

The information relayed to the communications specialist after the initial scene survey should include a confirmation of the nature of the incident; an estimated number of patients; and the need for further resources such as police, fire, or air support, and the priority of their responses.

ON-SCENE ACTIONS

Calm management and organization is the key to management of any emergency scene. Whether there is 1 patient or 100 patients, calm operation in an organized fashion facilitates appropriate care and timely transport of the patient(s).

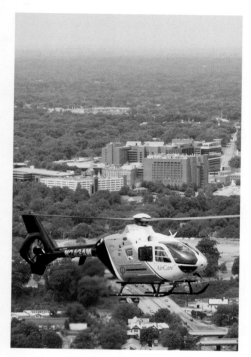

Figure 48.11 Air medical service can provide important, even lifesaving, skills and training at the scene of any emergency (Courtesy of Wake Forest University Baptist Medical Center, Winston-Salem, NC)

Street Smart

Occasionally, family members want to follow the ambulance to the hospital in a private vehicle. If the EVO is expecting to use the emergency warning lights and siren, the family should be advised not to follow the ambulance. A private vehicle following an ambulance through intersections is, at best, breaking the law and, at worst, risking a serious collision in the intersections.

ON-SCENE STABILIZATION

On every scene, the EMT has the responsibility to adequately assess every patient in a timely fashion. This assessment should follow previously outlined guidelines and should end with a determination of priority. Any necessary stabilization should be done, and plans for transport should be made as soon as is practical.

Often the EVO is responsible for preparing stretchers, stairchairs, and other means of conveyance for the EMT. This team approach reduces the time involved prior to transporting the patient.

TRANSPORTATION

Once appropriate stabilization techniques have been used, the patient should be prepared for transfer. The principles of patient movement are discussed in Unit 14. The transfer should be made as expediently as the patient's condition requires.

HELICOPTER TRANSPORT

The EMT will likely have occasion to call for air medical assistance at some point in her career. Helicopter transport has a significant role in prehospital emergency care for both trauma and medical patients (Figure 48.11). EMTs should be familiar with the capabilities of the air medical agencies that serve their area and should know how and when to contact them. Air medical transport will be discussed in more detail in Unit 54.

AMBULANCE TRANSPORT

Typically, the patient is transported to the hospital in an ambulance. The decision whether to use lights and sirens is dictated by the patient's condition. Thus, the EMT must make the decision and inform the EVO. It is important that the EMT and the EVO understand the reason for the decision. When a patient is potentially unstable, the EVO should be made aware that it may be necessary to "step up" the response to lights and sirens if the patient's condition should deteriorate.

Transport to Facility   Once the patient and the crew have been safely secured in the ambulance, the EVO should notify the communications specialist of the intended destination and the time of departure from the scene. Just as with the response to the scene, the EVO should plan the route prior to beginning the drive.

Most transports to a hospital are done without emergency lights and siren. The crew should weigh the risks associated with using these warning devices against the benefit of a potentially quicker transport time. If lights and sirens are used at all in this phase of response, they should be used only for high-priority patients. Extreme care should be used during this high-risk transport.

Often a family member wants to travel with the patient to the hospital. This may be appropriate if the family member is calm and can offer some support to the patient on arrival at the hospital or can provide hospital staff with useful information. The family member generally should ride in the front passenger seat of the ambulance, using a seat belt.

A family member who is hysterical and might create a distraction to the crew or the EVO during transport should not be allowed to ride in the ambulance. Instead, the crew should enlist the assistance of the police or a supervisor in transporting the distraught family member to the hospital.

As soon as possible during transport, the EMT in charge should contact the receiving facility and give them a brief verbal report. This report should include information that will help the receiving staff to properly prepare for the patient. This radio report is described in Unit 21.

ARRIVAL AT FACILITY

Immediately on arrival at the hospital, the EVO should notify the communications specialist. The ambulance should be safely positioned at the ambulance entrance. Often this requires backing up. It is always wise for an EVO to request a person to step out of the ambulance to watch the vehicle back up. This is insurance against unseen obstacles behind the ambulance. An emergency department entrance is a busy place. There is always a risk of inadvertently striking a person or another vehicle.

Once the vehicle is adequately parked, the EVO should assist the medical crew in taking the patient out of the ambulance and into the emergency department.

TRANSFER OF CARE

The patient should be transferred to the stretcher/bed that is designated by the triage staff at the emergency department. This should be done following principles of safe lifting and patient transfer discussed in Unit 14. Once the patient is safely on the hospital stretcher, any oxygen should be transferred to the hospital's oxygen supply. Any IV lines should be hung appropriately on IV poles or hangers, and the patient should be made comfortable.

Prior to leaving the bedside, the prehospital crew should raise the bedside rails on the stretcher/bed and lower the bed to its lowest position to prevent the patient from accidentally falling. A complete verbal report should be given to an appropriate staff member, usually a nurse, prior to leaving the patient's side (Figure 48.12). Any personal or other items belonging to the patient should be given to the receiving staff.

CHARTING

The written chart should be completed as soon as possible after patient care has been transferred to the hospital staff. Usually a written report with the details of the incident must be placed in the patient's hospital records before the EMT returns to service. The report enables hospital staff to refer to the Patient Care Report if any questions regarding prehospital care are asked. More information on documentation is contained in Unit 23.

CLEANING

The crew should turn its attention to cleaning and decontaminating the ambulance before returning to service. Specifics about decontamination and routine vehicle cleaning are covered in Unit 8.

RESTOCKING

The next order of business is to restock the ambulance in preparation for the next call. Some hospitals provide replacement items for equipment used, such as oxygen masks and IV supplies. Additionally, some hospitals may exchange clean for dirty linen. The linen on the stretcher should always be replaced with clean linen (Figure 48.13).

RETURN TO STATION

Once the necessary paperwork, cleaning, and restocking have been accomplished, the crew should return to the station to finish preparations for the next call. On their departure from the hospital, dispatch should be notified.

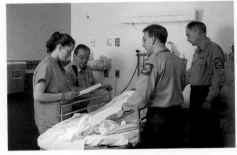

Figure 48.12 When transferring patient care to hospital staff, the EMT should give a complete verbal report to the accepting nurse and/or physician

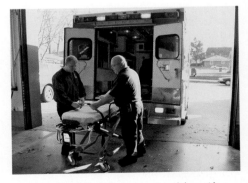

Figure 48.13 When restocking the ambulance after a call, the EMT should clean the stretcher of any visible contamination and make it up with clean linen (Courtesy of Clive Fire Department, Clive, IA)

When the vehicle has been completely cleaned and restocked, the crew should notify dispatch that the ambulance is in service, meaning the crew is ready to take another call.

RESTOCK AND REFUEL

Certain restock items, such as backboards and oxygen tanks, may not be available at the hospital. These items should be restocked as soon as possible on return to the station. Additionally, the vehicle should be refueled as needed. The fuel tank of an emergency vehicle should be maintained above one-half full at all times to ensure adequate fuel for prolonged emergency operations.

REPORTS

On return to the station, any further paperwork should be completed. It is always wise to complete any documentation that is relevant to the call as soon as possible after completion of the call. It is generally easier to recall specifics soon after the event than days later. Furthermore, events documented at the time of the event may be given more credence in a court of law than facts remembered days or even weeks later and may affect whether a document can even be received into evidence in court.

DEBRIEFING

Regardless of the nature of the event, it is a good idea for the crew to discuss the call. A brief discussion of any problems or concerns can be helpful in preventing similar incidents or problems on future calls. Concerns from any crew member should be addressed following the call. The crew should discuss or critique their actions to determine if they should do something differently, if presented with the same situation in the future. The post-call debriefing following each call should become routine. It allows issues to come to the surface quickly, rather than be hidden away until the problems are much larger.

CONCLUSION

The well-trained EMT not only will be an effective caregiver but also will understand the safety issues surrounding operation of emergency vehicles. Specifics of ground and air medical operations should be a part of any EMT training program.

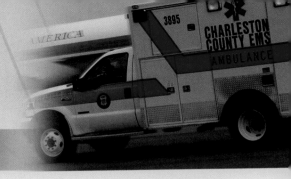

CASE STUDY Continued

As soon as they have completed the vehicle and equipment checks, Barney suggests to Tru they use the time before they get a call to help her get familiar with the EVO responsibilities and equipment in the driver's compartment. Tru is excited to begin familiarizing herself to the MWS and GPS system. Barney suggests she spend some time getting familiar with the location of the physical maps and other resource guides located in the container between the front seats.

Barney then walks Tru through the use of the mounted radio and because it is a slow day so far, they practice a couple of scenarios in which Tru receives and appropriately acknowledges the information sent over the MDT by the communications center.

Barney also uses scenarios to quiz Tru over safe driving practices, how to approach the scene, and where the ambulance should be staged on the scene of an MVC. Barney also has Tru recite the service's policies concerning the EVO's role and responsibilities. Barney is confident after working with Tru that she will be ready on Saturday to safely and efficiently perform the duties of the EVO.

Key Concepts Revisited

- Proper preparation prior to an emergency call ensures the vehicle will be roadworthy at all times.
  - Personnel
  - Equipment
    - SOP
  - Medical supplies
    - Jump kits
  - Nonmedical supplies
    - Mobile work stations
    - Maps
    - GPS
    - Radios
    - Cellular phones
- The EVO should be physically and mentally prepared for emergency responses.
  - Awake
  - Alert
  - No medication use

- The EVO must ensure the mechanical soundness of the emergency vehicle.
  - Mechanically sound
  - Fully fueled
- The EVO must understand the important considerations of each phase of an emergency call.
  - Alarm and alert
  - Departure
  - Driving
  - Arrival on scene
  - Ambulance transport
  - Arrival at facility
  - Transfer of care
  - Return to station
- The EVO has several specific considerations during an emergency response.
  - Reaction to unexpected action of other drivers on the road
  - Use of emergency lights and sirens
  - Right of way
  - Compensation for road and weather conditions

- Controlled intersections are the most common place for a crash involving an emergency vehicle.
- The EVO should be familiar with local laws and regulations governing the use of emergency warning devices and operation of emergency vehicles.
- The EVO must properly position the emergency vehicle on every scene.
    - Protection of scene
    - Allows exit
    - Stage upwind and uphill of any potential hazards
- The emergency vehicle must be cleaned, decontaminated, and restocked in preparation of the next call.
- Failure on the part of an EVO to anticipate, recognize, and respond appropriately to the dangers of the road is what leads to ambulance collisions.

Review Questions

1. Explain the importance of adequate preparation prior to an emergency call.
2. What personal considerations must every emergency vehicle operator take into account prior to driving?
3. Describe equipment considerations in daily EMS operations.
4. List the phases of an emergency call and the important considerations in each phase.
5. What should the EVO's considerations be during an emergency response?
6. What is meant by proper emergency vehicle positioning at the scene?
7. What activities should be completed when the crew returns to the station?
8. What is the four-second rule?

Key Terms

Controlled intersection
Covering the brake
Due regard
Emergency ambulance
Emergency ambulance service vehicle (EASV)
Emergency services vehicle (ESV)
Emergency vehicle operator (EVO)
Emergency Vehicle Operators Course (EVOC)
Flashback
Four-second rule

Mobile work stations
Panic stop
Right-of-way
Shorelines
Siren mode
Spotter
Wail
Wig-wags
Yelp

Further Study

Lindsey, J., and R. Patrick. *Emergency Vehicle Operations.* Upper Saddle River, NJ: Prentice Hall, 2006.

Morris, E. R., and R. W. Beach. *Emergency Vehicle Operations: A Line Officer's Guide.* Tulsa, OK: K&M Publishers, 2003.

U.S. General Services Administration. *Federal Specification for the Star-of-Life Ambulance.* Washington, DC: Author, 2002. Retrieved from http://www.upton.ma.us/media/EMS/ambulanc_1_R2FI5H_0Z5RDZ-i34K-pR.pdf.

UNIT (49) Incident Command and Multiple-Casualty Incidents

A response to a scene with multiple patients can be extremely stressful for the responding Emergency Medical Technician (EMT). These scenes are often confusing and chaotic. It is the EMT's responsibility to assist with establishing order in these situations. How these scenes are managed in the first few minutes often dictates the overall outcome of the entire incident.

National Education Standards

The Emergency Medical Technician (EMT) will demonstrate a fundamental depth and foundational breadth of understanding to establish and work within the Incident Management System and a simple depth and foundational breadth of understanding in managing a multiple-casualty incident.

Key Concepts

- A multiple-casualty incident places excessive demands on EMS personnel and equipment.

- National Incident Management System (NIMS) establishes management criteria enabling all responders to work together when disaster incidents occur.

- NIMS comprises specific components of preparedness working together to form a system for preparation, prevention, response, and recovery from disasters.

- The Incident Command System (ICS) is the standardized command structure for on-scene management of disasters and multiple-casualty incidents.

- The incident commander must delegate responsibilities to others while remaining in control of the incident.

- There are five tasks in a disaster or multi-casualty emergency.

- The objective of triage is to do the most good for the greatest number of patients.

- Patients are categorized into four classifications during the triage process.

- A triage tag is a shortened patient care document used during mass disaster to allow others to quickly identify the patient's condition.

- In a multiple-casualty incident EMTs ensure personal safety while systematically delegating the tasks they would normally perform themselves on an average call.

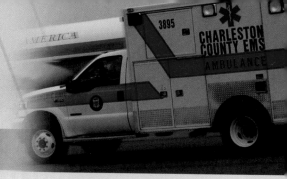

"Dispatch to Ambulance 83: MVC—School bus versus pickup truck, intersection of gravel roads Fox Ave and Buchanan Rd. Time out: 15:45."

Valene and Reece look at each other in surprise. They had just participated in a multiple-casualty drill two weeks ago with a scenario that involved a school bus collision. They had agreed at the time it was unlikely they would ever be faced with a real crash involving a school bus. Now they discuss the roles each of them will take initially on scene and the additional resources they will need. Reece mentions some of the lessons they learned from the drill two weeks ago and the methods they will use to determine patient priorities.

While en route to the scene, Valene listens to the radio traffic, noting the local fire department, police, and highway patrol are also en route. Valene calls into to the communications center and inquires if there is any further information on the number of occupants of the bus and pick-up and if additional ambulances have been dispatched.

The communications center states the driver of the pickup is on the phone and says the bus is on its side. He is unsure of how many children are on the bus. He says he can see the driver through the front window and can hear kids crying.

Critical Thinking Questions

1. What is the responsibility of the first-arriving emergency responder to the scene of a major incident?

2. How does a major incident compare to a typical EMS call?

3. How will the EMTs determine patient priority with multiple patients?

INTRODUCTION

Multiple-casualty incidents require the EMT to be able to organize and manage multiple patients, emergency responders, response vehicles, elements of the environment, and often the mechanism of the incident itself. Multiple-casualty incidents can result from the single motor vehicle crash (MVC) with several occupants to major disasters such as hurricanes, tornadoes, floods, earthquakes, and terrorist attacks, to name a few. Understanding and use of the basic fundamentals of incident command and multicasualty incident response will enable the EMT, partnered with other emergency responders, to competently manage and treat multiple patients. This unit discusses the incident management system and management of multiple-casualty incidents.

MULTIPLE PATIENT ENCOUNTERS

When an EMT arrives on a scene where there are many patients, he may feel overwhelmed by the sheer number of potential patients and people on the scene. However, it is important to keep in mind that the patient care approach for a hundred patients is the same as the patient care approach for one patient.

Someone has to be the leader to direct the activities of others on arrival and throughout the call. In some systems, this may be a crew chief or lieutenant. In a major incident, these responsibilies fall to the incident commander.

A crew chief is responsible for the safety of the crew and the patient. In a major incident, these responsibilities lie with the safety officer. (The responsibilities of the various officers are described later in this unit.)

The ambulance must be positioned in anticipation of transporting the patient to the hospital. Typically, the emergency vehicle operator (EVO) prepares the ambulance for the arrival of the patient. In a major incident, this would be the job of the staging officer.

First, someone has to approach and assess the patient, decide whether the patient is high or low priority, and then communicate that decision to the crew. Often this is the EMT in charge. In a major incident, the triage officer takes charge of these duties.

Next, someone has to treat the patient. This, again, is usually the EMT attendant or a team of EMTs and/or first responders. In a major incident, treatment officer's provide patient care.

Finally, someone has to notify the communications center, as well as the hospital, that the patient is being transported to the hospital. The EVO would normally perform these tasks. In a major incident, these tasks would be performed by the transportation officer.

On a routine call for EMS, each member of the crew assumes many roles in the course of providing patient care. When the number of patients increases, the roles must be distributed to other supporting personnel.

Yet, the tasks and objectives remain essentially the same. An EMT, with the assistance of supporting personnel, has a duty to provide emergency medical care to sick and injured patients.

An EMT must remember the tasks that need to be accomplished for many patients are the same as the tasks that need to be completed for one patient. The EMT must then delegate some of those responsibilities to others.

NATIONAL INCIDENT MANAGEMENT SYSTEMS

Lessons learned from disaster responses over the years identified a need for responders to be able to work together, but there was no system in place or standards to follow. The events of September 11, 2001, brought home the need for developing national standards for incident operations, including communications, personnel qualifications, resource management, information management, and supporting technology.

On February 28, 2003, Homeland Security Presidential Directive 5 (HSPD5) was signed by President George W. Bush authorizing the Secretary of Homeland Security to develop and manage a system that would provide for the consistent management of disasters by all emergency responders. The **National Incident Management System (NIMS)** established this management criteria for all responders—emergency responders as well as local, state, and federal government and nongovernmental agencies to work together when disaster incidents occur.

The purpose of NIMS is to provide improved coordination and cooperation ensuring interoperability between various groups and agencies. NIMS is based on two main components: flexibility and standardization. Any agency that may respond to a disaster was required to become NIMS compliant by September 2006 as a condition for receiving federal preparedness assistance. This required completion of training in basic incident command systems and NIMS. The purpose of this training is to ensure all responders understand and use the same terminology and incident command structure. Further NIMS

Table 49-1 Characteristics of the Incident Management System

- Agency autonomy: Each emergency service must still be able to operate under its command structure.
- Effective span of control: Supervisors must effectively oversee the individuals assigned to them.
- Modular organization: As the incident expands in either size or length of time, the system must be able to accommodate the change.
- Common terminology: Organizational position and tasks must have commonly recognized titles.
- Common action plan: Officers discuss approaches to avoid ending up at cross-purposes.
- Management by objective: Objectives must be clearly stated and achievable.
- Functional clarity: Each group must understand its specific purpose.
- Integrated communications: All emergency services officers must have a means to communicate with one another.
- Comprehensive resources management: Commanders and officers must share and save resources.
- Shared support: Common support staff by all emergency services, such as a public information officer, must be identified.

compliance required participation using the preparedness standardization components of planning, training, mutual aid agreements, and preparedness exercises involving a multiple agency response. Table 49-1 highlights the characteristics of the incident management system.

COMPONENTS OF NIMS

NIMS is composed of specific components of preparedness working together to form a system for preparation, prevention, response, and recovery from disasters. These components include command and management, preparedness, resource management, communications and information management, supporting technologies, and ongoing management and maintenance. Although NIMS has become well established, it will continue to evolve as lessons are learned with each response to a disaster.

COMMAND AND MANAGEMENT

The NIMS command and management component is based on three organizational systems: incident command system, multiagency coordination system, and public information system. The **Incident Command System (ICS)** defines operation and management components and the structure of incident management organizations throughout the incident. ICS will be discussed later in this unit.

The **multiagency coordination system** defines operating characteristics, management components, and the organizational structure of supporting organizations.

The **public information system** includes the procedures, process, and systems required for communicating timely and accurate information to the public during a disaster or emergency situation.

PREPAREDNESS

Incident management cannot be effective without participation in preparedness activities. Preparedness involves combining the essential activities of planning, training, exercises, personnel qualifications and standards, equipment acquisition and certification standards, publication management processes and activities, mutual aid agreements, and Emergency Management Assistance Compacts (EMACs). These activities must be developed, implemented, and evaluated in advance of any potential incident to be effective.

RESOURCE MANAGEMENT

Resource management includes standardized mechanisms and requirements for describing resources, as well as the inventory, mobilization, dispatch, tracking, and recovery of resources throughout the entire incident.

COMMUNICATION AND INFORMATION MANAGEMENT

Communication and the flow of information have long been identified as a critical element of disaster response needing improvement. NIMS identified the need for requiring that all incident management agencies must develop and implement effective interoperable communications processes, procedures, and systems across all agencies and jurisdictions involved in the incident. Information must flow efficiently through a commonly accepted structure, ensuring that information-sharing support exists at all levels of incident management. NIMS standardization of communication and information management criteria enhance the response and management of the incident by enduring informed decision making.

SUPPORTING TECHNOLOGIES

Technology and technological systems supporting capabilities necessary for implementing and refining NIMS include voice and data communications systems, data display systems, patient records and resource tracking systems, and supporting technologies capable of addressing unique situations requiring specialized technology.

ONGOING MANAGEMENT AND MAINTENANCE

The NIMS Integration Center was established by the Department of Homeland Security to provide ongoing strategic oversight and direction. Routine review and improvement of the system and the systems components are necessary to ensure the components of NIMS will continue to provide an efficient and effective template for incident management and command.

MULTIPLE-CASUALTY INCIDENTS

A **multiple-casualty incident (MCI)** can be defined as "more patients than EMTs." In other words, a multiple-casualty incident is an event that may overextend the EMS resources of personnel and equipment. In some systems, as few as three patients constitute an MCI. Some EMS systems make a distinction between a smaller and a larger number of patients, calling a smaller number of patients a **limited victim incident (LVI)** and a larger number of patients an MCI. This distinction is useful for assigning roles and responsibilities. The responsibilities do not change, just the number of people performing them.

For example, at a collision between a school bus and a passenger vehicle, where there are only minor injuries, it may be necessary only to establish a triage and treatment center. In other cases where there are sufficient ambulances immediately available, it may not be necessary to establish a treatment

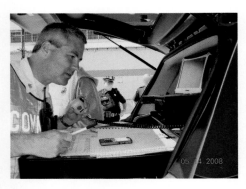

Figure 49.1 The incident commander establishes an incident command post (Courtesy of Clive Fire Department, Clive, IA)

area. These examples of an LVI can often be dealt with by establishing just the EMS sector described later in this chapter.

INCIDENT COMMAND SYSTEM

The Incident Command System (ICS) is the standardized command structure, in compliance with NIMS, for on-scene management of disasters and multiple-casualty incidents. In the incident command system there is an **incident commander (IC)** for every incident. (Figure 49.1) The IC is in command and has overall responsibility for the incident.

There are two forms of incident command: singular and unified. In a smaller incident involving just one agency, it makes sense that the head of the service, for example, the police chief, would be the incident commander.

In larger incidents or multijurisdictional incidents, several service leaders may share joint command. The advantages of a joint "unified" command are several. For example, when resources are limited, services can share assets.

There may be a fire chief, police chief, and EMS chief in the **command post.** The command post is a centralized location, often off site, where the heads of public safety agencies gather information and regulate on-scene operations. Each chief is responsible for his or her own service but all share the responsibility for incident management.

Often the leadership within a unified command rotates according to the incident needs. For example, in a house fire, initially fire suppression is the first priority. Naturally, the fire service takes prominence at this time. As victims are rescued, EMS may take dominance. Finally, after the fire is extinguished, the police arson investigators may have priority.

CHAIN OF COMMAND

The IC must delegate responsibilities to others and still remain in control of the incident. In other words, others are assigned roles and duties, but each reports to a supervisor, who ultimately reports to the incident commander. This reporting mechanism is called the **chain of command.**

The chain of command ensures that the IC and others in the chain of command have the best information about current conditions. The chain of command also permits the IC to stand back and look at the larger perspective. An IC cannot be giving detailed instructions for every activity, micromanaging, and still be able to comprehend the complexity of a large event.

The chain of command assumes delegation of authority. The IC delegates authority to others, who in turn assign tasks and duties. Borrowing from business management principles, a manager cannot supervise more than six or eight subordinates at one time. Limited supervisory responsibility is called span of control. By limiting span of control, the IC ensures the best supervision of personnel. Figure 49.2 illustrates the hierarchy of the chain of command.

COMMAND PERSONNEL

Several officers may be attached/assigned to the incident commander. These officers are charged with certain functional duties that are common to all services and all incidents.

SAFETY OFFICER

The safety officer (SO) is designated by the incident commander to be responsible for the safety of all personnel. The SO should be a trained person who understands the common hazards seen at an incident, as well as techniques to mitigate those hazards.

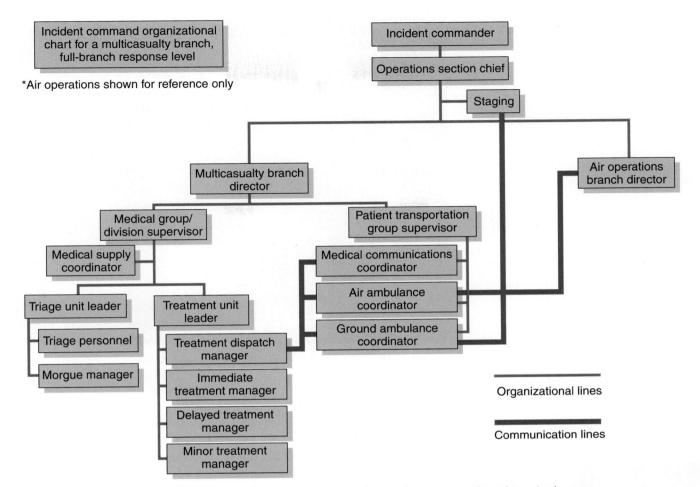

Incident command organizational chart for a multicasualty branch, full-branch response level

*Air operations shown for reference only

- Incident commander
- Operations section chief
- Staging
- Multicasualty branch director
- Air operations branch director
- Medical group/ division supervisor
- Patient transportation group supervisor
- Medical supply coordinator
- Medical communications coordinator
- Air ambulance coordinator
- Ground ambulance coordinator
- Triage unit leader
- Treatment unit leader
- Triage personnel
- Treatment dispatch manager
- Morgue manager
- Immediate treatment manager
- Delayed treatment manager
- Minor treatment manager

Organizational lines

Communication lines

Figure 49.2 The Incident Management System provides for both command and control

The SO should understand all applicable safety codes, including the Occupational Safety and Health Administration (OSHA) regulations and the National Fire Protection Association (NFPA) recommendations.

The SO has special emergency authority and can countermand any order given, including an order by the IC. The SO exercises that authority to stop unsafe actions and protect the lives of personnel on scene (Figure 49.3).

If the IC does not assign an SO, the IC retains the responsibility and liability for the safety of all personnel on the scene.

PUBLIC INFORMATION OFFICER

A public safety incident is a newsworthy event in most communities. Agents for the media will appear on almost any scene and ask for information about the incident. It is the responsibility of the incident commander to respond to these requests.

The IC may decide to assign a public information officer (PIO) to meet with the media and report the state of affairs at the incident (Figure 49.4). All information that is to be given to the public should only be provided by the designated PIO.

The IC may also decide to request that the highest elected official act as the PIO. Again, these highly visible officials divert the media's attention away from the IC, allowing the IC to concentrate on management of the incident.

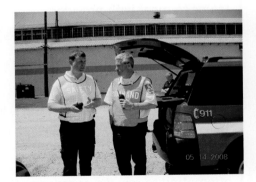

Figure 49.3 The safety officer reports directly to the incident commander and has responsibility for the safety of all personnel (Courtesy of Clive Fire Department, Clive, IA)

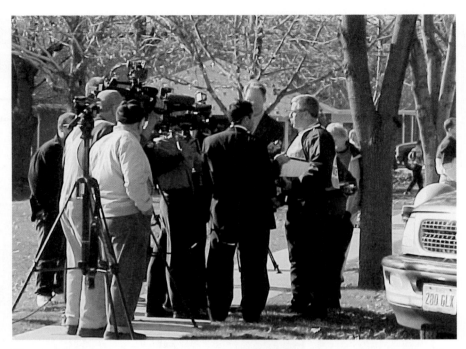

Figure 49.4 The public information officer interfaces with the media (Courtesy of Clive Fire Department, Clive, IA)

Street Smart

The very nature of most public safety incidents creates a great deal of stress in providers. When the incident is over, it is common for special critical incident stress debriefing (CISD) teams to meet with providers. However, these CISD sessions occur after the fact, after the damage has been done. In some systems, there is a special **trauma intervention program (TIP).** TIP teams operate in the field during an incident, identifying providers who are at risk and attempting to remove or reduce the stress on those individuals. These TIP teams operate freely throughout the arena with the permission of the IC.

ROLE OF THE EMT IN INCIDENT MANAGEMENT

The EMT is not expected to fully understand the complexities of the Incident Management System but should be familiar with the roles he may have during an incident. The objective of every EMT is to understand when to activate the IMS and how to participate in the IMS as a provider.

The following section details the steps involved in activating and participating in EMS operations.

EMS OPERATIONS SECTOR

From an EMS perspective, there are five tasks in a disaster or multicasualty emergency:

1. Take control of the situation—in other words, take command.
2. Assemble needed resources and personnel.
3. Locate and sort the patients according to the severity of their injuries.
4. Render needed medical care according to that severity.
5. Transport patients for further medical evaluation as soon as possible.

The IMS assigns a group of EMS officers within the operations sector who are charged with each of these tasks.

EMS DIRECTOR

The **EMS Director** has overall responsibility for EMS operations, as well as interfacing with other emergency services commanders. When an EMT is in charge of the first-arriving unit, he should establish his authority as the person in charge of EMS. The EMT would assume the title of EMS Director until relieved by another, higher-ranking EMS officer.

The next task is to establish a command post. Some systems use a flag or even a traffic cone to denote the command post, whereas others have command vehicles such as a paramedic supervisor's car. Establishing a command post

Table 49-2 Elements of the First-In Report

1. Incident location—with cross street if available

2. Type and cause of incident—as much as known

3. Is the incident open, with victims accessible, or closed, victims inaccessible and in need of rescue?

4. Is the incident contained, the cause ceased or continuing, the danger persistent?

5. What is the initial victim estimate?

6. What are the probable injuries?

7. What is the best access to the scene for other responders?

8. Where should staging be located?

9. What additional resources are needed?

10. What preplan is being used?

helps direct other responding chief officers to a central location. In many cases, a simple over-the-air declaration is all that is needed, for example, "Medcom, this is unit 24 establishing EMS command at the corner of Madison and Lark."

If a command post already exists—for example, the fire chief has established a command post—then the EMS director should link up with the fire chief and create a unified command post.

After determining the nature of the incident and perhaps the potential number of casualties, the IC should make a declaration. A declaration, often called the *first-in report*, communicates the problem present and the resources that may be needed to resolve the problem. An example of a first-in report might be: "Unit 24 reporting a school bus struck by a dump truck, possible 40 victims, smoke showing. EMS command is declaring an MCI and will be going to Plan B. Please send heavy rescue." Table 49-2 summarizes the elements needed in a declaration.

If a large number of resources is needed, a preplanned disaster response system may have to be activated. By declaring a "Plan B," as in the preceding example, the EMT knows which police, fire, and other EMS units will be dispatched to their location.

Some EMS systems have created **tactical command sheets.** These tactical command sheets provide specific instructions for how to proceed with managing a specific incident (Figure 49.5). Although these tactical command sheets can be useful, they are only a tool. The EMT must evaluate each scene individually and consider what resources may be needed.

TRANSFER OF COMMAND

To prevent any interruptions in operations and to decrease the likelihood of miscommunication, whenever another person such as an EMT or a high-ranking official assumes EMS command, they will need a **briefing.** A briefing is usually performed one on one, as one EMS commander provides the most up-to-date information about the current state of affairs (Figure 49.6). Any tactical command sheets that were used are reviewed, as well as any status

GUILDERLAND EMS Incident Tactical Work Sheet

Call Location_____ Medical Command Location_____

_____Establish unified command with Fire & Police _____Put on EMS Command bib _____Advise inbound units where to stage
_____Designate Triage Officer _____Advise crews to stay with units until given instructions
_____Advise units to switch radios to 7.15.(Level 2 & Level 3) **LEVEL 1, RESCUES & SIGNAL 30's STAY ON GEMS CHANNEL.**

Level 1 3-6 Patients	Level 2 7 - 15 Patients	Level 3 16 + Patients	Rehab & Rescues	Signal 30 (Major Fires)

_____ Declare MCI
_____ EMS All Call
_____ Request other units
_____ Cover Town ALS
_____ Cover Town BLS
_____ Roll Call Hospitals
	_____ Declare MCI
	_____ EMS All Call
	_____ Request other units
	_____ Cover Town ALS
	_____ Cover Town BLS
	_____ Roll Call Hospitals
	_____ Call in EMS Coordintor
	_____ Call in Medical Director
	_____ Medical Supply
	_____ Transport Officer
	_____ Treatment Officer
	_____ Staging Officer
	_____ Field Com.
		_____ Declare MCI
		_____ EMS All Call
		_____ Request other units
		_____ Cover Town ALS
		_____ Cover Town BLS
		_____ Roll Call Hospitals
		_____ Call in EMS Coordintor
		_____ Call in Medical Director
		_____ Medical Supply
		_____ Transport Officer
		_____ Treatment Officer
		_____ Staging Officer
		_____ Field Com.
			_____ Assess # and Types of
			    Units Needed. (With
			    Fire Command)
			_____ Establish Perimeter
			_____ Designate Triage Area
			_____ Designate Rehab Area
			_____ Second BLS Unit ?
			_____ Second ALS Unit ?
			_____ Medical Supply ?
				_____ Establish Perimeter
				_____ Designate Triage Area
				_____ Designate Rehab Area
				_____ Call in EMS Coordinator
				_____ Call in Medical Director
				_____ Second BLS Unit ?
				_____ Second ALS Unit ?
				_____ Medical Supply ?
				_____ Transport Officer ?
				_____ Treatment Officer ?
				_____ Staging Officer ?

3 - 5 Ambulances Needed	**6 - 10 Ambulances Needed**	**11 + Ambulances Needed**		

Hospital Roll Call	AMCH	ST. PETERS	MEMORIAL	VA	ELLIS	ST. CLARES	ST. MARYS	SAMARITAIN
CAN TAKE								
# PT. SENT								

NUMBER OF PATIENTS BY PRIORITY

1 (RED)	2 (YELLOW)	3 (GREEN)	0 (BLACK)	TOTAL

RESPONDING UNITS

GUILDERLAND	M15_____ M18_____ M19_____ M30_____ R1_____ R5_____ R40_____ R50_____ R60_____ MED. SUPPLY_____ EMS20_____ EMS5_____ EMS10_____	BETHLEHAM ONESQUETHAW RAVENA ROTTERDAM	5181_____ 5182_____ 2585_____ 2687_____ 2689_____ A10_____ A30_____
COLONIE	621_____ 622_____ 631_____ 632_____ 641_____ 642_____ 651_____ 652_____ 653_____		A40_____ A32_____
ALBANY COUNTY VOORHEESVILLE HELDERBURG DELMAR	M1_____ M2_____ M3_____ 5680_____ 5685_____ 5384_____ 5386_____ 5388_____ 0981_____	DUANSBURG MOHAWK CAPITAL DISTRICT	_____ _____

Figure 49.5 Tactical command sheets provide the EMT with a standardized approach that must be customized for each incident (Reprinted with permission of Guilderland Emergency Medical Services, Guilderland, NY)

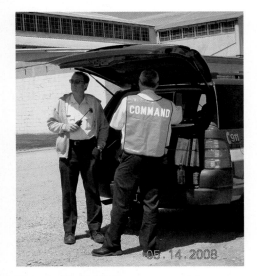

Figure 49.6 EMS command is transferred only after a complete situational briefing (Courtesy of Clive Fire Department, Clive, IA)

boards. A transfer of command and the responsibility of command are not completed until the new commander accepts the report. Often this acceptance of command is acknowledged over the air, for example, "Medcom, supervisor fifteen is assuming EMS command." The duties of the EMS commander are summarized in Table 49-3.

STAGING OFFICER

Without clear instructions, incoming units will proceed directly to the scene. Within minutes the scene may be a mass of emergency vehicles, each interfering with the other. To prevent this chaos, a staging area is usually established.

A **staging area** is an off-scene location where personnel and vehicles assemble and await assignment. A typical staging area is a parking lot or restaurant. The staging area should be close enough to the scene of the incident that units could be on scene within minutes.

As resources are needed, the IC or one of her officers would call the staging area and speak to the staging officer. A **staging officer** acts as a manager of the area, assembling and assigning equipment and personnel to specific duties or tasks (Figure 49.7). The duties of the staging officer are outlined in Table 49-4.

Table 49-3 EMS Director

Duties

1. Assesses the situation
2. Establishes command
3. Declares the emergency
4. Establishes a command post
5. Implements any preplans
6. Appoints officers
   Safety
   Staging
   Triage
   Treatment
   Transportation
7. Coordinates scene resources
8. Coordinates with chiefs of other services
9. Authorizes release of information
10. Terminates the incident
    Personnel
    Chief officer
    Public information officer
    Safety officer
    Trauma intervention team
    Clerical personnel
    Runners

Equipment

Radio
MCI plan
Command post identifier/vest

Table 49-4 Staging Officer

Duties

1. Establishes a safe assembly point
2. Assembles and inventories resources
3. Ensures support and services to personnel within staging area
4. Releases resources to meet operational needs
   Personnel
   Assistants
   Equipment
   Radio
   MCI plan
   Identifier/vest

EQUIPMENT STAGING

In some special operations, such as confined space rescue, or in larger incidents, there may be an equipment manager. An equipment manager assembles and maintains a stock of needed supplies.

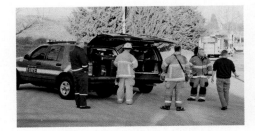

Figure 49.7 The staging officer assembles needed vehicles, personnel, and equipment (Courtesy of Clive Fire Department, Clive, IA)

One of the most disruptive influences on the scene of an MCI can be the arrival of nonrequested personnel. Although well meaning, these EMTs have not been assigned to a task or given a responsibility.

Rather than request that these potentially valuable human resources depart the scene, the IC could direct these EMTs to the staging area. Then the staging officer can assign these EMTs to other EMS units awaiting assignment.

TRIAGE OFFICER

During an MCI, the survival of some patients will depend on the effective utilization of limited resources. This utilization is best accomplished by prioritizing patients based on urgency, using a process called *triage*. Triage is a system of distribution of patients into treatment classifications according to their injury severity.

The objective of triage is to do the most good for the greatest number of patients. During an MCI, there are situations in which some patients who have serious injuries might survive, but only if a considerable amount of resources are expended. These resources are, quite simply, not available or are in high demand.

In those cases, the **triage officer** is in the unenviable position of deciding who will live and who will die. The triage officer oversees the triage process. If triage does not occur and resources are wasted on a patient in a hopeless cause, then others will die needlessly.

All EMTs can be trained to perform triage. In fact, at an MCI, several EMTs may be needed to triage all of the patients quickly. However, only one EMT, the triage officer, would report casualties to the IC. The duties of the triage officer are outlined in Table 49-5.

TRIAGE SYSTEMS

An evacuation triage is frequently the first triage performed. These evacuation triages are frequently two-tiered systems: The patient is either immediate or delayed. This triage determines which patients are removed by rescuers

---

Table 49-5 Triage Officer

Duties

1. Performs the first evacuation triage
2. Appoints assistants as needed
3. Performs second treatment/transportation triage as needed
4. Coordinates EMS activities on scene
5. Coordinates patient movement to triage and/or transportation

   Personnel

   Extrication officer

   Triage support personnel

   Patient handlers

   Equipment

   Radio

   MCI plan

   Identifier/vest

   Long backboards

   Triage tags

---

immediately. In some systems, surveyor's tape is used to identify the patient's status. Red is for immediate evacuation and green is for delayed.

As patients are evacuated, frequently to a forward triage point, a treatment or transport triage is performed. Once there, all patients are categorized into one of four classifications. Each classification has an assigned color that signifies the patient's condition.

The color red signifies that the patient is high priority or immediate. This patient is seriously injured but has a chance of survival, provided she gets immediate medical care.

The color yellow indicates that the patient is in need of medical attention but may wait or be delayed while more immediate patients are being treated.

The color green indicates that the patient has minor injuries. Often these patients are referred to as the "walking wounded." In a larger MCI, the assistance of these patients is sometimes requested to treat other more seriously injured patients.

Finally, the color black indicates that the patient is either dead or dying from mortal wounds. Sometimes termed *expectant,* these patients are extremely critical and will probably die. These patients are the last to be removed from scene.

START TRIAGE SYSTEM

Several triage systems have been developed. One system that has gained increasing popularity is the **START Triage System.** START stands for *simple triage and rapid treatment.* The START system's popularity is due to its simplicity.

A START triage begins with separating the walking wounded. Patients who are ambulatory are labeled green or delayed. If a patient is unable to walk, the EMT proceeds to assess the patient's breathing. If the patient is not breathing, the EMT manually opens the airway. If the patient takes a breath, she is classified as immediate. If the patient is still not breathing, she is classified as expectant or nonsalvageable.

The EMT then proceeds to assess the rate of respiration. If the patient's breathing is rapid, greater than 30 breaths per minute, the patient is classified as red or immediate. If the breathing is less than 30 breaths per minute or is slower than a breath every other second, the EMT assesses the patient's radial pulse. If there is no radial pulse, the patient is classified as immediate. Control of gross external bleeding is accomplished at this time.

If there is a pulse, the EMT proceeds to assess the patient's mental status. If the patient can follow simple commands, she is labeled delayed; otherwise, she is labeled immediate. This system is illustrated in Figure 49.8.

JUMPSTART PEDIATRIC TRIAGE

JumpSTART triage is a system that uses specific assessment techniques for infants and children to differentiate them from adults. Breathing is the key element on which triage decisions are based when using JumpSTART.

Initially JumpSTART was used for children 1–8 years of age or <100 pounds. However, attempting to estimate the age of a child is difficult on the scene of a multiple-casualty or disaster incident; therefore, the recommendation is to use JumpSTART on any patient who appears to be a child.

The JumpSTART triage systems should only take 15 minutes to perform and use the same categories as START triage: ability to walk (except infants), presence of spontaneous breathing, respirations less than 15 or greater than 45 breaths a minute, presence of pulses and appropriate response to painful stimuli (AVPU).

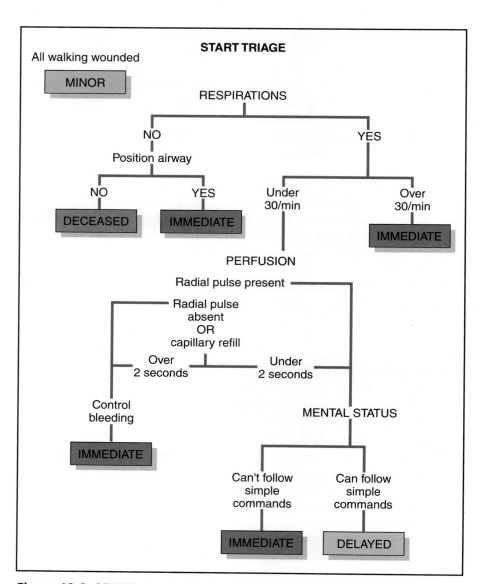

START TRIAGE

All walking wounded

MINOR

RESPIRATIONS

NO — Position airway
- NO → DECEASED
- YES → IMMEDIATE

YES
- Under 30/min → PERFUSION
- Over 30/min → IMMEDIATE

PERFUSION

Radial pulse present

Radial pulse absent OR capillary refill
- Over 2 seconds → Control bleeding → IMMEDIATE
- Under 2 seconds → MENTAL STATUS

MENTAL STATUS
- Can't follow simple commands → IMMEDIATE
- Can follow simple commands → DELAYED

Figure 49.8 START stands for Simple Triage And Rapid Treatment

JumpSTART Pediatric MCI Triage

Figure 49.9 JumpSTART Pediatric Triage System (Courtesy of Lou Romig, MD)

The triage color designations are the same as used in START triage in adults and based on the four triage categories (Figure 49.9).

Green is for minor patients who are able to walk around the scene and in no immediate need of treatment. Yellow is delayed treatment; patient is breathing spontaneously with pulses and appropriate pain response. Red is immediate and indicates intervention is needed; patient is in respiratory failure, initially not breathing but responsive to opening the airway or assisted ventilation, breathing but with no palpable pulses, or demonstrating an inappropriate response to painful stimuli. Finally, black is for the patient who is considered deceased or for whom death is likely—patients who are pulseless, breathless, or unresponsive to initial rescue breathing.

TRIAGE TAGS

Once a patient's classification has been determined, a triage tag is placed on either the wrist (more common) or the foot. A triage tag, also called a *disaster tag,* is a shortened patient care document used during times of mass disaster (Figure 49.10). The triage tag allows other EMTs to quickly identify the patient's condition and to prevent duplication of effort.

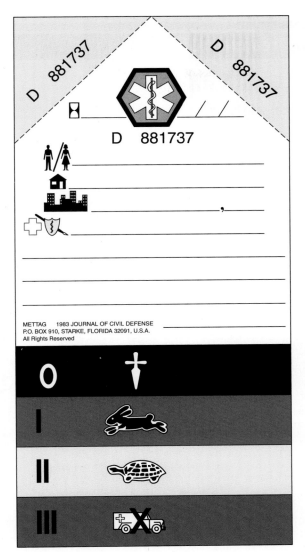

GREEN (bottom strip):
    Symbol: Ambulance–crossed out
    Meaning: No hospital treatment needed; first aid only
YELLOW (second strip from bottom):
    Symbol: Turtle
    Meaning: Nonurgent; hospital care
RED (third strip from bottom):
    Symbol: Rabbit
    Meaning: Urgent; hospital care
Black (fourth strip from bottom):
    Symbol: Cross/dagger
    Meaning: Dead or unsalvageable; no CPR

Figure 49.10 The triage tag provides a quick means of communication (Courtesy of American Civil Defense Association, Starke, FL)

There are a number of triage tag systems on the market. Most use the four-colored triage system. At the bottom, the tag has tear-off tabs. Every tag must have a means to attach the tag to the patient, as well as a stamped identification number for tracking the patient.

TREATMENT OFFICER

A treatment sector is set up whenever patients cannot be transported off scene immediately. The center of the treatment sector is the **field hospital.** The field hospital is a temporary on-site treatment facility. The field hospital is managed by the **treatment officer.** Typically, the incident commander assigns a paramedic to set up the field hospital and act as the treatment officer.

The first task of the treatment officer is to select a suitable area for the field hospital. In a large incident, a centralized area convenient to the scene is desirable. The treatment officer may also be concerned about inhospitable weather. Whenever possible, the treatment sector should be established uphill and upwind of the incident with unimpeded access for ambulances and other emergency vehicles.

Using the triage classification, patients would be distributed to corresponding areas within the field hospital according to their triage. For example,

Street Smart

Check with the incident commander before removing any deceased patients. Some of these scenes will become part of an investigation. Moving these patients interferes with that investigation. Of course, if the patient prevents an EMT from accessing another patient, then the patient must be moved.

Table 49-6 Treatment Officer

Duties

1. Establishes medical stabilization
2. Allocates advanced life support (ALS) resources
3. Reevaluates as necessary
4. Coordinates EMS activities within the field hospital
5. Coordinates patient movement to transportation

   Personnel

   Medical personnel (MD, PA, RN)

   Medical support personnel

   Patient handlers

   Clerical personnel

   Medical examiner

   Equipment

   Radio

   MCI plan

   Identifier/vest

   Stretchers

   Medical equipment

   Triage tags

a patient triaged urgent, or red, would be taken to the red section of the field hospital, yellow to the yellow section, and so on. The duties of the treatment officer are summarized in Table 49-6.

MORGUE

Patients tagged deceased should not be moved into the treatment area. The impact on patient morale would prohibit it. Instead, these patients should be placed in a separate area called a **morgue,** which is an area set aside for the collection of the deceased. This area should be shielded from public view and secured from unwanted intruders.

There are teams, usually made up of morticians or funeral directors, who will respond to a disaster and establish morgue services. The professionals on the team, called the D-Mort, are an invaluable aid to EMS operations.

TRANSPORTATION OFFICER

The **transportation officer** is responsible for the overall movement of patients from the scene to the appropriate hospitals. The transportation officer is also responsible for maintaining communications with the various hospitals, ensuring that no single hospital is being overloaded.

Table 49-7 Transportation Officer

Duties

1. Establishes and maintains ambulance loading area
2. Supervises patient evacuation
3. Coordinates with triage officer
4. Coordinates with staging officer
5. Supervises the hospital communication network

   Personnel

   Hospital liaison

   Clerical personnel

   Runners

   Equipment

   Radio

   MCI plan

   Ambulances

   Patient destination logs

The transportation officer is responsible for tracking the patients' whereabouts for all patients from the scene. He uses the identification number stamped on the triage tag to identify which patients are transported to the hospital. This information is entered on the transportation log.

Typically, patients are transported via an ambulance called up from the staging area. In some cases, it may be more efficient to transport patients with minor injuries aboard buses. The transportation officer may also be responsible for coordinating air medical evacuation. The duties of the transportation officer are summarized in Table 49-7.

CONCLUSION

A major incident need not be a disaster for an EMT. EMTs need to ensure personal safety while systematically delegating some of the tasks they would normally perform themselves on an average call. The first EMT would do a scene assessment and then delegate another EMT to perform multiple patient assessments or triage. Next, the EMT would institute treatment by establishing a field hospital and then commence transportation through the transportation officer. The standard approach to a major incident is much the same as the standard approach to any patient, only on a much greater scale.

Street Smart

When an MCI is declared and a hospital notified, the hospital may elect to implement its own emergency plan. When a hospital declares an emergency, extra staff is called into work and other patients are either discharged or diverted. After the last patient has been transported, either the transportation officer or the incident commander must notify the hospitals so that they can return to normal operations.

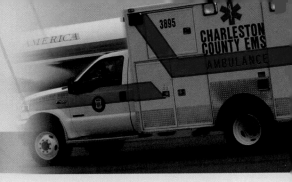

CASE STUDY Continued

Upon arrival, Valene and Reece note the presence of the fire department. A command vehicle is set up ahead of the scene, and a fire department staging officer instructs Reece on where to stage the ambulance.

Valene identifies herself to the incident commander as the first EMS personnel on scene. Valene is designated as EMS director as the incident commander briefs her on the incident.

After receiving her briefing, Valene instructs Reece to establish a triage area and designates him the triage officer. As more ambulances arrive, Valene designates the remaining officers, the treatment officer and transportation officer.

The fire department has removed the windshield of the bus and assisted the driver out. Reece begins the process of triage by addressing the individuals in the bus to walk out of the bus if able, so they can be taken to the treatment area.

The majority of the children are able to get out of the bus, and Valene delegates an EMT to lead them to the treatment area and to place a green triage tag on each of the "walking wounded."

Reece then enters the bus to find three more children inside. One child is crying and holding her leg, which is grossly deformed. Reece places a yellow tag on this child. Reece then approaches the other two children who appear unconscious. As Reece speaks to them, one opens his eyes and asks where he is. He looks blankly at Reece when asked where he is hurt. Reece applies painful stimulation to the other child who withdraws from pain but does not open her eyes or speak. Reece places a red triage tag on both of these children.

With the aid of the fire department, the EMTs package the children inside the bus to move to the triage area. Several ambulances are on scene at this time, and the transportation officer begins moving patients into ambulances, starting with the two children who have been designated as immediate, followed by the child who was designated delayed.

The remaining children are transported to the hospital for evaluation where their parents will meet them. Ten children and the driver of the school bus were all treated and transported, with only two children in serious condition.

Later that night, Valene and Reece join the rest of the responders to the incident to discuss the response. They determine by following the national incident management structure, they were able to work together and appropriately manage the multiple casualties.

Key Concepts Revisited

- A multiple-casualty incident places excessive demands on EMS personnel and equipment.
  - A limited victim incident (LVI) has a smaller number of patients than a multiple casualty incident.
- National Incident Management System (NIMS) establishes management criteria enabling all responders to work together when disaster incidents occur.
- NIMS comprises specific components of preparedness working together to form a system for preparation, prevention, response, and recovery from disasters.

  - Command and management
  - Preparedness
  - Resource management
  - Communications and information management
  - Supporting technologies
  - Ongoing management and maintenance
- The Incident Command System (ICS) is the standardized command structure for on-scene management of disasters and multiple-casualty incidents.

- o Singular command—one entity
- o Unified command—multijurisdictional agencies with command staff working together
- The incident commander must delegate responsibilities to others while remaining in control of the incident
  - o Chain of command
    - Several officers attached to the incident commander
    - Safety officer (SO)
    - Public information officer (PIO)
- There are five tasks in a disaster or multicasualty emergency:
  - o Take command.
    - Incident Commander
  - o Assemble needed resources.
    - Staging officer
  - o Locate and sort patients by injury severity.
    - Triage officer
  - o Render medical care.
    - Treatment officer
  - o Transport patients for further evaluation/care.
    - Transportation officer
- The objective of triage is to do the most good for the greatest number of patients.
  - o START Triage System
  - o JumpSTART Pediatric Triage System
- Patients are categorized into four classifications during the triage process.
- A triage tag is a shortened patient care document used in times of mass disaster that allows others to quickly identify the patient's condition.
- In a multiple-casualty incident, EMTs will ensure personal safety while systematically delegating the tasks they would normally perform themselves on an average call.

Review Questions

1. What is the initial role of an EMT on the scene of a multiple-casualty incident?
2. What is the National Incident Management System?
3. What is the chain of command?
4. What is the role of the incident commander?
5. When would a transfer of command occur?
6. What is the role of the safety officer?
7. Who should not be the public information officer?
8. What is the importance of staging?
9. What is triage?
10. What is the JumpSTART Triage System?
11. What is the START Triage System?
12. What is the responsibility of the transportation officer?

Key Terms

Briefing
Chain of command
Command post
EMS director/EMS incident commander
Field hospital
Incident commander (IC)
Incident command system (ICS)
JumpSTART Triage

Limited victim incident (LVI)
Morgue
Multiple-casualty incident (MCI)
Multiagency coordination system
National Incident Management System (NIMS)
Public information officer (PIO)
Public information systems
Staging area

Staging officer
START Triage System
Tactical command sheets
Transportation officer

Trauma Intervention Program (TIP)
Treatment officer
Triage officer

Further Study

Kean, T. H., and L. Hamilton. *The 9/11 Commission Report: Final Report of the National Commission on Terrorist Attacks Upon the United States.* New York: Norton, 2004.

Maniscalco, P. M., H. T. Christen, and H. T. Christen, Jr. *Security Officer's Terrorism Response Guide.* Boston: Jones and Bartlett, 2006.

Radvanovsky, R. *Critical Infrastructure: Homeland Security and Emergency Preparedness.* Boca Raton, FL: CRC Press, 2006. Wilson, W. C., C. M. Grande, and D. B. Hoyt. *Trauma: Critical Care, Volume II.* Boca Raton, FL: CRC Press, 2007.

UNIT (50) Hazardous Materials

Every Emergency Medical Technician (EMT) is responsible for the safety of herself and her crew. An EMT's ability to be safe is dependent on an ability to identify dangerous situations. Some situations are clearly dangerous, but many dangerous situations may not be evident until it is too late to prevent injury. To prevent these unfortunate circumstances, the EMT must be trained to be aware of the telltale signs in the environment that warn of a dangerous substance.

National Education Standards

The Emergency Medical Technician (EMT) will demonstrate a simple depth and breadth of understanding to be able to recognize a hazardous materials incident as well as the risks and responsibilities of operating in a cold zone of a hazardous materials incident.

Key Concepts

- An EMT's safety is dependent on an ability to identify dangerous situations, including the presence of hazardous materials.

- The EMT must be trained to recognize a hazardous materials incident and notify the appropriate authorities.

- The EMT should perform a thorough scene size-up, looking at the whole scene and using her senses to identify abnormalities indicating a potential hazardous material is present.

- Hazardous materials can be identified through a variety of means, including the type of vehicle in which they are transported.

- A placard is a hazardous materials identification using a system of symbols identifying what class of hazardous materials are being transported.

- Hazardous materials incidents can occur in fixed facilities, creating a widespread community incident.

- The Emergency Response Guidebook (ERG) provides instructions and information on how to handle the first 30 minutes of a hazardous materials spill.

- Perimeters are established once a hazardous material is identified to prevent further contamination.

- Decontamination corridors bridge the hot and cold zones, forming a warm zone where the hazardous material is washed off patients and rescuers.

- Care of patients exposed to hazardous materials focuses on removing the hazardous material and general first aid based on the identification of the chemical.

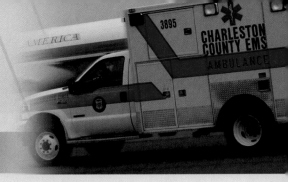

CASE STUDY

Gavin and Jin are cleaning the station when the tones sound. "Ambulance 43, Station 32 respond for an injury accident, car versus semi-truck, exit 225. Time out: 09:45."

En route to the scene, Jin asks the communications center if there is any further information. The communications center advises the semi-truck is a tanker truck. There are three potential patients, and law enforcement is en route.

As Gavin and Jin approach the exit, they suddenly notice a white fog rising from below with a pungent, heavy odor. They immediately close all windows as Gavin stops the ambulance above the scene, at the top of the exit ramp.

Grabbing the binoculars, Jin surveys the scene from where they have staged the ambulance, taking note of a tank trailer on its side at the bottom of the ramp. A white smoke or fog is billowing from its underside.

Gavin relays this information to the communications center, which advises fire engines are en route and the

hazardous materials unit has been notified. Gavin acknowledges the information and advises he and Jin will be staging at the top of the exit ramp, upwind from the smoke, until they receive further orders.

Jin notices, through the binoculars, that there are two individuals standing on the road on the other side of the street from the vehicle. She notes no one is visible in the car, which appears to be partially off the road, not far from the semi-truck. Jin has Gavin notify the communications center of the presence of the two individuals, possibly the drivers of the vehicles involved, walking around near the scene.

Critical Thinking Questions

1. What are the indications that this is a hazardous materials incident?

2. For what other signs should the EMT be looking?

3. What would be the EMT's initial priorities?

INTRODUCTION

A **hazardous material** can be defined as any substance that can cause injury or death to an exposed person. A hazardous material spill would, therefore, represent a dangerous situation for an EMT and the public. It is important that an EMT learn to identify spilled hazardous materials. Identifying a hazardous material affords an EMT the chance to avoid a potential exposure and subsequent injury. This unit discusses hazardous material awareness and response for the EMT.

FEDERAL REGULATION

The federal Hazardous Waste Operations and Emergency Response (HAZWOPER) regulation requires that EMTs and all other emergency responders be trained regarding hazardous materials. Specifically, section 29 of the Code of Federal Regulations (CFR), subsection 1910.120, requires that training be provided to "those likely to witness or discover a hazardous substance release and who have been trained to initiate the emergency response sequence by notifying the proper authorities of the release." (EPA 40 CFR 311 covers federal and local government employees.)

Those parties likely to discover a hazardous substance release are generally referred to as first responders. The term *first responder* does not refer to the level of medical training, but instead refers to who would arrive on the scene of such an incident first.

In many situations, the EMT may be a first responder. Therefore, an EMT must be trained to identify hazardous materials and notify proper authorities. This training is called the **first responder awareness level.** It should be noted that although EMTs are expected to be able to identify a potential hazardous material incident, they are not expected to take any action to stop the incident. The responsibility of an EMT trained at the first responder awareness level is strictly to identify the hazardous situation and retreat until properly trained personnel arrive.

When an EMT identifies a potential hazardous materials incident, other, more specially trained responders will be called to render the situation safe. The next responders, the **operations level responders,** are expected to act and minimize the spread of the spill as well as prevent further injuries. The actions of these operations level responders are primarily defensive. By establishing a perimeter and remaining at the periphery, these responders are primarily protected by distance.

Eventually, specially trained hazardous material technicians and specialists, usually part of a HazMat **emergency response team,** will arrive to rescue contaminated patients as well as control, confine, contain, and decontaminate the area. The EMT is the first link in the hazardous materials response and plays an important part in every hazardous materials response. Early identification of a spill and prompt notification of the proper authorities by an EMT improves the chances of a more favorable outcome.

ASSESSMENT

The assessment of the patient who has been exposed to potential hazardous materials starts by making sure the EMT is not the next patient. To do this, the EMT must proceed carefully and methodically through the steps of a patient assessment with a constant eye on personal safety.

SCENE SIZE-UP

When approaching a scene, the EMT should slow down or stop to assess the scene for obvious hazards. The EMT should try to look at the whole scene, not just the narrow setting surrounding the incident. The use of binoculars can improve an EMT's ability to observe the whole scene without getting dangerously close (Figure 50.1).

Smoke may indicate there is fire. Fire markedly increases the number of dangers present, including explosion as well as toxic vapors. Typically, smoke rises in the air. Spilled chemicals may release toxic vapors that tend to stay closer to the ground. In fact, more than 80% of toxic vapors are heavier than air. To protect themselves, EMTs should stage the ambulance far away from any smoke or vapors. The ambulance should be placed upwind and uphill of the vapors. These actions will decrease the chance of an accidental exposure.

The EMT should then assess the risk, preferably using binoculars to see the entire scene. Several signs or clues may indicate the presence of possible hazardous materials on scene. On the scene of a potential hazardous materials spill, the initial actions of the EMT are critical to the long-term impact of the event. To help the EMT remember which actions to take, the mnemonic SIN can be helpful.

The S in SIN stands for safety. First and foremost, the EMT must be concerned about safety. Staging the ambulance uphill and upwind, and at a safe distance, from the incident is the EMT's first priority.

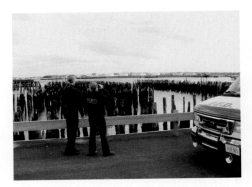

Figure 50.1 Using binoculars, the EMT should try to get the global picture (Courtesy of Larry Torrey and MEDCU, Portland, ME)

Once the EMT is in a safe area, an area called the *cold zone,* the EMT should turn her attention to the I in SIN. The I stands for isolation, or establishing a perimeter around the incident. The next section deals with hazardous material identification and the use of the Emergency Response Guidebook to establish an isolation zone and the borders of the perimeter.

Finally, the EMT should deny entry into the area until qualified personnel are on scene. No entry is the N in SIN and indicates the importance of establishing public safety.

HAZMAT IDENTIFICATION

Hazardous materials are transported every day by plane, boat, truck, and train. In some circumstances, the type and shape of the transporting vehicle give the EMT an idea of what type of hazardous materials may be involved. For example, when a train car derails and a tanker car is breached, it is probable that a large amount of fluid will be spilled.

Similarly, the name of the carrier may provide some clue to the cargo it contains. For example, a tanker truck, such as the one shown in Figure 50.2, may be marked "North Country Oil Company" is likely to be carrying petroleum products.

The shape of the container on the vehicle may also provide valuable additional information. Round containers with rounded ends are likely to be carrying materials such as gases or liquids, which may be under pressure. Any material under pressure is an explosive hazard.

HAZARDOUS MATERIALS PLACARDS

The U.S. Department of Transportation (USDOT) has adopted the United Nations (UN) standard for identifying a hazardous material using **placards.** A placard is a system of symbols placed on three sides of a container indicating the vehicle is carrying a certain class of hazardous materials. For an example of a placard for an explosive, see Figure 50.3.

Placards are usually 10¾-inch diamonds that are colored and numbered. Each placard has unique colors, symbols, and numbers to identify the class of the materials. The colors may also indicate the danger present. For example, an all-orange placard also indicates a danger of explosion. The placard in Figure 50.3 has both the orange color as well as the symbol for an explosive.

The symbol is also intended to provide a broad warning. A skull and crossbones, for example, indicates that the material is poisonous. A test tube with a liquid dripping onto a dissolving hand is indicative of a corrosive substance (Figure 50.4).

The numbers on a placard are perhaps more important than the colors and symbols. These numbers symbolize that a specific substance belongs to a certain classification of hazardous materials. When several different potentially hazardous materials are being carried, the primary hazard will be identified. While a placard number may not precisely identify the material, it does tell the EMT to what general class the most hazardous material belongs. This, in turn, can provide the EMT with some basic information on how to respond in the worst-case scenario.

FIXED FACILITY HAZARDOUS MATERIALS

Hazardous materials incidents can occur in situations other than in transit. Spills at a manufacturing plant or fires may create a hazardous materials incident. When arriving at any scene, the EMT should stop, look, and listen for signs of danger. The location of the call—for example, a chemical storage facility—should be an alert to the possibility of a hazardous materials

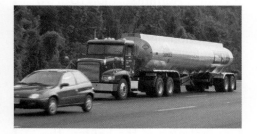

Figure 50.2 The name of the carrier may be a clue to the cargo

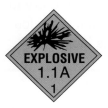

Figure 50.3 A placard indicates that hazardous materials may be aboard

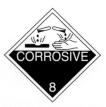

Figure 50.4 Symbols may also provide a clue to the nature of the cargo. A dripping test tube indicates a corrosive

incident. School chemistry labs and stores carrying chemicals for sale are also locations where a hazardous material spill or situation may occur. The nature of the plant, such as a petroleum distillation operation, may also be an alert to the type of hazardous materials.

Using binoculars, the EMT may observe large numbers of people exiting the building. There may also be clouds of smoke or the fog of a vapor. Instead of the UN placard system, the EMT might observe a diamond-shaped warning sign with four more diamonds inside. This is the National Fire Protection Association's **NFPA 704 symbol** (Figure 50.5). The NFPA recommends safety practices to the industry but cannot enforce these practices. The NFPA is an advisory group, not a law enforcement organization. Therefore, in some instances, a community may not have adopted the standard.

In many instances, local communities have adopted the NFPA recommendations and made them into legal ordinances under the fire or building codes. In those cases, the EMT will observe the diamond-shaped NFPA 704 symbol. Each diamond within the diamond represents a certain type of hazard. The red diamond represents a potential for fire. An EMT would be interested in the blue diamond, which represents health risk. At the bottom of the diamond is a white diamond. Special hazards, such as radioactive material, may be indicated by a spinning propeller (Figure 50.6).

Inside each of the diamonds is a number from 0 to 4. This number represents the nature of the most dangerous hazardous material within the facility. For example, a 4 in the health hazard would indicate a material that is "too dangerous to health to expose workers." According to the NFPA standards, the number 4 in the blue diamond represents a health hazard in which, "A few whiffs of the material could cause death."

PREPLANS AND MSDS

In many cases in which there is a high life hazard, public safety officials may have already planned for the potential of a disaster. This preplan often includes information about the substance as well as a general plan of approach. The health and safety information is often listed on a Material Safety Data Sheet (MSDS) that must be maintained by law at every site where dangerous or hazardous chemicals are stored. The EMT should ask to see the MSDS if it is available.

INCIDENT RESPONSE PLAN

Federal regulations (29 CFR 1910.120) require that every community have a plan of response for hazardous materials incidents. In many cases, Emergency Medical Services (EMS) and other public safety agencies have adopted the National Incident Management System (NIMS).

INITIAL ACTIONS

Once an EMT has identified a placard number, the EMT would refer to the *Emergency Response Guidebook* (Figure 50.7). The ERG provides responders with instructions and information on how to handle the first 30 minutes of a hazardous materials spill, also known as hazmat.

First, the placard numbers are cross-referenced in the yellow section of the ERG. Using the number, the EMT can find a reference directing to the **guides** in the orange section. These guides provide the EMT with instructions for evacuation distance, perimeter boundaries, and potential hazards. Every emergency vehicle should have an ERG readily available.

Small containers and quantities of hazardous materials may not be marked by the DOT UN placard. However, the contents of these small containers will

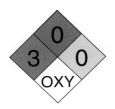

Figure 50.5 The NFPA 704 symbols are placed on fixed storage facilities

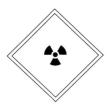

Figure 50.6 Symbols within the white diamond warn of special dangers

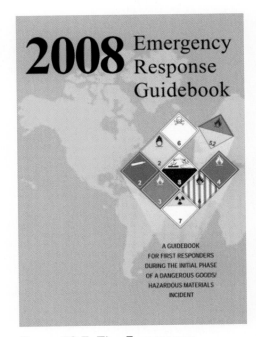

Figure 50.7 The Emergency Response Guidebook (ERG) is a valuable tool containing much-needed safety information

```
┌─────────────────────────────────────────────┐
│  SHIPPING PAPER                              │
├─────────────────────────────────────────────┤
│  PAPER 1 OF 1                                │
├─────────────────────────────────────────────┤
│  TO:     Wafers R Us                         │
│          88 Valley Street                    │
│          Silicon Junction, CA                │
├─────────────────────────────────────────────┤
│  FROM:  Essex Corporation                    │
│         5775 Dawson Avenue                   │
│         Coleta, CA 93117                     │
├─────────────────────────────────────────────┤
│  QT      HM                                  │
│  DESCRIPTION 1 Cyl                           │
│  WEIGHT        25 lbs                        │
├─────────────────────────────────────────────┤
│  RQ      Phosgene, 2.3, UN1076,              │
│          Poison, Inhalation                  │
│          Hazard, Zone CA                     │
├─────────────────────────────────────────────┤
│  This is to certify that the above named     │
│  materials are properly classified,          │
│  described, packaged, marked and             │
│  labeled, and are in proper condition for    │
│  transportation according to the applicable  │
│  regulations of the Department of            │
│  Transportation.                             │
├─────────────────────────────────────────────┤
│  Shipper:        Essex Corp                  │
│  Carrier:        Knuckle Bros.               │
│  Per:            Shultz                       │
│  Per:                                         │
│  Date:           6/27/00                      │
│  Date:                                        │
├─────────────────────────────────────────────┤
│  SPECIAL INSTRUCTIONS                         │
│              24 Hr. Emergency Contact         │
│              Ed Shultz, 1-800-555-555         │
└─────────────────────────────────────────────┘
```

Figure 50.8 Shipping papers also list the contents of a shipment

be listed on **shipping papers.** Shipping papers are required to accompany any hazardous material while it is in transit. Also called a *bill of lading,* shipping papers contain the chemical name of the materials, as well as the UN designation (Figure 50.8). These shipping papers may be found in the map pocket of a truck door or in the possession of the driver or pilot of the vehicle.

The shipping papers will also list a description of the material as well as immediate health hazards and the fire/explosion risk. The shipping papers must also list a telephone number to call for technical assistance. Many trucking companies use the services of **Chemical Transportation Emergency Center (CHEMTREC),** at 800-424-9300, for 24-hour technical assistance in the event of a chemical spill.

The EMT may also open the ERG to the blue section and, using the chemical name, find the cross-reference to the guide. Turning to the guide in the orange section, the EMT will find fundamental emergency response information. Figure 50.9 contains instructions for using ERG found on the inside cover of the book.

RESIST RUSHING IN !
APPROACH INCIDENT FROM UPWIND
STAY CLEAR OF ALL SPILLS, VAPORS, FUMES AND SMOKE

HOW TO USE THIS GUIDEBOOK DURING AN INCIDENT INVOLVING DANGEROUS GOODS

ONE **IDENTIFY THE MATERIAL** BY FINDING ANY **ONE** OF THE FOLLOWING:

THE 4-DIGIT ID NUMBER ON A PLACARD OR ORANGE PANEL

THE 4-DIGIT ID NUMBER (after UN/NA) ON A SHIPPING DOCUMENT OR PACKAGE

THE NAME OF THE MATERIAL ON A SHIPPING DOCUMENT, PLACARD OR PACKAGE

IF AN **ID NUMBER** OR THE **NAME OF THE MATERIAL** CANNOT BE FOUND, SKIP TO THE NOTE BELOW.

TWO **LOOK UP THE MATERIAL'S 3-DIGIT GUIDE NUMBER** IN EITHER:

THE ID NUMBER INDEX..(the yellow-bordered pages of the guidebook)

THE NAME OF MATERIAL INDEX..(the blue-bordered pages of the guidebook)

If the guide number is supplemented with the letter "P", it indicates that the material may undergo violent polymerization if subjected to heat or contamination.

If the index entry is highlighted, **LOOK FOR THE ID NUMBER AND NAME OF THE MATERIAL** IN THE TABLE OF INITIAL ISOLATION AND PROTECTIVE ACTION DISTANCES (the green-bordered pages). If necessary, **BEGIN PROTECTIVE ACTIONS IMMEDIATELY** (see the section on Protective Actions).

USE THE FOLLOWING GUIDES FOR ALL EXPLOSIVES:

DIVISION 1.1 (EXPLOSIVES A) - GUIDE 112
DIVISION 1.2 (EXPLOSIVES A & B) - GUIDE 112
DIVISION 1.3 (EXPLOSIVES B) - GUIDE 112
DIVISION 1.4 (EXPLOSIVES C) - GUIDE 114
DIVISION 1.5 (BLASTING AGENTS) - GUIDE 112
DIVISION 1.6 - GUIDE 112

THREE **TURN TO THE NUMBERED GUIDE** (the orange-bordered pages) **AND READ CAREFULLY.**

NOTE IF A NUMBERED GUIDE CANNOT BE OBTAINED BY FOLLOWING THE ABOVE STEPS, AND A PLACARD CAN BE SEEN, LOCATE THE PLACARD IN THE TABLE OF PLACARDS, THEN GO TO THE 3-DIGIT GUIDE SHOWN NEXT TO THE SAMPLE PLACARD.

IF A REFERENCE TO A GUIDE CANNOT BE FOUND AND THIS INCIDENT IS BELIEVED TO INVOLVE DANGEROUS GOODS, TURN TO **GUIDE 111** NOW, AND USE IT UNTIL ADDITIONAL INFORMATION BECOMES AVAILABLE. If the shipping document lists an emergency response telephone number, call that number. If the shipping document is not available, or no emergency response telephone number is listed, IMMEDIATELY CALL the appropriate **emergency response agency listed on the inside back cover of this guidebook.** Provide as much information as possible, such as the name of the carrier (trucking company or railroad) and vehicle number.

Figure 50.9 The inside cover of the Emergency Response Guidebook (ERG) provides information on how to use the book

EVACUATION DISTANCES

In some cases, the hazardous material is so dangerous that an evacuation of all civilians in the vicinity must take place immediately. When an EMT comes across a highlighted entry in either the yellow section, in the UN placard numbers, or in the blue section, the chemical names, she should immediately refer to the guide in the green section for evacuation information.

The green section of the ERG contains readily available information about isolation and evacuation distances for both day and night operations (Figure 50.10).

PERIMETERS

Once a hazardous material has been identified, a perimeter must be established to prevent further contamination of civilians and emergency responders. The immediate vicinity of the hazardous material spill that

TABLE OF INITIAL ISOLATION AND PROTECTIVE ACTION DISTANCES

ID No.	NAME OF MATERIAL	SMALL SPILLS (From a small package or small leak from a large package)						LARGE SPILLS (From a large package or from many small packages)					
		First ISOLATE in all Directions		Then PROTECT persons Downwind during-				First ISOLATE in all Directions		Then PROTECT persons Downwind during-			
		Meters	(Feet)	DAY Kilometers (Miles)		NIGHT Kilometers (Miles)		Meters	(Feet)	DAY Kilometers (Miles)		NIGHT Kilometers (Miles)	
2420	Hexafluoroacetone	60 m	(200 ft)	0.3 km	(0.2 mi)	1.0 km	(0.6 mi)	215 m	(700 ft)	0.8 km	(0.5 mi)	3.5 km	(2.2 mi)
2421	Nitrogen trioxide	60 m	(200 ft)	0.2 km	(0.1 mi)	0.5 km	(0.3 mi)	155 m	(500 ft)	0.5 km	(0.3 mi)	1.6 km	(1.0 mi)
2438	Trimethylacetyl chloride	60 m	(200 ft)	0.2 km	(0.1 mi)	0.5 km	(0.3 mi)	155 m	(500 ft)	0.5 km	(0.3 mi)	1.9 km	(1.2 mi)
2442	Trichloroacetyl chloride	60 m	(200 ft)	0.3 km	(0.2 mi)	1.0 km	(0.6 mi)	215 m	(700 ft)	0.8 km	(0.5 mi)	3.4 km	(2.1 mi)
2474	Thiophosgene	95 m	(300 ft)	0.3 km	(0.2 mi)	1.1 km	(0.7 mi)	215 m	(700 ft)	1.0 km	(0.6 mi)	4.2 km	(2.6 mi)
2477	Methyl isothiocyanate	60 m	(200 ft)	0.2 km	(0.1 mi)	0.6 km	(0.4 mi)	185 m	(600 ft)	0.6 km	(0.4 mi)	2.4 km	(1.5 mi)
2480	Methyl isocyanate	125 m	(400 ft)	0.5 km	(0.3 mi)	2.3 km	(1.4 mi)	305 m	(1000 ft)	1.9 km	(1.2 mi)	8.2 km	(5.1 mi)
2481	Ethyl isocyanate	185 m	(600 ft)	1.3 km	(0.8 mi)	6.1 km	(3.8 mi)	520 m	(1700 ft)	5.0 km	(3.1 mi)	11.0+ km	(7.0+ mi)
2482	n-Propyl isocyanate	155 m	(500 ft)	1.3 km	(0.8 mi)	5.8 km	(3.6 mi)	490 m	(1600 ft)	4.7 km	(2.9 mi)	11.0+ km	(7.0+ mi)
2483	Isopropyl isocyanate	155 m	(500 ft)	1.3 km	(0.8 mi)	5.8 km	(3.6 mi)	490 m	(1600 ft)	4.7 km	(2.9 mi)	11.0+ km	(7.0+ mi)
2484	tert-Butyl isocyanate	155 m	(500 ft)	1.1 km	(0.7 mi)	5.3 km	(3.3 mi)	460 m	(1500 ft)	4.3 km	(2.7 mi)	11.0+ km	(7.0+ mi)
2485	n-Butyl isocyanate	155 m	(500 ft)	1.1 km	(0.7 mi)	5.3 km	(3.3 mi)	460 m	(1500 ft)	4.3 km	(2.7 mi)	11.0+ km	(7.0+ mi)
2486	Isobutyl isocyanate	155 m	(500 ft)	1.1 km	(0.7 mi)	5.3 km	(3.3 mi)	460 m	(1500 ft)	4.3 km	(2.7 mi)	11.0+ km	(7.0+ mi)
2487	Phenyl isocyanate	155 m	(500 ft)	1.1 km	(0.7 mi)	4.8 km	(3.0 mi)	460 m	(1500 ft)	4.0 km	(2.5 mi)	11.0+ km	(7.0+ mi)
2488	Cyclohexyl isocyanate	155 m	(500 ft)	1.0 km	(0.6 mi)	4.7 km	(2.9 mi)	460 m	(1500 ft)	3.9 km	(2.4 mi)	11.0+ km	(7.0+ mi)
2495	Iodine pentafluoride	DANGEROUS: When spilled in water, see list at the end of this table.											
2521	Diketene, inhibited	60 m	(200 ft)	0.2 km	(0.1 mi)	0.6 km	(0.4 mi)	155 m	(500 ft)	0.5 km	(0.3 mi)	2.3 km	(1.4 mi)
2534	Methylchlorosilane	60 m	(200 ft)	0.2 km	(0.1 mi)	0.8 km	(0.5 mi)	185 m	(600 ft)	0.6 km	(0.4 mi)	2.9 km	(1.8 mi)

Figure 50.10 The green section of the Emergency Response Guidebook (ERG) provides minimum evacuation distances

is considered contaminated and a risk to rescue personnel is called the **hot zone.** Emergency services personnel, including EMS, are not allowed under any circumstances to enter the hot zone without special protective equipment.

The outermost perimeter beyond which it is considered safest for all emergency services providers is called the *cold zone.* EMS usually stages and sets up an aid station in the cold zone at the perimeter's edge. EMTs in this zone should not be at any risk for contamination. Figure 50.11 illustrates these zones.

MANAGEMENT

Before treatment can begin, the victim must be decontaminated. This process of decontamination can be lengthy. In the interim before the arrival of the first patient, the EMT should try to ascertain exactly what the contaminants are and then contact medical control for instructions on how to treat the patient.

DECONTAMINATION

Specially trained responders from an emergency response team, wearing proper protective equipment, will enter and rescue patients. These patients are then carried or moved into a **decontamination corridor** (Figure 50.12). The decontamination corridor bridges the hot zone and the cold zone in an area called the *warm zone.* The decontamination

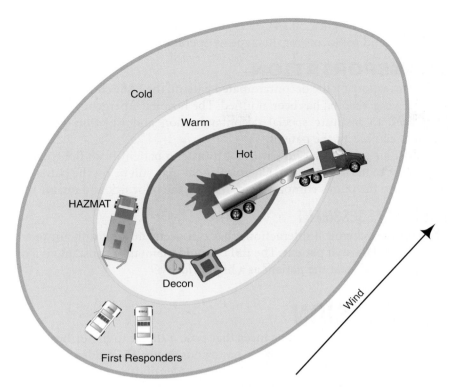

Figure 50.11 The area within the hot zone is contaminated

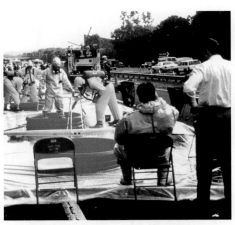

Figure 50.12 EMS usually awaits the arrival of patients at the end of the decontamination corridor in the cold zone (Courtesy of the Baltimore County Fire Department)

corridor is the area where the hazardous materials are cleaned off the rescuers and patients.

The usual method of decontamination involves dilution of the substance with large amounts of water and, perhaps, chemical degradation. The decontamination, or decon, area is usually clearly marked with cones and barrier tape. There is an entrance abutting the hot zone and an exit near the cold zone. EMTs transporting the patient for further medical evaluation would be at standby, at the exit in the cold zone.

TREATMENT

The care of a chemically exposed patient is the same as the care for a poisoned patient. First, the offending substance must be identified. In many cases, this is more difficult than one might anticipate. More than 100,000 known hazardous chemicals are used by industry. Many chemicals have similar spellings. It is critically important that the EMT obtain the correct spelling of the chemical.

General first aid information to treat the chemically exposed patient is provided in the ERG, but this is often insufficient for protracted medical operations. In those cases, other resources, including the Poison Control Center, must be contacted for further instructions. Many hazmat emergency response teams have a special **research officer.** The research officer is familiar with the computer databases and printed references available for the treatment of the chemically exposed patient (Figure 50.13). The research officer understands the mode of action of certain chemicals as well as the chemical effects and the critical exposure time frames.

Once the hazardous substance has been identified, the EMT would prepare to meet the patient at the end of the decontamination corridor. Despite the best efforts of the decon team, many patients still are not completely free of contamination. Many EMS agencies have EMTs wear a one-piece Tyvek suit, gloves, goggles, boots, and a mask to protect themselves from secondary

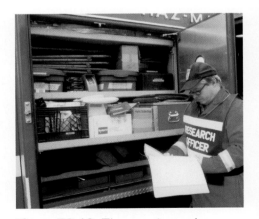

Figure 50.13 The great number of chemicals may require that a specialist, a research officer, be available to the incident commander

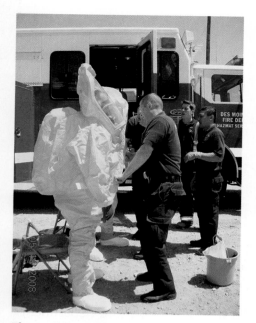

Figure 50.14 An EMT should wear appropriate personal protective equipment to prevent secondary contamination (Courtesy of Clive Fire Department, Clive, IA)

contamination (Figure 50.14). It is important that the EMT follow local guidelines and protocols for this type of operation.

TRANSPORTATION

Before transporting the decontaminated patient, the EMT should ensure that the receiving hospital has been notified. The hospital emergency department may need to institute special decontamination and isolation procedures before it can accept the patient.

Most air medical services will not transfer a patient from the scene of a hazardous materials incident. Chemicals that may still be on the patient can off-gas into the pilot's compartment, making the pilot sick and unable to fly.

ONGOING ASSESSMENT

The complex chemical interactions that can occur make it difficult to treat the poisoned hazmat patient. The EMT should maintain a constant vigil over the patient and treat the patient as a high priority.

CONCLUSION

Hazardous materials are substances that pose a threat to life or health. The EMT must be able to recognize a hazardous materials incident may exist, while protecting themselves and their crews. Identification of the hazardous material can be achieved through a number of methods, including identification markers, and is important for the notification of the appropriate authorities for management of the incident. The EMT will only treat patients once they have been decontaminated and moved into the cold zone. The EMT will provide first aid treatment of the chemical based on the recommendations provided in the ERG, local protocols, or on-line medical direction.

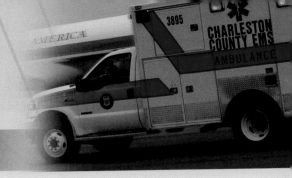

CASE STUDY Continued

As Gavin and Jin wait for the hazardous material response team to establish the perimeter and advise of the location of the cold zone, Jin continues to use the Emergency Response Guide to identify the chemical involved and what health issue the chemical may pose.

Noting the size and shape of the tank through the binoculars, Jin also looks for a placard on the tank. She identifies a diamond shaped placard on the rear of the truck that is white with a canister on the top, UN number 1005 and the number 2 on the bottom. Using the ERG, Jin indentified the chemical as anhydrous ammonia, a nonflammable gas used as a fertilizer. The ammonia that is being released from the spill is freezing the water in the air, causing the vapor to appear.

As Jin continues to consult the ERG for health-related issues and initial treatments, Gavin receives a radio update that a cold zone has been established and the patients are being taken there by the hazardous materials team after decontamination in the warm zone. Gavin is given directions to the cold zone that allows the ambulance to avoid any contact with the scene.

Upon arrival at the cold zone, Jin notes there are two patients, both walking and initially stating they do not want medical treatment. The driver of the truck states he put on a mask immediately prior to exiting the overturned truck and did not inhale the vapor. The driver of the car is coughing, stating his chest is a little tight but he doesn't want an ambulance.

Jin explains to the driver of the car, Mr. Dyson, that the chemical being spilled is irritating to the lungs. Mr. Dyson allows Jin to place oxygen by a non-rebreather mask at 12 lpm and explains that due to his exposure, he needs to be evaluated at the hospital. Mr. Dyson states the oxygen is making his chest feel a little better and agrees to being transported.

Gavin has had similar success with the truck driver, Mr. Blundon, explaining that even with the mask; he could have inhaled enough of the vapor to cause lung irritation and should be evaluated.

Mr. Blundon and Mr. Dyson are both transported to the local hospital, which has been advised of the hazardous materials spill by the transportation officer on scene of the incident and a patient report by Jin while en route to the facility.

Key Concepts Revisited

- An EMT's safety depends on an ability to identify dangerous situations, including hazardous materials.

- The EMT must be trained to recognize a hazardous materials incident and notify the appropriate authorities.

- The EMT should perform a thorough scene size-up, looking at the whole scene and using her senses to identify abnormalities indicating a potential hazardous material is present.

  ○ Colored smoke

  ○ Odors

- Hazardous materials can be identified through a variety of means, including the type of vehicle in which they are transported.

  ○ Tanker cars or trailers

  ○ Shape of the vehicle

  ○ Company identifications

  ○ Shipping papers

- A placard is a hazardous materials identification using a system of symbols identifying what class of hazardous materials are being transported.

  ○ Diamond shape

  ○ Unique colors and symbols

  ○ Number identifying the class of materials

- Hazardous materials incidents can occur in fixed facilities, creating a wide spread community incident.
  - Preplans
  - Material Safety Data Sheets (MSDS)
- The Emergency Response Guidebook (ERG) provides instructions and information on how to handle the first 30 minutes of a hazardous materials spill.
  - Placard number cross-references to the yellow section of the ERG
  - Orange section guides for fundamental emergency response information
- Perimeters are established once a hazardous material is identified to prevent further contamination.

- Evacuation distances are identified in the green section of the ERG.
- The hot zone is the vicinity immediately surrounding the hazardous material spill and a risk to rescuers without specialized protective equipment.
- The cold zone is the outermost perimeter of the area and considered safest for emergency responders and patient treatment.
- Decontamination corridors bridge the hot and cold zones, forming a warm zone where the hazardous material is washed off from the patient and rescuers.
- Care of patients exposed to hazardous materials focuses on removing the hazardous material and general first aid based on the identification of the chemical.

Review Questions

1. What are hazardous materials?
2. What is the role of a first responder awareness level responder?
3. What is the difference between a first responder awareness level responder and an operations level responder?
4. What are the indications of the presence of hazardous materials?
5. What is the role of an EMT on the scene of a hazardous materials incident?

6. How does an EMT use the *Emergency Response Guidebook*?
7. What is CHEMTREC?
8. What areas would be in the hot zone, cold zone, and warm zone?
9. How does the EMT determine the need for evacuation of civilians and how far they have to be evacuated?
10. What are the different hazardous materials identification systems in use for fixed facilities and transportation?

Key Terms

Chemical Transportation Emergency Center (CHEMTREC)
Decontamination corridor
Emergency response team
First responder awareness level
Guides
Hazardous material

Hot zone
NFPA 704 symbol
Operations level responders
Placards
Research officer
Shipping papers

Further Study

Brennan, J. A., J. R. Krohmer, and the American College of Emergency Physicians. *Principles of EMS Systems*. Boston: Jones and Bartlett, 2006.

Elling, B., and K. M. Elling. *Principles of Patient Assessment in EMS*. Clifton Park, NY: Thomson Delmar Learning, 2002.

McFee, R. B., and J. B. Leikin. *Toxico-terrorism: Emergency Response and Clinical Approach to Chemical, Biological, and Radiological Agents*. Columbus, OH: McGraw-Hill, 2007.

Radvanovsky, R. *Critical Infrastructure: Homeland Security and Emergency Preparedness*. Boca Raton, FL: CRC Press, 2006.

UNIT (51) Emergency Response to Terrorism

Emergency Medical Technicians (EMTs) understand that they potentially could be on the frontline following a terrorist attack. Emergency Medical Services (EMS), an integral part of the emergency response team, shares responsibility for crisis management and will be called on to respond to deal with the consequences of such an attack.

An EMT, in the capacity as a first responder to a terrorist attack, is also a potential target for terrorists. Hoping to disrupt emergency operations, terrorists have been known to place bombs, called **secondary devices,** that specifically target first-in emergency units. An EMT should never enter a dangerous situation; however, the potential for an ambush exists and the EMT must have an elevated awareness for the potential of a secondary device.

National Education Standard
The Emergency Medical Technician (EMT) will demonstrate a simple depth and breadth of understanding of the risks and responsibilities of operating on the scene of a natural or man-made disaster.

Key Concepts

- Terrorism is the illegal use of force against persons or property to intimidate the public or coerce a government.

- Domestic and international terrorists share a common purpose.

- EMTs must be trained to recognize the hallmarks of a terrorist attack, how to protect themselves from harm, and how to activate the emergency response plan.

- Weapons of mass destruction (WMD) are used to indiscriminately kill or maim large numbers of people at one time.

- The three major classifications of WMD are nuclear, biological, and chemical (NBC).

- The EMT must maintain a constant vigil for the presence of threats and plan for terrorist attacks by establishing and practicing an effective emergency response plan.

- The emergency response plan should outline additional resources that may be needed on the scene of a terrorist incident.

- Preparedness, assisted by understanding possible threats, can aid in reducing threats.

- Self-protection for the EMT is based on three concepts: time, distance, and shielding.

- The EMT's role is to communicate the nature of the incident and activate the emergency operations plan.

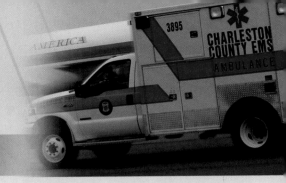

CASE STUDY

"Dispatch to Unit 98, Engine 59, Station 32, report of multiple sick persons, Jennet Office Building. Time out 08:45."

The course on emergency response to a terrorist attack Liz had taken recently comes to mind immediately when she hears the report of multiple sick persons. Liz asked her partner Enis, "Do you think this could be a terrorist attack? The building holds several federal offices."

Enis shrugs. "It could just be another building with poor ventilation like the last call that came out like this."

En route Liz and Enis discuss the incident command structure that will be in place by the time they arrive. Enis suggests that because it involves numerous agencies, it will most likely be a unified command structure. If that is the case, Enis says he will take on the role of EMS director as the senior EMT.

Upon arrival at the office building, Enis is directed by the fire department staging officer on where to park until they can determine the nature of the call. Enis parks in the staging area as directed and reports in with the

IC at the command center. Enis is informed this will be a unified command structure.

Once he is briefed on the situation, he informs Liz that no one will be entering the building. The initial patients had already reported to a hospital. A white powder was found in several envelopes in the mail room, after thee mail room employees became ill last night. The powder is being analyzed, and the search is on for additional contaminated mail that may have been delivered yesterday or this morning. Several individuals on each floor have been complaining of similar symptoms, including aching, cough, and fatigue, since yesterday.

Critical Thinking Questions

1. What information from the dispatch might suggest that this could be a terrorist attack?

2. What would be the approach to the scene of a potential terrorist attack?

3. What resources might be needed if this EMS call turns out to be a terrorist attack?

INTRODUCTION

EMTs must be able to identify the threat of terrorism, take measures to protect themselves from harm, and help keep others out of harm's way. Finally, they must know how to mitigate the effects of such an attack to save lives, decrease injury, and diminish the impact of the terrorist attack on the communities they serve.

TERRORISM DEFINED

The Federal Bureau of Investigation's (FBI) definition of **terrorism** is "the unlawful use of force against persons or property to intimidate or coerce a government, the civilian population, or any segment thereof, in the furtherance of political or social objectives." This definition sums up the three elements of a terrorist's activities: (1) they are illegal, (2) they involve the use of force, and (3) they are intended to intimidate the public.

Terrorists have one objective in general: to sow panic among the population by whatever means possible. The purpose of this panic is to cause the public to lose faith in the government or force the populace to accept the terrorist's political or social agenda.

INTERNATIONAL VERSUS DOMESTIC TERRORISM

The United States has enemies, both domestic and foreign, who would use violence to achieve their political means—the overthrow of the U.S. government or the American way of life.

Domestic terrorists are American citizens or "nationals," as defined by the Immigration and Nationality Act, who either have disputes with the way the U.S. government functions or who have quarrels with specific policies of the government. They often speak of conspiracies and deprivation of rights by the federal government. Rather than seek peaceful means to end these disagreements, these groups use violence to attempt to enact change. Some domestic terrorist groups, such as self-appointed "militias," are resolved to open armed conflict to advance their cause.

The 1995 Oklahoma City bombing, illustrated in Figure 51.1, is an example of a terrorist attack perpetrated by at least two Americans, Timothy McVeigh and Terry Nichols, against fellow Americans. Terrorists may operate in groups, such as the Aryan Nation or Ku Klux Klan, or alone as sole agents for a cause. An example of a lone terrorist is Theodore Kaczynski, the so-called "Unabomber" who mailed explosives to universities and airlines.

International terrorists, as opposed to domestic terrorists, are not citizens of the country whose government or values they oppose. International terrorists often cross another country's borders to initiate terrorist attacks and many times have subgroups, called cells, within other countries that are poised to attack when ordered. Typically, a common bond unifies these terrorists, such as hatred for America, which is the foundation of al Qaeda, the organization responsible for the attacks on September 11, 2001 (Figure 51.2). Some nations support these terrorists and are referred to as *rogue nations* in world opinion.

EMERGENCY RESPONSE TO TERRORISM

EMS providers, being proactive, need to assume that terrorism will occur in their community and start to plan for such inevitability. Training is the first step toward emergency preparedness from attacks by terrorists, both foreign and domestic, who would use violence to achieve their goals.

LEVELS OF TRAINING

Any person who is an emergency responder (i.e., law enforcement officer, EMS provider, firefighter, or industrial security officer) and who is likely to witness a terrorist event needs to be trained to identify that emergency as a potential terrorist act and to act accordingly.

Minimally, all emergency responders need to be trained to the **awareness level.** Emergency responders trained to the awareness level are able to recognize the hallmarks of a terrorist attack, know how to protect themselves from harm, and know how to activate the emergency response plan for such an event. All EMTs should be minimally trained to the awareness level.

More training is also available for command and control personnel, called *operations level training,* and for those personnel involved in decontamination, called *technician level training.* It should be noted that the EMT with awareness level training may only function in the cold zone, a relatively safe and uncontaminated area.

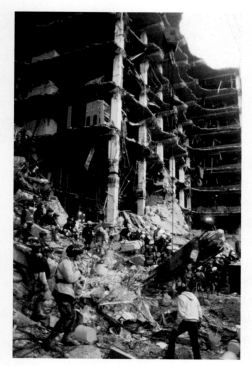

Figure 51.1 Terrorism can be domestic, as was the case with the Oklahoma City bombing (Courtesy of FEMA)

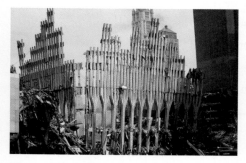

Figure 51.2 Terrorism can be foreign, as was the case with the September 11, 2001, attack on the World Trade Center (Courtesy of FEMA)

WEAPONS OF MASS DESTRUCTION

To instill the maximum amount of fear, or terror, among the populace, terrorists will use or threaten to use **weapons of mass destruction (WMD).** WMD were originally created to kill or maim large numbers of soldiers. These weapons are now being used by terrorists to kill or maim large numbers of civilians indiscriminately and to disrupt normal government operations. Nuclear, biological, and chemical (NBC) weapons represent the major classifications of WMD.

While the threat of WMD is always present, it should be noted that terrorists use explosives and incendiary devices for the majority of their attacks. Although technically not WMD, these devices can cause death and destruction on a large scale and could be grouped together with NBC weapons: nuclear, radiological, biological, chemical, and explosive.

NUCLEAR OR RADIOLOGICAL WEAPONS

A 5- to 18-kiloton nuclear bomb, a bomb as powerful as the one that destroyed Hiroshima, Japan, weighs only 60 pounds. A terrorist can carry one inside a briefcase and leave it in a busy airport, subway station, or at a mass gathering such as the local mall during the winter holidays. The likelihood of such a bomb being created is remote because of stringent international controls on the possession and transportation of fissionable weapons-grade nuclear materials, but the potential exists nevertheless.

What is more probable is that terrorists will encase a conventional explosive device, a bomb, in depleted nuclear materials, such as spent uranium from a nuclear reactor. This type of bomb would spread radioactive nuclear material across a wide area, causing widespread injury and illness. The proper name for this so-called "dirty bomb" is **nuclear dispersion device (NDD).**

Emergency responders should have a higher state of awareness that an NDD may be present when responding to a report of an explosion with multiple casualties. Although the majority of explosions in the United States are due to a natural gas mishap, the presence of chemical fuses, called blasting caps, electric switches, electronic timers, and mechanical trip wires should alert the emergency responder to the possibility of a terrorist attack and an NDD (Table 51-1).

Alternatively, terrorists could target a location that already stores nuclear materials or radiological materials in transit with a bomb or rocket. Examples of fixed locations include nuclear power plants, military installations, experimental reactors at universities, and nuclear research and development facilities.

Perhaps at great risk are nuclear materials in transit that do not have the protection of fences, guards, or other security defenses. Since 1964 more than 3,000 shipments of spent nuclear fuel rods have traveled more than 1.7 million miles in the United States. To protect these shipments, the U.S. Department of Transportation requires that they be transported in a special type B container, called a *cask*. A cask is difficult to penetrate and will not spill its contents even during a collision.

Nuclear materials are usually clearly marked with the international trefoil symbol, either in red or black, that looks like three propeller blades in the shape of the letter Y inside a white- or yellow-colored triangle. This symbol makes nuclear materials easy targets. Figure 51.3 is an illustration of this symbol.

PERSONAL PROTECTION

The three keys to radiological personal protection are (1) to limit the time of exposure to a radiation source, (2) to increase the distance from the radiation source to the EMT, and (3) to provide the EMT with shielding from the radiation. These are summarized as time, distance, and shielding.

Table 51-1 Evidence of a Nuclear Dispersion Device
1. Unusual debris such as lead shielding
2. Broken small metal containers
3. Dispersed powder or sand-like ceramic granules
4. Blue or purple glow from a powder or metal
5. Unexplained heat from a powder or metal

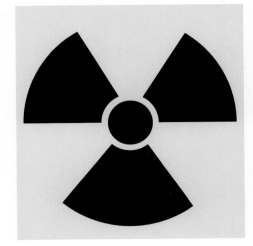

Figure 51.3 The trefoil hazard symbol warns of nuclear radiation

Once a material at an incident has been identified as a possible radioactive material, possibly by use of a **Geiger counter,** the EMT should immediately vacate the area and retreat to a safe distance. Geiger counters are portable or vehicle-mounted devices that detect radiation, creating a clicking sound in the process. Other radiation detection devices, such as a **radiation pager,** a device similar to a common pager that clips on the belt, measures the exact amount of exposure of the individual EMT so that appropriate treatments can be instituted immediately.

When considering where to stage ambulances, EMS equipment, and personnel, the EMT should first consider placing a significant distance between the source and the site. The Emergency Response Guidebook (ERG) can provide guidance in this matter as well as pre-established emergency evacuation plans.

The EMT should also endeavor to place a formidable object between the radioactive material and the EMS staging area. Ideal radiation barriers that act as a shield from radiation include man-made earthen works called *berms,* raised rail beds, or naturally occurring ridges, as well as thick concrete walls, basements, and even an engine block.

CONTAMINATION VERSUS IRRADIATION

Whenever a chemical or biological weapon is used by a terrorist, the EMT is potentially at danger of exposure to the chemical or biological agent through contact with contaminated clothing or other material. This is not always the case with a radiological incident.

A person who is a victim of a nuclear or radiological terrorist attack may have been exposed to the radiation (i.e., is irradiated) but has not necessarily been contaminated with the radiological material. In those cases of irradiation, the patient may become ill but does not present a danger to the EMT.

The person who has been contaminated is physically covered with the nuclear material, which continues to emit radiation. The key difference between irradiation and contamination is that the radiation during an irradiation ends and the patient sustains only the injury that the dose of radiation caused, whereas the radiation from contamination is ongoing and the patient will continue to suffer injury until he or she is decontaminated.

It is important that qualified personnel determine if the patient has been contaminated and thus needs decontamination or has been irradiated and needs treatment. Simple radiation exposure is not a danger to the EMT and should not impede the patient's care and transportation.

BIOLOGICAL WEAPONS

Biological weapons have been used in warfare for centuries. Stories are told of Scythian archers, ancient Euro-Asian mounted nomads who dipped their arrowheads into decomposing bodies in 400 B.C., and Tartar troops who flung plague-ridden bodies over the city walls during the siege of Kaffa. During the World War I, Germans made weaponized anthrax and cholera for use against the allies. One of the attractions of biological weapons for terrorists is that they are easy to acquire, synthesize, and distribute. Furthermore, it only takes a small quantity of the agents to kill hundreds or thousands of people. Unlike radioactive materials, which are relatively easy to detect with Geiger counters, biological agents are difficult to detect because they are often invisible, odorless, and tasteless.

Biological agents can be broken down into three classes: bacterial agents, viral agents, and biological toxins. Bacteria are microscopic single-celled organisms that cause disease and can multiply independently. Viral agents, including a subcategory called *rickettsia,* live inside a host cell in a parasitic relationship. These viral agents cannot live outside the host's body and depend on the host's living cells to multiply. Biological toxins are substances derived from a plant, animal, or even a microbe, and are very potent.

BACTERIAL AGENTS

Examples of bacterial agents—unicelled microbes abundant in the environment—that have been weaponized include *Bacillus anthracis* (anthrax), *Yersinia pestis* (plague), and *Burkholderia mallei* (glanders), among others.

Exposure to anthrax can start with symptoms similar to the flu, fever, fatigue, cough, and a mild chest discomfort within 1–6 days, which can progress to severe respiratory distress with stridor, cyanosis, and death within 24–36 hours of onset of serious symptoms.

Anthrax has already been weaponized by the United States and the former Soviet Union. Of the three diseases listed previously, anthrax presents unique challenges. Anthrax is a white powder that is highly resistant to sunlight, heat, and disinfectants, the typical means of infection control, and it is possible to aerosolize it so that it can be spread in the air. Furthermore, spores, a hardened capsule around the bacteria, allow anthrax to remain infectious within the soil or water for years. Figure 51.4A shows a microscopic view of *Bacillus anthracis*.

Plague, typically carried by flea-ridden rats, has been weaponized into an aerolized form. The plague is particularly troublesome because of its highly contagious nature. Like anthrax, the respiratory form of the plague, called *pneumonic plague*, begins with nonspecific flulike symptoms and progresses to respiratory distress, respiratory failure, and cardiovascular collapse. Figure 51.4B shows a microscopic view of *Y. pestis*, the caustic agent for the plague.

Glanders is a **zoonotic** disease, which is a disease of domestic animals, such as horses, that can be spread to humans. Once glanders is contracted, most likely through inhalation, the incubation period is about 10–14 days. Symptoms are similar to the flu: rigors or body chills, cold sweats, and unremitting headache, that rapidly progress to an acute systemic infection with resultant septic shock. The disease is fatal without treatment. Unlike other bacterial agents, there is no pre-exposure treatment, called *prophylaxis,* to prevent the infection. Fortunately, standard precautions, including cleansing surfaces with a hypochlorite solution, are effective in killing the bacteria. Figure 51.4C shows a microscopic view of *B. mallei,* the causative agent for glanders.

VIRAL AGENTS

A virus consists of a strand of RNA or DNA surrounded by a protein coat. It inserts itself into another cell within the host's body and reprograms that cell to stop what it normally does and instead reproduce more virus, eventually killing the host. Viruses of concern include smallpox and viral hemorrhagic fevers.

The World Health Organization declared that smallpox was eradicated around the world in May 1980. Shortly thereafter mass immunization programs to prevent smallpox were stopped. The threat of the use of smallpox has raised concerns because the majority of the population is not immunized. Smallpox starts with a rash similar to chickenpox except the rash is more concentrated on the face and extremities. Figure 51.5 illustrates smallpox infection. At present there is no effective treatment for smallpox, and all care remains supportive as the body tries to heal itself.

Ebola is perhaps the most widely known of the viral hemorrhagic fevers (VHF), yet there are four viral families with more than a dozen discrete diseases. VHF is easily spread by contact as well as airborne means. Flushing

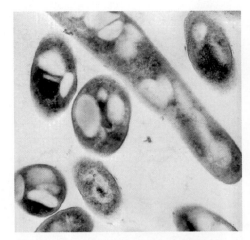

Figure 51.4A A microscopic view of *Bacillus anthracis*, the cause of anthrax (Courtesy of the Centers for Disease Control Public Health Image Library)

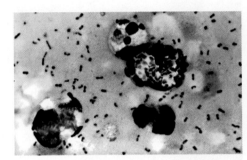

Figure 51.4B A microscopic view of the *Yersinia pestis* bacteria, the cause of bubonic plague (Courtesy of the Centers for Disease Control Public Health Image Library)

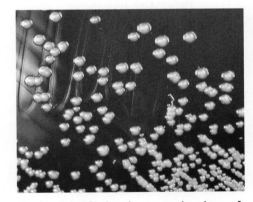

Figure 51.4C A microscopic view of *Burkholderia mallei,* the cause of glanders (Courtesy of the Centers for Disease Control Public Health Image Library)

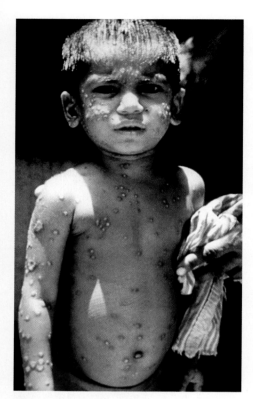

Figure 51.5 Smallpox is a highly contagious and potentially deadly infection (Courtesy of the Centers for Disease Control Public Health Image Library)

Table 51-2 SLUDGEM
S = Salivation (drooling)
L = Lacrimation (tearing)
U = Urination (excessive urine)
D = Defecation (diarrhea)
G = GI distress (abdominal pain)
E = Emesis (vomiting)
M = Muscle contractions (twitching)

of the face and chest associated with fever as well as the presence of petechiae, small ruptured capillaries under the skin, is suggestive of VHF. Subsequent disorders of bleeding, called **coagulopathy,** lead to hypoperfusion and shock and are treated accordingly.

BIOLOGICAL TOXINS

Biological toxins are not microorganisms themselves but rather harmful substances created by microorganisms, which differentiates them from chemical agents. Toxins such as botulinum (*Clostridium botulinum*) have been known for years and are more commonly the result of improperly canned foods. Botulinum is 275% more toxic than cyanide.

Another infamous toxin, ricin, has received recent attention in part because ricin is extracted from the castor bean, which is readily available worldwide. Fortunately, ricin, while toxic, is difficult to disperse over a wide area, limiting its use to attacks on individuals.

CHEMICAL WEAPONS

Chemical weapons saw their zenith during the First World War. Gases used to root troops out of trenches were invented by the Germans and used by the allies as well. More recently, gas warfare was used in the Iraq-Iran conflict and by Saddam Hussein to suppress the Kurdish tribes in northern Iraq.

Chemical weapons can be divided into five classifications: nerve agents, blister agents, blood agents, choking agents, and irritating agents.

The primary routes of exposure to these poisons are like all poisons: inhalation, ingestion, or absorption. While injection is possible, it is less likely. For a terrorist attack, the primary route of poisoning is likely to be inhalation.

NERVE AGENTS

Nerve agents were invented by the Germans in the First World War. Subsequently, many of these agents have abbreviations that start with the letter G, meaning German. An example of nerve agents is sarin (GB), used in a terrorist attack in a Tokyo subway and by Iraq against Iran.

Nerve agents stem from pesticides called organophosphates and are actually liquids that boil off at room temperature and create a gas. These pesticides were chemically altered to produce the characteristic symptom pattern represented in the mnemonic **SLUDGEM.** Table 51-2 explains each of the symptoms associated with a letter in SLUDGEM. Other associated symptoms include pinpoint pupils and blurry vision, involuntary muscle twitching to the point of convulsions, and chest pressure.

BLISTER AGENTS

The original blister agent was mustard gas, first used by the Germans in September 1917. Also called Yperite, for the place where it was used to great effect (Ypers), mustard gas was reportedly used in the 1980s against the Kurdish people of northern Iraq by Saddam Hussein's troops.

Mustard gas can have the characteristic smell of garlic and is readily absorbed in clothing and on the skin, where it can remain for weeks. Another blister agent, Lewisite, can have the characteristic smell of geraniums and is also readily absorbed in clothing and on the skin.

Blister agents are not as fatal as nerve agents but rather are intended to incapacitate a large number of people. Initial symptoms include reddened skin that eventually becomes covered with yellow, mustard-colored blisters. The most problematic effect of blister gases is eye irritation, with painful swelling and tearing, resulting in temporary blindness.

EMTs should be aware that blister agents rub off clothing very easily and can quickly contaminate the rescuer as well as the victim. Therefore, careful decontamination is mandatory to prevent further victims.

BLOOD AGENTS

The classic blood agent is cyanide, which interferes with the ability of cells to use oxygen. Cyanide is commonly used in many industrial processes, including photography, plastic manufacturing, and metallurgy, and thus can be easily obtained by terrorists.

A volatile chemical, cyanide, when it "off-gases," is a colorless gas with a faint, almond-like smell that some, but not all, people can smell.

Cyanide can rapidly lead to death at higher concentrations, and symptoms (vomiting, diarrhea, headaches) are nonspecific and therefore not helpful in the rapid determination of the causative agent.

CHOKING AGENTS

As the name implies, choking agents cause severe respiratory distress and eventual asphyxia. The classic choking agents are chlorine gas and phosgene gas. Chlorine gas is readily available and is used as a disinfectant for pools, as a cleaning agent for EMS (as hypochlorite solution or bleach), in paper manufacturing, and in many other uses. Thousands of tons of chlorine are manufactured and shipped in the United States annually. Phosgene (carbonyl chloride) is used in making plastics and pesticides and has the characteristic smell of freshly cut grass.

Chlorine gas, a heavier-than-air gas, converts to hydrochloric acid (HCl) when in contact with water. HCl causes burning of the eyes, severe paroxysms of coughing (coughing fits), and choking. The symptoms of exposure to phosgene are similar.

IRRITATING AGENTS

Irritating agents are used primarily for riot control and, as the name implies, are generally not lethal. Examples of irritating agents include tear gas (CS) and riot gas (CN). Pepper spray, first used by the U.S. Postal Service as a dog repellant, is oil (oleoresin capsicum) derived from cayenne peppers and is another example of an irritating agent. Although it is very difficult for a patient to overdose on these agents, their use can lead to widespread panic and injuries, including coughing, choking, shortness of breath, and nausea with vomiting.

PREPAREDNESS

Unfortunately, individuals or groups who have the means and the motive will commit acts of terrorism. EMS providers, in collaboration with and with the assistance of federal, state, and local law enforcement agencies, need to maintain a constant vigil for the presence of these threats that exist in their community and prepare for them through sharing of intelligence and open lines of communication.

The role of EMS in a terrorist attack is to reduce the number of losses, measured in death (mortality) and illness (morbidity). To be more effective, EMS must be proactive and prepare for a terrorist attack, assuming the inevitability of such an attack in their community. This goal is accomplished, in part, by establishing an **emergency operations plan (EOP)**. An EOP is an interagency document that assigns responsibilities to departments or organizations, establishing outlines of command (authority) and describing how emergency responders will protect people and property in the event of a terrorist attack and apprehend those who are responsible.

An EOP should be available at every level of government. At the federal level, Public Law 93-288 (Robert T. Stafford Disaster Relief and Emergency Assistance Act) provides for a **federal response plan (FRP).** The FRP is used whenever state and local authorities are overwhelmed and brings the immense resources of the federal government to their aid. For example, the FRP calls for the National Communication System to assist with communications and the Army Corps of Engineers to help with public works. For EMS, Congress has identified the American Red Cross as the lead federal agency. The federal government has identified 12 emergency support functions in which it can help local emergency responders with the mitigation of a terrorist attack. The agencies responsible for each emergency support function are listed in Table 51-3.

EMERGENCY OPERATIONS PLAN

Every emergency operations plan must first have a hazard vulnerability analysis, similar to a hazardous materials operations plan. High-risk hazards for terrorist attacks include government buildings (courthouses, post offices, etc.) as well as high life hazards (malls, schools, etc.). The plan should also contain a listing of potentially valuable resources as well as locations of equipment stockpiles, such as antidote kits. Also, facilities for mass decontamination should be prepared for just such an emergency.

EMS should also collaborate with local, state, and federal law enforcement agencies to share intelligence about terrorist groups that may be operating within the area. Groups that should be suspect include ethnic separatists, left- and right-wing radical organizations, survivalist groups, and foreign terrorist organizations.

EMERGENCY RESPONDERS AND THE EOP

For any plan to be effective, there must be training and regular drills. The mnemonic **LACES** can be used for EMS crews practicing scene safety.

Table 51-3 Emergency Support Functions Defined in the Federal Response Plan

Emergency Support Function	Responsible Federal Agency
1. Transportation	U.S. Department of Transportation
2. Communications	U.S. National Communications System
3. Public works	U.S. Department of Defense
4. Firefighting	U.S. Department of Agriculture
5. Information/planning	U.S. Federal Emergency Management Agency (FEMA)
6. Mass care	American Red Cross
7. Resource support	Government Supply Agency
8. Health and medical services	U.S. Department of Health and Human Resources
9. Urban search and rescue	FEMA
10. Hazardous materials	U.S. Environmental Protection Agency
11. Food	U.S. Department of Agriculture
12. Energy	U.S. Department of Energy

The L in LACES stands for lookout. Someone should be assigned as a lookout at any event that may be a target of a terrorist attack. That lookout is responsible for observing irregular or inconsistent behaviors as well as unattended packages. The lookout, as safety officer, should have a "stand back and observe" or big-picture attitude. Snipers, for example, depend on the emergency services focusing on the event and not taking their environment into account.

The A in LACES stands for awareness. Every EMT should be minimally trained to the awareness level for emergency response to terrorism. The federal Office of Domestic Preparedness, a part of Homeland Security, offers courses, as does the National Association of EMTs, to help EMTs identify potential hazards.

Communications, the C in LACES, is critical for on-scene operations. The mainstays of EMS scene communications are mobile and portable radios. These radios should be able to communicate with other emergency services, such as law enforcement, while on scene.

However, it may be hazardous to use portable radios for fear of triggering detonation of an explosive device by activating an electronic blasting cap designed to be triggered by radio signals from a safe distance. Secondary devices, intentionally left by terrorists to maim emergency services responders, may be designed to be triggered by emergency service radios in the near vicinity.

Personal safety is high on the list of responsibilities for an EMT. Therefore, an escape route, the E in LACES, must be available so that emergency responders can exit the scene quickly and with a minimum of confusion. Often this is as simple as positioning the emergency vehicle toward an exit and making sure that it is not blocked in.

Finally, the S in LACES stands for safety zones. The EMT should keep the principles of safety zones in mind, staying within the cold zone and avoiding the warm/hot zones. Typically, the cold zone is uphill, because many gases are heavier than air, and upwind, as well as a safe distance from the incident site. Table 51-4 lists all of the elements of LACES.

EMERGENCY RESPONSE

When responding to a suspect EMS call, the EMT must maintain a high index of suspicion that the call may be for a terrorist attack. Calls that should be considered suspect include unexplained explosions, multiple calls for the same or similar concern across a jurisdiction, called a *symptom cluster*, or the report of multiple casualties without a significant mechanism of injury.

Upon arrival, a scene size-up survey may reveal signs of an NBC attack. Indicators may include ground-level vapor clouds, dead foliage or dead wildlife such as birds, and objects such as a chemical sprayer that seem out of place.

Delaying entry in these cases may be the correct choice of action. The EMT should call for additional resources to help secure the scene and to bring detection equipment.

The EMT should also be suspicious of people and vehicles leaving the scene. License plate numbers or a brief description of persons on scene can be invaluable to investigators later. A rough sketch of the scene, as it was found, can also help investigators.

The EMT should consider this initial approach a reconnaissance mission, gathering data and then withdrawing to report the findings to the proper authorities.

EOP ACTIVATION

The actions of the first emergency responder can have critical importance on the number of civilian casualties and the effective mitigation of the terrorist attack.

Table 51-4 Elements of LACES	
L	= Lookout
A	= Awareness
C	= Communications
E	= Escape routes
S	= Safety zones

Street Smart

The EMT should consider wearing ballistic protection, also known as *body armor,* when responding to a potential terrorist attack. Body armor may save the EMT's life if a secondary device is used or a sniper remains on scene to disrupt emergency operations.

Street Smart

Every terrorist attack is, by definition, an illegal act and therefore a crime scene. It is important that the EMT leave things as they are found and only move those items that are absolutely necessary for patient care. If an object is moved, its position should be noted; if possible, a picture should be taken before it is moved.

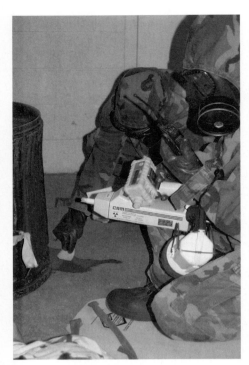

Figure 51.6 Military personnel using special chemical detection equipment, including M-8 paper

Of critical importance is the "first-in report." This report will put into motion the EOP and includes public warning and information and activating plans for evacuation and emergency shelters.

AIR MONITORING AND DETECTION DEVICES

The tactical use of detection devices can prevent needless illness or death. Many devices are available to help the EMT determine if WMD are present.

From simple Geiger counters to dosimeters, qualified and trained personnel can use special detection units to check for the presence of radioactive materials that may remain from an NDD.

Similarly, ionizing detection units and colorimetric sampling devices can test for the presence of toxic chemicals in the environment. The military has made available special field detection kits, such as M-8 and M-9 paper, that can detect liquid nerve and blister agents. These handheld points of detection devices should be used only by qualified personnel who have personal protective equipment in case of exposure (Figure 51.6).

SELF-PROTECTION

Upon establishing that a WMD attack may have occurred, EMTs should make efforts to protect themselves. Self-protection can be reduced to three concepts: time, distance, and shielding. Once the hazard has been identified, the EMT should spend the minimum amount of time in the area. A tactical withdrawal, even when casualties are present and evident, reduces the total number of casualties overall.

The next protection is distance. Using the Table of Initial Isolation and Protective Action Distances in the ERG, the EMT should withdraw to a minimum safe distance. This distance should be the edge of the cold zone, and the EMT should make efforts to secure the area, isolate the hazard, and deny entry to others who are not properly protected.

The final protection is shielding. Shielding can be in the form of concrete barriers, protection from snipers or radiation, or barrier devices such as gloves, masks, and gowns.

THREAT REDUCTION

Understanding what threats may be present can help the EMT prepare. The mnemonic **TRACEM** enumerates these hazards. The T in TRACEM stands for thermal harm. Explosive devices can produce harmful extremes of heat, causing burn injury. Fortunately, firefighting protective garments, from class A to standard issue equipment, can help protect against burn injury.

The harm created by a nuclear device, done at the cellular level, is via invisible alpha, beta, and gamma radiations (the R in TRACEM). The best protection among the cellular damage done by radiation is time, distance, and shielding.

The A in TRACEM represents asphyxiants, such as choking agents, which interfere with respiration and thus can be deadly. Gases are often asphyxiants, and most dangerous gases are heavier than air. Staging EMS uphill and upwind of these gases can prevent injury or death from asphyxiants.

Toxic or corrosive chemicals, the C in TRACEM, can also injure the EMT, causing painful chemical burns. To prevent exposure to these potentially lethal chemicals, the EMT should first delay assessment and treatment until the patient has been decontaminated. The EMT should then employ the use of barrier devices, such as gowns, gloves, and goggles, to prevent possible cross-contamination.

The average EMT works every day at risk for contracting a contagious disease, called an etiologic (The E in TRACEM). Use of common personal protective equipment, such as gloves and goggles, can eliminate the risk for an exposure to a potentially infectious material.

The last harm that can come to an EMT from WMD, and the last letter in TRACEM, is mechanical harm (M). Explosive devices, such as a secondary device, can produce serious life-threatening trauma. To prevent this harm or to reduce the amount of harm, the EMT should consider using ballistic protection, such as ballistic vests, for example. Table 51-5 outlines what TRACEM represents.

INCIDENTAL EXPOSURE TO NERVE AGENTS

Despite an EMT's best efforts, exposure to a nerve agent may occur. These nerve agents, as discussed earlier, are very potent and require immediate treatment.

Recognizing this fact, the military uses a special antidote kit called the *Mark I kit.* This kit is a pair of autoinjectors containing the antidotes atropine (equivalent 2 mg atropine sulfate) and 2-PAM Chloride (pralidoxime chloride) (Figure 51.7).

These autoinjectors work similarly to those that an EMT uses to administer epinephrine during an anaphylactic reaction. The Mark I kit should only be used by responders, one administering to the other; to patients, when the person is symptomatic (i.e., SLUDGE); or upon orders of medical control.

It is not necessary to remove clothing and expose the thigh to use these injectors, and the atropine is always given before the 2-PAM chloride. It may be necessary to give multiple doses, every 5 minutes, for a maximum of three or until the symptoms subside. The EMT should carefully read local and/or state guidelines for the use of these drugs.

CONCLUSION

In the current day and age, the EMT must have a heightened awareness of the potential for terrorist attacks and be prepared to act, within the established system, to bring order from chaos and to save as many lives as possible. For the EMT who is the first emergency responder, the task of communicating the nature of the incident and activating the emergency operations plan is of critical importance.

Table 51-5	TRACEM
T =	Thermal harm (burn trauma)
R =	Radiation harm (radiation burns)
A =	Asphyxiation
C =	Corrosive chemicals (chemical burns)
E =	Etiologic (infections)
M =	Mechanical (blast injuries)

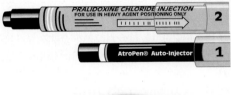

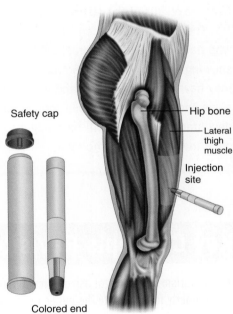

Figure 51.7 The atropine autoinjector is similar to the epinephrine autoinjector and can deliver lifesaving medications to contaminated patients, including EMTs

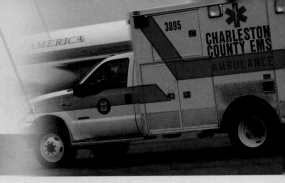

CASE STUDY Continued

As additional EMS units arrive, Enis completes his command staff assignments and instructs them to set up their needed areas of triage and treatment. Liz has been appointed the triage officer and, together with the treatment officer, proceeds to set up a triage/treatment area. There have not been any patients yet, but they will be ready for them when the time comes.

Enis continues to brief the EMS team on the status of the incident. The HazMat team has set up a potential decontamination corridor. The initial tests are indicating the white powder is not anthrax. They are currently waiting to hear the results of the testing for other biological agents.

The building has been evacuated of all personnel who have not been in contact with the white powder or showing signs of illness. The remaining 20 people who may have come in contact and are showing the same signs and symptoms as other individuals are undergoing decontamination and will be brought to the treatment area once that has been completed.

As the patients arrive at the triage and treatment area, they are all able to walk on their own. Liz classifies them as greens and turns them over to the treatment officer. All of the patients have vague concerns of flu-like symptoms, with two of the 20 having an additional concern of mild chest tightness. All 20 patients are transported to local hospitals for further evaluation.

Later that evening, Liz and Enis are sitting at the debriefing when the final report on the white powder is read. The white powder was a combination of flour and baking powder. There is an ongoing investigation to find the person responsible for a costly prank. The patients were all determined to have influenza, in various stages, that was unrelated to the white powder incident. However, the after-action report shows the emergency operations plan was successfully implemented and the incident was managed effectively and efficiently.

Key Concepts Revisited

- Terrorism is the illegal use of force against persons or property to intimidate the public or coerce a government.

- Domestic and international terrorists share a common purpose.

  ○ Domestic terrorists are American citizens or nationals who use violence to try to influence federal policy.

  ○ International terrorists are not citizens of the government they are attacking through the use of violence to try to influence governmental policies.

- EMTs must be trained to recognize the hallmarks of a terrorist attack, how to protect themselves from harm, and how to activate the emergency response plan.

  ○ Awareness level

  ○ Operations level

  ○ Technician level

- Weapons of mass destruction (WMD) are used to indiscriminately kill or maim large numbers of people at one time.

- The three major classifications of WMD are nuclear, biological, and chemical (NBC).

  ○ Nuclear or radiologic weapons

    • Nuclear dispersion device (NDD), a conventional explosive device used to disperse nuclear material or radioactive materials across a wide area, also known as *dirty bombs*

    • Conventional bombs

  ○ Biological agents

    • Bacterial agents: anthrax, plague, glanders (animal to human)

- Viral agents: smallpox, ebola
- Biological toxins: botulism, ricin
  - Chemical weapons
    - Nerve agents: sarin
    - Blister agents: mustard gas
    - Blood agents: cyanide
    - Choking agents: chlorine gas, phosgene gas
    - Irritating agents: tear gas, pepper spray, riot gas
- The EMT must maintain a constant vigil for the presence of threats and plan for terrorist attacks by establishing and practicing an effective emergency response plan.
  - Emergency operations plan (EOP): interagency document assigning responsibilities to departments or organizations
  - Federal response plan (FRP): federal emergency plan that can be activated when state and local authorities are overwhelmed
- The emergency response plan should outline additional resources that may be needed on scene of a terrorist incident.

- Preparedness, assisted by understanding possible threats, can aid in reducing threats.
  - TRACEM: enumerates the hazards possible with terrorist attacks
    - Thermal harm
    - Radiation harm
    - Asphyxiants
    - Corrosive chemicals
    - Etiologic
    - Mechanical
- Self-protection for the EMT is based on three concepts: time, distance, and shielding.
  - Time: tactical withdrawal—spend a minimum amount of time in the area
  - Distance: withdrawal to a minimum safe distance based on the ERG
  - Shielding: barrier devices
- The EMT's role is to communicate the nature of the incident and activate the emergency operations plan.

Review Questions

1. What is meant by the term *terrorism*?
2. Differentiate between domestic terrorism and international terrorism.
3. What are the levels of training for emergency response to terrorism?
4. What are weapons of mass destruction?
5. What does NBC stand for?
6. What are the elements of shielding?
7. What is an emergency operations plan?
8. Define the components of the mnemonic SLUDGEM.
9. What are some potential signs of a terrorist attack?
10. Describe how an EMT would "self-protect" from hazards on scene.

Key Terms

Awareness level
Biological agents
Chemical weapons
Coagulopathy
Domestic terrorist

Emergency Operations Plan (EOP)
Federal Response Plan (FRP)
Geiger counter
International terrorist
LACES

Nuclear Dispersion Device (NDD)
Radiation pager
Secondary device
SLUDGEM

Terrorism
TRACEM
Weapons of mass destruction (WMD)
Zoonotic

Further Study

Bevelacqua, Armando S. *Hazardous Materials Chemistry.* 2d ed. Clifton Park, NY: Delmar Cengage, 2006.

Bevelacqua, Amando S., and Richard H. Stilp. *Terrorism Handbook for Operational Responders.* 3rd ed. Clifton Park, NY: Delmar Cengage, 2010.

Bioterrorism: A Field Guide for First Responders. 2d ed. Clifton Park, NY: Delmar Cengage.

UNIT (52) Vehicle Extrication and Rescue Operations

A **rescue** is an attempt by one person to help another person who is incapable of freeing himself and who is in danger if he remains in that situation. If this incapacity is due to illness or injury, then an Emergency Medical Technician (EMT) may be involved in the rescue effort. In almost all rescues, the patient is in need of medical care, and an EMT should be immediately available.

If the patient has died as a result of his injuries, then the operation is not a rescue but a recovery—a recovery of the body. Without a live patient, there can be no rescue. Medical care provided by an EMT on scene can make the difference between a mission being a rescue or becoming a recovery.

National Education Standard
The Emergency Medical Technician (EMT) will be able to demonstrate a simple depth and breadth of understanding and ability to perform safe vehicle extrication.

Key Concepts

- Rescue is an attempt to help another person who is incapable of freeing himself or herself from confinement.

- The phases common to all rescues begin with establishing command.

- The common hazards encountered in confined space rescue is the low oxygen concentration, toxic fumes, and explosive gases.

- Hazards at a motor vehicle collision should be identified during the scene size-up.

- Motor vehicles must be stabilized before patients can be extricated and care provided.

- Heavy rescue is used when a patient must be disentangled from a vehicle.

- There are three common means of extrication from a vehicle using heavy rescue.

- The EMT should preplan for possible scenarios in operations involving water rescue.

- Scene size-up during a search and rescue must include a high life hazard assessment.

- Rescue situations can require the EMT to be creative and adjust plans of action to the situation.

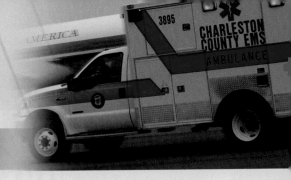

CASE STUDY

"Dispatch to Station 43: respond to an MVC, car versus pole, one entrapment. Time out 19:57."

The engine and rescue truck are first out of the station, with Ray and Kaelynn close behind in the squad. The lieutenant on the engine establishes command immediately, having the vehicle evaluated for stabilization. Ray will stage behind the engine and rescue vehicle.

On arrival, Kaelynn and Ray don the turnout gear they always wear whenever they respond to a motor vehicle crash. A small crowd has gathered, and law enforcement is working on clearing the scene.

As Kaelynn and Ray approach the vehicle, they visually assess the damage to get an initial idea of potential injuries. The car is a medium-sized, four-door sedan with the passenger side wrapped around a light pole. Firefighters are securing the vehicle and addressing the fluid leaking out from under the car.

Kaelynn can see a young male in the passenger seat and hear him crying out for someone to help. One of the firefighters has gained access to the vehicle from the back seat and is attempting to calm the patient while obtaining cervical spinal stabilization.

Critical Thinking Questions?

1. What are some of the hazards present on the scene of a motor vehicle collision?
2. What precautions must an EMT observe?
3. How can an EMT gain quick entry?
4. What can an EMT do to protect the patient while heavy rescue occurs?

INTRODUCTION

Many common hazards and rescue situations are seen in communities throughout the United States every day. Every community should have a plan for how to respond to these types of emergencies. The unit presents only an overview of rescue techniques; an EMT should not expect to be knowledgeable about rescue techniques after reading this text alone. Additional training, as well as extensive preparation, is required before an EMT should attempt any rescue. An EMT should always follow local procedures and protocols in rescues.

PHASES OF THE RESCUE

All rescues—whether an exciting wildlands search, a dramatic heavy rescue, or simply gaining access to a locked home to help an elderly person who is incapable of reaching the door—have phases similar to a routine emergency call. There is a scene assessment phase, a treatment phase, and a transportation phase. A few fundamental differences make rescues distinct from the average Emergency Medical Services (EMS) call.

A rescue typically takes place in an unusual environment or situation, such as the bottom of a cave or the top of a building. A rescue often requires special knowledge and/or equipment to access, disentangle, and rescue the patient.

Every EMT should have an awareness of which types of rescue situations may occur in her community and what special personnel and rescue equipment may be needed to rescue patients. No EMT should ever enter a rescue scene before she has been trained and is proficient at these special rescue techniques and the use of the equipment. Without a higher technical level of training, the EMT may endanger everyone on the scene needlessly while trying to help the patient. In the worst-case scenario, the EMT may become a victim. EMTs should obtain further training from qualified rescue instructors if they are interested in a particular area of rescue.

ESTABLISHING COMMAND

The first-arriving emergency services unit should immediately take control of the situation and establish scene command. In some jurisdictions, command and control are shared by several agencies in a unified command structure, with each emergency service commander supervising his or her own discipline. In other jurisdictions, a singular command structure identified by the presence of a single incident commander is used. More information regarding incident management can be found in Unit 49.

SCENE SIZE-UP

After arriving on scene, the EMT proceeds with a scene size-up. To help maintain a more global perspective and see the big picture, the EMT should start her observation from a distance. A pair of binoculars can help the EMT get the details of what is happening on scene without placing herself and her crew in harm's way (Figure 52.1). This environmental assessment, discussed more fully in Unit 15, provides the EMT with much-needed information.

The first part of a scene size-up is a risk assessment. A risk assessment prompts the EMT to think about hazards present on scene and how to control or mitigate those hazards.

Next, the EMT requests any additional resources that would be required to secure the scene and control the hazards. For example, the presence of smoke at a motor vehicle collision (MVC) should prompt the EMT to request assistance from the fire department. The request for additional assistance from heavy rescue may have come when the original dispatch information was obtained or when the first unit arrived. It is important that if additional resources are needed, they are called as soon as the need is identified. Often this moment occurs during the scene size-up.

If the scene poses a considerable number of hazards, the EMT should consider assigning a safety officer. The responsibility of the safety officer, outlined in Unit 49, is to ensure the well-being of rescuers.

Before crew members exit from the emergency vehicle, the EMT should ensure that everyone is wearing the personal protective equipment (PPE) that will be needed. Even if the EMT is not intimately involved in the rescue, special PPE, such as gloves and eye protection, may still be in order. It is not uncommon for bits of glass to fly during a vehicle rescue.

The nature of rescue also tends to draw emergency services providers into the scene. For instance, when a patient is being extricated and another pair of hands is needed, an EMT stationed at the outer perimeter will naturally step in to help out. For this reason, all emergency services personnel who are potentially at risk should be wearing appropriate PPE. Common hazards against which an EMT must protect herself are listed in Table 52-1. Either the officer in charge or the safety officer is responsible for ensuring all emergency personnel are wearing the appropriate PPE.

Next, the EMT must determine the number of patients and the severity of their injuries. This process is called *triage* and must be performed before extensive medical care is rendered to any single individual. In some cases, it is

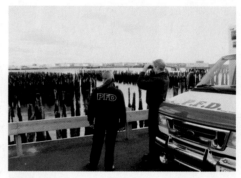

Figure 52.1 An EMT uses binoculars to check for hazards from a distance (Courtesy of Larry Torrey and MEDCU, Portland, ME)

Table 52-1	Hazards
Hazard	**Personal Protective Equipment**
Flash and flame	Turnout coat
Falling objects	Helmet
Sharp objects	Boots, gloves
Flying debris	Goggles
Poor visibility	Highway safety vest
Loud noises	Earplugs

Table 52-2 Examples of Confined Spaces

Grain bins

Wells

Sewers

Storage

Manholes

Drainage culverts

Natural caves

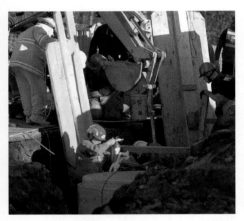

Figure 52.2 Entry into a confined space is limited to specially trained rescue personnel

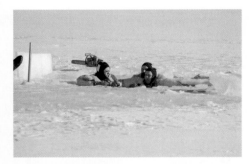

Figure 52.3 Technical rescue requires specialized equipment and training (Courtesy of Clive Fire Department, Clive, IA)

impossible to determine the number of patients immediately. In other cases, it is impossible to determine the severity of the patient's injuries because the patient is either trapped or inaccessible.

CONFINED SPACE RESCUE

A **confined space** is any area that has limited openings for entry or exit and is not typically designed for worker occupancy. Examples of confined spaces are listed in Table 52-2.

Confined spaces can be hazardous to workers who are trapped inside. Gases, such as methane, can accumulate and explode. Gases such as carbon monoxide and ammonia can poison a worker. In other cases, the worker who is in an oxygen-poor environment or engulfed in grain, for example, can be suffocated.

Confined space rescue is extremely dangerous. The National Institute of Occupational Safety and Health (NIOSH) reports that more than 60% of the fatalities in confined space rescue are fatalities of the rescuers.

An EMT needs to identify when a rescue is a confined space rescue and call appropriate rescue personnel (Figure 52.2). Under no circumstances should an EMT enter a confined space without special training and equipment. All confined space rescues are technical rescues by definition.

MANAGEMENT

Rescues may require special techniques to access the patient. Some rescues may be accomplished with simple tools, which should be available to every EMT. Other rescues are complex operations, called **technical rescues,** which require highly trained rescue technicians using specialized equipment (Figure 52.3).

Whenever there is a choice, the simpler means of rescuing the patient is better. Complex systems and elaborate equipment have a tendency to fail when they are needed most. An EMT might employ some simple rescue techniques while waiting for special or professional rescuers to arrive, protocols permitting. In other cases, an EMT might be standing by with simple tools, just in case the special rescue equipment fails.

In both cases, there is a backup plan. Having a backup plan in place in case the original plan fails is called **redundancy.** Whenever a human life is in danger, there should always be redundancy in the rescue plan. Redundancy decreases the chances of a catastrophic outcome should one critical piece of equipment fail.

ACCESS

The next task is to reach the patient. While this sounds easy, the reality is often quite different. The EMT should keep in mind that average persons will usually make extraordinary efforts to free themselves. The fact that the person is trapped should give the EMT an indication that ordinary efforts will not be sufficient.

If the EMT is trained, she should start to make preparations for a rescue. If the EMT is not trained, she must contact someone, such as a dive rescue team or a rope rescue team, who can rescue the patient. In the interim while waiting for the rescue to occur, the EMT should prepare or stage for the patient who will eventually be her responsibility.

RESIDENCE

When an elder person falls and is not able to get up to answer the door after calling for help through Lifeline, this person is essentially "trapped" in his own residence. This situation occurs so frequently in the United States that many EMS systems have a set of special protocols, a "preplan," on how to respond to these situations. Typically, these protocols for "gaining entry" dictate that the police are on scene and reasonable efforts have been made to gain entry before the EMT resorts to force.

After confirming the address and still getting no answer at the door, the EMT should circle the house. While circling the house, the EMT should call out the patient's name loudly and repeatedly. EMTs should also consider turning on all flashing emergency lights and sounding the siren to announce their presence.

As EMTs circle the perimeter of the house, they should try to open doors and windows. They should also be looking into the house trying to locate the patient. If the patient is found, the EMT should loudly announce who she is and explain that she is locked out. The EMT should ask the patient whether there is a hidden key or another means of entry.

It is also prudent for the EMT to ask whether there are any animals in the house. A frightened animal may attempt to protect an injured owner. If an animal is in the house, then the EMT should consider calling for the animal control officer.

Finally, the EMT should ask whether there is a security alarm system. Further efforts to gain entry will most likely set off the intruder alert. If a security alarm system is discovered, local law enforcement needs to be notified of a possible alarm trip.

The EMT needs to weigh the severity of the emergency against the time it will take to get a locksmith to the scene for disassembly of the door. If the patient is severely injured, the decision is always life before property. If time permits, the EMT should consider requesting law enforcement or fire department assistance. Both emergency services have training and tools for forcible entry.

Forcible entry, using special tools or brute force to overcome an obstacle to gain access, can be accomplished by a number of means (Figure 52.4). Prying a window open with a crowbar or smashing out a windowpane with a flashlight are two commonly used options. Forcing a door is a possibility, using special tools, but "kicking in" the door should be avoided. Kicking in the door frequently results in injury for the EMT, structural damage for the homeowner, and a door that is still left standing intact with a patient on the other side.

Usually a window or door farthest from the patient will be forced or broken. While this effort is going on, another EMT should be stationed with the patient, explaining what is going to happen and keeping contact with the patient.

RESCUE

Once the EMT reaches the patient, immediate lifesaving procedures should be performed and then the patient should be prepared for transport. In some cases, the transportation is simply a flexible stretcher whereas in other cases a complex high-angle rope rescue system must be created.

Each rescue situation usually requires a rescue system. Most of these rescue systems must be brought to the scene and set up. This process can be lengthy. A little forethought on the part of the EMT can decrease time lost on scene with this setup. The system can be set up ahead of time, while the patient is being accessed by other rescuers.

TREATMENT

In the majority of rescues, the patient has experienced some injury, whether it is a cold injury from exposure or a traumatic injury from an MVC. The severity of an injury is always time dependent. The longer the patient goes untreated, the greater the degree of injury. Problems such as crush injury and

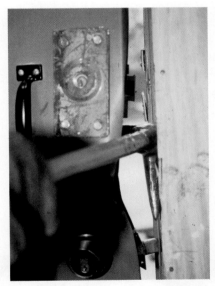

Figure 52.4 Using a crowbar or similar device, the EMT may be able to forcibly open a locked door

compartment syndrome can also occur. Units 37 and 38 contain more information on crush injury and compartment syndrome and should be reviewed. In most cases, the EMT can assume that the patient's injuries are more severe than usual based on the amount of time lost getting to the patient and getting the patient to definitive care.

TRANSPORT

While immediate medical care on scene is important, it is often more important to transport to definitive medical care as soon as possible. Once the patient has been moved to the ambulance, the EMT should consider a request for an advanced life support (ALS) intercept, if one has not already been arranged.

VEHICLE EXTRICATION

One of the most common rescues an EMT will encounter is that resulting from an MVC. Crushed cars and entrapped patients often result from heavy vehicles, traveling at high speeds, encountering a stationary object.

Many patients are easily rescued from a motor vehicle after a collision. The side door is opened, and the EMT extricates the patient from the vehicle. Other patients who are entangled and/or entrapped inside their vehicles require the use of special vehicle extrication equipment, called **heavy rescue,** to be freed.

PREPARATION

Not every MVC rescue situation can be presented in this text. However, an EMT should be aware of some of the more common scenarios and undergo training with heavy rescue technicians. An agreed-on plan of action, or a **preplan,** between rescuers can eliminate wasted time and confusion on an emergency scene.

Every community has slightly different rescue resources, but every community has MVCs within its jurisdiction. Combined training and preplanning are the keys to a successful rescue operation and an improved patient outcome.

COMMAND

As the first EMT approaches the scene, medical command should be established. In most cases, that is as simple as notifying the communications center of the EMT's arrival. In other cases, a more formal declaration is needed. Unit 49 provides a description of a first-in report.

The EMT's first and immediate concern is scene safety. In the case of an MVC, the greatest hazard may be traffic. Every possible protection should be taken to ensure the EMT's safety while on scene. The ambulance may be placed so that it becomes a physical barrier between the EMT and traffic (Figure 52.5).

In some systems, only rear-facing flashing lights are left on. Other revolving lights are turned off to prevent the EMT from being blinded and to prevent passing motorists from being distracted. Traffic cones, flashing lights, or flares may also help provide the EMT with a greater margin of safety. More details regarding scene safety measures can be found in Unit 48.

PERIMETERS

Every motor vehicle has two perimeters or circles. The first perimeter, where there is a greater danger of injury to the EMT, is called the *inner circle* or *action circle*. The outer circle is where equipment and personnel would be "staged" until needed in the inner circle or until the patient is brought out.

Every EMT who is within either the inner or outer circle should have appropriate PPE. The minimum PPE on scene of a vehicular rescue includes

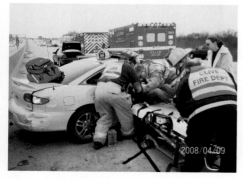

Figure 52.5 The ambulance may be used as a protective shield when on scene (Courtesy of Clive Fire Department, Clive, IA)

a safety helmet or bump cap, eye protection, a rip-resistant coat, and a pair of heavy-duty gloves. Even this PPE may not be sufficient within the action circle. The EMT should defer to the expert opinion of the rescue captain in decisions regarding PPE.

SCENE SIZE-UP

Other potential hazards on scene include those created by the motor vehicle itself. The EMT should carefully assess the motor vehicle before beginning to treat the patient. If there is any evidence of fire, the EMT should await the arrival of the fire department. Without proper training or equipment, an EMT should never approach a burning car.

Assuming the car is not on fire, the EMT should make a "walk around." By walking around the vehicle to conduct a 360-degree sweep, the EMT can assess for possible hazards amd examine the extent of damage created by the collision. The EMT checking the vehicle should be looking for spilled fluids (Figure 52.6). Spilled gasoline can ignite, burning the patient and EMT. Spilled antifreeze is extremely slippery. Walking on antifreeze with rubber-soled shoes or boots is akin to skating on ice. Absorbent materials, such as cat litter, placed on top of spilled antifreeze or oil, can decrease the chance of an accidental slip and fall.

More than 1 million air bags have deployed since these safety features were introduced, and air bags have been a leading factor in the reduction in mortality from vehicle collision. However, rescuers have also been injured by undeployed air bags. An undeployed air bag can be activated after a collision by heat from fire or by static electricity and can crush the head of an EMT between the air bag and the patient's chest.

EMTs should always keep about 20 inches between themselves and the air bag, in the event of accidental deployment. EMTs should never place a hard object, such as a shortboard, between themselves and the undeployed air bag before the battery is disconnected. As soon as possible, the battery cables should be disconnected, deactivating the air bag by allowing the capacitor to drain its power. In most cases, the capacitor that powers the air bag will be drained in less than 30 seconds. Lists of capacitor drain times are available from the United States Department of Transportation (USDOT) and automobile manufacturers. To disconnect battery power, the EMT should start with the negative terminal. If the negative cable is being cut, it should be cut twice to avoid arcing back to the battery. Then the positive cable should be cut to disconnect power to the capacitor, and the air bag capacitor should quickly drain its power.

If the motor vehicle has struck a utility pole, electric power lines may have fallen on top of the roof. If the motor vehicle drove over the top of an underground power splice, the entire car could be energized. The EMT should look above and below the motor vehicle for any contacts with electric power lines or transformers. If wires are down on the car, the fire department or utility company should be notified immediately, and the EMT should make a careful retreat.

Alternative fuel cars on the road today may pose different types of hazards. The EMT should be alert to placards or emblems indicating that the motor vehicle uses propane or is battery powered. These alternative fuel motor vehicles present unique hazards to the EMT.

HYBRID VEHICLES

Hybrid cars are motor vehicles that run on a combination of gas and electricity (Figure 52.7). They are extremely fuel efficient and are becoming widely popular today with the rising cost of gas. However, when hybrid cars are

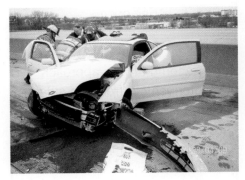

Figure 52.6 Spilled fluids such as antifreeze can be slippery and dangerous (Courtesy of Clive Fire Department, Clive, IA)

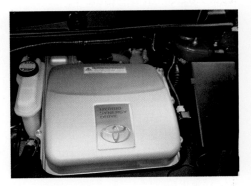

Figure 52.7 Hybrid car (Courtesy of Clive Fire Department, Clive, IA)

Cars have special impact bumpers that are designed to compress and reduce damage at low speeds. The majority of car manufacturers use a hydraulic device to absorb the energy of these low-speed impacts.

These hydraulic devices can be compressed and damaged, failing to release the bumper to its original position. The result is energy stored in the compressed bumper, with a bumper that is ready to spring open.

These *loaded bumpers* can be a danger to the EMT. An EMT should always approach a motor vehicle from the side to avoid a loaded bumper and then maintain a healthy distance of several feet from the bumpers at all times.

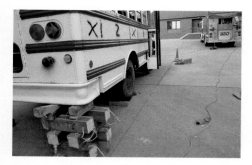

Figure 52.8 All unstable vehicles must be stabilized with cribbing before an EMT enters the passenger compartment (Courtesy of Clive Fire Department, Clive, IA)

involved in a crash, the car can remain charged with between 300 and 500 volts of electricity, which poses a hazard to EMTs and rescue personnel.

Most hybrids have a high-voltage battery located in the back of the vehicle with high-voltage lines encased in orange for easy identification. This battery must be disabled before continuing with the rescue operation and extrication of the patient. Even with the battery disabled, the lines can remain charged, providing additional challenges for rescue personnel who may need to cut into the vehicle during extrication.

The EMT must be able to recognize a hybrid car and have knowledge of the potential dangers it may present in an MVC. The EMT and other rescue personnel should never attempt to disconnect a battery or cut into a hybrid vehicle unless they have been trained in how to safely disable the battery and the location of the voltage lines.

STABILIZATION

Any movement of a damaged vehicle can cause the patient to also be moved within the vehicle. Any movement of the patient could potentially create additional injury, especially in the case of cervical spine injuries. Therefore, any vehicle with an injured patient inside that can be shifted or shaken is unstable and must be stabilized before patient care can proceed.

A vehicle that lands on its roof or is found on its side is unstable and must be stabilized. The stabilization of vehicles in these positions often requires chains, high-lift jacks, special tools, and/or cribbing. The EMT should leave stabilizing these vehicles to the rescue technicians.

Fortunately, most vehicles remain on their wheels after a collision. However, this does not necessarily mean that the vehicle is stable. Even a car on all four wheels can be shifted, creating movement of the passengers inside.

Several techniques have been developed to stabilize a vehicle that is still on its wheels. Essentially, all of these techniques use the same principle of isolating the wheels from the frame of the vehicle.

Blocks of wood, called **cribbing,** can be used to lift the vehicle's frame off the wheels and stabilize the vehicle. Using special prefabricated cribbing called *step-blocks,* a motor vehicle can quickly and effectively be stabilized (Figure 52.8).

As a last resort, provided no cribbing is available, the air can be let out of the tires. By cutting or pulling the air stem, the tire goes flat, and the car rests on its rims.

An EMT should never enter a motor vehicle unless it has first been stabilized. The EMT should advise the patient, if he is conscious, to remain seated with eyes straight ahead until the vehicle is stabilized and rescuers can safely enter the car.

ACCESS

Once the vehicle has been made safe, the EMT should determine the number of patients in the vehicle and their general condition. This first round of triage is not complicated. The patients are first classified as being either conscious or unconscious. An unconscious patient may be assumed to be high priority, while a conscious patient needs more assessment.

Access to the patient may be simple. The EMT may open the door and enter the passenger compartment. In some cases, a crowbar can be used to force a partially jammed door. Before using a tool, the EMT should try to open all the doors manually.

In some cases, the EMT must make her own entrance into a crushed motor vehicle. In many cases, a side or rear window can be quickly removed, and the EMT can enter or crawl through the opening that has been created.

The front windshield is made of special **safety glass,** or a piece of glass sealed between sheets of plastic. Safety glass is designed to remain in one piece after an MVC. It is difficult to remove quickly. Therefore, the EMT should consider using the front windshield for access into the vehicle as a last resort.

The rest of the glass in a motor vehicle is **tempered glass.** Tempered glass is special window glass designed to shatter into tiny fragments. This reduces the hazard from razor-sharp edges. However, the glass fragments can scatter over the patients and cause small lacerations. To avoid this danger, the EMT should choose the window farthest from the patient if a window must be broken.

Using a special glass-breaking tool called a **window punch,** the window is broken, and the EMT can now enter (Figure 52.9). The EMT should be wearing protective clothing, including eyewear and gloves, to prevent microlacerations from the broken glass fragments.

Once access has been obtained, the EMT should proceed to the driver first. Immediately after an MVC, the driver may have forgotten or may be unable to take the car out of gear and turn off the motor. If the EMT finds the car running or in gear, it should be put in park and the engine turned off.

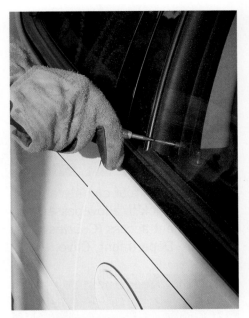

Figure 52.9 A window punch is a simple hand tool that can be carried in the pocket (Courtesy of Clive Fire Department, Clive, IA)

PRIORITIZATION

Once inside the motor vehicle, the EMT decides whether any patients are critical. Patients in critical condition require rapid extrication. The rapid extrication technique is described in Unit 35. In many cases, a critical patient is quickly extricated out the same entrance the EMT used to enter the vehicle.

In some cases, the opening the EMT created to gain entrance is too narrow for the EMT and the patient to exit. In those cases, the entrance must be widened quickly, using special extrication tools such as the Jaws of Life.

If the patient is not critically injured, the EMT proceeds to treat the patient while other rescuers create an adequate exit.

If the patient is trapped, heavy rescue will be needed to disentangle the patient from the vehicle. For example, the patient's feet may be caught under the gas or brake pedals, or the side door may be jammed up against the patient's pelvis, pinning him in the vehicle. In each of these cases, heavy rescue will need to disentangle the patient from the vehicle.

HEAVY RESCUE

A few basic approaches will extricate the patient in an MVC in most cases. If the door is jammed, rescuers will have to force the door open. The simplest method of extricating a patient is by **forcing the door,** using a tool to overcome the latching mechanism. Forcing the door usually involves using a crowbar, a Haligan tool, or similar device.

If the door is jammed because the lock is broken, the lock must be forced. A variety of tools can be used to overcome the door's locking mechanism.

All motor vehicles have a case-hardened pin, called the **Nader pin** that prevents the door from springing open in a crash. This pin is extremely difficult to cut. Often rescuers have to cut around the pin to open the door.

If the door is partially opened, it can be opened farther using both chains and a come-along or brute force (Figure 52.10). This creates an opening wide enough to insert a backboard and extricate a patient.

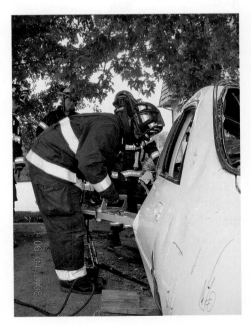

Figure 52.10 Heavy rescue may be required to force a jammed door (Courtesy of Clive Fire Department, Clive, IA)

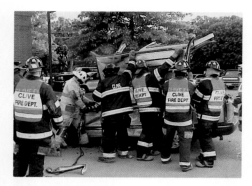

Figure 52.11 A roof can literally be peeled back to allow passenger compartment access (Courtesy of Clive Fire Department, Clive, IA)

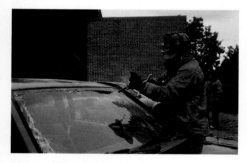

Figure 52.12 The glass from the windshield can be cut away and peeled back to gain access to the patient

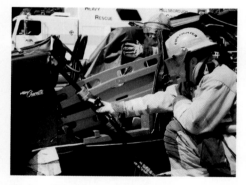

Figure 52.13 The patient should be protected from flying shards of glass by using a heavy oil tarp or the like

If the doors cannot be opened, the roof may have to be removed. **Flapping the roof** consists of cutting the uprights or posts that support the roof and peeling the roof back to allow access to the occupants in the vehicle (Figure 52.11).

The front windshield is special safety glass that can be removed in one piece. Using glass saws, chisels, and even axes, a window shield is literally carved out (Figure 52.12). The patient can then be extricated through the front of the vehicle.

If the patient is pinned under the dashboard or steering wheel, **rolling the dash** may be necessary. Rescuers simply peel the dashboard away from the patient using a variety of power tools, chains, block, and tackle.

PATIENT SAFETY

In every case, a rescuer, preferably an EMT, should remain inside the car with the patient while the heavy rescue is going on outside. The patient should be protected from flying debris, such as glass, and the crushing tips of cutting tools. A pair of goggles and even a helmet for the patient can significantly improve the patient's margin of safety. The patient and the EMT must also be protected from flying shards of glass. A heavy woolen blanket or a heavy oil tarp can be placed over both the patient and the EMT as a means of protection (Figure 52.13).

If heavy cutting tools are near the patient, a short wooden backboard should be placed between the tool and the patient. This board will effectively protect the patient if the tip of the tool should slip.

ASSESSMENT

Once the patient has been safely extricated and moved a reasonable distance from the vehicle, the EMT should complete the primary assessment, if it has not already been performed, followed by the rapid-method secondary assessment. Attention should be given to signs of internal injury, such as bruising and point tenderness, as well as obvious external injuries such as burns or lacerations.

Street Smart

An assumption is often made that if the person went into the vehicle through a door, then the quickest way to get the person out of the car is through the door. EMTs who can think "outside the box" quickly realize that there may be several alternatives for removing the patient from a vehicle. Seats that fold down, hatches that lift up, and convertible tops provide readily available alternative exits.

TRANSPORTATION

Based on the mechanism of injury and the length of time required to extricate, the EMT should have a high index of suspicion that injuries may have occurred and internal bleeding may be severe. Although it is possible for a patient to be trapped and not sustain any severe injuries, an EMT should always err on the side of caution and transport the patient to the closest appropriate facility, typically a trauma center, as soon as practical.

WATER RESCUE

Bodies of water exist in nearly every community. A body of water can be a stream, river, ocean, lake, pond, canal, or reservoir. Wherever there is water, there are people. Water tends to draw people. Water is used for recreation, such as swimming, boating, and fishing, and for the generation of hydroelectric power and other industry. Whenever people and water are together, there is a likelihood that a water emergency will occur.

A quick rescue by rescuers, including EMTs, can prevent a water emergency from becoming a drowning. Unfortunately, because of poor preparation and poor training, rescuers may end up as a drowning victim themselves. That is not to say that EMTs should not perform water rescue, but to prevent a rescue from becoming a tragedy, the EMT must know her limitations in both training and equipment.

The first question every EMT should ask on the scene is "Am I safe?" An EMT should never be in the position in which she may end up as the next victim.

ESTABLISHING COMMAND

Scenes of a water emergency, such as a drowning at a public beach, can be chaotic. Regardless of the scene's dynamic, the EMT must establish command. The EMT should work cooperatively with other emergency services, such as lifeguards and park rangers, to prepare for the rescue. Preseason water rescue drills can markedly improve the efficiency of responders on scene during an actual drowning and should be encouraged by EMS leaders.

SCENE SIZE-UP

A quick distinction between the two types of water hazards can help the EMT determine the type of rescue that will be needed. A body of water that has no current is considered **flat water.** A smooth surface does not equate with flat water. Rivers can be deceivingly calm on the surface and have tremendously powerful undercurrents. Typically, flat water is used for recreational swimming.

Rapidly moving water is considered **swift water.** By definition, swift water must have a current. Moving water can sweep people off their feet and hold them underwater. These powerful down-currents are called an **undertow.**

Natural or man-made dams, especially the low-head dam, can create powerful undertows at the base of the dam. These undertows can pull people underwater and keep them there, and they can also pull boats underwater. The undertows created by low-head dams are so powerful that professional swift water rescuers call these low-head dams "drowning machines."

An EMT should never underestimate the power of moving water. Every rescue in moving water is a technical rescue. When EMTs fail to identify swift water, they are placing themselves in danger of becoming a drowning victim.

MANAGEMENT

The EMT's role at a swift water rescue is primarily a supporting role. The objectives of the EMT are to locate the victim, attempt a shore-based rescue if protocols permit, and establish a base of operation for the dive rescue team in the event that a shore-based rescue is not possible.

Although this list of objectives may appear short, the tasks to accomplish these objectives are numerous. To become truly effective, the EMT must practice, as a part of the team, the different tasks involved in a water rescue.

ACCESS

The first priority is locating the victim. If the victim is underwater, special dive rescue teams will be needed. After calling for the dive rescue team, the

Every rescuer who is within 50 feet of shore must wear a personal flotation device (PFD), otherwise known as a life preserver. A PFD is usually a vestlike device or similar device that has positive buoyancy. A PFD is designed to help keep the rescuer afloat if she accidentally falls into the water. A Coast Guard–approved life preserver is recommended. The EMT should always follow local protocols established for water rescue.

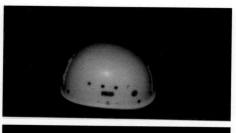
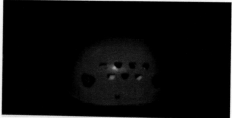
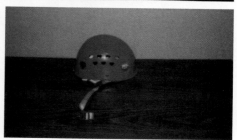

Figure 52.14 Closed helmets should not be worn when near water because they present a drowning hazard. Instead, using a vented helmet provides protection and reduces this hazard (Courtesy of Tim Strange)

EMT should determine the **point of contact (POC),** the point at which the person was last seen in the water. Friends, family, and witnesses can help the EMT determine the point of contact. Physical evidence such as clothing, footprints, boats, and vehicles can also be helpful.

If it is not known where the person was last seen or where he entered the water, it may be necessary to perform a shoreline search. If the POC is known, then a perimeter should be established around the area. At this point, if the person is found, a rescue is possible.

SHORE-BASED RESCUE—FLAT WATER

Flat water rescue efforts can be summarized by the maxim "reach, throw, row, and go." Each term denotes a specific activity that an EMT could perform to affect a rescue. Again, every EMT who is near water must wear a **personal flotation device (PFD).**

A pole or stick may be all that is needed to rescue victims if they are near the shoreline. The EMT simply reaches out with a pike pole, for example, and offers the pole's end to the victim.

After grabbing the pole, the victim can be pulled to shore by rescuers. If the victim is too weak to grab the pole, the patient's clothing can be hooked, and then the patient can be dragged to shore. The EMT should be prepared to drop the pole at any time if the patient starts to pull the EMT into the water.

A length of rope loosely coiled inside a cloth sack, called a **throw bag,** can be thrown to a victim. The victim, grasping the rope, would then be pulled to shore. The EMT should never tie the throw bag to herself. Instead, trees or other solidly anchored objects should be used as anchors for the throw bag.

If a throw bag is not available, sometimes a PFD can be thrown to the victim. The PFD might provide the victim a few more minutes of buoyancy until a more effective rescue can be effected. Seat cushions from a boat or even ice coolers can be used if a PFD is not available.

Use of a boat, such as a rowboat, or entering the water to rescue the patient requires special training and should be attempted only by a qualified lifeguard or similarly prepared person.

Finally, the EMT can enter the water. This last solution is dangerous and should be attempted only by those individuals who have received special training in water rescue. Lifeguards are typically trained in this type of rescue. However, this last option should be used only when the first three techniques have been exhausted. These techniques are demonstrated in Unit 39.

SHORE-BASED RESCUE—SWIFT WATER

An EMT is faced with a dilemma when called to the scene of a possible swift water rescue. Swift water rescue is dangerous, and numerous rescuers have drowned trying to save another person's life. On the other hand, it is difficult for an EMT to stand idly by while a victim drowns. A shore-based rescue attempt, while awaiting professional dive rescue, is a possible resolution to the dilemma that also prepares the scene for the arrival of dive rescue personnel.

Before approaching the water, all rescuers must be wearing a PFD. Closed helmets, such as fire helmets, should be removed. If the rescuer inadvertently falls into the water, the helmet could fill with water and drag the person's head underwater. Vented helmets should be considered instead (Figure 52.14). Similarly, high boots and fire boots should be discouraged for the same reason.

In a typical shore-based swift rescue plan, there are at least four teams. The first team, the upstream team, is usually dispatched to a river crossing, such as a bridge, to observe for hazards, such as logs floating downstream toward the victim and dive rescue team members.

The second team, a downstream team, usually strings two or more ropes diagonally across the water. These ropes, called **snag lines,** are the last line of rescue for anybody floating downstream. Water speed determines how far downstream a snag line is established. If the body of water is too wide for ropes—at a river, for example—then one or more boats may be launched to provide a recovery platform. Finally, two shore-based teams would proceed downstream from the point of last contact, searching the shoreline for the victim.

Dense underbrush can make shore-based rescue difficult. All members of the rescue team must be kept in constant contact at all times. When the victim is located, a signal is usually given and other rescuers respond to that location. Using throw bags and/or pike poles, a rescue is attempted. At no time does any rescuer enter the water who is not specially trained and prepared for water rescue. If the victim cannot be reached, rescuers should prepare for the arrival of the water rescue team.

TREATMENT AND TRANSPORT

Treatment should be started as soon as possible after the rescue has been accomplished. Rescuers often rescue someone who appears drowned but who can recover if aggressive treatment is started immediately. This is in part because of the effects of hypothermia on the nearly drowned person.

Hypothermia from the submersion in cold water may prolong the window of opportunity for recovery by slowing body functions and preserving the core organs, including the heart and brain. Victims who have been underwater for as long as 45 minutes have been recovered from near-drowning without serious neurologic impairment. More information on cold water immersion can be found in Unit 39 on environmental emergencies. Every effort should be made to save a near-drowning victim unless such efforts are obviously fruitless.

Many rescue plans call for an ambulance to be staged close by, ready to respond immediately once the patient has been rescued. In some cases, it may be appropriate to use air medical evacuation. In those cases, the patient may have to be transported from the remote shoreline to a landing zone to meet the helicopter.

SEARCH AND RESCUE

When the subject of search and rescue (SAR) is discussed, most EMTs think of wilderness SAR. SAR is not confined to the woods. SAR techniques are used whenever a person is lost. A search might have to be performed for a child lost in a mall.

SAR may have to be performed on the grounds of a building collapse or in an urban area. Modern urban SAR teams, commonly known as USAR, use high-tech equipment and specially trained scent dogs. The Oklahoma City bombing involved extensive use of urban search and rescue teams from across the country.

A common scenario for a full-scale SAR operation involves searching for a lost hiker or a person injured while in the backcountry.

SAR is evolutionary by nature. First, the person must be found. This is the search. Then the person must be carried out. This is the rescue. The person must also be treated for any injuries. Finally, the patient must be transported to an appropriate medical facility.

The danger that is consistent in all SAR operations is the length of time it takes to find the patient. The longer the person is lost, the greater the likelihood that some harm, such as exposure or hypothermia, will come to the person.

In some instances, such as in the National Park system, the incidence of search and rescue is so common that professional search and rescue teams exist. These professional rescuers prepare and plan for the SAR they know will come. These teams identify known dangerous conditions and hazardous places, called **high life hazards,** where a person could become injured or trapped, and they plan how they will respond in the event of an emergency.

ESTABLISHING COMMAND

Whenever a person has been reported lost or missing, the EMT, along with other emergency services, should establish a command post. This command post serves as a starting point for any rescue.

Many times a search goes on for days or even weeks. These extended operations should be established in a location that is well equipped to handle a long-term operation.

If local rescuers, including EMTs, are not familiar with SAR, then professional rescuers and search managers should be notified immediately.

SCENE SIZE-UP

Witnesses should be questioned about the last point of contact with the lost person, and detailed information must be obtained to help rescuers search efficiently. A standardized lost person questionnaire is often used to gather complete information about the person. An example of this form is shown in Figure 52.15.

Details such as the sex, height, weight, and clothing of the lost person need to be obtained. Details of the patient's medical history are also important. For example, a diabetic patient may need immediate treatment if he has gone without insulin for several hours.

ACCESS

Typically, large numbers of rescuers, often from diverse backgrounds, are assembled. As these resources arrive, they should be directed to a central staging area for assignment.

It is important that well-intentioned rescuers not be allowed to search freely. These so-called freelancers can inadvertently destroy valuable clues to the person's whereabouts. All rescue personnel must be directed to the staging area and assigned to teams.

HASTY SEARCH

A quick search of an area, called a **hasty search,** can be done while waiting for professional SAR personnel. A hasty search involves walking along trails, roadways, and shorelines, those areas where a person might reasonably be expected to be found. A hasty search does not include searching off road.

The EMT should not be concentrating on finding the person. Rather, the EMT should be looking for evidence that the person was in an area. Evidence or **clues** could be a wrapper from a candy bar or an article of clothing

MISSING PERSON QUESTIONNAIRE	TASK #	DATE PREPARED: TIME PREPARED:	PAGE # 1 OF 3

TASK NAME:	REVISED (DATE/TIME):	
SUBJECT # ___ OF ___	INTERVIEWED BY (PLANNING):	POLICE FILE #

INFORMANT IDENTIFICATION

FIRST NAME:	STREET ADDRESS:	
LAST NAME:	CITY:	
RELATIONSHIP TO SUBJECT:	**STATE:**	**ZIP** CODE:
HOME PHONE #:	ALT. PHONE #	

ADDITIONAL INFORMANTS/ WITNESSES	NAME:	NAME:	NAME:
	PHONE:	PHONE:	PHONE:

SUBJECT INFORMATION

FIRST NAME:	STREET ADDRESS:	
MIDDLE NAME:	CITY:	
LAST NAME:	**STATE:**	**ZIP** CODE:
ANSWERS TO:	HOME PHONE #:	
VEHICLE MAKE:	EMPLOYER:	
VEHICLE MODEL:	STREET ADDRESS:	
VEHICLE COLOR:	CITY:	
LICENSE PLATE #:	**STATE:**	**ZIP** CODE:
COMMENTS (e.g. **'CODE' NAME IF CHILD**):	WORK PHONE # :	
	WORK FAX #:	
	SUPERVISOR'S NAME:	

DATE OF BIRTH (Y/M/D):	AGE:	SEX:	HEIGHT:	WEIGHT:
HAIR COLOR:	EYES:	HAIRSTYLE/LENGTH:		
COMPLEXION:	FIRST LANGUAGE:			

DISTINGUISHING MARKS:
MEDICAL DISABILITIES:
MEDICATION REQUIREMENTS/QTY. ON HAND/DURATION OF SUPPLIES:
RECENT/CURRENT ILLNESS(ES):

FITNESS LEVEL:	SMOKER ❑ ( )	BRAND:	**ICS 302**

Figure 52.15 Missing person questionnaire

(continued)

MISSING PERSON QUESTIONNAIRE (CONT.)			PAGE # 2 OF 3
ALLERGIES:			
FEARS/PHOBIAS:			
MENTAL ATTITUDE:			
FINANCIAL SITUATION:			
CRIMINAL HISTORY:			
HOBBIES/INTERESTS:			
CLOTHING/EQUIPMENT			
SHOE TYPE:	COLOR:	SIZE:	
SHOE SOLE DESCRIPTION:			
SOCKS:	PANTS (TYPE & COLOR):		
TOP (TYPE & COLOR):	SWEATER (TYPE & COLOR):		
JACKET (TYPE & COLOR):			
RAINGEAR (TYPE & COLOR):			
HAT (TYPE & COLOR):	GLOVES (TYPE & COLOR):		
PACK (MAKE & COLOR):			
FOOD & DRINK (TYPE/BRAND/QUANTITY):			
POINT LAST SEEN			
DATE LAST SEEN:	TIME LAST SEEN:		
POINT LAST SEEN:			
MAP #	GRID REF:		

Figure 52.15 (Continued)

MISSING PERSON QUESTIONNAIRE (CONT.)

NAME OF OTHER PERSON(S) WHO SAW OR MIGHT HAVE SEEN THE SUBJECT AT OR NEAR THIS TIME:	#	NAME OF INFORMANT:	LOCATION SUBJECT SEEN:	TIME SEEN:
	1			
	2			
	3			
	4			
	5			

LOCATION OF VEHICLE (TRANSPORTATION):

INTENDED ROUTE:

WEATHER AT TIME LAST SEEN:

COMMENTS (DISPOSITION/PERSONALITY, RELATIONSHIP WITH SPOUSE/FAMILY/FRIENDS ETC.):

SUBJECT NEXT OF KIN			
FIRST NAME:	STREET ADDRESS:		
LAST NAME:	CITY:		
RELATIONSHIP TO SUBJECT:	STATE:	ZIP CODE:	
HOME PHONE #:	ALT. PHONE #		
ADDITIONAL INFORMANTS/ FRIENDS:	NAME:	NAME:	NAME:
	PHONE:	PHONE:	PHONE:
AVAILABILITY OF PHOTOGRAPH(S)?			

Figure 52.15 (Continued)

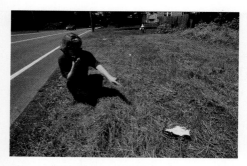

Figure 52.16 An EMT in a hasty search should look for clues

(Figure 52.16). Every clue represents an opportunity to find the person. Clues should not be moved. Instead, the clue should be left undisturbed and its location reported immediately to the command post.

Clues such as a piece of clothing may provide specially trained dogs with a scent trail that leads right to the person. Every effort should be made to try to preserve these scent trails whenever possible.

Law enforcement officers may be asked to search in local barns, abandoned buildings, and the like. A lost person is likely to approach a house or a business in search of help.

RESCUE

In most cases of backcountry rescue, for a variety of reasons, the patient is carried out by rescuers. It takes special training and practice to safely carry a patient out of the woods. Unit 14 reviews some of the more common carries that are used in the field.

At first glance, these carries appear easy. However, after 1 or 2 miles, the rescuers quickly realize how tiring these carries can be. Practice and physical conditioning are keys to a successful carry.

MANAGEMENT

After the person has been found, a medical evaluation is usually in order. In some cases, an emergency physician may be standing by at the trailhead. In other cases, the patient is transported to a local clinic for first-level assessment.

If the patient is seriously injured or there is a greater risk for serious injury, the patient should be airlifted from the scene and transported to an appropriate facility.

TRANSPORTATION

Helicopter evacuation from backwoods rescues is so common that many mountain communities have prearranged landing zones established. Unit 54 provides more information about helicopter operations. Before such a resource is called, the EMT should carefully consider the patient's condition and the advantage of an airlift versus ground transportation.

CONCLUSION

Rescues are often exciting. Unique conditions require an EMT to be creative and adjust her plan of action to the situation. However, reckless disregard of obvious dangers can change the role of an EMT from that of rescuer to that of patient. In every rescue, the EMT should participate only when she has had adequate training to proceed safely.

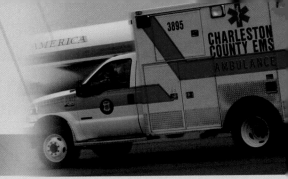

As Kaelynn and Ray watch the fire department stabilize the vehicle with cribbing, an officer approaches with a young woman who is crying.

"This is Niesha; she was in the vehicle, behind the driver. She says she's okay but I'd like to have her checked out. Her parents are on the way." Ray takes Niesha back to the ambulance to assess her for any injuries as Kaelynn is instructed that the vehicle is now stabilized.

Kaelynn approaches the car on the driver's side to access the patient. Jed is a 17-year-old male who is crying and says he cannot move his legs. He states his legs feel like they are twisted under the dash and the pain is horrible. Kaelynn is informed they are going to pull the roof back for better access and handed a heavy blanket to cover herself and the patient.

Kaelynn does a quick assessment of Jed's vital signs; blood pressure is 130/80, pulse 110, respirations 24. She explains to Jed what is going to happen. She tells him it will be noisy and she will cover them both with the blanket while they cut the roof.

Once the roof is removed, Kaelynn has better access to Jed. He tells her he has no other injuries other than to his legs, which he says "are killing me." Kaelynn does a quick physical assessment and finds no additional injuries. Jed's lower legs appear to be twisted at odd angles and his feet are not visible. He states he has a lot of pain in his ankles and feet but cannot move them.

Rescue decides they will need to roll the dash. As they are preparing to do that, Kaelynn has to move to the outside of the passenger side of the vehicle. She continues to talk with Jed, explaining everything that is happening. Once the dash is rolled up, Jed's legs are freed and he is able to move them both. He is secured to a long spine board and taken to the ambulance.

Kaelynn is repeating Jed's vital signs—blood pressure 118/68, pulse 112, respiration 22—as the ALS crew that had been requested due to the extended extrication time arrives. Ray has exposed Jed's lower legs, showing a deformity to the right ankle and left lower leg. Ray places vacuum splints on both extremities after ensuring pulses are present, while Kaelynn gives report and turns over patient care to the paramedic on the ALS crew.

Later that night as the crew discusses the call, the chief states that total extrication time had been 22 minutes. He further states law enforcement had found the driver, who was 17. He was uninjured, got scared, and ran home, approximately five blocks away. Ray reports the girl, Niesha, denied injury, and he didn't find anything on physical examination. She is 18 years old, and when her mother arrived, she refused to be transported. Her mother assured him she would be taking her to the hospital herself to be checked out.

Key Concepts Revisited

- Rescue is an attempt to help another person who is incapable of freeing himself or herself from confinement.
- The phases common to all rescues begin with establishing command.
  - Utilization of specialized resources may require a unified command.

- Scene size-up
  - Environmental assessment
  - Confined space rescue
- Management
  - Technical rescue: complex rescue operations performed by highly trained technicians using specialized equipment

- Redundancy of plans of action
- Access to patient
- Treatment
- Transport

- The common hazards encountered in confined space rescue are low oxygen concentration, toxic fumes, and explosive gases.

- Hazards at a motor vehicle collision should be identified during the scene size-up:
  - Power line
  - Loaded bumpers
  - Fire
  - Air bags

- Motor vehicles must be stabilized before patients can be extricated and care provided.
  - Cribbing

- Heavy rescue is used when a patient must be disentangled from a vehicle.
  - Extrication techniques
  - Patient safety

- There are three common means of extrication from a vehicle using heavy rescue.
  - Forcing the door
  - Flapping the roof
  - Rolling the dash

- The EMT should preplan for possible scenarios in operations involving water rescue.
  - Flat water
  - Swift water
    - Undertow
  - Access: point of contact (POC)

- Scene size-up during a search and rescue must include a high life hazard assessment.
  - Known dangerous condition that could injure or kill someone
  - Hasty search: quick search of the area

- Rescue situations can require the EMT to be creative and adjust plans of action to the situation.

Review Questions

1. When is a technical rescue needed?
2. What are the common phases seen in all rescues?
3. What are several situations of confined space?
4. What are the common hazards encountered in confined space?
5. How does the standard of care imply that an EMT must have special training for technical rescue?
6. What are the hazards common to a motor vehicle collision?
7. What is the importance of stabilizing a motor vehicle before rescue?
8. What are the three most common means of heavy rescue?
9. What is the difference between flat water and swift water?
10. What is the importance of searching for clues and not people?

Key Terms

Clues
Confined space
Cribbing
Flapping the roof
Flat water
Forcible entry
Forcing the door
Hasty search
Heavy rescue
High life hazard
Nader pin
Personal flotation device (PFD)
Point of contact (POC)

Preplan
Redundancy
Rescue
Rolling the dash
Safety glass
Snag lines
Swift water
Technical rescue
Tempered glass
Throw bag
Undertow
Window punch

Further Study

Brown, M. G. *Engineering Practical Rope Rescue Systems.* Clifton Park, NY: Thomson Delmar Learning, 2000.

Collins, L. *Technical Rescue Operations: Planning, Training, & Command.* Tulsa, OK: PennWell Books, 2004.

International Association of Fire Chiefs and National Fire Protection Association.

Fundamentals of Fire Fighter Skills. Sudbury, MA: Jones and Bartlett, 2008.

Veasey, D. Alan, Lisa Craft McCormick, Barbara M. Hilver, Kenneth W. Oldfield, Sam Hansen, and Theodore H. Kraver. *Confined Space Entry and Emergency Response.* Hoboken, NJ: Wiley-InterScience, 2006.

UNIT (53) Emergency Incident Rehabilitation

Regardless of the type of incident—be it a major fire, an earthquake, or even a bomb squad defusing a terrorist's bomb—an Emergency Medical Technician (EMT) will be needed to provided emergency medical care. Emergency incident rehabilitation is part of every disaster at the local, county, and statewide level. The EMT must be knowledgeable about emergency incident rehabilitation.

National Educational Standard

The Emergency Medical Technician (EMT) shall have a fundamental depth and foundational breadth of knowledge to establish and work within the Incident Management System and particularly Emergency Incident Rehabilitation.

Key Concepts

- There are several hazards to firefighters on the fire ground.
- Emergency incident rehabilitation is intended to mitigate those hazards.
- Emergency incident rehabilitation requires preplanning and adherence to standard operating guidelines.
- Medical monitoring is part of emergency incident rehabilitation.

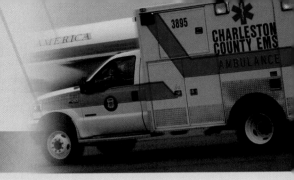

CASE STUDY

"Ladder ten, engine eleven, medic one, battalion chief, rehab unit 101, murmur, murmur." Kyle has almost tuned out the dispatcher as she seems to drone on endlessly with the list of responders to the emergency until he hears, "ambulance 24." "Well," Kyle announces to his partner as he puts on his seatbelt and flips on the lights, "It's showtime!"

They have been dispatched to a major fire. An abandoned factory has been torched. There is no sprinkler system, and there might not be enough water to extinguish the fire. Hydrants in the area are notorious for failing when you need them the most.

As they arrive on the scene, Kyle is listing for his new partner, Denis, their possible assignments. They might be assigned to watch the exposures, to look for downed firefighters, or to the rehabilitation sector.

"What is rehabilitation?" Denis asks. He is a new EMT, fresh from academy, and this is his first major working fire. "Kid," says Kyle, "look up rehab in the SOG, it should be listed under emergency incident rehabilitation and familiarize yourself with your duties."

The last time Kyle was at a major fire scene, he was assigned to medical monitoring and ended up transporting five firefighters with possible smoke inhalation or exhaustion.

Critical Thinking Questions

1. What is emergency incident rehabilitation?
2. What is medical monitoring?
3. What are the dangers of smoke inhalation?

INTRODUCTION

Firefighting is hard work. The excessive physiologic demand of firefighting puts firefighters at risk for illness, injury, and even death. The role of the EMT at the scene of an emergency incident is to provide care to stricken firefighters and relief to other firefighters in order to reduce illness and injury.

FIRE GROUND HAZARDS

The firefighters face threats to their health from both ordinary hazards and life-threatening hazards. Ordinary and expected hazards include personal injury from burning embers or falling objects, for example. Trip hazards may be the most common emergency incident hazard; the number one firefighter injury on a fire scene is a sprained ankle.

The more ominous life threats on the fire scene come from inhalation of toxic gases that contain carbon monoxide and hydrogen cyanide and from heat exhaustion aggravated by dehydration.

Although these hazards are always present on the fire ground, they are not unique to this form of emergency. These hazards can be found in confined space rescue, urban search and rescue, and trench rescue, to name a few. In fact, these hazards can be found at any emergency incident where responders are exposed to extreme conditions.

Fire rehabilitation is intended to monitor for the effects of these toxins and to prevent heat exhaustion. This unit discusses the role of the EMT in emergency incident rehabilitation.

EMERGENCY INCIDENT REHABILITATION

The stresses on firefighters can lead to stress, overexertion, and exhaustion. As a result of this stress firefighters are at greater risk for stress-related injury and illness. Exhaustion can impair reaction times, leading to a greater risk for injury. Overexertion and stress can lead to cardiovascular complications, including cerebrovascular accident and acute myocardial infarction. Half of all on-duty firefighter fatalities are due to heart attack.

To help mitigate the adverse impact of fire ground operations and increase the safety of the firefighters on scene, fire command officers have developed the concept of **emergency incident rehabilitation.** Emergency incident rehabilitation is an element of the operational plan that includes rest and rehydration as well as medical monitoring. Fire chiefs have long understood their responsibilities to provide for the safety and rehabilitation of their firefighters as emphasized under the Occupational Safety and Health Administration (OSHA) general duty clause (Section 5 (a)(1)). The general duty clause emphasizes that a workplace—in this case the fire grounds—be free from recognized hazards. Physical exhaustion and its impact on fire operations is a recognized hazard, as emphasized in the 1972 report "America Burning" and subsequent reports.

This responsibility was further emphasized under the OSHA regulations 29 CFR 1910.120 (g) (5) (x), as it pertains to hazardous materials operations. The use of special protective equipment, which has been estimated to increase the heat load by some 500%, and a toxic environment make these scenes particularly dangerous. Proper medical monitoring and responder rehabilitation is essential for the safety of responders on scene.

To provide guidance to incident commanders, the National Fire Protection Association (NFPA) has established the Standard 1584, entitled "Emergency Incident Rehabilitation." The standard outlines for incident commanders the process of establishing rehabilitation during both emergency operations and training exercises.

NFPA 1584 requires each department to develop and maintain a standard operating guideline (SOG) that outlines when, where, and how to establish a rehabilitation section on the scene of fire/emergency incident operations and training drills. Examples of prolonged emergency incidents that would require a rehabilitation section would include hazard materials operations, prolonged rescue operations such as urban search and rescue, or wildland fires.

The three recognized criteria used to justify establishing a rehabilitation section include a large incident, typically involving mutual aid or a multi-company response; a long duration event, such as a terrorist bombing; or a labor-intensive incident, such as a search and rescue incident following an earthquake.

Emergency rehabilitation can also be set up for smaller company-sized operations. Under operational command, be that a fire chief or search manager, the use of a rehabilitation sector permits responders to practice for larger scale incidents.

The rehabilitation section is also a recognized part of the National Incident Management System (NIMS). The incident commander, under NIMS, is responsible to ensure the establishment of a rehabilitation section. That section would be part of the logistics branch and, specifically, falls under the medical unit of the logistics branch. The medical unit of the logistics branch is not responsible for the care of victims at an incident, but for the responders.

FUNDAMENTALS OF EMERGENCY INCIDENT REHABILITATION

Once the decision has been made to establish an emergency incident rehabilitation section, also known as *rehab,* the officer in charge must create the rehabilitation unit. Typically a rehab unit has two sections. The first section is the

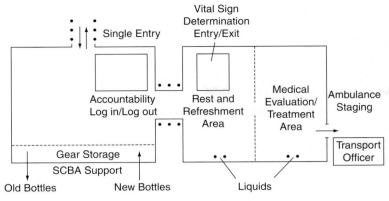

Figure 53.1 An ideal layout for a rehabilitation sector

rest and recovery area or sector, discussed in more detail shortly. The second section is the medical monitoring area or sector. At some incidents, such as a hazardous material incident, the medical monitoring area may be first.

The rehab sectors should ideally be located uphill and upwind of the incident. This prevents smoke and toxic fumes from entering the rehab area. It should be established in close proximity to the command post. This permits firefighters prompt reentry into the operation. In an emergency the incident commander could press the responders/firefighters in the rehab sector into service. From this perspective, the responders/firefighters in the rehab sector could be looked on as emergency reserves in case of disaster, such as a catastrophic building collapse. Like the command post, the rehab sector should not need to be moved except under extraordinary circumstances. Figure 53.1 shows an ideal layout for a rehabilitation sector.

PHYSICAL PLAN

The remaining circumstances focus on the practical. The rehab sector should be large enough to accommodate all responders. Many incidents tend to expand before the situation is brought under control. The rehab area should be free of smoke and exhaust. The exhaust of heavy diesel engines contains carbon monoxide and several known cancer-causing compounds. Therefore, it would be counterproductive to have diesel fumes permeate a rehab area where firefighters are recovering from smoke and fume inhalation.

The rehab unit should protect firefighters and responders from the elements. If the scene occurs during a hot summer day, firefighters should be protected from the sun. On the other hand, if the incident occurs during the dead of winter, firefighters will need an area to warm up.

The three models for rehab units are fixed facility, apparatus based, and portable shelters. A fixed facility is any building used for rehabilitation. Common examples of fixed facilities are fire stations in proximity to the incident, basements of churches, and even the store front of a department store. These facilities offer the convenience of protection, environmental control, and toilets.

An apparatus-based rehab unit has the advantage of portability. Some examples of apparatus-based rehab units include school buses, ambulances, and even the cabs of fire trucks. Using the latter, in the form of ambulances and fire trucks, may be problematic if the apparatus is needed later.

There is a growing trend toward using portable shelters. The military has long used portable shelters as temporary shelter for soldiers. Newer shelters are easy to erect and provide excellent shelter from the elements. Some of these shelters can be outfitted with portable heaters, or air conditioners, as well as lighting and even public address systems. If a shelter does not have heat, a portable electric or liquid propane gas (LPG) heater can be used. These units, sometimes called *salamanders,* can create a large amount of heat very quickly and are often used on industrial construction sites.

Whatever shelter is chosen should permit easy access and egress for emergency medical service units while permitting responders only one point of entry. This single point of entry permits control and facilitates accountability. With a single point of entry, the safety officer, or designee, can log in and out responders. Some fire companies use a tab system. The firefighters use unique personal identification tags to "tag in," just as they would if entering a building. Other fire companies prefer to log into the rehab area as an engine or truck company. This permits the entire engine or truck company to be called out as a unit.

Finally, firefighters and emergency responders should be allowed to relax free of intrusion. Therefore, the rehab officer should restrict media access to these areas. Unfortunately, if the rehab area is in close proximity of the command post and incident command is not forthcoming with details about the incident, the press may seek information from firefighters resting nearby.

REHABILITATION

The functions of the rehabilitation sectors can be summed up by the three Rs of restoration, rehydration, and refreshment. The first, restoration, speaks to operational preparedness. An exhausted firefighter will become clumsy, weak, and a risk to other firefighters. To return that firefighter to operational preparedness the rehab officer needs to ensure rest.

The first step of restoration is to recognize exhaustion. This decision has been simplified by the establishment of the "bottle rules." As company officers are required to assess a crew for operational readiness every 45 minutes, and most SCBA bottles last 30 to 45 minutes, it follows that the officer should assess firefighters at every SCBA bottle change. In fact, some rehab officers purposely set the rehab area next to the air bank, where SCBA bottles are exchanged, so that firefighters can easily be redirected to the rehab area.

Minimally, a firefighter/responder should be directed to the rehab area following the second bottle, or one bottle if the SCBA bottle has a 45- or 60-minute reserve. During nonfire operations, firefighters or responders should be directed to rehab after 40–45 minutes of intense work.

A major element of exhaustion is heat stress. The combination of endogenous heat, produced by intense labor, and exogenous heat sources, from smoke and fire, can leave the firefighter at greater risk for heat exhaustion. The extent of thermal exposure has been quantified. A small fire, below 140°F, is considered a class I thermal exposure. A class II thermal exposure, up to 200°F, might be encountered during overhaul operations. The higher levels of thermal exposure occur during active firefighting. Temperatures up to 480°F may be encountered in a class III thermal exposure, and temperatures up to 1,500°F may be encountered in extreme firefighting conditions, which occur during flashover or backdraft.

The EMT in the rehab sector caring for firefighters must also consider environmental stress. For example, hot humid temperatures defeat the body's cooling mechanisms. On a hot, humid day sweat does not evaporate and the body is not efficiently cooled. The heat stress index, also called the *misery index,* places these two factors along a continuum. Operations above a certain temperature and/or humidity place the firefighter at greater risk for heat exhaustion.

Conversely, wind and cold can defeat the body's ability to conserve heat. This cold stress is represented on the wind chill chart. Operations in cold temperatures with winds place a firefighter at greater risk for hypothermia.

However, the majority of risk to a firefighter is heat exhaustion secondary to heat stress. Therefore, the first task of the rehab officer is to get firefighters to remove helmet and turnout gear. The majority of heat from the body is radiated from the head and neck. Simply removing a helmet and opening a turnout coat can allow heat to escape and the body to cool. Under ideal conditions firefighters should remove helmets, coats, and bunker pants/boots. Other cooling techniques are discussed later.

A major component of rehabilitation is rehydration. Firefighters lose approximately one quart of body water per hour and more during labor-intensive operations. Loss of body fluids impairs the body's ability to cool and leaves the firefighter at risk for heat exhaustion.

Under ideal conditions, it is best to prehydrate before an operation. If the operation is a planned drill, firefighters should drink approximately 500 ml (16 ounces) one to two hours before the event. The same can be accomplished while en route to a fire scene.

While in the rehab area, the firefighter should replenish lost body fluids. The firefighter should drink approximately 12 to 32 ounces during the 10 to 20 minutes in the rehab area. It is optimal if the firefighter can drink a 50/50 solution of replacement electrolyte solution, or sports drink. Replacement drinks maintained around 40°F are preferred. This mixture is a neutral, or isotonic, drink, approximately 270–330 milliosmole (mOsm). Carbonated beverages, caffeinated beverages, and especially alcoholic beverages should be avoided.

Bottled water is often used by many fire services. Bottled water has the advantage of having a precise premeasured volume. Therefore, the rehab officer can estimate water needs based on the number of responders, the duration of the event, and responders' estimated fluid needs. NFPA 1584 offers the rehab officer some guidance regarding rehydration. Table 53-1 shows an example of prehydration recommendations from NFPA 1584.

At longer incidents it will be necessary to feed the firefighters and emergency responders. If the incident lasts from three to eight hours, simple quick sources of nutrition, such as fruits and soups are acceptable. Fruits, such as apples, oranges, and bananas, and soups, including broths and simple stews, are quick sources of energy.

For longer operations, those extending beyond eight hours, it will be necessary to have meal service. As with rehab, the three models of food service are fixed, mobile, and portable. Prepacked foods, such as MREs, are examples of portable foods that can be prepared on scene and stored for long periods of time in preparation of an incident. A canteen, such as that operated by the Red Cross, is an example of a mobile food service. Finally, fixed facilities include restaurants and mess halls.

Table 53-1 Prehydration		
16 oz	16 oz	16 oz
Water or	Sports Drink 50/50	Sports Drink
w/meal	moderate activity	high intensity
	event less than one hour	greater than one hour

Regardless of the model, it is imperative that sanitary codes be maintained. Hot foods should be kept at greater than 140°F continually, and cold foods should be maintained at less than 40°F. Any suspicious foods should be immediately discarded. In some cases, food inspectors from the local health department may come to the scene to ensure food safety and sanitation.

MEDICAL MONITORING

The other mission of a rehabilitation section is medical monitoring, which is among the safety officer's responsibilities. Following the death of several firefighters in the 1980s, safety became a top priority. The subsequent development of the NFPA 1500 safety standard helped establish safety as the primary concern of all firefighters, emergency responders, and command personnel.

It is the responsibility of the safety officer, and ultimately the incident commander, to ensure the health of firefighters and emergency responders. This responsibility has become more burdensome in light of the national trend toward obesity. Out-of-shape firefighters with preexisting medical conditions and taking prescribed medications that further complicate their situation are at greater risk for injury and illness on the fire grounds. Table 53-2 lists some common medications, by classifications, along with their use and impact on firefighters on the job.

The three threats to firefighters from fire ground operations are heat exhaustion, cyanide poisoning, and carbon monoxide poisoning. Fortunately, cyanide poisoning, carbon monoxide poisoning, and heat exhaustion all initially present with the same symptoms: tachypnea, tachycardia, and hypertension. Additionally, heat stress, leading to heat exhaustion and even heat stroke, presents with a high temperature.

The EMT needs to obtain a set of vital signs, including temperature, pulse, respirations, and blood pressure (TPR & B/P) to start the process of medical monitoring. If any of these vital signs are abnormally high or remain high despite rest and rehabilitation, then the patient should be transported; transportation criteria are discussed shortly.

SMOKE AND FIRE

Where there is smoke, there is fire, and firefighters are called to fight the fire. Hidden within the smoke are the products of partial combustion, including carbon monoxide and cyanide. These two by-products of combustion are particularly dangerous to the firefighter. These risks have been recognized by

Table 53-2 Medications That Affect Firefighter Fitness		
Medication	**Purpose**	**Impact**
1. Antihistamines	Allergy	Drowsiness
2. Tricyclic Antidepressants	Depression	Cardiac irregularities
3. Diuretics	Heart failure	Dehydration
4. Beta blockers	Hypertension	Prevent cardiac compensation

the fire service, and firefighters now use self-contained breathing apparatus (SCBA) to protect themselves from these hazards.

Despite their best efforts, firefighters are occasionally exposed to these toxins. That exposure may occur when an SCBA fails, when the firefighter exhausts the SCBA, or during an overhaul operation, for example. Therefore, the EMT should be aware of the signs and symptoms of exposure to these toxins.

Cyanide results from the partial combustion of many building materials. Most notably, hydrogen cyanide and its cousin isocyanate, can result from burning glass fibers used in insulation, synthetic nitrile rubbers used in tubing insulation, melamine found in countertop laminate, polyurethane rubber that makes the flexible foam for furniture upholstering, and even the adhesives in the particle board used as a base building material.

Cyanide, as a toxin, poisons the body at the cellular level. Cyanide interferes with the ability of cells to use oxygen, essentially suffocating the patient at the cellular level.

Carbon monoxide is even more ubiquitous. Carbon monoxide, a compound made of one oxygen and one carbon molecule, is a by-product of combustion of any natural carbon-based material, including wood and petroleum. Therefore, carbon monoxide is found not only at fires but wherever a gas-powered generator is in use.

Carbon monoxide, as a toxin, has 200 times more affinity to hemoglobin than does oxygen. Therefore, carbon monoxide replaces and binds to carbon monoxide, resulting in hypoxia. Carbon monoxide is thought to be the leading cause of poisoning death. Carbon monoxide is so common in the environment that the body has the ability to detoxify carbon monoxide, but that capacity is limited. The goal of the EMT is to support the patient's body while it detoxifies.

Fortunately, the symptoms of carbon monoxide and cyanide are similar, in part because both toxins cause hypoxia. The early symptoms of these poisons include headache, impaired judgment, and mild tachypnea and tachycardia.

As the effects of these poisons intensify, the patient will have an altered mental status manifested by confusion, and the patient may lapse into unconsciousness and coma. These patients may seize and eventually go into respiratory and then cardiac arrest.

These patients need respiratory support, including high-concentration oxygen, and advanced life support. Currently, there is an antidote available for cyanide poisoning, and hyperbaric oxygen (HBO) may be used to counteract carbon monoxide poisoning.

HEAT EXHAUSTION

Dehydration and increased heat stress lead to firefighter fatigue and heat exhaustion. To prevent heat exhaustion, it is important to assess for dehydration. Dehydration is a loss of body fluids and hypovolemia.

Any time the body loses fluids, be it from acute bleeding or excessive body sweat, the body compensates for that fluid loss by increasing the heart rate. The EMT should therefore carefully monitor the heart rate of firefighters in rehab to establish a baseline. If the heart rate is elevated from work, it will return to normal relatively quickly, usually within 10 to 20 minutes. If the heart rate is elevated from fluid loss (i.e., hypovolemia), it will stay elevated until the fluid volume is replaced. In some cases this fluid loss can be restored by simply drinking fluids. In other cases, it may be necessary to begin an intravenous administration of replacement fluid.

An EMT may choose to use a pulse oximeter to quickly obtain a heart rate. This tool is particularly useful if many firefighters need to be assessed

Street Smart

The EMT may smell an almond scent on the breath of the patient who is poisoned by cyanide. However, as much as 40% of the population cannot smell the almond scent. The ability to smell the almond scent of cyanide is genetic.

repeatedly. The EMT should remain skeptical about the oxygen saturation reading. The pulse oximeter may still give acceptable oxygen saturation readings even when the firefighter is poisoned by carbon monoxide. Therefore, an EMT should not depend on the pulse oximeter readings for assessing hypoxia. Instead he should assess the patient for other signs of carbon monoxide poisoning, including the use of a CO detector/monitor and hypoxia.

Another test for hypovolemia is the **tilt test.** To perform a tilt test, the EMT takes the patient's blood pressure lying or sitting, then standing. If the patient has lost a significant volume of body fluid, the heart rate will increase by 10–20 beats per minute while the blood pressure drops approximately 10–20 mmHg in the systolic pressure. These changes in vital signs indicate hypovolemia and suggest the patient should be treated. Of course, if the patient stands up and feels lightheaded, or even passes out, then the test is considered positive and the EMT does not need to do the vital signs. It also stands to reason that if the patient could pass out, then another EMT needs to be available to help support the patient and prevent the patient from falling.

PREVENTION OF HEAT EXHAUSTION

The key to the effective treatment of heat exhaustion is to prevent it by decreasing the heat stress via cooling. On-scene cooling is an effective means to help prevent heat exhaustion. The traditional method is the use of cooling fans that help evaporate sweat more quickly. This method works provided the humidity is not so high that it prevents evaporation.

An alternative method is the use of misting tents. These tents take advantage of the mechanism of sweat to accelerate heat loss. Often these misting tents are coupled with cooling fans; like the cooling fans, misting tents only work if the humidity is low.

A newer method of cooling the firefighter is called forearm immersion. First used by the British firefighters aboard navy ships, it was found that immersion of just the forearms in water between 50°F (10°C) and 86°F (30°C) resulted in significant cooling of the body's core. Research continues on the most effective means of cooling an overheated firefighter to prevent heat exhaustion.

TRANSPORT CRITERIA

The EMT at the entry point should be generally monitoring firefighters for signs of exhaustion. The firefighter may have problems with walking or gait, or problems with speech. These firefighters should be directed to the medical monitoring area immediately.

Any firefighter who complains of a headache, shortness of breath, chest pain, or nausea should also be directed to the medical monitoring area for evaluation. These four signs can be indicators of carbon monoxide poisoning, cyanide poisoning, heat exhaustion, or other potentially life-threatening conditions.

If the firefighter has an elevated heart rate or temperature, without the stated concerns, the firefighter should be allowed to rest in rehabilitation until his or her vital signs return to normal. Criteria for release for service vary, but generally a firefighter is allowed to return to service if the heart rate drops below 100 beats per minute, temperature is less than 100.6°F (38°C), and blood pressure is less than 130 systolic/90 diastolic.

If after one hour the firefighter's heart rate remains above 120 beats per minute, tachycardia persists, or temperature fails to go below 100.6°F, the firefighter should be transported to the emergency department for further evaluation.

If a firefighter's temperature is greater than 101°F, heart rate is greater than 150 beats per minute, systolic blood pressure is less than 90 mmHg or greater than 200 mmHg, or diastolic blood pressure is

Table 53-3 Criteria for Emergency Department Evaluation

Symptoms

a. Altered mental status

b. Shortness of breath not relieved with high-flow oxygen

c. Potentially cardiac-related chest pain

d. Unremitting nausea

Signs

a. Temperature greater than 101°F

b. Systolic blood pressure greater than 200 mmHg

c. Systolic blood pressure less than 90 mmHg

d. Diastolic blood pressure greater than 110 mmHg

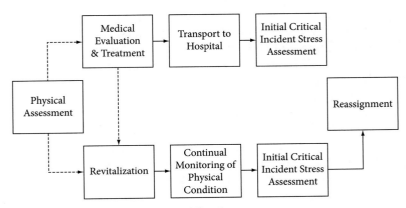

Figure 53.2 Triage tree for rehabilitation

greater than 110 mmHg, the firefighter should be transported to the emergency department for further evaluation.

Table 53-3 helps codify those signs and symptoms that require emergency department evaluation. Figure 53.2 illustrates the decision tree an EMT would use in triaging a firefighter or emergency responder coming into rehabilitation.

CRITICAL INCIDENT STRESS

Beyond physical stress, firefighters and emergency responders also experience mental stress. The EMT should observe for normal signs of stress, including venting and diffusing. The EMT should also observe for signs of psychological decompensation and psychic breakdown.

CONCLUSION

The objective of emergency incident rehabilitation is to prevent illness and injury. An organized plan of rehabilitation, with proper preparation of needed equipment and supplies, along with the assistance of EMTs who are trained in rehabilitation principles, can prompt a safer emergency operation.

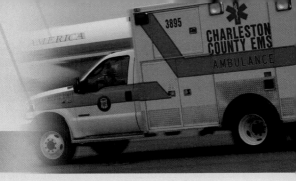

CASE STUDY Continued

The fire has been knocked down, and the firefighters are putting out a few hot spots. During this mop-up phase, a young firefighter is brought to rehab. He had been pulling down ceilings with his pike pole. His SCBA had run dry, but the operation was almost over and there was no visible smoke, so he thought it would be safe to remove his mask while he finished the job. As time progressed, he started to get weaker, he had trouble holding the pike pole up,

and then he vomited. After witnessing those symptoms, the lieutenant ordered him to immediately report to rehab.

It takes Kyle only one look to realize that the young firefighter has been poisoned. His heart rate is over 120 beats per minute, and his blood pressure is through the roof. Kyle immediately advises the rehab officer that the young firefighter is being sent to County General for an evaluation.

Key Concepts Revisited

- Fire ground hazards include heat exhaustion, cyanide poisoning, and carbon monoxide poisoning.
- Emergency incident rehabilitation is part of the National Incident Management System (NIMS).
- Heat stress and environment stress combine to create disease.
  - Medical monitoring of firefighters is part of the function of the EMT in emergency incident rehabilitation.
  - Smoke
    - Toxins
      - Carbon monoxide
      - Cyanide

  - Heat exhaustion
    - Hypovolemia
      - Dehydration
- Heat exhaustion can be treated through active cooling.
  - Cooling fans
  - Misting tents
  - Forearm submersion

Review Questions

1. What three hazards do firefighters face in fire ground operations?
2. List three emergency incidents in which emergency incident rehabilitation might be needed.
3. What three regulations or standards support the establishment of emergency incident rehabilitation?
4. What are three recognized incidents in which a rehabilitation sector would be needed?
5. In which part of the National Incident Management System (NIMS) does the rehabilitation sector fall?
6. What are three desirable characteristics for a rehabilitation area?

7. What are three models for a rehabilitation unit?

8. What are the criteria for firefighters to enter the rehabilitation area?

9. What signs or symptoms do cyanide poisoning, carbon monoxide poisoning, and heat exhaustion have in common?

10. What are three means of cooling a firefighter?

Key Terms

Emergency incident rehabilitation

Tilt test

Further Study

Dickinson, Edward V., and Michael A. Wieder. *Emergency Incident Rehabilitation.* 2d ed. Upper Saddle River, NJ: Brady/ Prentice Hall Health, 2004.

Federal Emergency Management Agency and U.S. Fire Administration. *Emergency Incident Rehabilitation.* Washington, DC: USFA Publications, 2008.

Ross, David, Peter McBride, and Gerald Tracy. "Rehabilitation: Standards, Traps, and Tools." *Fire Engineering,* May 2004.

UNIT (54) Air Medical Transport

Air Medical Services have become an integrated part of the Emergency Medical Services (EMS) in many areas. The expense and inherent risks associated with this mode of transport mandate appropriate utilization in all circumstances. This unit reviews the history of helicopter transport to help the Emergency Medical Technician (EMT) understand when it might be appropriate to request such a resource. Additionally, this unit emphasizes safety in all aspects of the EMT's interaction with an air medical service.

National Education Standards

The Emergency Medical Technician (EMT) will have a fundamental depth and foundational breadth of understanding of the safe and appropriate utilization of air medical resources within daily practice in an EMS system.

Key Concepts

- The progress of air medical services over the years has mirrored that of ground-based EMS, both with clear origins in military experiences.

- Air medical services are configured for the unique mission for which they are dedicated.

- Indications for air medical transport from a scene must be determined regionally.

- Interfacility transport of critically ill or injured patients may be best accomplished by an air medical team.

- Air medical services should not be used when benefit is not likely to be derived.

- Safety in all aspects of air medical operations is essential.

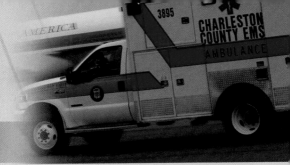

CASE STUDY

Danica notes the facial droop, slurred speech, and inability to raise one arm as she completes her assessment. Looking at her watch, she asks, "Mrs. Johnson, tell me the last time you saw your husband normal?" Knowing that the answer would mean the difference between destination hospitals, Danica calculates that the total time of symptoms was just under one hour. With at least an hour ground transport time to the nearest stroke center, Danica asks her partner to begin to move the patient to the ambulance while she steps outside to make a phone call. "Dr. Bradley, this is EMT 597. I am on the scene of a 48-year-old man with an acute stroke onset just under one hour ago. I would like permission to request a helicopter for rapid transport to the stroke center."

Critical Thinking Questions

1. What assessment findings caused Danica to believe she was dealing with a time-dependent illness?

2. What factors played into the request for helicopter transport?

3. If the symptoms had been present for a longer period of time, would the plan have changed?

INTRODUCTION

Emergency transport of critically ill and injured patients by air has become an expectation within the emergency medical community in the United States today. Although some areas of the country have some work to do to improve the integration of air medical services into the existing transport system, it is clear that progress has been made over the years (Figure 54.1).

HISTORY

As with ground-based EMS, air medical transport finds its origins in wartime rescue efforts. The first reported air transport of a patient was in 1915 when a French pilot reportedly evacuated an injured Serb in an unmodified fighter plane. Through progressive conflicts, airplane evacuation of ill and injured patients became more common. Although the first medical use of a helicopter was seen in 1944 in Burma, the first large-scale medical evacuation by helicopter was in Korea. This was accomplished largely with Sikorsky airframes outfitted with outboard stretchers. The UH-1H (Figure 54.2), or "Huey," was central to the medical efforts in Vietnam, with significant numbers of patients flown during this war. The use of helicopters to rapidly move injured patients was thought to contribute to the reduction in morbidity and mortality in subsequent conflicts. Not surprisingly, this improvement in care came to the attention of the American public.

CIVILIAN ADAPTATION

In the early 1970s, feasibility studies suggested tenuous economic viability of an air medical program. It was recognized that timely response would require a dedicated medical configuration in the airframe. Even in these early days of air transport, integration into the developing ground EMS systems was known to be an important part of a successful program.

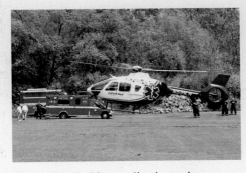

Figure 54.1 Air medical services work together with ground-based services to create an integrated approach to emergency medical care

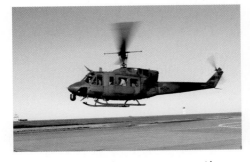

Figure 54.2 Helicopter evacuation was central to the rescue efforts during the war in Vietnam

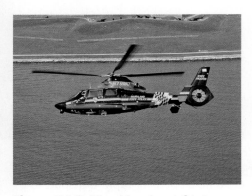

Figure 54.3 The Maryland State Police Aviation unit was the first dedicated air medical agency in the United States to provide emergency air transport from the scene of an accident

In 1970 the Maryland State Police Aviation unit was the first agency in the United States to provide emergency air transport from the scene of an accident (Figure 54.3). Two years later, St. Anthony's Hospital in Denver, Colorado, began its own civilian air medical transport program, offering both scene and interfacility transports. Although these two agencies were the first to pursue dedicated air medical agendas, other law enforcement and fire agencies developed aviation components that would offer air medical transport in addition to their primary mission.

GROUND EMS DEVELOPMENT

In much the same fashion, ground-based EMS developed as a result of wartime experiences. Multiple models of system operation were developed to meet the needs of different communities. These models included private contractors, EMS based in fire departments, private for-profit services, and municipal third service systems, to name a few.

In addition to multiple models for operation, multiple levels of providers were developed based on local needs. These tended to be regionally dependent and consisted of some form of Basic and, later, Advanced Life Support providers.

INTEGRATION OF GROUND AND AIR

While ground and air medical services were developing at much the same time with seemingly the same goal in mind, they developed more in parallel than in conjunction with one another. This may have been due to the fact that helicopter services were largely based at hospitals and ground-based EMS was run through the department of transportation. Whatever the reason, the result in many areas was air medical services and ground services coexisting but not necessarily cooperating as well as they could have. Significant work has been done in recent years to improve the integration of ground and air EMS with good results in many areas. It should be intuitive that the air service is an integral component of the emergency transport system in any area and should be used as such.

CURRENT STATE OF AIR MEDICINE IN THE UNITED STATES

The last decade has seen an incredibly rapid rise in the numbers of air medical services across the United States. This is likely due to many factors. An increased need for longer distance transports of more critically ill patients, more specialized time-dependent treatments offered at larger centers, and improved reimbursement rates all likely contributed to this expansion of programs. Today, helicopter transport is an expectation in appropriate circumstances in many communities. In 2006, the Association of Air Medical Services reported that there were 792 air medical helicopters providing this service across the United States, with more than a half-million patient transports completed annually. Compared to more than 16,000 ground EMS agencies, air medical agencies are still considered a limited resource and should be used appropriately.

PROGRAM TYPES

As the numbers of transport agencies increased, the most common model of operation involved a hospital-based program with some sort of cooperative effort between a helicopter vendor and hospital staff. Over the years, the structure of programs has continued to change with a community-based model becoming more and more common.

MISSION PROFILE

Nationally, the majority of air medical programs offer both scene and interfacility transports, with 30% to 50% of the transports being scene responses. Each community has a slightly different need based on geography and hospital capabilities.

Because helicopters are most often called to transport the more significantly injured or more critically ill patients, the staff usually has an expanded scope of practice when compared with typical ground transport agencies. They can be thought of as bringing the resources of the tertiary care hospital with which they are associated to the side of the patient—wherever the patient may be. This can be useful for both interfacility and scene medical care.

SPECIAL OPERATIONS

Some helicopter programs have special operations units that provide search and rescue or extraction services. These useful services should be integrated into the local system's response to a given situation.

STAFFING CONFIGURATION

The staffing configuration of an agency depends largely on the expected patient population. If an agency intends only to respond to scene requests and not offer interfacility services, it may staff with paramedics. On the other hand, if hospitalized patients will be included in the program mission, a nurse, physician, or respiratory therapist may be useful. The most commonly seen staffing pattern among U.S. programs is nurse/paramedic. Those that use this crew mix describe it as a useful mix of expertise for the expected mission profile of their agencies.

PARAMEDIC

Paramedics who staff a helicopter would benefit from training beyond the standard paramedic curriculum. This additional training will vary depending on local expectations and protocols, but at a minimum it must include flight physiology and flight safety. Typically, flight paramedics have some range of expanded skills and may have a more independent practice. This is necessary due to the critical nature of the patients they are likely to see and the remote situations in which they may find themselves. Skills such as rapid sequence intubation, surgical airway management, and advanced pharmacology may be useful when managing a patient in this environment.

Many advanced training programs are used by air medical agencies around the nation. The Air Medical Crew Curriculum, established by the Department of Transportation in conjunction with multiple air medical organizations, is a good resource for this education. A document created by the National Association of Flight Paramedics also outlines minimum guidelines for flight paramedic education. Close medical oversight to any advanced training program is imperative.

NURSE

A flight nurse must be capable of independent practice in the out-of-hospital environment. Typically flight nurses have background in a critical care environment and are provided with training regarding EMS operations. Skills provided by nurses in a helicopter often exceed those performed by in-hospital colleagues. Appropriate training must be provided to ensure competence.

RESPIRATORY THERAPIST

Their expertise in airway and pulmonary pathophysiology make respiratory therapists ideally suited to the patient population transported by helicopter services. A higher percentage of patients being transported by helicopter may require advanced airway management than those being moved by other means of transport. To ensure a broader experience base, some programs that staff respiratory therapists also require paramedic certification by these providers. If this is not the case, it would likely be necessary to expand the training of the respiratory therapist to best suit the flight environment and the expected patient population.

PHYSICIAN

Although in the minority, a few air medical programs continue to staff a physician on the aircraft. While it might logically appear more beneficial to have this highly trained provider on board the helicopter, there does not seem to be that much of a difference in the interventions they offer. Some feel that appropriately trained nurses, paramedics, or respiratory therapists can accomplish the same task at a fraction of the cost.

SPECIALTY TEAM

Specialized mission profiles may require special team configurations. Some services offer response to specialized patient populations such as neonatal or pediatrics. In these cases, the team comprises staff whose expertise lies in those areas of practice.

SCENE MISSIONS

When used appropriately, helicopter transport from the scene of an accident can potentially improve the patient's outcome. This may seem intuitive when the concept of the "golden hour" is considered; however, actual measured benefit continues to stimulate controversy.

INDICATIONS FOR AIR MEDICAL TRANSPORT

Given the relative scarcity of helicopters when compared with ground units, it is imperative that helicopters be used only in circumstances in which they are felt to offer the most benefit. Although every state and region should have guidelines to assist local providers with this determination, the National Association of EMS Physicians has put forth its own "Guidelines for Air Medical Dispatch." This document can be considered to be a national standard and can be used when creating local guidelines.

The two main advantages to using a helicopter are related to speed and capability. Helicopters can fly up to 150 mph in straight line travel—that is, they have no need to follow roads. This can offer significant benefit when environmental obstacles or traffic pose a significant delay to rapid ground transport. The second benefit many helicopter services offer is an advanced level of care provided by the flight team. As previously discussed, depending on the mission and staffing configuration, the interventions offered by the flight team may far supersede those available on the ground or even at small hospitals.

TRIAGE

The concept of triage is important to EMS providers. The most basic level provider is adept at determining whether certain criteria are met and what level of care is most likely needed for transport of a given patient. It is important to understand that triage is an inexact process completed in a rapid manner with limited information. This is necessary in the case of a critically ill or injured patient. However, it may result in some **overtriage.** That is, even when specific criteria are met, the patient may not actually have a level of injury that is considered severe. This will not be known until after a thorough Emergency

Department work-up is completed. No triage scheme is perfect, and it is always better to err on the side of overtriage than the opposite, undertriage. **Undertriage** would fail to use the helicopter for patients that do meet criteria and have real injuries that may benefit from its use. A certain percentage of overtriage is accepted as necessary to avoid unacceptable rates of undertriage.

DISPATCH

Once it is determined that a helicopter may be needed, the EMS Dispatch Center should initiate the request. Certain basic information must be provided to the helicopter dispatch center (Table 54-1).

Auto Launch   Early activation of a helicopter by responding personnel based on a potential expected need is commonly used. Another means to decrease the response time of the helicopter is to use an **auto launch** policy. This would involve simultaneous dispatch of the helicopter and the ground units based on dispatch information. Predesignated trauma and/or medical indications should be set up by a local or regional EMS system and can be used by the dispatchers to make these decisions. Depending on distances involved, some helicopter agencies will prepare the aircraft for response but not actually begin the flight until a confirmed need is reported.

In the case of either early activation or auto launch, if ground providers arrive on scene and realize that the helicopter is not actually needed, it should be cancelled immediately. There should be no penalty to the patient or provider in this case. There will likely be many such cancellations if an auto launch system is used, but this is often felt to be acceptable to offer faster response in those cases where it is needed. The Association of Air Medical Services distributed a position statement describing early activation and auto launch as effective means to decrease response time in certain circumstances. Criteria suggested in this position paper are listed in Table 54-2.

FIRST RESPONDER ARRIVAL

Although each air medical agency may have its own policy and local guidelines may define who may request a helicopter, it is common practice for helicopter dispatchers to accept flight requests from any provider on a scene. This may include law enforcement officials, firefighters, industrial safety officers, ski patrol, certified first responders, EMTs at any level, nurses, and physicians. The cancellation of a helicopter should be initiated by the highest level of medical provider on the scene. Cancellation should occur only after patient contact has been made and the patient condition has been determined not to warrant the helicopter response.

SPECIFIC CONDITIONS

Although no list can possibly include every possible condition that could benefit from helicopter response, creating a list of specific conditions is useful to guide prehospital providers in practice. Table 54-3 lists clinical traumatic conditions that, if suspected to be present in a given patient, might be appropriate indications for air medical transport from a scene. Local protocols must prevail as local conditions vary.

NONTRAUMA CONSIDERATIONS

Whereas the literature is certainly less robust in support of nontrauma indications for scene air medical transport, there are certainly situations in which access to rapid transport could offer significant patient benefit. Situations that may fall into this category include time-dependent conditions such as ST-segment elevation myocardial infarction (STEMI) and acute stroke. Local

---

Table 54-1 Information to Provide When Requesting Helicopter

Incident location

Requesting unit and designated landing zone officer

Radio frequency for contact

Nature of the incident

Number of patients

Ages of patients

Mechanism of injury

Vital signs

Specific injuries if known

Table 54-2 Air Medical Early Activation and Auto Launch Criteria

Flight distance >10 minutes or >29 miles

Patient location >20 miles from specialty hospital and condition is critical:

Including but not limited to:

Prolonged extrication time

Multiple victim incident

Ejection from vehicle/patient entrapped

Pedestrian struck with serious injury

Death of occupant in same vehicle

Critical burns >10% TBSA

Falls with serious injury

Deep penetrating injury to head, neck, or torso

Unstable vital signs

Acute stroke

Table 54-3 Trauma Criteria for Potential Air Medical Transport

Trauma

General and mechanism

    Unstable vital signs

    Significant trauma in young, old, or pregnant patients

    Multisystem injuries

    Ejection from vehicle

    Pedestrian struck by vehicle

    Death in same passenger compartment

    Penetrating trauma to abdomen, pelvis, chest, neck, or head

    Crush to abdomen, chest, or head

    Fall from significant height

Neurologic considerations

    GCS <10

    Deteriorating mental status

    Skull fracture

    Spinal cord injury

Thoracic considerations

    Major chest wall injury

    Pneumothorax/hemothorax

    Suspected cardiac injury

Abdominal/pelvic considerations

    Significant abdominal pain after blunt trauma

    Abdominal wall contusion

    Obvious rib fracture below nipple line

    Major pelvic fracture

Orthopedic/extremity considerations

    Partial or total ambulation of a limb (exclusive of digits)

    Finger/thumb amputation when emergent surgical evaluation is indicated and rapid surface transport is not available

    Fracture or dislocation with vascular compromise

    Extremity ischemia

    Open long bone fractures

    Two or more long bone fractures

Major burns

    >20% BSA

    Involvement of hands, feet, face, or genitalia

    Inhalation injury

    Electrical or chemical burns

    Burns with associated injuries

Patients with near drowning injuries

Street Smart

A good rule of thumb is to consider use of a helicopter if it would decrease the time to definitive care that would benefit the patient. This type of decision requires knowledge of local geography, travel times, and hospital capabilities. Development of local guidelines is imperative to guide decision making in a given region.

protocols will govern if patients with these conditions are to be selectively transported to certain hospitals. If so, helicopter transport should be considered if it would result in a more timely arrival at the most appropriate facility (Figure 54.4).

Additional situations might benefit from the advanced level of care brought by some helicopter services. These might include obstetric complications, neonatal emergencies, or other surgical or medical conditions in need of interventions not offered by local ground agencies. Another category of patients in need of rapid transport are those needing organ transplant when they have been called to respond to a transplant center or if they are having complications related to the transplant.

LOGISTICAL CONSIDERATIONS

Additional logistical issues might suggest benefit from helicopter transport. These might include patients in areas that are difficult to reach by surface transport or in areas so remote that ground transport would take too long. Other system considerations that might have an impact on the decision to use air medical services

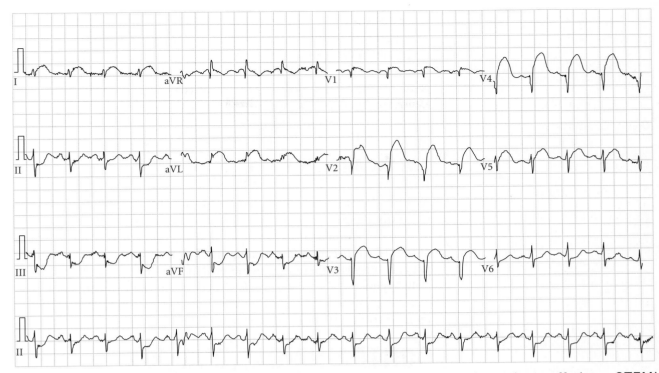

Figure 54.4 Some EMS protocols allow for helicopter transport in the case of a patient suffering a STEMI whose arrival at a cardiac center could be accelerated by this mode of transport

include a paucity of local ALS care or any other situation in which local services are threatened or overwhelmed. Once again, it is crucial to develop local protocols to guide providers in this decision making. Interregional cooperation on such protocols is wise because air medical services often cover more than one region.

INTERFACILITY MISSIONS

Patients who are in need of transfer from one facility to another may benefit from the use of air medical services in several circumstances. The most obvious would relate to the speed of travel, which is relevant in two circumstances. First, if the overall time to the receiving center can be minimized by use of a helicopter for transport, it should be considered. This is especially important in time-dependent conditions in which a crucial therapy awaits the patient at the destination facility. Second, the out-of-hospital time can almost always be shortened by helicopter transport when compared with ground travel. This can be extremely critical for patients who are unstable or whose conditions would not benefit from prolonged time in a moving vehicle.

Perhaps more commonly, air medical services are requested to transport patients between facilities for reasons related to the level of care they offer. Increasingly, hospitals are beginning advanced therapies as they work to stabilize patients prior to transfer. These therapies require trained hands to manage during the transport. The presence of a team with advanced capabilities in the transport vehicle is necessary. In many areas, the most advanced teams are found on helicopters. Some areas have ground-based critical care transport teams as well, and those should be considered if the travel time is less of an issue. Regardless of the vehicle used, it is imperative to realize that the level of care for the patient must be maintained from the sending to the receiving hospital. Care during transport is an important, but often neglected, consideration in patient care.

EMTALA

The Emergency Medical Treatment and Active Labor Act (EMTALA) is a section of the larger Consolidated Omnibus Budget Reconciliation Act (COBRA) that was originally passed in 1986 and, after several revisions, remains one of the most important pieces of health care legislation in the United States. A section of this legislation requires hospitals to make arrangements for transfers that are appropriate for the patient's needs. For critically ill or injured patients, air medical transport should be considered.

INDICATIONS FOR AIR MEDICAL TRANSPORT

As with the guidelines for scene air medical transport, there are nationally recognized indications for interfacility transport as well. These can be found in the NAEMSP position statement and are summarized in Table 54-4. The literature is most abundant in support of air transport of the critically injured patient; however, there is growing evidence of benefit in other situations as well. In general, if the level of care needed or the nature of the patient's illness would benefit from the speed of the aircraft or the skill level of the provider, then air transport should be considered.

CONTRAINDICATIONS FOR AIR MEDICAL TRANSPORT

As discussed previously, there are many fewer helicopters than ground ambulances. This fact, together with the increased cost and other risks involved, suggest that air transport should not be used when benefit is not likely to be derived. There are several circumstances in which use of a helicopter might be considered to be contraindicated. Of course, there could be exceptions to each of these circumstances and every situation should be evaluated individually.

If a patient is known to be terminally ill and has no correctable medical problems, when a move is necessary, ground ambulance would likely be more appropriate.

Similarly, the survival rates for patients who have suffered cardiac arrest who have not achieved return of spontaneous circulation after initial efforts would not likely achieve benefit from air transport. This is true of both medical and traumatic causes of arrest. A notable exception to these criteria may be the hypothermic drowning victim for whom invasive rewarming measures might be beneficial.

Patients who are likely to die or decompensate en route who are in a facility capable of definitively managing the condition should likely not be moved at all. In a similar line of thought, patients who are in active labor should not be removed from a hospital capable of a controlled delivery if delivery is expected during transport. This is sometimes difficult to predict; however, the risk for intra-transport delivery should be considered when deciding to transport a woman with ongoing contractions.

Patients who are prone to psychotic or violent behavior should not be placed into a transport vehicle without appropriate restraint in place.

OPERATIONS

The importance of safety in all aspects of air medical operations cannot be overstated. The EMT must understand not only appropriate utilization and triage criteria, but also how to prepare the patient and select an appropriate landing zone for an incoming aircraft.

Safety Tips

In some cases restraint of an uncontrollable patient may include chemical paralysis with intubation and appropriate sedation. This level of restraint obviously carries with it some degree of risk; therefore, the decision to embark on such a treatment pathway should be carefully considered by the appropriately trained ALS provider. The safety of the patient as well as the safety of the transport team should both be weighed against the risk of the procedure. At no time should a transport be initiated if it is felt to be potentially unsafe for any reason. Written policy and protocol should support this practice.

Table 54-4 Interfacility Indications for Air Medical Transport

Trauma

Any diagnositic consideration listed under the scene criteria that cannot be managed at the local hospital

Injuries or potential injuries that require evaluation or treatment beyond hospital capabilities

Cardiac

Acute coronary syndrome with time-critical need for urgent interventional therapy not available at local hospital

Cardiogenic shock

Cardiac tamponade

Mechanical cardiac disease

Critically ill medical or surgical patient

Pretransport cardiac/respiratory arrest

Continuous IV vasoactive medications or mechanical ventricular assist

Risk for airway deterioration

Acute pulmonary failure and/or requirement for sophisticated pulmonary intensive care during transport

Severe poisoning or overdose requiring specialized toxicology services

Urgent need for hyperbaric oxygen therapy

Requirement for emergency dialysis

Gastrointestinal hemorrhages with hemodynamic compromise

Surgical emergencies such as fasciitis, aortic dissection or aneurysm, or extremity ischemia

Pediatric patients for whom referring facilities cannot provide required evaluation and /or therapy

Obstetric (minimized out-of-hospital time must be weighed against risk of intratransport delivery)

Need for obstetric or neonatal care beyond capabilities of local hospital

Active premature labor

Severe preeclampsia or eclampsia

Third trimester hemorrhage

Fetal hydrops

Maternal medical conditions that may cause premature birth

Severe predicted fetal heart disease

Acute abdominal emergencies in third trimester

Neurologic

CNS hemorrhage

Spinal cord compression

Evolving ischemic stroke

Status epilepticus

Neonatal (consider using air transport to get specialized team to patient)

Gestational age <30 wks, body weight <2,000 grams, complicated neonatal course

Requirement for supplemental oxygen exceeding 60%, continuous positive airway pressure, or mechanical ventilation

Extrapulmonary air leak, interstitial emphysema, or pneumothorax

Medical emergencies such as seizure activity, congestive heart failure, or disseminated intravascular coagulation

Surgical emergencies such as diaphragmatic hernia, necrotizing enterocolitis, abdominal wall defects, intussusception, suspected volvulus, or congenital heart defects

Other

Transplant

Organ salvage

Organ recipient

LANDING ZONE SELECTION AND PREPARATION

If a helicopter is requested, the ground personnel must find a safe place for it to land. This area is usually referred to as a **landing zone.** A landing zone (LZ) is an area intended for the purpose of landing and taking off in the helicopter. One person who is familiar with the requirements of an LZ should take charge of its preparation. This person is referred to as the **LZ officer** and is the only person who should be in communication with the aircraft as it approaches.

Several issues must be considered in choosing an appropriate LZ. First, it should be located as close to the actual scene of the incident as possible while still being safe. Often, in the case of a car accident, the LZ can be in a field adjacent to the road or even in the road itself if traffic can be stopped. If a suitable area is not available close by, a more remote LZ may be chosen. In that case, the ground personnel should make arrangements to either bring the patient to the LZ or bring the helicopter crew to the patient.

Landing zones must be a certain size and have certain safety features. Most medical helicopters require a **touchdown area** of between 75 feet square and 100 feet square. The preference is 100 feet square, because that is large enough for both day and night operations and for landing the larger aircraft the military and many police agencies routinely use.

The touchdown area is the actual site where the aircraft will land. It should be fairly level and free of any obstacles such as trees, signs, posts, or markers. If the area is unpaved, shrubs, brush, grass, and weeds should not be higher than 24 inches. Any slope should not be more than 5 to 10 degrees.

The area above and around the touchdown area is called the **surrounding area** and should be free of any obstacles in which the helicopter could get tangled. When evaluating the surrounding area, the LZ officer should take note of any trees, poles, towers, signs, or wires that are in the surrounding area (Figure 54.5). These should be reported to the helicopter pilot as LZ hazards when the helicopter approaches the scene. The specific locations of such hazards must be made clear because sometimes it is difficult to see hazards such as wires from the air.

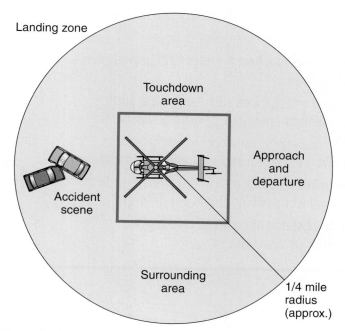

Figure 54.5 The LZ officer should choose a touchdown area that has a surrounding area and approach path free of obstacles

Additional information that is useful for incoming pilots includes a report of the wind direction and intensity and the condition of the touchdown area. For example, if there are moderate winds out of the southwest and the ground surface is muddy, the pilot should be made aware of these conditions when he or she is given the initial information about the LZ hazards.

APPROACH

Although a helicopter is capable of taking off and landing straight up and down, having a clear path for a more favorable approach angle is preferable. The approach path should be free of towers, poles, wires, trees, and so forth.

Because of the confusing nature of many accident scenes, it is often helpful to clearly mark the intended touchdown area with cones, flares, or other secured markers at its four corners (Figure 54.6). Any markers that are used should be carefully secured, because the wind created by the rotor blades can be quite forceful. This wind is called *rotor wash*.

If appropriate markers are not available, emergency vehicles can be used on two or four corners of the LZ. Headlights may be used to illuminate the LZ as shown in Figure 54.7, but lights must never be directed at the helicopter. Bright lights can temporarily blind the pilot, making a safe landing impossible.

LANDING ZONE SAFETY

As the touchdown area is prepared, the LZ officer must be sure to secure any loose debris, clothing, hats, or anything else that may blow around as the helicopter lands. A loose piece of debris can be blown into the rotor blades of the helicopter and cause significant damage, which may render the aircraft useless.

As the aircraft is approaching the touchdown area, any nearby personnel should wear goggles or face visors to protect their eyes from winds created by the helicopter's rotor until the helicopter has landed and shut down.

If the accident is near the LZ, the patient and any exposed crew members should be appropriately protected from blowing debris during the final approach of the aircraft. Doors and windows to nearby vehicles should be

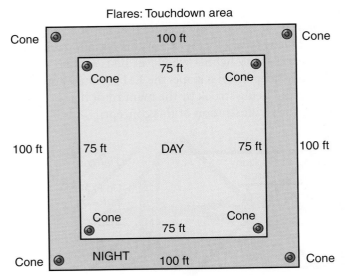

Figure 54.6 The marking of an LZ can be accomplished with cones, flares, or other secured markers that are clear to the pilot from the air

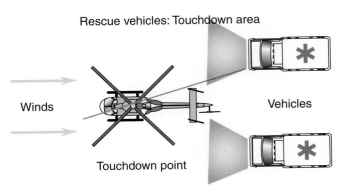

Figure 54.7 Emergency vehicle headlights can be used to mark a landing zone

kept closed, and any nearby traffic should be held if it has any potential for coming into contact with the aircraft in the LZ area.

Because it is certainly exciting to watch, rescues that involve helicopters often draw a crowd of onlookers. These people should be kept at a distance of at least 200 feet from the touchdown area for their safety.

As the aircraft approaches the touchdown area, the LZ officer should continue to observe its descent from a safe distance of at least 100 feet. Nobody should be within 100 feet of the touchdown area until it is safe to approach. The pilot of the aircraft will indicate when it is safe to approach the aircraft. If an unsafe situation develops during the final approach, the LZ officer should immediately and calmly contact the pilot with the information.

LZ HAND SIGNALS

The LZ officer needs to know only two hand signals to communicate with the pilot. While facing the pilot at the edge of the LZ, the LZ officer simply stands with her arms outstretched indicating that the aircraft approach is safe. The LZ officer should not be concentrating on how the aircraft is descending but should be looking around the aircraft for dangers.

If, for example, a wire strike suddenly seems possible, an individual runs out to meet the helicopter, or another danger under or around the helicopter arises, the LZ officer should signal to the pilot of the immediate danger, using a vigorous crossing and uncrossing of her arms over her head. This wave-off will cause the pilot to quickly abort the landing.

TOUCHDOWN

Operations around the helicopter while it is on the ground also have several rules. In general, nobody should ever approach the aircraft while it is running unless he is signaled to do so by the pilot. This includes the LZ officer as well. The pilot will usually direct the appropriate movement about the aircraft. If an EMT is signaled to approach the aircraft, she should always approach from the front, the twelve o'clock position, within clear view of the pilot. Personnel should never approach a helicopter from the rear, the six o'clock position. The danger zones around the aircraft are illustrated in Figure 54.8. On the rear of the aircraft tail is a tail rotor that spins very fast. It spins so fast that it is nearly invisible. The tail rotor is very dangerous. Being struck by a spinning tail rotor would cause serious, even fatal, injury.

The height of the main rotor blades may require that approaching personnel duck down to avoid being struck by them. For this reason, it is a good practice for an EMT to wear a safety helmet whenever he is around an aircraft. When approaching a helicopter on a slope, the EMT should approach from the downhill side to avoid being struck by the main rotor blades on the uphill side. See Figure 54.9 for an illustration of this concept.

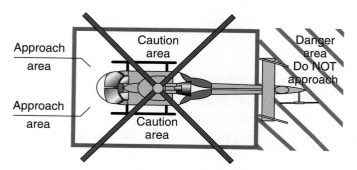

Figure 54.8 Ground personnel should be familiar with the danger zones around a helicopter

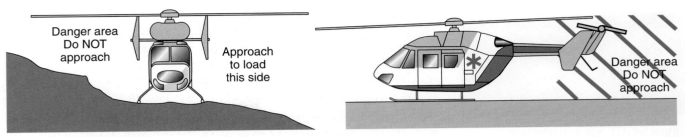

Figure 54.9 When approaching a helicopter that has landed on a slope, always approach from the downhill side to avoid injury. Never approach the aircraft from behind

Most helicopter crews will come to the patient, away from the aircraft, to quickly assess the patient. Any necessary treatment will be initiated, and then movement of the patient to the aircraft will be directed by the pilot and helicopter crew.

When carrying the patient to the waiting aircraft, the EMT should stay close to the patient's side, semi-crouched, and walk at a deliberate pace. The EMT should never run to the helicopter. The EMT should never carry anything, including IV fluids, over her head as she approaches the aircraft.

LIFTOFF

Once the patient has been safely loaded, all ground personnel should leave the landing zone in the direction indicated by the pilot or helicopter crew and should remain at least 200 feet away from the aircraft while it prepares to lift off. A great deal of rotor wash will be generated as the aircraft lifts off. Again, no bright lights or flashes should be aimed at the aircraft during this time, because they could create a vision problem for the pilot.

Although general safety issues surrounding operation around helicopters are similar between agencies, ground EMS personnel should routinely practice and train with their local helicopter agencies so that safe operation around the aircraft becomes second nature.

Safety Tips

It is common practice for the LZ officer to designate an assistant who takes a position opposite the LZ officer at the edge of the LZ. This assistant monitors activity in that area and radios problems to the LZ officer. The most dangerous place in the LZ is the area immediately behind the aircraft, near the tail rotor. No one should be allowed to approach the aircraft from that angle. It is the job of the assistant LZ officer to ensure no one does so.

Safety Tips

To save scene time, some helicopter pilots permit what is called a *hot load*. Whenever the rotors are still spinning and the engine is running during a hot load, the potential danger is increased. Therefore, only experienced crews should be permitted to hot load.

If the patient is being hot loaded, the patient's eyes must be protected by either safety glasses or a blanket folded over his eyes.

Street Smart

The landing team should remain assembled for about 5 minutes after liftoff. If an in-flight emergency should occur, the aircraft may need to return quickly to a secured landing zone.

AIRCRAFT CAPABILITIES

To determine the most appropriate aircraft for a particular patient, multiple factors must be considered. The patient's condition and the distance needed to travel will likely factor into the decision to use an air medical service. Within air transport, the choice of aircraft will depend on local availability and types of services offered as well as local geography, weather conditions, and aviation resources.

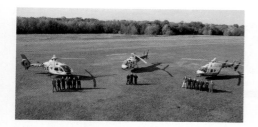

Figure 54.10 For a particular service, the type of airframe is chosen based on the geography covered and expected mission

ROTOR WING

The majority of the aircraft currently dedicated to emergency air medical transport are **rotor wing,** or helicopters. Many different types of helicopter are used depending on the geography covered and expected mission (Figure 54.10). They range from small single engine, single pilot aircraft up to extensively outfitted dual engine, instrument landing rated, dual pilot helicopters. It is important to realize that more is not always better. An airframe is chosen by a program based on its needs. Although there will always be controversy regarding what manufacturer or model aircraft is best, the Federal Aviation Regulations assure that all aircraft are safe to conduct the mission for which they are intended.

FLIGHT RULES

One feature that may distinguish the functionality of one helicopter from another from the EMS perspective is whether it is being operated under **Visual Flight Rules (VFR)** or **Instrument Flight Rules (IFR).** Visual flight rules refer to aviation regulations that essentially permit a pilot to fly only when environmental conditions allow him to actually see with his own eyes well enough to safely navigate the aircraft. The Federal Aviation Administration has established specific requirements for visibility, distance from clouds, and altitude to ensure safe operations. Many air medical programs have created limitations more stringent than those required by the FAA in the interest of safety. This means that there will be some weather and visibility situations in which a pilot operating a VFR helicopter will not be able to accept a mission.

Operating under IFR allows for planned operation of the aircraft by reference to the aircraft instruments with instruction from Air Traffic Control (ATC). Although IFR permits a planned flight in a broader range of environmental conditions, a flight plan must be filed and each part of the flight into controlled airspace must receive ATC clearance. In addition, an IFR rated program must maintain additional certifications held by the pilot and different equipment specifications for the aircraft.

Many VFR programs maintain pilot IFR credentialing and have equipment to allow for use of instruments when visibility unexpectedly deteriorates during a flight. This is a safety measure to allow the pilot to use every resource to safely navigate the aircraft to an appropriate landing zone.

Every air medical program is mandated to conduct every flight according to stringent safety regulations regardless of whether they are VFR or IFR rated. At the scene operation level, both VFR and IFR pilots must have sufficient visibility to allow for complete identification of the intended landing zone and any hazards.

WEIGHT AND BALANCE

An additional limitation that must be kept in mind when considering use of a helicopter is the issue of weight and balance. Every helicopter has a maximum lift capacity that requires accounting for the combined weight of the crew, patients, equipment, and fuel. Although larger aircraft may be less limited with regard to weight, it must always be considered when using this mode of transport.

SPEED

In general, rotor wing aircraft can travel at speeds two to three times faster than ground ambulances and have the advantage of straight line travel. That is, they can fly from point A to point B without having to overcome surface obstacles. In some areas where ground time is extensive due to such obstacles, the use of a helicopter may translate into even more time savings. Knowledge of the local area and estimated driving times in comparison to estimated flight times can help providers determine if use of a helicopter would be appropriate to consider in a given circumstance.

FIXED WING

Fixed wing, or airplanes, are also used in air medical transport (Figure 54.11). Although they can travel at greater speeds and their range of travel is significantly longer than their rotor-wing counterparts, the main disadvantage of fixed wing operations is the need to begin and end each transport at an airport. The need for alternative transport of the patient and team on both ends of the transport adds time to the trip. This sometimes negates the time saved with the faster aircraft. On the other hand, the main advantage of this form of transport is the ability to complete long-distance transports in a much shorter time than a ground vehicle. Transports that are greater than 100 miles in length in which there is an airport located within a reasonable distance to each end of the trip should be considered for fixed wing travel. Although many types of aircraft are used for fixed wing air medical transport, they are all instrument flight rated and most can travel in excess of 250 mph.

The cost of maintaining a fixed wing aircraft is more than for a rotor wing. However, the cost for each mile of travel on a transport is less, making an airplane a more economical choice for long-distance flights. Additionally, the larger cabin offers an obvious advantage for patient care and crew comfort when compared to most helicopters. Fewer restrictions with regard to weight and environmental conditions allow for a broader range of transports.

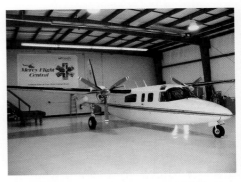

Figure 54.11 Fixed wing aircraft are useful for long-distance transports

COST AND REIMBURSEMENT

It would be impossible to have a discussion of air medical transport without addressing the issue of cost. It should be evident that the cost to operate a helicopter and the personnel associated with it is significantly more than for a neighboring ground ambulance. The cost of these operations is handled differently depending on the model of the program.

Although some large independent organizations operate programs throughout the country, the majority of the dedicated air medical programs remain based at, and at least partially supported by, hospitals or hospital systems. Regardless of the model or size of the program, the cost of business in air medicine can be significant.

Typically, the air medical program bills a patient or insurance company a standard rate made up of a base cost for lift-off plus a per mile fee for each loaded mile flown. Some programs have additional charges if high-priced items or services were used in patient care.

Many insurance companies set a rate for air transport they believe to be acceptable. If the flight is determined to have been warranted after an insurance own review, the program is reimbursed at the rate determined as appropriate.

Concerns regarding cost of this type of transport are appropriate. However, if air medical transport is the most appropriate means of transport for a given patient, fears about cost should not affect the decision to do what is right. It is possible that by deciding to use this method of transport up front, money can be saved in the long run through decreased length of stay in the hospital if the patient has a better outcome than if the transport had been completed in a different manner. This is probably most clearly seen in the case of a trauma patient flown from a distant scene directly to a trauma center as opposed to being taken to a nontrauma center first and then requiring additional transport for definitive care.

SAFETY

Safety during all phases of transport is essential. No matter the transport vehicle or the nature of the patient's illness, the priority of all involved must be to complete the task at hand in the safest manner possible.

SAFETY IN AIR MEDICAL TRANSPORT

In the early days of air medical transport and rapid growth within the industry, the rate of helicopter accidents was unacceptable. Regulatory changes led to a temporary improvement, but again in the late 1990s the number of helicopter accidents increased at an alarming rate. Given the nature of the vehicle, accidents in a helicopter tend to be more catastrophic than an accident in a ground transport vehicle. Although it is true that there are a greater number of ground ambulance accidents than air ambulance accidents, the air accidents tend to get more public attention. This attention and justified concern of the industry has led to increased regulation at the federal, state, and local levels as well as to a universal **culture of safety** within the air medical community.

REGULATION

The Federal Aviation Administration has imposed stringent regulatory requirements on air medical helicopter operators. These requirements are designed to create as safe an environment as possible within the industry. Equipment specifications, maintenance policies, training requirements, and risk assessment tools are among the measures required under the regulations.

CULTURE OF SAFETY

The Centers for Disease Control and Prevention (CDC) has defined a *culture of safety* as the shared commitment of management and employees to ensure the safety of the work environment. It is important to note that a true culture of safety involves the active participation of every team member with the overarching goal of risk reduction. In air medical services this means that both aviation and medical personnel are responsible to ensure the safety of the team. Support from management is integral. Obstacles to a culture of safety include imposed pressures, risks, distractions, poor communication, and complacency. Awareness of the potential for each of these factors to result in unsafe practices must be a part of the safety culture. Identification of errors or near-errors is mandatory; examination of the details of each situation by the entire team is one of the best methods of error prevention available.

AIR MEDICAL RESOURCE MANAGEMENT

Although the pilot in charge is given the ultimate responsibility over the aviation aspects of the flight, it is important to recognize that every member of the team can affect mission safety. This concept of entire team participation in a safety plan is fostered in the Air Medical Resource Management concept. This program involves training meant to foster open communications, teamwork, and an overall awareness and participation in risk reduction as a member of the crew on an aircraft.

Most accidents do not happen because of a single event, but rather result from a cumulative string or chain of events. Any of these events can be recognized by any member of the team and, if dealt with properly, can break the chain and hopefully prevent an accident.

SURVIVAL TRAINING

Although safe operations are the goal of every program, safe does not necessarily mean risk free. In the case of an unavoidable incident, the flight team can take measures to improve survivability. Protective equipment such as helmets, flight suits, and safety harnesses can help an individual survive an accident (Figure 54.12). Specific training meant to teach a provider how to best prepare to survive a survivable accident is useful and mandated by many programs.

CAMTS

In 1990, the Commission for Accreditation of Air Medical Services (CAAMS) was formed as an accrediting body developed by the industry to validate its members' standards regarding safety, medical care, and utilization review. With a name change to the Commission for Accreditation of Medical Transport Services (CAMTS) reflecting the broader range of services seeking accreditation, the self-imposed requirements reflected in the CAMTS standards are considered by many to be the national standard for practice in the air medical industry (Figure 54.13). Many states require air medical agencies operating within their borders to hold CAMTS accreditation or the equivalent. Excellence in patient care and safety of the transport environment are recognized as the pillars of the CAMTS standards. Continual review and revision as appropriate to these standards as well as the broad representation on the governing board lend to the credibility of the accreditation process.

PROFESSIONAL ORGANIZATIONS

As with other professional groups, organization on a national level has far-reaching benefits. In the case of the International Association of Flight Paramedics (IAFP), the group draws its members from a worldwide base. The IAFP was founded in 1986 (originally named the National Flight Paramedics Association) and lists the following as its mission statement: "The purpose of the IAFP is to maintain an international organization of paramedics which support and coordinate educational and research activities relating to its members and the flight paramedic industry at large, and establish standard levels of training and performance for safe, efficient and quality patient care." Holding true to that statement, the group has cosponsored numerous educational conferences, position statements, publications, and research endeavors. The IAFP continues to offer support to members through creation of a certification exam and legislative initiatives, among other activities.

CONCLUSION

When appropriately integrated into a well-organized EMS system, air medical programs may offer benefit to critically ill and injured patients. EMTs should understand the capabilities of air medical programs in their regions and always follow local protocols regarding their use. As with all aspects of EMS, a prominent culture of safety is crucial with air medical operations.

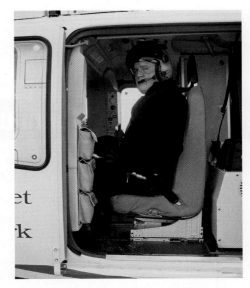

Figure 54.12 Protective clothing and equipment can improve the flight paramedic's chances of survival in a crash

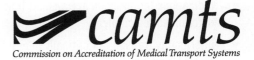

Commission on Accreditation of Medical Transport Systems

Figure 54.13 CAMTS accreditation is required in some states for air medical services

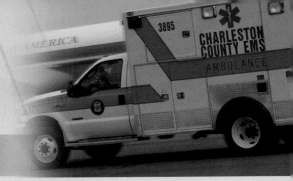

CASE STUDY Continued

Danica explains to her patient's wife that she has requested a helicopter to respond to provide rapid transport to a distant hospital that serves as the regional stroke center. The EMT explains that this hospital is the only center in the area that offers specific therapies for acute management of stroke. The treatment is extremely time dependent, making the air medical service a good option. While moving toward the arranged landing zone, Danica monitors her patient's vital signs and reassesses his neurologic status frequently.

Key Concepts Revisited

- The progress of air medical services over the years has mirrored that of ground-based EMS, both with clear origins in military experiences.

- Air medical services are configured for the unique mission for which they are dedicated.

- Indications for air medical transport from a scene must be determined regionally.

- Interfacility transport of critically ill or injured patients may be best accomplished by an air medical team.

- Air medical services should not be used when benefit is not likely to be derived.

- Safety in all aspects of air medical operations is essential.
  - Regulation
    - Equipment specifications
    - Maintenance policies
    - Training requirements
    - Risk management tools
  - Culture of safety
  - Flight Team Responsibility
    - Teamwork
  - Survival Training

Review Questions

1. Why should a helicopter service be integrated into the ground EMS system?
2. How is the team that staffs a medical helicopter determined?
3. Name some common indications for air medical transport from a scene.
4. Why might helicopter transport be useful for transfer of critically ill patients between hospitals?
5. Name some contraindications to air medical transport.
6. How many providers should be in contact with an helicopter inbound to a scene?
7. How large should a helicopter landing zone be?
8. Under what circumstances should an EMT approach a helicopter that is in operation?
9. What is a culture of safety?

Key Terms

Auto launch
Culture of safety
Fixed wing
Instrument Flight Rules (IFR)
Landing zone
LZ officer

Overtriage
Rotor wing
Surrounding area
Touchdown area
Undertriage
Visual Flight Rules (VFR)

Further Study

Air Medical Physicians Association. Web site: http://www.ampa.org.

American College of Emergency Physicians and National Association of EMS Physicians. "Guidelines for Air Medical Dispatch: Policy Resource and Education Paper." Approved January 2006. Available online at: http://www.acep.org/uploadedFiles/ACEP/Practice_Resources/issues_by_category/Emergency_Medical_Services/GuidelinesForAirMedDisp.pdf

Association of Air Medical Services. "Early Activation of an Air Medical Helicopter and Auto Launch Recommendations: Position Statement of AAMS." Available online at: http://www.aams.org/Content/NavigationMenu/PublicationsProducts/ResourceDocuments/EarlyActivation-FINAL.pdf

Association of Air Medical Services. Web site: http://www.aams.org.

International Association of Flight Paramedics. Web site: http://www.flightparamedic.org.

McGinnis, Kevin K., and others. "Air Medical Services: Future Development as an Integrated Component of the EMS System. A Guidance Document by the Air Medical Task Force of the National Association of State EMS Officials, National Association of EMS Physicians, and Association of Air Medical Services." *Prehospital Emergency Care,* October 1, 2007.

Three quarters of the land mass in the United States is considered rural (nonmetropolitan) and is home to approximately 50 million Americans. Much of this land is used for agricultural industries such as dairy farming, feed production, and the like. Historically, farming has been one of America's most dangerous occupations. Whereas farmers only represent 3% of the U.S. workforce, they account for 10% of all work-related deaths.

Key Concepts

- Most farm injuries are traumatic injuries involving diverse mechanisms of injury.

- The general principles of farm rescue begin with preplanning and local risk management.

- Dealing with livestock can pose a variety of dangers for the rescuer.

- The hazards of farm machinery range from heavy-duty machinery to power take off accessory machinery.

- Farm rescue principles begin with the general principles of technical rescue with adjustments for farm-specific mechanism of injury.

- The injuries from farm machinery can include avulsions, crush injuries, drowning, falls, and toxic exposures.

- Tractor accidents can be MVC involving other vehicles or rollovers.

- Power takeoff (PTO) shafts entangle any loose clothing or hair and can cause severe traumatic injuries with massive bleeding.

- The dangers of silo rescue involve the potential inhalation of toxic silo gas by the rescuer.

- Hazardous materials found on a farm can include farm chemicals used as insecticides and fertilizers.

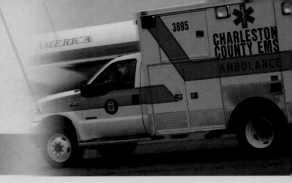

CASE STUDY

Christopher and Ahman are watching a training video on rescue techniques when the pager goes off: "Dispatch to Unit 76, respond to Barnstead Farms for an individual caught in a baler, conscious and breathing at this time. Time out: 14:32."

Christopher, having been raised on a farm, tells Ahman, "This could be bad. We need to be prepared for a serious injury with potentially heavy bleeding."

As Unit 76 goes en route, Christopher verifies the address with the communications center and programs it into the GPS. GPS indicates the farm is located approximately 16 miles from town. Christopher remembers the area as being remote with bad gravel roads. It has been raining for the past couple days, and Christopher hopes the baler is not in the middle of a soggy field.

Upon arrival they see a baler parked near the edge of the field, not too far from the field driveway. They are met by Janis who states she and her husband Roger had just finished baling. As she was climbing down from the wagon, she saw Roger begin to climb over the PTO shaft to get to the other side. The PTO was still spinning, and as he

stepped over, it grabbed his pant leg, throwing him to the ground as it began twisting his leg around the shaft.

Janis states she was able to disengage the clutch and after seeing that Roger's leg looked pretty bad, told him to lie still. Because their cell phones don't work well out here, Janis ran to the four-wheeler parked at the end of the row and then to the house to call 9-1-1. When she came back, she noticed Roger was acting like he wanted to go to sleep; even though there wasn't a lot of blood on the ground, she was worried he might be going into shock. She had thought to bring back blankets and had done her best to keep him warm, because it is only 50 degrees today and the ground is damp.

Critical Thinking Questions

1. What special hazard, unique to the rural environment, is presented in this case?
2. What are some of the barriers that rural EMS providers face?
3. What additional resources might be needed for this type of farm rescue?

INTRODUCTION

Farmers are independent and self-reliant out of necessity. When Emergency Medical Services (EMS) gets a call to respond to a farm, it can be assumed that a true emergency exists and that special circumstances, unique to rural EMS, may exist on scene. This unit discusses some of the special circumstances an EMT may encounter when called to respond to a farming emergency.

FARM EMERGENCIES

At one time the majority of farms were owned by private individuals or families, and these farms consisted of less than 500 acres of land. Approximately 8 million Americans operate these small farms. Farming has been considered a "family" business, requiring all family members to actively work on the farm, including children helping with the chores. Unfortunately, as many as 100,000 children are injured on farms annually.

Predictably, the majority (75%) of injuries on farms occur during the months of June, July, and August, when farming is at its peak. The case of a

97-year-old farmer killed in a tractor rollover only illustrates that many of the nation's farmers, like all Americans, are getting older.

Owing to the nature of a farm, most farm emergencies are traumatic in nature. The usual mechanisms of injury include machinery, tractor collisions, electrocutions, falling objects, and livestock. However, drowning is the second leading cause of death on the farm for children under 5 years of age.

FARM RESCUE

Farm rescue should be approached similarly to hazardous materials incident planning. A preplan serves as excellent preparation for future emergencies on a farm and should include detailed maps of the farm that outline building location, preplanned staging areas for heavy or special rescue, and Material Safety Data Sheets (MSDS) for chemicals used or stored on the farm.

After identifying farms within their jurisdiction, EMS providers should tour those farms and look for predictable health hazards, such as pesticide depots and feed silos. It can be helpful, especially at night, to have maps with premeasured mileage estimates from major intersections to the farm and global positioning satellite (GPS) coordinates for preplanned helicopter landing zones.

BASIC RESCUE PRINCIPLES

As in all EMS operations, the first rule for the Emergency Medical Technician (EMT) is not to become a victim. There are many cases of would-be rescuers who entered silos or feeding bins, only to become entrapped and suffocate. The EMT should approach every scene cautiously and observe for possible life threats.

When encountering unique situations, such as specialized heavy farm machinery or confined spaces, including open-feed bins, the EMT should call for trained rescue personnel immediately. Time may be critical, especially in a rural situation, and calling for help as early as possible improves the patient's chances for survival.

While awaiting the arrival of these specially trained rescue personnel, the EMT can attempt to reduce, or mitigate, life threats. In some cases, use of barn fans for ventilation of the area can reduce or eliminate toxic or explosive gas, for example, and shutting off power at a central electric panel can disable motors that power augers or belts.

The EMT should consider using an emergency move (Unit 14) such as a long axis clothing drag, to safely extricate the accessible patient. Once the patient is out of harm's way, then the EMT can complete a primary assessment, typically starting with manual stabilization of the cervical spine in cases of trauma.

LIVESTOCK

Many farms have cows, horses, sheep, and other livestock. Livestock has often been referred to as "dumb animals"; however, like all animals, they have a strong intuition for danger and can react unpredictably to avoid perceived harm. When scared or startled, livestock can unintentionally kick, pin, bite, or gore a person who is in their path of escape.

The EMT should never attempt to rescue a patient by getting between the animal and the patient. Animals that appear calm and distant will often suddenly charge without warning when they sense or see what they perceive as a new threat. The patient, who is down in a livestock area, should not be approached until the animal has been secured and is unable to reenter the scene.

As in all cases, the EMT's own safety comes first. Proper personal protective equipment (PPE) includes footwear with a slip-resistant tread, and the

EMT should consider steel-reinforced toes. Rubber firefighter's boots may not prevent falls due to slipping.

Animals also harbor many diseases that are "cross-species" communicable—that is, capable of being transmitted from animal to human—including salmonellosis, ringworm, and rabies. The EMT should consider wearing nonsterile gloves, the kind typically worn during patient care, under a pair of leather-palmed gloves, a pair that can withstand the wear and tear of moving or working with machinery or animals.

Shin guards are also helpful in preventing injuries to the EMT. Athletic shin guards, like the kind worn in soccer, can be put on quickly and may prevent unnecessary injuries.

The EMT should treat every barnyard emergency the same way as any patient encounter, including hand washing after either patient or animal encounter. With proper PPE in place, the EMT needs to remove the animal from the proximity of the patient. This can either be done by moving the animal, which is preferred when trained to do so safely or by removing the patient by using an emergency move.

Animal behavior is similar to human behavior—that is, animals are motivated by thirst, hunger, fear, and a maternal instinct to protect their young. Understanding these behaviors before approaching an animal can help to prevent a tragic mishap.

Animals also have species-specific differences. For example, cows and pigs are color blind and depend on changes in shades to differentiate objects and people. These animals tend to balk at shadows and are startled by sudden changes in light.

Furthermore, these animals lack depth perception. A cow may not even be aware that it has pinned an EMT against the side of a stall. A mature bull can weigh over 2,000 pounds.

The hindquarters of a cow are its blind spots. If an EMT were to approach a cow from the rear, an unexpected and often violent reaction might occur. It is better that the EMT announce his presence and approach the cow from the front. If it is necessary to approach a cow from the back, perhaps because it is tethered to the stall, the EMT should make his presence known in a manner that will not startle the cow. If it is necessary to move the cow, the EMT should get an individual trained in handling farm animals to help move it. Cows know their handlers and are often afraid of strangers. When possible, have the handler isolate and secure all animals away from the scene. Cows have a strong herd instinct and are more apt to follow the herd, as illustrated in Figure 55.1. The EMT should avoid loud sounds, including yelling or banging equipment, because this tends to startle and frighten the cows. The EMT should always have an escape route planned in case an animal charges. An escape route can help prevent the EMT from being pinned against a wall, trampled in a stampede, or gored by a frightened animal.

On the other hand, horses have a keen sense of hearing, are constantly scanning their environment, and will alert EMTs that they are aware of their approach by moving their ears in the direction of the individual approaching. The observant EMT knows when a horse is about to kick, usually rearward, or bite, because the horse will flatten its ears. The EMT should slowly back away from the animal. The EMT who is not familiar with working with horses should wait for someone with experience with horses to deal with the animal.

It is best to approach a horse from the left shoulder and move slowly but confidently toward the horse, all the time talking quietly, not shouting. The EMT should wait for the horse to turn and "address" him in recognition before proceeding any further.

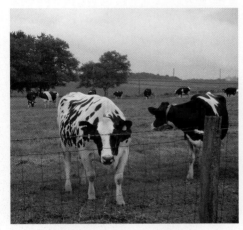

Figure 55.1 Cows are herd animals that can react unpredictably to strangers (Courtesy of Morguefile)

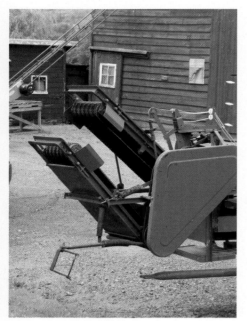

A.

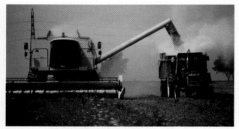

B.

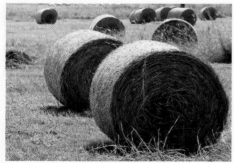

C.

Figure 55.2 A. Belts and pulleys can entangle and mangle limbs. B. Combines can cut a farmer's arm as easily as the crop being harvested (Courtesy of PhotoDisc). C. Hay bales, sometimes weighing hundreds of pounds, can easily crush an arm or leg (Courtesy of Morguefile)

Leading a horse is not difficult if the EMT follows a few simple rules. Always use the lead, not the halter to lead a horse. Grabbing ahold of the halter risks getting the EMT's fingers entrapped in the gear and then being dragged around the yard. With the lead firmly in hand and not wrapped around the fingers, about 8–10 inches away from the horse's head, the EMT should walk deliberately to lead the horse and not the other way around. Once the horse is following the EMT, he should take a position parallel to the horse; horses kick forward and rearward and walking parallel makes it difficult for the horse to kick the EMT.

FARM VEHICLE HEAVY RESCUE

Rescue personnel face many obstacles when managing a farm vehicle rescue. The first obstacle is usually in achieving a primary goal of trauma care—getting the patient to definitive care within an hour. In some cases, just getting to the scene within an hour may be a challenge. Farm accidents tend to happen in remote areas with poor road conditions that make gaining access to the site difficult.

Once on scene, the EMT may have trouble turning off diesel engines; stabilizing heavy equipment that weighs over one ton with standard cribbing; avoiding sharp cutting knives, rollers, and flails; and dealing with spilled fuel and battery acid.

Once the patient is disentangled from the machinery, the EMT must consider how to get the patient out. Although air medical evacuation would seem ideal, it may not be available in some rural areas or in adverse weather conditions, and ambulances have a difficult time traversing the rough terrain.

It should be noted that in some cases, the combination of these factors can change a patient rescue into a body recovery. If this is the case, medical control should be contacted as soon as possible to make on-the-scene decisions and to possibly prevent any injury of the rescuers who might work frantically to rescue a person who has no chance of survival.

MECHANISM OF INJURY

The typical mechanism of injury at a farm rescue involves entanglement in an exposed screw (auger), belt drive, or power takeoff (PTO) drive shaft; being struck by spinning crank handles; or being crushed by shifting loads.

The majority of these accidents are secondary to operator error. In many cases, these accidents could have been prevented by proper footwear preventing slips and falls or properly fitting clothing. Loose clothing, caught in augers, belts, and PTO shafts, is the cause of many farm accidents.

The injuries that an EMT might typically see on scene of a farm accident include severe lacerations, including partial or complete avulsions seen with limb entanglement in a PTO shaft, or limbs caught in exposed belts such as shown in Figure 55.2A. Other injuries are puncture wounds, secondary to impalements on conventional balers, or degloving injuries to hands caught within the rollers of a corn head or the cutting portion of a combine, such as the bean combine shown in Figure 55.2B. Crush injuries occur when heavy loads shift unexpectedly, like when the hay bale in Figure 55.2C is being lifted.

Although these injuries can be grotesque, the bleeding that accompanies them is usually more problematic and may be more life threatening. Therefore, the EMT should avoid focusing on the maimed limb but rather on the overall condition of the patient.

FARM RESCUE PRINCIPLES

Like in vehicle rescue, farm rescue is based on some general principles. First, the EMT should ensure that the scene is rendered as safe as possible and that a perimeter is established to prevent entry of unprotected personnel or bystanders into the scene. An inner action circle and an outer safety perimeter are commonly used. Only those EMTs and rescuers who are properly prepared with PPE are permitted within the inner action circle. The remaining EMTs and rescuers should stand outside the safety perimeter, along with bystanders, until summoned into either inside the outer safety perimeter or into the inner action circle. Needed equipment should be staged inside the outer safety circle, but outside the action circle, until needed.

Once the perimeter has been established, it is important that there be a plan for rescue. Fire rescue and EMS should confer and develop a plan as well as a backup plan in case of failure. Redundancy in planning—that is, a backup plan—helps ensure the overall success of the mission. Many rural emergency services implement the incident management system on the scene of a farm rescue. Refer to Unit 49 for information about incident management.

Often, special equipment may be needed on the scene of a farm rescue and must be requested early. For example, heavy timbers may be needed for cribbing and shoring; these timbers are heavier than the typical cribbing used in vehicular rescue. Special heavy-duty air bags or high-lift jacks may also be needed. In many cases, the availability of front-end loaders and tow trucks make them practical rescue tools. However, only experienced lift operators, in cooperation with trained heavy rescue personnel, should use this equipment.

As a rule, whenever a machine is being lifted, cribbing should be used to protect the patient and the rescuers from shifting loads. Generally, tractors and the like are never lifted by the wheels but rather a firm purchase is made on the frame of the machine directly.

If specialized farm equipment such as a baler or corn pickers are involved, the EMT should consider calling the local farm equipment dealer. These dealers are often expert at dismantling farm equipment; therefore, their emergency numbers should be maintained on board the ambulance or in the rescue truck.

In rare cases in which prolonged disentanglement could jeopardize the patient's life, it may be necessary to perform a field amputation. In those instances, a physician should be called to the scene to stand by and perform the necessary procedures.

It is important for the EMT to understand that disentanglement and extrication are only the first part of a rescue. The patient needs to be evacuated as soon as possible once extrication has occurred. Owing to the nature of these injuries, it is not uncommon to have air medical resources, such as a helicopter, standing by.

Depending on the location of the accident, such as a distant farm field, it may be necessary to have off-road vehicles, such as all-terrain vehicles, available to transport the patient to an awaiting ambulance.

TRACTOR ACCIDENTS

Tractors, first mass produced in 1916, have literally been the workhorse of the farm for almost a century. These machines often have different purposes and come in a variety of sizes and configurations. Many of these machines cost thousands of dollars; therefore, farmers keep these machines in service for many years.

Street Smart

Prolonged periods of compression on an extremity can lead to crush syndrome. The complications of crush syndrome can be eliminated or reduced by applying advanced life support measures before the object is removed.

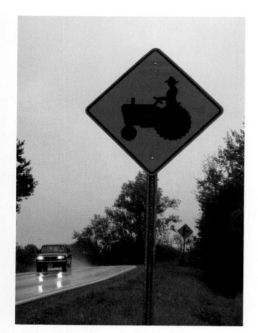

Figure 55.3 Slow-moving farm machinery is no match for high-performance engines in modern cars

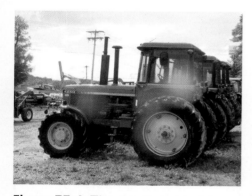

Figure 55.4 The tractor operator has a great deal more protection with a rollover protective structure (ROPS)

Tractor operation represents a dual hazard to the farmer. For one, tractors tend to be involved in collisions with other motor vehicles when they are on the highway. The other danger is that tractors can turn over, or roll over, pinning the driver in the process.

Car–tractor accidents are a reality of rural EMS. Automobile drivers sharing the road with the farmer fail to recognize the slow-moving tractor in time and tend to collide with it. Traveling at high speeds on country roads, the driver of a motor vehicle can suddenly, and unexpectedly, come upon a tractor in the roadway (Figure 55.3). The unfamiliar silhouette of the tractor may momentarily confuse the driver. In addition, the slow speed of the tractor, absent or poorly maintained lighting, or absent, bent, or worn slow-moving vehicle (SMV) emblems, can contribute to tractor/auto collisions.

Other contributing factors include the failure of tractor operators to signal their intentions (e.g., swinging right in a wide-turning radius to go left) and poor visibility. Many tractor accidents occur at dusk when lighting is poor or drivers are blinded by the setting sun.

TRACTOR ROLLOVERS

The single largest contributor to mortality on the farm is tractor rollovers. These rollovers can pin operators under the weight of the tractor and literally crush them.

The majority of tractor rollovers, about 85%, are sideways overturns that occur after the tractor strikes a hard unmovable object, or the tractor is operated on a steep slope where soils can unexpectedly shift.

Although less common, representing about 14% of tractor accidents, rear rollovers, sometimes called a *kickout,* account for more fatalities. When tractors flip in this manner, they tend to trap operators under the tractor or throw them off the tractor. Kickouts tend to occur when a tractor is forward facing a steep slope, such as driving over a hillock, or when a tractor is used to free another tractor that is stuck and a pull cable releases, overturning the tractor.

The advent of farm tractor safety regulations has decreased the incidence of these potentially deadly rollovers. Federal labor standards, for example, have required that new tractors, manufactured after 1976, have a **rollover protective structure (ROPS)** in place to protect the operator. ROPS is a protective bar or canopy, as shown in Figure 55.4, that prevents the driver from being crushed under the weight of the tractor.

Problems occur when older tractors, predating 1976, are still in service and in use by inexperienced operators or when the farmer has removed the ROPS. In many cases, these older tractors are being operated by younger, inexperienced operators who do not know how to respond when the tractor rolls or kicks back. A tractor without ROPS is shown in Figure 55.5.

When an EMT arrives on the scene of a tractor rollover, the first priority, in terms of scene safety, is fire suppression. Spilled fuels can easily ignite, causing a fire; a fire extinguisher or charged fire hose should be at standby at all times.

Next is to turn off the tractor. Many rescuers start by immediately blocking the wheels. Turning wheels can inadvertently restart a diesel engine. If the tractor engine operates on gasoline, then the engine can simply be shut off by the key. If the tractor engine operates on diesel fuel, then the injector pump stop rod should be engaged. If the diesel engine continues to idle, called *dieseling,* then it may be necessary to "choke" the engine. This can be accomplished by either stuffing a rag down the air intake or by discharging a carbon dioxide fire extinguisher into the air cleaner.

With the tractor turned off, the rescuers should turn their attention to the patient. The two options are to either lift the tractor off the patient or to dig the patient out. It usually takes a tow truck, hydraulic jacks, or heavy rescue air bags to lift a small tractor. In some cases, a small tractor can be lifted manually. The general rule of rescue is to "crib as you go"—that is, to build a frame of wooden blocks that prevents the tractor from shifting and falling back on the patient. These rescues should be performed only by trained farm rescuers who have practiced their techniques and know their equipment.

Alternatively, the rescuers may elect to dig the patient out. Digging the patient is used whenever a patient is entrapped under a heavy machine. Initially, the tractor must be firmly stabilized, similar to a motor vehicle, with cribbing, timbers, and the like. To prevent cave-ins, the "foot print" of the cribbing must be as wide as possible, and ancillary cribbing should be in place in case of soil shifting. Again, these rescue techniques should be used only by experienced and trained farm rescuers.

Once the patient has been disentangled and extricated, the EMT will often find a predictable injury pattern. Because of the mechanism of injury, a crushed pelvis is common; about 80% of tractor accidents result in a crushed pelvis. A crushed pelvis may be managed by either a pelvic sling or application of a pneumatic anti-shock garment (PASG), as noted in Unit 38.

Trauma to the chest may cause a collapsed lung, or pneumothorax, as well as massive contusions to the chest. Entrapped patients may also experience burns from the host of liquids present, including radiator fluids, hydraulic fluids, battery acid, and the calcium chloride mixture found in the tires. As much as 100–150 gallons of calcium chloride is placed inside the tractor's tires to provide weight (as much as 1,500 pounds) and therefore stability to the tractor. The EMT should take protective measures to prevent accidental exposure/contact.

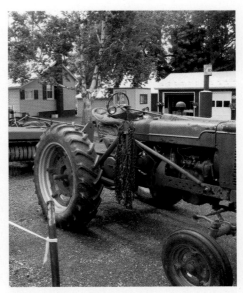

Figure 55.5 Operators of older tractors without ROPS, such as the one pictured here, are at risk for being entrapped and crushed

POWER TAKEOFF

The **power takeoff (PTO),** developed in the 1920s, permits farmers to use their tractor as a portable power supply. A PTO is a spinning shaft that transfers the tractor engine's power to another farm machine, such as a hay baler. The PTO is a versatile tool for providing power to augers that move manure or feed up elevators, to lift and move hay or feed, and to power post-hole diggers.

Traditionally, a PTO is found at the rear of the tractor, above the drawbars that are used to pull a machine behind the tractor. However, newer tractors may have a PTO at the front of the tractor as well.

A tractor PTO is not limited to farm use. Suburban landscapers, lawn maintenance workers, and everyday homeowners can own a tractor with a PTO. Snowblowers are powered by the engine via a PTO that is found in the front of the machine.

Early models of tractors had no shield over the PTO, and the operator could see the shaft and the universal joint connection spinning. These open PTOs presented a clear danger to the operator (Figure 55.6). Newer models had a U-shaped shield that protected the shaft from above while permitting access to the shaft, for service and maintenance, from below. The newest PTO has a circumferential shield that prevents accidental contact with the spinning shaft.

The PTO revolves in a clockwise fashion, facing the rear of the tractor, and has different speeds; in smaller tractors the PTO spins at 540 revolutions per minute (rpm), or 9 revolutions per second, and larger tractors at

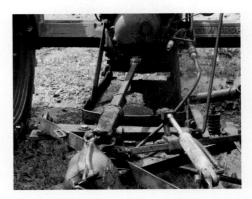

Figure 55.6 An unshielded power takeoff (PTO), spinning as fast as 1,000 rpm, can tear a limb off

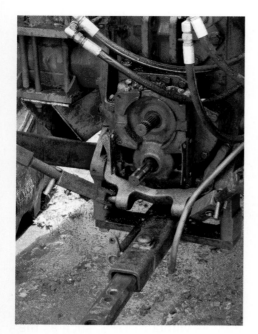

Figure 55.7 PTOs can spin at low speed (540 rpm) or high speed (1,000 rpm)

1,000 rpm. Figure 55.7 shows a tractor with two PTOs, one high speed and one low speed.

Accidents occur whenever a piece of clothing or hair becomes entangled in the PTO, when the operator either leans over the PTO or steps over it to get to the other side of the tractor.

The predictable injury pattern from this entanglement includes severe lacerations, particularly to the face if a beard becomes entangled; fractures of the arms and legs, as sleeves, pant legs, or boot laces become entangled and the operator is literally spun around the shaft, striking tractor hitches, equipment tongues, and the ground with terrific force with each revolution; or degloving injuries, where all or part of the genitals are avulsed when the operator steps over the PTO, a straddle injury. If the body is not heavy enough to stall the engine, then the body is repeatedly pounded against the ground, resulting in significant spine injuries.

The principles of farm rescue from a PTO are similar to a tractor rollover: secure the scene, turn off the tractor, and block the wheels to prevent rolling.

When these tasks have been accomplished, the EMT should then proceed with disentangling the patient from the PTO. To properly disentangle the patient often requires that the PTO be either disassembled, which is preferable and requires the expertise of the local farm agent, or cut. It is imperative that trained rescuers, with the proper tools, be called early.

In some cases it may be possible to disentangle the patient from the machine manually. In those cases, the PTO must be placed in neutral and disconnected from the tractor. Then a large pipe wrench or crowbar is placed inside the yoke of the PTO and turned counterclockwise. The rescuers should never use the power of the tractor to reverse the PTO.

If the rescuers are unable to disentangle the patient from the shaft or joints of the PTO, it may be necessary to cut the shaft. Solid shafts may be cut with power grinders or hacksaws. The use of the oxyacetylene cutting torch should be reserved to trained rescue specialists. These torches produce heat that can be transferred up the shaft to the patient, causing significant burns in the process.

Disentangling a patient from a PTO can be difficult. The PTO shaft that was under a load may suddenly release, further injuring the patient and possibly the EMT. Therefore, this type of rescue should be performed by trained farm rescuers.

SILOS

Silos are structures that store **silage** (forage, or food, typically stored in the silo) such as chopped corn, alfalfa, and chopped grass. Silos can be either horizontal, sometimes called bunker silos, or vertical. The vertical silo is the more traditional one that is seen in pictures of farms.

A traditional silo is between 12 and 14 feet in diameter, with large silos as large as 20–30 feet in diameter and up to 80 feet in height. A silo is actually rings of concrete blocks that raise one on top of another and are held in place by steel-retaining rings. The top of the roof is usually open with a weather cap, and feed is fed into the silo via a chute by a blower. Figure 55.8 shows a traditional silo.

New silage, depending on variables such as the time of year, feed, or weather may have between 45% and 70% moisture content. When stored in a confined space, this silage uses all of the available oxygen to ferment the sugar in it until it produces lactic acid, which stops the fermentation process and permits the silage to be stored for long periods of time. During this process certain gases, commonly referred to as silo gases, are created.

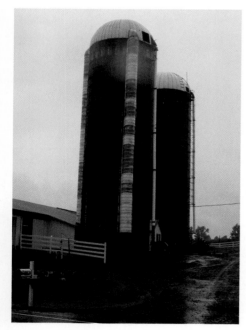

Figure 55.8 Traditional silos usually have an open roof with an aluminum weather cap

Chief among these silo gases is nitrogen dioxide (NO_2). NO_2 is an irritating brownish gas with a bleach-like odor that is heavier than air. The danger of NO_2 is greatest approximately 2 weeks after the silo is filled. The danger of NO_2 is that it is heavier than air and therefore tends to displace oxygen, in effect making the silo an oxygen-poor environment. A farmer who falls into a silo during this period is in danger of suffocating to death. Clues for the presence of NO_2 include dead birds at the chutes and brownish stains on the sides of the silos (Figure 55.9).

Newer silos may be constructed of steel and are glass-lined (Figure 55.10). These silos are built to eliminate or reduce the oxygen within a silo and are thus called oxygen-limiting silos. Although these oxygen-limiting silos eliminate the dangers of toxic silo gases seen in more traditional silos, they can be equally dangerous. As the name implies, an oxygen-limiting silo provides an oxygen-poor environment, similar to the type of environment encountered in confined space rescue.

Silo rescues, both traditional silos as well as oxygen-limiting silos, should be handled like a confined space rescue. There are cases of multiple victims during a silo rescue because each would-be rescuer who is not properly equipped with self-contained breathing apparatus (SCBA) becomes unconscious from the lack of oxygen and then suffocates.

Another common silo emergency is entrapment. Farmers may enter a silo to clean a chute or to loosen packed silage. Although settled silage can be firm enough to walk on, new silage has not compacted and the farmer is in danger of being engulfed in it.

On the scene of such an emergency, the EMT should first use any ventilation fans that are available to clear dangerous silo gases. The fact that the victim is still alive is a good indication that sufficient oxygen is available. However, the EMT should not take any chances and SCBA is strongly recommended.

If the victim is visible, it may be possible to drop a rope or reach him or her with a pike pole. The victim should be encouraged to self-rescue if possible. Under no circumstances should the EMT enter the silo without a

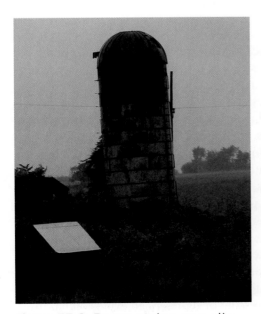

Figure 55.9 Brown stains on a silo can indicate the presence of nitrogen dioxide (NO_2)

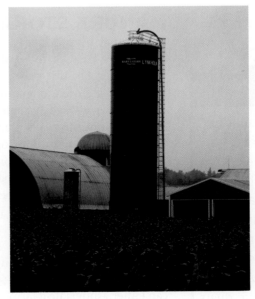

Figure 55.10 Steel blue silos may be oxygen-limiting silos and should be treated as confined space rescues

safety/recovery system in place. Only rescuers who are properly equipped and trained in silo rescue should enter a silo.

If the victim is firmly entrapped, it may be necessary to create cuts at the base of the silo to allow the silage to drain. These cuts, made with a corner of the bucket of a front-end loader, should be made perpendicular to one another to maintain the structural integrity of the silo. Otherwise, if too many holes are cut into the silo, there is a risk of collapse that would entrap the victim.

GRAIN BINS

Grain bins, while appearing open, are deceptive, and farmers can be entrapped in much the same way that they can be entrapped in a silo. Initially, the grain starts to flow, engulfing the farmer's feet. If the farmer is submerged up to the knees, there is little hope of escape and the farmer can be submerged in an avalanche of feed grain in as little as 10 seconds after that.

Like an avalanche, the EMT should assume that the victim is still alive, even if not visible, and continue to talk to the victim. Although this psychological first aid is important, it also helps identify where the victim is in the pile.

If the grain bin has gravity gates, do not open them. There is a danger that the victim will be entrapped in the gates as the river of grain flows out of the bin. Similarly, power augers should not be used to drain the grain bin because the victim may get entangled inside the auger mechanism.

If the victim is partially submerged and visible to rescuers, then self-rescue should be encouraged. A barrel, opened at both ends, can be lowered over the victim to act as a dam. Trained rescuers may create a plywood square that surrounds the victim, allowing him to dig his way out of the grain without danger of further entrapment.

If the victim is completely submerged, then pairs of rescuers, in a buddy system, who are tied in with safety harnesses and rope systems may enter the grain bin to attempt a rescue.

Under no circumstances should the EMT enter the grain bin without proper training and safety equipment. Grain can be unpredictable, sliding and shifting when least expected and entrapping the EMT.

MANURE STORAGE

A common by-product of livestock is manure. Animal manure, like most things on a farm, is not wasted; it is rich in nitrogen and is therefore a natural fertilizer. For this reason, manure is usually mixed with water to become slurry and is stored in a manure system.

Manure storage systems can be either above ground or below ground. Above-ground storage systems can include large manure storage tanks, silo-type storage structures, or open pools of manure called lagoons or manure ponds. These manure lagoons can be particularly dangerous. Over time the top of the manure lagoon hardens, sometimes to the point that grass grows over the top, and an unsuspecting person will walk on the cap, crumbling it, and the person will drown in the manure. For this reason manure lagoons should be fenced off.

Below-ground manure storage systems can be more dangerous than above-ground systems. Manure gases—that is, gases produced by bacteria breaking down the manure—can build to dangerous levels. These manure gases can either asphyxiate a farmer or a rescuer or represent an explosion hazard.

It is important that the EMT be aware of gases that may be present on scene and maintain a safe distance from the scene until adequate ventilation can ensure clearance of these gases. Until the gases are cleared, any source of ignition, either electronic (e.g., portable radios) or mechanical (e.g., cigarette lighters), should not be used in the vicinity.

If entry must be made into an underground storage facility, only those rescuers with SCBA should be permitted to enter. Standard N95 or dust/mist masks do not filter out gases and will not protect the EMT. Confined space rescue such as this should only be performed by trained rescuers who have SCBA and safety harnesses.

TOXIC MANURE GAS

The danger for explosion from manure gas is from methane, an odorless gas that is lighter than air, a by-product of decomposition of manure. Because methane is odorless, the EMT must have a high index of suspicion for its potential presence and take appropriate protective actions, including maintaining a safe distance, preventing ignition, and awaiting proper ventilation.

The danger of other manure gases is that they displace oxygen and asphyxiate the victim. These manure gases include hydrogen sulfide (H_2S), ammonia (NH_3), and carbon dioxide (CO_2). In 1989, a 28-year-old farmer went into a 10-foot-deep manure pit to repair an agitator shaft and was quickly overcome by manure gases. His 15-year-old nephew attempted to rescue him, only to meet the same fate. This pattern continued until the farmer, his nephew, and three other would-be rescuers lay at the bottom of the pit. The rescue squad arrived 20 minutes later, and all five family members were dead. This story helps to illustrate the clear danger that manure gases present to rescuers.

A common manure gas is hydrogen sulfate (H_2S), considered by many to be the most dangerous. H_2S has the characteristic smell of rotten eggs. Although it may seem obvious to the EMT that H_2S is present, the constant exposure to the smell, in small nonlethal quantities, dulls the farmer's awareness of its presence until the levels are dangerously high.

Another manure gas, NH_3, has effects similar to those of H_2S and its characteristic smell can be noted at much lower concentrations. CO_2 is odorless and simply displaces the oxygen in the environment.

All of these heavier-than-air gases displace oxygen, creating an oxygen-poor environment, and the patient, can become hypoxic and lose consciousness. Early symptoms of hypoxia can include headache, nausea, and dizziness. The key to survival is early recognition of these symptoms. Failure to do so can lead to collapse and worsening hypoxia as the patient is now lying at the level of the greatest concentration of toxic gases.

FARM CHEMICALS

Farmers use a large number of pesticides, herbicides, and fertilizers to improve production of foodstuffs. These products are all chemicals, and exposure to any one of them should be treated as a hazardous material exposure. For example, a few drops of methyl parathion on the skin can be deadly.

One of the more common farm chemicals is anhydrous ammonia. Anhydrous ammonia is infused into the soil as a ready source of nitrogen for plants. Anhydrous ammonia is a double danger: (1) it is a toxic substance, and (2) it is transported as a liquid under pressure. An accidental release of anhydrous ammonia into the environment and onto the skin of the farmer can instantly freeze the skin. It will also dehydrate the skin—*an-* means "without" and -*hydrous* means "water"—causing permanent damage to the skin. Treatment for an exposure to anhydrous ammonia includes flushing with copious volumes of water and then treating the exposed skin like a burn.

Other common farm chemicals are a class of chemicals called *organo-phosphates* (OP). Since their introduction as an insecticide by a chemist for the Bayer Pharmaceutical Company in the 1880s, these chemicals, including parathion, diazinion, and malathion, have been widely used as insecticides by many farmers. Unfortunately, OP was, like many other chemicals, weaponized during World War I into chemical gas compounds such as sarin, soman, and tabun. These chemical weapons have recently resurfaced, after a treaty banning their use was signed by major world governments, as a terrorist weapon. Sarin, for example, was used in a deadly terrorist attack by the Aum Shinrikyo sect in the Tokyo subway system.

The symptom pattern for OP exposure on the farm is the same as the one for exposure to chemical weapons. The mnemonic SLUDGEM, presented previously in Table 51-2, lists these common symptoms. Similarly, the treatment for exposure on the farm is the same, involving the use of atropine. Atropine use for OP chemical exposure is also described in Unit 51.

In every case in which an EMT is confronted with a patient who may have had an exposure to a farm chemical, the EMT should treat the exposure as a hazardous materials spill, including wearing appropriate protective equipment and attempting to identify the chemical. *The Emergency Response Guidebook* to hazardous materials can provide valuable information, and the EMT can also call the Poison Control Center, as local or regional protocols dictate.

CONCLUSION

Farming can be one of the most dangerous occupations in the United States. It can also be one of the most rewarding and important occupations, and for this reason farmers will always be a valued segment of the American workforce.

It is therefore predictable that farm accidents will occur and the EMT will be called to the scene. Although the majority of these EMS calls can be professionally managed with the training and skills of an average EMT, some instances require the assistance of specially trained rescuers. Any EMT whose primary jurisdiction includes farmland should consider taking a farm rescue course to be prepared for any situation that might arise.

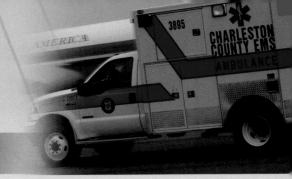

CASE STUDY Continued

Christopher has Ahman begin the primary assessment of Roger while he looks at the PTO shaft and the extent of the entanglement. Christopher has vast experience with PTO shafts, having been raised on the farm, and knows if Janis hadn't gotten the clutch disengaged as quickly as she did, Roger's leg might have been completely avulsed. Roger's leg is twisted at an angle that indicates it is probably fractured, but there is not a lot of external bleeding at this time. Christopher knows that will probably change when his leg is no longer compressed by the shaft.

Roger is answering questions appropriately and in obvious pain. Ahman had requested air medical immediately on arrival, and the local volunteer rescue squad has just arrived. Christopher knows several of them have experience with PTO rescue.

Ahman has one of the volunteer first responders maintain cervical spinal stabilization after applying a c-collar in preparation for moving Roger to a long spine board as soon as his leg is untangled. Janis is sitting on the ground next to her husband's head, holding his hand and talking quietly to him.

Christopher has himself positioned to stabilize the leg as soon as it is released. A couple rescuers begin turning the PTO shaft counterclockwise and Christopher can feel the leg beginning to become untangled. As the shaft continues to be turned, Roger's leg suddenly releases and Christopher immediately stabilizes the twisted leg so it doesn't move anymore than necessary.

As Roger is moved onto the long spine board, the flight crew arrives from the helicopter that landed farther down in the field. Christopher finds a weak pulse in Roger's foot and, after placing dressings on the exposed lacerations, stabilizes the leg in a vacuum splint to lessen movement of the exposed bone.

Roger is still conscious and talking, but weak at the time the air medical crew takes over care, quickly moving him to the helicopter to provide IV fluids and pain medication, as they transport him to the closest trauma center 20 minutes away by air. Christopher and Ahman are thankful the helicopter was able to come to the scene because it would have taken them well over an hour to get Roger to the trauma center by ground.

Key Concepts Revisited

- Most farm injuries are traumatic injuries involving diverse mechanisms of injury.
    - Machinery
    - Tractor collisions
    - Electrocutions
    - Falling objects
    - Livestock
    - Toxic inhalations
    - Drowning
- The general principles of farm rescue begin with preplanning and local risk management.
    - Identify farm jurisdictions
    - Locate specific hazards
    - Preplan helicopter landing zones
- Basic rescue principles involve calling for trained individuals as soon as possible.
    - Turn off power
    - Ensure ventilation
- Dealing with livestock can pose a variety of dangers for the rescuer.
    - Injuries from bites, kicks, pinning, or goring
    - Cross-species communicable diseases
    - Animal vision concerns

- The hazards of farm machinery range from heavy-duty machinery to power takeoff accessory machinery.
  - Heavy-duty machines
  - Cutting knives
  - Rollers
  - Hazardous fluids and fuels
- Farm rescue principles begin with the general principles of technical rescue with adjustments for farm-specific mechanism of injury.
  - Entanglement
    - Augers
    - Belt drives
    - Power takeoff shaft
  - Stuck by machinery objects
- The injuries from farm machinery can include avulsions, crush injuries, drowning, falls, and toxic exposures.
  - Severe lacerations
  - Partial or complete avulsions
  - Puncture wounds
  - Crush injuries
  - Massive bleeding
  - Fractures

- Tractor accidents can be MVC involving other vehicles or rollovers.
  - Road collisions with cars
  - Rollover with no rollover protection structure
  - Fire
  - Pinned under tractor
- Power takeoff (PTO) shafts entangle any loose clothing or hair and can cause severe traumatic injuries with massive bleeding.
- The dangers of silo rescue involve the potential inhalation of toxic silo gas by the rescuer.
  - Treat as confined space
  - Asphyxiation danger to rescuer
    - Hydrogen sulfate
    - Ammonia
    - Carbon dioxide
- Hazardous materials found on a farm can include farm chemicals used as insecticides and fertilizers.
  - Anhydrous ammonia
  - Organophosphates

Review Questions

1. What are some common mechanisms of injury on a farm?
2. When do most farm injuries occur?
3. What are the general principles of farm rescue?
4. What hazards do livestock represent?
5. What are the hazards of farm machinery?
6. What are the injuries that can be seen from entanglement with the power takeoff of a tractor?
7. What are the dangers of silo rescue?
8. How might rescuers be injured in grain bin rescues?
9. What gases may be found in a manure storage facility?
10. What dangerous chemicals can be found on a farm?

Key Terms

Power TakeOff (PTO)
Rollover protective structure (ROPS)
Silage

Silos
Toxic organic dust syndrome (TODS)

Further Study

Desafey Liller, Karen. *Injury Prevention for Children and Adolescents: Research, Practice, and Advocacy.* Washington, DC: American Public Health Association, 2006.

Glasgow, Nina, Nan Johnson, and Lois Wright Morton. *Critical Issues in Rural Health.* Hoboken, NJ: Wiley-Blackwell, 2004.

Jones, R. *Textbook of Primary Medical Care.* New York: Oxford University Press.

Glossary

A

abandoned infant protection act State law permitting mother to relinquish care of a newborn to a safe haven such as a fire station or rescue squad.

abandonment Situation in which a care provider assumes responsibility for an incapacitated person and then leaves the patient unsupervised.

ABCs Techniques involved in assessing airway, breathing, and circulation.

abdominal aortic aneurysm (AAA) A weakened area of the aortic wall resulting in a ballooning of the vessel within the abdomen.

abdominal cavity The space between the chest and the pelvis that contains the organs of digestion and elimination.

abdominal thrusts Forceful application of pressure to the upper abdomen, toward the chest, in an attempt to expel a foreign body from the airway.

abduction Movement away from the body.

abortion Premature termination of a pregnancy.

abrasion Superficial scrape to the skin.

absence seizure seizure characterized by a blank or vacant (absent) stare lasting a few seconds.

acceleration/deceleration Injuries caused by the brain continuing to move back and forth inside the skull after the head has come to a sudden stop.

accessory muscles of respiration Neck, chest, and abdominal muscles that can be used to assist in respiration in times of distress.

accessory muscle use Muscles of the shoulder girdle and chest wall used in addition to the intercostal muscles and the diaphragm in an attempt to improve the flow of air in and out of the lungs in respiratory distress.

acetabulum The socket in the pelvis where the proximal femur meets the pelvis.

acme When an infection reaches its peak.

acquired immunodeficiency syndrome (AIDS) A group of symptoms, or syndrome, that results from the HIV infection.

acrocyanosis Cyanosis of the extremities.

acromioclavicular (A/C) dislocation Separation of the shoulder and clavicle.

action The effect of a medication on the person who takes it.

activated charcoal Suspension of charcoal in a liquid that has the ability to bind most ingested toxins and prevent their absorption.

active listening An effort to listen for the meaning of a patient's statements.

active rewarming Actions taken to increase body temperature.

activities of daily living (ADLs) Normal functions of self-care that people must be able to perform to live on their own, such as eating, toileting, and dressing.

acute coronary syndrome (ACS) Continuum of conditions affecting blood flow to the heart, including angina and acute myocardial infarction.

acute mountain sickness (AMS) Adverse reaction to high altitude in unacclimated individuals.

acute myocardial infarction (AMI) The death of heart muscle due to an inadequate supply of oxygen-rich blood (hypoperfusion).

acute stress Single event that creates a stress response.

acute stress reaction: Exaggerated response due to sympathetic stimulation

adenosine triphosphate (ATP) High-energy fuel molecule the cells need to function

addiction Physical need the body has developed for a drug.

adduction Movement toward the body.

advance directive A method to make a patient's wishes about resuscitation known to family and health care providers before the patient becomes incapacitated.

advanced cardiac life support (ACLS) Complex procedures used to treat sudden cardiac death or acute coronary syndrome; typically performed by an ALS provider (i.e., advanced EMTs and paramedics).

Advanced Emergency Medical Technician (AEMT) Emergency Medical Technician who can provide basic emergency care but can also provide some advanced emergency medical care such as advanced airway management, intravenous therapy, and basic medications.

advanced life support (ALS) A broad term applied to emergency medical care rendered beyond basic life support, the hallmark of which is usually special tools and procedures.

advanced lividity Pooling of blood in the dependent portions of the body with a clear line of demarcation.

AEIOU TIPS Mnemonic used to remember the causes of altered mental status: alcohol, epilepsy, insulin, oxygen/overdose, uremia, trauma, infection, psychiatric, and stroke.

aerobic metabolism Process of metabolizing glucose using oxygen that produces large amounts of energy for the cells to use.

affidavit Written testimony.

afterdrop Drop in core body temperature as a result of peripheral vasodilation and shunting of cool blood to the body center during active rewarming of the severely hypothermic patient.

afterload Amount of force the ventricle must overcome to provide blood flow through the circulatory system.

against medical advice (AMA) Patient's refusal of medical care despite a great risk of loss of limb or life.

age of majority Age at which a person may act without parental permission and is generally treated as an adult.

agitated delirium (AD) or excited delirium Combination of agitation, violent or bizarre behavior, insensitivity to pain, elevated body temperature, or increased strength.

air embolism Air that has gotten into a blood vessel, resulting in a blockage of blood flow.

air hunger The feeling a person may have if his or her oxygen level is low or he or she is unable to effectively breathe; indicated by mouth breathing.

airway The passageway for air movement into and out of the lungs.

alert Term used to describe the mental status of a patient who is awake and interacting with his or her environment.

all clear An order that means that nothing, not even the bag-valve-mask, should touch the patient.

allergen A substance that causes an exaggerated response of the immune system (allergic reaction).

allergic reaction An exaggerated response of the immune system upon exposure to a particular substance.

altered mental state A change in behavior due to illness or disease.

alveolar-capillary gas exchange The movement of gases between alveoli and adjacent capillaries.

alveolar ventilation Amount of inhaled air that reaches the alveoli in the lungs for gas exchange.

alveoli Tiny air sacs in the lungs that allow exchange of carbon dioxide and oxygen.

Alzheimer's disease A progressive, irreversible deterioration of intellectual function.

ambulances volante Literally meaning "flying ambulances," these vehicles, considered to be the first ambulances, were used by Baron Larrey in the Napoleonic War era to retrieve injured soldiers.

American Academy of Emergency Physicians (ACEP) Association of physicians, specializing in emergency medicine, that was formed in 1968.

American Ambulance Association (AAA) National group that represents ambulance service owners that provide service to 75% of the American population.

American Heart Association (AHA) National group of citizens, physicians, and allied health care professionals dedicated to reducing death and disability from cardiovascular disease.

American Red Cross (ARC) Relief organization founded by Clara Barton in the Civil War era; has played a large role in training civilians and rescuers in first aid and CPR.

amniotic sac The membranous sac that surrounds the fetus and placenta within the uterus.

amputation Cutting off of an extremity.

amyotrophic lateral sclerosis (ALS) Neuromuscular disease caused by the degeneration of motor neurons; also known as Lou Gehrig's disease.

anabolism Process of metabolism requiring energy that builds larger molecules by combining smaller molecules.

anaerobic metabolism Process of metabolizing glucose without oxygen that produces minimal energy.

anaphylactic shock Allergic reaction to an allergen characterized by a severe inflammatory response.

anaphylaxis Exaggerated allergic reaction that can result in life-threatening airway, breathing, or circulatory compromise.

anatomy Study of the structure of an organism.

angina Pain or discomfort that results from insufficient oxygenated blood flow to the heart muscle.

angle of Louis The bony ridge where the manubrium meets the body of the sternum; also called the sternal angle.

anisocoria Unequal pupils.

anoxeria Absence of appetite.

anoxia No oxygen.

antecubital fossa Anterior surface of the elbow, in the bend of the arm.

anterior Directional term referring to a location toward the front.

antibodies Specialized defense particles within the blood that help to protect against foreign material.

anticonvulsant Any drug intended to control or prevent seizures.

antidote Substance that counteracts or neutralizes the effects of a poison or toxic substance.

antioxidants Photochemical metabolite found in plants that deactivates free radicals.

anus The end of the digestive tract, which allows for exit of solid wastes.

anxiety disorder Inappropriate or exaggerated response that is abnormal in relation to the situation, formerly called *neurosis*.

aorta Largest artery in the body, which carries blood from the left ventricle of the heart out to the rest of the body.

aortic valve Final valve in the heart that regulates blood flow from the heart into the aorta and the systemic circulation.

apex The point of a triangle; a directional term used to describe the top of the lungs or the bottom tip of the heart.

Apgar Predictive score for measuring the health of newborns at 1 and 5 minutes immediately following birth.

apnea Lack of breathing; breathlessness.

appendicitis Inflammation/infection of the appendix often characterized by the presence of right lower quadrant pain.

appendicular skeleton Bony extremities composed of the shoulder girdle, arms, pelvic girdle, and legs.

appendix Small saclike portion of the large intestine that may become inflamed in a condition called appendicitis.

arachnoid Weblike middle protective membrane covering the brain and spinal cord.

arm pull Patient movement technique in which the EMT grasps the wrists of the patient, pulls the arms to the patient's chest, and drags the patient by the arms.

arterial bleeding Bleeding from an artery, usually under pressure that can be life threatening.

arteries Vessels that carry blood away from the heart; with the exception of the pulmonary artery, they carry oxygenated blood.

arterioles Smaller arteries that supply blood to the capillaries.

arteriorvenous (AV) shunt Bridge or shunt between the artery and vein, usually in the arm, which permits access several times a week to be connected to the hemodialyzer, the machine used to clean the blood.

arteriosclerosis Group of diseases characterized by a loss of elasticity and thickening of artery wall.

arthritis Decrease in the flexibility of joints along with an inflammation within those joints.

artificial pacemaker Man-made electronic device that creates the electrical impulse signaling the heart to beat.

artificial ventilation Method of providing oxygen to a patient who is not effectively breathing; also known as *rescue breathing*.

ascending spinothalmic tracts Nerve fiber bundles that send sensations to the brain.

aspiration Term meaning "to draw into"; refers to foreign material inadvertently being drawn into the airway during inspiration.

aspirin-induced asthma (AIA) Sensitivity to aspirin that some patients exhibit that can progress to an asthma attack.

assault In civil law, refers to placing a person in fear of being touched through an attempt at treatment without the person's having given consent to do so.

asthma Condition consisting of bronchospasm and inflammation in response to multiple stimuli; also known as *reactive airway disease*.

asystole Flatline ECG of the heart in cardiac standstill.

atheromas: Deposits of fat; also called plaques.

atherosclerosis Disease of arteriosclerosis characterized by plaque build-up on the walls of arteries causing narrowing and potential occlusion of blood flow.

atlanto–occipital dislocation Movement of the head off of the neck.

atlantoaxial instability First two cervical vertebrae are unstable due to weak ligaments, which can cause neck pain and weakness (commonly seen in individuals with Down Syndrome).

atlas The first cervical vertebrae that holds the head.

atrial fibrillation Unorganized impulses in the atrial of the heart.

atrioventricular (AV) node Node of specialized cardiac conduction fibers that slow the electrical impulse as it moves from the atria to the ventricles to allow for the mechanical contraction of the heart to catch up to its electrical activity; primarily influenced by the vagus nerve of the parasympathetic nervous system.

atrium Small receiving chamber, one on each side of the heart, that empties blood into its corresponding ventricles to be pumped out of the heart; plural: atria.

auditory hallucination A false perception of the sensation of the ears; hearing something that is not actually there.

aura Sensation or awareness that a seizure is about to begin.

auscultate Term that means to listen.

autism Part of a group of disorders (Autism Spectrum Disorders) characterized by social interaction deficit, impaired communication (verbal and nonverbal),severely limited range of activities and interests of play, and repetitive, obsessive behaviors.

auto launch Practice of a helicopter launching toward a scene based on certain dispatch criteria.

autolysis Biological self-destruction of cells.

automated external defibrillator (AED) Defibrillator that can "read" the ECG using a logic algorithm stored in a microprocessor; advise the EMT to "shock," or defibrillate; and then deliver that shock to the patient.

automatic implantable cardioverter/defibrillator (AICD) Defibrillator that can be placed within the body.

automatic transport ventilator (ATV) Positive pressure ventilation device that delivers ventilations automatically.

automaticity Ability of the myocardium to self-pace.

autonomic nervous system Collection of nerves that originates in the brainstem and transmits impulses to many organs to allow for many basic body functions.

AVPU Abbreviation to remember the classifications of mental status: alert, voice, pain, and unresponsive.

avulsion Forceful separation of an extremity.

awareness level Ability of EMTs to recognize a hazard, know how to protect themselves, and know how to activate the emergency preplan for such an event.

axial distraction Separation of the spinal vertebrae.

axial loading Compression of the spine by force from above.

axial skeleton Bony skeleton that forms the axis of the support structure of the body; includes the skull, spinal column, and thoracic cage.

axilla Armpit.

axis Second cervical vertebra around which the atlas sits and may rotate.

B

back care Regular back exercises along with practice in proper lifting techniques and use of certain lift assist devices.

back injury Any injury of the muscles, tendons, or ligaments that arms to form a seat.

back slaps Firm blows administered to an infant's upper back in an attempt to expel a foreign body from the airway.

bacteremia Bacteria in the blood.

bag-valve-mask (BVM) Device consisting of a refilling bag, a one-way valve, and a mask that is used to ventilate a patient.

bandage Strip of cloth applied to a wound.

bariatric medicine The branch of medicine that deals with the diagnosis and treatment of problems of obesity.

bariatric stretchers Special ambulance stretchers designed to carry patients over 700 pounds.

baroreceptors Stretch receptors located in the carotid arteries and aortic arch that send messages to increase or decrease systemic vascular resistance and cardiac output based on the change in blood pressure.

barotraumas Trauma caused by rapid or extreme changes in air pressure.

base Directional term used to describe the bottom of an object, such as a triangle.

base station Main radio transmitter used in a system, frequently located at the base of operations.

baseline vital signs First set of vital signs obtained, used to compare the following sets.

basic life support (BLS) Broad term applied to those skills that can be performed by either a citizen or an EMT with a minimum of specialized equipment.

basilar skull fracture Break at the base of the skull (the area behind the face).

basket stretcher Type of stretcher, such as the Stokes basket, that will allow complete immobilization of the patient and protection during a move over rough terrain.

battery In civil law, refers to touching a person without his or her consent.

battle's sign Bruising behind the ears on the mastoid process; indicates a fracture of the skull.

beats per minute (bpm) Measurement of the rate of the heart.

bedroll Stretcher linens wrapped around the patient during transport.

behavioral disability Condition that affects how a child interacts with people, things, and his or her environment.

behavioral emergency Any situation in which a patient exhibits a behavior that is unacceptable or intolerable to one's self, family, or the community.

biceps muscle The muscle that allows flexion of the arm at the elbow; antagonist to the triceps muscle.

bilateral Directional term used to describe points on both sides of the body.

biohazard Short for "biological hazard," refers to any material that is considered unsafe because of contamination with body fluids.

biological agents Live organisms or natural substances that can kill or incapacitate.

bipolar disorder Psychiatric disorder characterized by cyclic mood changes, ranging from extreme elation to severe depression; also known as manic-depressive disorder.

bipolar traction splint Traction splint with a double shaft.

black widow spider Poisonous spider that is black with a red hourglass mark on the abdomen.

bladder Organ in the pelvis that stores urine as it is made by the kidneys.

blading Defensive sideways stance that minimizes body exposure.

blanket drag Method of moving patient in which the EMT logrolls the patient onto a blanket, sheet, or drape, then grasps a handful of blanket and drags the patient to safety.

blood Made of several types of cells; fluid that carries fuels and wastes around the body for distribution and removal as appropriate.

blood pressure Pressure placed on the walls of blood vessels by the circulatory system.

blood vessels Structures through which blood travels around the body.

bloody show Expulsion of a small amount of bloody mucus from the cervix as the cervix begins to thin in preparation for childbirth.

body habitus The shape and condition of a person's body as a result of a chronic health condition.

body language Unspoken message conveyed by body position.

body mass index A clinical classification that takes into account height and weight.

body mechanics The proper or most efficient way to perform physical activities that are safe and energy conserving and help prevent the physical strains that may cause injury.

body substance isolation Protecting oneself from unnecessary exposure to potentially infectious body substances by avoiding direct contact with any body substance that may be infected.

bowel obstruction Blockage of flow through the intestine that results in proximal distension, abdominal pain, and vomiting.

Boyle's law Scientific principle that explains that the volume of a gas varies indirectly with the surrounding pressure.

bradycardia Decreased heart rate.

bradypnea Slow breathing.

brain contusion Bruising and swelling of brain tissue.

brain laceration Laceration (cut) to brain tissue caused by a penetration in an open head injury or bone fragments in a closed skull fracture.

brainstem The most basic part of the human brain, which acts as a junction box from the body to the rest of the brain structures and back.

Braxton-Hicks contractions Random contractions that occur in the third trimester that are not associated with cervical effacement or dilation; also known as "false labor."

breach of confidentiality A situation in which a person divulges information about a patient without having the patient's permission to do so.

breech presentation The presentation of the buttocks or a limb instead of the fetal head during birth.

briefing Meeting or consultation in which a commander provides the most up-to-date information about the current state of affairs at the incident.

bronchi Cartilaginous tubes that carry air into the lungs; singular: bronchus.

bronchioles Small muscular tubes with cartilaginous rings that carry air from bronchi into smaller air spaces in the lungs.

bronchodilator Medication that specifically opens up narrowed airways.

bronchospasm Constriction of the lower airways in the lungs.

brown recluse spider Poisonous spider that is brown with a classic violin-shaped mark on its back.

bundle branches Part of the heart's specialized conduction system; they receive electrical impulses from the bundle of His and transmit them to the Purkinje fibers in the ventricles.

bundle of His Part of the heart's specialized conduction system; it receives an electrical impulse from the AV node and transmits it to the bundle branches.

burn Injury caused by significant heat applied to the skin.

burnout Condition that exists when an EMT no longer feels able to perform his duties because of the effects of chronic stress.

C

calcaneus The largest bone in the foot, the heel bone.

call sign An identifying name or number assigned to a particular radio or person.

capillaries Tiny blood vessels that receive blood from arteries and pass it into adjacent veins.

capillary bleeding Slow, oozing type of bleeding, easily controlled and usually not life threatening.

capillary refill time The time it takes to see refill (evidenced by a return to normal color) of a capillary bed after blanching (loss of color in area of skin when pressed).

carbon dioxide (CO_2) Gas found in the air and created within the body.

cardiac contusion Bruising of the heart.

cardiac output The amount of blood pumped from the left ventricle in one minute.

cardiac standstill Condition in which the heart lies flaccid and unable to respond to any stimulus.

cardinal movements of labor The series of natural movements the infant makes upon descent through the birth canal.

cardiogenic shock A hypoperfused state resulting from inadequate cardiac pumping, usually due to multiple heart attacks.

cardiopulmonary resuscitation (CPR) Life-preserving technique involving chest compressions and artificial respiration that has been widely taught to both civilians and health care providers since the late 1950s.

cardioversion Process of restoring the heart's normal rhythm through controlled electric shock or medication.

caregiver Person who assists in the identification and treatment of an illness and helps to alleviate mental and physical suffering.

carina Point at which the trachea ends and the right and left bronchi begin.

carpal bones The eight bones of the wrist.

carrier Someone who carries an infectious microorganism; a carrier does not necessarily become ill from it, but can transmit it to someone else.

carry transfer A means of moving a patient from one stretcher to another by lifting and carrying the patient.

catabolism Process of cellular metabolism in which energy is released to break down large molecules into smaller molecules.

caterpillar pass To overcome an obstacle by passing the patient hand over hand over the obstacle to waiting EMTs on the other side.

cellular respiration (cellular metabolism) Process that describes the chemical changes that take place within the cell to produce energy.

central chemoreceptors Sensors located in the medulla for carbon dioxide levels and the pH of blood.

Centers for Disease Control and Prevention (CDC) U.S. federal agency charged with monitoring infectious disease outbreaks; typically the CDC provides a supportive role to state and local health departments.

central Directional term used to describe points toward the center of the body.

central nervous system Consists of the brain and spinal cord and is involved in the initiation and transmission of all control-oriented messages throughout the body.

central venous catheter An intravenous tube that may be left in for long periods of time and may be used for intravenous medication administration or blood sampling.

cephalocaudal Head to toe.

cerebellum The part of the brain that controls muscular coordination and complex actions; sometimes called the *athletic brain*.

cerebral circulation Supplies the brain with oxygen and nutrients and removes waste.

cerebrospinal fluid (CSF) The nutrient-rich fluid that bathes and protects the spinal cord and brain.

cerebrospinal fluid shunt A special catheter used to drain excess CSF off the brain and into the abdomen, where it can be easily absorbed.

cerebrovascular accident (CVA) Injury to the brain tissue that occurs as a result of disruption of blood flow to part of the brain; also known as *stroke*.

cerebrum The largest and most highly evolved area of the brain.

certification Recognition of the EMT having attained a certain level of competency as recognized by his or her peers.

cervical dilation Progressive opening of the cervix that occurs as the fetal head descends into the pelvis.

cervical immobilization device (CID) A device intended to assist in maintaining the cervical spine in a natural neutral position.

cervical spine The uppermost section of the spinal column, made up of seven vertebrae in the neck; it protects the cervical spinal cord.

cervix The opening to the uterus at the bottom.

cesarean section The surgical removal of a newborn from the uterus through an abdominal incision.

chain of command Assignment of roles and duties to individuals in a multiple-casualty incident with a specific order of reporting to supervisors.

chain of infection Three essential parts that must exist for an infection to occur: reservoir, transmission, and host.

chain of survival A concept embraced by the American Heart Association that refers to the multiple elements needed in a response system to have a successful resuscitation. As in a chain, each element is connected with the others and the strength of the entire chain depends on the strength of each link.

chair carry The use of a standard kitchen chair to move a patient.

channel guard A device that prevents extraneous interference from radio transmissions from outside the base station; also called a *private line*.

CHART Acronym that stands for chief complaint/concern of the patient, history (including the history of present illness and the patient's past medical history), the physical assessment of the patient, the plan of patient care, and treatment and/or transportation.

CHEATED Acronym to help recall the outline of a completely documented patient record: chief complaint, history, exam, assessment of situation, treatment, evaluation, and disposition.

chemical restraint The use of medications to keep the patient calm or sedated.

Chemical Transportation Emergency Center (CHEMTREC) A 24-hour technical assistance phone number (1-800-424-9300) about hazardous materials.

chemical weapons Poisons that can kill or incapacitate.

chemoreceptors Sensors that measure the chemical changes in the body.

chest thrusts Firm compressions delivered at midchest in an attempt to expel a foreign body from the airway.

Cheyne-Stokes Characterized by periods of shallow, slow breathing increasing to rapid, deep breathing and then returning to shallow, slow breathing followed by a short apneic period.

chief complaint (CC) The patient's main problem and reason for seeking medical services.

chilblains Painful, inflamed skin lesions resulting from excessive exposure of skin to cool, windy, damp weather.

child abuse Any act, or failure to act, on the part of responsible adults that results in death, serious physical or emotional harm, sexual abuse or exploitation, or an act or failure to act that presents an imminent risk of serious harm.

childbirth The act of delivering a child.

child neglect When an adult with custodial responsibilities fails to provide legally mandated care for the child.

children with special health care needs (CSHCN) Children who are at risk of having chronic physical, developmental, behavioral, or emotional conditions requiring health and other related services that would not be required by children developing normally.

cholecystitis Infection of the gallbladder often characterized by fever, abdominal pain, and jaundice.

chronic obstructive pulmonary disease (COPD) Group of diseases characterized by chronic airway obstruction and bronchospasm.

chronic stress Repeated stressors that affect an EMT over a period of time.

cilia Hair-like projections from cells lining the airways that keep a thick mucous blanket constantly moving upward and out of the lungs.

Cincinati Prehospital Stroke Scale A three-item scale used to identify patients with likelihood of stroke.

circulation The action of blood flowing in the circuit of blood vessels and the heart.

clavicle The collarbone; located at the top of the chest, connecting the shoulder to the sternum.

clonic phase The stage in a seizure in which the body paroxysmally stiffens and relaxes.

closed fracture A broken bone in which the bone ends remain roughly in line and do not break the skin.

clothing drag The technique of pulling a patient to safety using the clothing he or she is wearing.

clues Evidence a person was in an area.

coagulation The process of blood clotting.

coagulopathy A blood-clotting disorder caused by disease or chemical exposure.

coccyx The tailbone, or last portion of the spinal column.

cochlear implant Surgically placed hearing device that converts sounds to electrical impulses, sending them directly to the auditory nerve.

cognitive The mental processes of comprehension, judgment, memory, and reasoning.

cognitive impairment Alteration in any of the mental processes of comprehension, judgment, memory, and reasoning.

cold zone Area without any risk of contamination to rescue personnel.

Colles' fracture A broken wrist that is shaped like a silver fork.

combining form Used when two or more roots are placed together.

command hallucination An auditory hallucination, coming from a false or imaginary figure or person that tells the individual what to do.

command post A centralized location, often off site, where the heads of public safety agencies gather and regulate on-scene operations.

Commission for the Accreditation of Ambulance Services (CAAS) Independent organization that sets minimum standards for ambulance services.

communicable Passed from person to person.

communications center A central dispatch point.

communications specialist (COMSPEC) A specially trained radio operator.

compartment syndrome A buildup of pressure from swelling within muscle cavities.

compassion Ability to be aware of another person's suffering and to have a wish to help relieve it.

compensated shock A hypoperfused state that the body is compensating for by increasing heart rate, increasing respiratory rate, and shunting blood from certain organs.

competent Able to act in a responsible manner and comprehend the decision at hand.

complex partial seizure Begins with a vacant or blank stare, followed by a repetitive, random activity such as lip smacking or chewing.

compress Cotton dressing integrated into a two-tailed bandage.

computer-aided dispatch (CAD) Use of computers to assist emergency medical dispatchers with control and command of emergency services.

concussion Closed head injury caused by blunt force trauma in which mild stretching, tearing, and shearing of brain tissue occurs.

conduction Transfer of heat from a warm object to a cool object by direct contact.

conductor Material that easily carries a current.

confidentiality Privacy; maintaining confidentiality means ensuring that medical information is provided only to the patient's health care providers.

confined space Any area that has limited openings for exit and access and is not designed for worker occupancy.

congenital heart defects (CHD) Structural or functional anomaly of the heart or great vessels present at birth.

congestive heart failure Condition in which the heart does not pump adequately, creating a buildup of fluids in the lungs and eventually the rest of the body.

consensual response Both pupils will have the same response when light is shined in only one of them.

consent A voluntary agreement by a person to allow something to take place.

contagious The state of an illness when the affected person can transmit it to others.

continuing education Training beyond the initial certification requirements.

continuous positive airway pressure (CPAP) Positive pressure applied to the upper airway by machine splinting the airway open and preventing collapse.

continuous quality improvement (CQI) Process by which an organization monitors and addresses areas in need of improvement.

contraindications Reasons why a medication should not be administered.

controlled intersection An intersection with a traffic control device.

contusion Bruising of tissue, caused by blunt forces.

convection Heat loss to air currents passing by a warm surface.

convalescence The body starts to recover and repair itself.

coral snake A venomous snake identified by its red and yellow bands directly opposed.

coronary arteries The two arteries that supply blood to the heart muscle.

costal arch The umbrella-appearing arch at the lower portion of the front of the thoracic cage.

costovertebral angle The angle formed by the tenth rib as it meets the thoracic spine.

coup-contrecoup Characterized by damage to brain tissue at the point of the initial impact to the head and also damage on the side opposite point of the initial impact, where the brain impacts the skull on the opposite side.

covering the brake Placing one foot over the brake pedal in anticipation of stopping.

crackles A popping sound heard in the lungs that is created as tiny air spaces that are stuck together by abnormal fluid accumulation pop open.

cradle carry An emergent means of moving a patient involving lifting the patient up and cradling him in the arms for a rapid move from the dangerous environment.

cranium The bony skull.

cravat A simple cotton triangular bandage useful in many circumstances.

crepitus The sound of bone ends grinding against one another; the feeling of air under the skin; it feels like Rice Krispies popping under the fingertips.

cribbing Blocks of wood used to stabilize a vehicle.

cricoid pressure A technique of applying pressure to the cricoid ring during ventilation to occlude the esophagus and prevent regurgitation.

critical incident stress debriefing (CISD) Structured sessions facilitated by trained personnel meant to review the incident in detail and encourage the involved group of providers to discuss their experience during and after the incident. Such a debriefing can help participants effectively deal with the stress of the incident.

cross-fingered technique Technique whereby the EMT places the thumb against the upper incisors and the fore forefinger against the lower incisors to gently force the mouth open in a scissors maneuver.

croup A swelling and inflammation of the larynx, trachea, and to some extent the bronchi, usually caused by a viral infection.

crowing Sound like a crow cawing that occurs when the muscles around the larynx spasm and the opening into the trachea narrows.

crowning The term used to describe the appearance of the fetal head at the vaginal opening when delivery is imminent.

crumple zone Automobile fenders designed to absorb energy while compacting.

crush injury Prolonged pressure on the skin and underlying tissues.

CSF otorrhea Leaking of cerebrospinal fluid from the ear.

CSF rhinorrhea Leaking of cerebrospinal fluid from the nose.

cultural competency The ability to positively interact with—and in the case of an EMT, care for—persons of many cultures.

culture A system of symbols, icons, and activities that is important to a group of people.

culture of safety Shared commitment of management and employees to ensure the safety of the work environment.

current The passage of electricity through an object.

cushing's reflex Hypertension and bradycardia associated with serious head injury.

Cushing's triad Hypertension, bradycardia, and an altered respiratory pattern seen in serious head injuries.

cyanosis A bluish discoloration to the skin seen with poor oxygen content of the blood.

D

dangerous instruments Things capable of producing death or serious bodily injury when used in certain circumstances.

dead air space Volume of air that stays in the respiratory tract.

dead space The space in the respiratory tract that is not in contact with pulmonary capillaries and cannot participate in gas exchange with the blood.

deadly weapon Any device that, by its nature, is intended to produce death.

deafness Indicates the loss of hearing prior to learning to talk.

debriefing An organized discussion among personnel involved in a difficult situation in an attempt to prevent an unnecessary buildup of stress.

decompensated shock Hypoperfused state for which the body is no longer able to compensate, with resulting hypotension.

decompression sickness A diving injury that occurs during rapid ascent resulting in expansion of gases that become trapped in tissues; also known as *the bends*.

decontamination Removal of potentially hazardous substances by either chemical or physical means.

decontamination corridor Area where the hazardous materials are cleaned off the rescuers and patients; also referred to as the *warm zone*.

deep Term used to describe an injury that extends far into the injured structure.

defamation Information spoken or written about an individual that can be seen as damaging to that person's character or reputation.

defibrillation Process of applying an electrical shock to the heart to stop an abnormal rhythm, ventricular fibrillation, or pulseless ventricular tachycardia and restore normal rhythm.

deformity Misshapen or not in the usual position.

degloving avulsion The forceful separation of just the skin from an extremity.

dehydration Loss of too much body fluid causing an imbalance of the elements affecting muscle activity and body fluid levels.

delirium Alteration in the level of consciousness exhibited by a sudden erratic change in behavior, usually caused by an acute medical problem.

delirium tremens (DTs) Symptoms associated with the sudden withdrawal of alcohol from an alcohol-dependent person.

deltoid muscle Triangular muscle covering the shoulder and upper arm; a site commonly used for intramuscular injections.

Department of Transportation (DOT) Federal agency responsible for traffic safety; considered the starting point for modern EMS.

dementia Syndrome characterized by a progressive decline in intellectual function that usually leads to deterioration of occupational, social, and interpersonal functions.

dentures False teeth.

dependency The psychological need the person has for a drug.

depression Psychiatric condition characterized by persistent sadness and lack of interest in usual life pleasures.

dermatome An area of movement or sensation that corresponds with a nerve root.

dermis The layer of skin just beneath the surface, or epidermal, layer; contains capillaries and specialized nerve endings.

descending corticospinal tract Nerve fiber bundles that send motor instructions to the muscles and organs of the body.

diabetes mellitus Disease in which the pancreas fails to produce insulin.

diabetic coma Condition of an unconscious, hyperglycemic diabetic patient.

diabetic ketoacidosis (DKA) The result of excessive fat metabolism seen in diabetic patients with hyperglycemia.

diamond stretcher carry A technique in which four EMTs carry a patient on a stretcher, with one EMT at either end and one on each side.

diaphoretic Exhibiting excessive perspiration due to stress or pain.

diaphragm The specialized muscle that separates the chest from the abdomen and is the main muscle of breathing.

diastolic The lower number in the blood pressure; the pressure in the vessels when the heart is resting between contractions.

diastolic blood pressure Pressure exerted on blood vessels when the heart is at rest.

diet-controlled diabetes Condition of a person whose blood sugar is controlled by diet modification.

diffusion Movement of oxygen and carbon dioxide across a membrane from an area of higher concentration to an area of lower concentration.

direct carry Lifting a patient and carrying him a short distance directly to the stretcher.

direct contact Actually coming into contact with the infectious material on a person by touching.

direct current (DC) A unidirectional electrical current.

direct force The transfer of energy to the point of impact of violence.

direct laryngoscopy Use of a laryngoscope to directly visualize the airway structures.

direct lift A technique that allows three EMTs to lift a patient from the ground without using assistive devices.

direct pressure Constant firm pushing on the bleeding site.

disease Condition characterized by abnormal symptoms.

dislocation A bone that slips out of joint and out of alignment.

disorder Pathological condition or deficiency of the body or mind.

displacement Avoiding painful emotions by transferring one's emotions to others.

distal Directional term used to describe points farther from the core of the body (trunk).

distracting painful injury A severe injury that occurs when the patient focuses on the injury to the exclusion of everything and everyone else.

diversionary techniques Activities such as physical exercise, deep breathing, or creative imagery that are useful in dissipating the effects of an acutely stressful event.

diverticula Sac or pouch in the colon that can become packed with fecal matter, causing inflammation.

diverticulitis Inflammatory disease caused by impacted diverticula that may lead to an obstructed colon, perforation, and hemorrhage; often associated with left-side abdominal pain.

domestic terrorists Groups of "nationals," as defined by the U.S. Immigration and Nationality Act, that have disputes with the way the U.S. government is operated or with specific U.S. policies.

domestic violence An act of violence against a partner, spouse, family member, or member of the household.

Don Juan syndrome A predictable injury pattern from a fall resulting in broken heel, lumbar injuries, and cervical spine injuries.

do not resuscitate order (DNR) A medical-legal order to restrain health care providers from providing invasive procedures and resuscitation such as CPR.

dormant In a state of biological rest.

dorsal Directional term referring to the top or back surface of a structure such as the hand.

dorsiflexion Movement of the toes upward, toward the nose.

dose The amount of a substance; usually refers to the amount of a medication given.

Down syndrome Also known as trisomy 21, a disorder caused by the presence of three 21st chromosomes, characterized by similar physical features and varying levels of cognitive impairment.

draw sheet Either a regular bed sheet folded over in half or a sturdy linen of equal length used to move a patient from a bed to a stretcher, or vice versa.

draw sheet transfer Use of a draw sheet to move a patient from one stretcher to another.

dressing A sterile absorbent cloth used to cover a wound.

due regard Respect and consideration for others.

duplex A radio that allows the EMT to both speak and listen at the same time, like a telephone.

durable power of attorney-health care (DPOA-HC) A legal document that extends authority of one person to control the legal affairs of another—in this case, the health care issues of a patient.

dura mater (tough mother) Tough, fibrous outer layer of the meninges, lining the cranial vault.

duty to act An obligation to provide care to a patient who requires it.

dysarthria Difficulty speaking resulting in garbled or slurred speech.

dyspnea The feeling or appearance of respiratory distress.

dysrhythmia Abnormal change in the electrical rhythm of the heart.

E

ecchymosis A wider collection of blood under the skin like a contusion (bruise).

eclampsia A convulsive disorder seen only during pregnancy.

ectopic pregnancy A pregnancy that develops outside the uterus.

edema Fluid seeping out of the bloodstream and into the tissues.

effacement Thinning of the cervix that occurs as a pregnancy nears its conclusion.

elder abuse An act of violence toward or neglect of an elderly person who is dependent on the other person.

electrocardiogram (ECG) A recording of the electrical activity of the heart graphically displayed on an oscilloscope or printed on paper; also abbreviated EKG.

elevate Raising the bleeding site above the level of the heart.

emancipated minor A person who is not the age of majority but who is no longer under the control of a parent or guardian and is legally responsible for his or her decisions and any consequences that result from those decisions.

embolism A physical blockage in the bloodstream.

embolus Debris that travels through blood vessels until it lodges and occludes blood flow.

emergency ambulance A vehicle specifically designed for patient transportation in an emergency.

emergency ambulance service vehicle (EASV) A vehicle used in service to EMS and staffed by EMS personnel.

emergency carry A technique used if the patient must be moved in an emergency over a greater distance.

emergency department (ED) A division or portion of a hospital designated to care for emergency medical problems or trauma; in some countries called an accident room.

emergency dispatch (EMD) A trained person who answers 9-1-1 emergency telephone calls from the public and provides public safety assistance through communication with emergency services such as fire, law enforcement, and EMS.

emergency doctrine A legal principle that allows for emergency treatment of prisoners or children if they are incapable of giving consent.

emergency drag A technique used by a single EMT to move a patient quickly in an emergency.

emergency incident rehabilitation An element of the operational plan that includes rest and rehydration as well as medical monitoring.

emergency medical dispatch (EMD) Specially trained dispatch call takers who are trained to provide specific pre-arrival medical care instructions to callers while emergency crews respond.

emergency medical responder (EMR) Person who has advanced training for first responders that includes basic assessment, simple airway management, oxygen administration, bleeding control, rescuer CPR, and defibrillation.

emergency medical services (EMS) Coordinated network of professionals whose function is to provide a variety of medical services to people in need of emergency care.

emergency medical services system (EMSS) An organization of equipment, such as ambulances, and personnel, such as the EMTs, created to respond to medical emergencies within a community.

emergency medical technician (EMT) Person who has completed the basic entry level of training for prehospital care that includes airway maintenance, oxygen administration, bleeding control, CPR, defibrillation, patient assessment, and limited medication administration.

Emergency Medical Treatment and Active Labor Act (EMTALA) Federal legislation that ensures that patients receive medical treatment regardless of their ability to pay.

emergency move The technique that an EMT uses to quickly remove a patient from danger.

emergency operations plan (EOP) An interagency document that assigns responsibilities to U.S. government departments and organizations, thereby setting lines of command (authority). It describes how emergency responders will protect people and property in the event of a terrorist attack as well as apprehend those responsible.

emergency physician Medical doctor specially trained in rapid assessment and diagnosis of acutely ill or traumatically injured patients.

Emergency Response Guidebook (ERG) A guidebook that provides responders instructions and information on how to handle the first 30 minutes of a hazmat spill.

emergency response team A group of people who arrive and rescue contaminated persons and control, confine, contain, and decontaminate the area.

emergency services vehicle (ESV) A vehicle used by an emergency service, including law enforcement, fire service, and EMS.

emergency vehicle operator (EVO) A driver of a vehicle used for emergency service.

emergency vehicle operators course (EVOC) A training course for drivers of vehicles used for emergency service.

EMS director/EMS incident Commander assigning unit leaders for triage, transport, staging, treatment, and morgue.

endocarditis Inflammation of the inside of the heart.

endocrine system Assists the nervous system in maintaining control over the body by producing hormones that act upon certain organs.

endothelial cells Cells that line the circulatory system.

endotoxin Fragments of bacteria cell wall membranes released following the death of the bacteria.

end-to-end stretcher carry Grasping the litter/stretcher at the head and the feet to carry.

enteral Ingested route of medication administration; sublingual, oral.

entrance wound Damage created as an object or electricity enters the body.

environmental assessment An EMT's visual overview of an entire scene while identifying potential hazards.

Environmental Protection Agency (EPA) Federal agency charged with maintaining the quality of the environment; typically concerned with pollution.

epidermis The outermost layer of skin.

epidural hematoma A collection of blood between the skull and the dura mater, often arterial in nature.

epiglottis Located above the larynx, a cartilaginous structure that protects the trachea from aspiration of foreign bodies.

epiglottitis A bacterial infection, characterized by a swollen, inflamed epiglottis, that can cause upper airway obstruction.

epilepsy A disease characterized by recurrent seizures of a similar nature.

epinephrine A medication that dilates the airways and constricts the blood vessels.

escape rhythm The special ability of the myocardium to function independently when the electrical system fails.

esophageal varices Dilated veins within the lining of the lower esophagus that may bleed profusely if they rupture.

esophagus A collapsible muscular tube that directs food from the mouth into the stomach.

ethnocentrism A natural bias toward one's own culture.

etiology Cause or origin of a disease.

evaporation Transfer of heat into body fluids, such as sweat, for dissipation into the environment.

eversion An outward movement, such as when the foot twists outward and strains the ankle; the opposite of inversion.

evidence conscious Awareness of the importance of preserving items that may be considered evidence of a crime and conditions that pertain to a crime.

evisceration An abdominal wound with abdominal contents protruding through the wound.

excited delirium A state of hyperactive irrational behavior.

excited utterance A spontaneous statement during a stressful time.

exhalation Breathing out.

exit wound Damage created as a foreign object or electricity exits the body.

exotoxin Poisonous protein produced by organisms such as bacteria.

expected time of arrival (ETA) The anticipated arrival of either the patient or the EMT to the scene.

expiration date The last day that a medication is guaranteed by the manufacturer to be safe and effective as expected.

express consent The act of verbally advising a medical provider to proceed with treatment.

expressive aphasia Difficulty forming words often seen when a stroke affects the brain's speech center.

extension A movement that widens the angle at a joint between two bones; the opposite of flexion.

extremity lift A lifting technique whereby one EMT stands behind a seated patient and grasps him under the shoulders, while a second EMT grasps him under the knees so they can lift and carry him.

extrinsic By external causes.

F

facial droop One-sided facial muscle weakness that indicates focal brain or nerve injury.

fallopian tube Tiny muscular tube that allows an egg to travel from the ovary to the uterus.

false imprisonment The intentional confinement of a patient without the patient's consent and without an appropriate reason.

false motion Movement in the bone where there is not supposed to be movement.

false ribs The eighth through tenth ribs, which are not attached directly to the sternum; rather, they are attached anteriorly to the seventh rib by cartilage.

fasciotomy A surgical procedure whereby skin is cut to relieve pressure.

febrile seizure A seizure that results from a rapid rise in body temperature.

Federal Communications Commission (FCC) Federal agency that regulates radio communications.

federal response plan (FRP) A plan used when state and local authorities are overwhelmed; it brings the immense resources of the federal government to their aid.

feedback A return conversation that helps the EMT enssure that the message sent was correctly understood by the patient.

feeding tube A soft, flexible tube that is placed into the stomach, either through the nose or through the anterior abdominal wall, to allow nutritional supplementation.

femur The single bone in the thigh, the longest and strongest bone in the body.

fetal circulation Temporary circulation between the mother and fetus during pregnancy.

fetus The ovum after it is implanted in the uterine wall.

fibrinolytics (to divide the fibrin) Formerly called *thrombolytics*, is a class of drugs often used in the treatment of AMI.

fibula The laterally placed bone in the lower leg.

Fick Principle Equation That explains the process of cellular perfusion through five elements: oxygenation, ventilation, respiration, circulation, and cellular respiration.

field hospital A temporary on-site treatment facility.

fight-or-flight response Describes the reaction of the body to a stressor by preparing to fight to defend itself or to run away.

figure-of-eight A roller bandage that turns across itself.

firefighter's carry A technique that involves lifting a supine patient up onto the EMT's shoulder to quickly move the patient from a dangerous environment.

firefighter's drag A carrying technique that uses a simple cotton triangular bandage (cravat) tied around the patient's wrists; the patient's arms are around the EMT's neck and the EMT crawls on hands and knees, dragging the patient underneath him.

first responder (FR) The first person who arrives on the scene of an incident; also may refer to the level of medical training provided to persons who expect to be put in this position during their daily routine, such as firefighters, police officers, and security guards.

first responder awareness level A person trained to identify and report a hazardous materials incident.

first stage of labor The process of cervical effacement and dilation at the beginning of childbirth.

fixed wing Airplanes.

flail chest Segment of at least two ribs are broken in at least two places.

flail segment Two or more ribs fractured in two or more places where the underlying segment is unstable and moves in a paradoxical motion to the rest of the chest wall.

flapping the roof Cutting the uprights or posts to peel back the roof in a motor vehicle.

flashback The strobe of the emergency lights bouncing back into the emergency vehicle operator's eyes.

flat water A body of water without current.

flexible splint Any material that can be formed to fit any angle and then made rigid.

flexible stretcher A lightweight plastic stretcher that may be rolled up when not in use; commonly used in confined space and cave rescue.

flexion A movement at a joint that decreases the angle between the two bones on either side of it; opposite of extension.

floating ribs The last two pairs of ribs in the thoracic cage; they are unattached anteriorly.

flow-restricted oxygen-powered ventilation device (FROPVD) A device that can deliver oxygen to a patient at restricted flow rates.

focused physical examination A physical exam focused upon the medical patient's chief complaint.

fomite Pathogen contaminated surface.

fontanel Soft, flexible fibrous region in an infant's skull that allow for skull growth; also known as soft spots.

Food and Drug Administration (FDA) Federal agency responsible for drug purity and safety.

footdrop A loss of nervous control that results in a flaccid foot.

foramen magnum Large opening at the base of the skull through which the spinal cord passes.

forcible entry Using special tools or brute force to overcome an obstacle to gain entrance.

forcing the door Using a tool to overcome a latching mechanism.

foreign body airway obstruction (FBAO) Any ingested object that is capable of causing suffocation by blocking the trachea.

four corners carry A patient transportation technique in which four or more EMTs carry a stretcher over a distance.

four-second rule Determining the amount of time between when the vehicle in front of the emergency vehicle passes a landmark and when the emergency vehicle passes it; for safety reasons this time should be greater than 4 seconds.

Fowler's position Position in which a person is sitting at a 45-degree to 60-degree angle.

fracture A sudden breaking of a bone.

Frank-Starling law (Starling law) Contractility of cardiac muscle relative to the amount of stretch placed on the muscle by additional blood volume.

free radicals By-product of incomplete metabolism that can cause cellular injury.

French catheter A flexible suction catheter meant to suction through endotracheal tubes or via the nasopharynx.

frontal bone The strong anterior-most bone in the skull that makes up the forehead.

frostbite Tissue damage resulting from exposure to freezing and subfreezing temperatures.

frostnip A mild local skin injury resulting from exposure to freezing temperatures.

full-thickness burn A burn that affects all three layers of the skin.

fundus The top of the uterus.

G

gag reflex The protective response that a person has when the back of the throat is stimulated by the presence of a foreign substance.

gallbladder A small pouchlike organ that lies underneath the liver and stores bile to be used in digestion.

gastrocnemius muscle The muscle in the back of the calf that enables a person to stand on his toes.

gastroenteritis A condition characterized by vomiting and diarrhea, usually caused by a viral illness.

gauze dressing Sterile cotton weave cloth.

Geiger counter A device used to detect radiation.

general impression The initial feeling, based on observation, of how seriously ill or injured the patient is.

generalized seizure A seizure that involves the entire brain and results in loss of consciousness; also known as a *grand mal seizure*.

generic name The initial name given to a drug that is shorter than the actual chemical name and is listed in the U.S. Pharmacopeia.

geriatrics The study of the diseases of elderly adults.

gestational diabetes A form of diabetes that occurs only in pregnant women and usually only for the duration of the pregnancy.

gestational diabetes mellitus (GDM) Diabetes that occurs during pregnancy, usually disappearing follow birth.

glands Specialized organs that respond to and produce hormones of the endocrine system.

Glasgow Coma Scale (GCS) A scale that is used to quantify a patient's level of responsiveness.

global assessment The EMT's general feeling of the entire scene; should involve thoughts of safety and need for additional rescuers.

global positioning satellite (GPS) A constellation of geo-synchronized satellites that are used to determine position, speed, and time of any object on earth.

glucose A substance used by the body for fuel.

gluteus muscles Strong muscles in the buttock that are important in allowing proper leg movement.

goblet cell Cells that produce a mucous designed to entrap particles and microorganisms, such as bacteria, and prevent them from entering the alveoli.

gonads Organs of reproduction; testes (male) and ovaries (female).

Good Samaritan laws Laws that protect certain classes of people, such as physicians, who volunteer to assist others; laws vary from state to state.

grand mal seizure The old term for a generalized seizure.

gravidity The total number of pregnancies a woman has had.

grunting A noise made on exhalation during periods of respiratory distress.

guardian A person who has authority to act on behalf of another individual and to give consent for medical care.

guarding Muscular tension created by a patient to protect an underlying injury.

guides Instructions for evacuation distance, perimeter boundaries, and potential hazards found in the *Emergency Response Guidebook*.

gunshot wound (GSW) An injury created by a projectile fired by a gun.

gurgling Sound of liquid moving; if heard at the airway, indicates a need for suctioning.

H

hailing frequency The channel used to call a particular agency or hospital.

hallucination A sensation or perception that has no basis in reality.

halo test Observing for a ring of blood around CSF spilled from the ears or nose in a head-injured patient.

hard of hearing Some hearing ability is present, usually with the use of hearing aids.

hard palate The bony structure that forms the roof of the mouth.

hasty search A quick search of an area.

hazardous material Any substance that can cause an exposed person injury or death.

hazardous waste operations and emergency response (HAZWOPER) Legislation that pertains to toxic waste management.

head-tilt, chin-lift Maneuver used to open the airway, involving tilting the head back and lifting the jaw up; used only in nontrauma patients.

health care proxy A person chosen to make medical decisions on behalf of another in the event the person becomes incapable of making such decisions.

Health Insurance Portability and Accountability Act (HIPAA) An act of Congress that protects health insurance coverage for workers and their families when they change or lose their jobs; regulates national standards for electronic health care transactions and the security and privacy of health data.

healthy lifestyle A lifestyle that includes exercise, a balanced diet, and avoidance of unhealthy habits such as smoking.

hearing impairment Reduction in the ear's responsiveness to loudness and pitch.

heart Four-chambered muscular organ that pumps to provide the body with nutrient-rich blood.

heat cramps Painful, involuntary muscle spasms caused by dehydration and exposure to heat.

heat exhaustion The mildest form of generalized heat-related illness, characterized by multiple symptoms and often by dehydration.

heat stroke A life-threatening form of heat illness that involves a rise in body temperature and altered mental status.

heavy rescue The use of special vehicle extrication equipment.

Heimlich maneuver A series of forceful upward abdominal thrusts that force air out of the lungs and the trachea.

hematochezia Passage of bright red blood from the rectum.

hematoma An accumulation of blood.

hemetemesis Vomitus that consists mostly of blood.

hemoglobin Protein molecule found on the surface of red blood cells responsible for carrying oxygen in blood.

hemoglobin saturation Amount of oxygen-rich hemoglobin in the blood.

hemophilia Rare, inherited bleeding disorder in which there is a deficiency or absence of specific clotting factors preventing blood from clotting normally.

hemoptysis Spitting up or coughing up blood.

hemorrhage Medical term for bleeding.

hemorrhagic shock A hypoperfused state resulting from loss of blood.

hemorrhagic stroke Injury to brain tissue as a result of rupture of a vessel that supplies it with blood.

hemostatic dressing Contains powders or substances that promote blood clotting when placed on an open wound.

hemostasis The process of controlling bleeding.

hemothorax Bleeding between the lung and the chest wall.

hepatitis B virus (HBV) The virus responsible for hepatitis B infection, which attacks the liver.

high-altitude cerebral edema (HACE) Swelling of the brain as a result of hypoxia at high altitudes; characterized by altered mental status, difficulty walking, and decreased level of consciousness.

high-altitude pulmonary edema (HAPE) Pulmonary edema as a result of hypoxia at high altitudes; characterized by dry cough and dyspnea on exertion.

high-efficiency particulate air filter (HEPA) A filtration device intended to remove very small airborne contaminants.

high index of suspicion Based on the noted mechanism of injury, the feeling that there is a high likelihood of injury.

high life hazard Known dangerous conditions that could injure or kill someone.

high-Fowler's position Position in which a person is sitting upright at a 90-degree angle.

history of present illness (HPI) An account of the course of an illness; typically done as a narrative from witnesses such as family members.

hobble restraint The tying of wrists to ankles behind the patient's back.

homeostasis The body's ability to maintain a steady optimal state for growth and development and to resist any influence, internal or external, that would upset this balance.

hormones Chemicals that are excreted into the bloodstream by specialized organs called glands.

hospice A facility with a team of health care professionals who care for dying patients.

host The target of an infection.

hot zone The immediate vicinity of the hazardous material spill that is considered contaminated and a risk to rescue personnel.

hot-load Placing a patient aboard a running helicopter.

human immunodeficiency virus (HIV) The virus that causes AIDS (acquired immunodeficiency syndrome).

humerus The single long bone of the upper arm.

humidification The process of adding moisture to the inspired air.

hydrochloric acid (HCl) A strong acid that can cause serious burns.

hydrogen sulfide (H₂S) A chemical with the smell of rotten eggs.

hyperbaric chamber A device that creates a simulated dive to allow for recompression of air in a diver suffering from decompression sickness or other diving-related illnesses.

hypercarbic High carbon dioxide.

hyperemia Increased blood flow.

hyperextension Excessive backward bending.

hyperflexibility Loose-jointedness

hyperflexion Excessive forward bending.

hyperglycemia A high amount of sugar in the blood.

hyperosmolar hyperglycemic non-ketonic coma (HHNK) Condition of diabetes that can lead to coma; different than keto-acidosis.

hypertension Abnormally high blood pressure.

hyperthermia Overall heat gain greater than heat loss, resulting in a rise in body temperature.

hyperventilate To breathe faster and more deeply than usual.

hyphema A collection of blood in the anterior part of the eye.

hypoglycemia A condition of low blood glucose levels.

hypoperfusion Inadequate supply of oxygenated blood to a tissue or organ.

hypopnea Slow, shallow breathing.

hypothermia Condition in which the body temperature drops below 95 degrees Fahrenheit.

hypotonia Low muscle tone.

hypoventilation Breathing more slowly than normal or less effectively than usual.

hypovolemia A state of decreased blood volume.

hypovolemic shock A hypoperfused state resulting from low fluid levels.

hypoxemia Insufficient oxygen in circulation blood for perfusion.

hypoxia Lack of oxygen in the body.

hypoxic drive Process of respiration to increase oxygen levels, not to reduce carbon dioxide levels.

I

idiopathic Unknown etiology or cause for an illness or disease.

iliac bones The main component of the bony pelvis, the hip bones, sometimes described as "wings" because of their shape.

illiteracy The inability to read or write or understand the spoken word.

immunity Insusceptibility to a specific illness, usually as a result of prior exposure or immunization.

immunity statute A law that protects a specific group of people from having to pay civil damages as a result of occurrences during job performance.

immunization The process of exposing the body to or inoculating it with weakened pathogens to allow it to create specific antibodies.

immunocompromise Lack of disease resistance.

impaled object A foreign object embedded in the skin.

implied consent The legal presumption that a patient who is unable to verbally express agreement to treatment would agree to be treated in certain circumstances.

incident commander (IC) The person in command who has overall responsibility for the entire incident.

Incident Command System (ICS) A system of command and control that defines operation and management components and the structure of incident management organizations throughout the incident.

incision A cutting of the skin.

incontinence Loss of bowel and/or bladder control.

indication The reason to use a drug to treat a specific condition.

indirect contact Exposure to an infectious agent that is on a nonhuman surface.

indirect force A transfer of energy as a result of violence away from the point of impact.

individual factors Elements such as allergies, medications, tobacco use, alcohol use, diet, and living environment that may be factors for a person's health status.

infarction Death of cells as the result of prolonged lack of oxygen.

infection control Taking preventive measures to lessen the likelihood of disease transmission.

infection control officer Designated officer of a company or department that is assigned to monitor infection control practices and act as a liaison to the hospital's infection control department.

inferior Lower than the reference point.

Infirmity Patient incapacitated by infection.

inflammation The body's attempt to prevent infection and begin healing.

informed consent Consent given following explanation of the risks and benefits of treatment.

initial assessment The first evaluation performed on every patient to address life-threatening problems.

initial report The first emergency responder's first radio report of scene conditions; includes hazards, number of patients, and requests for additional resources.

in loco parentis Someone who has authority to act on behalf of a minor in place of the parent.

innervate Nerves that connect to muscles and organs of the body.

inspiration Breathing in.

instrument flight rules (IFR) Aviation regulations that allows for planned operation of the aircraft by reference to the aircraft instruments with instruction from Air Traffic Control (ATC).

insulator Material that resists the passage of electrical current.

insulin A hormone produced by the pancreas that allows glucose utilization by the body.

insulin-dependent diabetes A condition for which the diabetic patient must inject insulin into the body to survive.

insulin shock Condition resulting from low blood sugar due to either too much insulin or too little sugar.

integumentary system The skin and skin structures that cover and protect the body.

intercostal muscles Muscles between the ribs.

intercostal retraction A retraction of skin and muscle between the ribs with each breath, as seen in a child with respiratory distress.

interference Factors that affect the quality of a transmission.

international terrorists Terrorist groups that cross over national borders and often have subgroups, called cells, in other countries to perform terrorism.

International Association of Fire Fighters (IAFF) An international group representing more than 263,000 firefighters in more than 3,500 communities in the United States and Canada.

intermammary line The imaginary horizontal line that runs between the nipples.

interoperability Cross-jurisdictional standardization of emergency medical care at each level of practice.

intervertebral disk The fibrous pad that cushions each vertebra from the others.

intonation Changes in pitch, volume, and cadence of voice.

intracranial pressure (ICP) The pressure within the skull.

intramuscular Referring to administration of medication into the muscular layer under the subcutaneous layer of soft tissue.

intrauterine fetal demise A fetus who has died while still in the uterus, occurring after the 20th week of gestation and/or a fetal weight of 500 grams (1.1 lb).

intravenous (IV) Referring to administration of medication into the veins.

intrinsic By internal causes.

inversion Turning something inward; opposite of eversion.

irreversible shock Hypoperfusion that has progressed to a point where survival is highly unlikely.

ischemia Injury of tissue resulting from a blockage of the vessel that normally supplies that tissue with blood.

ischemic stroke Injury to brain tissue as a result of blockage of the vessel that supplies it with blood.

ischium The portion of the bony pelvis that supports body weight while in the sitting position.

J

jaundice A yellow discoloration of the skin caused by excess bilirubin in the bloodstream.

jaw thrust A technique that lifts the mandible and tongue up and away from the pharynx, often effective in opening the airway; is used on trauma patients with suspected spinal injury.

jugular vein A large vein in the side of the neck that is situated rather close to the surface of the skin.

jugular venous distention (JVD) Bulging veins in the side of the neck.

jumpSTART Triage A triage system that uses the specific assessment techniques for infants and children to differentiate them from adults.

K

keto-acid An organic acid that is the by-product of ineffective metabolism; also called ketone.

kidney A solid organ in the retroperitoneal space that filters toxins from the blood and makes urine to dispose of such toxins and excess salts or water.

kidney stone Particulate material crystallizes in the urine, resulting in a formed piece of solid material.

killing zone Area controlled by hostile gun fire.

kinematics of trauma Science of analyzing the mechanism of injury.

kinetic energy The energy possessed by a body because of its motion.

kinetics The mechanics dealing with the motions of material objects.

knee The joint that joins the upper leg and the lower leg.

Kussmaul's respiration Deep, almost sighing, respiration.

kyphosis Severe outward curvature of the upper back.

L

labor The childbirth process by which the uterus expels the fetus and placenta.

laceration A type of wound characterized by a full-thickness tear in the skin.

LACES A mnemonic for first responders on the scene of a potential terrorist attack; L stands for lookout, A for awareness, C for communications, E for escape, and S for safety zone.

landing zone (LZ) An area intended for the purpose of landing and taking off in a helicopter.

lap belt syndrome A phenomenon in which a misplaced seatbelt causes liver and spleen injuries.

large intestine Hollow digestive organ that encircles the abdominal cavity and receives digested food from the small intestine.

laryngoscope A tool that is used to view the lower airway structures during endotracheal intubation.

laryngoscopy The use of a laryngoscope to view the lower airway structures.

larynx A cartilaginous structure in the midline of the neck that contains the vocal cords and is the beginning of the trachea, or windpipe.

lateral Directional term used to describe the side of a structure; points farther from the midline.

lateral bending Forced sideways motion.

law enforcement officer (LEO) The broad category including police officers, state police, deputy sheriffs, FBI agents, and DEA agents, who have the responsibility to uphold the law.

leadership Quality of causing others to follow in one direction to accomplish a goal.

left lateral recumbent position Position in which the person is lying on his or her left side; also known as the *recovery position*.

legal duty to act The requirement that an EMT respond to calls whether as an employee under contract or as a volunteer.

liability The legal responsibility for one's own actions.

libel Statement that makes a false claim, expressively stated or implied to be factual, that may harm the reputation of an individual.

lifelong learning Education that a person continues throughout life by keeping current on new information and maintaining competence in skills.

lift teams Specialty teams of EMTs trained to lift heavy patients.

ligament Connective tissue that connects bone to bone.

light-emitting diode (LED) An electronic device that shines light using small amounts of electricity.

limited victim incident (LVI) A smaller number of patients than multiple-casualty incident (MCI).

linear A straight course.

lipids Substances such as a fat, oil, or wax that dissolve in alcohol but not in water.

liquid oxygen (LOX) Compressed oxygen in liquid form; it takes up an extremely small volume and is thus more portable.

liters per minute (lpm) A measurement of the rate of flow of a liquid.

litter A stretcher or other means of patient conveyance that does not have wheels and must be carried.

liver Large, solid organ in the right upper abdomen that creates bile for digestion, produces special factors to help in blood clotting, and filters blood from the intestines to rid the body of specific toxins.

living will A document signed by a patient that informs the reader of what types of treatment and under what conditions that patient would want or would not want medical treatment.

loaded bumper A vehicle's front or rear bumper that, when compressed and locked, is able to suddenly and unexpectedly spring forward.

locked A bone that is unable to return to its natural position.

lower extremities Term used to refer to the legs.

lumbar vertebrae The five vertebrae that make up the lower back and support the weight of the entire upper body.

lumen Hollow center of blood vessels.

lymph Straw-colored fluid similar to plasma that carries white blood cells.

lymph node Solid glandlike bodies, such as the tonsils, where white blood cells destroy microorganisms.

lymphatic system Part of the immune system that carries microorganism-laden white blood cells in a fluid, called lymph, to lymph nodes for removal. Also assists the circulatory system by draining the body's tissues of excess fluids and returning that fluid to the central circulation.

LZ officer A designated person on the scene of an incident responsible for choosing a landing zone (LZ) for the helicopter and ensuring its safety.

M

malaise Feeling of weakness or exhaustion.

malfeasance Action or failure to act that causes intentional damage.

malleolus Bony prominences at the medial and lateral aspects of the ankles.

malpractice Act or omission by a health care provider that deviates from accepted standards of practice in the medical community and that causes injury to the patient.

Mandated child abuse reporter Individuals within certain groups such as daycare providers, educators/teachers, law enforcement and EMTs, who are required to report suspected child abuse.

mandated reporter Individual who comes into contact with certain situations, such as child abuse, and is required by law to report these situations to the proper authorities.

mandible Bony lower jaw.

manubrium Upper section of the bony sternum.

mass Weight of an object.

mastoid process Bony prominence behind the ear.

mastoid sinus Air-filled space within the mastoid bone, behind the ears.

material safety data sheet (MSDS) Reference list of the health and safety information for a chemical substance.

maturation Positive mental, physical, or psychosocial growth or change.

maxilla One of the two fused bones that form the upper jawbone; plural, maxillae.

McGill forceps A pair of special long, curved pinching tongs.

mechanical ventilator Machine that provides artificial ventilation for a patient who cannot breathe effectively on his or her own.

mechanism of action How a drug works on the body.

mechanism of injury (MOI) The instrument or event that results in harm to a patient.

meconium Fetal stool.

med channel Radio frequency used by paramedics and EMTs to speak to base hospital physicians.

medial Directional term used to describe points closer to the midline of the body.

medial malleolus Bony prominence on the tibia side of the ankle.

mediastinum Hollow area between the right and left lungs that houses the trachea.

MedicAlert Emergency medical information service that provides a directive worn on the patient's body.

medicalese Unique medical terms and phrases used in the practice of medicine.

medical direction Advice provided by a higher medical authority, usually a physician.

medical director A physician who acts as a medical expert, consultant, and educator.

medical protocols Set of written regulations that specify the proper procedures for patient care.

medically necessary restraint Used when a patient must be confined to prevent him or her from harming himself or herself or others.

megahertz (MHz) Frequency band of radio wave transmission.

melena Dark, tarry stool containing digested blood caused by bleeding in the upper gastrointestinal tract.

meninges Three membrane layers covering the brain, brain stem, and spinal cord.

meningitis An infection and inflammation of the lining around the brain and spinal cord.

menstruation Monthly flow that rids the uterus of its lining when fertilization of an egg does not occur.

mental illness Any disorder that impairs the brain's function that is without a firm physical (organic) cause.

metabolism Chemical and physical reactions taking place within the cells.

metabolites Small molecules left over from chemicals after the cells have reacted with them.

metacarpals The five bones that connect the carpal bones in the wrist to the phalanges in the fingers.

metered dose inhaler (MDI) Handheld device that carries a form of medication that may be aerosolized on discharge of the inhaler device.

microorganism Tiny living creature visible only by microscope.

midaxillary line Imaginary line drawn from the center of the armpit down the side of the chest.

midclavicular lines Imaginary lines drawn from the middle of each clavicle, or collarbone, down the front of the chest.

midline Imaginary line drawn down the center of the body, splitting it equally into a right half and a left half.

miles per hour (mph) Measurement of the speed of a vehicle.

military anti-shock trousers (MAST) Device that is inflated over the lower extremities and pelvis to attempt to increase blood flow to the core organs; also called *pneumatic antishock garment (PASG)*.

millimeters of mercury (mmHg) The measurement of the height of mercury that is an indirect measurement of a pressure, such as blood pressure.

minimum data set The specific pieces of information required on a patient care report.

minute volume Amount of air breathed in and out in one minute.

miscarriage Spontaneous, unintentional termination of a pregnancy.

misfeasance Perform the duty inadequately or poorly.

mitral valve Bicuspid valve that prevents blood flow backward from the left ventricle into the left atrium.

mobile radio Radio unit mounted inside a vehicle.

mobile work stations Computerized device in emergency vehicles that communicates with a central dispatch or communications center.

modified Trendelenburg position in which a person is lying supine with legs elevated 12–16 inches; also known as *shock position*.

molding The shaping of a neonate's head to pass through the birth canal.

morbidly obese Patients with potentially life-threatening weight-related health problems.

morgue An area set aside for the collection of the deceased.

motion artifact A false ECG reading created by vibration.

motor neurons Nerve cells that control voluntary muscle movement.

motor nerves Nervous tissue that carries impulses that initiate muscular contraction.

motor vehicle collision (MVC) Formerly referred to as a car accident; when a vehicle forcefully strikes another vehicle or object, often leading to trauma.

mottling Skin discoloration similar to cyanosis but in a blotchy pattern.

mucous membrane Porous tissue lined with blood vessels that creates a liquid that serves to wash away the surface of the respiratory and gastrointestinal tracts that are regularly in contact with the outside environment.

multiagency coordination system Defines operating characteristics, management components, and the organizational structure of supporting organizations.

multi-drug resistant organism Pathogens that have adapted to and developed the ability to resist antibiotics that would normally be prescribed to treat them.

multiparous Term used to describe a woman who has previously given childbirth.

multiple-casualty incident (MCI) Incident involving multiple injured patients, often overwhelming the initial responding units.

multiplex radio Multiple-channel radio that allows for complex data such as ECGs and spoken messages to be transmitted simultaneously.

Murphy eye Opening on the side of the distal end of the endotracheal tube.

myocardium Heart muscle.

N

9-1-1 Three-digit phone number for accessing emergency services in the United States.

Nader pin Case-hardened pin designed to prevent the vehicle door from springing open in a motor vehicle collision.

Narcan (naloxone) Reduces the effects of a narcotic, as seen with heroin overdose.

nasal cannula (NC) Device placed in the patient's nose to deliver between 24% and 44% oxygen.

nasal flaring Widening of the nostrils during breathing; a sign of increased respiratory effort commonly seen in children.

nasogastric tube Small-diameter, flexible plastic tube placed through the nose and the esophagus and into the stomach.

nasopharyngeal airway (NPA) A flexible tube that may be passed through the nose into the pharynx that can help to hold the tongue off the back of the throat and keep the airway open; also called a *nasal airway*.

nasopharynx Back of the throat immediately behind the nose; the nasal passage.

National Association of Emergency Medical Services Physicians (NAEMSP) National organization of physicians and EMS professionals dedicated to providing leadership in EMS and promoting excellence in EMS care.

National Association of Emergency Medical Technicians (NAEMT) National organization that represents EMS practitioners to the public and government.

National EMS Education Standards Broad educational statements that state the objective of EMS education and recognize that EMS is a rapidly changing profession that requires flexibility within limits.

National Fire Protection Agency (NFPA) Advisory board of fire service experts who publish standards and advocate for improved emergency services.

National Highway Traffic Safety Administration (NHTSA) Division of the U.S. Department of Transportation that has taken a leading role in establishing standards for training for emergency services.

National Incident Management System (NIMS) Management criteria enabling all responding agencies to work together when disaster incidents occur.

National Institute of Occupational Safety and Health (NIOSH) Federal agency charged with studying causes and prevention of work-related illness or injury.

National Registry of EMTs (NREMT) National EMS certification organization that provides a valid, uniform process to assess the knowledge and skills required for competent practice required by EMS professionals throughout their careers and maintains a registry (list) of certification status.

nature of the illness (NOI) Explanation of the character and history of an illness, analogous to MOI in trauma.

near-drowning Water submersion that does not result in death within a 24-hour period.

nebulizer Device that creates a fine mist of a liquid medication so that it can be inhaled.

necrosis Tissue death.

necrotic Dead tissue.

necrotizing fasciitis "Flesh-eating disease," an aggressive soft tissue infection associated with streptococcal bacteremia.

negative pressure ventilation Change of pressure inside the lungs compared to the pressure outside the atmosphere.

negligence Delivery of care in a manner considered to be below the accepted standard.

neonatal Life from birth to the end of the first month.

neonate Newborn infant up to 1 month old.

nephrons The functional parts of the kidney.

nerve roots Where nerves enter and exit the spinal column between the spinal vertebrae.

nervous system Body system made up of the brain, spinal cord, and nerves that controls and coordinates all body functions.

neurogenic shock Hypoperfused state resulting from injury to the spinal cord and generalized vasodilation.

neutral inline alignment Natural anatomical position of the neck.

NFPA 704 symbol Diamond-shaped warning sign with four more diamonds inside designating the presence of hazardous material on a truck or tank.

nitrogen dioxide (NO$_2$) Airborne pollutant that can cause severe respiratory irritation.

nitrogen narcosis Reversible condition caused by the anesthetic effect of nitrogen at high partial pressures seen in divers at depth; commonly referred to as *the bends*.

nitroglycerin Medication that dilates, or opens, blood vessels.

nonfeasance Fail to perform the duty at all.

non-insulin-dependent diabetes Condition of a diabetic patient whose blood sugar is controlled by diet or drugs and not by insulin injections.

noninvasive blood pressure monitor (NIBP) Mechanical blood pressure device that automatically obtains serial blood pressures.

non-rebreather mask (NRB) Device that when used with oxygen at 10–15 lpm can deliver up to 100% oxygen.

nonverbal information Information gathered through observation, including body language and position.

normal saline solution (NSS) Commonly used intravenous solution that consists of 0.9% sodium chloride.

normal sinus rhythm (NSR) Predominant natural pacemaker of the heart.

nothing by mouth (NPO) Prohibition against ingestion to prevent aspiration secondary to vomiting; acronym stands for the Latin "nil per os."

nuchal rigidity Stiff and painful neck condition.

nuclear dispersion device (NDD) Conventional bomb that spreads radioactive material across a wide area.

O

objective information Obtained by the EMT through direct observation or assessment.

obsessive-compulsive disorder (OCD) Psychiatric disorder characterized by repetitive behaviors.

obstetrics (OB) Medical practice involving pregnancy and childbirth.

occipital bone The most posterior bone in the skull.

occlusion Blockage.

occlusive dressing Bandage secured on three sides that allows air to escape from the open wound but prevents air from entering the open wound.

Occupational Safety and Health Administration (OSHA) Federal organization that regulates safety requirements for businesses.

off-line medical control Concept that physician does not have to be physically present while the EMT is caring for a patient but, through protocols and procedures, has control over each patient's care.

onboard oxygen Large oxygen tank kept on an ambulance for purposes of administering oxygen to a patient in the ambulance.

ongoing assessment Continuing observation of the patient throughout contact.

on-line medical control Direct communication between the EMT and physician while care is being rendered in the field.

open fracture Broken bone in which the bone ends erupt through the skin.

open-ended questions Questions that cannot be answered with simple yes or no, or automatic answers.

operations level responder Person expected to minimize the spread of a hazardous materials spill and to prevent further injuries.

OPQRST Abbreviation used to prompt questions related to a patient's complaint: onset; provocation; quality; region, radiation, relief; severity; time.

optical character recognition (OCR) Computer-based system for translating written documents into digital computer language.

oral Route of medication administration by the mouth.

orbit The bony cavity that houses the eyeball.

organic disorder Any disease or condition that causes the brain to malfunction.

organophosphates (OP) Class of chemicals used to make fertilizers and chemical weapons.

oropharyngeal airway (OPA) Plastic device that may be placed in the mouth to assist in keeping the tongue off the back of the throat and keeping the airway open; also called an *oral airway*.

oropharynx Section of throat that is visible from the mouth.

orthopedic back support Wide cloth belt, or back brace, used to prevent injury during heavy lifting.

orthopedic "scoop" stretcher Stretcher that splits in two halves and can be placed under the patient one half at a time.

orthopedics Study of the musculoskeletal system.

orthostatic vital signs Heart rate and blood pressure measured in different positions, usually lying, then standing.

osteopenia Loss of bone mineral density.

osteoporosis Progressive loss in the calcium content of the bones seen commonly in elderly women.

out-of-hospital DNR Do not resuscitate order that is binding in the prehospital setting in specifying that lifesaving measures should not be started.

ovary Primary female gonad, located in the pelvis; produces female sex hormones.

overdose Intentional exposure to, usually ingestion of, a potentially harmful substance.

over-the-counter (OTC) Nonprescription medication self-administered by the patient and readily available at a pharmacy.

overtriage Use of a resource based on set criteria when the end result is not as severe as initially predicted.

ovulation Release of an egg from the ovary.

ovum Female egg released from the ovary.

oxygen Colorless gas the body needs in adequate amounts to function normally.

oxygenation Amount of available oxygen in a medium, such as the air.

P

pack strap carry Carrying technique whereby the EMT steps in front of a standing patient and, using the patient's arms, hoists the patient onto his or her back with the patient's feet dragging.

palliation Alleviation of or improvement in pain, discomfort, or a condition.

pallor Pale skin color.

palmar Directional term used to describe the palm of the hand.

palmar method Method of determining the percentage of burned skin using the patient's palm.

palpate To feel with one's hands.

pancreas Organ located in the retroperitoneal space that produces both digestive enzymes and hormones such as insulin.

pancreatitis Inflammation of the pancreas characterized by abdominal pain and often vomiting.

pandemic Global disease outbreak.

panic stop Emergency stop for an unexpected obstacle.

paradoxical motion Movement of a flail chest segment in a direction opposite to that of the rest of the chest wall.

paralysis Inability to move a limb.

paramedic Highest level of EMS provider; paramedics are typically educated in rigorous college-level courses covering comprehensive patient assessment, advanced airway management, intravenous access techniques, expanded medication administration, and cardiac arrest management.

paraplegia Paralysis of the lower extremities, typically due to a spine injury below the cervical spine.

parenteral Inhaled or injected route of drug administration.

paresis Muscular weakness.

paresthesia Decreased ability to feel in extremities.

parietal bone The largest of the bones in the skull, located in the lateral part of the cranium.

parietal pain Localized, intense, sharp, constant pain associated with irritation of the peritoneum; also called *somatic pain.*

parietal pleura The thin covering adhering to the inside of the chest wall.

parity Total number of children born to a woman.

partial seizure Malfunction in the brain isolated to a small portion of the brain; formerly known as *petit mal.*

partial-thickness burn Burn that affects the epidermis and dermal layers of skin.

passive rewarming Treatment geared toward preventing any further body heat loss.

patella Small bony island over the knee joint, known as the kneecap.

pathogens Microorganisms or agents that cause disease, including bacteria, viruses, and fungi.

pathogenesis The beginning and progression of disease.

pathology Study of disease.

pathophysiology Study of the functional changes associated with or resulting from disease or injury

patient care report (PCR) Document on which an EMT records the evidence of the patient encounter.

patient history Detailed investigation of the present illness or injury and the patient's current health status and pertinent past medical history.

patient refusal form Specific form a patient must sign if he or she refuses to allow care or transport.

Patient Self-Determination Act Federal law that provides protections to a patient's right to decide on matters of life and death.

patient's bill of rights The rights and privileges to which a patient is entitled.

pattern of injury Injuries characteristic of a particular mechanism of injury.

pectoralis major muscles Muscles that cover the upper part of the anterior chest and help to lift the sternum and upper ribs.

Pediatric Assessment Triangle (PAT) A quick look assessment tool used to assessment the patient's appearance, work of breathing, and circulation to the skin to help form a general impression.

Pediatric Glasgow Coma Scale (PGCS) Adult assessment tool modified for assessing the neurological status of infants and children.

pelvic girdle The bones of the pelvis and the attached legs.

pelvic wrap technique Encircling the injured pelvis with an elasticized bandage or commercial device to stabilize fractures and prevent further damage.

penis Male organ that serves as a conduit for the passage of urine and semen.

penumbra Group of brain cells that surround an area of infarct.

perfusion Supply of oxygenated blood to an organ or tissue throughout the body.

pericardial tamponade Blood within the pericardial sac around the heart.

perimeter Imaginary boundary created that divides safe areas from dangerous areas.

peripheral Directional term used to describe points farther from the core of the body (trunk).

peripheral chemoreceptors Located in the carotid arteries and aortic arch, arterial oxygen level sensors.

peripheral nervous system Composed of nerves that originate in the spinal cord and transmit messages to and from the body's organs and tissues.

PERRL Acronym to report an eye exam: pupils equal, round, and reactive to light.

personal flotation device (PFD) Device that has positive buoyancy such as a life jacket or life preserver.

personal protective equipment (PPE) Gear that may be used by a health care provider to protect against exposure or injury.

personal safety The assurance that no hazards are present that might endanger the EMT.

pertinent negatives When the patient denies the specific signs and symptoms that could normally be seen in with the condition the patient is experiencing.

pertinent past medical history Relevant information concerning past illness or injuries the patient has experienced that are pertinent to the current condition.

petechiae Small pinpoint hemorrhages under the skin.

petit mal seizure The old term for a partial seizure.

phalanges Fingers and toes.

pharmacology The study of medications and their interactions.

pharynx The back of the throat.

photophobia Abnormal sensitivity to light.

phrenic nerve Located in the third, fourth, and fifth cervical segments of the spinal cord.

physical restraint Restriction of a patient's freedom of movement by use of ties, cravats, or other means.

physician's assistant (PA) An allied health care professional, sometimes referred to as a *mid-level provider*, who generally has authority to write medical orders that are later reviewed by a physician.

physiology Study of the function of an organism.

pia mater Innermost membrane covering the spinal cord and brain.

pit viper Venomous snake that can be recognized by characteristic pits in front of each eye.

placard Sign established by the U.S. Department of Transportation (USDOT) to identify the presence of a hazardous material.

placenta Interface between the uterus and the fetus.

placenta previa Condition in which the placenta grows over the cervical opening.

placental abruption Condition in which the placenta prematurely detaches from the uterine wall.

plantar Directional term used to describe the bottom surface of the foot.

pleural cavity/potential space Tiny space between lungs and chest wall.

plural form When more than one thing is being described by the medical term.

pneumatic anti-shock garment (PASG) Another name for military anti-shock trousers (MAST), a device that is inflated over the lower extremities and pelvis to attempt to increase blood flow to the core organs.

pneumatic lift pads Airbag lift devices.

pneumatic splint Splint that conforms to the shape of the injury by either inflation or vacuum.

pneumothorax Air in the pleural space potentially causing collapse of the lung.

pocket mask Dome-shaped plastic tool used as a barrier device for artificial ventilation.

point of contact (POC) Location where the person was last seen.

point tenderness Finite area that is painful when pressed.

poison A potentially deadly substance, solid, liquid, or gas, that is detrimental to an individual's health or causes death.

poison control center Regional center that serves as a resource for laypeople and health care providers on poisons and the management of the poisoned person.

poisoning Exposure to a substance that results in illness.

polypharmacy Use of multiple medications by a single patient.

portable radio Small handheld radio unit that typically has power output of 1–5 watts.

portal of entry Route an organism uses to enter the body.

position of function Natural relaxed position of a hand or foot.

positional asphyxia Suffocation that results from the patient's inability to take a deep breath when in a particular position.

positive pressure ventilations (PPV) Method of artificial ventilations by forcing air into the lungs.

posterior Directional term referring to a location toward the back.

posterior tibial pulse Easily palpable pulse created by blood flow through the posterior tibial artery behind the medial malleolus of the ankle.

postictal phase Recovery period immediately after a seizure.

post-traumatic seizure Seizure that may occur after head trauma.

post-traumatic stress disorder (PTSD) Psychiatric disorder that is the result of mental shock to the patient (e.g., witnessing a horrific trauma).

postural hypotension Drop in blood pressure associated with a change in position, usually from lying to standing.

pounds per square inch (psi) Measurement of pressure applied to a surface.

power grip Technique of lifting with the palms up to provide better grip.

power lift Technique used to lift a heavy object, such as a patient on a backboard, from the ground; also called *squat lift*.

power of attorney (POA) Designated person who makes decisions on behalf of another who is incapacitated.

power takeoff (PTO) Spinning shaft that transfers the tractor engine's power to another farm machine.

pox Small blisters filled with virus.

precipitous delivery Occurs when the birth of the fetus takes place less than 3 hours after labor begins

prefix Complements a root word; placed at the beginning of the root and adds meaning to the word.

prehospital health care team Multidisciplinary team composed of medical personnel, firefighters, and police officers who care for patients before their admittance to the hospital.

preload Volume of blood returning to the heart.

premature delivery Delivery that occurs prior to 36 weeks of gestation.

premature ventricular complex (PVC) A small group of irritated cells in the ventricles that fire earlier than expected.

preoxygenation Providing high-concentration oxygen to a patient for a period of time before a procedure, such as endotracheal intubation or suctioning, is performed.

preplan Agreed-on response that is planned before an emergency occurs.

pressure points Specific areas over major arteries where if compressed, bleeding from that artery can be halted.

preventive maintenance (PM) Program of replacing and repairing vehicles or equipment before they fail.

priapism A painful, sustained erection that is the result of spinal cord injury.

primary assessment Rapid, systematic assessment and management of life-threats of the patient mental status and airway, breathing, and circulatory status.

primary brain injury Direct trauma to the brain and associated vascular structures.

primary spinal cord injury Spinal cord injury that occurs at the time of the trauma.

primiparous Term used to describe a woman who is in her first pregnancy.

prodrome Nonspecific signs of an infection.

professional conduct Behavior demonstrating a caring, confident, and courteous demeanor; expected from all health care providers.

prognosis Expected or predicted outcome of a disease.

projection When one person attributes his or her thoughts or feelings to another.

prolapsed umbilical cord Presentation of the umbilical cord prior to the infant, resulting in compression of the cord.

pronation Action of turning something, such as the hand, downward.

pronator drift A test of neurological function that involves raising both arms straight out in front of the body, palms up, eyes closed; a positive test involves one arm drifting and indicates weakness in that arm.

prone Position in which a person is lying facedown.

prophylaxis Doing something to prevent an unwanted outcome.

prostate gland Male organ that produces a fluid that assists in the transport of sperm.

protected health information (PHI) Personal patient information protected from accidental disclosure or discovery by HIPAA.

provocation Aggravating or making the pain, discomfort, or condition worse.

proximal Directional term used to describe points on the body that are closer to the core of the body (trunk).

pruritus Itching sensation.

psychiatry The medical study of mental illness.

psychogenic shock (vasovagal shock) Form of neurogenic shock in which the vagal nerve is stimulated (by sudden fright or severe pain), resulting in a quick dilation of the peripheral blood vessels, causing a sudden loss of consciousness.

pubus The front of the bony pelvis.

public access defibrillation (PAD) Public training in the use of an AED.

public address system (PA) An electronic device designed to project a voice loudly.

public information officer (PIO) An individual designated by the incident commander to meet with the media and report the state of affairs at the incident.

public information systems Procedures, process, and systems required for communicating timely and accurate information to the public during a disaster or emergency situation.

public safety access point (PSAP) A local dispatch office that receives 9-1-1 calls from the public. A PSAP may be local fire or police department, an ambulance service, or a regional office covering all emergency services.

pulmonary artery Large artery that transfers blood from the right ventricle to the pulmonary circuit for oxygenation.

pulmonary circuit Blood vessels that pass through the lungs and allow oxygenation and removal of carbon dioxide.

pulmonary circulation Circulation of blood through the lungs for gas exchange.

pulmonary contusion Bruising of the lungs.

pulmonary edema Swelling of the pulmonary blood vessels.

pulmonary embolism Occurs when the blockage breaks free from a lower extremity and lodges in the arteries of the lungs.

pulmonary embolus Blockage in the pulmonary arterial circulation resulting in an area of lung that does not allow alveolar capillary gas exchange.

pulmonary overpressurization syndrome (POPS) Expanding air within the lungs as pressure decreases and the volume of air proportionally increases, resulting in rupture of alveoli.

pulmonary valve A semilunar valve that prevents the backflow of blood from the pulmonary artery back into the right ventricle.

pulmonary vein The large vessel that takes oxygenated blood from the pulmonary circuit and delivers it to the left atrium.

pulse The palpable feeling of blood flow through a superficial artery; count of the heartbeat.

pulse, movement, sensation (PMS) Assessment of distal neuro-vascular function to assess for injury.

pulse oximeter Tool that allows noninvasive measurement of the blood's oxygen saturation.

pulse pressure The difference between systolic and diastolic blood pressures.

pulseless electrical activity (PEA) Situation in which a pulse is not created but the ECG will show a rhythm.

puncture A hole created in the skin by a sharp, pointed object.

pupil The black center of the eye.

purkinje fibers Specialized cardiac conduction fibers within the ventricles.

pursed lip breathing Exhaling past partially closed lips.

pyelonephritis A urinary tract infection (UTI) that involves the kidneys.

Q

quadriceps muscle The strong muscle in the anterior thigh that permits leg extension.

quadriplegia Paralysis of all four extremities, typically caused by high cervical spine injury.

quality assurance (QA) A review of care to ensure minimum standards are met.

quickening First movements of the fetus that a mother senses.

R

raccoon's eyes Bruising around the eyes that may be indicative of a skull fracture.

radiation The transfer of heat from the warm body into the cooler environment just by the fact that a temperature gradient exists.

radiation pager A portable device that clips to the belt and measures radiation in the environment, alarming the wearer when dangerous levels of radiation are present.

radio head The main section of a mobile radio, often located in the driver's compartment of the vehicle.

radius The more lateral of the two bones in the forearm.

rales A bubbly or soft crackling sound, like hair rubbed between the fingers next to the ear.

range of motion (ROM) The movement that a bone, or limb, is allowed in a joint.

rapid extrication Technique for quickly removing an unstable potentially spine injured patient.

rapid physical examination A quick head-to-toe examination done on a patient who is unable to provide a history owing to a decreased level of consciousness.

rapid trauma assessment A quickly performed head-to-toe examination of a seriously injured trauma patient to discover hidden or suspected injuries.

rationalizations Patient develops a logical explanation to events in order to avoid dealing with painful emotions.

receptive aphasia Inability to comprehend language often seen when a stroke affects the speech center in the brain.

recovery Return to health with no remnant of the disease.

recovery position Position in which the patient is on the side so that secretions may spontaneously drain from the airway; also known as the *coma position* or *left lateral recumbent position*.

rectum End of the large intestine where stool is stored before it is eliminated via the anus.

recurrent bandage Bandage that is laid back and forth across the tape of a dressing and then anchored.

red blood cells Hemoglobin-carrying blood cells whose function is to deliver oxygen to tissues.

redundancy Having two plans of action in place in case one of them fails.

Reeves stretcher Commercially available, long, flat litter with handles on all corners that can be wrapped around the patient; allows for easy movement of the patient who has not suffered a spinal injury.

referred pain Pain felt in a body part away from the point where the pain originates.

refusal of medical assistance (RMA) When a patient refuses medical care and understands the risk and possible consequences of such action; generally there is not a great risk for loss of life or limb.

regulator Device placed on an oxygen tank to regulate the flow of the gas; also called a *flowmeter*.

reinforce Brace or strengthen a bandage.

remission Nonactive state.

renal stone The accumulation of solid material in the kidney that may become lodged in the ureter during passage to the bladder.

repeater Radio receiver/transmitter that picks up the signal from a mobile unit and increases, or boosts, the signal to the base station receiver.

repetitive persistence Repeating a message several times until it is evident that the point has been taken.

repression When a person subconsciously eliminates all thoughts of a painful situation from his or her mind.

rescue Helping another person who is incapable of freeing himself or herself from confinement.

rescuer assist The use of one EMT on one side of a walking patient for assistance with walking.

research officer A person familiar with the computer and reference resources that are available for chemical exposures.

reservoir The source for an infection.

residuals Physical or chemical changes left behind after recovery from a disease.

respiration The exchange of gases, such as oxygen and carbon dioxide, at the capillary level.

respiratory rate Number of breaths in one minute.

respiratory syncytial virus (RSV) Infectious form of bronchiolitis seen more commonly in children than adults.

responsive to painful stimuli Term used to describe the mental status of a patient who is aroused only by uncomfortable action of touch.

responsive to voice Term used to describe the mental status of a patient who is aroused by verbal stimuli but is not spontaneously awake and interactive.

resuscitate To attempt to revive a patient by way of medical therapies.

retroperitoneal cavity The most posterior section of the abdomen, containing organs, such as kidneys, pancreas, and aorta.

return of spontaneous circulation (ROSC) Pulses returning with just CPR or defibrillation.

revised trauma score Standard method of trauma scoring that uses results of the Glasgow Coma Scale and the patient's respiratory rate and systolic blood pressure, assigning a number to each element.

rhonchi Coarse sounds that are heard over the lungs when mucus or other foreign material accumulates in the larger airways.

rhythm A regularly repeating ECG pattern.

rib cage Bony ribs that surround the organs of the chest like a protective cage.

right-of-way Privilege of proceeding ahead of others on a roadway.

rigid splint Any firm material that can provide support for a limb.

rigor mortis Generalized stiffening of the body following death.

riot gas (CS) Noxious gas used to disperse crowds.

risk factors Predisposing factors that can make a person more susceptible to disease.

risk management Actions geared toward protection from hazard.

Risk Mitigation process of identifying hazards and ensuring protection.

risk profile Likelihood of the presence of a disease in a person or group of people.

roller bandage Cotton cloth rolled into a cylinder for easier control when unwrapping.

rolling the dash Pulling the vehicle's dashboard off the patient.

rollover protective structure (ROPS) A protective bar or canopy that prevents the driver from being crushed under the weight of the tractor.

root word Sometimes called the *stem*, relates to the main idea and serves as the foundation of the word.

rotor wash Wind created by the cycling of a helicopter's rotors.

rotor wing Helicopters.

route Where a drug is administered, i.e., enteral (ingested, sublingual and oral) and parenteral (inhalation and injection).

rule of nines Formula to determine the percentage of burnt skin.

Ryan White law Regulation that states that a hospital is required to notify an EMS agency if its staff identifies an infectious illness to which the agency's employees may have been exposed.

S

sacral vertebrae Five strong bony vertebrae that close the pelvic ring posteriorly.

safety corridor Zone of protection, created by a barrier, that permits the EMT to work safely.

safety glass Piece of glass sealed between two sheets of plastic designed to remain in one piece if damaged.

safety officer (SO) Designated person who is charged with knowledge of relevant regulations and standards regarding responder and patient safety.

saliva Normally occurring secretions from the mouth.

SAMPLE Acronym to remember the most important basic history questions: signs and symptoms, allergies, medications, past medical history, last oral intake, events leading up to the incident/illness.

scalene muscles Responsible for lifting the sternocleidomastoid muscle.

scanner Electronic device that may be used to listen to various radio frequencies.

scapulas Strong bony prominences on the back, also known as the *shoulder blades*.

scene survey Procedure used to initially evaluate a situation for potential dangers.

sciatic nerve The primary sensory and motor nerve of the legs.

scope of practice Legal description of the limits of care that an EMS provider can offer to a patient.

scrotum Externally located sac that encloses the male testes.

search and rescue (SAR) Organized and disciplined approach to the rescue of injured, ill, or lost persons.

seat carry Technique of carrying a conscious patient in which two EMTs join arms and allow the patient to sit on their arms as if they formed a seat.

second stage of labor Phase of childbirth that begins when the cervix is completely dilated and ends with the delivery of the infant.

secondary brain injury Extension of the primary brain injury, such as hypoxia and hypotension.

secondary device Explosive device intended to harm emergency services responders and delay emergency operations.

secondary spinal cord injury Spinal cord injury that occurs after the trauma, often as a result of mishandling.

seizure Event that begins within the brain and results in involuntary movements and sometimes loss of consciousness.

self-contained breathing apparatus (SCBA) Equipment that permits the wearer to have an independent air supply, used in hazardous environments.

self-splint When a patient uses his or her body to protect and stabilize a limb.

Sellick maneuver Cricoid pressure.

sensory nerves Nervous tissue that carries impulses of feelings such as pressure or pain.

sentinel PCR Report that requires special review by the medical director or a risk management group.

septic shock Hypoperfused state resulting from overwhelming infection and generalized vasodilation.

sexual abuse Any sexual activity with a child in which consent is not or cannot be given.

sexual assault Physical and psychological trauma of a sexual nature.

sexual molestation Form of sexual abuse that is performed for the sexual gratification of the parent or caregiver.

shaken baby syndrome Shaking an infant violently and causing a head injury.

sharps Instruments with a sharp point, such as needles, syringes, and sharp blades.

sharps container Puncture-proof container used to dispose of needles and other sharp instruments; the container is usually red with a biohazard label on the side.

shingles Adult chicken-pox.

shipping papers Paperwork that accompanies hazardous material while in transit; it contains the chemical name of the materials, as well as the UN designation of the substance being transported.

shock State in which the body is hypoperfused, resulting in inadequate oxygenation of cells, tissues, and organs.

shock position Position in which the body is hypoperfused, resulting in inadequate oxygenation of cells, tissues, and organs.

shoreline An electrical extension linking an ambulance with a building's electricity.

short spine immobilization device (SSID) Interim device used to stabilize a patient's spine while transferring him or her to a long backboard.

shoulder dislocation Separation of the scapula and the humerus.

shoulder dystocia Shoulders become wedged against the pubic bone and sacrum during birth.

shoulder girdle The scapula, clavicle, and attached arms.

show of force Demonstration of determination.

side effect Effect of a medication that was not the intended effect.

sign Something the examiner can objectively see.

signs of circulation Responsiveness, breathing, coughing, and movement.

silage Forage (food) typically stored in a silo.

silent myocardial infarction Death of heart tissue that occurs without the patient experiencing classic cardiac symptoms such as chest pain.

silo Structure that stores silage.

simple partial seizure Seizure in which the patient is awake but experiencing jerky movements, usually in only one area of the body, which are not controlled.

simplex A type of radio that can only receive or transmit at one time; allows only one-way communication.

sino atrial (SA) Point at the top of the heart, at the atria, where a collection of nervous tissue is found; this nervous tissue is the primary pacemaker of the heart.

sinoatrial (SA) node Specialized cardiac conduction fibers that serve as the primary pacemaker of the heart.

siren mode Characteristic patterns of sound to alert motorists of the vehicle's presence.

size-up Rapid determination of the situation, including hazards, at the scene of an emergency.

slander False statements spoken with malicious intent or reckless disregard, which injure a person's reputation or good name.

sling A loop of webbing used to help balance the load when carrying a litter or a basket.

sling and swathe (S/S) The use of a cravat and a triangular bandage to splint a limb.

slippery sheets Specially coated sheets reduce friction between the patient and the bed and allow for an easier transfer.

slow-moving vehicle (SMV) Any vehicle, typically farm machinery, that is incapable of maintaining posted highway speeds.

SLUDGEM Characteristic symptom pattern seen with nerve agents; acronym represents salivation, lacrimation, urination, defecation, GI distress, emesis, and muscle contractions.

small intestine Long, hollow organ that takes up much of the abdominal cavity and is responsible for much of the absorption of nutrients from food.

small volume nebulizer (SVN) Methods of delivering humidified oxygen.

snag lines Rescue ropes slung over a stream or river.

snoring Sound made when a partial upper airway obstruction, such as the tongue, exists in the supine patient.

social distancing Public health practice of limiting the number of people an infected person can infect by banning public gatherings.

social history Patient's housing environment, occupation, economic status, travel history, and high-risk behaviors.

special incident report (SIR) Specific document upon which the EMT writes the details of a defined special incident, such as equipment failure.

sperm Male reproductive material responsible for fertilization of the female egg.

sphygmomanometer A device that is used to measure blood pressure; a blood pressure cuff.

spinal canal Passageway in the vertebrae through which the spinal cord passes.

spinal column Series of bones that support the back and protect the spinal cord.

spinal cord The collection of nerves that run from the brain through the spinal column and branch out as peripheral nerves to body organs and tissues.

spinous process The centrally palpable posterior element of each vertebrae.

spiral bandage A roller bandage wrapped around a limb.

spleen Solid, highly vascular organ, located in the left upper quadrant of the abdomen that serves to store blood, destroy old red blood cells, filter foreign substances from the blood, and produce lymphocytes.

spontaneous abortion Loss of a pregnancy, also known as *miscarriage*.

spontaneous reduction A bone that returns to its natural position, within a joint, without assistance.

spotter A person who assists the driver with backing up the vehicle.

sprain A stretch of a ligament or tendon beyond its range of motion resulting in tissue injury.

sputum Secretions formed in the airway.

squat lift Technique used to lift a heavy object, such as a patient on a backboard, from the ground; also known as the *power lift*.

staging Designating a specific area for emergency vehicles and providers entering a scene.

staging area An off-scene location where personnel and vehicles assemble and await assignment.

staging officer A manager of an area who assembles and assigns equipment and personnel to specific duties or tasks.

stairchair A specially designed chair that has handles on the back and on the front that a patient may be secured into and then carried down a flight of stairs by two EMTs.

stand by Radio terminology meaning "hold on a minute."

standard anatomical position Facing forward, legs slightly apart, with feet pointing forward, arms straight and extended a few inches away from the side, with palms facing forward.

standard comfort measures Treatments that are provided to ease suffering but that do not include resuscitation of a patient.

standard of care Level of care recognized as being appropriate for a particular level of training and certification.

standard precautions Refers to the personal protective equipment used routinely in certain circumstances.

standing orders Off-line medical control consisting of procedures that are to be followed by the EMT for specific injuries or illness.

standing takedown Technique in which rescuers use a rigid backboard to gently move a patient from the standing upright position to a horizontal supine position.

star of life Six-pointed star with staff and serpent in the center; recognized as the symbol of EMS; each point on the star represents a key component of the EMS system: detection, reporting, response, on-scene care, care in transit, and transfer to definitive care.

START Triage System Standardized system for triage; acronym stands for simple triage and rapid treatment.

status epilepticus One continuous seizure or one or more seizures without an intervening period of consciousness.

stellate Starlike pattern of broken skin.

stenosis Constriction or narrowing of a duct or passage, such as a vessel or valve; a stricture.

step blocks Prefabricated cribbing designed for use in rapidly stabilizing a vehicle.

sterilization Thorough cleaning of an item so that all microorganisms have been completely removed.

sternal angle The bony ridge where the manubrium meets the body of the sternum; also called the *angle of Louis*.

sternal body The largest center piece of the bony sternum, or breastbone.

sternal retraction Sternal depressions with each breath seen in a child with severe respiratory distress.

sternal rub Technique used to assess a patient's response to a painful stimulus; with this technique the knuckles are rubbed against the patient's sternum.

sternocleidomastoid muscle Important accessory muscle of respiration and the main muscle that moves the head; a triangular muscle that connects the sternum with the clavicle and mastoid process; also called the *strap muscle*.

sternum The bony island in the center of the chest, also known as the *breastbone*.

steward Someone who cares for the affairs of another in their absence.

stimming Humming or repetitive body movements, such as hand flapping seen in individuals with an autistic disorder, believed to self-stimulate one or more senses to self-regulate or self-soothe.

Stokes basket Type of basket stretcher that allows complete immobilization and protection of the patient during a move over rough terrain.

stoma Surgically created hole at the base of the neck to allow breathing in patients with severe upper airway diseases.

straddle injury Damage to the perineal area.

stress Physical, emotional, and behavioral response of the body to changing external conditions.

stress management program Means of dealing effectively with acute and chronic stress.

stressors Events that trigger stress.

stridor Harsh, high-pitched sound heard during inspiration characteristic of an upper airway obstruction due to swelling in the larynx.

stringer Nylon webbing loop tied with a half-hitch through the handhold or rail.

stroke Injury to brain tissue that occurs as a result of disruption of blood flow to part of the brain; also known as a *cerebrovascular accident*.

stroke volume Amount of blood the heart pumps out with each beat.

subarachnoid space Space between the dura mater and arachnoid layers of the meninges, filled with cerebrospinal fluid.

subclinical An infected patent who does not have symptoms.

subcutaneous Space just under the skin, made up of fat and tiny blood vessels.

subcutaneous emphysema Air under the skin and above the chest wall.

subcutaneous tissue The fatty tissue beneath the dermis of the skin; connects the skin to the underlying muscle.

subdural hematoma A collection of blood between the surface of the brain and the dura mater, often venous in nature.

subjective information the patient or family members tell an EMT.

subjective, objective, assessment plan (SOAP) A system of organizing medical information, called charting, into an organized and coherent document.

subjective, objective, assessment plan, intervention, evaluation (SOAPIE) Additional EMS-specific information added to the SOAP format of charting.

sublingual Under the tongue.

subluxation Partial dislocation at a joint.

substance abuse Misuse of a drug to alter perception or mood.

sucking chest wound Wound on the chest through which air can enter the pleural space, making a sucking sound.

sudden cardiac death (SCD) Death of a patient early in the course of a heart attack, usually due to an arrhythmia.

sudden infant death syndrome (SIDS) The sudden, unexplained death of an infant in the first year of life.

suffix Complements a root word when it is placed behind the root and changes the meaning of the term.

suicide Voluntary taking of one's own life.

superficial Term used to describe something at or close to the top, or surface.

superficial burn A burn affecting only the uppermost layer of skin.

superior A directional term referring to a location toward the top of an object.

supination The action of turning something, such as the hand, upward.

supine Position in which a person is lying faceup with the spine to the ground.

supine hypotensive syndrome Compression of the vena cava when a pregnant woman lies flat, resulting in a loss of blood pressure.

suppression Voluntary elimination of a painful thought.

suprasternal notch The notch formed where the clavicles meet the manubrium.

surge capacity Ability of a healthcare system, including EMS systems, to care for a sudden increase in the number of patients.

surrounding area The space above and around the touchdown site where a helicopter will land.

suspension A powder suspended in a liquid so that it may be more easily ingested.

sutures Immovable joints, composed of connective tissue, in the skull where the cranial bones meet; these joints begin to fuse as a child gets older and are completely fused in an adult.

swelling An increase in soft tissue size due to inflammation.

swift water A rapidly moving body of water.

symbiotic A mutually beneficial relationship between a microorganism and its host.

symphysis pubis The joint at the center of the front of the pelvis where the two pubis bones meet.

symptom Sign of illness or injury reported by a patient or discovered on examination.

syndrome Group of features, including certain signs, symptoms, and characteristics that occur together.

systemic circuit Refers to the circuit of blood vessels providing blood to the body's many systems; includes all of the vessels from the aorta through to the vena cava.

systemic circulation Supplies blood to the organs of the body's systems.

systemic vascular resistance (SVR) Resistance to flow blood must overcome to move through the circulatory system.

systolic The top number in a blood pressure; refers to the pressure in the vessels when the heart is contracting.

systolic blood pressure pressure exerted against the vessel walls when the heart contracts.

T

tachycardia Increased heart rate.

tachypnea Respiratory rate faster than normal.

tactical channel A designated channel for special operations that permits efficient scene coordination.

tactical command sheets Document that provides specific instructions for how to proceed with managing a specific incident.

tactile hallucination A false perception of a sensation of the skin; a false feeling.

Takedown procedure Planned orderly restraint of a patient for a medical purpose.

target organs Specific organs upon which hormones are intended to work.

tarsals Small bones within the foot, corresponding to the carpal bones of the wrist.

tattooing A peppering of gunpowder to the skin.

teachable moment Ability to affect the patient's behaviors in the future because the patient's mind is receptive to suggestion today.

tear gas (CN) Noxious gas used to disperse crowds.

technical assistance program (TAP) Federal aid and support for EMS operations, typically offering expertise and financial assistance to specific targeted goals.

technical rescue Complex rescue operations performed by highly trained technicians using specialized equipment.

telemetry Sending an ECG rhythm strip to the base hospital for physician interpretation.

tempered glass Special glass designed to shatter into fragments.

temporal bone Cranial bone that forms the base of the skull, behind and at the sides of the face.

tender Referring to an area that is sensitive or painful upon palpation.

tendon The connective tissue that attaches the muscle to the bone.

tension pneumothorax Air in the pleural space under tension, causing complete collapse of the affected lung and shift of the heart and other intrathoracic structures.

teratogens Chemicals that affect fetal development in the womb.

terminal A patient who is at the end of a disease that will result in death.

terminal bronchioles The smallest tubular airways leading to the alveoli.

terrorism The unlawful use of force against persons or property to intimidate or coerce a government, the civilian population, or any segment thereof, in the furtherance of political or social objectives.

testes Male gonads.

therapeutic communications Communication techniques demonstrating compassion and caring, that can have a positive effects on the patient's health.

therapeutic effect Desired effect the drug was administered to achieve.

thermoregulation Attempt to balance the amount of heat lost and heat gained to maintain a constant body temperature.

third stage of labor Final stage of labor during which the placenta is delivered.

thoracic cavity The space enclosed within the rib cage, bordered inferiorly by the diaphragm; otherwise known as the *chest cavity*.

thoracic vertebrae The 12 vertebrae that are found below the cervical spine and above the lumbar spine; these are attached to the 12 sets of ribs.

thrombus An accumulation of platelets and other blood components that locally occlude a vessel; a blood clot.

throw bag A length of rope loosely coiled in a sack.

tibia The larger of the two bones in the lower leg; the shinbone.

tidal volume Volume or amount of air inhaled and exhaled in one breath.

tilt test Test for hypovolemia that is considered positive if the heart rate goes up by 10 to 20 beats per minute and the systolic blood pressure drops by 10–20 mmHg with a change of position from sitting or lying to standing.

tonic phase The stage in a seizure in which the entire body stiffens.

tonsils Pillars of soft tissue on each side of the back of the throat.

topical On the surface; refers to administration of medication by placing it on the surface of the skin so it can be slowly absorbed.

topographic anatomy The study of the relationship of one body part to another.

tort law Area of law involving civil wrongs against another and a finding of liability in a civil case, typically only resulting in the award of monetary damages.

total peripheral resistance See *systemic vascular resistance*.

touchdown area Actual site where the aircraft will land; most medical helicopters require a touchdown area of between 75 feet square and 100 feet square.

tourniquet (TK) A tight, constricting band that stops blood flow to a limb.

toxic organic dust syndrome (TODS) Special respiratory hazards caused by organic dust that can be inhaled, leading to fever, headache, and malaise.

toxic substance Any substances that are poisonous to the human body.

toxicology The study of toxins, antidotes, and the effects of toxins on the body.

toxin Any drug or substance poisonous to the human body that can affect cellular respiration by internal and external means, causing a decline in health and ultimately leading to death.

TRACEM Mnemonic used to indicate the threats created by a terrorist attack; T stands for thermal harm, R for radiation harm, A for asphyxiation, C for corrosive chemicals, E for etiologic, and M for mechanical.

trachea The cartilaginous tube that is the passageway for air to get from the upper airway to the lungs; also known as the *windpipe*.

tracheal deviation Movement of the trachea from the mid-line.

tracheostomy The surgical creation of a hole in the anterior neck into the trachea to allow more effective ventilation in patients with upper airway problems or chronic lung disease.

tracheostomy tube Rigid tube placed into a tracheostomy to maintain a patent airway.

traction The application of a steady pull in line with an axis.

traction splint A splint that provides a continuous pull along the axis of the bone.

trade name The brand name given to a medication by the manufacturer.

transfer board A smooth, flat device used when transferring a patient from one stretcher to another to reduce friction and the work involved in the transfer; also called a *slide board*.

transfer sheets Special heavy-duty vinyl sheets reinforced with webbing to carry extra weight

transient ischemic attack (TIA) Temporary disruption of blood flow to part of the brain that results in signs and symptoms of a stroke, yet resolves within minutes to hours.

transmission The transfer of an infectious agent from one source to another.

transportation officer The individual responsible for the overall movement of patients from the scene to appropriate hospitals.

trapezius muscle Triangular muscle that covers the upper back and helps to lift the shoulders.

trauma Physical injury or wound caused by external forces.

trauma center A specially designated hospital that is experienced in and capable of caring for patients with severe injuries.

trauma dressing A large cotton dressing placed over a major open wound.

trauma intervention program (TIP) A team of people who operate in the field, during an incident, identifying providers who are at risk and attempting to remove or reduce the stress on those individuals.

traumatic asphyxia A crushing blow that forces air and blood out of the chest.

traumatic brain injury (TBI) Injury to the brain due to a direct cause (penetrating trauma), indirect cause (blow to the skull), or secondary cause (hypoxia).

treatment officer The person responsible for setting up the field hospital.

trench foot An injury to tissue resulting from prolonged exposure of the skin to cool, wet conditions.

trend Identification of a pattern over a period of time.

triad Three signs that are characteristic of a disease.

triage A system of distribution of patients into treatment classifications according to their injury severity.

triage officer The individual responsible for the distribution of patients into treatment classification according to their injury severity.

triage tag A special document that is used in multiple-casualty incidents to indicate the priority of each patient.

triangular bandage A 36-by 42-inch triangular piece of muslin cloth.

triceps muscle The muscle in the back of the upper arm that allows elbow extension; antagonist to the biceps muscle.

tricuspid valve The three-cusped valve between the right atrium and right ventricle that prevents backflow of blood.

trigger words Words that remind the patient of a painful past experience.

tripod position The three-legged position maintained by a person with severe difficulty breathing; with the upper body leaning slightly forward, arms straight, and hands supporting the upper body by resting on the upper legs.

true ribs The first seven pairs of ribs, which attach directly to the sternum anteriorly.

trunked line A truncated frequency made possible by the use of computers; used to prioritize messages.

tuberculosis (TB) The bacterium responsible for the disease tuberculosis, which typically attacks the lungs.

tunica adventitia Outer layer of blood vessels walls made of white fibrous connective tissue.

tunica intima Inner layer of the walls of blood vessels.

tunica media Smooth muscle middle layer of the walls of blood vessels.

tunics Layer or coats of vessel walls.

twelve-lead ECG tracing the heart's electrical activity from 12 different views.

twisting force Turning force of violence.

two-way radio Wireless electronic device that permits the transmission of messages to distant radio receivers as well as receipt of signals from those distant radios.

U

UHF Ultrahigh frequency radio signal.

ulcer Erosion of the lining of the stomach that can lead to pain and/or bleeding.

ulna The more medial bone in the forearm.

undertow A powerful downward current in bodies of water.

undertriage Failing to use a resource based on set criteria when the end result is more severe than originally predicted.

unilateral Directional term used to describe a point on only one side of the body.

unipolar traction splint A traction splint with a single shaft.

United States Fire Academy (USFA) The federal training organization for firefighters.

universal dressing A 9-by 36-inch gauze dressing.

unresponsive Term used to describe the mental status of a patient who cannot be aroused with verbal or even painful stimuli.

unstable angina Injured heart muscle that creates pain, generally due to a narrowing of the coronary artery.

unwind time Time that is designated in an EMT's personal life to relax, spend leisure time with family and friends, and participate in hobbies, sports, or exercise.

upper extremities Term used to refer to the arms.

ureters Muscular tubes that carry urine from the kidneys to the bladder.

urticaria Raised, red rash that results from localized dilation and leaking of blood vessels resulting in red, warm swelling to the surface of the skin; also known as hives.

U.S. Pharmacopeia The national drug reference that includes drug indications, contraindications, and side effects.

uterus Muscular chamber that holds the products of conception; also known as the *womb*.

uvula Small piece of tissue that is seen hanging off the roof of the mouth in the pharynx.

V

vagina Part of the female genitalia that allows passage of menstrual flow or a baby during labor and serves as the conduit for the acceptance of the male penis during coitus.

vallecula Space posterior to the base of the tongue, anterior to the epiglottis.

vector Organism, such as an animal, that carries a disease from one source to another, where it can result in infection.

veins Vessels that carry blood back to the heart, usually with deoxygenated blood.

velocity Speed.

vena cava The largest vein in the body.

venous bleeding Bleeding from the oxygen-poor veins; can be severe and life threatening.

ventilation The process of moving air into and out of the lungs; breathing.

ventral Directional term referring to points located in the front of the body.

ventricles Primary pump chambers of the heart.

ventricular fibrillation Uncoordinated and spontaneous contraction of individual heart muscle fibers.

ventricular tachycardia A cardiac event in which a small group of irritated cells in the ventricles start to fire automatically at rates of 100–250 beats per minute (bpm).

ventriculo-peritoneal (VP) A shunt that diverts extra cerebrospinal fluid from the brain to the abdomen, thereby preventing increased intracranial pressure.

venules Tiny vessels that connect the capillaries and veins.

verbal communication Communication through the use of speech.

verbal report A spoken account of the patient encounter given to the accepting health care provider.

vernix caseosa A cheese-like, white substance found on a newborn.

vertebrae Individual bones of the spine.

vertebral foramen A canal, formed by a ring of bone that houses the spinal cord.

VHF Very-high-frequency radio signal.

viral hemorrhagic fever (VHF) Disease that causes bleeding as well as severe fever.

vial of life Complete patient history documented and stored in a designated spot marked in a patient's home.

visceral pain Poorly localized, intermittent, crampy, dull or achy pain originating with an organ.

visceral pleura The membrane lining the surface of the lungs.

visual flight rules (VFR) Aviation regulations that essentially permit a pilot to fly only when environmental conditions allow him or her to actually see with his or her own eyes well enough to safely navigate the aircraft.

visual hallucination False perception of the sensation of the eyes; a false visualization.

W

wail Long and steady sound that ascends and descends.

wave-off The rigorous crossing and uncrossing of the landing zone officer's hands alerting the pilot that it has become unsafe to land.

weapons of mass destruction (WMD) Weapons created to indiscriminately kill or maim large numbers of civilians and to disrupt normal government operations.

wheezing High-pitched expiratory sound heard when lower airway narrowing exists.

white paper Detailed or authorization report on any subject; the National Academy of Sciences' article titled "Accidental Death and Disability: The Neglected Disease of Modern Society," written for President Kennedy, laid the groundwork for EMS legislation.

wig-wags Alternating headlights on an emergency vehicle.

window punch A special tool for breaking window glass.

wire strikes The impact of a helicopter's rotors against overhead wires.

withdrawal symptoms The unpleasant physical and/ or psychological effects experienced by a drug-addicted patient when the drug is kept from him or her.

Wong-Baker FACES scale Card that uses faces to indicate pain levels.

wound Damage to the skin as a result of trauma.

X

xiphoid process The inferior portion of the sternum.

Y

Yankauer A rigid suction catheter that has a curvature meant to follow the pharyngeal curve and a large open suction tip.

yelp A sharp, quick, fast-paced, almost chirping sound.

Z

zoonoses Diseases shared by animals and humans.

zoonotic Diseases that humans have in common with animals.

zygomatic bones The facial bones that extend anteriorly from the temporal part of the skull on each side to form the prominence of the cheeks.

Index

airway control and, 210
alveolar, 131–132, 132f
exhalation. See Exhalation
head injuries and, 743
inhalation. See Inhalation
obstructive disease of, 132–133
respiratory rate, 131
Ventolin, 298t, 311
Ventral, 80, 80f, 496t
Ventricle, 89–90
Ventricular fibrillation, 145f, 528, 532, 534b, 535–536, 882. see also Automated external defibrillator (AED)
Ventricular septal defect (VSD), 1008t
Ventricular tachycardia (VT), 144–145, 145f, 531, 532f
Ventriculo-peritoneal (VP) shunts, 1006
Ventro/- prefix, 492t
Venturi mask, 235
Venules, 138
Verbal persuasion, 629
Verbal report, 484–485
Verbal response, trauma scoring and, 713t, 714
Vernix caseosa, 933
Vertebrae, 107–108, 324
Vertebral arch, 108f
Vertebral body, 107–108, 108f, 751f
Vertebral column, 106f, 850f
Vertebral foramen, 108
VHF (very high frequency), 477
Viagra, 431–432
Vietnam War, history of EMS and, 8
Violence. see also Crime scenes; Gunshot wounds (GSW)
domestic, 166
legal responsibilities regarding threat of, 47–48
safety in potentially-violent situations, 627–628
Viral agents, 1114–1115, 1115–1116
Viral hemorrhagic fevers (VHF), 1115–1116
Viruses, 672
Visceral pain, 648–649
Visceral pleura, 95, 95f, 129
Vision, in infancy, 161
Visual Flight Rules (VFR), 1172
Visual hallucinations, 638
Visual impairments, 438
Vital signs. see also Baseline vital signs

of abdominal pain patient, 655–656
firefighter, 1154–1155
head injury assessment, 741–742
obese patient, 663–664
pediatric, 954t
reassessing, 466
respiratory, 581
of respiratory distress patient, 584
Vital systems, 83–96
circulatory system, 87–93
nervous system, 83–87
respiratory systems, 93–96
Vitreous humor, 727
Vocal cords, 93
Voice box, 93
Voice, responsive to, 398
Volunteers, 18
Vomiting
head immobilization and, 769
head injuries and, 740
with head trauma, 976–977

W

Wail siren, 1061, 1063b
"Walking wounded," 1085
Warm zone, 1100
Warning lights
array of, 382
color of, 382, 1059
flashback, 1060
patterns, 1060
safety and, 383
used on highways, 1060b
used when arriving at the scene, 1065–1066
used with caution, 1062
Waste disposal, 188–189, 194f
Water, heat conduction and, 877, 877b
Water-related emergencies, 886–890
Water rescue, 1135–1137
Wausau, Wisconsin, 9
Weak pulse, 281
Weapons of mass destruction (WMD), 1113–1117
Weather conditions, 388–389
Weed, Lawrence, 507
Weight measurements, 446
Wernicke's area, 413b
West Nile Virus Map, 177f
Wet chemicals, 841
Wet dressings, 838, 838f, 839

Wheezing, 280, 581, 691
White lights, 1059
"Whooping cough," 959
Wig-wags, 1059
Wilderness EMT (WEMT), 852b
Window punch, 1133, 1133f
Windpipe, 93
Windshields, vehicle damage survey and, 386
Withdrawal, alcohol, 641
Withdrawal symptoms, 640, 641
Wong-Baker FACES scale, 436
World Health Organization, 1115
Worms, 672
Wounds. see also Bandages; Bleeding; Dressings (wound); Gunshot wounds (GSW)
abrasions, 821
amputations, 822, 830–831
avulsions, 822, 830
bandaging for, 823–831
defined, 815
entrance, 822
exit, 822
incisions, 821–822
neck, 829
ongoing assessment of, 831
open chest, 797–798
punctures, 822
sucking chest, 797, 798f, 829
transporting patient with, 831
types of, 821–822
Wrist, injury of the, 861–862

X

Xiphoid process, 106f, 110
-x plural form, 495t

Y

Yankauer suction catheter, 214, 214f
Yellow lights (warning lights), 382, 1059
Yelp siren, 1061, 1063
Yersinia pestis (plague), 1115, 1115f
Young infant, 948
Yperite, 1116
-y plural form, 495t

Z

Zoonoses, 673, 673t, 676
Zoonotic disease, 1115
Zygomatic bone, 107f
Zygomatic bones, 106